Krugman's

INFECTIOUS DISEASES
OF CHILDREN

Krugman's
INFECTIOUS DISEASES
OF CHILDREN

SAMUEL L. KATZ, M.D.

Wilburt C. Davison Professor and Chairman Emeritus,
Department of Pediatrics
Duke University Medical Center
Durham, North Carolina

ANNE A. GERSHON, M.D.

Professor of Pediatrics
Division of Infectious Diseases
Columbia University
College of Physicians and Surgeons
New York, New York

PETER J. HOTEZ, M.D., Ph.D

Associate Professor of Pediatrics and
Epidemiology and Public Health
Yale University School of Medicine
New Haven, Connecticut

TENTH EDITION

*with **184** illustrations and **22** color illustrations in **9** plates*

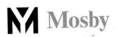 Mosby

St. Louis Baltimore Boston Carlsbad Chicago Naples New York Philadelphia Portland
London Madrid Mexico City Singapore Sydney Tokyo Toronto Wiesbaden

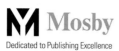

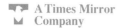

Editor: Laura DeYoung
Senior Developmental Editor: Sandra Clark Brown
Project Manager: Patricia Tannian
Senior Production Editor: Melissa Mraz Lastarria
Book Design Manager: Gail Morey Hudson
Manufacturing Manager: Dave Graybill
Cover Design: Teresa Breckwoldt

Printed in the United States of America
Composition by The Clarinda Company
Lithography/color film by Color Dot Graphics, Inc.
Printing/binding by Maple-Vail Book Manufacturing Group

Mosby–Year Book, Inc.
11830 Westline Industrial Drive
St. Louis, Missouri 63146

International Standard Book Number 0-8151-5251-5

97 98 99 00 01/9 8 7 6 5 4 3 2 1

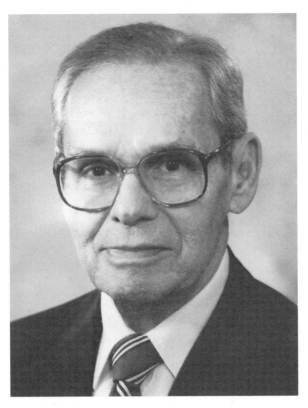

To

SAUL KRUGMAN

(1911-1995)

Clinician, teacher, investigator, mentor, and friend whose
wisdom, knowledge, enthusiasm, energy, candor, pragmatism, generosity, and spirit
have guided and nurtured this book since its first edition in 1958.

To my husband

Dr. Michael Gershon, and our children

AAG

To my wife

Ann Hotez, and our children

Matthew, Emily, Rachel, and **Daniel**

PJH

To my wife

Dr. Catherine Wilfert, and all our children

SLK

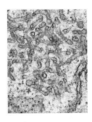

CONTRIBUTORS

STUART P. ADLER, M.D.
Professor and Division Chairman,
Department of Pediatrics
Medical College of Virginia
Virginia Commonwealth University
Richmond, Virginia

PAULA WINTER ANNUNZIATO, M.D.
Assistant Professor
Department of Pediatrics
Columbia University
College of Physicians and Surgeons
New York, New York

CAROL J. BAKER, M.D.
Professor of Pediatrics, Microbiology, and Immunology
Head, Section of Infectious Diseases
Department of Pediatrics
Baylor College of Medicine
Houston, Texas

WILLIAM BORKOWSKY, M.D.
Department of Pediatrics
New York University Medical Center
New York, New York

KENNETH BOYER, M.D.
Department of Pediatrics,
Rush Presbyterian St. Lukes
Chicago, Illinois

KENNETH BROMBERG, M.D.
Associate Professor of Pediatrics
Associate Professor of Medicine
Associate Professor of Microbiology/Immunology
Co-Director of Pediatric Infectious Disease
Director of Vaccine Study Center
State University of New York Health Science Center at Brooklyn
Brooklyn, New York

DENNIS A. CLEMENTS, M.D., Ph.D.
Associate Professor
Primary Care and Infectious Diseases
Duke Children's Hospital
Durham, North Carolina

EMILY DiMANGO, M.D.
Assistant Professor of Clinical Medicine
Columbia University
College of Physicians and Surgeons
New York, New York

MORVEN S. EDWARDS, M.D.
Professor, Department of Pediatrics
Baylor College of Medicine
Houston, Texas

ANNE A. GERSHON, M.D.
Professor of Pediatrics
Division of Infectious Diseases
Columbia University
College of Physicians and Surgeons
New York, New York

LAURA GUTMAN, M.D.
Duke Vaccine Unit
Duke University Medical Center
Durham, North Carolina

CAROLINE BREESE HALL, M.D.
Professor of Pediatrics and Medicine in Infectious
    Diseases
Departments of Pediatrics and Medicine
University of Rochester School of Medicine and
    Dentistry
Rochester, New York

MARGARET R. HAMMERSCHLAG, M.D.
Professor of Pediatrics and Medicine
Department of Pediatrics
Co-Director of Pediatric Infectious Disease
State University of New York
Health Science Center at Brooklyn
Brooklyn, New York

DAVID S. HODES, M.D.
Professor of Pediatrics
Department of Pediatrics
Mount Sinai School of Medicine
New York, New York

PETER J. HOTEZ, M.D.
Associate Professor of Pediatrics and Epidemiology and
    Public Health
Yale University School of Medicine
New Haven, Connecticut

SHIRLEY JANKELEVICH, M.D.
HIV and AIDS Malignancy Branch
National Cancer Institute
National Institutes of Health
Department of Health and Human Services
Besthesda, Maryland

EDWARD L. KAPLAN, M.D.
Professor of Pediatrics
World Health Organization Collaborating Center for
    Reference and Research on Streptococci
University of Minnesota Medical School
Minneapolis, Minnesota

BEN Z. KATZ, M.D.
Associate Professor
Department of Pediatrics
Northwestern University Medical School
Attending Physician, Children's Memorial Hospital
Chicago, Illinois

SAMUEL L. KATZ, M.D.
Wilbert C. Davison Professor and
Chairman Emeritus, Department of Pediatrics
Duke University Medical Center
Durham, North Carolina

JEROME O. KLEIN, M.D.
Department of Pediatrics
Boston University School of Medicine
Maxwell Finland Laboratory for Infectious Diseases
Boston Medical Center
Boston, Massachusetts

WILLIAM C. KOCH, M.D.
Assistant Professor
Department of Pediatrics
Medical College of Virginia
Virginia Commonwealth University
Richmond, Virginia

KEITH KRASINSKI, M.D.
Professor of Pediatrics and Environmental Medicine
New York University Medical Center
New York, New York

PHILIP LaRUSSA, M.D.
Division of Infectious Diseases
Columbia University
College of Physicians and Surgeons
New York, New York

LINDA L. LEWIS, M.D.
Staff Physician
Infectious Diseases Division
DuPont Hospital for Children
Wilmington, Delaware

GEORGE H. McCRACKEN, Jr., M.D.
Professor of Pediatrics
The Sarah M. and Charles E. Seay Chair in Pediatric
    Infectious Diseases
University of Texas Southwestern Medical Center
Dallas, Texas

RIMA McLEOD, M.D.
Department of Ophthalmology
Visual Sciences Center
The University of Chicago
Chicago, Illinois

MARIAN MELISH, M.D.
Department of Pediatrics
University of Hawaii
Honolulu, Hawaii

GEORGE MILLER, Jr., M.D.
John F. Enders Professor of Pediatric Infectious
    Diseases
Professor of Epidemiology and Molecular Biophysics
    and Biochemistry
Department of Pediatrics
Yale University School of Medicine
New Haven, Connecticut

DOUGLAS K. MITCHELL, M.D.
Assistant Professor of Pediatrics
Center for Pediatric Research
The Children's Hospital of the King's Daughters
Eastern Virginia Medical School
Norfolk, Virginia

EDWARD A. MORTIMER, M.D.
Elisabeth Severance Prentiss Professor Emeritus
Department of Epidemiology and Biostatistics
Case Western Reserve University
School of Medicine
Cleveland, Ohio

LARRY K. PICKERING, M.D.
Professor of Pediatrics
Children's Hospital of the King's Daughters
Chair in Pediatric Research
Director, Center for Pediatric Research
Eastern Virginia Medical School
Norfolk, Virginia

PHILIP A. PIZZO, M.D.
Thomas Morgan Rotch Professor of Pediatrics
Harvard Medical School;
Physician-in-Chief and Chair
Department of Medicine
Children's Hospital
Boston, Massachusetts

STANLEY A. PLOTKIN, M.D.
Medical Scientific Director
Pasteur Merieux Connaught
Marnes-la-Coquette, France

ALICE S. PRINCE, M.D.
Professor of Pediatrics
Columbia University
College of Physicians and Surgeons
New York, New York

SARAH A. RAWSTRON, M.B.B.S.
Assistant Professor
Department of Pediatrics
State University of New York Health Science Center at
    Brooklyn
Brooklyn, New York

FIONA ROBERTS, M.D.
Department of Pathology
Western Infirmary, NHS Trust
Glasgow
United Kingdom

HARLEY A. ROTBART, M.D.
Professor of Pediatrics and Microbiology
Pediatric Infectious Diseases
University of Colorado Health Sciences Center
Denver, Colorado

XAVIER SÁEZ-LLORENS, M.D.
Professor of Pediatrics
University of Panama School of Medicine
Head, Division of Pediatric Infectious Diseases
Hospital del Nino
Panama

LISA SAIMAN, M.D.
Division of Infectious Diseases
Columbia University
College of Physicians and Surgeons
New York, New York

EUGENE D. SHAPIRO, M.D.
Professor of Pediatrics and of Epidemiology
Department of Pediatrics
Yale University School of Medicine
New Haven, Connecticut

JEFFREY R. STARKE, M.D.
Associate Professor of Pediatrics
Department of Pediatrics
Baylor College of Medicine
Houston, Texas

MELINDA WHARTON, M.D., M.P.H.
National Immunization Program
Centers for Disease Control and Prevention
Atlanta, Georgia

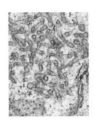

PREFACE

The goals of this book have changed little since its first publication in 1958. The format of the book, however, has changed since it was originally written by the late Robert Ward and the late Saul Krugman. This change in format was necessitated for two reasons. First, no one today could possibly have the breadth of knowledge and creativity of those two giants in the field, Ward and Krugman, who were among the few individuals who founded the subspecialty of Pediatric Infectious Diseases in the late 1950s. Second, the explosion of knowledge in the subspecialty now precludes the possibility of even two exceptional individuals to write such a book. Consequently, this 10th edition was edited by a group of 3 and written by a group of 34. But the aims of the book are unchanged. The preface to the initial edition stated that "the purpose of this book is to provide a concise and handy description of certain common infectious diseases of children. It is written primarily for pediatricians, general practitioners, and medical students who deal with children." We continue to resist the temptation to enlarge the volume to an encyclopedia of infectious diseases, which has been successfully accomplished in a number of other textbooks. Our goal continues to be to produce a concise, handy, and readable volume.

The 10th edition has experienced an evolution in editors and contributors. Dr. Saul Krugman's death on October 25, 1995, left a major void and saddened us all. We, the current editors, have chosen to name the book in Saul Krugman's honor and memory and therefore the title of the book has become *Krugman's Infectious Diseases of Children.* The loss of Dr. Catherine Wilfert as an editor was also difficult, but her departure has enabled her to concentrate her energies on AIDS in a number of roles, including Chair of the Pediatric AIDS Foundation. We continue to miss her intellectual energy and devotion, but we have also had the privilege of welcoming a member of the talented younger generation, Dr. Peter Hotez of Yale University, as a new editor.

New developments that are highlighted in this edition include updates on the rapidly moving field of HIV infection and AIDS; changes in the epidemiology of *H. influenzae* infections as a result of widespread immunization; new information on herpesviruses 6, 7, 8; the expanded current pathologic spectrum of streptococcal infections; and the latest information on tuberculosis. There are also several entirely new sections, including chapters on endocarditis, cystic fibrosis, parasitology, and wound and anaerobic infections. A number of new authors have participated in developing this 10th edition. They include Drs. Stuart Adler, Paula Annunziato, Carol Baker, Morven Edwards, Laura Gutman, Caroline Breese Hall, David Hodes, Shirley Jankelevich, Douglas Mitchell, Stanley Plotkin, Harley Rotbart, Lisa Saiman, Eugene Shapiro, Jeffrey Starke, and Melinda Wharton. The editors are deeply grateful to them and their other respected colleagues who have made this new format of the book possible. We hope that this 10th edition will contribute to the medical education of many and will result in improvements in the lives of children everywhere.

Samuel L. Katz
Anne A. Gershon
Peter J. Hotez

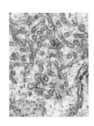

CONTENTS

COLOR PLATES

(can be found after page 370)

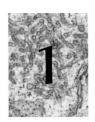

Acquired Immunodeficiency Syndrome (AIDS) and Human Immunodeficiency Virus (HIV)

1

William Borkowsky

In 1980 an outbreak of community-acquired *Pneumocystis carinii* pneumonia (PCP) was recognized in California and New York, and, simultaneously, Kaposi's sarcoma was recognized to be occurring at 50 times the expected rate in male homosexuals. These events combined to define an immunodeficiency syndrome never before described. This syndrome was soon observed in intravenous drug users, recipients of standard blood products (both male and female), and non–drug-using female sex partners of individuals with the disease.

In 1982 an *acquired immunodeficiency syndrome* (AIDS) was recognized in children (Centers for Disease Control, CDC, 1982) and was described in New Jersey (Oleske et al., 1983), New York (Rubinstein et al., 1983), San Francisco (Ammann et al., 1983), and Miami (Scott et al., 1984). In less than a decade a previously unknown disease became the single most important communicable disease in the United States and many other nations, a position it still holds today. Although pediatric HIV infection makes up only 2% of the total number of reported cases of AIDS in the United States, the rapid increase in reported cases in children and its emergence as a cause of death in young infants and children are clear.

ETIOLOGY

The causative agents of AIDS were isolated from the blood of patients and were described in both France (Barre-Sinoussi et al., 1983) and the United States (Gallo et al., 1984; Levy et al., 1984). They were referred to as the *lymphadenopathy-associated viruses* (LAV), the *human T-cell lymphotrophic viruses* (HTLV-III), and the *AIDS-related retroviruses* (ARV) by the respective groups. By consensus these agents now are termed the *human immunodeficiency viruses* (HIVs). These enveloped RNA viruses are in the lentivirus

subfamily of retroviruses and are 80 to 120 nm in diameter. Characteristics of HIV that resemble those of lentiviruses include (1) the long incubation period; (2) the ability to establish latent or persistent infection; (3) the ability to produce immune suppression; (4) tropism to lymphoid cells, particularly macrophages; (5) the ability to affect the hematopoietic system; (6) tropism to the central nervous system (CNS); and (7) the ability to produce cytopathic effects observed in appropriate cell types (Bryant and Ratner, 1991). The major targets of HIV are CD4-antigen–bearing cells such as helper T cells, monocytes and macrophages, Langerhans' cells, and glial cells of the CNS. HIV has also been reported as capable of infecting non–CD4-bearing cells such as enterocytes and certain neuronal cells. Virtually all individuals with primary HIV infection have viruses, isolated from peripheral blood mononuclear cells, which are monocytotropic and do not multiply in T-cell leukemia cell lines. As the infection progresses over the years and immune function fails, viruses capable of multiplying in T-cell lines such as HUT-76 and CEM emerge. These viruses that grow very rapidly in tissue culture and to high titer have been termed *syncytium-inducing* (SI) and *rapid-high* isolates. The monocytotropic isolates are referred to as *non–syncytium inducing* (NSI).

In vivo, virus production from infected lymphocytes continues for a relatively short period of time (i.e., a viral half life of 1.6 days) (Ho et al., 1995), 99% of virus production coming from recently infected cells (30% to 50% of virions in the plasma having come from a CD4 T cell infected the previous day).

HIV has a cylindrical eccentric core, or nucleoid, that contains the diploid RNA genome (Fig. 1-1). A nucleic acid–binding protein and reverse transcriptase are associated with the genome. Nucleocapsid

1

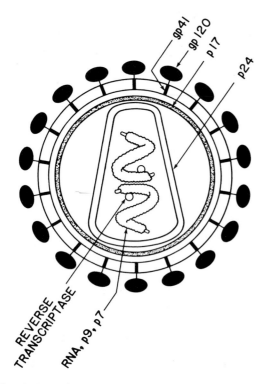

Fig. 1-1 Schematic representation of the morphologic structure of HIV-1. ENV gene products, gp120 and gp41; gag gene products, p24, p17, p9, and p7; pol gene product, RT.

structure is completed by the capsid antigen (p24), which encloses the nucleoid components. Surrounding the core of the virus is p17, the matrix antigen, which lines the inner surface of the envelope. Knoblike projections formed by the envelope glycoprotein, gp120, are on the surface of the virus. An associated intermembranous portion of the envelope, gp41, anchors the gp120 component.

A portion of the gp120 domain of the envelope binds to the CD4 molecule of human cells with high affinity, and a segment of the gp41 plays a crucial role in the fusion of the viral envelope with the host cell (Fig. 1-2). Several non-CD4 antigens also play an important role in viral entry. These include the recently described fusin molecule (C × CR4) in T cells (Feng et al., 1996) and a chemokine receptor (CCR-5) on monocyte/macrophage lineage cells (Deng et al., 1996) and activated T cells. After viral entry and uncoating, the reverse transcriptase characteristic of all retroviruses produces double-stranded virally encoded DNA that enters the nucleus and integrates randomly in the host genome by using the long-terminal-repeat (LTR) segments that flank the other genes of the virus. The virus is then in a latent state, in which it may remain indefinitely. A variety of stimuli—including antigens, mitogens, ultraviolet light, heat shock, hypoxia, and proteins derived from other viruses—are capable of initiating the transcription of HIV messenger

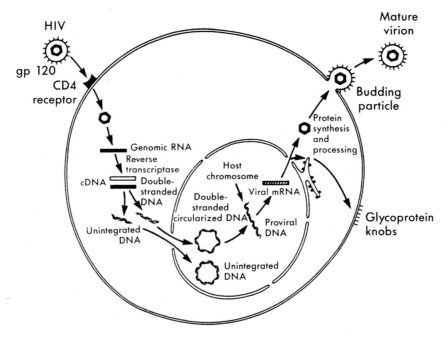

Fig. 1-2 The life cycle of the human immunodeficiency virus. (From Pizzo P, Wilfert CM, [eds]. Pediatric AIDS. Baltimore: Williams & Wilkins, 1991.)

RNA, which is first translated into complex spliced messages. These encode a group of regulatory molecules that ultimately govern the production of HIV messenger RNA capable of producing full-length transcripts and the associated structural proteins. The ribonucleoprotein core buds from the cellular membrane and acquires a coat of viral envelope glycoprotein and the lipid bilayer from the host cell. A viral enzyme (protease) completes the maturation of the virion by cleaving specific internal core components.

The individual isolates of HIV-1 from different persons vary a great deal. There is also considerable variation between sequential isolates obtained from the same infected person. HIV can spread from cell to cell independent of release of virus from the cell. This spread may occur through fusion or syncytium formation of an infected cell with uninfected cell(s).

PATHOGENESIS

HIV infection in children is characterized by an incubation period or asymptomatic interval that may be much shorter than it is in adults, but is not always so. The inevitable consequence of infection with HIV is profound immunosuppression, which leaves the host susceptible to the development of infections and neoplasms.

T4 Cells

The depletion of helper T cells (CD4) in symptomatic patients has been noted since 1981. HIV is capable of causing a profound cytopathic effect in T4 cells in vitro. However, only a small proportion of cells are infected with the virus, and not all are killed. Uninfected cells also die by a process of programed cell death, such as apoptosis, or are dysfunctional, perhaps mediated by the binding of gp120 to CD4 and thus interfering in its essential association with major histocompatibility complex (MHC) class II molecules. The virus is capable of establishing latency or a low level of replication in some cells.

T4-cell depletion is due in part to direct virus-induced damage, and there is some indication that "memory" helper T cells are more selectively depleted than "virgin" cells as a result of selective replication in the former cell type. The budding of large numbers of virus particles disrupting the external cell membrane contributes to destruction of the cell by creating osmotic disequilibrium. HIV replication results in the accumulation of a number of foreign products, including viral DNA, RNA,

and core proteins, which may interfere with normal cellular function and contribute to the death of the cell. Syncytia, or multinucleated giant cells, are observed in vitro with HIV replication. Such syncytia can form when CD4 molecules of uninfected T4 cells bind to the gp120 expressed on the surface of HIV-infected T4 cells. It is unknown whether syncytial formation contributes to cell death. The functional abnormalities of T4 cells from HIV-infected individuals are numerous despite the fact that the virus is present in only a small percentage of circulating T4 cells. These abnormalities include (1) defective helper interaction with B cells for immunoglobulin production; (2) defective proliferative responses to antigenic stimuli; (3) diminished expression of interleukin (IL-2) receptors; and (4) defective lymphokine production in response to antigenic stimuli, particularly of IL-2 and gamma interferon. These defects would be expected to predispose infected persons to infections with intracellular pathogens.

In the course of a normal immune response the CD4 molecule binds to the class II MHC molecules on the surface of an antigen-presenting immune cell. However, the CD4 molecule binds to gp120 of HIV with a greater affinity than for its normal ligand (class II MHC molecules). This high-affinity binding of gp120 to CD4 may contribute to the impaired T-cell responses and may also be the basis of autoimmune reactions destroying T4 cells. The gp41 of the virus possesses a region of homology with the class II MHC molecule. Anti-gp41 HIV antibodies from AIDS patients can react with class II MHC antigens and may therefore be involved in cytotoxicity or complement-mediated cell killing of uninfected target cells carrying only the class II MHC molecule. Antibody-dependent cellular cytotoxicity (ADCC) may contribute to cell death of both infected cells and uninfected cells. If an uninfected T4 cell binds free gp120 to its surface, the cell can be mistakenly identified as infected and subsequently be destroyed by ADCC or by gp120-specific, CD4-positive cytotoxic T cells. It has also been noted that HIV-infected T4 cells can kill adjacent uninfected T4 cells in vitro. It is estimated that as many as 2 billion cells (i.e., 5% of the total CD4 T-cell population) are destroyed daily. To maintain constant CD4 T-cell numbers, comparable numbers of cells must be produced daily.

T8 Cells

Soon after HIV infection, CD8+ T cells increase in frequency and number. In addition, these cells appear to be activated (Plaeger-Marshall S et al., 1993), most likely by HIV (Landay et al., 1993) but perhaps also by herpes viruses. Some of these cells may perform as cytotoxic T cells (Koup et al., 1994); others may inhibit viral replication in the absence of cytotoxicity (Walker et al., 1986).

Monocyte, Macrophage, and Dendritic Cells

HIV also infects cells of the CD4-expressing monocyte-macrophage lineage. The virus is not cytopathic to these cells but may interfere in their ability to present antigens to helper T cells. Intact virus particles may replicate to high numbers in these cells and may also be disseminated to tissues—such as the brain, spinal cord, lung, bone marrow, liver, heart, and gut—where soluble virus products may produce organ dysfunction. Alternatively, the virus may be borne to tissues wherein they replicate directly, thereby producing cell damage. These infected cells may also produce increased quantities of IL-1, IL-6, prostaglandins, and other molecules that may affect adjacent cell functions.

HIV has been shown to adhere to antigen-processing dendritic cells at high concentration but not to replicate in them. This probably serves as an important source of infection to T4 cells that come in contact with them.

B Cells

No spontaneously infected B cells have been observed in vivo, although some B lymphocytes bear CD4 on their surface and can be infected in vitro. Nevertheless, HIV infection results in profound effects on B-cell function. In vitro the HIV envelope can induce polyclonal B-cell activation (Pahwa et al., 1985). It may also produce increased IL-6 production by other cells, with resulting hypergammaglobulinemia. In spite of the observed hypergammaglobulinemia that is commonly seen, both primary and secondary antibody responses to some antigens may be impaired (Bernstein et al., 1985b), contributing to the high incidence of infection with common bacterial pathogens. The B-cell impairment often is observed in association with impaired T-cell responses to the same antigens (Borkowsky et al., 1987), and these findings are correlated with a poorer clinical outcome (Blanche et al., 1986).

Neutrophils

Although neutrophils are not directly infected by HIV, autoimmune neutropenias have been observed and neutrophil dysfunction has been described (Roilides et al., 1990). This defect may contribute to the immunodeficiency-related infections that occur.

PATHOLOGY

The primary pathologic effects of HIV infection are seen in the lymphoreticular system in which marked cell depletion is the end-stage pathology. HIV probably infects the epithelial cells of the thymus, and thymitis has been described. This initial inflammatory response is characterized by multinucleated giant cells in the medulla of the thymus or by diffuse lymphoplasmocytic or lymphomononuclear infiltrates of the cortex and medulla. These changes precede the involution noted in end-stage disease. The involution is characterized by depletion of lymphocytes, loss of corticomedullary differentiation, and microcystic dilation of Hassall's corpuscles (Joshi, 1991). In a few instances a reduction of Hassall's corpuscles has also been described, and this constellation is termed *dysinvolution.* The severe effects of the virus on the thymus of the young infant or fetus may contribute to the more rapid progression of the immunologic compromise. It is likely that thymic dysfunction continues to contribute to illness in adult life.

Lymphoproliferation in lymph nodes, the gastrointestinal tract, and lungs has been observed. It is now known that the concentration of HIV in these nodes vastly exceeds that seen in peripheral blood lymphocytes. Multinucleated giant cells are present. Late in the disease, lymph nodes are depleted of lymphocytes in the paracortex, ultimately progressing to marked lymphocyte depletion of the entire lymph node. Atrophic changes of the spleen, appendix, and Peyer's patches are also described in late stages. The pathologic features in the brain include atrophy; sclerosis; microglial nodules; and necrosis, with or without an inflammatory cell infiltrate, loss of myelin, vasculitis, and calcification of vessels and basal ganglia (Sharer, Cho, Epstein, 1985; Sharer et al., 1986). The virus has been localized by in situ hybridization in macrophages, microglia, and giant cells and less frequently in glial cells and neurons (Shaw et al., 1985; Stoler et al., 1986). Brain atrophy with compensatory ventricular dilatation is a common finding in children with clinically evident encephalopathy.

Opportunistic infections and malignancies of the CNS are infrequently seen in children. Pathologic findings associated with a broad spectrum of infectious agents—including *P. carinii* in the lungs,

Candida infection of the mucous membranes, *Mycobacterium avium-intracellulare* in almost all tissues, and cryptosporidirosis of the gastrointestinal tract—are seen in biopsy and autopsy specimens. Viruses that are common causes of infection include herpes simplex virus (HSV), cytomegalovirus (CMV), Epstein-Barr virus (EBV), and varicella-zoster virus (VZV). In contrast to adults, infections with human herpes virus 8 (HHV8), the probable agent causative of Kaposi's sarcoma, is rarely found in HIV-infected children.

Other findings of undetermined pathogenesis appear frequently in tissue examinations. Dilated cardiomyopathy is observed with microscopic hypertrophy of myocardial fibers, focal vacuolation, interstitial edema, small foci of fibrosis, and endocardial thickening. Unusually sparse inflammatory infiltrates are seen.

Clinically important renal disease is accompanied by microscopic findings of focal segmental glomerulosclerosis and mesangial proliferative glomerulonephritis (Connor et al., 1988). Immunoglobulin and complement deposits are evident by immunofluorescence. It is speculated that circulating immune complexes may contribute to the pathogenesis of the renal disease. P24 antigen has been demonstrated by in situ hybridization in tubular and glomerular epithelial cells in renal biopsy specimens of adults.

Hepatobiliary disease is not uncommon. Unfortunately, a variety of causes (i.e., HIV, EBV, CMV, HCV, drug toxicity) have been implicated, and it is rare that the liver histologic findings can clarify the process. Fatty infiltration, portal inflammation, lymphoplasmacytic inflammation, and cholestasis can be seen. Infection with CMV or cryptosporidium have also been associated with cholecystitis and sclerosing cholangitis-like conditions.

A variety of neoplastic disorders of the gastrointestinal tract—including lymphoma, leiomyosarcoma, and Kaposi's sarcoma (rarely)—have been described. The first two appear to have EBV genome in the tumor cells. Longer survival of children may result in more frequent occurrence of malignancies.

LABORATORY DIAGNOSIS

Antibody to HIV can be measured accurately and is the mainstay of laboratory diagnosis of HIV infection in adults, in children perinatally infected who are more than 15 months old, and in children of any age who have acquired HIV infection through transfusion or blood products. Enzyme-linked immunosorbent assay (ELISA) and Western blot assays measure antibodies to the major structural proteins or antigens of the virus and are commercially available. A positive ELISA must be confirmed by a second determination plus a positive Western blot assay on the same specimen to reduce the rate of false positives to approximately 1 in 100,000. Because all newborns receive maternal antibodies during the latter part of pregnancy through the placenta, any infant born to a mother with antibodies to HIV will also test positive, regardless of whether actually infected with HIV. The titer of maternal antibodies is usually high and may be detected of a dilution of 1 to several million. Because the half-life of IgG1, the predominant maternally transmitted immunoglobulin, is approximately 3 to 4 weeks, maternally derived anti-HIV antibody may persist for up to 15 or more months. Consequently, standard antibody assays for HIV may be misleading for the diagnosis of HIV infection in the infant less than 18 months of age. Assays that measure IgA subclass HIV-specific antibodies may facilitate the serologic diagnosis of HIV infection in young infants between 2 months and 1 year of age.

HIV can be grown in tissue culture from the majority of HIV-infected adults and children. HIV is detected in peripheral blood mononuclear cells and as cell-free virus in plasma and cerebrospinal fluid. These cultures may prove positive as early as 3 days after initiation but may require as long as 4 to 6 weeks for the diagnosis of low levels of virus. Early experience with attempts to isolate HIV from newborn or cord-blood lymphocytes suggests that no more than half of infected children are culture positive for HIV in the neonatal period. The HIV recovery rate increases substantially during the ensuing months, and almost all infected infants can be diagnosed by culture within the first 2 to 3 months of life. HIV core (p24) antigen can be detected in body fluids by ELISA. This antigen appears early after HIV infection and then often becomes undetectable, associated with the appearance of anti-p24 antibody in most infected adults. The antigen reappears as the HIV infection progresses and can be found with increasing frequency in more symptomatic individuals. This antigen can be found in more than half of HIV-infected infants during the first year of life but in substantially fewer babies during the first months of life and in only 10% of infected newborns (Borkowsky et al., 1989). The measurement of p24 antigen may also help identify the 10% of HIV-infected hypogammaglobulinemic children who are anti-HIV ELISA negative (Borkowsky et al., 1987). Dissociation of anti-p24 antibodies from p24 antigen may increase the sensitivity of the assay during the first month of life (Smiles et al.; Chandwani et al, 1993).

One of the most sensitive diagnostic techniques is the polymerase chain reaction (PCR), a method by which the viral DNA can be amplified a million times. Virus culture and detection of virus DNA by PCR in infant blood appear to be equally sensitive as tests to diagnose infection in an infant. The sensitivity of PCR in early diagnosis of infection of infants born to HIV-infected mothers was first shown in a study conducted by the CDC, in collaboration with the New York City Department of Health and several hospitals in New York (Rogers et al., 1989). Many subsequent studies have verified the sensitivity of PCR and have shown that it is comparable to HIV culture for early diagnosis. The technical problems with PCR relate to the extreme sensitivity of the test. If there is the smallest amount of contaminating DNA in the material tested, it can be amplified and give either ambiguous or false-positive results. Modifications of the assay have made these inaccuracies less likely to occur. The test can be completed in 1 to 2 days. A recently licensed test to measure HIV RNA copy numbers can also be completed within this period of time and may prove even more sensitive than DNA PCR for early diagnosis.

Other nonspecific laboratory parameters that may be helpful in the diagnosis of infection include immunologic measurements. The classic hallmark of infection is a low CD4 cell count and an altered CD4:CD8 ratio. Age-appropriate normal values must be used for comparison. Elevated serum immunoglobulin levels are characteristic of infection. A minority (approximately 10%) of children may have hypogammaglobulinemia.

Other assays for early detection of HIV infection in babies use measurement of antibody production by the infant. Several approaches have been used. Peripheral blood lymphocytes have been harvested and stimulated with pokeweed mitogen or Epstein-Barr virus and the supernatant fluids tested for the production of specific HIV antibody (Amadori et al., 1988; Pahwa et al., 1989; Pollack et al., 1993). Alternatively, peripheral blood mononuclear cells have been placed into cell culture wells containing HIV antigens. When labeled antihuman globulin is used, the cells producing antibody are identified by "spots" in the wells (Lee et al., 1989). Maternal

IgA antibody does not cross the placenta, so the presence of HIV-specific antibody of this subclass describes an infant who is infected. Detection of specific IgA antibody is being evaluated as a means of making an early diagnosis of HIV infection in young infants, and it has been demonstrated by 6 months of age in cohorts of infected infants (Mann et al., 1994). The ability to make HIV-specific antibody does not become fully developed until a few months of age, well after HIV antigen or nucleic acid can be detected.

EPIDEMIOLOGY AND NATURAL HISTORY

The World Health Organization (WHO) estimates that, as of 1996, 18 million adults and adolescents and 1.5 million children had been infected with HIV. Sub-Saharan Africa has 11 million people who are infected, but the disease is spreading most rapidly in South and Southeast Asia, where there are an estimated more than 3 million infected adults. By the year 2000, 30 to 40 million individuals are expected to be infected, the majority from developing countries. Sexual transmission is the major mode of spread of HIV-1 infection in most developing countries. In some African and Caribbean cities 5% to 20% of pregnant women are HIV seropositive. Bidirectional heterosexual transmission has been well documented. The role of heterosexual transmission is steadily increasing in the United States. Perinatal transmission parallels heterosexual transmission because a substantial proportion of these infected persons are women of reproductive age. The male/female ratio of reported AIDS cases approaches 1 when heterosexual transmission of infection predominates, and the percentage of pediatric AIDS cases increases dramatically with this ratio (CDC, 1995).

The risk factors associated with the development of AIDS among women are also risk factors for the transmission of HIV to infants and children. They include (1) intravenous drug use, which is an admitted risk behavior in 50% of HIV-infected women in the United States; (2) heterosexual contact with a person who is HIV infected, which is the risk behavior for 40% of infected women in the United States (two thirds of the partners are admitted intravenous drug users; sexual exposure in prepubertal children may occur in the context of childhood sexual abuse [Gutman et al., 1991]); and (3) receiving blood products (whole blood and its components, including clotting factor concentrates). Although the screening of blood products for HIV antibody as of May 1984 has largely eliminated any transmission of HIV by blood products in the United States, such transmission continues to plague developing countries and countries such as Russia and Romania.

Perinatal Infection

In the United States the major risk for pediatric HIV infection is a child born to an infected mother. Black and Hispanic populations are disproportionately infected. In 1995, 84% of children reported with AIDS were in these categories. In the U.S. population, lower socioeconomic status is also disproportionately represented (CDC, 1995). It is unknown whether HIV infection is transmitted predominantly in utero or during parturition. HIV transmission probably can occur by more than one mechanism. There is evidence that in utero infection occurs, based on the recovery of HIV in cell culture from fetuses that have been aborted between 9 and 20 weeks of gestation (Sprecher et al., 1986; Kashkin et al., 1988; Jovais et al., 1985; Di Maria et al., 1986). Evidence of severe thymic depletion has been seen in such abortuses. These and other observations suggest that a portion of the cohort found to be infected perinatally is infected in utero. In Africa, studies of placentas demonstrated chorioamnionitis in placentas of women who delivered infected babies. These women had advanced HIV disease, and it is not possible to determine whether this inflammatory response is a result of secondary infection or a direct consequence of the severity of the HIV infection. Recovering HIV from placental tissue has been difficult, but HIV has been found in placentas by in situ hybridization (Chandwani, 1991) and by PCR (Andiman and Modlin, 1991). HIV has been demonstrated in placental macrophages (Hofbauer cells) in fetal villi. These cells could serve either as a barrier to or as a means of fetal HIV infection. The detection of HIV in the placenta does not predict whether an infant has acquired infection.

In spite of the timing of perinatal infection, virtually all newborns of HIV-infected mothers are born without obvious signs of clinical or immunologic abnormalities. Studies performed worldwide have found that 15% to 30% of children born to infected women will prove to be infected with HIV, even in the absence of breast-feeding. Yet half of this group cannot be shown to have evidence of HIV infection at birth using current virologic, immunologic, and molecular biological techniques.

A variety of factors have been found to correlate with increased HIV transmission to the fetus or young infant. These include (1) maternal blood viral burden (Weiser et al., 1994; Borkowsky et al., 1994); (2) exposure to high levels of vaginal HIV burden (Minkoff et al., 1995); (3) low maternal CD4 level (Goedert et al 1989); (4) high maternal CD8 level (St. Louis et al., 1993); and (5) vaginal delivery (Tovo et al., 1995).

The increase in HIV transmission to the first (twin A) of multiple births with discordant HIV infection has been used to suggest that exposure to vaginal HIV is an important risk factor (Duliege et al., 1995). However, this pattern was also seen in those delivered by cesarean section. In addition, a perinatal intervention trial in Malawi that studied the effect of vaginal cleansing on HIV transmission failed to show an effect. Nevertheless, prolonged (>4 hours) ruptured membranes (Landesman et al., 1996) appears to be a risk factor for HIV transmission.

Several reports (Devash et al., 1990; Goedart et al., 1989; Rossi et al., 1989) have suggested that the frequency of perinatal HIV transmission is decreased in those women who have antibodies directed at gp120. More specifically, women with antibody (particularly of "high affinity") to the third variable region (V3 loop) of the HIV envelope were far less likely to transmit HIV to their offspring. Unfortunately, there has been a great deal of disagreement about the actual site recognized by these antibodies. There have also been discrepant findings when sera were shared and analyzed by these and independent investigators. With the finding that combined treatment of an HIV-infected mother during the last trimester of pregnancy and her offspring for 6 weeks with a nucleoside analog, zidovudine (ZDV), resulted in a reduction of transmission from 26% to 8% (Connor et al., 1994), this regimen with ZDV has become the standard of care.

Thus it remains likely that some HIV transmission occurs at the time of parturition, as in the model of hepatitis B transmission. Although some studies have suggested that children infected at this time are more likely to have a better clinical outcome than children infected in utero (Dickover et al., 1994; Mayaux et al., 1996), the effect of the timing of infection on outcome as an isolated high-risk factor has been disputed, and it has been suggested that the extent of viral replication in the first months of life may be a better correlate (Arlievsky et al., 1995; Papaevangelou et al. 1996).

Data suggest that maternal HIV infection results in lower birth weights for infants. Many of the studies have been complicated by the high rate of illegal drug use in HIV-I seropositive women, and infants born to cocaine- or heroin-using women have significantly lower birth weights and higher mortality rates than non–drug-using women (Selwyn et al., 1989). Studies in developing nations have been free of the confounding effects of illegal drug use, but women having babies in these nations have more advanced HIV disease. In both Africa and Haiti the birth weights of infants born to HIV-I–seropositive women are significantly lower than the birth weights of infants born to seronegative women (Ryder et al., 1989; Halsey et al., 1990). In addition, the mortality rates in both Africa and Haiti are higher in infants born to seropositive women. This may be due to an increased exposure to other infectious agents or to decreased accessibility to medical care. Mortality rates in infants born to HIV-negative women are substantially higher in these areas than in developed nations, and it is apparent that HIV and AIDS are increasing the overall perinatal mortality rate. A prospective natural history study in the United States showed that HIV-infected infants were 0.28 kg lighter and 1.64 cm shorter than uninfected infants at birth (Moye et al., 1996). The children maintained their decrease in height and weight and had a sustained decrement in head circumference by 18 months of age. In this study, zidovudine therapy was not associated with improved growth. Results have also shown diminished stature in HIV-infected newborns (Pollack et al., 1996), with catch-up growth in those who demonstrate limited HIV viral burden as measured by RNA copy number, but sustained short stature and diminished weight in those with high viral burden.

The majority of infected children become symptomatic during the first 6 (median of 5.2, range of 0.03 to 56) months of life, with the development of lymphadenopathy as the initial finding (Galli et al., 1995). The most common signs in the first year of life are lymphadenopathy (70%), splenomegaly (58%), and hepatomegaly (58%), with only 19% of infected children remaining asymptomatic for a year. Some HIV-infected children develop a severe failure to thrive or encephalopathy during the first year of life. These children appear to have exceptionally high levels of HIV in their blood during the first few months of life (Arlievsky et al., 1995). Survival in such children, as well as in those who develop symptoms before 5 months of age, is significantly lower than in those with a later onset of symptoms when assessed at both 1 year and 5 years of age.

Transfusion and Coagulation Factor Acquired Disease

Approximately one half (or 10,000) of Americans with hemophilia are seen regularly in treatment facilities. The largest cohort study reported to date indicates that the prevalence of HIV antibodies in those with severe factor VIII deficiency is 76.5%; in those with moderate disease, 46.3%; and in those with mild disease, 25.4% (Eyster, 1991). In a smaller population of persons with Christmas disease (factor IX deficiency) the prevalence is 41.9% in those with severe disease, 26.9% in those with moderate disease, and 8.3% in those with mild disease (Eyster, 1991). Exposure to coagulation factor deficiency now represents fewer than 10% of all cases of pediatric and adolescent AIDS. The use of recombinant factors and methods that effectively eliminates the possibility of HIV survival in today's products should make this risk factor extraordinarily rare as a cause of pediatric HIV infection.

Screening of blood products for HIV, initiated in 1984, has made this risk factor a rare cause of HIV infection for children, adolescents, and adults. A recent study estimates the risk for infection as 1 in 493,000 (95% confidence interval of 202,000 to 2,778,000; Schreiber et al., 1996). Antibody screening alone will not detect blood products from donors who have acute HIV infection. The use of assays that detect actual virus should prevent the likelihood that such blood will be used for transfusion.

Adolescents

The absolute number of cases of AIDS among adolescents 13 to 19 years of age is smaller than that reported in children less than 13 years of age, but this number underestimates acquisition of HIV in teenagers. The incubation period is sufficiently long that adolescents who have acquired infection may not become ill until an older age (i.e., in their twenties and thirties). The steady rate of increase of reported AIDS in adolescents has paralleled that recorded in adults and children.

Transmission in adolescents results from the same routes as in adults. Initially, the largest proportion of reported adolescent AIDS cases was composed of those resulting from transfusion of blood products for coagulation disorders. Currently a large category comprises those resulting from homosexual or bisexual contact. Among young adolescents 13 to 14 years old, exposure to HIV through the transfusion of blood products for hemophilia accounts for 70% of the cases and blood transfusions for an additional 21%; in this age subset almost 90%

of AIDS cases are among boys. However, the proportion of cases attributable to transfusion with blood or blood products decreases in the older teens. The proportion of cases caused by behavior-related exposure increases from 9% among 13 and 14 year olds to 24% among 15 and 16 year olds and to 69% among 17 to 19 year olds. The single largest exposure category is sexual contact between males, which accounts for 36% of the cases.

The number of infected adolescent girls is now approaching the number of infected adolescent boys. Among female adolescents the most frequent exposure category is heterosexual contact, which accounts for 44% of cases. Male intravenous drug users are reported as partners in 60% of the female heterosexually acquired cases. Intravenous drug use by the girl accounts for 28% of the female cases. Therefore a total of 8% of reported female cases are related to intravenous drug use. Estimates of HIV seroprevalence in adolescents and young adults are accumulating as part of the CDC Comprehensive Family of Serosurveys. The median seroprevalence is highest in the sexually transmitted disease (STD) clinics for adolescents and

ranges from 0% to 4.6%, with a median of 0.5% (Gayle and D'Angelo, 1991). Several studies of adolescents have been performed, indicating seroprevalences ranging from 0.37% in Washington, D.C., to 7% in homeless adolescents in New York City (Gayle and D'Angelo, 1991). The variability is obvious, as is the fact that the number of reported AIDS cases does not accurately reflect the number of HIV infections in this population.

CLINICAL MANIFESTATIONS

Children with HIV infection have a broad spectrum of clinical manifestations. The original classification was a useful way to categorize illness, and it demonstrates the array of infectious agents and organ systems that may be involved. Using the original classification system, however, only clinical problems were used to to stage HIV infection with regard to natural history and prognosis. Table 1-1 presents the new modified classification system for HIV in children developed by the CDC in 1994 (MMWR Sept. 30). This new classification system incorporates both clinical (Boxes 1-1 and 1-2) and immunologic variables (Table 1-2) to stage in-

Table 1-1 Pediatric human immunodeficiency virus (HIV) classification*

Immunologic categories	Clinical categories			
	N: No signs/ symptoms	A: Mild signs/ symptoms	B:† Moderate signs/ symptoms	C:† Severe signs/ symptoms
1: No evidence of suppression	N1	A1	B1	C1
2: Evidence of moderate suppression	N2	A2	B2	C2
3: Severe suppression	N3	A3	B3	C3

From Centers for Disease Control: MMWR 1994;43:1-10
*Children whose HIV infection status is not confirmed are classified by using the above grid with a letter E (for perinatally exposed) placed before the appropriate classification code (e.g., EN2).
†Both Category C and lymphoid interstitial pneumonitis in Category B are reportable to state and local health departments as acquired immunodeficiency syndrome.

Table 1-2 Immunologic categories based on age-specific CD4+ T-lymphocyte counts and percentage of total lymphocytes

Immunologic category	Age of child					
	<12 mos		1-5 yrs		6-12 yrs	
	μl	(%)	μl	(%)	μl	(%)
1: No evidence of suppression	≥1,500	(≥25)	≥1,000	(≥25)	≥500	(≥25)
2: Evidence of moderate suppression	750-1,499	(15-24)	500-999	(15-24)	200-499	(15-24)
3: Severe suppression	<750	(<15)	<500	(<15)	<200	(<15)

From Centers for Disease Control: MMWR 1994;43:1-10

BOX 1-1

CLINICAL CATEGORIES FOR CHILDREN WITH HUMAN IMMUNODEFICIENCY VIRUS (HIV) INFECTION

Category N: Not Symptomatic

Children who have no signs or symptoms considered to be the result of HIV infection or who have only one of the conditions listed in Category A.

Category A: Mildly Symptomatic

Children with two or more of the conditions listed below but none of the conditions listed in Categories B and C.
- Lymphadenopathy ($\geq$0.5 cm at more than two sites; bilateral = one site)
- Hepatomegaly
- Splenomegaly
- Dermatitis
- Parotitis
- Recurrent or persistent upper respiratory infection, sinusitis, or otitis media

Category B: Moderately Symptomatic

Children who have symptomatic conditions other than those listed for Category A or C that are attributed to HIV infection. Examples of conditions in clinical Category B include but are not limited to the following:
- Anemia (<8 gm/dl), neutropenia (<1,000/mm^3), or thrombocytopenia (<100,000/mm^3) persisting $\geq$30 days
- Bacterial meningitis, pneumonia, or sepsis (single episode)
- Candidiasis, oropharyngeal (thrush), persisting (>2 months) in children >6 months of age
- Cardiomyopathy
- Cytomegalovirus infection, with onset before 1 month of age
- Diarrhea, recurrent or chronic
- Hepatitis
- Herpes simplex virus (HSV) stomatitis, recurrent (more than two episodes within 1 year)
- HSV bronchitis, pneumonitis, or esophagitis with onset before 1 month of age
- Herpes zoster (shingles) involving at least two distinct episodes or more than one dermatome
- Leiomyosarcoma
- Lymphoid interstitial pneumonia (LIP) or pulmonary lymphoid hyperplasia complex
- Nephropathy
- Nocardiosis
- Persistent fever (lasting >1 month)
- Toxoplasmosis, onset before 1 month of age
- Varicella, disseminated (complicated chickenpox)

Category C: Severely Symptomatic

Children who have any condition listed in the 1987 surveillance case definition for acquired immunodeficiency syndrome (10), with the exception of LIP (Box).

From Centers for Disease Control: MMWR 1994;43:1-10

fected children. A comparison of the old classification system and the new one is shown in Table 1-3. In addition to characterizing clinical syndromes, the classification system has proved useful for determining who should receive prophylaxis against PCP.

PCP is the most commonly reported AIDS-indicator disease in children. Infants presenting with PCP are usually less than 1 year of age. In adults with AIDS there is a correlation between the CD4 count and the subsequent occurrence of PCP. Seven percent of adults with a CD4

BOX 1-2

CONDITIONS INCLUDED IN CLINICAL CATEGORY C FOR CHILDREN INFECTED WITH HIV

Category C: Severely Symptomatic*

- Serious bacterial infections, multiple or recurrent (i.e., any combination of at least two culture-confirmed infections within a 2-year period), of the following types: septicemia, pneumonia, meningitis, bone or joint infection, or abscess of an internal organ or body cavity (excluding otitis media, superficial skin or mucosal abscesses, and indwelling catheter-related infections)
- Candidiasis, esophageal or pulmonary (bronchi, trachea, lungs)
- Coccidioidomycosis, disseminated (at site other than or in addition to lungs or cervical or hilar lymph nodes)
- Cryptococcosis, extrapulmonary
- Cryptosporidiosis or isosporiasis with diarrhea persisting >1 month
- Cytomegalovirus disease with onset of symptoms at age >1 month (at a site other than liver, spleen, or lymph nodes)
- Encephalopathy (at least one of the following progressive findings present for at least 2 months in the absence of a concurrent illness other than HIV infection that could explain the findings): (a) failure to attain or loss of developmental milestones or loss of intellectual ability, verified by standard developmental scale or neuropsychological tests; (b) impaired brain growth or acquired microcephaly demonstrated by head circumference measurements or brain atrophy demonstrated by computerized tomography or magnetic resonance imaging (serial imaging is required for children <2 years of age); (c) acquired symmetric motor deficit manifested by two or more of the following: paresis, pathologic reflexes, ataxia, or gait disturbance
- Herpes simplex virus infection causing a mucocutaneous ulcer that persists for >1 month; or bronchitis, pneumonitis, or esophagitis for any duration affecting a child >1 month of age
- Histoplasmosis, disseminated (at a site other than or in addition to lungs or cervical or hilar lymph nodes)
- Kaposi's sarcoma
- Lymphoma, primary, in brain
- Lymphoma, small, noncleaved cell (Burkitt's), or immunoblastic or large-cell lymphoma of B-cell or unknown immunologic phenotype
- *Mycobacterium tuberculosis,* disseminated or extrapulmonary
- *Mycobacterium,* other species or unidentified species, disseminated (at a site other than or in addition to lungs, skin, or cervical or hilar lymph nodes)
- *Mycobacterium avium* complex or *Mycobacterium kansasii,* disseminated (at site other than or in addition to lungs, skin, or cervical or hilar lymph nodes)
- *Pneumocystis carinii* pneumonia
- Progressive multifocal leukoencephalopathy
- Salmonella (nontyphoid) septicemia, recurrent
- Toxoplasmosis of the brain with onset at >1 month of age
- Wasting syndrome in the absence of a concurrent illness other than HIV infection that could explain the following findings: (a) persistent weight loss >10% of baseline OR (b) downward crossing of at least two of the following percentile lines on the weight-for-age chart (e.g., 95th, 75th, 50th, 25th, 5th) in a child ≥1 year of age OR (c) <5th percentile on weight-for-height chart on two consecutive measurements, ≥30 days apart PLUS (a) chronic diarrhea (i.e., at least two loose stools per day for ≥30 days) OR (b) documented fever (for ≥30 days, intermittent or constant)

From Centers for Disease Control: MMWR 1994;43:1-10
*See the 1987 AIDS surveillance case definition (10) for diagnosis criteria.

Table 1-3 Comparison of the 1987 and 1994 pediatric human immunodeficiency virus (HIV) classification systems

1987 Classification	1994 Classification
P-0	Prefix "E"
P-1	N
P-2A	A, B, and C
P-2B	C
P-2C	B
P-2D1	C
P-2D2	C
P-2D3	B
P-2E1	C
P-2E2	B
P-2F	B

From Centers for Disease Control: MMWR 1994;43:1-10

count of $<200/\text{mm}^3$ will develop PCP within 6 months, 15% within 12 months, and 30% within 36 months (Phair et al., 1990). Infection correlates with the degree of immunocompromise, and CD4 counts are predictive of risk of PCP. Correlations with CD4 counts in children can also be made, although infants normally have much higher CD4 levels than adults. CD4 counts of $<1500/\text{mm}^3$ have been observed in 90% of reported cases of PCP younger than 12 months (CDC, 1991).

PCP may occur in children 1 to 2 years old when CD4 counts are $<750/\text{mm}^3$ and in children 2 to 6 years old when CD4 counts are $<500/\text{mm}^3$. These values reflect the higher numbers of CD4 cells normally present in young children. Thus prophylaxis for PCP can be empirically based on the CD4 values and be offered to all children with "severe suppression" (category 3).

In the original classification of HIV disease in children, multiple or recurrent serious bacterial infections were included as a prominent manifestation of AIDS. Two or more serious infections in a 2-year period met the case definition of AIDS in a young HIV-seropositive infant. When AIDS was first identified in children, bacteremia appeared to occur in almost half of the children who were diagnosed. More recent estimates of the frequency of bacteremia suggest that it occurs less often, particularly if only community-acquired infections are evaluated. The relative risk for invasive bacteremia with community-acquired organisms is about threefold to twelvefold higher (with about 1 infection per 100 person-months) than that seen in HIV-uninfected children born to infected mothers (Andiman et al.,

1994; Felowyn et al., 1994). This decrease may in part be attributable to the ability to diagnose HIV infection before such severe complications bring a child to medical attention. Children less than 2 years old have an evolving immunologic ability to identify polysaccharide antigens. Thus even normal infants are susceptible to pathogens such as pneumococcus and *Haemophilus influenzae* type B. Children with HIV infection are not only susceptible, but, with their compromised immune system, their susceptibility is prolonged. Hypergammaglobulinemia is a common development in children with HIV infection because of polyclonal activation of B cells. These antibodies are largely nonspecific, and children do not recognize antigens or respond well as their disease progresses. Thus elevated IgG levels in these children indicate an abnormal host response and one that is functionally antibody deficient. The major bacterial diseases in HIV-infected children are bacteremia and sepsis; but meningitis, cellulitis, wound infection, gastroenteritis, and pneumonia also occur frequently. A primary focus of infection is not uniformly identified in bacteremic children; more than half may have no known focus. Several reports (Krasinski et al., 1988; Bernstein et al., 1985a) have indicated that *Streptococcus pneumoniae* is the most common pathogen in bacteremic disease and is reported in approximately 30% of infections. A National Institute of Child Health and Human Development (NICHD) study has estimated that pneumococcal bacteremia in untreated symptomatic patients occurs at a rate of 37 per 1,000 patients per year. Infections with *Haemophilus influenzae, Salmonella* species, staphylococci, and a variety of other encapsulated organisms have been reported. Unfortunately, many of these children have had community- and hospital-acquired gram-negative bacteremias. Upper-respiratory infections, including sinusitis and otitis media, are very common. Recurrent episodes of these infections are frequent sources of chronic fever and require vigorous antibiotic therapy. Chronic sinusitis may require prolonged intravenous antibiotic therapy or aggressive surgical drainage.

Chronic Pneumonitis

Lymphoid interstitial pneumonitis (LIP), or pulmonary lymphoid hyperplasia, is a common occurrence and was reported in 28% of children with AIDS in 1988 and 1989. The etiology of this syndrome is unknown, with both EBV and HIV being implicated in the disease process (Andiman et al., 1985; Chayt et al., 1986). However, EBV is not always found, and HIV may be isolated from bronchoalveolar fluid and lung tissue even in the absence of LIP.

LIP usually is diagnosed in children with perinatally acquired HIV infection who are more than 1 year of age. It often begins as an asymptomatic pulmonary infiltrate but can progress to severe pulmonary compromise with superimposed complications of disease such as pneumonia or congestive heart failure. The chronic illness and hypoxemia can be similar to that with chronic bronchiectasis. Children with LIP tend to have a longer survival time than children with encephalopathy or a history of PCP. The entity frequently is associated with chronic parotitis, hypergammaglobulinemia, and lymphadenopathy. A possible adult equivalent of LIP has been described and appears to occur exclusively in individuals with a particular HLA class II haplotype (Itescu et al., 1989). As children with LIP develop progressive T4 lymphopenia with advanced age, the LIP syndrome appears to improve, although their overall HIV disease actually worsens.

Encephalopathy and Myelopathy

CNS involvement is frequent in children with HIV infection. Studies reporting children with advanced HIV disease suggest that up to 60% will have neurologic manifestations (Belman et al., 1988; Epstein et al., 1986). Reported neurologic findings include impaired brain growth, generalized weakness with pyramidal signs, pseudobulbar palsy, ataxia, seizures, myoclonus, and extrapyramidal rigidity. Approximately 40% of HIV-infected children may develop progressive encephalopathy, resulting in the loss of developmental milestones or subcortical dementia. However, some preliminary natural history studies suggest that progressive encephalopathy may be present in a smaller proportion (i.e., 9% to 20%) of children (European Collaborative Study, 1988; Blanche et al., 1989; Mok et al., 1987). These children were observed to a mean age of 18 months and included those with mild and asymptomatic disease. It has also been reported that approximately 25% of children have an encephalopathy that does not progress (Epstein et al., 1988). A recent study of children who were evaluated at a mean age of 9.5 years revealed that two thirds had normal IQs. However, 54% had abnormal results on visual-spatial and time orientation tests. Children with normal school achievement had higher CD4+ cells during the first years of life (Tardieu et al., 1995). Although the manifestations

of CNS involvement with HIV may vary considerably, it is agreed that the virus does infect the CNS and that the young infant with an immature CNS is uniquely susceptible to damage, resulting in an array of developmental deficits and neurologic abnormalities such as spastic paraparesis. In addition to the harmful effects of HIV infection per se on the CNS, HIV-infected children can develop additional CNS complications, including neoplasm, stroke, and infections with other pathogenic organisms.

Wasting Syndrome and Diarrhea

The gastrointestinal tract is also a source of invasive pathogens, and children with HIV infection sustain symptomatic infections with the common bacterial organisms such as *Salmonella, Shigella, Campylobacter,* and *Clostridium difficile. Salmonella* species occur more commonly than in normal children and cause invasive disease. Relapse of symptomatic illness has been reported. Adult studies have suggested that ceftriaxone may be more successful in eradicating *Salmonella* species than more commonly used forms of therapy such as ampicillin or trimethoprim-sulfamethoxazole (Rolston et al., 1989). In children with exceptionally low T4 counts ($<50/mm^3$ absolute), disseminated *M. avium-intercellulare* may produce a profound wasting disease. Anemia, daily fever, and leukopenia are also commonly seen in such cases. Treatment with multiple drugs—including ethambutol, long-acting macrolides, rifabutin, quinolones, and aminoglycosides—may result in transient improvement.

Gastrointestinal tract infections with protozoal organisms are usually of short duration in normal persons. However, in persons with a compromised immune system, such as children with AIDS, the clinical course often is protracted. *Cryptosporidium, Isospora belli, Giardia lamblia,* and *Microsporida* infection have been reported in AIDS patients. *Cryptosporidium* species are probably the most common parasitic causes of diarrhea in adult AIDS patients and have produced similar chronic disease, although less frequently, in children. Failure to thrive, or the HIV wasting syndrome, may be due to a complex array of infectious agents, including HIV. HIV-infected adult patients may have malabsorption even when no opportunistic infections are present. HIV infection can be associated with abnormal small bowel mucosa, and the histologic conditions vary from normal to villous atrophy with crypt hypoplasia. HIV RNA has been demonstrated in macrophages and lymphocytes in the lamina propria of intestinal biopsies (Fox et al.,

1989; Nelson et al., 1988). A child may have acute diarrhea, chronic nonspecific diarrhea, or failure to thrive. In addition to these problems, HIV-infected individuals apparently are in a hypermetabolic state, which probably increases normal caloric and fluid requirements.

Opportunistic Infections

Opportunistic infections are a common complication in HIV-infected children but are somewhat different from those in adults. Oral *Candida* infection is extremely common in immunocompetent infants because they may acquire the organism as early as parturition. It is thought that 80% of infants are colonized by 4 weeks of age (Russell and Lay, 1973). It is estimated that 15% to 40% of children with HIV infection have oral candidiasis. In the normal child, oral *Candida* infection is often mild and readily treated. *Candida* infection in children with HIV infection appears as oral mucosal candidiasis, gingivostomatitis, and periodontitis. Although it may respond initially to simple therapy such as oral nystatin solution, the hallmark of HIV infection is the persistence of *Candida* species.

Children who develop severe *Candida* infection are likely to have diminished numbers of CD4 cells. Candidiasis may extend to the esophagus and the larynx. Esophageal candidiasis is an indicator disease of AIDS, and it can occur without obvious oral pharyngeal candidiasis. Disseminated candidiasis is an unusual occurrence in HIV-infected children. Infections with agents of the herpesvirus group—including HSV, CMV, and VZV—are among the reported manifestations of HIV infection in children. These are ubiquitous pathogens of children, and their ability to establish latency and the potential to induce severe infections in immunocompromised hosts are manifest as both severe and chronic infection in children with HIV infection.

Hematologic Syndromes

Although cervical lymphadenopathy is a very nonspecific sign, the presence of axillary and inguinal nodes in a young infant should arouse suspicion of HIV infection. Hepatosplenomegaly may accompany the lymphadenopathy. CD4+ cell numbers may remain normal at this time. The most common abnormality is microcytic or normocytic anemia, which occurs even with elevated erythropoietin levels. Thrombocytopenia resulting from the clearance of immune-complex–coated platelets by the reticuloendothelial system occurs in approximately 10% of patients. This syndrome can be differenti-

ated from idiopathic thrombocytopenic purpura (ITP) by the presence of complement on the platelet surface, but it may respond to standard therapies effective in treating ITP. Treatment with antiviral medications that inhibit HIV replication may be the treatment of choice for this disorder. Alternate therapies include high dose monthly infusions of IVIG, intermittent treatment with anti-D immunoglobulin (Rhogam), and splenectomy. Lupus anticoagulants are seen in HIV-infected adults and are probably also found in HIV-infected children.

Anemia and leukopenia are common manifestations of advanced HIV disease. In some cases these have been associated with infections (e.g., disseminated MAI, CMV, parvovirus), whereas in others toxicity from multidrug therapy has been implicated (e.g., ZDV, trimethoprim-sulfa). HIV may also directly interfere with hematopoietic stem cell maturation.

Hepatitis Syndrome

Liver transaminase and alkaline phosphatase levels are often elevated in HIV-infected children. Hyperbilirubinemia occurs infrequently, but obstructive jaundicelike conditions have been seen in young infants (Persaud et al., 1993). Although this hepatitis may be due to infection with secondary pathogens or may be a reaction to drugs such as trimethoprim-sulfamethoxazole and fluconazole, it is often intrinsic to HIV infection alone. HIV can replicate in hepatoma cell lines and can be found in liver macrophages. Chronic hepatitis B infection is usually milder in HIV-infected immunocompromised individuals than in those not infected, reaffirming the theory that chronic active hepatitis is immunologically mediated. Hepatitis C virus (HCV) infection is often present in HIV-infected women and may be transmitted to their offspring at increased frequency (15% to 50%), often in the absence of anti-HCV antibody in coinfected children (Papaevangelou et al., unpublished). The contribution of HCV to the hepatitis syndrome remains to be elucidated.

Renal Syndrome

Some children with HIV infection may present with a rapidly progressive glomerulopathy. Light microscopy demonstrates focal segmental glomerulosclerosis and mesangial glomerulonephritis (Connor et al., 1988). Immunoglobulin and complement deposits are evident by immunofluorescence. It is speculated that circulating immune complexes may contribute to the disease. HIV p24 antigen has been demonstrated by in situ hybridization in tubular and glomerular epithelial cells in renal biopsy specimens of adults. Increased production of IL-6, a lymphokine associated with other glomerulopathies, may also play a role in pathogenesis.

Cardiac Syndrome

Abnormalities, including progressive left ventricular dilatation and poor myocardial contractility with compensatory hypertrophy, may occur early in children with HIV disease without obvious clinical consequences (Lipshultz et al., 1992). The progression of this disease and the occurrence of myocarditis, pericardial effusion, and the effects of LIP on function of the right side of the heart may ultimately produce congestive heart failure. EBV coinfection is strongly correlated with chronic congestive failure (Luginbuhl et al., 1993). As children progress to a diagnosis of AIDS, significant cardiac dysfunction is seen with tachycardia, bradycardia, hypertension, hypotension, and dysrhythmias. Secondary agents such as CMV, enteroviruses, and *M. avium-intracellulare* may contribute to this syndrome. HIV RNA has been found in macrophages infiltrating myocardial tissue in children with this disorder.

Malignancies

Although Kaposi's sarcoma, recently associated with HHV8 infection, is the most common neoplasm in adults with AIDS, it occurs very rarely in children, possibly because of relative infrequent infection of young children with HHV8. Lymphoreticular malignancies are being reported with increasing frequency in both HIV-infected adults and children. These tumors can appear as both Hodgkin's and non-Hodgkin's lymphomas. The latter is most often a B-cell malignancy (e.g., Burkitt's lymphoma) but may also be a T-cell lymphoma. The lymphomas may be discrete or disseminated and commonly present in the CNS. The risk is increased in individuals who have lived with fewer than 50 CD4+ cells/mm^3 for more than 2 years. Rarely, eiomyosarcomas and progressive giant papillomas may also occur.

DIFFERENTIAL DIAGNOSIS

HIV infection can both mimic a host of other disorders and predispose a patient to certain of them. These disorders include the following:

1. Maturational immunodeficiency of newborns, resulting in neonatal sepsis and severe infection with herpesviruses (especially CMV)
2. Congenital infections, with associated lymphadenopathy and hepatosplenomegaly
3. Congenital immunodeficiency states
   a. Severe combined immunodeficiency
   b. DiGeorge's syndrome
   c. Wiskott-Aldrich syndrome
   d. Agammaglobulinemia or hypogammaglobulinemia
   e. Ataxia telangiectasia
   f. Neutrophil defects in mobility or killing
   g. Chronic mucocutaneous candidiasis
4. Inflammatory bowel diseases
5. Hereditary encephalopathies and neuropathies
6. ITP
7. Chronic allergies with sinusitis, otitis, and dermatitis
8. Cystic fibrosis or α_1-antitrypsin deficiency
9. Primary lymphoreticular malignancy

TREATMENT
Specific Retroviral Therapy

Primary infection with HIV results in HIV copy numbers in excess of a million/ml of plasma. Eventually this level of viremia decreases to a "set point" that is unique to each individual, ranging from 100 to several million copies/ml, remaining stable for months and occasionally years. There appears to be an inverse correlation between the set point HIV copy number and survival.

The ideal goal of treatment would be to eradicate all virus-infected cells and cure the infection. This is currently becoming feasible as more potent antiretrovirals become available, in spite of the fact that 1 to 10 billion viral particles are produced daily. Available therapeutic agents (Table 1-4) suppress viral multiplication by 0.5 log to 3 log titers and improve or reverse some of the symptoms, improving the quality and duration of life.

Azidothymidine (AZT), or ZDV, was the first antiretroviral agent approved for use in children. The recommended dosage for children is 60 to 180 mg/m^2 administered every 6 hours. ZDV was shown to increase the rate of the patient's growth, decrease p24 antigen levels in the serum and cerebrospinal fluid, and decrease serum immunoglobulin levels (McKinney et al., 1991). ZDV, at higher doses and given intravenously, also improved the neurobehavioral status of children with HIV infection (Brouwers et al., 1994). The survival of ZDV-treated children with AIDS appears longer than that of historical controls. Prolonged use of ZDV is lim-

Table 1-4   Available therapeutic agents to suppress viral multiplication

Generic name	Trade name	Dose	Preparation	Administration	Side effects	Drug interaction
Nucleoside Agents						
zidovudine (AZT, ZDV)	Retrovir	90-180 mg/m^2 tid or qid	Syrup: 10 mg/ml Tablet: 100 mg		Bone marrow suppression elevated liver transaminases	acetaminophen ganciclovir fluconazol pentamidine rifampin
didanosine (DDI)	Videx	100 mg/m^2 bid	Liquid: 10 mg/ml Powder: 100 mg pack Chewable: 100 mg	Empty stomach or 30′ before meal	Pancreatitis, peripheral neuropathy bone marrow suppression	dapsone ketoconazole itraconazole ethambutol, INH zalcitabine metronidazole
lamivudine (3TC)	Epivir	3 mo-12 yr 4 mg/kg bid	Liquid: 10 mg/ml Tablets: 150 mg		Pancreatitis (8-14%) peripheral neuropathy (12%) rash (9%)	bactrim
stavudine (D4T)	Zerit	1.25-2 mg/kg/ day <60 kg: 30 mg bid >60 kg: 40 mg bid	Liquid: 1 mg/ml Tablets: 15, 20, 30, 40 mg	With or without food	Peripheral neuropathy increased liver transaminases	dapsone ethambutol, INH metronidazole foscarnet pentamidine
zalcitabine (DDC)	Hivid	0.005 or 0.01 mg/kg q8h adult: 0.75 mg q8h	Syrup: (investi-gational) 0.1 mg/ml Tablets: 0.375 mg 0.75 mg		Peripheral neuropathy oral ulcers	foscarnet phenytoin metronidazol ganciclovir
Nonnucleosides						
nevirapine	Virimune	60 mg/m^2 bid adult: 200 mg bid	Liquid: 10 mg/ml Tablets: 50, 100, 200 mg	Empty stomach 1 hr before food	Rash (17%) severe rash (4%) fever increased liver transaminases thrombo-cytopenia	erithromycin cimetidine augmentin timentin
Protease Inhibitors						
saquinavir	Invirase	adult: 600 mg bid	Capsules: 200 mg	2 hrs after food	Diarrhea (4%) nausea (2%) rash (1%) mucositis (2.5%)	ketoconazol rifampin rifabutin

Table 1-4   Available therapeutic agents to suppress viral multiplication—cont'd

Generic name	Trade name	Dose	Preparation	Administration	Side effects	Drug interaction
Protease Inhibitors—cont'd						
indinavir	Crixivan	500 mg/m² tid adult: 800 mg tid	Capsules: 200, 400 mg	Empty stomach or light meal 2 hrs after meal	Nephrolithiasis (9%) flank pain increased bilirubin increased liver transaminases nausea (12%) taste perversion hematuria	ketoconazol rifabutin rifampin
ritonavir	Norvir	400 mg/m² bid	Capsules: 100 mg Liquid: 80 mg/ml	Full stomach Heavy meal	Nausea vomiting diarrhea increased liver transaminases increased cholesterol	ketoconazol rifabutin meperidine diazepam versed
nelfinavir	Viracept	400-500 mg/m² tid or 20-30 mg/kg/dose	Capsules: 500, 750 mg	8-12 oz of water	Loose stools diarrhea	ketoconazol rifabutin meperidine diazepam versed

ited by bone marrow toxicity to erythroid and myeloid elements. Some of the toxicity can be modified by dose reduction. ZDV-resistant HIV isolates emerge after 6 to 12 months of therapy and limit its usefulness as a single agent.

Other nucleoside derivatives, including didanosine (DDI), zalcitabine (DDC), and stavudine (D4T) have also proven effective in adults and children. Initial treatment with DDI was found to be superior to that of ZDV alone and equivalent to that of DDI and ZDV in children (Englund et al., 1997). Peripheral neuropathy and pancreatitis are recognized toxicities of DDI. Mutations in single bases in the reverse transcriptase molecule are sufficient to produce resistant virus. A given mutation (e.g., codon 184) may also result in cross resistance to other nucleoside RT inhibitors. The use of drug combinations will likely result in a decrease in the emergence of resistant viruses. In adults, lamivudine (3TC), another nucleoside analog, has proven clinically more efficacious, when combined with ZDV, than monotherapy alone (Eron et al., 1995).

Nonnucleoside reverse transcriptase inhibitors (NNRTI) such as niverapine and delaveridine appear to be more potent (resulting in a 2-log reduc-

tion of viral RNA levels) than the nucleosides but also fraught with the likelihood of the appearance of highly resistant HIV isolates emerging within weeks of treatment initiation. In contrast to the nucleoside analogs, which are incorporated into nascent viral DNA and cause chain termination, the NNRTI drugs bind to the viral reverse transcriptase and inhibit its function. The combination of these drugs with several other anti-HIV drugs, including the nucleoside reverse transcriptase inhibitors, may result in a delay in the appearance of resistant virus.

The introduction of HIV protease inhibitors such as saquinavir, ritonavir, indinavir, and nelfinavir to the therapeutic armamentarium has resulted in far more dramatic reductions (1 log to 2.5 log) of HIV burden than any of the isolated nucleosides (0.5 log to 1.5 log) (Carpenter et al. 1996). Unfortunately, HIV resistance often develops rapidly in an environment of insufficient drug concentration. Although several mutations appear to be necessary to produce resistant virus, cross-resistance to other protease inhibitors (e.g., indinavir resistance may render a virus resistant to ritonavir) although not always (e.g., indinavir/ritonavir resistant virus remains sensitive to saquinavir). The combination of

Antivirals. HIV-infected children may develop overwhelming or chronic secondary viral infections. VZV may produce disseminated disease and death, or it may result in a necrotizing ulcerating zoster skin lesion. Varicella-zoster immune globulin (VZIG) should be used prophylactically to prevent or modify VZV infection when a known exposure occurs in a child susceptible to varicella. Acyclovir therapy may be used to modify VZV infection. Prolonged high-dose oral acyclovir therapy is often used to heal and prevent exacerbations of the skin ulcers (Jura et al., 1989). Measles may produce a fulminating and fatal disease in HIV-infected children (Krasinski et al., 1988). Gamma globulin may modify the clinical appearance of the disease but has not prevented measles. All HIV-infected children, even if vaccinated, should receive gamma globulin if a known exposure to measles occurs. Some limited experience with ribavirin, given parenterally, has suggested that it may be an effective antimeasles agent.

Respiratory syncytial virus (RSV) infection in the HIV-infected infant results in delayed eradication of this respiratory pathogen. It also produces a modified clinical picture, with only the rare occurrence of wheezing and the more common appearance of pneumonia (Chandwani et al., 1990). Aerosolized ribavirin has not been systematically studied in this situation.

Immunizations. HIV-seropositive and HIV-infected children should receive all of their recommended childhood immunizations. Inactivated poliovirus vaccine should be substituted for oral poliovirus vaccine in both the children and their household contacts who are receiving vaccine, although this may not be possible in developing nations. In particular, HIV-seropositive infants should receive measles, mumps, and rubella (MMR) vaccines. Studies done in Africa have shown that protection attributable to vaccine in these children is substantial but less than that achieved in healthy children (Oxtoby et al., 1988).

There has been some concern raised about the potentially adverse effects of immune stimulation by vaccines, resulting in increased HIV RNA levels. Thus far, these increases appear to be limited to the immediate postvaccination period, with a return to baseline levels by 4 weeks (Rosok et al., 1996). The clinical consequences of such transient elevation in viremia remain to be elucidated.

General Nutrition. Many children with HIV infection are unable to sustain a positive nutritional balance. Some drugs, such as the steroid Megace, may improve appetite and increase patient weight. It should be noted that such increases are largely a result of fat and not protein. Protein and caloric support can be provided with tube feedings and/or total parenteral nutrition. It has, however, been shown that the risk of catheter infections is considerably higher in HIV-infected children than in other children requiring such intravenous support (e.g., those with malignancies), necessitating an individualized approach to choosing this option for any patient.

MEDICAL MANAGEMENT

Infants born to HIV-seropositive women should be identified so they can receive optimal medical care. Access to care is of critical importance. Ideally, identification of infected women would occur before or during pregnancy so that they too could receive optimal medical care. The recommendation by the U.S. Public Health Service is for seropositive women not to breast-feed because of the undefined risk of viral transmission in the postpartum period. However, in developing nations the benefits of breast-feeding are clearly more important than the small risk of transmission of the virus, and those women should breast-feed their infants. The care of HIV-seropositive infants in the first year of life is very much the same as that for healthy infants. However, these infants should have a CD4 count and HIV culture done every 1 to 3 months if possible. Depending on the resources available, a PCR should be performed along with viral culture for diagnosis. Supportive care provided to children known to be seropositive is of critical importance. The response to an unknown febrile illness or the suspicion that pulmonary disease may be PCP can be lifesaving for these infants. Finally, the institution of PCP prophylaxis is probably the single most important lifesaving part of their medical management at the present time. It is possible that early administration of retroviral therapy may provide even greater benefit than its administration to symptomatic children; thus infected infants must be identified as early as possible.

PROGNOSIS

The epidemiologic and circumstantial data suggest that there are two groups of children who have different responses to HIV infection. The first group, who present with illness during the first year of life, has a more rapid progression of disease and death. These children may have been infected in utero (Dickover et al., 1994), although this remains controversial (Papaevengalou et al., 1996). Other infants may be infected in the first year but present with symptoms later; they appear to have a more sustained course of illness.

The diagnosis of PCP in an HIV-infected child carries a poor prognosis. The survival rate after diagnosis of PCP is shown in Fig. 1-4 (Borkowsky, unpublished data based on 294 perinatally infected children seen at Bellevue Hospital). The 50% survival for this group is less than 2 years. This is in marked contrast to those perinatally infected children without PCP, with a 50% survival in excess of 12 years. Improved methods for early HIV diagnosis—coupled with earlier implementation of primary and adjunctive therapies, including prophylactic measures against PCP—should dramatically improve future survival.

PROPHYLAXIS
Vertical Transmission

The institution of antiretroviral therapy during the late stages of pregnancy of an HIV-infected woman and the continuation for the first weeks of infancy have resulted in a dramatic reduction of HIV transmission, from over 20% to under 10% (Connor et al., 1994). Although it appears reasonable that this

effect was due to a reduction in maternal viral load, this was not the case in the original study (ACTG 076) (Spelling et al., 1996).

The regimen employed in ACTG 076 was maternal AZT 500 mg/day after 14 weeks of gestation. During labor a loading dose of AZT was intravenously given (2 mg/kg over 1 hour) followed by a continuous infusion of 1.5 mg/kg. Infants were begun on AZT within 8 to 12 hours of age, either orally (2 mg/kg q6h) or intravenously (1.5 mg/kg q6h) and treated orally for 6 weeks, with close follow up of hemoglobin levels for the presence of anemia, the major adverse event encountered.

Postexposure Needle Stick

Exposure to HIV by needle stick in a nosocomial setting or in the community unfortunately occurs all too often. Fortunately, the average risk for HIV infection from all types of percutaneous exposure is estimated to be only 0.3%. Guidelines have been drafted by the Centers for Disease Control and Prevention Task Force (Centers for Disease Control 1996;45:468-72). These guidelines, based on a case-control study demonstrating a 79% reduction in HIV transmission in treated individuals and presumptions of relative antiviral efficacy, suggest that therapy with multiple antiretroviral drugs be initiated as soon as possible and continued for 4 weeks (or 2 weeks if 3 or more drugs are given simultaneously) if percutaneous exposure to blood from high- or increased-risk source material occurs. The definition of high risk would include a large volume of inoculum with a high titer of HIV in the inoculum (e.g., blood from a symptomatic individual). Increased risk would be a large volume of inoculum *or* a high-titer inoculum.

Mucous Membrane and Skin Exposure

The risk following exposure to HIV-containing fluids is estimated to be <0.1% and probably depends on the titer of HIV in the fluid. The risk increases if the duration of exposure is long or if there is a loss of integrity in the skin or mucous membrane barrier. ZDV plus another antiretroviral may be offered if the risk is felt to be increased. Urine and saliva are not likely to transmit HIV.

Sexual Exposure

In the absence of data, physicians should discuss the potential risk and unknown benefits of prophylactic antiretroviral intervention with those exposed to semen from an HIV-infected individual.

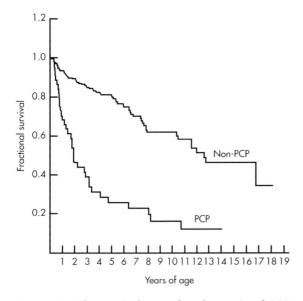

FIG. 1-4 The survival rate after diagnosis of PCP. (Borkowsky, unpublished data based on 294 perinatally infected children seen at Bellevue Hospital.)

BIBLIOGRAPHY

Amadori A, De Rossi A, Giacquinto C, et al. In vitro production of HIV-specific antibody in children at risk for HIV infection. Lancet 1988;1:852-854.

Ammann AJ, Cowan MJ, Wara DW, et al. Acquired immunodeficiency in an infant: possible transmission by means of blood products. Lancet 1983;1:956-958.

Andiman W, Eastman RN, Martin K, et al. Opportunistic lymphoproliferations associated with EBV DNA in infants and children with AIDS. Lancet 1985;2:1390-1393.

Andiman WA, Mezger J, Shapiro E. Invasive bacterial infections in children born to women infected with human immunodeficiency virus type 1. J Pediatri 1994;124:846-852.

Andiman WA, Modlin JF. Vertical transmission. In Pizzo P, Wilfert CM (eds). Pediatric AIDS. Baltimore: Williams & Wilkins, 1991.

Arlievsky NZ, Pollack H, Rigaud M, et al. Shortened survival in infants with human immunodeficiency virus with elevated p24 antigenemia. J Pediatr 1995;127:538-543.

Barre-Sinoussi F, Cherman JC, Rey F, et al. Isolation of a T-lymphotrophic retrovirus from a patient at risk for acquired immunodeficiency syndrome (AIDS). Science 1983;220:868-871.

Belman AL, Diamond G, Dixon D, et al. Pediatric acquired immunodeficiency syndrome: neurologic syndromes. Am J Dis Child 1988;149:29-35.

Bernstein LJ, Krieger BZ, Novick B, et al. Bacterial infection in the acquired immunodeficiency syndrome of children. Pediatr Infect Dis 1985a;4:472-475.

Bernstein LJ, Ochs HD, Wedgwood RJ, Rubinstein A. Defective humoral immunity in pediatric acquired immunodeficiency syndrome. J Pediatr 1985b;107:352-357.

Biggar RJ, Miotti PG, Taha TE, et al. Perinatal intervention trial in Africa: effect of a birth canal cleansing intervention to prevent HIV transmission. Lancet 1996;347:1647-1650.

Blanche S, Le Deist F, Fischer A, et al. Longitudinal study of 18 children with perinatal LAV/HTLV III infection: attempt at prognostic evaluation. J Pediatr 1986;109:965-970.

Blanche S, Rouziouz C, Moscato ML, et al. A prospective study of infants born to mothers seropositive for human immunodeficiency virus type 1. N Engl J Med 1989;320:1643-1648.

Borkowsky W, Krasinski K, Paul D, et al. Human immunodeficiency virus infections in infants negative for anti-HIV by enzyme linked immunoassay. Lancet 1987;1:1168-1171.

Borkowsky W, Krasinski K, Paul D, et al. Human immunodeficiency virus core protein antigenemia in children with HIV infection. J Pediatr 1989;114:940-945.

Borkowsky W, Kaul A. Cholestatic hepatitis in children with HIV infection. Ped Infect Dis 1993;12:492-497.

Borkowsky W, Krasinski K, Cao Y, et al. Correlation of perinatal transmission of human immunodeficiency virus-1 with maternal viremia and lymphocyte phenotypes. J Pediatr 1994;125:345-351.

Brouwers P, Decarli C, Tudorwilliams G, et al. Interrelations among patterns of change in neurocognitive, CT brain imaging, and CD4 measures associated with anti-retroviral therapy in children with symptomatic HIV infection. Adv Neuroimmunol 1994;4:223-231.

Bryant ML, Ratner L. Biology and molecular biology of HIV. In Pizzo P, Wilfert CM (eds). Pediatric AIDS. Baltimore: Williams & Wilkins, 1991.

Carpenter C, Fischl MA, Hammer S, et al. Antiretroviral therapy for HIV infection in 1996. JAMA 1996;276:146-154.

Centers for Disease Control. Unexplained immunodeficiency and opportunistic infections in infants: New York, New Jersey, California. MMWR 1982;31:665-667.

Centers for Disease Control. Update: acquired immunodeficiency syndrome—United States, 1989. MMWR 1990;39:81-86.

Centers for Disease Control. Pneumocystis carinii pneumonia prophylaxis in children. MMWR 1991;40:1-14.

Centers for Disease Control. 1994 Recommendations of the U.S. Public Health Service Task Force on the use of zidovudine to reduce perinatal transmission of human immunodeficiency virus. MMWR 1994;43:1-20.

Centers for Disease Control. 1994 Revised classification system for human immunodeficiency virus infection in children less than 13 years of age. MMWR 1994;43:1-10.

Centers for Disease Control. 1995 Revised guidelines for Prophylaxis against Pneumocystis Carinii pneumonia for children infected with or perinatally exposed to human immunodeficiency virus. MMWR 1995; 44:1-11.

Centers for Disease Control. HIV/AIDS Surveillance Report. MMWR 1995;7:1-38.

Chandwani S, Borkowsky W, Krasinski K, et al. Respiratory syncytial virus infections in human immunodeficiency virus infected children. J Pediatr 1990;117:251-254.

Chandwani S, Greico A, Mittal K, et al. Pathology and human immunodeficiency virus expression in placentas of seropositive women. J Infect Dis 1991;163:1134-1138.

Chandwani S, Moore T, Krasinski K, Borkowsky W. Early diagnosis of HIV-1 infected infants by plasma p24 antigen assay after immune complex dissociation. Pediatr Infect Dis J 1993;12:96-97.

Chayt K, Harper M, Marselle L, et al. Detection of HTLV-III RNA in lungs of patients with AIDS and pulmonary involvement. JAMA 1986;256:2356-2359.

Connor E, Gupta S, Joshi V, et al. Acquired immunodeficiency syndrome: associated renal disease in children. J Pediatr 1988;113:38-44.

Connor EM, Sperling RS, Gelber R, et al. Reduction of maternal-infant transmission of human immunodeficiency virus type 1 with zidovudine treatment. N Engl J Med 1994;331:1173-1180.

Deng HK, Liu R, Ellmeier W, et al. Identification of a major coreceptor for primary isolates of HIV-1. Nature 1996;381:661-666.

Devash Y, Calvetti TA, Wood DG, et al. Vertical transmission of human immunodeficiency viruses correlated with the absence of high affinity/avidity maternal antibodies to the GP 120 principal neutralizing domain. Proc Natl Acad Sci USA 1990;87:3445-3449.

Dickover RE, Dillon M, Gillette SG, et al. Rapid increases in load of human immunodeficiency virus correlate with early disease progression and loss of CD4 cells in vertically infected infants. J Infect Dis 1994;170:1279-1284.

Di Maria H, Courpotin C, Rouzioux C, et al. Transplacental transmission of human immunodeficiency virus. Lancet 1986;2:215-216.

Duliege AM, Amos CI, Felton S, et al. Birth order, delivery route, and concordance in the transmission of human immunodeficiency virus type 1 from mothers to twins. J Pediatr 1995;126:625-632.

Englund JA, Baker CJ, Raskino C, et al. Diadanosine and combination zidovudine/didanosine are superior to zidovudine monotherapy for the initial treatment of symptomatic children infected with human immunodeficiency virus. N Engl J Med 1997;326:1704-1712.

Epstein LG, Sharer LR, Goudsmit J. Neurologic and neuropathological features of HIV infection in children. Ann Neurol 1988;23:S19-S23.

Epstein LG, Sharer LR, Oleski JM, et al. Neurologic manifestations of human immunodeficiency virus infection in children. Pediatrics 1986;78:678-687.

Eron JJ, Benoit SL, Jemsek J, MacArthur RD. Treatment with lamivudine, zidovudine, or both in HIV-positive patients with 200 to 500 CD4+ cells per cubic millimeter. N Engl J Med 1995;333:1682-1689.

European Collaborative Study. Mother to child transmission of HIV infection. Lancet 1988;2:1039-1042.

European Collaborative Study. Children born to women with HIV-1 infection: natural history and risk of transmission. Lancet 1991;337:253-260.

Eyster ME. Transfusion and coagulation factor acquired disease. In Pizzo P, Wilfert CM (eds). Pediatric AIDS. Baltimore: Williams & Wilkins, 1991.

Felowyn PA, Farley JJ, King JC, et al. Invasive pneumococcal disease among infected and uninfected children of mothers with human immunodeficiency virus infection. J Pediatr 1994;124:853-858.

Feng Y, Broder CC, Kennedy PE, Berger E. HIV-1 entry cofactor: functional cDNA cloning of a seven-transmembrane, G protein-coupled receptor. Science 1996;272:872-877.

Fox CH, Kotler D, Tierney A, et al. Detection of HIV-1 RNA in the lamina propria of patients with AIDS in GI disease. J Infect Dis 1989;159:467-471.

Galli L, de Martino M, Tovo PA, et al. Onset of clinical signs in children with HIV-1 perinatal infection. AIDS 1995;9:455-461.

Gallo RC, Salahuddin SZ, Popovic M, et al. Frequent detection and isolation of cytopathic retroviruses (HTLV-3) from patients with AIDS and at high risk for AIDS. Science 1984;224:500-503.

Gayle HD, D'Angelo LJ. The epidemiology of AIDS and HIV infection in adolescents. In Pizzo P, Wilfert CM (eds). Pediatric AIDS. Baltimore: Williams & Wilkins, 1991.

Goedert JJ, Mendez H, Drummond JE, et al. Mother to infant transmission of human immunodeficiency virus type 1: association with prematurity or low anti-gp 120. Lancet 1989;2:1351-1354.

Gutman LT, St.-Claire K, Weedy C, et al. Human immunodeficiency virus transmission by sexual abuse. Am J Dis Child 1991;145:137-141.

Halsey NA, Boulos R, Holt E, et al. Transmission of HIV-1 infections from mothers to infants and babies. Impact on childhood mortality and malnutrition. JAMA 1990;264:2088-2092.

Ho DD, Neumann AU, Perelson AU, et al. Rapid turnover of plasma virions and CD4 lymphocytes in HIV-1 infection. Nature 1995;373:123-126.

Hutto C, Parks WP, Lai S, et al. A hospital-based prospective study of perinatal infection with human immunodeficiency virus type 1. J Pediatr 1991;118:347-353.

Itescu S, Brancato LJ, Winchester R. A sicca syndrome in HIV infection: association with HLA-DR5 and CD8 lymphocytosis. Lancet 1989;2:466-468.

Joshi VV. Pathologic findings association with HIV infection in children. In Pizzo P, Wilfert CM (eds). Pediatric AIDS. Baltimore: Williams & Wilkins, 1991.

Jovais E, Koch MA, Schafer A, et al. LAV/HTLV-III in a 20-week fetus (letter). Lancet 1985;2:1129.

Jura E, Chadwick E, Joseph S, et al. Varicella-zoster virus infections in children infected with human immunodeficiency virus. Pediatr Infect Dis 1989;8:586-590.

Kashkin JM, Shliozberg J, Lyman WD, et al. Detection of human immunodeficiency virus (HIV) in human fetal tissues. Pediatr Res 1988;23(2):355A.

Koup RA, Safrit JT, Cao Y, et al. The initial control of viremia during primary HIV-1 syndrome is temporally associated with the presence of cellular immune responses. J Virol 1994;68:4650-4655.

Krasinski K, Borkowsky W, Bonk S, et al. Bacterial infections in human immunodeficiency virus infected children. Pediatr Infect Dis 1988;7:323-328.

Landay AL, Mackewicz CE, Levy JA. An activated CD8+ T cell phenotype correlates with anti-HIV activity and asymptomatic clinical status. Clin Immunol Immunopath 1993; 69:106-116.

Landesman SH, Kalish LA, Burns DN, et al. Obstetrical factors and the transmission of human immunodeficiency virus type 1 from mother to child. N Engl J Med 1996;334:1617-1623.

Lee FK, Nahmias AJ, Lowery S, et al. ELISPOT: a new approach to studying the dynamics of virus-immune system interaction for diagnosis and monitoring of HIV infection. AIDS Res Hum Retrovir 1989;5:517-523.

Levy JA, Hoffman AD, Kramer SM, et al. Retroviruses from San Francisco patients with AIDS. Science 1984;225:840-842.

Lipshultz SE, Orav EJ, Sanders SP, et al. Cardiac structure and function in children with human immunodeficiency virus infection treated with zidovudine. N Engl J Med 1992;327:1260-1265.

Luginbuhl LM, Orav J, McIntosh K, and Lipshultz SE. Cardiac morbidity and related mortality in children with HIV infection. JAMA 1993;269:2869-2675.

Mann DL, Hamlin-Green G, Willoughby A, et al. Immunoglobulin class and subclass antibodies to HIV proteins in maternal serum: association with perinatal transmission. J AIDS 1994;7:617-622.

Mayaux MJ, Burgard M, Teglas JP, et al. Neonatal characteristics in rapidly progressive perinatally acquired HIV-1 disease: the French Pediatric HIV Infection Study Group. JAMA 1996;275:606-610.

Minkoff H, Burns DN, Landesman S, et al. The relationship of the duration of ruptured membranes to vertical transmission of human immunodeficiency virus. Am J Obstet Gynecol 1995;173:585-589.

Mok JG, Gianquinto C, Derossi A, et al. Infants born to mothers seropositive for human immunodeficiency virus: preliminary findings from the multicenter European study. Lancet 1987;1:1164-1168.

Moye J, Rich KC, Kalish LA, et al. Natural history of somatic growth in infants born to women infected by human immunodeficiency virus. J Pediatr 1996;128:58-69.

Nelson JA, Wiley CA, Reynolds-Kohler C, et al. Human immunodeficiency virus detected in bowel epithelium from patients with gastrointestinal symptoms. Lancet 1988;1:259-262.

Oleske J, Minnefor A, Cooper R, et al. Immune deficiency in children. JAMA 1983;249:2345-2349.

Oxtoby MS, Mvula M, Ryder R, et al. Measles and measles immunity in African children with HIV (abstract 1353). Interscience Conference on Antimicrobial Agents and Chemotherapy, Los Angeles, 1988.

Pahwa S, Pahwa R, Saxinger C, et al. Influence of the human T-lymphotropic virus/lymphadenopathy virus on functions of human lymphocytes: evidence for immunosuppressive effects and polyclonal B-cell activation by banded viral preparations. Proc Natl Acad Sci USA 1985;82:8198-8202.

Pahwa S, Chirmule N, Leombruno C, et al. In vitro synthesis of human immunodeficiency virus–specific antibodies in peripheral blood lymphocytes of infants. Proc Natl Acad Sci 1989;86:7532-7536.

Papaevangelou V, Pollack H, Rigaud M, et al. The amount of early p24 antigenemia and not the time of first detection of virus predicts the clinical outcome of vertically HIV-1 infected infants. J Infect Dis 1996;173:574-578.

Persaud D, Bangaru B, Greco MA, et al. Cholestatic hepatitis in children with HIV infection. Ped Infect Dis 1993;12:492-499.

Plaeger-Marshall S, Hultin P, Bertolli J, et al. Activation and differentiation antigens on T cells of healthy, at-risk, and HIV-infected children. J AIDS 1993;6:984-993.

Pollack H, Glasberg H, Lee E, et al. Neurodevelopment, growth, and viral load in HIV-infected infants. Brain Behav, Immun 1996;10:298-312.

Quinn TC, Ruff A, Halsey N. Special considerations for developing nations. In Pizzo P, Wilfert CM (eds). Pediatric AIDS. Baltimore: Williams & Wilkins, 1991.

Roilides E, Mertins S, Eddy J, et al. Impairment of neutrophil chemotactic and bactericidal function in children infected with HIV-1 and partial reversal after in vitro exposure to granulocyte-macrophage colony stimulating factor. J Pediatr 1990;117:531-540.

Rolston K, Rodriquez S, Mansell P. Therapy of salmonella infection in AIDS patients (abstract). Fifth international conference on AIDS, Montreal, June 1989.

Rossi P, Moschese V, Broliden PA, et al. Presence of maternal antibodies to human immunodeficiency virus 1 envelope glycoprotein gp120 epitopes correlates with the uninfected status of children born to seropositive mothers. Proc Natl Acad Sci USA 1989;86:8055-8058.

Rosok B, Voltersvik P, Bjerknes R, et al. Dynamics of HIV-1 replication following influenza vaccination of HIV+ individuals. Clinical & Experimental Immunology 1996;104:203-207.

Rubinstein A, Sicklick M, Gupta A, et al. Acquired immunodeficiency with reversed T4/T8 ratios in infants born to promiscuous and drug-addicted mothers. JAMA 1983;249:2350-2356.

Russell C, Lay K. Natural history of Candida species of the yeast in the oral cavities of infants. Arch Oral Biol 1973;18:957-962.

Ryder RW, Nsaw W, Hassigs E, et al. Perinatal transmission of the human immunodeficiency virus type 1 to infants of seropositive women in Zaire. N Engl J Med 1989;320:1637-1642.

Schreiber GB, Busch MP, Kleinman SH, et al. The risk of transfusion-transmitted viral infections. N Engl J Med 1996;334:1685-1690.

Scott GB, Buck BE, Leterman JG, et al. Acquired immunodeficiency syndrome in infants. N Engl J Med 1984;310:76-81.

Selwyn PA, Schoenbaum EE, Davenny K, et al. Prospective study of human immunodeficiency virus infection and pregnancy outcomes in intravenous drug users. JAMA 1989;261:1289-1294.

Sharer LR, Cho ES, Epstein LG. Multinucleated giant cells and HTLV/III in AIDS encephalopathy. Hum Pathol 1985;16:760.

Sharer LR, Epstein LG, Cho ES, et al. Pathologic features of AIDS encephalopathy in children: evidence for LAV/HTLV-III infection of brain. Hum Pathol 1986;17:271-284.

Shaw GM, Harper ME, Hahn BH, et al. HTLV/III infection of brains of children and adults with AIDS encephalopathy. Science 1985;227:117-182.

Sperling RS, Shapiro DE, Coombs RW, et al. Maternal viral load, zidovudine treatments, and the risk of transmission of human immunodeficiency virus type 1 from mother to infant. N Engl J Med 1996;335:1621-1629.

Sprecher S, Soumenkoff G, Puissant F, Degueldre M. Vertical transmission of HIV in 15-week fetus. Lancet 1986;2:288-289.

St. Louis ME, Kamega M, Brown C, et al. Risk for perinatal HIV-1 transmission according to maternal immunologic, virologic, and placental factors. JAMA 1993;269:2853-2859.

Stoler MH, Eskins TA, Benn S, et al. Human T-cell lymphotrophic virus type 3 infection of the central nervous system. A preliminary in situ analysis. JAMA 1986;256:2360-2364.

Tardieu M, Mayaux MJ, Seibel N, et al. Cognitive assessment of school-age children infected with maternally transmitted human immunodeficiency virus type 1. J Pediatr 1995;126:375-379.

Tovo PA, de Martino M, Gabiano C, et al. Mode of delivery and gestational age influence perinatal HIV-1 transmission: Italian register for HIV infection in children. J AIDS & Hum Retrovirol 1995 Jan 11:88-94.

Uetmann MH, Belman WL, Ruff HA, et al. Developmental abnormalities in infants and children with acquired immune deficiency syndrome (AIDS) and AIDS-related complex. Dev Med Child Neurol 1985;27:563-571.

Walker CM, Moody DJ, Stites DO, Levy JA. CD8+ lymphocytes can control HIV infection in vitro by suppressing viral replication. Science 1986;234:1563-1566.

Weiser B, Nachman S, Tropper P, et al. Quantitation of human immunodeficiency virus type 1 during pregnancy: relationship of viral titer to mother-to-child transmission and stability of viral load. PNAS (USA) 1994;91:8037-8041.

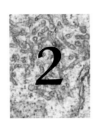

2 BOTULISM IN INFANTS

Since the first case report in 1976 (Pickett et al.) describing two infants with a clinical illness attributed to in vivo formation of *Clostridium botulinum* toxin, more than 1,200 similar cases have been found among infants in the United States. Between 60 and 90 cases are reported annually to the CDC (Fig. 2-1). Although most of the cases initially came from California, almost all states have now reported patients with infantile botulism. California, Utah, Hawaii, and Pennsylvania have the highest rates. Additional reports have come from all continents except Africa. These infants have had constipation followed in varying degrees by lethargy, weakness, difficult feeding, general floppiness, descending paralysis, and oculomotor dysfunction; some progress to life-threatening respiratory failure. The detection of clostridial organisms and specific toxin in the infants' stools has led to the term *infant botulism,* in contrast with the previously more frequently recognized form of botulism, which is a "food poisoning" resulting from ingestion of food contaminated by preformed toxin.

ETIOLOGY

C. botulinum organisms, most often serotypes A and B, have been isolated from feces of affected infants. The same fecal specimens contained the specific toxin of the botulinal serotype (Midura and Arnon, 1976). Toxin has rarely been detected in serum samples. Apparently, ingested vegetative cells or spores germinate and multiply in the infant gastrointestinal tract and then release their neurotoxin, which causes the clinical manifestations. *C. botulinum* toxin binds irreversibly to the presynaptic cholinergic nerve terminals and prevents the release of acetylcholine, blocking neuromuscular synaptic transmission and resulting in autonomic dysfunction and flaccid paralysis. No evidence has

been found that these infants ingested preformed toxin, the usual mechanism for botulism of adults and older children. Those factors that permit the sequence of toxin formation in the infant gastrointestinal tract are not yet defined. Of the seven distinct serotypes of *C. botulinum* (A to G), types A and B have been responsible for more than 90% of cases of botulism in infants.

PATHOLOGY

Because nearly all identified patients have recovered after provision of supportive therapy, no published autopsy studies are available. However, an early investigation of postmortem specimens from 280 California infants who died in the first year of life revealed *C. botulinum* organisms or toxin in 10 infants (Arnon et al., 1981). Of the 10 deaths, 9 had been classified as resulting from sudden infant death syndrome (SIDS). Among the SIDS infants with positive *C. botulinum* organisms or toxin, the study reported intrathoracic organ petechiae, alveoli and airways filled with frothy fluid, and extramedullary hepatic erythropoiesis. Arnon et al. have postulated that infant botulism may be one cause of SIDS. In contrast, a study of 248 SIDS patients in Australia (Byard et al., 1992) failed in all cases to implicate *C. botulinum.*

EPIDEMIOLOGIC FACTORS

The age of patients at onset has ranged from 1 week (Thilo et al., 1993; Hurst and Marsh, 1993) to 1 year, and there has been no sex predilection. Of the affected infants, 70% have been predominantly breast-fed (Morris et al., 1983). There was an interesting association of the type B cases in California with the use of honey as a carbohydrate source in infant feeding (Arnon et al., 1979), and up to 27% of subsequent patients had been fed honey before their illness. The full extent of the disease is not yet

Botulism (infant) – by year, United States, 1975-1995

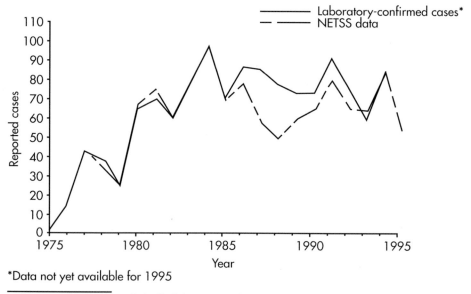

*Data not yet available for 1995

In the United States, nearly half of the reported cases of infant botulism occur in California.

FIG. 2-1   Number of cases of infant botulism reported annually to the CDC. (From CDC and Prevention: Summary of notable diseases: United States, 1995. MMWR 1995;44[53][suppl]:25.)

known, but it is safe to assume that many mild cases continue to go unrecognized. Less severely affected infants with moderate hypotonia, transient feeding difficulties, and failure to thrive are not hospitalized and escape detection because stool cultures and toxin assays are not performed. In association with their study of a possible relationship between infant botulism and SIDS, Arnon et al. (1978) pointed out the similar age distribution curves of patients with the two conditions in the first 6 months of life.

CLINICAL MANIFESTATIONS

Constipation (no spontaneous stools for 3 or more days) has been the initial manifestation in most cases. Within a few days this may be followed by lethargy; poor sucking; slow feeding; feeble cry; weakness; loss of head and neck control; generalized floppiness; swallowing difficulties; pooling of oral secretions; and, in some, respiratory arrest. On examination there is loss of muscle tone and diminished deep tendon reflexes. Additional cranial nerve findings may include ptosis, sluggish pupillary light reflexes, decreased extraocular motility, lack of facial movement, and decreased gag reflex (Berg, 1977; Long et al., 1985; Long, 1985; Spika et al., 1989 Glatman-Freedman, 1996). The symptoms and signs have been variable in degree and

duration, resolving spontaneously over a period ranging from 10 days to 8 weeks. The most serious complication has been respiratory arrest, occurring in nearly one half of hospitalized patients within the first 2 to 5 days. For this reason, admission to an intensive care unit where prompt respiratory support can be provided is crucial. Recovery has been gradual and complete, but rare relapses have been observed. Recovery is initiated by the regeneration of terminal endings, inducing growth of new motor end plates. The only deaths reported have been caused by respiratory arrests.

Box 2-1 lists a number of the relevant clinical features and findings.

DIAGNOSIS

The clinical suspicion of infant botulism should lead to diagnostic studies initiated while supportive care is underway (Hatheway and McCroskey, 1987). Electromyography may demonstrate a somewhat characteristic pattern of brief, low-amplitude, overabundant (BSAP) motor reaction potentials (Clay et al., 1977). Confirmation of precise diagnosis requires isolation of *C. botulinum* or detection of heat-labile botulinal toxin in the patient's stool. Appropriate reference laboratories are available (state health department or Centers for Disease Control) if local facilities are unable to per-

> ## BOX 2-1
> ## INITIAL FEATURES OF CLINICAL HISTORY AND PHYSICAL FINDINGS IN INFANT BOTULISM
>
> | | |
> |---|---|
> | Constipation | Hypotonia |
> | Floppiness | Ptosis |
> | Decreased activity | Pupillary dilatation |
> | Poor sucking | Facial paresis |
> | Slow feeding | Ophthalmoplegia |
> | Weakness | Decreased gag reflex |
> | Poor cry | Shallow respirations |
> | Loss of head control | Decreased deep tendon reflexes |

form the isolation and identification techniques. Midura and Arnon (1976) have described the appropriate tests and their application to fecal specimens. Polymerase chain reaction (PCR) assays have been adapted for detection of the organism in infant stool specimens and appear to correlate well (95.6%) (Szabo et al., 1994) with the more tedious mouse bioassay.

DIFFERENTIAL DIAGNOSIS

Other conditions considered on the initial presentation of these infants have included sepsis, poliomyelitis, myasthenia gravis, brain tumor, failure to thrive, drug or chemical poisoning, metabolic disorders, infantile polyneuropathy, Werdnig-Hoffmann disease, Reye's syndrome, congenital myopathy, and Leigh disease. With appropriate cultures and screening tests to exclude many of the others, a specific diagnosis should be achieved. Cerebrospinal fluid and peripheral blood studies in infant botulism have been normal.

COMPLICATIONS

As noted in the discussion of clinical manifestations, the most serious complication in infant botulism is respiratory failure that requires mechanical ventilation. The lengthy hospitalization of affected infants (a few weeks to a few months) may also result in secondary infections (otitis media, pneumonia, urinary tract infection) and nutritional failure resulting from inability to feed normally. Inappropriate overproduction of antidiuretic hormone has also been reported.

TREATMENT

The difficulties that may arise in handling oropharyngeal secretions and the unpredictability of sudden respiratory arrests require the level of support-

ive care usually available only in an intensive care unit. If the infant's course is a prolonged one, supplementary nutritional support also will become essential (Schreiner et al., 1991). No benefit has been demonstrated from the use of equine antitoxin, antibiotics, or cholinomimetic drugs. Infants treated with antibiotics have continued to excrete organisms and toxins for weeks or months after clinical recovery. The use of aminoglycoside antibiotics is specifically contraindicated because they may augment neuromuscular blockade and produce respiratory arrest (L'Hommedieu et al., 1979; Santos et al., 1981). A current trial of human-derived botulinus antitoxin botulinus immune globulin [BIG]) is in progress in California. To enroll patients, phone 510-540-2646 (Schwarz and Arnon, 1992).

PREVENTION

Although the prevention of infantile botulism is not clearly defined, avoiding known food sources of *C. botulinum* spores during the first year of life is epidemiologically justified. This would entail the discontinuation of honey and corn syrup as sources of calories and sweeteners for infant feeding.

BIBLIOGRAPHY

Arnon SS, Damus K, Chin J. Infant botulism, epidemiology of and relation to sudden infant death syndrome. Epidemiol Rev 1981;3:45-66.

Arnon SS, Midura TF, Damus K, et al. Intestinal infection and toxin production by *Clostridium botulinum* as one cause of sudden infant death syndrome. Lancet 1978;1:1273-1278.

Arnon SS Midura TF, Damus K, et al. Honey and other environmental risk factors for infant botulism. J Pediatr 1979;94:331-336.

Berg BO. Syndrome of infant botulism. Pediatrics 1977;59:322.

Byard RW, Moore L, Bourne AJ, et al. *Clostridium botulinum* and sudden infant death syndrome: a 10-year prospective study. J Pediatr Child Health 1992;28:156-157.

Centers for Disease Control and Prevention. Summary of notable diseases: United States, 1995. MMWR 1995;44 (53)(suppl):25.

Clay SA, Ramseyer JC, Fishman LS, Sedgwick RP. Acute infantile motor disorder: infantile botulism? Arch Neurol 1977;34:236-243.

Ferrari ND, Weisse ME. Botulism. Adv Pediatr Infect Dis 1995;10:81-91.

Glatman-Freedman A. Infant botulism. Pediatr Rev 1996;17:185-186.

Hatheway CL, McCroskey LM. Examination of feces and serum for diagnosis of infant botulism in 336 patients. J Clin Microbiol 1987;25:2334-2338.

Hurst DL, Marsh WW. Early severe infantile botulism. J Pediatr 1993;122:909-911.

L'Hommedieu C, Stough R, Brown L, et al. Potentiation of neuromuscular weakness in infant botulism by aminoglycosides. J Pediatr 1979;95:1965.

Long SS. Epidemiologic study of infant botulism in Pennsylvania: report of the infant botulism study group. Pediatrics 1985;75:928-934.

Long SS, Gajewski JL, Brown LW, Gilligan PH. Clinical, laboratory, and environmental features of infant botulism in southeastern Pennsylvania. Pediatrics 1985;75:935-941.

Midura TF, Arnon SS. Infant botulism: identification of *Clostridium botulinum* and its toxins in faeces. Lancet 1976;2:934-936.

Morris JG Jr, Snyder JD, Wilson R, Feldman RA. Infant botulism in the United States: an epidemiologic study of cases occurring outside of California. Am J Public Health 1983;73:1385-1388.

Pickett J, Berg B, Chaplin E, et al. Syndrome of botulism in infancy: clinical and electrophysiologic study. N Engl J Med 1976;295:770-771.

Santos JI, Swensen P, Glasgow LA. Potentiation of *Clostridium botulinum* toxin by aminoglycoside antibiotics: clinical and laboratory observations. Pediatrics 1981;68:50-54.

Schreiner MS, Field E, Ruddy R. Infant botulism: a review of 12 years' experience at the Children's Hospital of Philadelphia. Pediatrics 1991;87:159-165.

Schwarz PJ, Arnon SS. Botulism immune globulin for infant botulism arrives: one year and a Gulf war later. West J Med 1992;156:197-198.

Spika JS, Shaffer N, Hargrett-Bean N, et al. Risk factors for infant botulism in the United States. Am J Dis Child 1989;143:828-832.

Szabo EA, Pemberton JM, Gibson AM, et al. Polymerase chain reaction for detection of *Clostridium botulinum* types A, B, and E in food, soil, and infant feces. J Appl Bact 1994;76(6):539-545.

Thilo EH, Townsend SF, Deacon J. Infant botulism at 1 week of age: report of two cases. Pediatr 1993;92:151-153.

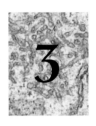

3   CYSTIC FIBROSIS

EMILY DiMANGO AND ALICE PRINCE

Cystic fibrosis (CF) is the most common autosomal recessive disorder in whites, affecting approximately 30,000 persons in the United States, with a carrier rate of 1 in 25 (Fitzsimmons, 1993). The primary cause of morbidity and mortality in patients with cystic fibrosis is persistent bacterial infection of the airways, with subsequent bronchiectasis, fibrosis, and obstructive lung disease. Chronic respiratory infection with resultant respiratory failure accounts for over 90% of fatalities in this disease (Abman et al., 1991; Konstan and Berger, 1993). The disorder was first recognized in 1938 by Dorothy Anderson, who described a syndrome in children that resulted in pancreatic insufficiency, malnutrition, and chronic respiratory infections (Anderson, 1938). At that time 70% of babies with CF died within the first year of life. Data from the Cystic Fibrosis Foundation patients registry of 1994 show median survival of 28.3 years among CF patients in the United States, largely as a result of the development of effective antibiotics and improved nutritional status (Fitzsimmons, 1994).

The disease is caused by a mutation in a single gene on the long arm of chromosome 7 that encodes the cystic fibrosis transmembrane conductance regulator (CFTR) (Collins, 1992). CFTR has multiple functions involving fluid and electrolyte balance across epithelial cells. It acts as a chloride channel activated by adenosine triphosphate (ATP).

PATHOGENESIS

Lung infection in CF is primarily endobronchial and chronic with superimposed acute exacerbations. Localized infections at nonpulmonary sites or systemic infections are rare. The spectrum of bacteria, viruses, and fungi associated with CF respiratory infection is comparatively restricted (Gilligan, 1991; Govan and Deretic, 1996; Karem et al.,

1990). The microbial pathogens most commonly isolated include *S. aureus, H. influenzae,* and particularly *P. aeruginosa,* which infects more than 80% of CF patients.

The earliest observed morphologic lesions are mucous obstruction of small airways and inflammation of the bronchiolar walls (Konstan and Berger, 1993). Concomitant with the persistent infection is chronic neutrophil dominated airway inflammation, which contributes greatly to lung damage (McElvaney et al., 1992). Bronchoalveolar lavage studies demonstrate neutrophil-rich inflammation in airway lining fluid of infants with CF in the first year of life (Armstrong et al., 1995). Mediators released by these inflammatory cells overwhelm the normal antiinflammatory defense screen of the epithelial surface and contribute directly to lung damage (Birrer et al., 1994).

Several abnormalities in the CF lung have been proposed as possible explanations for the chronic infection seen in this disease. As a consequence of the viscid nature of airway secretions in CF, mucociliary clearance of bacteria from the lungs is impaired (Konstan and Berger, 1993). Bacteria are loosely enmeshed in the viscous endobronchial mucous layer that contains large amounts of cellular debris. Epithelial defensins, naturally occurring bactericidal peptides that serve as one of the first local lines of defense against inhaled organisms, do not function effectively in the high-salt environment of the CF lung, contributing to the inability to clear inspired organisms (Smith et al., 1996). Once infected with *P. aeruginosa,* despite a seemingly normal immune response, organisms cannot be cleared, suggesting a problem with local clearance, perhaps phagocytosis (Cabral et al., 1987). As the organisms persist within the CF lung, mutants adapted for this milieu are selected. A unique feature of CF patients chronically infected with *P.*

aeruginosa is the recovery of an unusual mucoid morphotype of *Pseudomonas* from respiratory secretions (Baker and Svanborg-Eden, 1989; Bayer et al., 1990). These strains overproduce alginate, a polymer of guluronic and mannuronic acid as a result of mutations in any of several *alg* genes. Approximately 80% of *P. aeruginosa* isolates from CF patients are mucoid, whereas only 3% of *P. aeruginosa* respiratory tract isolates from non-CF patients. Therefore the *P. aeruginosa* strains that infect the airways of CF patients are not necessarily unique, but rather the environment of the CF lung facilitates selection of the mucoid phenotype.

Several factors may contribute to the selection of *P. aeruginosa*. There are an increased number of *Pseudomonas* receptors available on CF epithelial cells, compared to normal epithelial cells, as a direct result of a sialylation defect in CF (Barasch et al., 1991; Saiman and Prince, 1993). CFTR mutations are associated with undersialylation of glycolipids and glycoproteins on the apical membranes of epithelial cells. These asialylated glycoconjugates provide receptors for the major *P. aeruginosa* adhesins, pilin. Pilin-mediated attachment to these receptors directly stimulates epithelial cytokine expression and the ensuing inflammatory response (DiMango et al., 1995).

The sequence of events leading from the defective CFTR protein to bacterial colonization and inflammation of the airway is not yet well understood.

ETIOLOGIC AGENTS

Pulmonary infection in CF is primarily restricted to the airways rather than the lung parenchyma and typically occurs in an age-related sequence. *S. aureus* colonization occurs in young infants; *H. influenzae* appears in early childhood, with *P. aeruginosa* following, although infants with *P. aeruginosa* infection are being recognized with increasing frequency (Armstrong et al., 1995; Gilligan, 1991; Govan and Deretic, 1996). Other organisms found include *Burkholderia cepacia* and other glucose nonfermenters, such as *Stenotrophomonas maltophilia* and *Alcaligenes* sp. (Baltimore et al., 1982; Marks, 1981). At the present time, it is unclear if these organisms behave as true pathogens or whether their presence is simply a marker for end-stage lung disease (Box 3-1 and Table 3-1).

S. aureus was the first organism recognized to cause chronic lung infections in young CF patients and was the leading cause of mortality in the preantibiotic era. It continues to be an important pulmonary pathogen, especially in CF patients who are less than 10 years old. Methicillin-resistant *S. aureus* has been isolated with increasing frequency from the CF lung, though it does not appear to be

---

BOX 3-1

RESPIRATORY MICROBIOLOGY RESULTS IN PATIENTS WITH CYSTIC FIBROSIS

Patients Cultured:

Sputum	69.2%
Throat	29.4%
Bronchoscopy	1.4%
TOTAL	16,955
	(91% of all patients seen in clinic)

Cultured Positive:

Pseudomonas aeruginosa:	60.1%
Staphylococcus aureus:	36.4%
Hemophilus influenzae - any species:	15.0%
Aspergillus:	6.1%
Burkholderia cepacia:	3.6%
Stenotrophomonas maltophilia:	3.4%
Other pseudomonas species:	2.2%
Non-tuberculous mycobacterium:	0.6%

From Cystic Fibrosis Foundation, National Cystic Fibrosis Patient Registry, 1995.

associated with worse outcome (Bauernfeind et al., 1988; Boxerbaum et al., 1988).

Once a chronic infection with *P. aeruginosa* is established, organisms are rarely, if ever, eradicated, and infection with mucoid *P. aeruginosa* heralds the onset of progressive decline in pulmonary function. (Bedard et al., 1993). The immune response to the organism makes a significant contribution to the tissue damage seen in the lungs of infected CF patients. CF patients with high levels of circulating immune complexes have poorer lung function than those with lower levels (Wheeler et al., 1984). Besides immune complex–mediated damage to the lung, there are very high levels of elastase and protease of phagocytic cell origin in the lungs of CF patients infected with *P. aeruginosa*. These proteases contribute to lung damage and airway inflammation by stimulating secretion of inflammatory cytokines (McElvaney et al., 1992).

During the early 1980s *Burkholderia cepacia* emerged as a pathogen of importance in patients with CF. This organism has been associated with significant mortality at CF centers in the United States and Canada, often in the setting of epidemic spread within institutions (Millar-Jones et al., 1992). In addition to its potential virulence, epidemiologic evidence for patient-to-patient transmission both in hospital and through social contacts has emerged. Ribotyping, a method of strain identification based on analysis of bacterial genomic RFLPs, proved person-to-person transmission of *B. cepacia* in the setting of an educational camp (LiPuma et al., 1988). There is also evidence that transmission may be strain dependent, with some strains being more virulent and more likely to cause epidemics.

Factors that lead to colonization by *B. cepacia* are just beginning to be understood. The risk for *B. cepacia* colonization is increased by the severity of underlying pulmonary disease, having a sibling with CF who has also been colonized, increasing age, and hospitalization in the previous 6 months (Millar-Jones et al., 1992). The characteristic multidrug resistance of *B. cepacia* to potent antipseudomonal agents makes antimicrobial therapy difficult, and aggressive therapy seldom results in significant clinical improvement or even reduction in the numbers of bacteria cultured from sputum (Pitt et al., 1996).

The disease usually follows one of three clinical courses (Pitt et al., 1996). In some CF patients, long-term colonization occurs without adversely affecting lung function. In others, chronic infection associated with slowly declining lung function is seen. Finally, in about 20% of patients, acute fulminant lung infection with necrotizing pneumonia, fever, bacteremia, elevated ESR, and leukocytosis leads to death in weeks to months. The 1994 CF Registry found the overall prevalence of the organism to be less than that seen in specific centers, with an overall mean isolation rate of 6.1% (Fitzsimmons and Brooks, 1994).

OTHER PATHOGENS

In addition to the bacterial agents mentioned in the preceding section, there are several microorganisms that seem to have a high predilection for the CF lung. Cystic fibrosis patients are frequently colonized with *Aspergillus fumigatus*, with some centers reporting up to 57% of patients being colonized (Mroueh and Spock, 1994). The high rate of colonization in CF patients is due to the propensity of *A. fumigatus* to grow in thick secretions in diseased lungs. Colonization leads to chronic antigenic stimulation, which may lead to sensitization in a susceptible host, resulting in allergic bronchopulmonary aspergillosis (ABPA), reported to occur in up to 10% of patients with CF. The clinical course is characterized by wheezing, episodic pulmonary infiltrates, and bronchiectasis occurring most commonly in the upper lobes. The diagnosis of ABPA in patients with CF is difficult because the signs and symptoms of each disease mimic each other. Skin prick testing, elevated total serum IgE, *A. fumigatus* in respiratory secretions, eosinophilia,

Table 3-1 Concurrent infections

Infections	Number of cystic fibrosis patients (1995)
Pseudomonas aeruginosa	10,185
also infected with:	
B. cepacia	333
S. aureus	3,389
Methicillin Resistant *S. aureus*	12
S. maltophilia	343
other pseudomonads	252
H. influenzae	1,156
Klebsiella species	111
Alkaligenes	47
other gram negative organisms	747
Aspergillus	777

From Cystic Fibrosis Foundation, National Cystic Fibrosis Patient Registry 1995.

and the presence of *A. fumigatus* serum precipitins are used as diagnostic criteria for ABPA.

Atypical mycobacteria, particularly *Mycobacterium avium* complex, have also been isolated with increased frequency from the sputum of CF patients, with some centers reporting an incidence of up to 30% in their adult patients. Though there are well reported cases where this organism is demonstrated to be a true pathogen in the CF lung, it is often felt to be a colonizer, with a tendency to affect those patients with mild lung disease. Treatment for patients who have this organism recovered usually involves intensive bronchial hygiene, including antibacterial antibiotics, in an attempt to rid the lung of this colonizer.

Later in the course of disease, multiply resistant gram-negative organisms including *Stenotrophomonas maltophilia* and *Alcaligenes* spp. are recovered from the lung; the contribution of these organisms to progression in lung disease has not been established (Marks, 1981).

CLINICAL MANIFESTATIONS

The major clinical manifestations of CF are due to the progressive lung disease. Pancreatic insufficiency is adequately treated with pancreatic enzyme supplements and replacement of the fat-soluble vitamins A, D, E, and K (Ramsey et al., 1992). The inability to eradicate bacterial pathogens from the airways results in chronic pulmonary symptoms. Patients have cough with expectoration of thick, purulent sputum and progressive deterioration in pulmonary function (Karem et al., 1990). Acute episodes of clinical exacerbations are superimposed on chronic pulmonary symptoms. Because of wide variation in the severity of underlying manifestations, it is often difficult to define a pulmonary exacerbation on clinical criteria alone. Rather than new symptomatology, more often an exacerbation is heralded by a quantitative change in ongoing symptoms: an increase in frequency and intensity of cough or in the quantity and purulence of sputum. The acute and chronic symptoms are largely the result of the vigorous inflammatory response to endobronchial infection. Increased airway disease is manifest by tachypnea and increased work of breathing (retractions, use of accessory respiratory muscles, and wheezing). Systemic manifestations of pulmonary exacerbation include malaise, myalgia, anorexia, weight loss, and occasionally low-grade fever (Karem et al., 1990).

Decline in pulmonary function is the most accurate and objective indicator of a pulmonary exacerbation. Unfortunately, most patients younger than 5 years cannot perform pulmonary function tests reproducibly, making the diagnosis of an exacerbation more difficult. The appearance of a new pulmonary infiltrate on chest radiograph may be helpful; however, most pulmonary exacerbations, especially in patients with advanced disease, are unassociated with significant radiographic changes.

Sputum culture can accurately identify the bacterial pathogens colonizing lower airway secretions; oropharyngeal culture (a suggested alternative in the nonexpectorating patient) is a relatively insensitive measure of lower airway pathogens (Ramsey et al., 1991). A study comparing oropharygeal cultures with bronchoalveolar cultures showed that oropharyngeal cultures yielding *P. aeruginosa* or *S. aureus* are highly predictive, but such cultures lacking these organisms do not rule out the presence of these pathogens in the lower airways. The use of selective media and quantitative culturing methods to identify infecting organisms in sputum may also be useful, particularly when mucoid strains of *P. aeruginosa* obscure the growth of more fastidious organisms such as *H. influenzae* (Bauernfeind et al., 1987).

Other laboratory studies that may be helpful in defining a pulmonary exacerbation include white blood cell count with differential and acute phase reactants, such as erythrocyte sedimentation rate and C-reactive protein. Bacteremia is seen rarely in patients with CF, except in a subpopulation of patients with *B. cepacia.* It is hypothesized that the low incidence of bacteremia is due to the relatively low virulence of the infecting organism; intense antibody response; and endobronchial, rather than parenchymal, location of the infectious process (McCarthy et al., 1980).

In addition to pulmonary disease, almost all patients with CF have chronic sinusitis, often associated with nasal polyps (Ramsey and Richardson, 1992). This is likely to be the result of the CFTR defect affecting the lining cells of the sinuses. Etiologic agents include the usual sinus pathogens plus the organisms that colonize the lower airways in this population. In addition to causing acute and chronic disease, sinuses may serve as a reservoir for antibiotic-resistant organisms in patients undergoing lung transplantation (Flume et al., 1994).

Nonpulmonary symptoms of cystic fibrosis that can mimic infection include immune complex–mediated manifestations such as vasculitic skin rashes and arthritis. In addition to pancreatic insufficiency, gastrointestinal manifestations include severe constipation, intestinal obstruction, and unrecognized or unusual presentations of acute appendicitis.

TREATMENT

Current therapy for lung disease in CF requires a multidisciplinary approach of outpatient and inpatient care. Outpatient therapy includes postural drainage and chest percussion performed daily to help expectorate the inspissated secretions; along with administration of antibiotics, bronchodilators, and recombinant human DNase (Webb, 1995). Optimizing nutritional status has been shown to have a positive impact on pulmonary function and should be aggressively addressed, sometimes necessitating gastrostomy feeds (Ramsey et al., 1992). Intravenous antibiotic therapy is often necessary and is frequently performed as outpatient therapy, particularly in older children and adults; hospitalization is required for severe exacerbations or complications such as hemoptysis, pneumothorax, respiratory failure, pulmonary hypertension, or cor pulmonale.

Effective antibiotics administered to CF patients are thought to act by decreasing the sputum bacterial density and hence the ensuing inflammatory response (deGroot and Smith, 1987). Antibiotics are typically directed against the major pathogens isolated from the sputum, with attention to antibiotic sensitivity (Table 3-2). One important consideration in the treatment of CF patients is antibiotic dosing. Cystic fibrosis patients have increased total body clearance of β-lactams and aminoglycosides as a result of an increased rate of elimination by the kidney (deGroot and Smith, 1987). As a result, CF patients often require higher doses of antibiotics to achieve therapeutic levels. Because sputum concentration is dependent on the peak serum concentration, CF subjects require larger doses of most antibiotics.

During the last two decades, chronic *P. aeruginosa* lung infection has emerged as the most difficult therapeutic problem in patients with CF. There is no universal agreement on how or when to treat this infection, and, regardless of the regimen used, *P. aeruginosa* is seldom permanently eradicated. Infections are typically treated with two antipseudomonal antibiotics: an aminoglycoside in addition to a second drug, usually a β-lactam antibiotic (deGroot and Smith, 1987). The intravenous administration of antibiotics is the currently accepted treatment for pulmonary exacerbations of CF in patients infected with *P. aeruginosa*. After 14 days of administration of intravenous antibiotics, the forced expiratory volume in 1 second (FEV1) typically increases approximately 20%, and the density of *P. aeruginosa* in sputum decreases substantially (Redding et al., 1982).

Some physicians treat patients only when there is evidence of a clinical deterioration, whereas others treat at regular intervals regardless of symptoms. A single study of Danish CF patients followed between 1971 to 1980 showed that patients treated every 3 months with anti-*Pseudomonas* antibiotics had improved 5-year survival (82% in the regularly treated group versus 54% in the as-needed group) and improved pulmonary function compared with those patients treated only during an exacerbation (Jensen et al., 1989; Szaff et al., 1983).

Table 3-2   Intravenous treatment of pathogens associated with pulmonary exacerbations of cystic fibrosis (treatment often depends on sputum sensitivity testing)

Organism	Drug	Dosage mg/kg	Interval
S. aureus	Nafcillin	25-50	q6h
	Cephalothin	25-50	q6h
	Vancomycin	15	q6h
H. influenzae	Ticarcillin/clavulanate	100/3.3	q6h
*P. aeruginosa**	Ticarcillin/clavulanate	100/3.3	q6h
	Tobramycin	3	q8h
	Amikacin	5-7.5	q8h
	Ceftazidime	50-75	q8h
	Ciprofloxacin	15	q12h
	Aztreonam	50	q6h
	Piperacillin	100	q6h
	Imipenem	15-25	q6h

*Use two agents simultaneously; aminoglycoside + β-lactam or quinolone.

Another approach is the institution of early and aggressive anti-*Pseudomonas* treatment as soon as organisms are recovered from sputum, via oral or inhaled antibiotics (Valerius et al., 1991). The use of direct aerosol delivery of aminoglycosides such as tobramycin to the lower airways has been shown to result in improved lung function, decreased density of *P. aeruginosa* in sputum, and decreased use of systemic antibiotics (Ramsey et al., 1993).

Treatment for allergic bronchopulmonary aspergillosis (ABPA) usually includes administration of corticosteroids. The efficacy of amphotericin B for treatment of this problem has not been established.

RECENT ADVANCES

Although life expectancy for CF patients has increased dramatically over the past two decades, mainly through the development of better anti-*Pseudomonas* drugs and improved nutrition, airway obstruction resulting from chronic infection remains the main cause of mortality (Fig. 3-1). Extracellular DNA released by disintegrating inflammatory cells, particularly polymorphonuclear leukocytes, is present in infected CF sputum in very high concentrations and likely contributes to the increased viscosity of the sputum (Shak et al., 1990). Aerosolized recombinant human DNase, an enzyme that cleaves high–molecular-weight DNA, has been shown to result in improvement of mean FEV1 to 10% to 15% over baseline in some patients (Fuchs et al., 1994).

Bilateral lung transplantation for cystic fibrosis was first performed in 1983. Ion transport in the lung is corrected after transplantation; however, since CF transport abnormalities persist in the native proximal airways and sinuses, it has been suggested that the presence of airway pathogens before lung transplantation may place CF patients at a higher risk for infectious complications after transplant (Flume et al., 1994). However, 5-year survival of CF patients after lung transplantation is the same as that for patients undergoing transplant for other diseases (Flume et al., 1994).

With the knowledge that the clinical manifestations of CF are predominantly a result of abnormalities on the epithelial surface of the airways, combined with the discovery of the CFTR gene, there is a major research effort to develop methods to deliver the normal CFTR gene to respiratory epithelial cells. Different vectors—including recombinant viruses, liposomes, and other vector systems—are presently being investigated.

It is presently unclear how many epithelial cells need to be corrected or which cells are the proper target. Though effective transfer of the gene to epithelial cells has been achieved, the transfer is not long-lived, and many of the vectors themselves result in airway inflammation. Current work involves modification of the vectors and potentially altering the host immune response to these vectors. Though still in its infancy, human gene therapy remains a hope for cure of the respiratory manifestations of cystic fibrosis.

Approaches to the prevention of *P. aeruginosa* colonization in patients with CF have included the development of antipseudomonal vaccines for use in uncolonized patients. Preliminary studies have demonstrated that a polyvalent *P. aeruginosa* conjugate vaccine is safe and immunogenic; but effica-

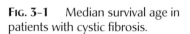

FIG. 3-1   Median survival age in patients with cystic fibrosis.

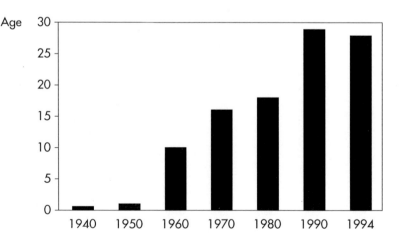

cy has not been demonstrated (Cryz et al., 1994). Cystic fibrosis patients should receive routine childhood immunizations (including *H. influenzae* type B vaccine). In addition, patients and their families should receive influenza vaccine annually because of the excess morbidity associated with infection. There is no indication for routine administration of pneumococcal vaccine.

BIBLIOGRAPHY

Abman SH, Ogle JW, Harbeck RJ, et al. Early bacteriologic, immunologic, and clinical courses of young infants with cystic fibrosis identified by neonatal screening. J Pediatr 1991;119:211-217.

Anderson, DH. Cystic fibrosis of the pancreas and its relation to celiac disease: a clinical and pathologic study. Am J Dis Child 1938;56:344-399.

Armstrong DSK, Grimwood R, Carzmo JB, et al. Lower respiratory infection and inflammation in infants with newly diagnosed cystic fibrosis. Br Med J 1995;310:1571-1572.

Baker NR, Svanborg-Eden C. Role of alginate in the adherence of *Pseudomonas aeruginosa*. Antibiot Chemother 1989;42:72-79.

Baltimore RS, Rudney-Baltimore K, van Graevenitz A, et al. Occurrence of nonfermentative gram negative rods other than *P. aeruginosa* in the respiratory tract of children with cystic fibrosis. Helv Paediat Acta 1982;37:547-554.

Barasch J, Kiss B, Prince A, et al. Defective acidification of intracellular organelles in cystic fibrosis. Nature 1991;52:70-73.

Bauerfeind A, Berlete RM, Harms K, et al. Quantitative and qualitative microbiological analysis of sputa of 102 patients with cystic fibrosis. Infection 1987;15:270-277.

Bauernfeind A, Rotter K, Weisslein-Pfister CH. Selective procedure to isolate *H. influenzae* from sputa with large quantities of *P. aeruginosa*. Infection 1987;15:278-280.

Bauernfeind A, Hurl G, Przyklenk G. Microbiologic and therapeutic aspects of *S. aureus* in CF patients. Scand J Gastroenterol 1988;143:99-102.

Bayer ASF, Eftekhar J, Nast CC, Speert D. Oxygen dependent up-regulation of mucoid exopolysaccharide (alginate) in *Pseudomonas aeruginosa*. Infect Immun 1990;58:1344-1349.

Bedard M, McClure D, Schiller NL, et al. Release of IL-8, IL-6, and colony stimulating factor by upper airway epithelial cells: implications for cystic fibrosis. Am J Respir Cell Mol Biol 1993;9:455-462.

Birrer P, McElvaney NG, Ruderberg A, et al. Protease-antiprotease imbalance in the lungs of children with cystic fibrosis. Am J Respir Crit Care Med 1994;150:207-213.

Boxerbaum B, Jacobs MR, Cechner RL. Prevalence and significance of methicillin resistant *Staphylococcus aureus* in patients with cystic fibrosis. Pediatr Pulmon 1988;4:159-163.

Brett MM, Ghonei TM, Littlewood JM. Prediction and diagnosis of early *Pseudomonas aeruginosa* infection in cystic fibrosis: a follow-up study. J Clin Microbiol 1988;26:1565-1570.

Cabral DA, Loh BA, Speert DP. Mucoid *Pseudomonas aeruginosa* resists nonopsonic phagocytosis by human neutrophils and macrophages. Pediatr Res 1987;22:429-431.

Collins FA. Cystic fibrosis: molecular biology and therapeutic implications. Science 1992;256:774-777.

Crystal RG, McElvaney NG, Rosenfeld MA. Administration of an adenovirus containing the human CFTR cDNA to the respiratory tract of individuals with cystic fibrosis. Nat Genet 1994;8:42-51.

Cryz SJ, Wedgwood J, Lang AB, et al. Immunization of noncolonized cystic fibrosis patients against *P. aeruginosa*. J Infect Dis 1994;169:1159-1164.

de Groot R, Smith AL. Antibiotic pharmacokinetics in cystic fibrosis: differences and clinical significance. Clinical Pharmacokin 1987;13:228-253.

DiMango E, Zar H, Bryan R, and Prince A. Diverse *Pseudomonas aeruginosa* gene products stimulate respiratory epithelial cells to produce IL-8. J Clin Invest 1995;2204-2210.

Fitzsimmons SC. The changing epidemiology of cystic fibrosis. J Pediatr 1993;122:1-9.

Fitzsimmons SC, Brooks M. Annual Cystic Fibrosis Patient Registry Report. Bethesda, MD: Cystic Fibrosis Foundation, 1994.

Flume PA, Egan TM, Paradowski LJ, et al. Infectious complications of lung transplantation. Am J Respir Crit Care Med 1994;149:1601-1607.

Fuchs HJ, Borowitz DS, Christiansen DH, et al. Effect of aerosolized recombinant human DNase on exacerbations of respiratory symptoms and on pulmonary function in patients with cystic fibrosis. N Engl J Med 1994;331:637-642.

Gilligan PH. Microbiology of airway disease in patients with cystic fibrosis. Clin Microbiol Rev 1991;4:35.

Govan JRW, Deretic V. Microbial pathogenesis in cystic fibrosis: mucoid *Pseudomonas aeruginosa* and *Burkholderia cepacia*. Microbiol Rev 1996;60:539-574.

Jensen T, Pedersen SS, Hoiby N, et al. Use of antibiotics in cystic fibrosis. Antibiot Chemother 1989;42:237-246.

Karem E, Corey M, Gold R. Pulmonary function and clinical course in patients with cystic fibrosis after pulmonary colonization with *Pseudomonas aeruginosa*. J Pediatr 1990;116:714.

Konstan MW, Berger M. Infection and inflammation of the lung in cystic fibrosis. In Davis PB (ed). Cystic fibrosis. New York: Marcel Dekker, 1993.

LiPuma JL, Mortensen JE, Dasen SE, et al. Ribotype analysis of *Pseudomonas cepacia* from cystic fibrosis treatment centers. J Pediatr 1988;113:859-862.

Marks MI. The pathogenesis and treatment of pulmonary infections in patients with cystic fibrosis. J Pediatr 1981;98:173-179.

McCarthy MM, Rourke MH, Spock A. Bacteremia in patients with cystic fibrosis. Clinical Pediatrics 1980;19:746-748.

McElvaney NGH, Nakamura B, Birrer CA, et al. Modulation of airway inflammation in cystic fibrosis. J Clin Invest 1992;90:1296-1301.

Millar-Jones L, Paull A, Saurnelers Z, et al. Transmission of *Pseudomonas cepacia* among cystic fibrosis patients. Lancet 1992;340:491.

Mroueh S, Spock A. Allergic bronchopulmonary Aspergillosis in patients with cystic fibrosis. Chest 1994;105:32-36.

Pitt TL, Govan JRW. *Pseudomonas cepacia* and cystic fibrosis. Microbiol Dig 1993;10:69-72.

Pitt TL, Kaufmann P, Patel BS, et al. Type characterization and antibiotic susceptibility of *Burkholderia cepacia* isolates from patients with cystic fibrosis in the United Kingdom and the Republic of Ireland. J Med Microbiol 1996;44:203-210.

Ramsey BW, Dorkin HL, Eisenberg JD, et al. Efficacy of aerosolized tobramycin in patients with cystic fibrosis. N Engl J Med 1993;328:1740-1746.

Ramsey BW, Farrel PM, Pencharz P. Nutritional assessment and management in cystic fibrosis: a consensus report. Am J Clin Nutr 1992;55:108-116.

Ramsey BW, Wentz KR, Smith AL, et al. Predictive value of oropharyngeal cultures for identifying lower airway bacteria in cystic fibrosis patients. Am Rev Respir Dis 1991;144:331-337.

Ramsey B, Richardson M. Impact of sinusitis in cystic fibrosis. J Allergy Clin Immunol 1992;90:547-552.

Redding GJ, Restuccia R, Cotton EK. Serial changes in pulmonary functions in children hospitalized with cystic fibrosis. Am Rev Respir Dis 1982;126:31-36.

Saiman L, Prince A. P. aeruginosa pili bind asialoGM1 which is increased on the surface of cystic fibrosis epithelial cells. J Clin Invest 1993;92:1875-1880.

Shak I, Capon DJ, Hellmiss R, et al. Recombinant human DNase reduces the viscosity of CF sputum. Proc Natl Acad Sci USA 1990;87:9188-9192.

Smith JJ, Travis SM, Greenberg EP. Cystic fibrosis airway epithelia fail to kill bacteria because of abnormal airway surface fluid. Cell 1996;85:229-236.

Szaff M, Hoiby N, Flensborg EW. Frequent antibiotic therapy improves survival of cystic fibrosis patients with chronic P. aeruginosa infection. Acta Pediatr Scand 1983;72:651-657.

Valerius NH, Koch C, Hoiby N. Prevention of chronic P. aeruginosa colonization in cystic fibrosis by early treatment. Lancet 1991;338:725-726.

Webb AK. The treatment of pulmonary infection in cystic fibrosis. Scand J Infect Dis 1995;96:24-27.

Wheeler WB, Williams M, Matthews WJ, et al. Progression of cystic fibrosis lung disease as a function of serum immunoglobulin G levels: a 5-year longitudinal study. J Pediatr 1984;104:695-699.

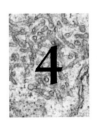

4   Cytomegalovirus

Infections of newborn infants caused by cytomegalovirus (CMV) were first recognized in the latter part of the nineteenth century. It was believed that these infections were caused by a protozoan or represented a form of syphilis, and the salivary glands were believed the major pathologic site. By the 1950s it was known that the clinical signs and symptoms of this disease in infants were hepatosplenomegaly, thrombocytopenia, jaundice, intracerebral calcifications, chorioretinitis, poor growth, and eventual development of microcephaly and mental retardation. These infants were said to have "cytomegalic inclusion disease" or infection with "salivary gland virus," because by then the causative agent had been isolated in tissue culture and identified (Rowe et al., 1956; Smith, 1956; Weller et al., 1957). In 1960 Weller, Hanshaw, and Scott proposed the term *cytomegalovirus infection* for the illness because it better reflected the nature of the disease. At that time it was thought that CMV infection of infants was rare, but it is now known that the illness is not uncommon and that infants with obvious CMV infection represent the proverbial "tip of the iceberg." Devastating congenital CMV infections, however, are unusual; a far greater number of inapparent infections are acquired in the perinatal period because of maternal shedding of CMV in genital secretions and breast milk. Recent studies of the epidemiology of CMV infections in the United States reveal that 1% to 2% of newborns and 5% to 25% of pregnant women harbor occult infections with CMV.

Another significant cause of morbidity and mortality as a result of CMV occurs in the immunosuppressed host, in particular in patients with an underlying malignancy, those who have had organ transplantation, and persons with coexisting human immunodeficiency virus (HIV) infection. Infections in immunologically normal hosts beyond the newborn period are frequent but are also usually without symptoms or sequelae. Thus, as with many other agents whose initial association was with only a limited clinical syndrome, CMV has emerged as a ubiquitous virus with host interactions ranging over the full spectrum of health and disease.

ETIOLOGY

Despite initial confusion concerning the cause of cytomegalic inclusion disease, some investigators suspected this illness was caused by a virus long before the agent itself was identified. Similarities observed in pathologic specimens between cytomegalic inclusion cells (Goodpasture and Talbot, 1921) and those in herpetic lesions (von Glahn and Pappenheimer, 1925) are remarkable in the light of modern evidence classifying human CMV in the herpesvirus group. In 1954 Smith was the first to carry out serial propagation of murine CMV in mouse tissue cultures, after which human CMV was isolated (Rowe et al., 1956; Smith, 1956; Weller et al., 1957). Subsequently, it became possible to develop serologic tests to delineate a broader understanding of the epidemiology of this common viral infection.

The genome of CMV is composed of double-stranded DNA of 230 kbp, which is the largest of the human herpesviruses. Virions (Fig. 4-1) consist of an inner core with a diameter of 65 nm, an icosahedral capsid composed of 162 capsomeres with a diameter of 110 nm, a tegument, and an envelope with a diameter of 200 nm. Virions are similar in appearance to those of the other human herpesviruses exemplified by herpes simplex virus (HSV). The CMV genome, however, is more complex than that of HSV, consisting of over 208 open reading frames (ORFs) (Baldick and Shenk, 1996). Replication of CMV occurs in a regulated sequence

37

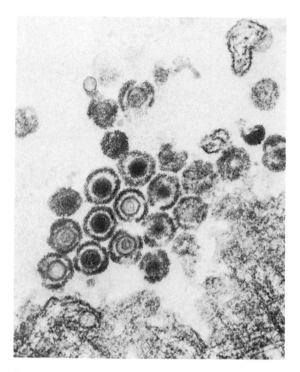

Fig. 4-1 A group of negatively stained cytomegalovirus particles propagated in human lung fibroblasts. The core, a typical hexagonal capsid (actually icosahedral in three dimensions) of a herpesvirus surrounded by a tegument and double-layered envelope, can be seen. (×155,000.) (Courtesy Janet D Smith, PhD.)

with immediate early alpha gene products controlling subsequent transcription and translation of early beta and late gamma gene products (Merigan and Resta, 1990; Plotkin et al., 1990; Baldick and Shenk, 1996). CMV DNA encodes for at least 30 proteins, some of which are structural and others of which are nonstructural. The envelope glycoproteins, which are antigenic, are believed to play an important role in generating immune responses on the part of the infected host, and undoubtedly they also play roles in viral infectivity. Although only 4 glycoproteins of human CMV have been identified, there are undoubtedly additional ones because 54 ORFs that encode for glycoproteins have been identified. Two of the glycoproteins, gB and gH, are believed to play major roles in viral pathogenesis and generation of host immune responses. In addition, tegument proteins, some of which are structural and others of which are nonstructural regulatory proteins, may also play an important role in the host response to CMV. One of these is tegument protein pp 65 (Kozinowski et al., 1987; Plotkin et al., 1990; Baldick and Shenk, 1996).

A great many strains of human CMV exist; it has been possible to distinguish between them both by analyzing their DNA with restriction enzyme technology and antigenically (Chou, 1989a, 1989b). There is extensive homology between strains, however, so that, although reinfections with CMV may occur, primary infection may provide at least partial immunity against other strains (Plotkin et al., 1990). Viral antigens may be identified in infected cells by immunological means such as fluorescent-labeled antibody assays. Cultivation of CMV in human fibroblasts reveals characteristic cytomegaly with nuclear and cytoplasmic inclusions containing viral antigenic structures.

In the cell, human CMV causes both permissive infections, in which viral progeny are produced, and abortive infections, in which there are no progeny but there is DNA replication and formation of some viral antigens. Although CMV also causes oncogenic transformation in some tissue culture systems (Heggie et al., 1986), no specific malignancies of humans have been related to this virus. All of the herpesviruses share the characteristic of causing latent infection, as well as primary infection and reinfections. The site of latency of CMV probably is one or more cells of lymphoid origin, possibly including granulocytes (Merigan and Resta, 1990) and monocytes (Taylor-Wiedeman et al., 1994). The virus has been detected in mononuclear blood cells from healthy seropositive donors (Schrier et al., 1985; Spector and Spector, 1985; Taylor-Wiedeman et al., 1994) and may be inadvertently transmitted by blood transfusions. It has been postulated that latent CMV in white blood cells may account for transmission of the virus by organ transplantation (Merigan and Resta, 1990). In general, primary infections with CMV are potentially more serious than secondary infections, although this is not necessarily so in highly immunocompromised hosts.

PATHOGENESIS

The natural history of CMV infections is exceedingly complicated, with the possibility of primary infection, reactivation of latent infection, and reinfection with a new strain of virus. These potential events are diagrammed in Fig. 4-2.

Primary Infection

A susceptible (immunologically inexperienced) host may be infected during the prenatal, perinatal, or postnatal period. Prenatal, or congenital, infection presumably is acquired transplacentally.

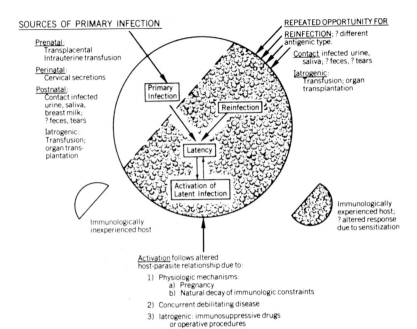

FIG. 4–2 Natural history of human cytomegalovirus infection. (From Weller TH: N Engl J Med 1970;285:203.)

Viremia during pregnancy may be the most common source of prenatal CMV infection. Perinatal infection is probably caused by exposure to CMV-infected cervical secretions. The presence of CMV in cervical secretions is well documented (Alexander, 1967; Diosi et al., 1967). Postnatal infections most commonly are acquired by contact with various secretions known to be infected with CMV such as urine, semen, saliva, and tears (Lang and Hanshaw, 1969; Lang and Kummer, 1975). The exact route of postnatal transmission is unknown; it may be by the oral route, the respiratory route, or both. Breast milk is a recognized vector for transmission of CMV to infants despite the presence of transplacental maternal CMV antibody. Acquisition of CMV by the infant from breast milk has been associated with prolonged viral shedding, but rarely do symptoms occur. Sexual transmission of CMV is probably a major route of spread in adult life (Chandler et al., 1985, 1987). Day-care settings in which there are many children in diapers who may be teething and drooling are also recognized as foci for potential spread of CMV to other children, their parents, and the staff (Adler, 1988a, 1988b; Pass et al., 1986; Adler 1991). Other sources of postnatal CMV infection include transfusions with CMV-infected blood and transplantation of organs that harbor the virus (Yeager et al., 1972, 1981; Whitley et al., 1976; Stagno et al., 1981; Meyers et al., 1986; Merigan and Resta, 1990).

Secondary Infection: Reactivation of and Reinfection with Cytomegalovirus

Hosts with prior immunologic experience with CMV may be exposed to exogenous or endogenous sources of infection. Reactivation of latent CMV infection may stem from various physiologic, pathologic, or iatrogenic mechanisms such as pregnancy, concurrent malignancy, and/or transplantation with concomitant administration of immunosuppressive therapy. The frequent detection of IgM antibodies in healthy individuals suggests that reactivation infections with CMV occur often in immunocompetent individuals (McEvoy and Adler, 1989). CMV infections in seropositive individuals may also be secondary to reinfection with a new strain of virus (Huang et al., 1980). In a study of women attending a clinic for sexually transmitted diseases, four of eight (50%) were infected with more than one strain of CMV as evidenced by analysis of viral DNAs by restriction enzymes. Two were simultaneously shedding different strains of CMV from different body sites (Chandler et al., 1987). Simultaneous viral shedding of two different strains of CMV in other healthy persons (McFarlane and Koment, 1986) and in immunocompromised persons (Spector et al., 1984; Chou, 1986) has also been reported. Finally, more than one strain of CMV can establish latent infection in one host, and new viral strains may emerge as a result of recombination of these strains (Chou, 1989a).

Since secondary infection with CMV is possible as a result of either reactivation of latent virus or reinfection, it is obvious that immunity to this virus is often only partial. Therefore it is not surprising that seropositive women may transmit a congenital CMV infection to their offspring. Stagno et al. (1977b) found that intrauterine infection with CMV occurred in 3.4% of seropositive mothers. However, the birth of a second symptomatic congenitally infected infant to one mother is exceedingly rare, which probably reflects at least partial immunity to CMV in most seropositive women (Ahlfors et al., 1981; Rutter 1985). In a study of 3,712 pregnant women reported by Stagno et al. (1982), approximately one third were seronegative and had no evidence of prior experience with CMV before pregnancy. Infants with symptomatic CMV infection were born only to women in this group. Some women who had been seropositive before pregnancy gave birth to congenitally infected infants, but their babies were asymptomatic at birth and also at 1 year of age. An extension of this study (Stagno et al., 1986) involving 16,218 pregnant women confirmed the importance of gestational primary infection as a risk factor for development of symptomatic congenital CMV infection in the infant. The risk to the infant was greatest when maternal infection occurred in the first half of pregnancy. There was a 30% to 40% rate of transmission of CMV in utero for women with primary CMV infection. Although there were fewer seronegative results among women from low-income than from high-income families, women in low-income families were more likely to experience a primary infection during pregnancy than women from high-income families. It may be that older, multiparous women are more likely to be infected from their preschool-age children who attend day-care centers and that low-income, primiparous mothers are more likely to acquire CMV sexually (Istas et al., 1995).

The rates of CMV excretion by seropositive women increase in the later months of pregnancy. One factor in the failure of immune mothers to restrict spread of CMV to their infants despite the presence of positive antibody titers may be the specific impairment of cell-mediated immunity to CMV (Rola-Pleszczynski et al., 1977; Reynolds et al., 1979; Starr et al., 1979). On the other hand, since fetal infection is not invariably the result of depressed maternal cellular immunity to CMV, the exact role of cellular immunity in modulating transmission of congenital infection is unclear

(Faix et al., 1983). It is believed that antibody affords the infant considerable protection from the adverse effects of the virus (Fowler et al., 1992; Bratcher et al., 1995). Clinically apparent maternal CMV infections in which there is a greater viral burden are more likely to result in transmission of CMV to the fetus (Alford et al., 1988).

PATHOLOGY

The histologic lesion of CMV infection is characterized by enlarged cells that contain intranuclear and cytoplasmic inclusion bodies. The intranuclear inclusion body appears reddish purple after being stained with hematoxylin and eosin and is surrounded by a halo, the "owl's eye" appearance. The paranuclear cytoplasmic inclusion or dense body is more granular and more basophilic in appearance.

Inclusion-bearing cells may be widely disseminated in the rare fatal infection. Involvement of almost every tissue and organ in the body has been described. Infection of the kidneys and lungs may induce chronic interstitial nephritis and pneumonitis, with focal areas of infiltration of mononuclear cells in the interstitial tissue. In the liver, focal areas of necrosis may occur. The brain may show necrotizing granulomatous lesions and extensive calcifications in congenital infections (Fig. 4-3), and the liver and spleen may display evidence of extramedullary hematopoesis. In patients with acquired immunodeficiency syndrome (AIDS), the retina, gastrointestinal tract (especially the colon), and lungs are most frequently invaded by CMV. In AIDS patients, CMV may be isolated from even more body sites than in transplant patients (Ho, 1990). In patients with colitis caused by CMV the presence of inclusion bodies and thrombi in endothelial cells in the submucosa and muscle wall, indicative of vasculitis, has been observed (Tatum et al., 1989), and CMV has also been implicated in the pathologic conditions leading to some instances of atherosclerosis (Melnick et al., 1983). CMV also expresses gene products that result in evasion of the immune system of the host (Gilbert et al., 1993).

CLINICAL MANIFESTATIONS

The clinical manifestations of congenital and postnatal CMV infections cover a broad spectrum. Both types of infection may range from an asymptomatic process associated with viruria and presence of specific antibody to a severe, widely disseminated disease involving virtually every organ in the body. The great majority of CMV infections, however, is totally inapparent.

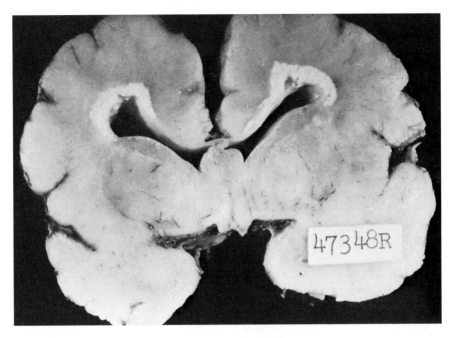

FIG. 4-3   Brain of an infant with congenital cytomegalovirus infection. Note extensive periventricular necrosis and calcification.

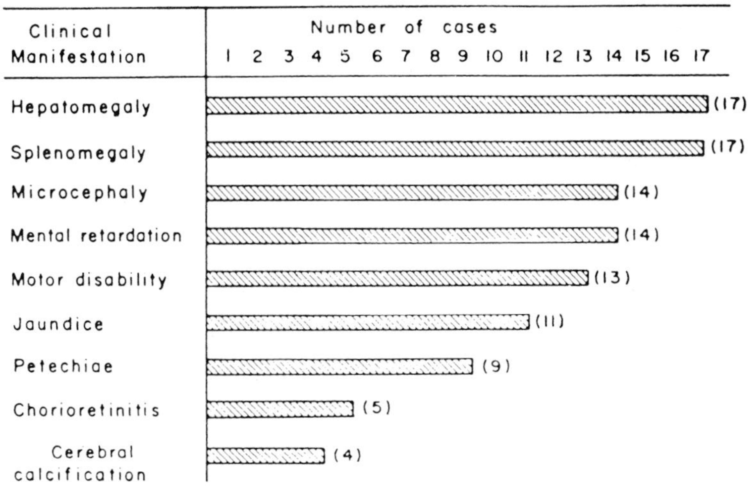

Clinical Manifestation	Number of cases 1 2 3 4 5 6 7 8 9 10 11 12 13 14 15 16 17
Hepatomegaly	▨▨▨▨▨▨▨▨▨▨▨▨▨▨▨▨ (17)
Splenomegaly	▨▨▨▨▨▨▨▨▨▨▨▨▨▨▨▨ (17)
Microcephaly	▨▨▨▨▨▨▨▨▨▨▨▨▨ (14)
Mental retardation	▨▨▨▨▨▨▨▨▨▨▨▨▨ (14)
Motor disability	▨▨▨▨▨▨▨▨▨▨▨▨ (13)
Jaundice	▨▨▨▨▨▨▨▨▨▨ (11)
Petechiae	▨▨▨▨▨▨▨▨ (9)
Chorioretinitis	▨▨▨▨ (5)
Cerebral calcification	▨▨▨ (4)

FIG. 4-4   Clinical features in 17 infants with congenital cytomegalovirus infection. (From Weller TH, Hanshaw JB: N Engl J Med 1962;266:1233.)

Congenital Infection

The typical clinical manifestations of severe generalized CMV infection are listed in Fig. 4-4, the skull roentgenogram of such a child with congenital CMV is shown in Fig. 4-5, and a child with severe congenital CMV is shown in Fig. 4-6. This fulminating illness is characterized by jaundice, hepatosplenomegaly, and a petechial rash; it occurs several hours or days after birth in a newborn infant, who usually is premature. Early onset of lethargy, respiratory distress, and convulsive

seizures may be followed by death at any time from a few days to many years later.

In infants who survive, jaundice may subside in as few as 2 weeks, or it may persist for months. The hemorrhagic phenomena subside rapidly. The hepatosplenomegaly may increase for the first 2 to 4 months and persist for a prolonged period (Boppana et al., 1992). Chorioretinitis is common (Istas et al., 1995).

Laboratory findings usually include anemia and thrombocytopenia. The cerebrospinal fluid (CSF) may show pleocytosis and increased concentration of protein. Roentgenograms of the skull may reveal cerebral calcifications (Fig. 4-6). The virus can be isolated from many body fluids, including urine, blood, and saliva. Examination of a fresh urine specimen sometimes reveals the inclusion bodies in cells in the urinary sediment. Recovery of virus is a more sensitive technique than cytology, which on occasion may give repeatedly negative results even in the presence of large quantities of virus isolated from the urine. As indicated in Fig. 4-4, many affected infants have severe neurological sequelae. Mental retardation and motor disability are common. In many infants, microcephaly either is present at birth or becomes apparent in a few months.

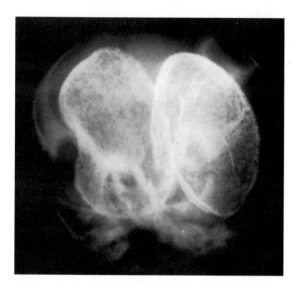

FIG. 4-5 Skull roentgenogram demonstrating massive intracranial calcifications of a 1-week-old infant with severe congenital cytomegalovirus infection.

Other manifestations of cerebral damage include spasticity, diplegia, epileptiform seizures, and blindness. A classic review by Hanshaw (1970) includes a summary of cerebral, ocular, and extraneural abnormalities associated with congenital CMV infection of 260 infants from birth to 12 months of age. These defects may occur singly or in combination.

Deafness, which may become increasingly apparent with increasing age of the child, is a major sequela of congenital CMV infection (Stagno et al., 1977a; Peckham et al., 1987). A study by Stagno et al. (1977a) reported on ten patients with sensorineural hearing loss caused by congenital CMV, seven of whom had been clinically well at birth. The defect was bilateral and moderate to profound in eight of the ten, and it was progressive in two. Immunofluorescent studies of the inner ear in the infants who died revealed widespread viral invasion of cochlear structures.

In contrast to rubella virus, CMV is believed to have only weak teratogenic capabilities. Reported structural abnormalities caused by congenital CMV infection include inguinal hernia in males, abnormalities of the first brachial arch, hypoplasia or agenesis of central nervous system (CNS) structures, and defects of enamel of primary dentition (Reynolds et al., 1986). Malformations associated with CMV infection probably are mainly the result of tissue necrosis rather than interference with organogenesis.

Extensive overt disease presenting in the neonatal period as just described is by far the exception in congenital CMV infection. More than 95% of congenitally infected infants are totally asymptomatic in the neonatal period (Alford et al., 1975). Approximately 90% have benign infections that re-

FIG. 4-6 Four-month-old child with symptomatic congenital infection manifesting severe failure to thrive, hepatitis with hepatosplenomegaly, bilateral inguinal hernias, and micropenis. (From Stagno S: Curr Prob Pediatr 1986;16:646.)

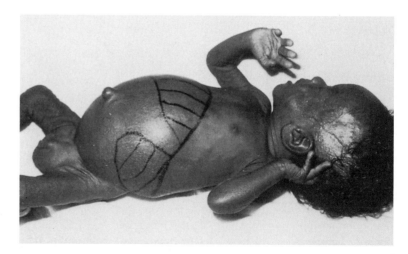

main inapparent; many result from secondary maternal CMV infection caused by reactivation of latent virus or reinfection with CMV during pregnancy. Even the majority of CMV-infected infants whose mothers had primary CMV infections during early pregnancy never develop sequelae.

Approximately 20% to 25% of asymptomatic, congenitally infected infants whose mothers have primary CMV infection during pregnancy can be expected to develop sequelae such as deafness and mental retardation (Stagno et al., 1986; Fowler et al., 1992). Since transmission from mother to fetus occurs in only approximately 40% of women, the risk of having a child damaged by CMV even after a primary infection during pregnancy is low— about 10%. Moderate-to-profound bilateral sensorineural deafness and increased school failure rates associated with low intelligence quotients in 8% to 20% of children congenitally infected with CMV have been observed (Reynolds et al., 1974; Hanshaw et al., 1975; Stagno et al., 1977a; Fowler et al., 1992). Unfortunately, there is still no reliable, widely available means to prospectively identify these high-risk infants.

Perinatal Infection

Infants may be infected at the time of birth, despite the presence of maternal CMV antibody, during passage through the maternal cervix, where secretions harbor reactivated CMV. Perinatal infections, although common, are considered of little significance; approximately 2% to 5% of all newborn infants are so infected. The infants develop viruria at approximately 1 month of age, but they remain asymptomatic. All are seropositive both before and during infection. Infants may also be infected after birth from either a maternal or nonmaternal source. Maternally derived infections usually are contracted through breast milk, presumably by lymphocytes infected with latent CMV. These infections usually are not accompanied by symptoms or sequelae.

On the other hand, when CMV is acquired by a seronegative infant from a nonmaternal source, a severe infection may occur. Yeager et al. (1972) described two low birth weight infants with CMV infections believed to have been acquired from blood transfusions. Subsequently, Yeager (1974) determined that CMV infections occurred in nineteen of seventy-seven (25%) of high-risk infants who were transfused and in only seven of seventy-four (11%) of those who were not. It is now recognized that premature infants who were seropositive to CMV

at birth but whose transplacental maternal antibodies have waned over time are also at increased risk to acquire severe CMV infections.

Others have also reported CMV infections in small premature infants who received multiple blood transfusions in the first week of life (Ballard et al., 1979). At approximately 6 weeks of age they developed hepatosplenomegaly, gray pallor, respiratory deterioration, lymphocytosis with atypical lymphocytes, and thrombocytopenia. Of fourteen such infants, three died. Prospective studies indicated that these infants had acquired CMV infection in the intensive care nursery, most likely as a result of multiple blood transfusions (mean of 21 separate blood units per infant). Unpasteurized banked breast milk is also a potential source of such infection, especially for low birth weight infants.

Acute respiratory disease with cough, pneumonitis, and abnormalities of pulmonary function and chest roentgenogram have been ascribed to CMV infection in young infants; often this occurs in conjunction with other pathogens such as *Chlamydia trachomatis* or *Ureaplasma urealyticum* (Brasfield et al., 1987). According to a study of thirty-two infants and thirty-two matched controls, CMV infection of low birth weight infants may also play a role in subsequent development of bronchopulmonary dysplasia (Sawyer et al., 1987). Intestinal infection by CMV in young infants has also been associated with symptoms of an acute surgical abdomen (Kosloske et al., 1988). It is unknown whether these syndromes are the result of perinatal infection, a postnatal infection, or both.

Postnatal Infection

Postnatal CMV infection in children and infection in adults are usually inapparent and asymptomatic. The clinical manifestations, when present, may be associated with specific involvement of the liver and with a mononucleosis-like syndrome.

Evidence of a relationship between a spontaneously occurring illness resembling infectious mononucleosis and CMV was reported by Kääriäinen et al. (1966a). A significant rise of antibodies to CMV was described in four adult patients and one child, all of whom had a negative heterophil agglutination test. Illness in the four adults was characterized by fever lasting 2 to 5 weeks, cough, headache, or pain in the back or limbs, a large number of atypical lymphocytes in the peripheral blood, and abnormal liver function tests. There was no exudative pharyngitis or lymphadenopathy. A 22-month-old child exhibited fever; migratory polyarthritis in the knees, fingers, and toes; a maculopapular skin rash; and pneumonia. The pneumonia and arthritis cleared completely, and the child was well 2 months after discharge from the hospital. None of nineteen control patients with heterophil-positive infectious mononucleosis showed a significant rise in titer of antibodies to CMV.

Subsequently, it was recognized that this syndrome could also follow blood transfusion (Kääriäinen et al., 1966b). An illness resembling infectious mononucleosis with fever, rubelliform rash, atypical lymphocytes, and a negative heterophil antibody test was reported in a 28-year-old woman 3 weeks after open heart surgery, during which she received fresh blood from fourteen donors. CMV was isolated from the urine 40 days after onset of illness, and the antibody titer rose from a titer of less than 1:4 at onset to 1:512 on the fortieth day. Moreover, a significant rise in antibodies to CMV was demonstrated in the absence of clinical manifestations of disease in eight of twenty successive patients after open heart surgery associated with fresh blood transfusions (Kääriäinen et al., 1966a, 1966b). These findings were confirmed by Lang and Hanshaw (1969), who also recognized the association of the syndrome with transfusion of fresh but not stored blood and implicated the leukocytes in viral transmission.

A more recent study is that of Horwitz et al. (1986), who reported eighty-two previously healthy individuals with a mononucleosis-like syndrome caused by CMV. None of these patients had received recent blood transfusions. These investigators emphasized the difficulty of making an accurate diagnosis in these patients, many of whom were initially thought to have serious diverse entities such as leukemia, systemic lupus erythematosus, and autoimmune hemolytic anemia. CMV infection has been implicated as a trigger for autoimmunity leading to type 1 diabetes in children (Pak et al., 1988). Using a molecular probe, CMV DNA was identified in the lymphocytes of 22% of fifty-nine children within 1 month of diagnosis of diabetes and in only 2.6% of thirty-eight control subjects, suggesting that persistent CMV infections may be involved in the pathogenesis of some cases of diabetes.

Systemic overt disease caused by CMV is more likely to occur in immunocompromised persons than in those who are immunologically normal. These infections are well recognized in patients who have had organ transplantation, who are being treated for malignant disease, or who have infection with HIV. These patients may manifest fever, lymphadenopathy, hepatitis, pneumonia, gastritis, colitis, arthralgia, arthritis, encephalopathy, retinitis, and leukopenia. Risk factors for infection in seronegative patients are transplantation with an organ from a seropositive donor and blood transfusion (including granulocytes) from a seropositive individual.

The presence of acute graft-versus-host disease is a significant risk factor for both CMV-seronegative and CMV-seropositive patients. In general, the severity of CMV infection is higher in seronegatives than in seropositives, but highly immunocompromised CMV seropositive patients may become ill because of reactivation of or reinfection with CMV. Receipt of antithymocyte globulin (OKT3 antibodies) is an additional risk factor for infection (Meyers et al., 1986; Singh et al., 1988; Pollard, 1988). In patients with AIDS, CMV has been the cause of colitis, encephalitis, pneumonia, and progressive retinitis leading to blindness (Drew, 1988). In leukemic children, CMV infection has been reported to cause fever, pneumonia, and chorioretinitis (Cox and Hughes, 1975). A growing body of clinical and experimental evidence indicates that CMV is itself immunosuppressive (Grundy, 1990). Patients with CMV mononucleosis have depressed in vitro cell-mediated immune responses to mitogens and other antigens (Ho, 1981). The virus also depresses natural killer cell activity and T-cell proliferation in vitro (Schrier et al., 1986). In a series of forty-nine recipients of heart transplants the incidence of pulmonary bacterial and *Pneumocystis* infections was higher in eleven patients with primary CMV infection after transplantation than in nineteen patients with evidence of CMV infection before transplantation (Rand et al., 1978). It is also possible that CMV may contribute to the immunosuppression in patients with HIV infection. Although it was suspected at one time that primary CMV infections in childhood might predispose children to serious bacterial infections, this has not been substantiated (Adler, 1988a).

The effects of CMV on the immune system, however, are far from simple. Despite the belief that CMV is immunosuppressive, its frequent association with graft rejection in transplanted patients has led to the hypothesis that CMV plays a significant role in this process. Interestingly in this regard, the virus enhances both cytoplasmic and surface expression of HLA class I antigens in vitro (Grundy et al., 1988), and it also induces a variety of autoantibodies (Grundy, 1990). It remains controversial, however, whether CMV plays a central role in triggering rejection or is simply activated as a result of prophylaxis or treatment of rejection (Grundy, 1990; Merigan and Resta, 1990). Similarly, in HIV-infected patients it remains unclear whether progressive immunodeficiency allows the emergence of CMV disease or whether CMV disease causes HIV infection to progress rapidly (Chandwani et al., 1996).

DIAGNOSIS

Serious infection with CMV should be strongly considered in a newborn infant with enlargement of the liver and spleen, jaundice, petechial rash, microcephaly, thrombocytopenia, and cerebral calcifications. Microcephaly, mental retardation, and motor disability may become evident in older infants.

In older children and adults the possibility of CMV infection should be kept in mind (1) in instances of pneumonia in immunocompromised patients or in those with chronic debilitating diseases such as malignant tumors and leukemia, (2) in unexplained liver disease, (3) in illnesses similar to infectious mononucleosis in which heterophil antibody tests are normal, (4) in febrile patients who have received organ transplants, and (5) in those

patients with risk factors for HIV infection or those with AIDS (Scott et al., 1984).

The diagnosis of CMV disease may be extremely difficult to make with certainty. It is helpful to analyze tissue (e.g., from a lung biopsy) for the presence of viral invasion. Isolation of CMV in tissue culture and/or histologic, immunologic, or molecular evidence of the presence of virus from tissue (or fluid) presumed infected may be diagnostic. However, CMV may be a bystander or coexist with other pathogens and may not necessarily cause disease, even if its presence is documented, since shedding of CMV by apparently healthy persons can occur.

It is often useful for diagnostic purposes to perform serologic analyses for detection of CMV antibodies such as complement fixation, indirect immunofluorescence anticomplement assay, or enzyme-linked immunosorbent assay (ELISA) in addition to attempts to detect the virus (Drew, 1988). Antibody titers to CMV, however, are known to fluctuate even in the absence of disease, making interpretation of results of antibody titers very difficult (Waner et al., 1973). In some patients a negative antibody test may be helpful in ruling out CMV infection.

As indicated in Fig. 4-7, CMV may persist in urine for prolonged periods of time. Urinary excretion of CMV by ninety-nine congenitally infected

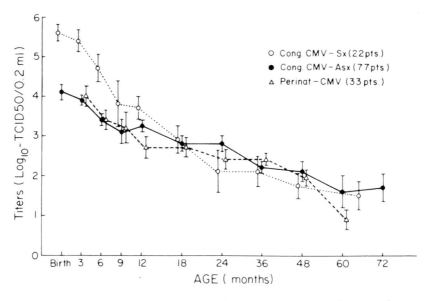

Fig. 4-7 Quantitative assessment of cytomegalovirus excretion in subjects with congenital symptomatic *(open circles)*, congenital asymptomatic *(closed circles)*, and perinatal *(triangles)* infections. (From Stagno S et al: Semin Perinatol 1983;7:34-42.)

infants, of whom twenty-two were symptomatic, and thirty-three perinatally infected infants is shown in Fig. 4-7 (Stagno et al., 1983). Symptomatic, congenitally infected infants shed the greatest amount of virus, an observation that may have diagnostic implications in selected situations. Infants with perinatal infections usually began to shed the virus between 4 to 8 weeks of age; in one such infant, shedding began at 3 weeks of age. Practically speaking, therefore, culture of urine for CMV during the first 2 weeks of life is necessary to distinguish between congenital and perinatal infection. Since prolonged viral shedding by all infected infants is the rule, diagnosis of congenital infection by urine culture may be problematic. A positive culture of urine or saliva is conclusive in the newly born infant with obvious symptoms of congenital CMV infection and no evidence of other congenital infections. Urinary shedding of CMV in infants with other congenital infections has been documented (Florman et al., 1973). Diagnosis of CMV in the infant who is asymptomatic at birth but later manifests developmental problems—statistically the most likely situation—is virtually impossible because congenital infection cannot be distinguished from postnatal CMV infection by urine culture after the neonatal period. Isolation of CMV from a site such as CSF is considered significant, although rather unusual (Jamison and Hathorn, 1978).

Antibody titers to CMV may also be difficult to interpret. Specific IgM has been detected in sera from healthy patients who presumably are experiencing an asymptomatic episode of viral reactivation (McEvoy and Adler, 1989), and IgG titers may also increase significantly without disease (Waner et al., 1973). There are few differences in titers from babies with congenital and perinatal infections. Interestingly, however, levels of specific IgG antibodies in maternal and infant sera are higher in babies with clinically apparent CMV infection with multiple system involvement than in babies with subclinical CMV infection (Britt and Vugler, 1990).

Presumably any specific IgM present in an infant's serum is diagnostic of infection, but the methodology is often questioned. An indirect immunofluorescence test for CMV IgM, described by Hanshaw et al., (1968), was positive only in infants with congenital CMV infections. This test has yielded false-positive and false-negative results in some other laboratories, however, and it is not generally available. A radioimmunoassay (RIA) for CMV IgM has been developed and tested by Griffiths et al. (1982a, 1982b). These investigators found CMV IgM in seventeen of seventeen (100%) infants with symptomatic CMV infections; however, sixty-six of seventy-six (87%) infants with asymptomatic infections also had detectable CMV IgM.

With this same assay, primary and recurrent maternal CMV infections were studied, since only mothers with primary CMV developed CMV IgM. CMV IgM was detected by RIA in sixteen of twenty-nine (55%) women with primary CMV and in none of eighteen women with recurrent infection. It was thus possible to identify high-risk pregnancies and infants with a high likelihood of symptomatic congenital CMV (Griffiths et al., 1982a, 1982b). Unfortunately, it is unlikely that this test will ever become widely available because of technical difficulties involved in the assay.

In addition, more data are required to confirm that IgM develops only in primary CMV infection. The observation that CMV-specific IgM is detectable in more than 90% of homosexual men suggests that, as has been found for other herpesvirus infections, IgM is produced in secondary, as well as primary, infections and therefore is not a specific indicator for primary infection except in the newborn infant (Drew, 1988).

An ELISA procedure for CMV IgM has been developed. Data thus far suggest that it compares favorably with RIA but only in serum obtained beyond the neonatal period (Demmler et al., 1986c). Other studies have found that, although CMV IgM may be detected by ELISA in congenitally infected infants, this test is less sensitive and specific than RIA (Stagno et al., 1985). Because some ELISA results are reported as an optical density reading rather than as a titer, it is necessary to check with the laboratory for the range of normal values.

Diagnosis of CMV may be suggested by detection of virus in urine, other body fluids, or white blood cells by molecular techniques. CMV has been detected in clinical samples using DNA hybridization (Chou and Merigan, 1983; Spector and Spector, 1985; Schrier et al., 1985; Jenson and Robert, 1987). Although low levels of CMV DNA can be detected in urine from some patients with asymptomatic shedding of virus, those with disease caused by CMV excrete much greater quantities of virus; therefore this assay may identify patients with illness caused by CMV (Chou and Merigan, 1983). With this same technique, CMV has also been detected in buffy coat cells from bone marrow transplant patients (Spector et al., 1983). In this study, DNA hybridization was more sensitive than culture of buffy coat for CMV, which often yielded negative results on patients who obviously were infected with CMV. In older patients, including AIDS patients in whom CMV pneumonia is suspected, bronchiolar lavage specimens have been useful for diagnosis of CMV (Stover et al., 1984, Springmeyer et al., 1986; Drew, 1988). The major advantage of DNA hybridization procedures, however, is the rapidity with which results can be reported, rather than the sensitivity of the test. These techniques, moreover, are usually only available on a research basis.

Another molecular test for demonstration of CMV, currently available mainly on a research basis, is polymerase chain reaction (PCR). With this methodology, minute amounts of viral nucleic acid are specifically amplified and then detected with molecular probes. Although highly subject to the possibility of nonspecificity PCR has been highly successful, when performed carefully, in rapid identification of CMV in urine and serum from congenitally infected newborns (Demmler et al., 1988; Nelson et al., 1995). Detection of CMV DNA by PCR in CSF in infants with congenital infection is highly predictive of a poor neurological outcome (Atkins et al., 1994). It is predicted that with time this assay will become clinically readily available for diagnosis.

In most hospitals, culture for CMV is performed in the diagnostic virology laboratory, and amplification methods for viral growth in tissue culture are used to speed the time for identification of CMV. Amplification procedures include centrifugation of the inoculum into tissue culture cells and early identification of positive cultures by staining for the presence of early antigens of CMV with fluorescent-labeled monoclonal antibodies after several days of incubation (shell vial technique) (Alpert et al., 1985; Drew, 1988). Thus a positive culture may be reported within days rather than weeks. The presence of high titers of virus in clinical specimens shortens the interval necessary for viral growth, which is also correlated with significant CMV infection; thus a rapid report of a positive culture may be indicative of CMV infection rather than asymptomatic viral shedding.

In summary, although diagnosis of CMV infection may not be difficult, proving that the virus is actually causing a disease is more problematic. In general, a significant increase in CMV antibody titer and/or positive IgM determination associated with evidence of viral invasion or excretion in urine or other body fluids, if accompanied by symptoms consistent with CMV infection, is considered presumptive evidence of CMV-induced disease.

DIFFERENTIAL DIAGNOSIS

In children, CMV infection may be confused with various forms of hepatitis, Epstein-Barr virus (EBV) infections, and toxoplasmosis. Congenital symptomatic CMV infection must be distinguished from a variety of infections and diseases that are characterized by jaundice, hepatosplenomegaly, and purpura in the neonatal period.

Congenital Toxoplasmosis

The clinical picture of congenital toxoplasmosis is remarkably similar to that of generalized congenital CMV. Both are characterized by jaundice, hepatosplenomegaly, chorioretinitis, and cerebral calcifications. Petechial and purpuric eruptions, which are common in patients with symptomatic congenital CMV infections, are rare with toxoplasmosis. When toxoplasmosis involves the CNS, elevated protein levels and pleocytosis are often detected in CSF, findings much less frequently associated with CMV infections. The precise diagnosis is established by serologic evidence of congenital toxoplasmosis or virologic and serologic evidence of CMV infection.

Congenital Rubella Syndrome

The consequences of fetal infection with rubella virus during the first trimester of pregnancy, which in the aggregate has been termed the *congenital rubella syndrome,* include features also seen in infants with CMV, such as hepatosplenomegaly, jaundice, petechial and purpuric rashes, thrombocytopenia, microcephaly, abnormalities of long bones on x-ray film, and mental retardation (Jenson and Robert, 1987). The diagnosis of the congenital rubella syndrome, suggested by a history of maternal infection in the first 3 to 4 months of pregnancy, should be confirmed by virologic and serologic evidence (See Chapter 26).

Erythroblastosis Fetalis

The jaundice, purpura, and lethargy in an infant with erythroblastosis fetalis are associated with a positive Coombs' test. The serum alanine aminotransferase (ALT) activity, which is increased in patients with CMV hepatitis, is within normal limits in those with erythroblastosis fetalis. A similar syndrome with prominent congestive heart failure and edema is also caused by parvovirus B19 infection (see Chapter 18).

Disseminated Herpes Simplex Virus Infection

Vesicular skin lesions, which may be found in 80% of babies with perinatal HSV infection, are rare in CMV infection. Cerebral calcifications generally have not been observed in patients with perinatal HSV, but a few cases have been reported. Isolation of HSV or detection of HSV antigens in skin lesions or other tissues is usually required to confirm a diagnosis of HSV (See Chapter 12).

Sepsis of the Newborn

Sepsis of the newborn may be characterized by lethargy, jaundice, and hepatomegaly. A blood culture usually reveals the causative organism.

Congenital Syphilis

Congenital syphilis, which is becoming much more common in the United States, can be differentiated from CMV infection by serologic tests and roentgenographic evidence of syphilitic osteitis.

EPIDEMIOLOGIC FACTORS

CMV infections are worldwide in distribution. Virologic and serologic studies have contributed to knowledge of the epidemiology of CMV infection. Surveys of unselected newborn infants in the United States and England have revealed a startling 1% to 2% incidence of viruria, indicative of congenital infection. Surveys of virus shedding in pregnant women from various countries have revealed incidences ranging from 1.9% to 5.6%. Based on an estimate of 4 million births each year, therefore, it could be estimated that 40,000 infants with CMV infection are born each year in the United States. Approximately 20%, or 8,000, will eventually manifest symptoms such as deafness and varying degrees of mental retardation (Fowler et al., 1992). These findings indicate that CMV infection is the most common congenital infection of humans.

The incidence of CMV infection is related to age, geographic location, and economic status. Serologic evidence of CMV infection increases with advancing age, reaching levels of 80% in various parts of the world. In general, infection is acquired at an earlier age by children who live in crowded, unhygienic conditions that may be prevalent in slum areas; institutions for mentally re-

tarded children; and day-care centers with more than twenty children in daily attendance. The epidemiology of CMV infection in the United States apparently is changing, since more and more children of middle and upper socioeconomic status are placed in day care and since breast-feeding is becoming more common in our society. Both would tend to increase the incidence of CMV infections in young children and to increase the incidence of disease in seronegative adults with whom they have contact (Yow et al., 1987). In a study of 1,989 pregnant women of middle to upper socioeconomic status, seropositivity was associated with nonwhite race, less than 16 years of education, being breast-fed in infancy, presence of children in the home, and being more than 30 years of age (Walmus et al., 1988). In the large study by Stagno et al. (1986) 65% of young women of upper socioeconomic status and 23% of young women of lower socioeconomic status lacked detectable antibodies against CMV. The incidence of primary CMV during pregnancy was higher in women from low-income families than in upper-middle-class women (Stagno et al., 1986). In this large study the annualized rate of primary CMV infection was 6.8% in the former and 2.5% in the latter.

The incidence of symptomatic congenital CMV infection is greater in highly industrialized countries than in developing nations. Acquisition of CMV in girls may be thought of as a natural form of immunization that later prevents symptomatic CMV infection in offspring.

Intrauterine transmission of CMV after primary infection is thought to occur in approximately 40% of cases (Stagno et al., 1986). More than 35% of postpartum women excrete reactivated CMV in breast milk, vaginal secretions, urine, or saliva. Approximately 20% of breast-fed infants become infected with CMV (Stagno et al., 1983).

Infection of children in day-care centers in the United States is very common. Variables concerning whether infection will occur include the number of children in the center, age of the child, and the time spent in the setting. After an 18-month interval, approximately 50% of seronegative children below the age of 3 years who are in a day-care center with more than fifty children will be infected. In children in day care who are 12 to 36 months of age the rate of excretion of CMV is very high—between 25% and 100% (Adler, 1988a, 1991b). No data are available on transmission for children who are cared for in smaller groups. CMV has been isolated from many potential sources of spread such as saliva, urine, toys, hands, and diapers (Demmler et al., 1987; Adler, 1988a, 1988b). It is likely that there is significant transmission of CMV from infants and small children. Taber et al. (1985) noted that an important risk factor for maternal acquisition of CMV was an infected child in the home. Pass et al. (1986) observed an increased incidence of CMV infection among sixty-seven parents whose children attended day care. In this study, susceptible parents whose children were infected had an infection rate of 30%. If only parents whose children were less than 18 months old were analyzed, the parental infection rate increased to 45%. There were no CMV infections in twenty-one parents whose children were in day care and not shedding CMV, nor in twenty-one children cared for at home. Other observers have also found that the risk of parental infection, particularly maternal, is increased as a result of exposure to infected children; in some cases transmission has been proven because the virus isolated from both parent and child has been identical on analysis of DNA (Spector and Spector, 1982; Pass et al., 1987; Adler, 1988a, 1988b). Although infection at day care is not particularly harmful to children, their parents may become infected as a result, which may have serious consequences if the mother is pregnant.

It is difficult to assess whether hospital workers are at increased risk of infection with CMV through contact with their patients. One study of the risks of 122 seronegative pediatric healthcare workers acquiring a primary CMV infection revealed an annual attack rate of approximately 3%, similar to that of young women in the community (Dworsky et al., 1983a). This low risk of nosocomial transmission in nurses exposed to patients who were shedding CMV was confirmed by Balfour and Balfour (1986). However, another study of 842 female employees in a pediatric hospital revealed that five of forty-five (10.9%) intensive care nurses, two of eleven (18.2%) intravenous team nurses, and three of eighty-one (3.7%) ward nurses seroconverted to CMV after 1 year (Friedman et al., 1984).

During a 2-year period, Demmler et al. (1987) investigated patient-to-caretaker, patient-to-patient, and caretaker-to-patient transmission of CMV in two pediatric settings, a chronic care unit and a neonatal nursery. In two years of study, two of sixty-nine (3%) nurses in the neonatal nursery seroconverted, and none of the nurses in the chronic care facility seroconverted. Of 188 personnel and 630 patients, there was one instance of pos-

sible patient-to-patient spread and one instance of patient-to-caretaker spread. Analysis of CMV isolates by restriction enzymes revealed that one additional presumed instance of patient-to-caretaker spread was actually a case of spread from husband to wife (Demmler et al., 1986b). This observation illustrates a significant point: the source of transmission cannot be identified by antibody assays; viral isolates taken from both the presumed source and the secondary case in question must have identical DNA before it can be concluded that transmission actually occurred. Using this criterion, it can be said that nosocomial transmission of CMV from a patient to a hospital worker has yet to be proven, although it undoubtedly occurs on occasion. The development of restriction endonuclease "fingerprinting" techniques has made it possible to prove various transmissions of CMV and thus clarify routes of transmission. For example, transmission from mother to fetus has been documented (Huang et al., 1980; Wilfert et al., 1982; Pass et al., 1987; Adler, 1988a, 1988b), as has transmission from infant to mother (Spector and Spector, 1982; Dworsky et al., 1984; Pass et al., 1987; Adler, 1988a,b). Nosocomial transmission from infant to infant has been demonstrated (Demmler et al., 1987; Spector, 1983), although it is apparently an unusual phenomenon (Adler et al., 1986).

Transmission among infants in a day-care setting has been proven (Adler, 1985; Murph et al., 1986; Adler, 1988b), as has transmission from husband to wife (Demmler et al., 1987). On the other hand, three medical staff personnel known to have been exposed to a patient with CMV were shown to have been infected with CMV from a different source (Wilfert et al., 1982; Yow et al., 1982; Dworsky et al., 1984). Data from one of these cases are shown in Fig. 4-8. A pregnant physician who contracted CMV while caring for a baby with CMV had her pregnancy terminated. As indicated in Fig. 4-8, DNA of the CMV isolated from the physician-mother and her fetus were similar but different from the DNA isolated from the presumed index case, indicating that the source of the physician's infection was not her patient.

There is increasing evidence for iatrogenic CMV disease in certain individuals. Some of these infections are undoubtedly reactivation syndromes that occur when immunosuppressive drugs are given to patients for underlying malignancy or organ transplantation. Others are primary infections caused by transfusions containing white blood cells harboring latent CMV or by transplantation of a kidney from

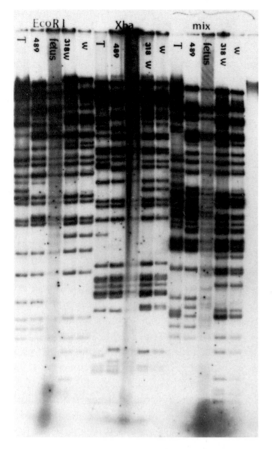

FIG. 4-8 DNA analysis by restriction endonucleases obtained from *T,* Towne (control) strain of CMV; *489,* mother's cytomegalovirus (CMV); *fetus,* fetal CMV; *318W* and *W,* CMV of index case. Fetus and 489 are similar but different from 318W and W.

a CMV-seropositive donor to a CMV-seronegative recipient (Ho et al., 1975). Although the risk of CMV infection in renal transplant patients is higher when the recipient is seronegative, infection may also occur in seropositive recipients (Chou, 1986). The risk of acquiring CMV from transfusion rises as increasing units of transfused blood and numbers of donors are used (Adler, 1983).

PROGNOSIS

Infants who survive generalized severe congenital CMV infection usually have significant neurological sequelae such as microcephaly, mental retardation, and motor disability. Of sixteen patients followed by Weller and Hanshaw (1962), only two failed to show residual damage. Of thirty-four patients with congenital symptomatic CMV infections followed for 9 months to 14 years, ten died, sixteen (47%) had microcephaly, fourteen (41%)

had mental retardation, seven (21%) had hearing loss, eight (24%) had neuromuscular disorders, and five (15%) had chorioretinitis or optic atrophy (Pass et al., 1980). No strains of CMV with a predilection to cause neurological damage have been identified (Griller et al., 1988).

The many infants who have symptomatic congenital CMV infection may show no effects until later childhood, when some manifest hearing loss and school failure (Reynolds et al., 1974; Hanshaw et al., 1975; Stagno et al., 1977a). Current studies suggest that this may occur in as many as 10% of congenitally infected children. With approximately 4 million births annually in the United States, this could involve 8,000 school children each year. Interestingly, a follow-up study of thirty-two children with symptomatic congenital CMV infection showed no correlation between the sequela of deafness and low intelligence (Conboy et al., 1987). On the other hand, chorioretinitis, in particular, but also microcephaly and neurological abnormalities, manifested by 1 year of age were all associated with development of severe mental retardation. These investigators have therefore stressed the wide range of possible outcomes of primary congenital infection that may not be generally appreciated. They have pointed out, for example, that an infant with hepatosplenomegaly, thrombocytopenia, jaundice, prematurity, and hearing loss might be expected to attain intellectual and developmental outcomes that are nearly normal.

Infants infected in the perinatal period rarely if ever manifest sequelae, with the exception of seronegative premature infants inadvertently infected with CMV by blood or banked breast milk containing latent virus. The long-term prognosis for these particular infants is unknown.

Evaluation of the prognosis of CMV infection in immunocompromised patients, including older children, is often complicated by the underlying condition and its therapy. Transplant patients who acquire CMV may develop illnesses caused directly by CMV, such as pneumonia; retinitis; and bacterial, protozoal, and fungal superinfections. In a series of 545 individuals who had undergone bone marrow transplantation, CMV infection occurred in approximately one third of seronegative patients and in two thirds of seropositive patients (Meyers et al., 1986). In general, however, the prognosis is better in patients who are seropositive at the time of infection than in those who are seronegative. Pneumonia caused by CMV carries a very high case/fatality ratio, although recently, with the availability of ganciclovir and high-titered immune globulin, the prognosis has improved somewhat.

The long-term prognosis of CMV infection in HIV-infected infants, including those with congenital or perinatal infections with both viruses, is not known, nor is it known whether congenital infection with one of these viruses predisposes to infection with the other. Similarly, the long-term prognosis of HIV-infected children infected with CMV in early infancy, as might occur in a day-care setting, has not been determined.

PREVENTION

A number of approaches to prevention of severe CMV infections in immunocompromised patients are being explored. They include active and passive immunization and administration of antiviral compounds on a prophylactic basis. It is conceivable that one day a vaccine will be used to prevent congenital CMV infection, as is done to prevent congenital rubella.

Experimental live CMV vaccines were evaluated by various investigators. Studies by Plotkin et al. (1976) have revealed that it is possible to prepare a live CMV vaccine that is well tolerated and antigenic. Questions that have been raised about a live CMV vaccine include (1) the degree of its attenuation, (2) its potential to become oncogenic, (3) its potential to induce a persistent infection, (4) the duration of immunity, and (5) whether it will protect against disease.

Placebo-controlled studies in ninety-one renal transplant patients indicated that, although infection was not prevented by prior immunization, illness caused by CMV was modified in those immunized in comparison to those who received a placebo (Plotkin et al., 1984). Immunized patients do not excrete vaccine type of CMV in their urine, and it is believed that the vaccine virus does not result in reactivation of latent infection (Plotkin et al., 1984, 1985; Plotkin and Huang, 1985). Studies in healthy human volunteers have indicated that the vaccine is attenuated in comparison to wild strains of CMV and that prior inoculation with the vaccine strain prevents disease after challenge with wild virus (Plotkin et al., 1985; Plotkin et al., 1987). In a study of Towne vaccine in CMV-seronegative women of childbearing age, immunized women had neutralizing antibody titers tenfold to twentyfold lower than after wild type of infection, and they were not protected against primary CMV infection (Adler et al., 1995). A subunit glycoprotein

CMV vaccine that would avoid the theoretical problems of viral latency is also being evaluated currently (Plotkin et al., 1990). Subunit vaccines that have been proposed and are under investigation in animal models include recombinant gB, gH, and pp65; a DNA vaccine is also being studied (Harrison et al., 1995; Pande et al., 1995).

Several approaches to prevention of CMV infection may be taken in low birth weight, hospitalized infants. Breast-fed infants may be given milk from only their own mothers, frozen or pasteurized banked human breast milk, or a prepared formula (Stagno et al., 1980; Dworsky et al., 1983b). Unfortunately, any cellular immunity present in milk that is theoretically of potential benefit to the infant will be destroyed along with the virus by pasteurization or freezing. The infectivity of CMV is lost after freezing (except at very low temperatures, such as $-70°$ C) or heating to $62°$ C (pasteurization).

Probably the most important method of prevention of CMV in low birth weight infants is by transfusion with blood that does not contain latent CMV. One approach is to transfuse these infants with blood from CMV-seronegative donors; another is to use frozen deglycerolized red blood cells (Yeager et al., 1981; Adler, 1983). Unfortunately, infection with CMV cannot be prevented by transfusion of saline-washed red blood cells, which are much simpler to prepare (Demmler et al., 1986a). Identification of potentially CMV-infected donor blood by DNA hybridization has not been proven successful (Jackson et al., 1987). Although it has been possible to identify blood that is unlikely to transmit CMV by testing it for the presence of CMV IgM antibodies, the assay is neither generally available nor consistently accurate and is therefore impractical (Lambertson et al., 1988).

Although only CMV-seronegative infants are at risk, most hospitals do not test babies for CMV antibodies. Appropriate preventive measures are therefore best carried out for all low birth weight infants unless CMV antibody determinations are performed.

Hyperimmune globulin has been found to reduce the incidence of severe CMV infections in some studies of bone marrow transplant patients (Meyers et al., 1983; Condie and O'Reilly, 1984), but not in others (Bowden et al., 1986). Hyperimmune globulin decreased the incidence of CMV disease in approximately two thirds of renal transplant patients in controlled studies (Snydman et al., 1987). Treated patients also experienced fewer fungal and bacterial superinfections. Hyperimmune globulin has been approved for use by the Food and Drug Administration (FDA) and is commercially available. Although hyperimmune globulin contains four to eight times as much CMV antibody as regular gamma globulin for intravenous use, many experts believe that use of the more expensive hyperimmune globulin provides no clinical advantage (Adler, 1991a).

Performing serologic screening of women to determine if they are susceptible to CMV and therefore at risk to have a primary infection during pregnancy is controversial. Those who advocate testing point out that knowledge of susceptibility is helpful for counseling, particularly for women at increased risk of infection, such as those with small children in day care or hospital workers (Walmus et al., 1988). Women who are seropositive against CMV may be reassured. However, Pass et al. (1987) and Adler (1988a, 1988b) have emphasized the difficulties of diagnosis of maternal infection, the futility of trying to prevent CMV infection in susceptible individuals, and the problem of deciding whether to continue a pregnancy if CMV is diagnosed. Until a means of prevention of CMV is developed, serologic screening of pregnant women for antibodies to CMV is probably of little use. At this time, experts seem to agree that there is not enough information to indicate the exact risk of CMV infection to the infant; therefore termination of pregnancy, even if a primary maternal infection is documented during the first trimester, is usually not routinely recommended (Stagno et al., 1986; Adler, 1988a, 1988b).

Administration of acyclovir (ACV) on a prophylactic basis has been reported to decrease the incidence of serious CMV infections in renal transplant patients (Balfour et al., 1989). These results were controversial. Ganciclovir, recently licensed and to which CMV is more sensitive, is the preferred prophylactic medication (Merigan et al., 1993).

THERAPY

Specific therapy is not indicated for normal hosts. Whether specific therapy could improve the outcome of congenital infection is not known. In immunocompromised patients, nonspecific measures such as decreasing the dosage of immunosuppressive drugs is recommended if possible (Pollard, 1988). Fortunately, CMV infections in immunocompromised patients have apparently been less severe since the introduction of cyclosporine (Pollard, 1988). CMV immunoglobulin in conjunction with ganciclovir has been used to treat CMV pneumonia (Reed et al., 1988).

Ganciclovir, which is structurally similar to ACV but has greater activity against CMV, has been used with success to treat severe CMV infections in immunocompromised patients. The drug has been licensed in the United States for treatment of severe CMV infections, such as those that occur in renal transplant patients and patients with AIDS. Although most of the studies of this drug have been uncontrolled, it appears that patients with retinitis and colitis caused by CMV generally respond well, but the outcome in those with pneumonia is less positive (Collaborative DHPG Study Group, 1986; Keay et al., 1987; Laskin et al., 1987; Lim et al., 1988). In some instances the virologic response is more prominent than the clinical response. Latent infection with CMV is neither cured nor prevented; the drug is not curative. Iatrogenically immunosuppressed patients who have had organ transplantation seem to respond better than patients with underlying AIDS (Keay et al., 1987; Laskin et al., 1987). In patients with AIDS, CMV relapses are common after therapy, such that long-term administration of ganciclovir is required. The recommended therapeutic dose of ganciclovir is 7.5 mg/kg/day intravenously (IV); 5 mg/kg IV 5 to 7 times per week is recommended for maintenance dosage. Ganciclovir for oral administration to CMV-infected AIDS patients has been approved by the FDA for use in adults with HIV retinitis (1g tid po). The dosage for children is not known. Reported adverse effects of ganciclovir include neutropenia and leukopenia. Because of drug toxicity, zidovudine (AZT) and ganciclovir cannot be administered simultaneously. Other approaches in immunocompromised patients include administration of foscarnet for CMV retinitis in HIV-infected patients, as well as interferon.

BIBLIOGRAPHY

Adler SP. Transfusion-associated cytomegalovirus infections. Rev Infect Dis 1983;5:977-993.

Adler SP. The molecular epidemiology of cytomegalovirus transmission among children attending a day care center. J Infect Dis 1985;152:760-768.

Adler SP. Cytomegalovirus transmission among children in day care, their mothers, and caretakers. Pediatr Infect Dis 1988a;7:279-285.

Adler SP. Molecular epidemiology of cytomegalovirus: viral transmission among children attending a day care center, their parents, and caretakers. J Pediatr 1988b;112:366-372.

Adler SP. Cytomegalovirus hyperimmune globulin: who needs it? Pediatr Infect Dis J 1991a;11:266-269.

Adler SP. Molecular epidemiology of cytomegalovirus: a study of factors affecting transmission among children at three daycare centers. Ped Infect Dis J 1991b;10:584-590.

Adler SP, Baggett J, Wilson M, et al. Molecular epidemiology of cytomegalovirus in a nursery: lack of evidence for nosocomial transmission. J Pediatr 1986;108:117-123.

Adler SP, Starr S, Plotkin SA, et al. Immunity induced by primary human cytomegalovirus infection protects against secondary infection among women of childbearing age. J Infect Dis 1995;171:26-32.

Ahlfors D, Harris S, Ivarsson S, et al. Secondary maternal cytomegalovirus infection causing symptomatic congenital infection. N Engl J Med 1981;305:284.

Alexander ER. Maternal and neonatal infection with cytomegalovirus in Taiwan. Pediatr Res 1967;1:210.

Alford CA, Hayes K, Britt W. Primary cytomegalovirus infection in pregnancy: comparison of antibody responses to virus-encoded proteins between women with and without intrauterine infection. J Infect Dis 1988;158:917-924.

Alford CA Jr, Reynolds DW, Stagno S. Current concepts of chronic perinatal infections. In Gluck L (ed). Modern perinatal medicine. Chicago: Year Book Medical Publishers, 1975.

Alpert G, Mazeron M-C, Colimon R, Plotkin S. Rapid detection of human cytomegalovirus in the urine of humans. J Infect Dis 1985;152:631-633.

Atkins JT, Demmler GJ, Williamson WD, et al. Polymerase chain reaction to detect cytomegalovirus DNA in the cerebrospinal fluid of neonates with congenital infection. J Infect Dis 1994;169:1334-1337.

Baldick CJ, Shenk T. Proteins associated with purified human cytomegalovirus. J Virol 1996;6097-6105.

Balfour CL, Balfour HH Jr. Cytomegalovirus is not an occupational risk for nurses in renal transplant and neonatal units: results of a prospective surveillance study. JAMA 1986;256:1909-1914.

Balfour HH, Chace BA, Stapleton JT, et al. A randomized placebo-controlled trial of oral acyclovir for the prevention of cytomegalovirus disease in recipients of renal allografts. N Engl J Med 1989;320:1381-1387.

Ballard RA, Drew WL, Hufnagle KG, et al. Acquired cytomegalovirus infection in preterm infants. Am J Dis Child 1979;133:482.

Boppana S, Pass RF, Britt WJ, et al. Symptomatic congenital cytomegalovirus infection: neonatal morbidity and mortality. Ped Infect Dis J 1992; 11:93-99.

Bowden RA, Sayers M, Fluornoy N, et al. Cytomegalovirus immune globulin and seronegative blood products to prevent primary cytomegalovirus infection after bone marrow transplantation. N Engl J Med 1986;314:1006-1010.

Brasfield DM, Stagno S, Whitley RJ, et al. Infant pneumonitis associated with cytomegalovirus, Chlamydia, Pneumocystis, and Ureaplasma: follow up. Pediatrics 1987;79:76-83.

Bratcher DF, Bournae N, Bravo, FJ, et al. Effect of passive antibody on congenital cytomegalovirus infection in guinea pigs. J Infect Dis 1995;172:944-950.

Britt WJ, Vugler LG. Antiviral antibody responses in mothers and their newborn infants with clinical and subclinical congenital cytomegalovirus infections. J Infect Dis 1990;161:214-219.

Chandler SH, Alexander ER, Holmes KK. Epidemiology of congenital viral infection in a heterogenous population of pregnant women. J Infect Dis 1985;152:249-256.

Chandler SH, Handsfield HH, McDougall JK. Isolation of multiple strains of cytomegalovirus from women attending a clinic for sexually transmitted diseases. J Infect Dis 1987;155:655-660.

Chandwani S, Kaul A, Bebenroth D, et al. Cytomegalovirus infection in human immunodeficiency virus type 1–infected children. Pediatr Infect Dis 1996;15:310-314.

Chou S. Acquisition of donor strains of cytomegalovirus by renal transplant recipients. N Engl J Med 1986;314:1418-1423.

Chou S. Reactivation and recombination of multiple cytomegalovirus strains from individual organ donors. J Infect Dis 1989a;160:11-15.

Chou S. Neutralizing antibody responses to reinfecting strains of cytomegalovirus in transplant recipients. J Infect Dis 1989b;160:16-21.

Chou S, Merigan TC. Rapid detection and quantitation of human cytomegalovirus in urine through DNA hybridization. N Engl J Med 1983;308:921-925.

Collaborative DHPG Treatment Study Group. Treatment of serious cytomegalovirus infections with 9-(1,3dihydroxy-2-propoxymethyl) guanine in patients with AIDS and other immunodeficiencies. N Engl J Med 1986;314:801-805.

Conboy TJ, Pass RF, Stagno S, et al. Early clinical manifestations and intellectual outcome in children with symptomatic congenital cytomegalovirus infection. J Pediatr 1987;111:343-348.

Condie RM, O'Reilly RJ. Prevention of cytomegalovirus infection by prophylaxis with an intravenous, hyperimmune, native, unmodified cytomegalovirus globulin. Am J Med 1984;76:134-141.

Cox F, Hughes WT. Cytomegalovirus in children with acute lymphatic leukemia. J Pediatr 1975;87:190.

Demmler GD, Brady M, Bijou H, et al. Posttransfusion cytomegalovirus infection in neonates: role of saline-washed red blood cells. J Pediatr 1986a;108:762-765.

Demmler GD, Buffone GJ, Schimbor CM, May RA. Detection of cytomegalovirus in urine from newborns by using polymerase chain reaction. J Infect Dis 1988;158:1177-1184.

Demmler GD, O'Neil GW, O'Neil JH, et al. Transmission of cytomegalovirus from husband to wife. J Infect Dis 1986b;154:545-546.

Demmler GD, Six HR, Hurst M, et al. Enzyme-linked immunosorbent assay for the detection of IgM-class antibodies to cytomegalovirus. J Infect Dis 1986c;153:1152-1155.

Demmler GD, Yow MD, Spector S, et al. Nosocomial cytomegalovirus infections within two hospitals caring for infants and children. J Infect Dis 1987;156:9-16.

Diosi P, Babusceac L, Nevinglovschi O, et al. Cytomegalovirus infection associated with pregnancy. Lancet 1967;2:1063.

Drew LW. Cytomegalovirus infection in patients with AIDS. J Infect Dis 1988;158:449-456.

Dworsky M, Lakeman A, Stagno S. Cytomegalovirus transmission within a family. Pediatr Infect Dis J 1984;3:236-238.

Dworsky M, Stagno S, Pass RF, et al. Persistence of cytomegalovirus in human milk after storage. J Pediatr 1982;101:440-443.

Dworsky M, Welch K, Cassady G, et al. Occupational risk for primary cytomegalovirus infection among pediatric healthcare workers. N Engl J Med 1983a;309:950-953.

Dworsky M, Yow M, Stagno S, et al. Cytomegalovirus infection of breast milk and transmission in infancy. Pediatr 1983b;72:295-299.

Faix RG, Zweig SE, Kummer JF, et al. Cytomegalovirus-specific cell-mediated immunity during pregnancy in lower socioeconomic class adolescents. J Infect Dis 1983;148:621-629.

Florman AL, Gershon AA, Blackett PR, et al. Intrauterine infection with herpes simplex virus. JAMA 1973;225:129-132.

Fowler KB, Stagno S, Pass R, et al. The outcome of congenital cytomegalovirus infection in relation to maternal antibody status. N Engl J Med 1992;326:663-667.

Friedman HM, Lewis MR, Nemerofsky DM, et al. Acquisition of cytomegalovirus infection among female employees at a pediatric hospital. Pediatr Infect Dis 1984;3:233-235.

Gilbert MJ, Riddell SR, Li CR, Greenberg PD. Selective interference with class I major histocompatibility complex presentation of the major immediate-early protein following infection with human cytomegalovirus. J Virol 1993;67:3461-3469.

Goodpasture EW, Talbot FB. Concerning the nature of "protozoan-like" cells in certain lesions of infancy. Am J Dis Child 1921;21:415.

Griffiths PD, Stagno S, Pass RF, et al. Infection with cytomegalovirus during pregnancy: specific IgM antibodies as a marker of recent primary infection. J Infect Dis 1982a;145:647-653.

Griffiths PD, Stagno S, Pass RF, et al. Congenital cytomegalovirus infection: diagnostic and prognostic significance of the detection of specific immunoglobulin M antibodies in cord serum. Pediatrics 1982b;69:544-549.

Griller L, Ahlfors K, Ivarsson S, et al. Endonuclease cleavage pattern of cytomegalovirus DNA of strains isolated from congenitally infected infants with neurologic sequelae. Pediatrics 1988;81:27-30.

Grundy JE. Virologic and pathologic aspects of cytomegalovirus infection. Rev Infect Dis 1990;12(suppl):S711-S719.

Grundy JE, Ayles HM, McKeating JA, et al. Enhancement of class I HLA antigen expression by cytomegalovirus: role in amplification of virus infection. J Med Virol 1988;25:483-495.

Hansfield HH, Chandler SH, Caine VA, et al. Cytomegalovirus infections in sex partners: evidence for sexual transmission. J Infect Dis 1985;151:344-348.

Hanshaw JB. Developmental abnormalities associated with congenital cytomegalovirus infection. Adv Teratol 1970;4:64.

Hanshaw JB, Steinfeld HJ, White CJ. Fluorescent-antibody test for cytomegalovirus macroglobulin. N Engl J Med 1968;279:566.

Hanshaw JB et al. CNS sequelae of congenital cytomegalovirus infection. Infections of the fetus and the newborn infant. Prog Clin Biol Res 1975;3:47.

Harrison CJ, Britt WJ, Chapman NM, et al. Reduced congenital cytomegalovirus (CMV) infection after maternal immunization with a guinea pig CMV glycoprotein before gestational primary CMV infection in the guinea pig model. J Infect Dis 1995;172:1212-1220.

Heggie AD, Wentz WB, Reagan JW, Anthony DD. Roles of cytomegalovirus and Chlamydia trachomatis in the induction of cervical neoplasia in the mouse. Cancer Res 1986;46:5211-5214.

Ho M. The lymphocyte in infections with Epstein-Barr virus and cytomegalovirus. J Infect Dis 1981;143:857-862.

Ho M. Epidemiology of cytomegalovirus infections. Rev Infect Dis 1990;12(suppl):S701-S710.

Ho M, Suwansirkul S, Dowling JM, et al. The transplanted kidney as a source of cytomegalovirus infection. N Engl J Med 1975;293:1109.

Horwitz CA, Henle W, Henle G, et al. Clinical and laboratory evaluation of cytomegalovirus-induced mononucleosis in previously healthy individuals: report of 82 cases. Medicine 1986;65:124-134.

Huang ES, Alford CA, Reynolds DW, et al. Molecular epidemiology of cytomegalovirus infections in women and their infants. N Engl J Med 1980;303:958-962.

Hutto C, Little A, Ricks R, et al. Isolation of CMV from toys and hands in a day-care center. J Infect Dis 1986;154:527-530.

Istas AS, Demmler GJ, Dobbins JG, et al. Surveillance for congenital cytomegalovirus disease: a report from the national congenital cytomegalovirus disease registry. Clin Infect Dis 1995;20:665-670.

Jackson JB, Orr HT, McCullough JJ, Jordan C. Failure to detect human cytomegalovirus DNA in IgM-seropositive blood donors by spot hybridization. J Infect Dis 1987;156:1013-1016.

Jamison RM, Hathorn AW. Isolation of cytomegalovirus from cerebrospinal fluid of a congenitally infected infant. Am J Dis Child 1978;132:63-64.

Jenson HB, Robert M. Congenital cytomegalovirus infection with osteolytic lesions: use of DNA hybridization in diagnosis. Clin Pediatr 1987;9:448-452.

Kääriäinen L, Klemola E, Paloheimo J. Rise of cytomegalovirus antibodies in an infectious mononucleosis-like syndrome after transfusion. Br Med J 1966a;2:1270.

Kääriäinen L, et al. Cytomegalovirus-mononucleosis. Isolation of the virus and demonstration of subclinical infections after fresh blood transfusion in connection with open heart surgery. Ann Med Exp Biol Fenn 1966b;44:297.

Keay S, Bissett J, Merigan TC. Gancyclovir treatment of cytomegalovirus infections in iatrogenically immunocompromised patients. J Infect Dis 1987;156:1016-1021.

Kosloske AM, Jewell PF, Florman AL, et al. Acute abdominal emergencies associated with cytomegalovirus infection in the young infant. Pediatr Surg 1988;3:43-46.

Kozinowski UH, Reddehase MJ, Keil GM, Schieckedanz J. Host immune response to cytomegalovirus: products of transfected viral immediate-early genes are recognized by cloned cytolytic T lymphocytes. J Virol 1987;61:2054-2058.

Kumar ML, Nankervis GA, Jacobs IB, et al. Congenital and postnatally acquired cytomegalovirus infections: long-term follow up. J Pediatr 1984;104:674-679.

Lambertson HV, McMillan JA, Weiner LB, et al. Prevention of transfusion-associated cytomegalovirus (CMV) infection in neonates by screening blood donors for IgM to CMV. J Infect Dis 1988;157:820-823.

Lang DJ, Hanshaw JB. Cytomegalovirus infection and the postperfusion syndrome: recognition of primary infections in four patients. N Engl J Med 1969;280:1145.

Lang DJ, Kummer JF. Cytomegalovirus in semen: observations in selected populations. J Infect Dis 1975;132:472.

Laskin O, Cederberf D, Mills J, et al. Gancyclovir for the treatment and suppression of serious infections caused by cytomegalovirus. Am J Med 1987;83:201-207.

Lim W, Kahn E, Gupta A, et al. Treatment of cytomegalovirus enterocolitis with gancyclovir in an infant with acquired immunodeficiency syndrome. Pediatr Infect Dis 1988;7:354-357.

McEvoy MA, Adler S. Immunologic evidence for frequent age-related cytomegalovirus reactivation in seropositive immunocompetent individuals. J Infect Dis 1989;160:1-10.

McFarlane ES, Koment RW. Use of restriction endonuclease digestion to analyze strains of human cytomegalovirus isolated concurrently from an immunocompetent heterosexual man. J Infect Dis 1986;154:167-168.

Melnick JL, Petrie BL, Dreesman Gr, et al. Cytomegalovirus antigen within human arterial smooth muscle cells. Lancet 1983;2:644-647.

Merigan T, Renlund D, Keay S, et al. A controlled trial of ganciclovir to prevent CMV disease after transplantation. N Engl J Med 1992;326:1182-1186.

Merigan T, Resta S. Cytomegalovirus: where have we been and where are we going? Rev Infect Dis 1990;12(suppl):S693-S700.

Meyers JD, Flournoy N, Thomas ED. Risk factors for cytomegalovirus infection after human marrow transplantation. J Infect Dis 1986;153:478-488.

Meyers JD, Leszczynski J, Zaia JA, et al. Prevention of cytomegalovirus infection by cytomegalovirus immune globulin after marrow transplantation. Ann Intern Med 1983;98:442-446.

Murph JR, Bale JF, Murran JC, et al. Cytomegalovirus transmission in a midwest day-care center: possible relationship to child care practices. J Pediatr 1986;109:35-39.

Nelson CT, Istas AS, Wilkerson MK, Demmler GJ. PCR detection of cytomegalovirus DNA in serum as a diagnostic test for congenital cytomegalovirus infection. J Clin Micro 1995;33:3317-3318.

Pak CY, Eun HM, McArthur RG, et al. Association of cytomegalovirus infection with autoimmune type I diabetes. Lancet 1988;2:1-4.

Pande H, Campo K, Tanamachi B, et al. Direct DNA immunization of mice with plasmid DNA encoding the tegument protein pp65 (ppUL83) of human cytomegalovirus induces high levels of circulating antibody to the encoded protein. Scand J Infect Dis Suppl 1995;99:117-120.

Pass RF, Hutto C, Ricks R, et al. Increased rate of cytomegalovirus infection among parents of children attending day-care centers. N Engl J Med 1986;314:1414-1416.

Pass RF, Little EA, Stagno S, et al. Young children as a probable source of maternal and congenital cytomegalovirus infection. N Engl J Med 1987;316:1366-1370.

Pass RF, Stagno S, Myers G, et al. Outcome of symptomatic congenital cytomegalovirus infection: results of long-term longitudinal follow-up. Pediatr 1980;66:758-762.

Peckham CS, Stark O, Dudgeon JA, et al. Congenital cytomegalovirus infection: a cause of sensorineural hearing loss. Arch Dis Child 1987;62:1233-1237.

Plotkin SA, Farquhar J, Hornberger E. Clinical trials of immunization with the Towne 125 strain of human cytomegalovirus. J Infect Dis 1976;134:470-475.

Plotkin SA, Friedman HM, Fleischer GR, et al. Towne-vaccine–induced prevention of cytomegalovirus disease after renal transplants. Lancet 1984;1:528-530.

Plotkin SA, Huang ES. Cytomegalovirus vaccine virus (Towne strain) does not induce latency. J Infect Dis 1985;152:395-397.

Plotkin SA, Starr SE, Friedman HM, Gonczol E. Comparison of vaccine-induced and natural immunity to human cytomegalovirus (abstract #951). Pediatr Res 1987;21:332A.

Plotkin SA, Starr SE, Friedman HM, et al. Vaccines for the prevention of human cytomegalovirus infection. Rev Infect Dis 1990;12(suppl):S827-S838.

Plotkin SA, Weibel RE, Alpert G, et al. Resistance of seroposi-

tive volunteers to subcutaneous challenge with low-passage human cytomegalovirus. J Infect Dis 1985;151:737-739.

Pollard RB. Cytomegalovirus infections in renal, heart, heart-lung, and liver transplantation. Pediatr Infect Dis J 1988;7:S97-S102.

Rand KH, Pollard RB, Merigan TC. Increased pulmonary superinfections in cardiac-transplant patients undergoing primary cytomegalovirus infection. N Engl J Med 1978;298:951.

Reed EC, Bowden RA, Dandliker PS, et al. Treatment of cytomegalovirus pneumonia with gancyclovir and intravenous cytomegalovirus immunoglobulin in patients with bone marrow transplants. Ann Intern Med 1988;109:783-788.

Reynolds DW, Dean PH, Pass RF, Alford CA. Specific cell-mediated immunity in children with congenital and neonatal cytomegalovirus infection and their mothers. J Infect Dis 1979;140:493-499.

Reynolds DW, Stagno S, Alford C. Congenital cytomegalovirus infection. In Reynolds DW, Stagno S, Alford C (eds). Teratogen update: environmentally induced birth defect risks. New York: Alan R Liss, 1986.

Reynolds DW, Stagno S, Stubbs G, et al. Inapparent congenital cytomegalovirus infection with elevated cord IgM levels: causal relation with auditory and mental deficiency. N Engl J Med 1974;290:291-296.

Rola-Pleszczynski M, Frenkel L, Fuceillo DA, et al. Specific impairment of cell-mediated immunity in mothers of infants with congenital infection due to cytomegalovirus. J Infect Dis 1977;135:386-391.

Rowe WP, et al. Cytopathogenic agent resembling human salivary gland virus recovered from tissue cultures of human adenoids. Proc Soc Exp Biol Med 1956;92:4181.

Rutter D, Griffiths P, Trompeter RS. Cytomeglic inclusion disease after recurrent maternal infection. Lancet 1985;2:1182.

Sawyer MH, Edwards DK, Spector SA. Cytomegalovirus infection and bronchopulmonary dysplasia in premature infants. Am J Dis Child 1987;141:303-305.

Schrier RD, Nelson JA, Oldstone MBA. Detection of human cytomegalovirus in peripheral blood leucocytes in a natural infection. Science 1985;230:1048-1051.

Schrier RD, Rice GPA, Oldstone MBA. Suppression of natural killer cell activity and T cell proliferation by fresh isolates of human cytomegalovirus. J Infect Dis 1986;153:1084-1091.

Scott GB, Buck BE, Leterman JG, et al. Acquired immunodeficiency syndrome in infants. N Engl J Med 1984;310:76-81.

Singh N, Dummer JS, Kusne S, et al. Infections with cytomegalovirus and other herpesviruses in 121 liver transplant recipients: transplantation by donated organ and the effect of OKT3 antibodies. J Infect Dis 1988;158:124-131.

Smith MG. Propagation of salivary gland virus of the mouse in tissue cultures. Proc Soc Exp Biol Med 1954;86:435.

Smith MG. Propagation in tissue cultures of a cytopathogenic virus from human salivary gland virus (SGV) disease. Proc Soc Exp Biol Med 1956;92:424.

Snydman DR, Werner BG, Heize-Lacey B, et al. Use of cytomegalovirus immune globulin to prevent cytomegalovirus disease in renal transplant recipients. N Engl J Med 1987;317:1049-1054.

Spector SA. Transmission of cytomegalovirus among infants in hospital documented by restriction-endonuclease-digestion analyses. Lancet 1983;1:378-381.

Spector SA, Hirata KK, Neuman TR. Identification of multiple cytomegalovirus strains in homosexual men with acquired immunodeficiency syndrome. J Infect Dis 1984; 150:953-956.

Spector SA, Rua LA, Spector DH, et al. Rapid diagnosis of CMV viremia in bone marrow transplant patients by DNA-DNA hybridization (abstract 914). Las Vegas: Twenty-Third Interscience Conference in Antimicrobial Agents and Chemotherapy, 1983.

Spector SA, Spector DH. Molecular epidemiology of cytomegalovirus infections in premature twin infants and their mother. Pediatr Infect Dis 1982;1:405-409.

Spector SA, Spector DH. The use of DNA probes in studies of human cytomegalovirus. Clin Chem 1985;31:1514-1520.

Springmeyer SC, Hackman RC, Holle R, et al. Use of bronchoalveolar lavage to diagnose acute diffuse pneumonia in the immunocompromised host. J Infect Dis 1986;154:604-610.

Stagno S, Brasfield DM, Brown MB et al. Infant pneumonitis associated with cytomegalovirus, chlamydia, pneumocystis, and ureaplasma: a prospective study. Pediatr 1981;68:322-329.

Stagno S, Pass R, Cloud G, et al. Primary cytomegalovirus infection in pregnancy. Incidence, transmission to fetus, and clinical outcome. JAMA 1986;256:1904-1908.

Stagno S, Pass RF, Dworsky ME, et al. Congenital cytomegalovirus infection: the relative importance of primary and recurrent maternal infection. N Engl J Med 1982; 306:945-949.

Stagno S, Pass R, Dworsky M, et al. Congenital and perinatal cytomegalovirus infections. Semin Perinatol 1983;7:31.

Stagno S, Reynolds D, Amos CS, et al. Auditory and visual defects resulting from symptomatic and subclinical congenital cytomegaloviral and toxoplasma infections. Pediatr 1977a; 59:699-678.

Stagno S, Reynolds DW, Huang ES, et al. Congenital cytomegalovirus infection. Occurrence in an immune population. N Engl J Med 1977b;296:1254-1258.

Stagno S, Reynolds DW, Pass RF, Alford CA. Breast milk and the risk of cytomegalovirus infection. N Engl J Med 1980;302:1073-1076.

Stagno S, Tinker M, Elrod C, et al. Immunoglobulin M antibodies detected by enzyme-linked immunosorbent assay and radioimmunoassay in the diagnosis of cytomegalovirus infections in pregnant women and newborn infants. J Clin Micro 1985;31:930-935.

Starr SE, Tolpin MD, Friedman HM, et al. Impaired cellular immunity to cytomegalovirus in congenitally infected children and their mothers. J Infect Dis 1979;140:500-505.

Stover DE, Zaman MB, Hajdu SI, et al. Bronchoalveolar lavage in the diagnosis of diffuse pulmonary infiltrates in the immunosuppressed host. Ann Intern Med 1984;101:1-7.

Taber LH, Frank Al, Yow MD, et al. Acquisition of cytomegaloviral infections in families with young children: a serologic study. J Infect Dis 1985;151:948-952.

Tatum ET, Sun PC, Cohn DJ. Cytomegalovirus vasculitis and colon perforation in a patient with the acquired immunodeficiency syndrome. Pathology 1989;21:235-238.

Taylor-Wiedeman J, Sissons P, Sinclair J. Induction of endogenous human cytomegalovirus gene expression after differentiation of monocytes from healthy carriers. J Virol 1994; 1597-1604.

von Glahn WC, Pappenheimer AM. Intranuclear inclusions in visceral disease. Am J Pathol 1925;1:445.

Walmus BF, Yow MD, Lester JW, et al. Factors predictive of cytomegalovirus immune status in pregnant women. J Infect Dis 1988;157:172-177.

Waner JL, Weller TA, Kevy SV. Patterns of cytomegalovirus complement fixing antibody activity: a longitudinal study of blood donors. J Infect Dis 1973;127:538-543.

Weller TH, Hanshaw JB. Virologic and clinical observations on cytomegalic inclusion disease. N Engl J Med 1962;26:1233.

Weller TH, Hanshaw JB, Scott DE. Serologic differentiation of viruses responsible for cytomegalic inclusion disease. Virology 1960;12:130.

Weller TH, Macaulay JC, Craig JM, et al. Isolation of intranuclear inclusion agents from infants and illnesses resembling cytomegalic inclusion disease. Proc Soc Exp Biol Med 1957;94:4.

Whitley RJ, Brasfield D, Reynolds DW, et al. Protracted pneumonitis in young infants associated with perinatally acquired cytomegaloviral infection. J Pediatr 1976;89:16-22.

Wilfert CM, Huang ES, Stagno S. Restriction endonuclease analysis of cytomegalovirus deoxyribonucleic acid as an epidemiologic tool. Pediatr 1982;70:717-721.

Yeager AS. Transfusion-acquired cytomegalovirus infection in newborn infants. Am J Dis Child 1974;128:478-483.

Yeager AS, Grumet FC, Hafleigh EB, et al. Prevention of transfusion-acquired cytomegalovirus infections in newborn infants. J Pediatr 1981;98:281-287.

Yeager AS, Jacobs H, Clark J. Nursery-acquired cytomegalovirus infection in two premature infants. J Pediatr 1972;81:332-335.

Yow MD, Lakeman AD, Stagno S, et al. Use of restriction enzymes to investigate the source of a primary cytomegalovirus infection in a pediatric nurse. Pediatr 1982;70:713-716.

Yow MD, White N, Taber L, et al. Acquisition of cytomegalovirus infection from birth to 10 years: a longitudinal serologic study. J Pediatr 1987;110:37-42.

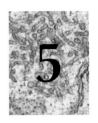

5   DIPHTHERIA

MELINDA WHARTON

Diphtheria is a preventable acute disease caused by *Corynebacterium diphtheriae.* The microorganism produces an exotoxin that is responsible for many of the severe manifestations of diphtheria. The disease is characterized clinically by a sore throat and a membrane that may cover the tonsils, pharynx, and larynx. Diphtheria is rare today in developed areas of the world and is seldom considered in differential diagnosis. Nevertheless, sporadic cases still occur, and epidemic diphtheria reemerged in the Soviet Union in the early 1990s. In addition, it is still prevalent in many developing countries, and importation of cases into the United States and other developed countries may occur.

HISTORY

The recognition of diphtheria as a disease probably dates back to the second century. It was in 1826, however, that Bretonneau named the illness *la diphthérite* and accurately described the clinical manifestations. He distinguished scarlet fever from diphtheria and identified membranous croup as a form of diphtheria.

The diphtheria bacillus was discovered by Klebs in 1883 and was isolated in pure culture by Löffler. It was called the Klebs-Löffler bacillus, and its etiologic relationship to the disease was demonstrated in 1884. In 1888 Roux and Yersin showed that the bacillus produced an exotoxin that was responsible for the various clinical manifestations of the disease such as myocarditis and neuritis. In 1890 von Behring showed that the toxin stimulated the production of antitoxin. Subsequently, in 1894 Roux and Martin used equine antitoxin for treatment of diphtheria in children at one hospital, with a reduction in mortality from 51% to 24%. In the same year, von Behring used toxin neutralized by antitoxin to induce immunity in animals and man. A large-scale immunization program to protect children was initiated by Park in 1922. Finally, in 1923

Ramon showed that formalin-treated toxin, currently known as *toxoid,* was superior to toxin-antitoxin as an immunizing agent. A century of progress culminated in 1923 in the development of a safe and effective vaccine capable of preventing the disease.

EPIDEMIOLOGY

Diphtheria is worldwide in distribution. The extensive use of diphtheria toxoid in industrialized countries in the 1940s and 1950s has led to a marked decrease in diphtheria incidence. Since 1980 no more than five cases of respiratory diphtheria have been reported each year in the United States (Fig. 5-1). Although some cases may be unrecognized, the low level of reported disease likely reflects the near absence of respiratory diphtheria in this country.

In developing countries with effective childhood immunization programs, diphtheria incidence has decreased dramatically, but the proportion of cases among older adolescents and adults has increased. Because immunity induced by diphtheria toxoid is not lifelong, additional doses of diphtheria toxoid are needed to extend protection into adolescence and adulthood. In some developing countries that have achieved high levels of vaccination among children, diphtheria epidemics have occurred among older children, adolescents, and adults, highlighting the importance of vaccination of these age groups (Galazka and Robertson, 1995).

In 1990 a diphtheria epidemic began in Russia that by 1994 had spread to all the New Independent States (NIS) of the former Soviet Union. From 1990 to 1995 approximately 125,000 cases and 4,000 deaths resulting from diphtheria were reported in the NIS. Lack of routine vaccination of adults and delayed vaccination of children may have led to increased susceptibility of the population; socioeconomic instability and population movement may have been contributing factors

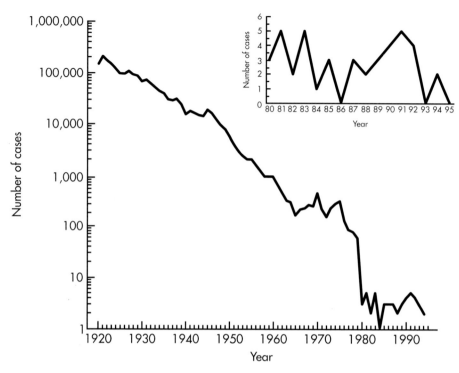

FIG. 5-1 Reported cases of diphtheria, United States, 1920-1995. Since 1980, only respiratory diphtheria has been reportable in the United States.

(Hardy et al., 1996). Adults who never received a full primary series of diphtheria toxoid in childhood were at increased risk of severe disease and death. Outbreak control strategies included achieving and maintaining high immunization coverage among children and administering a single dose of diphtheria toxoid to adults; additional doses were recommended for age cohorts that had not necessarily received a full primary series in childhood. With implementation of these strategies, reported cases of diphtheria are now decreasing.

Diphtheria is acquired by contact with an ill person with the disease or with an asymptomatic carrier of the organism. Persons with cutaneous diphtheria serve as a reservoir of *C. diphtheriae*. In tropical countries, cutaneous infection is common among children and results in naturally acquired immunity. Milk-borne epidemics have been reported. The organism can also be spread by fomites.

In temperate climates the highest seasonal incidence occurs during the autumn and winter months and epidemics of respiratory diphtheria occur in susceptible populations. Increased disease incidence among school-age children during the first few months of the school year has been reported

(Naiditch and Bower, 1954). In the prevaccine era, achieving high vaccination coverage among school-age children, combined with moderate coverage among preschool-age children, was associated with control of epidemics, suggesting that children of school age may play an important role in spread of diphtheria. In tropical climates, seasonality is less distinct, and cutaneous infections are more common.

ETIOLOGY

C. diphtheriae is the only major human pathogen of the corynebacterial group. These organisms are taxonomically related to the mycobacteria and *Nocardia* species.

Morphology

C. diphtheriae organisms are slender gram-positive rods that measure 2 to 4 μm by 0.5 to 1 μm. When grown on suboptimal media, the bacteria are pleomorphic. The cells vary in diameter, and the ends are broader than the center, producing a typical club-shaped appearance. A beaded or bandlike appearance is produced by the metachromatic granules, which are accumulations of polymerized polyphosphates. As a result of cell division the bacteria appear in palisades or as individual cells at sharp angles to each other.

Cultural Characteristics

C. diphtheriae is an aerobe requiring complex media for isolation and characterization. Tellurite-containing medium (e.g., cystine-tellurite or modified Tinsdale medium) selectively inhibits a number of potentially contaminating organisms and allows three colony types of *C. diphtheriae*—gravis, mitis, and intermedius—to be distinguished. No constant relationship exists between colonial type and disease severity.

Other Corynebacterial Species Associated with Respiratory Disease

Pseudomembranous pharyngitis clinically indistinguishable from respiratory diphtheria has been reported in association with infection with both *Corynebacterium pseudodiphtheriticum* and *Corynebacterium ulcerans*. Although an uncommon cause of human infection, strains of *C. ulcerans* have been demonstrated to produce diphtheria toxin. Susceptible patients with disease associated with toxigenic *C. ulcerans* can develop severe disease.

PATHOGENESIS AND PATHOLOGY

Diphtheria toxin is responsible for many of the serious clinical manifestations of the disease. It is extremely unstable and is easily destroyed by heat (75° C for 10 minutes), light, and aging. Toxin is produced by strains of *C. diphtheriae* that are lysogenic for a bacteriophage carrying the *tox* gene (Freeman and Morse, 1953). Thus a person may harbor *C. diphtheriae,* and the organism may acquire beta corynebacteriophage, converting the bacterium to a toxin producer. Toxin production does not require lytic growth of the phage. The tox gene is thought to confer an advantage in survival both to the phage and to *C. diphtheriae* in the human host. In vitro, diphtheria toxin is maximally produced when there is a limited amount of iron present. When adequate iron is present, a repressor-iron complex binds to the phage tox gene and prevents toxin formation. When the iron concentration is lowered, dissociation of the repressor complex from the tox gene occurs, and toxin is produced.

The toxin is synthesized on membrane-bound polysomes and is released extracellularly as a single inactive precursor polypeptide chain. Cleavage exposes the active enzymatic site of toxin, and the biologically active toxin consists of two functionally distinct polypeptides, A and B, linked by a disulfide bond. Fragment A is extremely stable, enzymatically active, and responsible for the toxic effects, which are due to inhibition of cellular protein synthesis. Fragment A inactivates elongation factor 2, which is a protein common to all eukaryotic cells. This protein is essential for translocation of peptidyl transfer RNA on ribosomes. Fragment B is unstable, is not enzymatically active, and is required for attachment of the activated toxin molecule to receptors of sensitive host cells. All human cells have receptor sites for fragment B, and the binding is rapid and irreversible. The attachment of B is necessary for penetration of fragment A into the cell. Both A and B are necessary for cytotoxicity.

Following attachment of the diphtheria organism to the nasopharyngeal mucosa of a susceptible person, the toxin is elaborated and absorbed locally. The toxic effect on the cells causes tissue necrosis, which provides the environment for growth of the organism and production of more toxin. In addition to the necrosis, an inflammatory and exudative reaction is induced by the toxin. The necrotic epithelial cells, leukocytes, red blood cells, fibrinous material, diphtheria bacilli, and other bacterial inhabitants of the nasopharynx combine to form the typical membrane. The superficial epithelial cells of the mucosa form an integral part of this membrane and cause it to adhere; attempts to separate it are followed by bleeding and the formation of a new membrane, which sloughs off during the recovery period.

The toxin produced at the site of the membrane is distributed through the bloodstream to tissues all over the body. The size of the membrane usually reflects the amount of toxin produced. The toxin reaches the circulation more readily from the pharynx and tonsils than from the larynx and trachea. Consequently, laryngotracheal diphtheria produces less toxemia than pharyngotonsillar involvement, but the obstruction of the airway by the laryngotracheal membrane may be life threatening.

Differential effects on various tissues are not well understood. The most striking clinical manifestations are seen in the heart and the nervous system, but other organs may also be affected. Pathologic changes associated with diphtheria myocarditis include hyaline degeneration and necrosis, associated with inflammation in the interstitial spaces. The maximal pathologic effects of fatty degeneration and fibrosis occur after the first week of illness, consistent with the observation that myocarditis usually develops 10 to 14 days after onset of illness.

In the nervous system, segmental demyelination of nerve fibers within the sensory ganglia is found, along with demyelination of adjacent parts of peripheral nerves and anterior and posterior roots. Degeneration is limited to short segments of the myelin sheath (Fisher and Adams, 1956). Macrophages ingest myelin; otherwise, there is little inflammation. It has been suggested that Schwann's cells are sensitive to toxin, with resulting inhibition of synthesis of myelin basic protein, leading to development of segmental lesions. When myelinization is resumed, recovery occurs.

Although diphtheria toxin is the most important virulence factor of *C. diphtheriae,* colonization of mucous membranes can be accomplished by both toxigenic and nontoxigenic strains. The well-documented occurrence of pseudomembranous pharyngitis in persons infected with nontoxigenic strains suggests that there are important virulence factors other than diphtheria toxin. The organisms have a toxic glycolipid and a cord factor, which is considered necessary for virulence; in addition, other virulence factors may exist.

CLINICAL MANIFESTATIONS

Diphtheria usually develops after a short incubation period of 2 to 4 days, with a range of 1 to 5 days. For clinical purposes the disease may be classified by the anatomic location of infection. More than one anatomic site may be involved at the same time.

Nasal Diphtheria

The onset of nasal diphtheria is indistinguishable from that of the common cold. It is characterized by a nasal discharge and a lack of constitutional symptoms. Fever, if present, is usually low grade. The nasal discharge, which at first is serous, subsequently becomes serosanguineous. In some cases there may be frank epistaxis. The discharge, which may be unilateral or bilateral, becomes mucopurulent, and the anterior nares and upper lip usually have an impetiginous appearance. The discharge may obscure the presence of a white membrane on the nasal septum. The poor absorption of toxin from this site accounts for the mildness of the disease and the paucity of constitutional symptoms. In the untreated patient the nasal discharge may persist for many days or weeks. This rich source of diphtheria bacilli becomes a menace to all susceptible contacts.

Tonsillar and Pharyngeal Diphtheria

Tonsillar diphtheria usually begins insidiously with malaise, anorexia, sore throat, and low-grade fever. Within 24 hours a patch of exudate or membrane appears in the faucial area. In vaccinated persons the membrane may be limited, resembling tonsillitis, but in susceptible persons it may spread rapidly and within 12 to 24 hours involve the anterior and posterior faucial pillars, the soft palate, and the uvula. It is smooth, adherent, and white or gray (Color Plate 1); in the presence of bleeding it may be black. Forcible attempts to remove it are followed by bleeding. Pharyngotonsillar involvement is characterized by a variable amount of cervical adenitis, and in severe cases the marked swelling produces a "bull-neck" appearance.

The course of the illness is variable, but disease is usually mild in previously vaccinated persons. The temperature remains either normal or slightly elevated, but the pulse is disproportionately rapid. In mild cases the membrane sloughs off between the seventh and tenth day and the patient has an uneventful recovery. In moderately severe cases, convalescence is slow, with the course frequently complicated by myocarditis and neuritis. Severe cases are characterized by increasing toxemia manifested by severe prostration, striking pallor, rapid thready pulse, stupor, coma, and death within 6 to 10 days.

Laryngeal Diphtheria

Laryngeal diphtheria most often develops as an extension of pharyngeal involvement. Occasionally, however, it may be the only manifestation of the disease. The illness is ushered in by fever, hoarseness, and cough, which develops a barking quality. Increasing obstruction of the airway by the membrane is manifested by inspiratory stridor followed by suprasternal, supraclavicular, and subcostal retractions. The membrane may extend downward to involve the entire tracheobronchial tree.

The clinical picture of laryngeal diphtheria is dominated by the consequences of the mechanical obstruction to the air passages caused by the membrane, congestion, and edema. In mild cases or in those modified by antitoxin therapy the airway remains patent and the membrane is coughed up between the sixth and tenth day. A sudden acute and fatal obstruction may occur in a mild case in which a partially detached piece of membrane blocks the airway. In very severe cases there is increasing obstruction followed by progressive hypoxia, which is manifested by restlessness, cyanosis, severe prostration, coma, and death.

Signs of toxemia are minimal in primary laryngeal involvement because toxin is poorly absorbed from the mucous membrane of the larynx. In most instances, however, the laryngeal involvement is associated with tonsillar and pharyngeal diphtheria. Consequently, the clinical manifestations are those of both obstruction and severe toxemia.

Cutaneous Diphtheria

Cutaneous diphtheria classically has been described as a deep, rounded, "punched out" ulcer with sharply demarcated edges and a membranous base; the ulcer does not extend into the subcutaneous tissue. However, other clinical presentations occur; because *C. diphtheriae* can colonize preexisting skin lesions (wounds, dermatitis, and insect bites, for example), the clinical presentation may be highly variable (Höfler, 1991). Cutaneous diphtheria may be important epidemiologically; chronic skin infection may serve as a reservoir of the organism. Because toxin is absorbed slowly from cutaneous sites, complications are relatively uncommon following cutaneous infection.

Unusual Types of Diphtheria

Diphtheritic infections occasionally develop in sites other than the respiratory tract or the skin. Conjunctival, aural, and vulvovaginal infections may occur. The conjunctival lesion primarily involves the palpebral surface, which is reddened, edematous, and membranous. Involvement of the external auditory canal is usually manifest by a persistent purulent discharge. Vulvovaginal lesions are usually ulcerative and confluent.

DIAGNOSIS

An early diagnosis of diphtheria is essential because delay of administration of antitoxin may impose a serious and preventable risk to the patient. Accurate bacteriologic confirmation by means of culture requires special media, a proficient laboratory, and a minimum of 15 to 20 hours; smears are not reliable. Consequently, the initial diagnosis, as a basis for therapy, must be made on clinical grounds alone.

The diagnosis of diphtheria is confirmed by the demonstration of diphtheria bacilli cultured from material obtained from the site of infection. Care should be exercised in obtaining the culture. The swab should be rubbed firmly over the lesion or, if possible, should be inserted beneath the membrane; if it can be obtained, a fragment of the membrane should be submitted for culture. Swabs should also be taken from the nasopharynx and from any wounds or other skin lesions in patients with suspected diphtheria. Lesions should be cleaned with sterile normal saline, crusted material removed, and the swab applied firmly to the base of the lesion. The physician must notify the laboratory that diphtheria is suspected to have correct media used. If swabs must be shipped to a reference laboratory, silica gel transport medium should be used. A Löffler's slant, a blood agar plate, and a tellurite plate should be streaked with the swab. The slant and plates should be placed in the incubator without delay. After incubation, the organisms on the plates should be identified by an experienced laboratorian.

Diphtheria bacilli that are isolated on culture should be classified by biotype (mitis, gravis, or intermedius) and tested for toxigenicity. Although the original assays for toxigenicity were performed in vivo, the method now most commonly used for determining toxigenicity is the Elek immunoprecipitation test. Because diphtheria has become a rare diagnosis in most developed countries, many laboratories are not proficient in performing the test, and specimens will need to be forwarded to a reference laboratory for toxigenicity testing. A polymerase chain reaction (PCR) assay detecting the A and B subunit and the tox regulatory gene, which correlates well with the Elek test, has also been developed. PCR may be performed directly on clinical specimens, allowing rapid confirmation of the presence of toxigenic *Corynebacterium*.

DIFFERENTIAL DIAGNOSIS

The differential diagnosis of diphtheria varies with the particular anatomic site of involvement. The presentation of nasal diphtheria may be clinically indistinguishable from that of a foreign body in the nose. Tonsillar and pharyngeal diphtheria may resemble streptococcal infection; coinfection with both toxigenic *C. diphtheriae* and group A streptococcus is well documented. Other diagnoses that may be considered in patients with diphtheria of these sites are infectious mononucleosis, nonbacterial membranous tonsillitis, primary herpetic tonsillitis, and thrush. Laryngeal diphtheria may present with signs and symptoms resembling laryngotracheitis or epiglottitis.

COMPLICATIONS

The most common and most serious complications are those caused by the effect of the toxin on the heart and central nervous system.

Myocarditis

Myocarditis occurs frequently as a complication of severe diphtheria, but it may also follow milder forms of the disease. The more extensive the local lesion is and the more delayed the institution of antitoxin therapy is, the more frequently myocarditis occurs. In most instances the cardiac manifestations appear during the second week of the disease. Occasionally, myocarditis may be noted as early as the first week and as late as the sixth week of the disease. Abnormal electrocardiographic findings include flattening and inversion of T waves; elevation of the ST segment; and conduction abnormalities, including complete heart block. The myocarditis may be followed by cardiac failure.

Neuritis

Neuritis also is generally a complication of severe diphtheria. The manifestations of neuritis appear after a variable latent period, are predominantly bilateral, and usually resolve completely. Neuropathy affecting cranial nerves typically occurs early in the course of illness, during the first 4 weeks after the onset of disease; peripheral neuropathy occurs later, 5 to 8 weeks after onset of disease. Cranial nerve involvement rarely if ever occurs as a complication of cutaneous diphtheria without respiratory involvement. Paralysis of the limbs has been reported following cutaneous infection, and the latent period may be quite prolonged.

Paralysis of Soft Palate. Soft-palate paralysis is the most common manifestation of diphtheritic neuritis. It may occur as early as the first week after onset of illness. It is characterized by a nasal quality to the voice and nasal regurgitation. The paralysis usually subsides completely within 1 to 2 weeks.

Ocular Palsy. This palsy usually occurs between the third and fifth week and is characterized by paralysis of the muscles of accommodation, causing blurring of vision. Less commonly there may be involvement of the extraocular muscles, causing strabismus. Involvement of the lateral rectus muscle, causing an internal squint, may also occur.

Paralysis of Diaphragm. Paralysis of the diaphragm may occur between the fifth and seventh week as a result of neuritis of the phrenic nerve.

Death occurs if mechanical respiratory support is not provided.

Paralysis of Limbs. Limb paralysis may occur between the fifth and tenth week. Both sensory and motor nerves are involved. Paresthesias are followed by weakness of the extremities and loss of deep tendon reflexes. Nerve conduction studies show slowing of conduction; prolongation of distal motor latency; and, in severe cases, conduction block. The absence of deep tendon reflexes, bilateral symmetric involvement, and the presence of an elevated level of spinal fluid protein make this complication clinically indistinguishable from the Guillain-Barré syndrome.

Other Complications

In severe diphtheria, thrombocytopenia and coagulation abnormalities are not uncommon. The peripheral blood smear may show evidence of microangiopathic hemolytic anemia, and frank disseminated intravascular coagulation may occur. These abnormalities are thought to be a result of the effects of diphtheria toxin on the vascular endothelium. Likewise, proteinuria is commonly found in severe disease, and renal failure may occur.

PROGNOSIS

Before the turn of the century the mortality rate of diphtheria was 30% to 50%. The advent of diphtheria antitoxin in 1894 and the beginning of large-scale active immunization programs in 1922 led to a dramatic reduction in the mortality rate to approximately 10%. In spite of subsequent improvements in the care of critically ill patients, case-fatality ratios of 5% to 10% have been reported in most series. Extensive disease and delays in seeking medical care, diagnosis, and receipt of diphtheria antitoxin are risk factors for death resulting from diphtheria. Mortality rates are consistently lower for cases receiving antitoxin within the first 2 days of illness. The susceptibility of the patient is also critical; illness is usually mild in vacinated persons.

The prognosis in the individual case of diphtheria must be guarded. Sudden death may be caused by a variety of unpredictable events, including the sudden complete obstruction of the airway by a detached piece of membrane, the development of myocarditis and heart failure, or the late occurrence of respiratory paralysis caused by phrenic nerve involvement. Patients who survive myocarditis or neuritis generally recover completely. Occasionally, however, diphtheritic myocarditis may be followed by permanent damage to the heart.

IMMUNITY

Antibody to diphtheria toxin (antitoxin) confers protection from severe clinical manifestations of diphtheria. Antitoxin levels of 0.01 to 0.09 IU (international unit)/ml are thought to confer some protection, and, with levels of ≥0.1 IU/ml, protection is considered reliable. However, persons with "protective" levels of antitoxin have developed diphtheria (Ipsen, 1946). Antibodies to other components of *C. diphtheriae* may also play a role in immunity.

Antitoxin levels are most commonly measured by in vitro neutralization in tissue culture. Both enzyme-linked immunosorbent assays (ELISA) and passive hemagglutination have been used, but both are unreliable at low concentrations of antitoxin (<0.1 IU/ml). The poor correlation between results of ELISA and in vitro neutralization at low antitoxin concentrations is thought to be caused by the binding of nonneutralizing antibodies.

Passive Immunity

Passive immunity may be acquired either by transplacental transfer of antibody from an immune mother or by parenteral inoculation with diphtheria antitoxin. Congenitally acquired passive immunity persists for approximately 6 months. Protection after injection of diphtheria antitoxin disappears after 2 to 3 weeks.

Active Immunity

Active immunity may be induced either by previous infection with *C. diphtheriae* or, more commonly today, by vaccination with diphtheria toxoid. The toxin is more toxic than immunogenic; thus reliable immunity is produced only by vaccination. Persons with diphtheria should therefore be immunized. Recurrent attacks of the disease frequently occurred in the prevaccine era, but by late adolescence most of those persons were immune.

Immunization with diphtheria toxoid can be relied on to prevent serious or fatal disease. The widespread and routine immunization of infants and children has had a profound effect on the immune status of the population at large. Fully immunized individuals have antibody to toxin but do not have antibody to the organism and may become nasopharyngeal carriers or, uncommonly, may develop mild disease.

TREATMENT
Antitoxin Therapy

Diphtheria antitoxin must be given promptly and in adequate dosage (Table 5-1). Any delay increases the possibility that myocarditis, neuritis, or death may occur. During an infection, diphtheria toxin may be present in three forms: (1) circulating or unbound; (2) bound to the cells; or (3) internalized in cytoplasm. Antitoxin will neutralize circulating toxin and may affect bound toxin but will not affect internalized toxin. Because bacteriologic confirmation of the diagnosis cannot be obtained immediately, the decision to administer diphtheria antitoxin must be made on clinical and epidemiologic grounds.

Currently available diphtheria antitoxin is of equine origin, and, like any heterologous serum, its administration may be followed by an immediate reaction, such as acute anaphylactic shock, or a delayed type of reaction, such as serum sickness. Any history regarding previous horse serum injections or possible allergy should be obtained before administering the product, and the patient must be tested for hypersensitivity by skin or eye tests. When testing for hypersensitivity or administering diphtheria antitoxin, health-care workers should always have a syringe loaded with a 1:1,000 solution of epinephrine ready and available for emergency use.

Skin Test. An injection of 0.1 ml of a 1:100 dilution of diphtheria antitoxin in physiologic saline solution is given intracutaneously. The test is read in 20 minutes and is positive if a wheal 1 cm or more in diameter is present. In persons with a history of allergy to equine serum the dose should be reduced to 0.05 ml of a 1:1,000 dilution intracutaneously. The use of undiluted antitoxin will invariably cause a false-positive reaction; dilution is

Table 5-1 Dosage of antitoxin recommended for treatment of diphtheria

Type of diphtheria	Dosage (units)
Anterior nasal	10,000-20,000
Tonsillar	15,000-25,000
Pharyngeal ≤48 hours duration	20,000-40,000
Laryngeal ≤48 hours duration	20,000-40,000
Nasopharyngeal	40,000-60,000
Extensive disease of ≥3 days duration or any patient with brawny swelling of the neck	80,000-120,000

Table 5-2   Desensitization to serum: intradermal, subcutaneous, and intramuscular routes

Dose number*	Route of administration	Dilution of serum in normal saline	Amount of injection (ml)
1	Intradermal	1:1,000	0.1
2	Intradermal	1:1,000	0.3
3	Subcutaneous	1:1,000	0.6
4	Subcutaneous	1:100	0.1
5	Subcutaneous	1:100	0.3
6	Subcutaneous	1:100	0.6
7	Subcutaneous	1:10	0.1
8	Subcutaneous	1:10	0.3
9	Subcutaneous	1:10	0.6
10	Subcutaneous	Undiluted	0.1
11	Subcutaneous	Undiluted	0.3
12	Intramuscular	Undiluted	0.6
13	Intramuscular	Undiluted	1.0

From the 1997 Red Book: Report of the Committee on Infectious Diseases, ed 24, American Academy of Pediatrics, Elk Grove Village, IL.
*Administer at 15-minute intervals.

therefore mandatory. A negative skin test does not preclude the occurrence of serum reactions.

Conjunctival Test. One drop of a 1:10 dilution of the serum in physiologic saline solution is instilled inside the lower lid of one eye; 1 drop of physiologic saline solution is used as a control for the other eye. The test is read in 20 minutes and is positive if conjunctivitis and lacrimation are present. If a positive reaction occurs, the eye should be treated with 1 drop of a 1:100 solution of epinephrine.

If the history and sensitivity tests are negative, the total recommended dose of antitoxin should be given without delay. The precise dose and route of administration of antitoxin is determined by the location and extent of the membrane, the degree of toxemia, and the duration of the illness. Dosage does not vary by the patient's age and weight. The dosages shown in Table 5-1 are recommended for the various types of diphtheria.

To neutralize toxin as rapidly as possible, the preferred route of administration is intravenous; antitoxin may also be administered by intramuscular injection, but peak antitoxin levels may not be reached for several days. If intravenous therapy is indicated, antitoxin should be diluted in 500 ml of saline and administered by intravenous drip. The rate should be very slow over the first half hour to allow for desensitization; the entire dose should be administered within 90 minutes. The patient must be carefully monitored, and the infusion must be stopped if signs of shock appear. The addition of

0.1 to 0.3 ml of 1:1,000 dilution of epinephrine to the solution is a useful precaution. If administered by intramuscular injection, antitoxin is injected undiluted into the buttocks.

If a patient is sensitive to horse serum, the indications for the diphtheria antitoxin should be reevaluated because of this potential risk. If the antitoxin is administered, it can be given as described in Tables 5-2 and 5-3. Signs of acute anaphylaxis call for the immediate intravenous injection of 0.2 to 0.5 ml of 1:1,000 epinephrine solution.

In the United States, diphtheria antitoxin is no longer commercially available, but it is available from the Centers for Disease Control and Prevention as an investigational agent. Physicians caring for patients with suspected diphtheria should contact their state health department for assistance in obtaining diphtheria antitoxin.

Antibacterial Therapy

Penicillin and erythromycin are effective against most strains of diphtheria bacilli. Penicillin is the preferred drug and may be given as aqueous procaine penicillin G (25,000 to 50,000 units per kilogram of body weight per day for children, with a maximum dosage of 1.2 million units per day, in 2 divided doses). Patients who are sensitive to penicillin should be given parenteral erythromycin in a daily dosage of 40 to 50 mg per kilogram, with a maximum dosage of 2 g per day. When the patient can swallow comfortably, oral erythromycin in 4 divided doses or oral penicillin V (125 to 250 mg 4 times daily) may be substituted for a recommended

Table 5-3 Desensitization to serum: intravenous route

Dose number*	Dilution of serum in normal saline	Amount of injection (ml)
1	1:1,000	0.1
2	1:1,000	0.3
3	1:1,000	0.6
4	1:100	0.1
5	1:100	0.3
6	1:100	0.6
7	1:10	0.1
8	1:10	0.3
9	1:10	0.6
10	Undiluted	0.1
11	Undiluted	0.3
12	Undiluted	0.6
13	Undiluted	1.0

From the 1997 Red Book: Report of the Committee on Infectious Diseases, ed 24, American Academy of Pediatrics, Elk Grove Village, IL.
*Administer at 15-minute intervals.

total treatment period of 14 days. Antimicrobial therapy is not a substitute for antitoxin treatment.

Eradication of the organism should be documented by culture. Persons who continue to harbor the organism after treatment with either penicillin or erythromycin should receive an additional 10-day course of erythromycin, and follow-up cultures should be obtained.

Supportive Treatment

Bed rest is more important in the management of diphtheria than in most other infectious diseases. It should be enforced for at least 12 days because of the possibility of complicating myocarditis. The patient's activity subsequently is guided by the results of the daily physical examinations, the serial electrocardiograms, and the presence or absence of complications. In addition to requiring antitoxin, penicillin, and other supportive measures, patients with laryngeal diphtheria may require treatment for the relief of airway obstruction. Intubation and/or tracheostomy may be necessary. Steroid therapy did not prevent myocarditis or neuritis in one controlled trial (Thisyakorn et al., 1984).

Treatment of Complications

Myocarditis and neuritis are the most important complications requiring therapy. In general the management of diphtheritic myocarditis and its sequelae is the same as that used for any other type of acute myocardial damage. Bed rest and inactivity

may be beneficial. Sudden death caused by myocardial failure may be precipitated by excessive activity. The administration of digitalis is controversial; however, it should not be withheld if there is evidence of cardiac decompensation. Conduction abnormalities may require use of a temporary pacemaker.

Palatal and pharyngeal paralysis may be complicated by aspiration because of the tendency for regurgitation and difficulty in swallowing. Under these circumstances, gastric or duodenal intubation is indicated. Mechanical ventilation may be required in patients with paralysis of the diaphragm resulting from phrenic nerve involvement.

Treatment of Diphtheria Carriers

A carrier is an individual who has no symptoms and harbors virulent diphtheria bacilli in the nasopharynx. The eradication of these microorganisms may be extremely difficult. A single dose of intramuscular benzathine penicillin G (600,000 units for children <6 years of age and 1.2 million units for those ≥6 years of age) or a 7- to 10-day course of oral erythromycin (40 mg/kg/day for children, 1 g/day for adults) is recommended. Although there is some evidence that erythromycin may be more effective in eradicating the carrier state, intramuscular penicillin is preferred if compliance is in doubt. Because neither regimen is 100% effective and bacteriologic relapse may occur, specimens should be obtained for repeated culture a minimum of 14 days after completion of therapy. Persons who continue to harbor the organism after treatment with either penicillin or erythromycin should receive an additional 10-day course of oral erythromycin, and follow-up cultures should be obtained (Farizo et al., 1993). Occasionally an undetected foreign body in the nose may be responsible for persistence of a carrier state.

ISOLATION AND QUARANTINE

The patient is infective until diphtheria bacilli can be no longer cultured from the site of the infection. Isolation should be maintained until elimination of the organism is demonstrated by negative cultures of two samples obtained at least 24 hours after completion of antimicrobial therapy.

Care of Exposed Persons

Close contacts of the patient should be identified, evaluated, and maintained under surveillance for 7 days. Close contacts include household members and other persons with a history of direct contact with a case (e.g., caretakers, relatives, or friends who regularly visit the home), as well as medical staff exposed to oral or respiratory secretions of the case. Both nasal and pharyngeal swabs should be obtained for culture from close contacts, regardless of vaccination status. As soon as specimens are obtained, antimicrobial prophylaxis is recommended, using either a single dose of intramuscular penicillin (600,000 units for children <6 years of age and 1.2 million units for those ≥6 years of age) or a 7- to 10-day course of oral erythromycin (40 mg/kg/day for children, 1 g/day for adults). If compliance is in question, intramuscular penicillin is preferred.

The diphtheria vaccination status of contacts should be reviewed, and persons who have not been vaccinated should receive an immediate dose of diphtheria toxoid and complete the series in accordance with the recommended schedule for vaccination. In addition, contacts who have not received a booster dose within the last 5 years should receive a booster. If the contact has received diphtheria toxoid within 5 years, no additional vaccine is needed (Farizo et al., 1993).

Notification of Public Health Authorities

If the diagnosis of diphtheria is suspected, local or state public health authorities should be notified immediately. Measures to prevent additional cases should be undertaken promptly. In the United States, diphtheria antitoxin is available through state health departments. Notification is mandatory in all states and in most countries.

PREVENTIVE MEASURES

The dramatic decline in the incidence of diphtheria since 1922 can be attributed for the most part to mass immunization programs and routine immunization of infants and children. Diphtheria toxoid is prepared by formaldehyde treatment of diphtheria toxin. The limit of flocculation (Lf) content of each toxoid (quantity of toxoid as assessed by flocculation) varies between products. The concentration of diphtheria toxoid used in preparations intended for adult use is reduced because adverse reactions to diphtheria toxoid are directly related to the quantity of antigen and to the age or previous vaccination history of the recipient, and because a smaller dosage of diphtheria toxoid produces an adequate immune response in adults. Diphtheria toxoid is administered in combination with pertussis vaccine (either whole cell or acellular) and

tetanus toxoids, DTP or DTaP, or with tetanus toxoid, DT or Td. Pediatric formulations of diphtheria toxoid (DTP, DTaP, and DT) are for use among infants and children <7 years of age. Each 0.5 ml dose is formulated to contain 6.7 to 25 Lf units of diphtheria toxoid. Adult formulation diphtheria and tetanus toxoids (Td) is for use among persons ≥7 years of age; each 0.5-ml dose is formulated to contain ≤2 Lf units of diphtheria toxoid. The vaccine is administered by intramuscular injection. In infants the anterolateral aspect of the thigh provides the largest muscle mass and is the recommended site for intramuscular injection. In toddlers and older children the deltoid may be used if the muscle mass is adequate.

In the United States the routine diphtheria, tetanus, and pertussis vaccination schedule for children <7 years of age comprises 5 doses of vaccine containing diphtheria, tetanus, and pertussis antigens. Three doses should be administered during the first year of life, generally at 2, 4, and 6 months of age. The fourth dose is recommended for children 15 to 18 months old to maintain adequate immunity during the preschool years. The fourth dose should be administered at least six months after the third. The fifth dose is recommended for children 4 to 6 years of age to confer continued protection against disease during the early elementary school years. A fifth dose is not necessary if the fourth dose in the series is administered on or after the fourth birthday.

For children <7 years of age in whom pertussis vaccine is contraindicated, DT should be used instead of DTP or DTaP. To ensure that there is no interference with the response to DT antigens from maternal antibodies, previously unvaccinated children who receive their first DT dose when <1 year of age should receive a total of 4 doses of DT as the primary series, the first 3 doses at 4- to 8-week intervals, and the fourth dose 6 to 12 months later. If additional doses of pertussis vaccine (DTP or DTaP) become contraindicated after the series is begun in the first year of life, DT should be substituted for each of the remaining scheduled DTP or DTaP doses. If a child develops acute anaphylaxis following a dose of DTP or DTaP, further doses of the vaccine or any of its components should be deferred. Because of the importance of tetanus vaccination, referral to an allergist for evaluation and possible desensitization should be strongly considered.

Unvaccinated children 1 to 6 years of age for whom pertussis vaccine is contraindicated should receive 2 doses of DT 4 to 8 weeks apart, followed by a third dose 6 to 12 months later to complete the primary series. Children who have already received 1 or 2 doses of DT or DTP after their first birthday and for whom further pertussis vaccine is contraindicated should receive a total of 3 doses of DT (if <7 years of age) or Td (≥7 years of age), with the third dose administered 6 to 12 months after the second dose. Children who complete a primary series of DT before their fourth birthday should receive a fifth dose of DT before entering kindergarten or elementary school. This dose is not necessary if the fourth dose was given after the fourth birthday.

Diphtheria infection may not confer immunity; therefore vaccination should be initiated at the time of recovery from the illness, and arrangements should be made to ensure that all doses of a primary series are administered on schedule.

Because immunity induced by both diphtheria and tetanus toxoids wanes with time, booster vaccination with Td is recommended at 10-year intervals throughout life, following administration of a primary series. Administering the first Td booster vaccination at an adolescent immunization visit at 11 to 12 years of age is now recommended to increase compliance and thereby reduce the susceptibility of adolescents to tetanus and diphtheria.

BIBLIOGRAPHY

Belsey MA. Skin infections and the epidemiology of diphtheria: acquisition and persistence of *C. diphtheriae* infections. Am J Epidemiol 1975;102:179-184.

Centers for Disease Control and Prevention. Immunization of adolescents: recommendations of the Advisory Committee on Immunization Practices, the American Academy of Pediatrics, the American Academy of Family Physicians, and the American Medical Association. MMWR 1996;45(No. RR-13):1-16.

Centers for Disease Control and Prevention. Pertussis vaccination: use of acellular pertussis vaccines among infants and young children. Recommendations of the Advisory Committee on Immunization Practices (ACIP). MMWR 1997; 46(No. RR-7):1-25.

Clarridge JE, Spiegel CA. *Corynebacterium* and miscellaneous irregular gram-positive rods, *Erysipelothrix,* and *Gardnerella.* In Murray PR, Baron EJ, Pfaller MA, et al. (eds). Manual of Clinical Microbiology, ed 6, Washington, D.C.: American Society for Microbiology, 1995.

Collier RJ. Diphtheria toxin: mode of action and structure. Bacteriol Rev 1975;39:54-85.

Committee on Infectious Diseases. 1994 Red Book: Report of the Committee on Infectious Diseases. Elk Grove Village, Ill.: American Academy of Pediatrics, 1994.

Dobie RA, Tobey DN. Clinical features of diphtheria in the respiratory tract. JAMA 1979;242:2197-2201.

Dolman CE. Landmarks and pioneers in the control of diphtheria. Can J Public Health 1973;64:317-336.

Efstratiou A, Maple PAC. Manual for the Laboratory Diagnosis of Diphtheria. WHO Regional Office for Europe, 1994.

English PC. Diphtheria and theories of infectious diseases: centennial appreciation of the critical role of diphtheria in the history of medicine. Pediatrics 1985;76:1-9.

Farizo KM, Strebel PM, Chen RT, et al. Fatal respiratory disease due to *Corynebacterium diphtheriae:* case report and review of guidelines for management, investigation, and control. Clin Infect Dis 1993;16:59-68.

Fisher CM, Adams RD. Diphtheritic polyneuritis: a pathological study. J Neuropathol Exp Neurol 1956;15:243-268.

Freeman VJ, Morse U. Further observations on the change of virulence of bacteriophage-infected avirulent strains of *Corynebacterium diphtheriae.* J Bacteriol 1953;63: 407-414.

Galazka AM, Robertson SE. Diphtheria: changing patterns in the developing world and the industrialized world. European J Epidemiol 1995;11:107-117.

Godfrey ES. Study in the epidemiology of diphtheria in relation to the active immunization of certain age groups. Am J Public Health 1932;22:237-256.

Hardy IRB, Dittman S, Sutter RW. Current situation and control strategies for resurgence of diphtheria in newly independent states of the former Soviet Union. Lancet 1996;347:1739-1744.

Höfler W. Cutaneous diphtheria. Int J Dermatol 1991;30:845-847.

Ipsen J. Circulating antitoxin at the onset of diphtheria in 425 patients. J Immunol 1946;54:325-347.

Liebow AA, MacLean PD, Bumstead JH, Welt LG. Tropical ulcers and cutaneous diphtheria. Arch Intern Med 1946;78:255-295.

Mikhailovich VM, Melnikov VG, Mazurova IK, et al. Application of PCR for detection of toxigenic *Corynebacterium diphtheriae* strains isolated during the Russian diphtheria epidemic, 1990 through 1994. J Clin Microbiol 1995;33:3061-3063.

Morgan BC. Cardiac complications of diphtheria. Pediatrics 1963;32:549-557.

Naiditch MJ, Bower AG. Diphtheria: a study of 1,433 cases observed during a ten-year period at the Los Angeles County Hospital. Am J Med 1954;17:229-245.

Neubauer C. Clinical signs of diphtheria in inoculated children. Lancet 1943;2:192-194.

Solders G, Nennesmo I, Persson A. Diphtheritic neuropathy, an analysis based on muscle and nerve biopsy and repeated neurophysiological and autonomic function tests. J Neurol Neurosurg Psych 1989;52:876-880.

Tao X, Schiering N, Zeng H, et al. Iron, DtxR, and the regulation of diphtheria toxin expression. Mol Microbiol 1994; 14:191-197.

Thisyakorn U, Wongvanich J, Kampeng V. Failure of corticosteroid therapy to prevent diphtheritic myocarditis or neuritis. Pediatr Infect Dis 1984;3:126.

Wesley AG, Pather M, Chrystal V. The hemorrhagic diathesis in diphtheria with special reference to disseminated intravascular coagulation. Ann Trop Paediatr 1981;1:51-56.

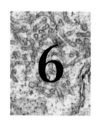

6 ENDOCARDITIS

LISA SAIMAN

The diagnosis and management of endocarditis in children present considerable challenges. Classically, endocarditis had been divided into two distinct categories: (1) subacute, chronic infection of valves damaged by rheumatic fever; and (2) acute, fulminant infection of normal hearts. However, numerous changes in medical and surgical practices during the past 25 years have led to new risk factors and more subtle presentations for endocarditis in children. These risk groups include children with increasingly complex cyanotic heart disease, often with shunts and prosthetic valves; premature infants and older critically ill children in intensive care units, often with central venous catheters and thus at risk for nosocomial endocarditis with less common pathogens; and adolescents who use intravenous drugs or have mitral valve prolapse (Table 6-1). In addition, although certain clinical presentations are caused by predictable pathogens, the widespread problem of antibiotic resistance has had a substantial impact on the management of endocarditis.

RISK FACTORS
Rheumatic Carditis

The relationship between rheumatic carditis and endocarditis has been understood for decades (Feinstein, 1964a). Carditis develops in approximately one third of patients with rheumatic fever and, although the majority of persons recovers uneventfully, some patients experience recurrent episodes of rheumatic fever and progressive cardiac damage (Feinstein, 1964b). Approximately 5% of patients with rheumatic carditis develop endocarditis (Griffiths and Gersony, 1990). Series describing cases of pediatric endocarditis from 1940 to the 1960s implicated rheumatic carditis as the underlying lesion in up to one third of children (Blumenthal, 1960; Johnson, 1975). However, as the incidence of rheumatic fever has declined, the importance of rheumatic carditis as a risk factor for endocarditis has declined. Series from the 1970s implicated rheumatic carditis in 10% of the cases (Kramer, 1983; Stanton, 1984; Van Hare et. al., 1984), and during the past decade this percentage declined even further (Normand, 1995; Saiman, 1993). Several endemic pockets of rheumatic fever were observed in the United States during the 1980s; these episodes were notable for high rates of associated carditis ranging from 50% to 90% (Wald, 1987; Veasy, 1987; Hosier, 1987). It remains to be seen whether these outbreaks will have a great impact on the epidemiology of endocarditis.

Congenital Heart Disease and the Impact of Cardiac Surgery

For over 150 years the link between endocarditis and congenital heart disease has been known. Studies from the 1940s and 1950s first described the pathophysiology and anatomic defects noted during autopsies performed on children with congenital heart disease (Cutler, 1958; Gelfman and Levine, 1942; Johnson, 1975). It is striking to note that, among 181 such children, endocarditis was observed in 16.5% during autopsy (Cutler, 1958). Ventricular septal defects (VSDs), patent ductus arteriosus (PDAs), and tetralogy of Fallot (TOF) were the most common lesions associated with endocarditis in these early series. Atrial septal defects were rarely associated with endocarditis. This epidemiology reflected the increased risk of endocarditis associated with turbulent blood flow created by these lesions, as well as the relatively prolonged life expectancy associated with these lesions before the advent of cardiac surgery (Van Hare, 1987).

Other instructive series described the impact of early surgical attempts at palliation and correction of congenital heart disease on the epidemiology of endocarditis (Linde and Heins, 1960; Johnson

Table 6-1 Risk factors associated with endocarditis

Lesion	Historical importance
Rheumatic carditis	More common in earlier series
Congenital heart disease	Early series: PDA,* VSD,† TOF‡
	Later series: complex cyanotic lesions
Postoperative endocarditis	Early: Within 3 mo of surgery
	Late: >3 mo of surgery
Nosocomial endocarditis	Premature infants
	Central venous catheters
	Dialysis catheters
Mitral valve prolapse	
Intravenous drug abuse	Well described in adults

*Patent ductus arteriosus.
†Ventricular septal defect. ‡Tetralogy of Fallot.

1975, 1982; Geva 1988). These studies demonstrated that cardiac surgery (i.e., PDA ligation or construction of a palliative shunt for TOF) was a risk factor for endocarditis because early surgical techniques were imperfect; equipment, the operating field, and the operative site became contaminated. However, the frequency of cyanotic lesions increased as improvements in cardiac surgery led to prolonged life expectancy for such children. This increase was highlighted in a large series of endocarditis in children; from 1930 to 1952 only 5% of patients in this series had TOF, whereas 33% of patients had this lesion from 1953 to 1972 (Johnson, 1975). Because surgical techniques have greatly improved, endocarditis in the period immediately following surgery has become uncommon. Today cardiac surgery can actually be protective for endocarditis. The Natural History Study prospectively observed patients with VSDs, aortic stenosis, and pulmonic stenosis and demonstrated that by 30 years of age the risk of endocarditis in unrepaired VSDs was 9.7%, compared with 2% after surgery (Gersony and Hayes, 1977). Interestingly, the diagnosis of previously undetected VSDs and mitral valve prolapse may first be made when endocarditis presents (Saiman 1993).

Premature Infants

Endocarditis can develop in infants hospitalized in neonatal intensive care units and can be associated with high mortality rates. Most of these infants have normal cardiac anatomy; catheter tips, turbulent blood flow from PDAs, and persistent fetal circulation can cause endovascular damage, which can lead to sterile thrombus formation (Blieden et al., 1972; Edwards et al., 1977; Morrow et al., 1982; Symchych et al., 1977; Oelberg et al., 1983). Prolonged use of indwelling central venous catheters and frequent instrumentation are suggested as the portals of entry for infection. Broad spectrum antibiotics are thought to be risk factors for infection caused by nosocomial pathogens such as antibiotic-resistant bacteria and fungi. Partly as a result of endocarditis being increasingly diagnosed in these neonates, the proportion of children less than 2 years of age with endocarditis is also increasing.

Nosocomial Endocarditis

The frequency of nosocomial endocarditis has been increasing in patients with and without structural heart disease (von Reyn et. al., 1981; Terpenning et al., 1988). Seriously ill patients on broad spectrum antibiotics with prolonged hospitalization and central venous catheters or dialysis catheters are at increased risk of nosocomial endocarditis. It has been reported that these children were found to have endocarditis only at autopsy (Saiman et al., 1993). In addition, their infections were caused by organisms not generally associated with endocarditis (e.g., gram-negative pathogens) or organisms not generally cultured from blood (e.g., *Aspergillus* species) (Barst 1981).

Mitral Valve Prolapse

Mitral valve prolapse is also a risk factor for endocarditis (Danchin 1989). Because this lesion occurs in about 5% of children (Greenwood, 1984), a case-control study was performed that firmly established MVP as a risk factor for endocarditis (Clemens et al., 1982). The indications for prophylaxis of this lesion are discussed later in the chapter, but it is estimated that the risk of endocarditis occurring in persons with mitral valve insufficiency caused by prolapse is 1.5% to 3% over 20 years (McNamara, 1982).

PATHOGENESIS
Subacute Endocarditis

Our understanding of the pathogenesis of subacute endocarditis has been derived from animal models (Durack et al., 1973) and from human studies of rheumatic carditis (Bleich and Bovo, 1974; Scheld, 1984). Whereas generalized pancarditis occurs during an episode of rheumatic fever, valvular involvement leads to the most sequelae. Initially, an immunopathogenic process that is still not completely understood leads to thickening of the valves with fibrin and inflammatory cells. This organizes to fibrosis, stenosis, and calcification, which is generally limited to the mitral and aortic valve. The tricuspid and pulmonary valves are rarely involved. Valvular stenosis leads to turbulent blood flow and resultant endothelial damage. Fibrin and platelets are deposited on the collagen beneath the damaged mural or valvular endothelium, and a sterile thrombus is created. Transient bacteremia from endogenous oral flora such as viridans streptococci colonize the thrombus, and more platelets and fibrin are deposited over the microbes. Thus a critical early event in the pathogenesis of endocarditis is adherence to the thrombus by the microorganisms. Adherence can occur by several bacterial factors, including dextran, the platelet-aggregating ability of *Streptococci* and *Staphylococci* spp., and the teichoic acid of staphylococci (Scheld, 1984). The continuous antigenic stimulation of relatively less virulent microorganisms associated with subacute endocarditis leads to circulating immune complexes (Bleich and Boro, 1974). These deposit in the skin, kidney, and retina and cause the classic clinical manifestations of subacute endocarditis, which is discussed later in the chapter.

Acute Endocarditis

Our understanding of the pathogenesis of acute endocarditis is derived from clinical correlations with autopsy findings (Bleich and Boro, 1974; Arnett and Roberts, 1976). Approximately 50% to 60% of cases occur in patients with normal cardiac anatomy. It is generally thought that the infection originates in an extracardiac site and spreads to involve the heart. The mechanism of bacterial adherence to normal cardiac tissue is not well understood. *S. aureus* has been shown to bind to collagen, fibronectin, laminin, vitronectin, and fibrinogen, but the bacterial adhesins responsible are largely unknown (Heinz et al., 1996). *S. aureus* can cause extensive valvular destruction and intracardiac extension with abscesses. Extracardial disease is caused by embolic phenomenon, which are more frequent in acute endocarditis because of the bulky friable vegetations caused by the organisms associated with this entity (Bile, 1995).

Postoperative Endocarditis

As described earlier, cardiac surgery has been known to be a risk factor for endocarditis since the 1960s. Postoperative endocarditis is divided into early and late postoperative infection. Early postoperative endocarditis is caused by intraoperative contamination of the surgical site, the prosthesis, the bypass pump, or indwelling catheters or is spread from extracardial infection. A capsular polysaccharide adhesin has been implicated in the pathogenesis of prosthetic valve endocarditis caused by *S. epidermidis* (Shiro et al., 1995).

The pathogenesis of late postoperative endocarditis is different, since the postoperative site is almost completely endothelialized by 6 months (Arnett and Roberts, 1976). Late postoperative infections are similar to those of subacute endocarditis in that endogenous bacteria colonize prosthetic material such as valves, patches, and shunts. Patients with prosthetic valves are at particular risk for endocarditis; 1% to 4% of valve recipients develop endocarditis in the year following valve replacement and an additional 1% do so during subsequent years (Bayer, 1993).

CLINICAL PRESENTATION
Subacute Endocarditis

The clinical presentation of subacute endocarditis is typified by fever, including fever of unknown origin, malaise, splenomegaly, regurgitant valvulitis, weight loss, and fatigue of weeks to months in duration (Herman, 1982). The classic immunologic phenomena, though diligently taught, are rarely seen today. These include Roth's spots, Janeway's lesions, Osler's nodes, and glomerulonephritis (Bleich, 1974; Scheld, 1984; Neugarten, 1984). Thus meticulous and repeated examination of the skin, conjunctiva, and retina should always be performed in patients with suspected endocarditis.

Acute Endocarditis

Acute endocarditis is a fulminant process that typically presents with fever, a new murmur, congestive heart failure caused by valvular destruction, sepsis, and systemic emboli. Left-sided endocarditis leads to embolic events in the central nervous system; the extremities; the kidney, liver, and spleen; and occasionally the coronary arteries. Emboli to the central nervous system can cause stroke symptoms. In the extremities, loss of pulses or the appearance of a cool or cyanotic limb or digit can be the first sign of an embolus. Hematuria and sterile pyuria are the usual presentations of emboli to the kidneys, and emboli to the coronary arteries can cause congestive heart failure. Right-sided endocarditis most commonly causes embolic phenomena in the lungs, unless a right-to-left shunt exists. The classic manifestations of emboli to the lungs are shortness of breath and chest pain. Patients are at risk of embolic events before, during, or following antibiotic treatment, although, as reported in adults, embolization is more common before effective antimicrobial treatment has begun (Bayer, 1993). Thus daily physical examinations must be performed, including the evaluation of neurologic status.

Nosocomial Endocarditis

Nosocomial endocarditis in the neonate, in the early postoperative period, or in critically ill patients may initially be misdiagnosed. Although such children almost always have positive blood cultures, it can be difficult to distinguish between endocarditis and more common clinical entities, such as bacteremia or sepsis. Persistently positive blood cultures, a new murmur, embolic phenomenon, and cardiac failure are obvious clues for the diagnosis of endocarditis. However, endocarditis is at times less convincingly diagnosed in a child with congenital heart disease whose presentation is limited to fever, positive blood culture(s), and no other explanation for fever.

DIAGNOSIS

Thus the diagnosis of endocarditis is not always straightforward and often requires a high index of clinical suspicion. Two sets of criteria have been developed to diagnose endocarditis in adults: von Reyn's criteria, published in 1981 (von Reyn), and Duke University's criteria, described in 1994 (Durack). In each, the diagnosis of endocarditis is based on a combination of diagnostic evaluations such as histopathologic findings, autopsy findings, blood cultures, and supportive laboratory data. The likelihood of endocarditis is graded as definite, probable, possible, or unlikely based on the strength of the evidence gathered by the diagnostic evaluation.

There have been major criticisms of the earlier criteria published by von Reyn. These authors did not address the role of echocardiograms in diagnosing endocarditis, only declared the diagnosis of endocarditis definite if documented by intraoperative histopathologic or autopsy findings, and ignored intravenous drug abuse as a risk factor. In clinical practice echocardiograms are far more widely employed in the diagnosis of endocarditis than surgery and autopsy. The incorporation of this diagnostic test by Duke's criteria is an important addition. Duke's criteria have been independently validated by other investigators and found to have a high degree of predictive value (Bayer, 1994; Hoen). Unfortunately, neither set of criteria has been validated in children, but they serve as useful guidelines for pediatric cases.

Blood Cultures

Blood cultures are the most important diagnostic test for endocarditis. Ninety percent of patients with endocarditis have a positive blood culture. It is recommended that three sets of blood cultures be obtained at different times from patients not receiving antibiotics, and five sets be obtained from those patients on antibiotics, or in whom subacute endocarditis is suspected (Washington, 1982). Arterial blood cultures are not better at recovering organisms than venous blood cultures. Although a positive blood culture in the correct setting may be highly suggestive of endocarditis, extracardial infection such as uncomplicated bacteremia, wound infections, colonization of central venous catheters, or contamination of the blood culture must also be considered in the differential diagnosis.

Approximately 10% of pediatric patients have culture-negative endocarditis (Walterspiel and Kaplan, 1986). Antecedent antibiotics are the most common cause of negative blood culture. However, it has been shown that most patients previously treated with oral antimicrobials still had positive blood cultures (Saiman et al., 1993). In addition, some organisms may be difficult to culture because of their unique growth requirements (Walterspiel and Kaplan, 1986). Some organisms are slow growing and others require special media, vitamin or amino acid supplements, or specialized growth conditions. It is imperative to inform the clinical microbiology laboratory that endocarditis is being considered to ensure adequate handling of the specimens.

Echocardiography

Transthoracic echocardiography (TTE) revolutionized the diagnosis of endocarditis over two decades ago both by visualizing vegetations and by diagnosing valvular abnormalities. However, only approximately 70% of children diagnosed with endocarditis have vegetations observable by echocardiogram (Bricker et al., 1985; Webb et al., 1983; Geva and Frand, 1988; Kavey et al., 1983; Yokochi et al., 1986). There are numerous reasons for negative TTE results. It is thought that TTEs are most commonly negative because this methodology cannot visualize vegetations smaller than 2 mm. Preexisting valvular abnormalities or palliative shunts may obscure visualization of a vegetation.

Transesophageal echocardiography (TEE) has been used with increasing frequency in adult populations in recent years. There are few reports using TEE in children, as a result of technical limitations for very small children and the relative invasiveness of the procedure. TEE is thought to improve the visualization of intracardiac abscesses; periannular complications; and intracardiac anatomy in patients with chest wall abnormalities, obesity, recent cardiothoracic surgery, or prosthetic valves (Rohman et al., 1995; Bayer, 1993; Lindner et al., 1996). TEE can also aid in determining the significance of valvular abnormalities such as thickening or in visualizing vegetations less than 5 mm.

Ancillary Tests

Several ancillary tests may be useful to diagnose endocarditis and to monitor response to treatment. Every child with endocarditis should have a complete blood count, a sedimentation rate, a urine analysis, liver function tests, and an electrocardiogram. Complement and rheumatoid factor may be obtained, although their use was promoted more during the era before TTE.

MICROBIOLOGY

Although the microbiologic factors associated with endocarditis have been very well described, there have been changes in the past decade in the organisms associated with this infection, since the lesions at risk have changed. An understanding of the different risk factors that are associated with different pathogens can be used both diagnostically and therapeutically (Table 6-2).

The most common cause of subacute, community-acquired endocarditis in children with congenital or rheumatic heart disease is viridans streptococci (Roberts et al., 1979). Many clinical microbiology laboratories are now speciating these streptococci to *S. sanguis, S. mitis, S. salivaris, S. mutans, S. oralis,* and others.

Staphylococci have become increasingly common and in some series have replaced streptococci as the most common cause of endocarditis. *S. aureus* is the most common cause of acute bacterial endocarditis. Yet it has been shown that *S. aureus* can also cause a surprisingly indolent course in children with congenital heart disease (Saiman et al., 1993). Infection can occur on normal heart valves, especially those of intravenous drug abusers, patients with mitral valve prolapse, or prosthetic valves.

Table 6-2 Association of microorganisms and risk factor

Pathogen	Risk factor
Viridans streptococci	Rheumatic fever
	Late postoperative infection
Staphylococcus aureus	Normal heart–extracardial foci
	Mitral valve prolapse
	Nosocomial endocarditis
	Intravenous drug use
Coagulase-negative staphylococci, esp. *S. epidermidis*	Prosthetic valve endocarditis
	Early postoperative endocarditis
Enterococci	Congenital heart disease
	Postoperative endocarditis
Fungi	
Aspergillus spp.	Intraoperative contamination
Candida spp.	Postoperative endocarditis
	Premature infants
Gram-negative rods	Nosocomial infection
	Central venous catheter
Culture-negative endocarditis HACEK* organisms *Aspergillus* spp. Nutrionally variant streptococci *Brucella* spp.	Pretreatment with antibiotics

Haemophilus, Actinobacillus, Cardiobacterium, Eikenella, and *Kingella* spp.

The most common causes of early postoperative endocarditis are nosocomial pathogens. These include coagulase-negative staphylococci, generally *S. epidermidis* (Karchmer et al., 1983), and, more rarely, Enterobacteriaceae or fungi such as *Aspergillus* or *Candida* spp. Methicillin-resistant *S. aureus, S. epidermidis,* and fungi have all been causes of endocarditis in premature infants. Late postoperative endocarditis is generally caused by those organisms associated with subacute endocarditis, that is, viridans streptococci. In general, there has been a trend toward more unusual pathogens causing endocarditis (Normand et al., 1995).

TREATMENT OF ENDOCARDITIS
General Principles

Medical management with parenteral antimicrobials remains the cornerstone of therapy (Fleming,

1987; Besnier and Choutet, 1995). Daily monitoring of hemodynamic status, careful observation of the patient for evidence of embolic complications, and, when indicated, timely surgical intervention are critical to ensure the best possible outcome for patients with endocarditis. Thus optimal therapy depends on collaboration between several subspecialists, including cardiologists, infectious disease physicians, cardiothoracic surgeons, neurologists, and the clinical microbiology laboratory staff.

An understanding of the basic principles of antibiotic therapy for endocarditis incorporates knowledge of the pathology of the thrombus, as well as the differences between infection of the native valve and infection of prosthetic material. Bactericidal, not bacteriostatic, antibiotics are imperative because (1) the organisms within the infected thrombus grow slowly; (2) antibiotics do not diffuse well into the thrombus; and (3) complement, antibodies, and inflammatory cells are often excluded from the avascular thrombus. Thus adequate therapy necessitates higher and more predictable blood levels. In addition, the growing problem of antibiotic resistance has had an enormous impact on the treatment of endocarditis.

Initial antimicrobial management is often empiric until a causative agent is isolated. The choice of antimicrobials is guided by (1) the risk factors of the infected patients, (2) the clinical presentation, (3) the presence of prosthetic material, and (4) patterns of antibiotic susceptibilities for organisms in specific settings. Subsequent modifications in antibiotic therapy are made when the pathogen is identified and the antimicrobial susceptibilities are determined. Treatment for pediatric patients with endocarditis is extrapolated from recommendations for adults with endocarditis, although adults often have a different spectrum of risk factors, such as calcified valves, or higher rates of prosthetic valves, intravenous drug abuse, and rheumatic heart disease.

For years, many experts recommended obtaining peak antibiotic serum cidal levels when treating a patient with endocarditis. However, this recommendation has fallen out of favor since standardized laboratory methods have not been developed and results have generally not been correlated with clinical outcome. Serum cidal levels do not replace measuring peak and trough antibiotic levels. Weekly vancomycin or gentamicin levels need to be determined if these antibiotics are used, especially in patients with renal insufficiency.

Empiric Antibiotic Therapy

In the hemodynamically stable patient with subacute endocarditis, antimicrobial treatment can be delayed until blood cultures are obtained over 24 to 48 hours. Subacute endocarditis in a child with rheumatic heart disease can be treated initially with penicillin and low-dose gentamicin. Streptomycin is not used today, since it is difficult to obtain and is associated with a greater risk of ototoxicity than with gentamicin.

Empiric antimicrobial therapy for community-acquired endocarditis in a child with congenital heart disease should include three agents; penicillin; a semisynthetic β-lactam agent, such as oxacillin (or nafcillin); and low-dose gentamicin. Methicillin should not be used because of the higher incidence of interstitial nephritis. Community-acquired methicillin-resistant *S. aureus* has been described but is rare in children. Vancomycin can be used in place of penicillin and oxacillin in penicillin-allergic patients, but it is critical that allergy be well documented. Vancomycin should be used with caution. Vancomycin has been shown to be less effective against *S. aureus* than semisynthetic penicillins when treating endocarditis (Wilson et al., 1995). Overuse of vancomycin in the hospital setting has also been strongly associated with the growing problem of vancomycin-resistant enterococci.

Empiric antibiotic therapy for early postoperative endocarditis generally consists of vancomycin and gentamicin because of the high incidence of methicillin-resistant staphylococci in many hospitals.

DRUG REGIMENS FOR SPECIFIC PATHOGENS

Following identification and susceptibility testing of the pathogen, antibiotic therapy can be modified. These modifications also take into account the underlying lesion. In general, endocarditis of prosthetic material is treated longer, using more agents to provide synergy (Kaye, 1996). Many of the following recommendations are a synopsis of the most recent recommendations of the Committee on Rheumatic Fever, Endocarditis, and Kawasaki Disease, sponsored by the American Heart Association (Wilson et al., 1995). It should be noted that these treatment recommendations are for adults, since treatment trials have not been conducted in children. However, these recommendations are generally suitable for children, as supported by anecdotal experience.

Streptococci

Viridans streptococci are the α-hemolytic and non-hemolytic flora of the oral cavity and gastrointestinal tract. Treatment guidelines take into account the minimum inhibitory concentration (MIC) to penicillin (Table 6-3). These organisms can be quite sensitive to penicillin, with MIC of less than 0.1 μg/ml. Traditional treatment regimens include both penicillin G and low-dose gentamicin for 2 weeks, and penicillin G alone for 4 weeks. Uncomplicated endocarditis of natural valves caused by highly penicillin-susceptible strains of streptococci has been successfully treated with a once-daily ceftriaxone outpatient regimen (Francioli et al., 1992). Studies with ceftriaxone have only been performed in adults but most likely would be effective in children. Cure rates of 98% have been obtained with all three medical regimens. These recommendations also apply to *S. bovis,* but this is a very infrequent cause of pediatric endocarditis. It should be emphasized that these recommendations are only applicable to uncomplicated endocarditis (i.e., they do not apply to intracardial extension or abscesses). Courses of intravenous antibiotics may be completed at home in the very stable patient with close monitoring of hemodynamic status and possible antimicrobial toxicity.

Streptococci are considered relatively resistant to penicillin when the MIC is greater than 0.1 μg/ml and less than 0.5 μg/ml. Patients infected with these organisms should be treated with 4 weeks of penicillin G and 2 weeks of low-dose gentamicin. There are not adequate data to support the use of single daily dosing of aminoglycosides for treatment of endocarditis. Streptococcal infection of prosthetic valves should be treated for 6 weeks with penicillin G, and gentamicin is added for the first 2 weeks. Resistant streptococci, including nutritionally variant streptococci defined as having an MIC of ≥0.5 μg/ml, should be treated

like enterococcal endocarditis, as is described in the following discussion (Besnier and Choutet, 1995).

S. pneumoniae, S. pyogenes, group B, C, F *streptococci*

Streptococcal species such as *S. pneumoniae, S. pyogenes,* and group B streptococci are relatively rare causes of endocarditis in children. To date, there have been no treatment trials in adults, and management is guided by the antimicrobial susceptibilities. Pneumococci are becoming increasingly resistant to penicillin and cephalosporins; knowledge of the MICs to penicillin is necessary to manage infection caused by this pathogen. Susceptible pneumococci have an MIC to penicillin less than 0.1 μg/ml, and these strains can be treated with penicillin alone. Intermediately resistant strains have an MIC between 0.1 and 1.0 μg/ml and can be managed with high-dose penicillin or a third-generation cephalosporin, such as ceftriaxone or cefotaxime. Resistant strains with an MIC equal to or greater than 2 μg/ml that cause central nervous system involvement should be managed with vancomycin and a third-generation cephalosporin (Friedland and McCracken, 1994). Clearly, management of endocarditis caused by *S. pneumoniae* should be done in consultation with an infectious diseases subspecialist. Some experts recommend the addition of an aminoglycoside for treatment of group B, C, and G streptococci.

Enterococci

Treatment of enterococcal endocarditis is also becoming more complex; multiply resistant strains with high levels of resistance to penicillin, gentamicin, and most recently vancomycin have been documented (Centers for Disease Control, 1993). Enterococcal endocarditis caused by strains susceptible to penicillin should be treated with 6

Table 6-3 Antibiotic management of common causes of endocarditis

Organism	Minimum inhibitory concentration (MIC)	Antibiotic and duration
Viridans streptococci	<0.1 μg/ml	Penicillin 4 wk
		Penicillin + gentamicin 2 wk
		Ceftriaxone 4 wk
	0.1 to 1 μg/ml	Penicillin + gentamicin 4 wk
Staphylococci	Methicillin-susceptible	Oxacillin 4-6 wk
		+
		Gentamicin + rifampin
	Methicillin-resistant	Vancomycin + gentamicin + rifampin 5-7 day

weeks of penicillin (or ampicillin) and low-dose gentamicin. If the strain exhibits high-level resistance to gentamicin, susceptibility to streptomycin should be determined, since resistance is encoded by different enzymes. Strains resistant to penicillin are generally susceptible to vancomycin, but vancomycin resistance is increasing. Management of vancomycin-resistant endocarditis is limited to case reports and animal models and suggests that multidrug regimens may be successful (Francioli, 1995; Landman et al., 1995, 1996).

Staphylococcus aureus

Treatment of *S. aureus* endocarditis is also complex and is guided by several considerations, including the antibiogram, right sided–versus–left sided disease, the presence of prosthetic valves or material, and the presence of embolic events or intracardiac extension (Bile, 1995). In general, gentamicin in synergistic doses is used for 1 to 2 weeks or until blood cultures are negative, after which most authors would discontinue gentamicin. Rifampin can be added, usually after discontinuation of gentamicin, especially if a myocardial or peripheral abscess is suspected.

The duration of treatment can also vary considerably. There are uncontrolled data to suggest that intravenous drug addicts with right-sided endocarditis caused by methicillin-susceptible *S. aureus*, generally regarded as a milder disease, can be successfully treated in 2 weeks (Chambers, 1988). Uncomplicated endocarditis can be treated with oxacillin (or nafcillin) for 4 weeks if there is a rapid clinical response. Antimicrobial therapy should be continued for 6 weeks or occasionally longer in the patient with a slow clinical response or with complications such as persistently positive blood cultures, intracardiac extension, valve replacement, or embolic phenomena. For humans, there are only limited data to suggest that combination therapy is better than monotherapy and that the subsequent shortened duration of bacteremia improves clinical outcome. Throughout treatment, urinalysis and liver function tests are monitored closely because of the risk of interstitial nephritis and hepatitis from the antimicrobial agents. For patients taking vancomycin and gentamicin, weekly peak and trough levels must also be assessed.

Endocarditis caused by methicillin-resistant staphylococci has become an increasingly common problem. Methicillin resistance is defined as growth of the organism on an agar plate containing 6 μg/ml of oxacillin and resistance to imipenem and augmentin (Hindler and Warner, 1987). These organisms are not sensitive to cephalosporins or the macrolides erythromycin, clarithromycin, azithromycin, and clindamycin. Methicillin-resistant strains of *S. aureus* are treated with vancomycin for 6 weeks and low-dose gentamicin for 1 to 2 weeks. Rifampin may be added if blood cultures are persistently positive or if an abscess is suspected. Methicillin-resistant strains have not been associated with increased morbidity and mortality when compared with methicillin-sensitive strains. Clinical cure in early postoperative endocarditis often requires removal of the prosthetic valve or shunt.

Coagulase-negative staphylococci

Treatment recommendations for coagulase-negative staphylococci parallel those for *S. aureus* (Wilson et al., 1995; Bile, 1995). The majority of cases occurs in the postoperative setting and is associated with infection of a prosthetic valve. Choice of oxacillin or vancomycin is guided by the antimicrobial susceptibilities of the organism, and treatment generally lasts for 6 weeks. Aminoglycosides and rifampin are added to the treatment regimens of methicillin-resistant strains.

Fungal spp.

Endocarditis caused by fungi may be very difficult to diagnose and treat effectively (Rubinstein and Lang, 1995). Blood cultures can be negative, especially with *Aspergillus* spp., and a high index of suspicion is required for diagnosis. Fungal endocarditis should be suspected in the early postoperative period, especially if a large friable vegetation is present without a positive blood culture or if the patient fails to respond clinically to antibacterial agents.

Management of fungal endocarditis requires both medical treatment and surgical intervention. Amphotericin B is used to treat either *Candida* or *Aspergillus* spp. endocarditis. The toxicities of amphotericin are considerable, and the patient's renal function and blood counts must be carefully monitored during the prolonged 6- to 8-week course. There are no clinical data suggesting that liposomal amphotericin is more effective than conventional amphotericin in the treatment of endocarditis. Liposomal amphotericin is very costly and should be reserved for patients who either cannot tolerate intravenous amphotericin or who are failing to respond and appear to require higher dosages. Surgical excision of the vegetation and removal of the prosthetic valve have been widely recommended by the vast majority of experts. There are, however, rare case reports of premature infants with inoperable fungal endocarditis who have survived medical management alone (Sanchez et al., 1991). There is increasing support for using fluconazole "indefinitely" after apparent cure of endocarditis caused by *Candida* spp. to prevent relapse by presumed residual foci of fungi (Muehrcke et al., 1995). Even when managed both surgically and medically, fungal endocarditis carries a mortality rate of 50% to 90%.

Culture-Negative Endocarditis

Culture-negative endocarditis occurs in an estimated 5% to 15% of cases of pediatric endocarditis and is most often secondary to pretreatment with antibiotics (Pesanti and Smith, 1979). Blood cultures must be held for 4 weeks to ensure growth of the nutritionally fastidious streptococci and the HACEK *(Haemophilus, Actinobacillus, Cardiobacterium, Eikenella,* and *Kingella)* organisms. Fungi, chlamydiae, rickettsiae, *Bartonella* spp., *Legionella* spp., and *Brucella* spp. may also cause culture-negative endocarditis. With the exception of fungi, these pathogens are very infrequent causes of pediatric endocarditis. A high index of suspicion is needed to recover these rare pathogens from blood cultures because they frequently require special culture techniques.

Therapy of community-acquired, culture-negative endocarditis should include ampicillin, oxacillin, and low-dose gentamicin. If the patient has undergone recent cardiac surgery, vancomycin should be used instead of oxacillin. Gram stain and subculture of the original blood cultures, culture of peripheral emboli or the resected valve, teichoic acid antibodies that measure a cell wall component of *S. aureus,* and bacterial antigen detection of *S. pneumoniae* may occasionally reveal a pathogen, although generally these studies are not helpful. If all these ancillary tests remain negative, continual surveillance of the clinical course is imperative to demonstrate response to the initial choice of antimicrobials (Oakley, 1995).

SURGICAL MANAGEMENT

Surgical intervention may be necessary to effectively manage endocarditis (Box 6-1). The indications for surgery include correcting valvular dysfunction, excising tissue that cannot be sterilized, removing intracardiac abscesses, closing interven-

tricular fistulas, and removing vegetations that are sources of emboli (Acar et al., 1995). Surgery is most likely to be needed during the acute episode of endocarditis but may occur later, after treatment is complete (Acar et al., 1995). It is important to note that approximately 15% to 25% of adult patients who have been cured with medical management alone eventually require cardiac surgery to repair damaged valves (Vlessis et al., 1996).

The literature has generally divided surgery into two categories: absolute indications and relative indications. Absolute indications for surgery include intractable heart failure secondary to valvular obstruction, prosthetic valve dehiscence, fungal endocarditis, or persistently positive blood cultures for more than 1 week despite appropriate antibiotics. In general, bacteriologic indications for surgery are accompanied by signs of heart failure resulting from valvular dysfunction. Intracardiac extension causing myocardial abscess, rupture of the papillary muscles, chorda tendineae, and ventricular septum are also clear indications for emergent surgical intervention. Early postoperative prosthetic valve endocarditis is usually an indication for surgery, since cure cannot be achieved by medical management alone.

One of the most difficult management decisions is whether or not to surgically remove a vegetation. The presence of a large vegetation, even when found on the left side of the heart, is not an absolute indication for surgery. Several studies have ad-

---

BOX 6-1

INDICATIONS FOR SURGERY

Absolute Indications

Intractable heart failure
Valvular obstruction
Intracardiac extension*
Prosthetic valve dehiscence
Fungal endocarditis
Persistently positive blood cultures

Relative Indications

≥2 embolic events†
Central nervous system emboli

---

*Rupture of papillary muscles, chordae tendineae, ventricular septum; myocardial abscess; purulent pericarditis.
†Excluding pulmonary emboli.

dressed whether size is predictive of future embolization and have generally concluded that size alone is not an indication for removal of the vegetation (Alsip et al., 1985; Erbel et al., 1995). Likewise, with the exception of fungal endocarditis, the type of organism does not dictate surgery. The timing of embolization is also somewhat variable, in that vegetations can embolize at presentation, during therapy, or even following the successful completion of therapy. Pulmonary emboli, even when multiple, do not necessitate surgical excision of the vegetation. Left-sided embolic events, usually to the central nervous system, do represent relative indications for surgery. However, because of the enormous surgical risks associated with these patients, many researchers recommend waiting until a second embolic event occurs before proceeding with surgery. In adults, surgery associated with infection of prosthetic valves has the highest mortality rate.

PROGNOSIS

The outcome for patients diagnosed with endocarditis appears to be improving, but it largely depends on the pathogen. Mortality rates in the 1950s and 1960s were as high as 38% (Zakrzewski, 1965). In the late 1970s and 1980s the mortality rates in published series of endocarditis in pediatrics patients ranged from 14% to 22%, and more recent studies have shown mortality rates ranging from 5% to 11% (Normand et al., 1995; Saiman et al., 1993). Streptococcal endocarditis is associated with excellent outcomes and minimal morbidity. Children with endocarditis caused by *S. aureus* have a higher risk of morbidity and mortality, as do younger children and those with fungal endocarditis and gram-negative endocarditis. In a small study of long-term follow-ups of children after endocarditis, the majority was hemodynamically stable as long as 27 years after the episode of endocarditis (Fisher et al., 1985). Relapse can occur, however, most often in patients with complex cyanotic heart disease who have prosthetic valves and shunts. Children who have had one episode of endocarditis have about a 5% to 10% chance of a recurrent infection; therefore blood culture specimens should be obtained during subsequent febrile illnesses.

PROPHYLAXIS

The most recent recommendations for prophylaxis by the American Heart Association attempt to simplify the regimens; clarify the types of lesions; and shorten the list of dental, gastrointestinal, genitourinary, and cardiac procedures for which prophylaxis is indicated (Durack, 1995). These recommendations are continually being updated, and physicians should review the literature periodically (Box 6-2). There have been several studies documenting lack of compliance with prophylaxis (Brooks, 1980; Brooks et al., 1988). The rationale for antimicrobial prophylaxis for patients at risk for endocarditis is based on animal models (Glauser et al., 1982) and many assumptions that may be flawed (Kaye, 1986). Most importantly, it is assumed that endocarditis is preceded by an antecedent event that can be identified so that the patient can receive prophylaxis. However, most of the episodes of endocarditis are not caused by a known event. Furthermore, adequate prophylaxis can fail to prevent endocarditis (Durack et al., 1983), and only the streptococci and enterococci are sensitive to the oral antimicrobials used. An adequate clinical trial to prove the efficacy of prophylaxis will most likely never be done. Yet, despite these limitations, antimicrobial prophy-laxis to prevent endocarditis has been established as routine medical practice (De Gevigney et al., 1995).

BOX 6-2

LESIONS AT RISK FOR ENDOCARDITIS

Higher Risk

Ventricular septal defect
Patent ductus arteriosus
Tetralogy of Fallot
Previous endocarditis
Prosthetic valve
Coarctation of aorta
Mitral stenosis or insufficiency
Mitral valve prolapse with regurgitant murmur

Intermediate Risk

Mitral valve prolapse without regurgitation
Triscuspid valve disease
Pulmonary valve disease
Idiopathic hypertrophic subaortic stenosis

Very Low/Negligible Risk

ASD
Coronary artery disease
Pacemakers
Surgically corrected lesions without prosthetic implants

BIBLIOGRAPHY

Acar J, Michel PL, Varenne O, et al. Surgical treatment of infective endocarditis. Europe Heart J 1995;16:94-98.

Alsip SC, Blackstone EM, Kirklin JW, Cobbs CG. Indications for cardiac surgery in patients with active infective endocarditis. Amer J Med 1985;78(suppl 6B):138-148.

Arnett EN, Roberts WC. Prosthetic valve endocarditis: clinicopathologic analysis of 22 necropsy patients with comparison of observations in 74 necropsy patients with active endocarditis involving natural left-sided valves. Amer J Cardiol 1976;38:281-292.

Barst R, Prince A, Neu HC. Aspergillus endocarditis in children: case report and review of the literature. Pediatrics 1981;68:73-78.

Bayer AS. Infective endocarditis. Clin Infect Dis 1993;17:313-322.

Bayer AS, Ward JI, Ginzton LE, Shapiro SM. Evaluation of new clinical criteria for the diagnosis of infective endocarditis. Amer J Med 1994;96:211-219.

Besnier JM, Choutet P. Medical treatment of infective endocarditis: general principles. Eur Heart J 1995;16(suppl B):72-74.

Bile J. Medical treatment of staphylococcal infective endocarditis. Europ Heart J 1995;16(suppl B):80-83.

Bisno AL, Dismukes WE, Durack DT, et al. Antimicrobial treatment of infective endocarditis due to streptococci, enterococci, staphylococci, and HACEK microorganisms. JAMA 1995;274:1706-1713.

Bleich HL, Boro ES. Pathoanatomic, pathophysiologic, and clinical correlation in endocarditis. N Eng J Med 1974; 291:832-837.

Blieden LC, Morehead RR, Burke B, et al. Bacterial endocarditis in the neonate. Amer J Dis Child 1972;124:747-749.

Blumenthal S, Griffiths SP, Morgan BC. Bacterial endocarditis in children with congenital heart disease. Pediatrics 1960;26:993-1016.

Bricker JT, Latson LA, Huhta JC, Gutgesell HP. Echocardiographic evaluation of infective endocarditis in children. Clin Pediatr 1985;24:312-317.

Brooks SL. Survey of compliance with American Heart Association guidelines for prevention of bacterial endocarditis. J Amer Dent Assoc 1980;101:41-43.

Brooks RG, Notario G, McCabe RE. Hospital survey of antimicrobial prophylaxis to prevent endocarditis in patients with prosthetic heart valves. Amer J Med 1988;84:617-621.

Centers for Disease Control. Nosocomial enterococci resistant to vancomycin: United States 1989-1993. Monthly Morbidity and Mortality Review 1993;42:597-599.

Chambers HF, Miller T, Newman MD. Right-sided *Staphylococcus aureus* endocarditis in intravenous drug abusers: two-week combination therapy. Ann Intern Med 1988;109:619-624.

Clemens JD, Horowitz RI, Jaffe CC, et al. Controlled evaluation of the risk of bacterial endocarditis in persons with mitral valve prolapse. N Eng J Med 1982;307:776-781.

Cutler JG, Ongley PA, Shwachman H, et al. Bacterial endocarditis in children with heart disease. Pediatrics 1985; 22:706-714.

Danchin N, Brianchon S, Mathieu P. Mitral valve prolapse as a risk factor for infective endocarditis. Lancet 1989;1:743-745.

Dajani AS, Bisno AL, Chung KJ, et al. Prevention of bacterial endocarditis: Recommendations by the American Heart Association. JAMA 1990;264:2919-2922.

De Gevigney G, Pop C, Delahaye JP. The risk of infective endocarditis after cardiac surgical and interventional procedures. Europe Heart J 1995;16(suppl B):7-14.

Durack DT. Prevention of infective endocarditis. N Eng J Med 1995;332:38-44.

Durack DT, Beeson PB, Petersdorf RG. Experimental endocarditis: III. production and progress of the disease in rabbits. Brit J Exp Pathol 1973;54:142-150.

Durack DT, Kaplan EL, Bisno AL. Apparent failure of endocarditis prophylaxis: analysis of 52 cases submitted to a national registry. JAMA 1983;250:2318-2322.

Durack DT, Lukes AS, Bright DK, Duke Endocarditis Service. New criteria for diagnosis of infective endocarditis: utilization of specific echocardiographic findings. Amer J Med 1994;96:200-209.

Edwards K, Ingall D, Czapek E, Davis AT. Bacterial endocarditis in 4 young infants. Clin Pediatr 1977;16:607-609.

Erbel R, Liu F, Ge J, et al. Identification of high-risk subgroups in infective endocarditis and the role of echocardiography. Europe Heart J 1995;16:588-602.

Feinstein AR, Spagnuolo M, Wood HF, et al. Rheumatic fever in children and adolescents: A long-term epidemiologic study of subsequent prophylaxis, streptococcal infections, and clinical sequelae: VI. clinical features of streptococcal infections and rheumatic recurrences. Ann Intern Med 1964a;60(suppl 5):68-86.

Feinstein AR, Harrison HF, Spagnuolo M, et al. Rheumatic fever in children and adolescents: a long-term epidemiologic study of subsequent prophylaxis, streptococcal infections, and clinical sequelae: VII. cardiac changes and sequelae. Ann Intern Med 1964b;60(Suppl 5):87-122.

Fisher RG, Moodie DS, Rice R. Pediatric bacterial endocarditis: long-term follow-up. Cleve Clin Q 1985;52:41-45.

Fleming HA. General principles of the treatment of infective endocarditis. J Antimicrob Chemother 1987;20(suppl A):143-145.

Francioli P, Etienne J, Hoigne R, et al. Treatment of streptococcal endocarditis with single daily dose of ceftriaxone for 4 weeks: efficacy and out-patient treatment feasibility. JAMA 1992;267:264-267.

Francioli P. Antibiotic treatment of stuptococcal and enterococcal endocarditis: an overview. Evr Heart J 1995;16(5):75-79.

Friedland IR, McCracken GH. Management of infections caused by antibiotic-resistant *Streptococcus pneumoniae*. N Eng J Med 1994;331:377-382.

Gelfman R, Levine SA. The incidence of acute and subacute bacterial endocarditis in congenital heart disease. Amer J Med Sci 1942;204:324-333.

Gersony W, Hayes CJ. Bacterial endocarditis in patients with pulmonary stenosis, aortic stenosis, or ventricular septal defect. Circulation 1977;56(suppl):184-187.

Geva T, Frand M. Infective endocarditis in children with congenital heart disease: the changing spectrum, 1975-1985. Europe Heart J 1988;9:1244-1249.

Glauser MP, Bernard JP, Moreillon P, et al. Successful single-dose Amoxicillin prophylaxis against experimental streptococcal endocarditis: evidence for two mechanisms of protection. J Infect Dis 1982;147:568-575.

Greenwood RD. Mitral valve prolapse: incidence and clinical course in a pediatric population. Clin Pediatr 1984;23:318-320.

Griffiths SP, Gersony WE. Acute rheumatic fever in New York City (1969 to 1988): a comparative study of two decades. J Pediatr 1990;116:882-887.

Heinz SA, Schennings T, Heimdahl A, Flock JI. Collagen binding of *Staphylococcus aureus* is a virulence factor in experimental endocarditis. J Infect Dis 1996;174:83-86.

Herman PE. The clinical manifestations of infective endocarditis. Mayo Clin Proc 1982;57:15-21.

Hindler W, Warner NL. Effect of source of Mueller Hinton agar on detection of oxacillin resistance in *Staphylococcus aureus* using a screening methodology. J Clin Microbiol 1987; 25:734-735.

Hoen B, Selton-Suty C, Danchin N, et al. Evaluation of the Duke criteria versus the Beth Israel criteria for the diagnosis of infective endocarditis. Clin Infect Dis 1995;21:905-909.

Hosier DM, Craenen JM, Teske DW, et al. Resurgence of acute rheumatic fever. Amer J Dis Child 1987;141:730-733.

Johnson CM, Rhodes KH. Pediatric endocarditis. Mayo Clin Proc 1982;57:86-94.

Johnson DH, Rosenthal A, Nadas AS. A forty-year review of bacterial endocarditis in infancy and children. Circulation 1975;51:581-588.

Karchmer AW, Archer GL, Dismukes WE. *Staphylococcus epidermidis* causing prosthetic valve endocarditis: microbiologic and clinical observations as guides to therapy. Ann Intern Med 1983;98:447-455.

Kavet JEW, Frank DM, Byrum CJ, et al. Two-dimensional echocardiographic assessment of infective endocarditis in children. Amer J Dis Child 1983;137:851-856.

Kavey K, Frank DM, Byrum CJ, et al. Two-dimensional echocardiographic assessment of infective endocarditis in children. Amer J Dis Child 1983;137:851-856.

Kaye D. Prophylaxis for infective endocarditis: an update. Ann Intern Med 1986;104:419-423.

Kaye D. Treatment of infective endocarditis. Ann Intern Med 1996;124:606-609.

Kramer H, Bourgeois M, Liersch R, et.al. Current clinical aspacts of bacterial endocarditis in infancy, childhood, adolescence. Eur J Pediatr 1983;140:253-259.

Landman D, Quale JM, Burney S, et al. Treatment of experimental endocarditis caused by multidrug resistant *Enterococcus faecium* with ramoplanin and penicillin. J Antimicrob Chemother 1996;37:323-329.

Landman D, Quale JM, Mobarakai N, Zaman MM. Ampicillin plus ciprofloxacin therapy of experimental endocarditis caused by multidrug-resistant *Enterococcus faecium*. J Antimicrob Chemo 1995;36:253-258.

Liepman MK, Jones PG, Kauffman CA. Endocarditis as a complication of indwelling right atrial catheters in leukemic patients. Cancer 1984;64:804-807.

Linde LM, Heins HL. Bacterial endocarditis following surgery for congenital heart disease. N Eng J Med 1960;263:65-69.

Lindner JR, Case RA, Dent JM, et al. Diagnostic value of echocardiography in suspected endocarditis: an evaluation based on the pretest probability of disease. Circulation 1996;93:730-736.

Mansur AJ, Grinberg M, da Luz P, Bellotti G. The complications of infective endocarditis: a reappraisal in the 1980s. Arch Intern Med 1992;152:2428-2432.

McNamara DG. Idiopathic benign mitral leaflet prolapse. Amer J Dis Child 1982;136:152-156.

Morrow WB, Haas JE, Benjamin DR. Nonbacterial endocardial thrombosis in neonates: relationship to persistent fetal circulation. 1982;100:117-122.

Muehrcke DD, Lytle BW, Cosgrove DM. Surgical and long-term antifungal therapy for fungal prosthetic valve endocarditis. Ann Thorac Surg 1995;60:538-543.

Neugarten J, Baldwin DS. Glomerulonephritis in bacterial endocarditis. Amer J Med 1984;77:297-304.

Normand J, Bozio A, Etienne J, et al. Changing patterns and prognosis of infective endocarditis in childhood. Europ Heart J. 1995:16(suppl B):28-31.

Oakley CM. The medical treatment of culture-negative endocarditis. Europ Heart J 1995;16(suppl B):90-93.

Oelberg DG, Fisher DJ, Gross DM, et al. Endocarditis in high-risk neonates. Pediatrics 1983;71:392-397.

Pesanti EL, Smith IM. Infective endocarditis with negative blood cultures: an analysis of 52 cases. Amer J Med 1979;66:43-50.

Roberts RB, Krieger AG, Schiller NL, Gross KC. Viridans streptococcal endocarditis: the role of various species, including pyridoxal-dependent streptococci. Rev Infect Dis 1979;1:955.

Rohman S, Erbel R, Mohr-Kahaly, Meyer J. Use of trans-esophageal echocardiography in the diagnosis of abscess in infective endocarditis. Europ Heart J 1995;16(suppl B):54-62.

Rubinstein E, Lang R. Fungal endocarditis. Europe Heart J 1995;16(suppl B):84-89.

Saiman L, Prince A, Gersony W. Pediatric infective endocarditis in the modern era: a review of 62 cases from 1977-1992. J Pediatr 1993;122:847-853.

Sanchez PJ, Siegel JD, Fishbein J. *Candida* endocarditis: successful medical management in three preterm infants and a review of the literature. Pediatr Infect Dis J 1991;10:239-242.

Scheld WE. Pathogenesis and pathophysiology of infective endocarditis. In Sande MA, Kaye D, Root RK (eds). Endocarditis: contemporary issues in infectious disease. New York: Churchill Livingstone, 1984.

Shiro H, Meluleni G, Groll A, et al. The pathogenic role of *Staphylococcus epidermidis* capsular polysaccharide/adhesin in a low inoculum rabbit model of prosthetic valve endocarditis. Circulation 1995;92:2715-2722.

Smchych PS, Krauss AN, Winchester P. Endocarditis following intracardiac placement of umbilical venous catheters in neonates. J Pediatr 1977;90:287-289.

Stanton BF, Baltimore RS, Clemens JD. Changing spectrum of infective endocarditis in children: analysis of 26 cases, 1970-1979. Amer J Dis Child 1984;138:720-725.

Terpenning MS, Buggy BP, Kaufmann CA. Hospital-acquired infective endocarditis. Arch Intern Med 1988;148:1601-1603.

Van Hare GF, Ben-Sachar G, Liebman J, et al. Infective endocarditis in infants and children during the past 10 years: a decade of change. Amer Heart 1984;138:1235-1240.

Van Hare GF, Soffer LJ, Sivakoff MC, Liebman J. Twenty-five year experience with ventricular septal defect in infants and children. Amer Heart J 1987;114:606-614.

Veasy LG, Wiedmeier SE, Orsmond GS, et al. Resurgence of acute rheumatic fever in the intermountain area of the United States. N Eng J Med 1987;316:421-426.

Vlessis AA, Hovaguimian H, Jaggers J, et al. Infective endocarditis: ten-year review of medical and surgical therapy. Ann Thorac Surg 1996;61:1217-1222.

von Reyn CF, Levy BS, Albeit RD, et al. Infective endocarditis: an analysis based on strict case definitions. Ann Intern Med 1981;94(part 1):505-518.

Wald ER, Dashefsky B, Feidt C, et al. Acute rheumatic fever in western Pennsylvania and the tristate area. Pediatrics 1987;80:371-374.

Walterspiel JN, Kaplan SL. Incidence and clinical characteristics of "culture-negative" infective endocarditis in a pediatric population. Ped Infect Dis J 1986;5:328-332.

Washington JA. The role of the microbiology laboratory in the diagnosis and treatment of infective endocarditis. Mayo Clin Proc 1982;57:22-32.

Webb RE, Frank DM, Byrum CF, et al. Two-dimensional echocardiographic assessment of infective endocarditis in children. Amer J Dis Child 1983;137:851-856.

Wilson WR, Karchmer AW, Dajani AS, et al. Antibiotic treatment of adults with infective endocarditis due to streptococci, enterococci, staphylococci, and HACEK microorganisms. JAMA 1995;274:1706-1713.

Yokochi K, Sakamoto H, Mikajima T, et al. Infective endocarditis in children: a current diagnostic trend and embolic complications. Jpn Circ J 1986;50:1294-1297.

Zakrzewski T, Keith JD. Bacterial endocarditis in infants and children. J Pediatr 1965;67:1179-1193.

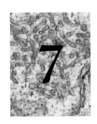

7   ENTEROVIRUSES

HARLEY ROTBART

The enteroviruses (EVs) comprise nearly 70 serotypes of closely related pathogens that cause a wide spectrum of human illness—ranging from asymptomatic infection to common upper-respiratory infections, aseptic meningitis, severe myocarditis, encephalitis, and paralytic poliomyelitis. No single serotype is associated with any one clinical syndrome, and no clinical syndrome is unique to a single serotype; significant overlap exists in the clinical manifestations of the various EVs. The EVs hold a pivotal place in the history of clinical virology and continue to be important in our understanding of the role of viruses in human disease.

HISTORY

Sporadic cases of paralytic disease are as old as recorded history. The term *poliomyelitis* was derived from the Greek for "gray marrow of the spinal cord" and the Latin *(-itis)* for "inflammation." The first isolation of poliovirus was achieved in 1908 by the intracerebral inoculation of CNS tissue into susceptible monkeys. In 1949 Enders, Weller, and Robbins reported their classic experiments on the cultivation of poliovirus in tissue cultures of nonneural human cells (Enders et al., 1949). This Nobel Prize–winning accomplishment, the first successful propagation of viruses in continuous cell lines, allowed for the preparation of high quantities of polioviruses and the subsequent development of poliovirus vaccines.

The histories of the other EVs are relatively recent. In 1948 Dalldorf and Sickles isolated an agent from the stool of a patient with paralytic illness from Coxsackie, New York (Dalldorf and Sickless, 1948). Subsequently, a large group of antigenically related viruses have been designated *coxsackievirus A* and *coxsackievirus B*. Isolation of echoviruses was accomplished from fecal specimens and frequently from patients without overt disease. *Echovirus* is an acronym: *E,* enteric; *C,* cy-topathic; *H,* human; *O,* orphan. Echoviruses have since been associated with a wide variety of illnesses and are no longer "orphans." Since 1969 new EVs have been assigned "enterovirus numbers" rather than being designated coxsackieviruses or echoviruses.

ETIOLOGY

The EVs are members of the family *Picornaviridiae* ("pico" meaning small; "rna" for ribonucleic acid). The original subclassification of the EVs (Box 7-1) was based on the ability of individual serotypes to grow in various cell culture and animal systems. Hence coxsackievirus A serotypes were characteristically able to replicate in suckling mice, with resultant diffuse myositis and flaccid paralysis; however, these viruses were not readily grown in tissue culture cells derived from monkey or human tissues. In contrast, coxsackievirus B serotypes grow readily in tissue cultures of both simian and human origin, as well as in suckling mice. The pathology in the latter differs from the coxsackievirus A serotypes in that the myositis with B serotypes is more focal; and direct infection of brain, myocardium, pancreas, and liver also occurs. Neither group of coxsackieviruses is pathogenic for monkeys. The echoviruses were defined by their ability to grow in simian-derived tissue culture cells but not at all in animal systems. The polioviruses grow most prolifically in cells of human and simian origin and in monkeys; they fail to grow in murine models. Since these original distinctions were observed, they have been significantly blurred by the identification of new strains and new tissue culture cell lines, resulting in crossover patterns of EV growth. For that reason, recent serotypes have simply been numbered (enteroviruses 68 through 71) (Melnick et al., 1974).

Like other picornaviruses, EVs are small (27- to 30-nm diameter; 1.34-g/ml buoyant density), con-

---

---

sisting of a simple viral capsid and a single strand of positive (message) sense RNA. The capsid contains four proteins, VP1 through VP4, arranged in sixty repeating protomeric units of an icosahedron. Variations within capsid proteins VP1 through VP3 are responsible for the antigenic diversity among the EVs; neutralization sites are most densely clustered on VP1. VP4 is not present on the viral surface; rather, it is in close association with the RNA core functioning as an anchor to the viral capsid. Destabilization of VP4 results in viral uncoating (see following section); this may occur during experimental treatment with heat or alkali and following virion binding to a specific cell receptor (see below). The atomic structure of two poliovirus serotypes, types 1 and 3, have been resolved by computerized crystallographic studies (Hogle et al., 1985) and reveal a deep cleft or canyon in the center of each protomeric unit, into which the specific cellular receptor for the EVs fits when the virus encounters a susceptible host cell (Racaniello, 1995). A similar canyon configuration has been shown for another major genus of picornaviruses, the rhinoviruses.

The encapsidated RNA is approximately 7.4 kb in length and serves as a template for both viral protein translation and RNA replication. A single reading frame, coding for a single polyprotein, begins at approximately nucleotide 740 from the 5′ end and terminates at approximately nucleotide 7370, leaving 740 bases at the 5′ end and 70 bases at the 3′ end (just upstream from the poly A tail) untranslated; these untranslated sequences are involved in viral regulatory activities such as replica-

tion and translation. Posttranslational modification of the polyprotein is accomplished by virus-coded proteases and results in generation of the four separate capsid proteins, as well as other functional proteins.

Although genetic differences in the capsid coding regions result in the wide variety of EV serotypes, great similarities exist among the genomes of many of the EVs in a number of other regions along the RNA. Numerous EV serotypes have been fully or partially sequenced at the genomic level, including poliovirus types 1, 2, and 3; coxsackieviruses A2, A9, A16, A21, A24, B1, B3, B4, and B5; echoviruses 6, 9, 11, and 12; and enteroviruses 70 and 71 (Hellen and Wimmer, 1995). The virus formerly known as *enterovirus 72,* or hepatitis A, has been reclassified on genetic grounds and is no longer considered an EV. Similarly, echoviruses 22 and 23, for which substantial genomic sequence information has been determined, are likely to be reclassified as non-EV picornaviruses.

PATHOGENESIS AND PATHOLOGY

The pathogenesis of EV infections has been studied at molecular, cellular, and organ system levels (Rotbart and Kirkegaard, 1992). EVs are acquired by fecal-oral contamination and, less commonly, by respiratory droplet. Although some replication occurs in the nasopharynx with spread to upper-respiratory tract lymphatics, most of the viral inoculum is swallowed. The EVs distinguish themselves from the rhinoviruses (which are also picornaviruses) by being stable at acid pH, the characteristic responsible for the ability of the EVs to traverse the stomach en route to the site of primary infection in the lower gastrointestinal tract— specifically, the Peyer's patches in the lamina propria, where significant viral replication occurs. A minor viremia ensues, seeding numerous organ systems, including the central nervous system (CNS), liver, lungs, and heart. More significant replication at these sites results in a major viremia associated with the signs and symptoms of viral infection. If the CNS has not been seeded with the initial viremic episode, spread there may occur with the major viremia. Although fairly well established, viremia as the source of CNS infection has been long debated, with direct neural spread suggested as an alternate hypothesis. The mechanism by which EVs leave the blood and enter the CNS is entirely unknown. In the case of poliomyelitis, evidence using a transgenic mouse model (Ren and

Racaniello, 1992) supports earlier hypotheses about the importance of muscle infection. Polioviruses may spread to skeletal muscle viremically, reaching neuromuscular end plates, from which the viruses ascend along nerves to the spinal cord and from there may widely disseminate within the CNS. During clinical infections, EVs have been recovered from both the cellular and plasma fractions of the blood, and the more important of the blood compartments for establishing specific organ system infection is not known.

At the cellular level the events of infection with polioviruses are well studied; nonpolioviruses likely have analogous cellular pathogenesis. The virus binds a specific cell receptor at a single viral capsid canyon site (Racaniello, 1995): this likely occurs first in the intestine and, with subsequent progression of infection, at other target tissue sites. The human cellular receptor for poliovirus and certain other enteroviruses maps to chromosome 19. The poliovirus receptor has been well characterized and represents a unique molecule within the "Ig superfamily" (Mendelsohn et al., 1989). At least one echovirus serotype (echovirus 1) binds to a cellular receptor that is a member of the integrin family of surface molecules. Other echovirus serotypes appear to bind to the cell surface molecule known as the "decay-accelerating factor," a glycoprotein that protects cells from complement-mediated lysis. Still other echovirus serotypes do not bind to either the integrin or the decay-accelerating factor molecules. Preliminary binding studies also have revealed putative specific receptors for coxsackievirus A and B serotypes (Racaniello, 1995). Following attachment of the virus, recruitment of additional cellular receptors occurs, and the virion is enveloped by cell membrane, bound now at multiple viral protomers. A steric shift in the capsid conformation occurs, resulting in extrusion of the VP4 viral protein and destabilization of the capsid structure. The now "uncoated" RNA is released freely into the cellular cytoplasm, where it rapidly binds to ribosomes and begins protein synthesis. Within as little as 2 hours of infection, all host cell protein synthesis has been shut down by the EV, and the cell has become a factory for viral production. Infectious virions are released by cell lysis and spread to neighboring and distant cells via the surrounding growth media in vitro and via the blood in vivo.

Molecular determinants of pathogenesis are increasingly being investigated, in attempt to understand the phenotypes of specific EV serotypes and subgroups. Whereas all three serotypes of the wild type of polioviruses are neurotropic and neurovirulent, specific tropisms and virulence patterns vary widely among the nonpolio EVs, with certain serotypes consistently reported as causes of specific organ system disease and others only rarely so. The determinants of neurotropism and neurovirulence have been investigated extensively for the polioviruses. The viral RNA of both neurovirulent and attenuated (vaccine) strains has been sequenced, and only a few differences exist between them. At least two single-base changes are felt to be responsible for the attenuation of previously neurovirulent polioviruses (Hellen and Wimmer, 1995). Following vaccination with attenuated strains, "back-mutation" to virulence has been observed in the fecally shed virions recovered from normal children within a few days of vaccination; it is this revertant genotype that is presumed to be responsible for cases of vaccine-associated poliomyelitis. Molecular neurovirulence determinants among the nonpolio EVs are now being studied in hopes of finding a genomic explanation for the increased frequency of aseptic meningitis and encephalitis observed with certain serotypes and the virtual absence of those diseases with others. Studies of the echoviruses have identified specific base changes in the 5' nontranslated region of the EV genome that are unique to serotypes that rarely cause CNS disease; neurotropic echoviruses, in contrast, have base sequences identical to the polioviruses in these regions (Romero and Rotbart, 1995). Coxsackie B4 strains with pancreatic tropism and virulence are distinguished from avirulent coxsackievirus B4 strains by a single amino acid residue in the VP1 capsid protein. Genotypic determinants of myocarditis remain to be elucidated; cardiovirulent strains of coxsackievirus B have been sequenced and demonstrate mutations throughout the genome, suggesting that tertiary structures, rather than specific base changes, are virulence determinants (Martino et al., 1995).

The host immune system and/or genetic makeup may importantly contribute to EV pathogenesis. Myocarditis, for example, represents an intricate interplay between virus and host genetics and immunity in which direct viral injury and "innocent-bystander" damage as a result of the immune response both probably affect the ultimate outcome of disease (Martino et al., 1995). Similar interactions between EVs and host response have been implicated in the pathogenesis of chronic dilated cardiomyopathy, juvenile-onset diabetes mellitus, and inflammatory muscle diseases (discussed later).

The benign nature of most EV infections has made human pathologic data somewhat sparse. In patients dying of acute poliomyelitis, mixed inflammatory infiltrates (lymphocytes and neutrophils) and neuronal necrosis are found within the gray matter of the spinal cord's anterior horn and motor nuclei of the hindbrain (Bodian, 1949). Small hemorrhages and edema are associated with the inflammation. Involvement of the cerebellum, cerebrum, and midbrain may also be found. Only occasional pathologic descriptions of nonpolio EV meningitis have been reported. A child who died of coxsackievirus B5 myocarditis with concomitant meningitis was noted to have inflammation of the choroid plexus of the lateral and fourth ventricles, fibrosis of the vascular walls with focal destruction of the ependymal lining, and fibrotic basal leptomeninges. Parenchymal findings were limited to moderate, symmetric dilation of the ventricles and an increase in number and size of subependymal astrocytes. The inflammatory reaction at the choroid plexus supports the concept of viremic spread to the CNS. A second patient presenting with a similar constella-

tion of findings died of systemic coxsackievirus B3 infection. The dura was grossly distended, with swelling also of the pia, arachnoid, and brain parenchyma. Microscopically, round cell infiltrates were noted in the meninges overlying the cerebellum; the brain parenchyma was congested with increased numbers of oligodendrocytes. Lymphocytic infiltration was most prominent around blood vessels in the cerebral white matter and in the basal ganglia, again suggesting viremic access to the CNS; focal areas of necrosis and hemorrhage were also seen. The pathologic findings in EV myocarditis, as with myocarditis resulting from other etiologies, are classified according to criteria established in 1984 and known as the "Dallas criteria" (Aretz, 1987). Inflammation with mononuclear cells, usually in the interstitium (Fig. 7-1), is associated with widespread myocardial necrosis. With resolution, fibrosis may replace most inflammatory changes. Findings may be quite focal, with a wide spectrum of severity in the inflammatory response and resultant myocardial damage. Fatal newborn infection with EVs has shown nonspecific but extensive dam-

Heart   Liver

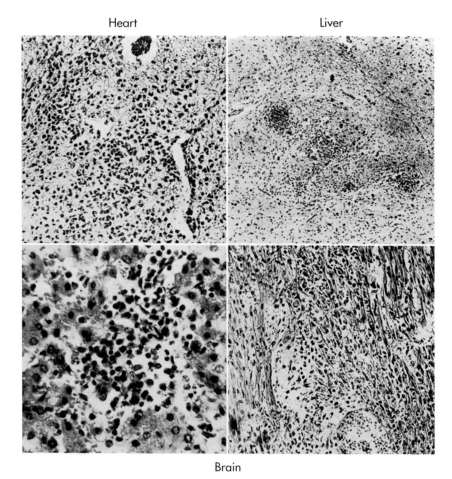

FIG. 7-1 Histologic appearance of the heart, liver, and brain in coxsackievirus infection, showing diffuse and focal cellular infiltration. (From van Crevald S, de Jager H: Ann Pediatr 1956; 187:100.)

Brain

age of infected tissues; echoviruses are associated with hepatic necrosis, progressing to cirrhosis, and disseminated intravascular coagulation in multiple organs. Neonatal coxsackievirus infections are similarly systemic in distribution of tissue damage, but with myocarditis often the dominant manifestation (see Fig. 7-1).

CLINICAL ILLNESS

The broad spectrum of clinical disease produced by the enteroviruses overlaps among groups. A list of the various syndromes and the serotype groups most commonly associated with them is in Table 7-1. The more common manifestations associated with infection are discussed briefly.

Nonspecific Febrile Illnesses

It is estimated that between 10 and 15 million people in the United States annually develop minor EV infections characterized by fever and nonspecific symptoms, with or without rashes (Strikas et al., 1986). These illnesses are of significance mainly for other diseases that they mimic, including bacterial sepsis, other viral exanthematous diseases, and herpes simplex infections; also, their age distribution makes them of great practical concern to the clinician. Most affected patients are young infants in whom differentiation of viral illness from the more alarming causes of nonspecific fevers and rashes is extremely difficult. In a prospective study of newborn infants in Rochester, New York, as many as 13% of infants born in the summer months were infected with enteroviruses during the first month of life; 21% of the infected infants were admitted to the hospital with suspected bacterial sepsis and received unnecessary antibiotics or antiherpes therapy (Jenista et al., 1984). It has been calculated that, during the months of seasonal prevalence, about 7 infants per 1,000 live births require hospitalization for neonatal enteroviral infection. Clinical manifestations include abrupt onset of fever, usually ≥39° C, with accompanying irritability; the fever may be biphasic. Additional symptoms, in order of decreasing frequency, include lethargy, anorexia, diarrhea, vomiting, rash (23% of patients), and respiratory symptoms. Aseptic meningitis may accompany the nonspecific symptoms of EV infection in infants, and there are no clinical features that distinguish between EV-infected infants with and without meningitis. The systemic, global nature of this illness results in hospitalization of many of these infants to rule out bacterial sepsis. The duration of symptomatic illness in young infants beyond the neonatal period is usually 4 to 5 days.

Respiratory Illnesses

Many EV infections are accompanied by nonspecific respiratory signs and symptoms, usually mild in nature. In a recent 10-year review of EV-associated respiratory illnesses, 46% of cases pre-

Table 7-1 Clinical manifestations of enterovirus infections

| Clinical syndrome | Poliovirus | Coxsackievirus | | Echovirus | Enteroviruses 68 to 71 |
		A	B		
Asymptomatic infection	X*	X	X	X	
Nonspecific febrile illness	X	X	X	X	
Respiratory disease		X	X	X	
Exanthems		X	X	X	
Enanthems		X			
Hemorrhagic conjunctivitis		X			X
Pleurodynia			X		
Orchitis					
Myocarditis			X		
Pericarditis			X	X	
Aseptic meningitis and meningoencephalitis	X	X	X	X	X
Disseminated neonatal infection			X	X	
Transitory muscle paresis	X	X	X	X	
Paralytic disease	X	X	X	X	X

*X, May be a result of multiple serotypes.

sented with URIs; 13% with respiratory distress or apnea; 13% with pneumonia; 12% with otitis media; and fewer cases with bronchiolitis, wheezing, croup, and pharyngotonsillitis (Chonmaitree and Mann, 1995). The clinical manifestations of EV-associated respiratory illnesses are indistinguishable from those resulting from other respiratory viruses. Pneumonia resulting from the EVs, although less common than other respiratory manifestations, has been associated with numerous serotypes. Several distinctive syndromes of EV respiratory illness have been well described and are discussed in the following paragraphs.

Hemorrhagic Conjunctivitis. From 1969 to 1971 acute hemorrhagic conjunctivitis was pandemic in Asia and Africa. More than 60,000 cases occurred in Singapore alone in September and October of 1970. In 1981 similar cases were reported in an outbreak in Florida. Enterovirus 70 was the responsible agent in all of these cases. Outbreaks of coxsackievirus A24v have also been widespread and temporally overlapped with EV70 outbreaks. The illnesses caused by the two serotypes are indistinguishable from each other. After an incubation period of about 24 hours, rapid onset of swelling of the eyelids—with congestion, lacrimation, and pain in the eyes—occurs. A minority of patients develop characteristics of subconjunctival hemorrhages, varying from petechiae to large blotches. Epithelial keratitis is common, transient, and seldom followed by subepithelial opacities. Preauricular adenopathy is frequent. Occasionally, a mucopurulent discharge from the eyes is found. The illness is generally nonsystemic, although transient lumbar radiculomyelopathy was encountered in Bombay, occurring 2 to 4 weeks after onset of the conjunctivitis. A poliomyelitis-like illness was described in some cases in Thailand (Wadia et al., 1983). Recovery is usually complete within 1 to 2 weeks of onset. Other EV serotypes have been known to cause outbreaks of acute conjunctivitis or keratoconjunctivitis, usually without hemorrhagic manifestations (Cherry, 1992).

Herpangina. Coxsackievirus A is the most common cause of herpangina, but the syndrome has also been reported with coxsackievirus B and the echoviruses. The highest incidence is among children 1 to 7 years old, but infection has also been described in neonates and adults. There is usually an abrupt onset of fever, associated with a sore throat, dysphagia, and malaise. One fourth of the patients may have vomiting and abdominal pain. Early in the illness, grayish-white vesicles measuring 1 to 4 mm in diameter appear over the posterior portion of the palate uvula and tonsillar pillars and occasionally on the oropharynx. These vesicles are discrete, are surrounded by erythema, and usually number fewer than twenty. The vesicles usually rupture, leaving punched-out ulcers that may enlarge slightly, and new vesicles may appear. The fever lasts 1 to 4 days; local and systemic symptoms begin to improve in 4 to 5 days, and recovery is usually complete within a week of onset (Cherry and Jahn, 1965).

Hand-Foot-and-Mouth Disease. Although hand-foot-and-mouth disease is one of the more common syndromes associated with coxsackievirus A16 (Robinson et al., 1957), other serotypes are sometimes isolated. In outbreaks, the highest attack rates are among children younger than 4 years old, but adults are also frequently affected, and intrafamilial spread is common. The disease is usually mild, and the onset is associated with a sore throat with or without a low-grade fever. Scattered vesicular lesions occur randomly on the oral structures, the pharynx, and the lips; these ulcerate readily, leaving shallow lesions with red areolae. About 85% of patients also develop sparse grayish vesicles (3 to 5 mm in diameter, surrounded by erythematous areolae) on the dorsum of the fingers, particularly in periungual areas, and on the margins of heels. Occasionally, palmar, plantar, and groin lesions may appear, particularly in young children.

Pleurodynia. Pleurodynia is primarily a disease of muscle that masquerades as pleuritic disease, although pleural involvement can occur; hence pleurodynia is often discussed as a respiratory manifestation of EV infection. Various members of the coxsackievirus B group are the usual causes of pleurodynia (also known as *epidemic myalgia, Bornholm disease, devil's grip*). The onset is abrupt in about three fourths of patients, with the remainder first developing prodromal symptoms of headache, malaise, anorexia, and vague myalgia lasting 1 to 10 days. The major symptom is severe paroxysmal pain referred to the lower ribs or the sternum. Deep breathing, coughing, and other movement accentuate the pain, which is described as knifelike stabbing, smothering, or catching. The pain may radiate to the shoulders, neck, or scapula and is characteristically lacking between paroxysms. Other symptoms include fever, headache, cough, anorexia, nausea, vomiting, and diarrhea. Fever is usually about 38° C, but temperature may vary from 37° C to 40° C. The mean duration of the illness is 3½ days, ranging from 1 to 14 days. Muscle tenderness is ordinarily not prominent, nor is frank myositis or muscle swelling, but some patients experience marked cutaneous hyperesthesia over the affected areas. A pleural friction rub may be heard in 25% of patients. There may be splinting and tenderness on abdominal examination, especially in the upper quadrants and periumbilical area. The chest roentgenogram is typically normal.

Exanthems

Nonspecific febrile illnesses and respiratory syndromes caused by the enteroviruses are frequently associated with rashes (Cherry, 1992). Younger children are more likely to develop exanthems, which vary widely in their characteristics. Macular and maculopapular eruptions indistinguishable from rubella have been observed with a number of coxsackieviruses and echoviruses. Petechiae have accompanied some rashes, especially with echovirus 9. The presence of virus has occasionally been demonstrated in skin lesions themselves.

Orchitis

Although viral orchitis most often is due to mumps, it has accompanied infections with coxsackievirus B.

Acute Myocarditis

The EVs are among the most commonly identified etiologies of myocarditis, although most cases of that disease may be undiagnosed (presenting as sudden death without autopsy) or, if diagnosed, have no identifiable cause. EVs may cause between 25% and 35% of cases of myocarditis for which a cause is found based on serology, nucleic acid hybridization, and/or PCR studies of endomyocardial biopsies and autopsy specimens (Martino et al., 1995). Neonates and young infants (≤6 months of age) are particularly susceptible to coxsackie B virus–associated myocarditis accompanying systemic infection with those serotypes (see congenital and neonatal infections). Most cases occur in young adults between the ages of 20 and 39 years. Rigorous exercise is anecdotally reported as a precedent to many cases of myocarditis, but it has never been systematically studied as a risk factor, except in animal models, where exercise does increase the incidence and severity of myocardial disease during EV infections.

Clinically, myocarditis reflects the regions and extent of the cardiac involvement. Symptoms include palpitations and chest pain, often with accompanying fever or a history of recent viral respiratory illness. Arrhythmias and sudden death reflect a prominent involvement of the conducting system, which may be of very recent onset; congestive heart failure or myocardial infarction–like presentation suggests more significant necrosis of myocytes and, most likely, longer-standing disease. Pericardial friction rub indicates a myopericarditis. Electrocardiographic findings include an evolution from early stage S-T segment elevation and T-wave inversion to intermediate-stage normalization to late-stage recurrence of T-wave inversion. Myocardial enzyme elevations are detected in the blood. Although most patients recover uneventfully from clinically apparent myocarditis, many have residual electrocardiographic or echocardiographic abnormalities for months to years. Smaller percentages of patients develop congestive heart failure, chronic myocarditis, or dilated cardiomyopathy (Martino et al., 1995).

Aseptic Meningitis and Encephalitis

The clinical disease observed during EV meningitis varies with the host's age and immune status. Neonates are at risk for severe systemic illness (see following section), of which meningitis or meningoencephalitis is commonly a part. EV meningitis outside of the immediate (≤2 weeks of age) neonatal period is rarely associated with severe disease or poor outcome. Onset is usually sudden, and fever of 38° to 40° C is the most consistent clinical finding, occurring in 75% to 100% of patients (Wilfert et al., 1983). The fever pattern may be biphasic, appearing first with nonspecific constitutional symptoms, followed by resolution and reappearance with the onset of meningeal signs. Nuchal rigidity is found in more than half of the patients, particularly in children older than 1 to 2 years of age. Headache is nearly always present in adults and children old enough to report it, and photophobia is also common. Nonspecific and constitutional signs and symptoms of viral infection, in decreasing order of occurrence, include vomiting, anorexia, rash, diarrhea, cough and upper-respiratory findings (particularly pharyngitis), diarrhea, and myalgias. Symptoms other than fever may also be biphasic, a presentation observed more often in adults than children. Neurologic abnormalities are unusual. The duration of illness resulting from EV meningitis is usually less than 1 week, with many patients feeling better immediately after the lumbar puncture, presumably because of the transient reduction of intracranial pressure with fluid removal. Adult patients may have symptoms that persist for several weeks, an observation not frequently made in children. The prognosis for young children with EV meningitis early in life appears to be good, without strong evidence of long-term sequelae (Rorabaugh et al., 1992).

Encephalitis caused by EVs is well known but is nonetheless thought to be an unusual complication. Unlike aseptic meningitis, encephalitis caused by an EV may have more profound acute disease and long-term sequelae. In contrast to the typical focal disease seen with herpes simplex virus encephalitis, EVs have been more commonly associated with global encephalitis and generalized neurologic depression. The illness usually begins like aseptic meningitis, with a prodrome of fever, myalgias, and upper-respiratory symptoms. Onset of CNS signs and symptoms is often abrupt, with confusion, weakness, lethargy, drowsiness, or irritability. Progression to coma or generalized seizures may occur. When meningeal signs and CSF pleocytosis accompany these findings, *meningoencephalitis* is the appropriate term. Focal EV encephalitis is less commonly reported than global disease, but its incidence may be underappreciated. As evidenced in the NIAID antiviral studies, EVs are demonstrable by brain biopsy in 13% of patients suspected of having herpes simplex encephalitis, the most commonly identified cause of focal encephalitis (Whitley et al., 1989).

The unique situation of a child or adult with absent or deficient humoral immunity illustrates an important "experiment of nature" with regard to EV infections of the CNS. Unlike other viruses, which are largely contained by cellular immune mechanisms, the EVs are cleared from the host by antibody-mediated mechanisms. Agammaglobulinemic individuals infected with the EVs may develop chronic meningitis or meningoencephalitis lasting many years, often with fatal outcome (McKinney et al., 1987). Approximately 50% of these infected patients also develop a rheumatologic syndrome, most often dermatomyositis, which is also felt to be a direct result of EV infection of the affected tissues. Treatment with antibody preparations intravenously and intrathecally or intraventricularly has resulted in stabilization of some of these patients; however, viral persistence has been documented during therapy. With the availability of intravenous preparations of immune globulin and the early recognition of this illness, fewer patients appear to be progressing according to the classic description of this disease, and atypical neurologic presentations have appeared (Webster et al., 1993).

Congenital and Neonatal Infections

The infected neonate appears to be at greatest risk for severe morbidity and mortality when signs and symptoms develop in the first days of life, suggesting a possible transplacental acquisition (Abzug et al., 1993). Maternal illness has been reported in 59% to 68% of infected neonates. Even in the youngest patients, fever is ubiquitous, accompanied early by nonspecific signs such as vomiting, anorexia, rash, and upper-respiratory findings. Neurologic involvement may or may not be associated with signs of meningeal inflammation, including nuchal rigidity and bulging anterior fontanelle. As the neonatal disease progresses, major systemic manifestations such as hepatic necrosis, myocarditis, and necrotizing enterocolitis may develop. Disseminated intravascular coagulation and other findings of sepsis result in a patient with illness that may be indistinguishable from that caused by overwhelming bacterial infection. The CNS disease may progress to a more encephalitic picture, with seizures and focal neurologic findings suggestive of herpes simplex virus. The incidences of morbidity and mortality resulting from perinatal EV infections are not precisely known, but they may be as high as 74% and 10%, respectively (Kaplan et al., 1983; Modlin, 1986). When death occurs, it is typically a result of hepatic failure (echoviruses) or myocarditis (coxsackieviruses).

Poliomyelitis

Poliovirus infections range from asymptomatic to paralytic illness. The ratio of inapparent infection to paralytic infection variously is estimated as 100:1 to 850:1. Even with overt infection, most persons have a mild and brief illness, starting abruptly and lasting from a few hours to a few days. The illness is characterized by fever, uneasiness, sore throat, headache, nausea, anorexia, vomiting, and pain in the abdomen; one or more of these symptoms may occur. Except for slight redness of the throat, there usually are no physical findings, and there are no signs of involvement of the CNS. This may be the entire self-limited illness (minor illness). These nonspecific symptoms may also occur as the initial presentation of aseptic meningitis or paralytic disease.

Nonparalytic Poliomyelitis. Nonparalytic poliomyelitis (aseptic meningitis) is characterized by many of the features just listed and by pain and stiffness of the neck, back, and legs. Headache is more severe, the temperature is higher, and the patient is sicker than with minor illness. Hyperesthesia and sometimes paresthesia may occur. The CSF shows a pleocytosis with a slight predominance of polymorphonuclear leukocytes, with subsequent increase in the proportion of lymphocytes. The protein level is slightly elevated. As the protein level rises later in illness, the cell count declines.

Paralytic Disease. Poliovirus infection, especially type 1, is responsible for most of the paralytic disease caused by EVs. Occasional cases of transient paralysis and muscle weakness have been noted with other EVs, particularly the coxsackievirus B agents. Enteroviruses 70 and 71 have been associated with paralytic disease and encephalitis (Hayward et al., 1989; Wadia et al., 1983). Three of five children with enterovirus 71 paralysis had residual weakness and muscle wasting.

With classic paralytic polio, there is a 2- to 6-day incubation period with an initial nonspecific febrile illness. This period probably coincides with early replication of virus in the pharynx and gastrointestinal tract. With the subsequent hematogenous spread of virus, CNS involvement may result in meningitis and anterior horn cell infection. From 1% to 4% of susceptible patients infected with polioviruses develop CNS involvement. The spectrum of paralytic disease is enormously variable and may involve the denervation of an isolated muscle group or extensive denervation and paralysis of all extremities. Characteristically, the picture is one of asymmetrical distribution, with the lower extremities more frequently involved than the upper. Large muscle groups are affected more often than the small muscles of the hands and feet. Involvement of cervical and thoracic segments of the spinal cord may result in paralysis of the muscles of respiration. Infection of cells in the medulla and cranial nerve nuclei results in bulbar polio with compromise of the respiratory and vasomotor centers.

Studies have indicated that tonsillectomy and adenoidectomy within a month of infection predispose to paralytic poliomyelitis including bulbar involvement. Strenuous exercise and fatigue occurring at the onset of the major illness have often been followed by severe paralysis. Intramuscular injections of vaccines—especially combinations of diphtheria, tetanus, and pertussis—have been associated with subsequent paralysis in the injected extremity. With the return of the patient's temperature to normal, the progress of paralysis ceases, and the subsequent weeks and months reveal a variable spectrum of recovery ranging from full return of function to significant residual paralysis. Atrophy of involved muscles becomes apparent after 4 to 8 weeks. Recovery may be exceedingly slow, and its full extent cannot be judged for 6 to 18 months.

On clinical grounds it is impossible to distinguish nonparalytic and preparalytic poliomyelitis from aseptic meningitis of another cause. Paralytic poliomyelitis has been confused with infectious polyneuritis, or Guillain-Barré syndrome. Since the striking decrease in incidence of poliomyelitis in the postvaccine era, the most commonly recognized causes of aseptic meningitis are coxsackieviruses and echoviruses.

In the United States in the vaccine era fewer than ten paralytic cases of poliomyelitis are reported per year. The majority is associated with receipt of attenuated vaccine or contact with a vaccine. The differential diagnosis should consider paralysis caused by other enteroviruses, Guillain-Barré syndrome, and transverse myelitis.

As many as 25% of individuals who recover from paralytic disease may develop the syndrome of postpoliomyelitis muscular atrophy (Dalakas et al., 1995). Characterized by recurrent weakness, pain, and atrophy 25 to 30 years after the initial acute infection, the clinical course of this manifestation is usually a gradual one that seldom results in total disability of the affected areas. Although ongoing viral infection or reactivation has been postulated, most researchers believe that the postpoliomyelitis syndrome is a result at least in part of aging and neuronal dropout in already compromised neuromuscular connections.

Bulbar Poliomyelitis. Bulbar poliomyelitis is characterized by damage to the motor nuclei of the cranial nerves and other vital zones in the medulla concerned with respiration and circulation. It may occur in the absence of clinically recognized involvement of the spinal cord. Bulbar poliomyelitis is potentially the most life-endangering form. The incidence of bulbar involvement varies from 5% to 10% of the total number of paralytic cases. In a Minnesota group of 107 cases, cranial nerve nuclei were affected in descending frequency, with the tenth nerve affected in 90%, seventh in 66%, eleventh in 37%, sixth and twelfth in 14%, third in 11%, and fifth in 9%.

The most ominous form of bulbar poliomyelitis results from spread of infection to the respiratory and vasomotor centers. Damage to the respiratory center causes breathing to become irregular in rhythm and depth. Respirations are shallow and are associated with periods of apnea. The pulse rate and temperature increase. The blood pressure, at first elevated, may drop rapidly to shock levels. The patient becomes confused, delirious, and comatose, and then respiration stops. When the vasomotor center is involved, the pulse becomes extremely rapid, irregular, and difficult to palpate. The blood pressure fluctuates from high to low levels, with a small pulse pressure.

Possible Enterovirus Diseases

Juvenile-onset diabetes mellitus, dermatomyositis or polymyositis, and chronic fatigue syndrome have been postulated to be the result of an initial enterovirus infection followed by an aberrant host immune response. Persistence of virus during the chronic phases of these illnesses has been purported based on PCR studies, but similar assays by other investigators fail to find evidence of acute or persistent infection. The actual role of enteroviruses in these illnesses remains to be determined.

EPIDEMIOLOGY

The epidemiology of all human enteroviruses is quite similar. The pattern is most clearly defined for the polioviruses because paralytic disease has been identifiable. As early as 1916, the epidemiologic features were defined on the basis of an outbreak that occurred that year in New York City. These principles were (1) that poliomyelitis is exclusively a human infection, transmitted from person to person; (2) that the infection is far more prevalent than is apparent from the incidence of clinically recognized cases; (3) that the most important sources of infection are asymptomatic or mild illnesses escaping recognition; and (4) that an epidemic of 1 to 3 recognized cases per 1,000 infects the general population to such an extent that the outbreak declines spontaneously.

Enteroviruses have a worldwide distribution, with increased prevalence during the warm months of the year in temperate climates. In the United States it is estimated that the enteroviruses cause 10 to 15 million symptomatic infections each year; some variation in geographic distribution of infections may be due to importation of viruses from other countries. Epidemics occur between May and October in the United States and other areas of the Northern temperate zone, but sporadic infections are identified throughout the year. The seroepidemiology of enteroviral infections demonstrates an increased transmission of infection at a young age among persons of lower socioeconomic status. Crowded living conditions and poor hygiene enhance the fecal-to-oral transmission of these agents. Surveillance data on isolates obtained from March through May have been successfully used to predict the serotypes that will predominate from July to December.

Among the nonpoliovirus EVs, each EV season in each part of the world is dominated by only a few serotypes. In the United States, the fifteen most commonly occurring EVs account for more than 80% of all U.S. EV isolates (Strikas et al., 1986). The predominant serotypes cycle with varying periodicity, a reflection of the availability of new susceptible host populations, especially children, within a community. Serotypes with "endemic" patterns (i.e., occurring with significant incidence every year) are most likely to affect only the youngest children. They are the most susceptible to these serotypes for the same reason that they are most susceptible to many common infections—the absence of previous exposure and immunity. Older children and adults are more likely to predominate in an outbreak of a serotype that has not been present in a community for several years, creating a reservoir of susceptibles among children born since the last appearance of that serotype. Overall, enteroviral illness is most commonly reported in children 1 to 4 years old. The infections may occur more frequently in infants, and recognition and reporting of disease may reflect an enhanced concern over any illness at that age. Nevertheless, when specific outbreaks occur within a community, persons of all ages may be infected.

The clinical epidemiology of these infections suggests that respiratory excretion of virus is not as important a means of spread as is fecal-to-oral transmission. Intimate human contact is important in transmission of virus, and communicability within households is greatest between children. Diapered infants apparently are more efficient disseminators of infection than other individuals. In the current era of day-care centers and nursery school it already has been shown that hepatitis A virus, a nonenteroviral picornavirus, is transmitted in this setting and, if present, is transmitted to virtually all children in the nursery. It is likely that outbreaks of infection caused by enteroviruses are also occurring in these facilities.

Community outbreaks of enteroviral infection can spread to hospital nurseries. A newborn who acquires a virus from his mother or from nursery personnel may spread it throughout the nursery. The viruses can be introduced into intensive care units by patients or personnel. Recognition of such infections imposes a need to institute isolation precautions such as cohorting of infants and personnel to minimize spread of infection.

IMMUNITY

Enteroviruses induce secretory and humoral antibody responses. The humoral responses initially are predominantly IgM antibodies, followed by IgA and IgG antibodies that persist for months to years. Coproantibodies, primarily IgA, have been studied as a response to administration of poliovirus vaccines or to natural infection. Local secretory immunoglobulin A production occurs at the site of contact of the virus with lymphoid cells. Development of type-specific antibody provides lifelong protection against clinical illness caused by the same agents. Local reinfection of the gastrointestinal tract may occur, but this is accompanied by an abbreviated period of viral replication without clinical illness.

In experimental poliovirus infection, specific IgG antibody-producing cells and measurable antibodies can be demonstrated in areas of the CNS where virus is replicating. Local CNS antibody production is independent of systemic humoral antibody production. Although specific CNS enteroviral antibodies are probably produced primarily within the CNS, some passive transfer of serum antibody to the CSF may occur as permeability is increased by inflammation. Evidence for the extreme importance of CNS antibody is deduced from agammaglobulinemic patients who are unable to eliminate enteroviruses from the CNS. Administration of extraordinarily large quantities of parenteral globulin or plasma with specific antibody is necessary to achieve measurable antibody levels in the CSF (Weiner et al., 1979).

Cellular immunity against enteroviral infection is not well defined. Circulating peripheral white blood cells have been a source of viral isolation during acute illness. Recognition of virus by lymphocytes occurs in experimental models using coxsackieviruses. As noted earlier, cell-mediated mechanisms may actually facilitate the develop-

ment of certain enteroviral illnesses, such as myocarditis.

DIAGNOSIS

Isolation of EVs in cell culture remains the standard for laboratory diagnosis. The commercial availability of increasing numbers and types of continuous cell lines has provided numerous options for routine EV culturing; however, no single cell line is optimal for all EV serotypes. The most sensitive method for diagnosis of some coxsackievirus A infections—isolation in suckling mice—is now rarely performed because of the difficulty of the technique and of the animal maintenance.

There are numerous compelling reasons for seeking a rapid direct diagnostic assay for the EVs. Isolation of EVs in cell culture and recognition of cytopathic effect require a high level of expertise and may be quite labor-intensive. Some EV serotypes, particularly within the coxsackievirus A group, do not grow at all in cell culture. Of greater significance, 25% to 35% of specimens from patients with characteristic EV infections of any serotype are negative by cell culture because of antibody neutralization in situ; because of inadequate collection, handling, and processing of the samples; or because of insensitivity intrinsic to the cell lines used. EVs that do grow in cell culture may do so slowly. Reported mean isolation times for EVs from cerebrospinal fluid range from 3.7 to 8.2 days; EVs from other sites, where viral titers are higher, often grow more rapidly.

The absence of a widely shared antigen has hampered the development of immunoassays for the EVs. The greatest success has been with assays limited to a particular subgroup of EV serotypes (e.g., coxsackievirus B) that share a common antigen. Recent reports of polyclonal and monoclonal antibodies that cross-react with multiple EV serotypes are promising, but further testing is required to determine the clinical relevance of those observations (Yousef et al., 1987).

The most promising development in direct detection of the EVs has been the application of the polymerase chain reaction (PCR). Several sets of PCR primers and probes that detect the majority of EV serotypes have been described. All are directed at highly conserved regions of the 5′ noncoding region of the viral genome and designed for reverse transcription combined with PCR (RT-PCR). Enteroviral RT-PCR using these primer/probe sets has now been tested in clinical settings by numerous investigators and has been found to be consistently more sensitive than culture and virtually 100% specific (Rotbart, 1990; Sawyer et al., 1994). A colorimetric, microwell titer–based PCR assay for the EVs has been developed and is in clinical trials; preliminary results show high sensitivity and specificity for this assay in aseptic meningitis, nonspecific febrile illnesses, and neonatal enterovirus infections.

Acute and convalescent serum samples obtained 7 to 21 days apart help define quantitative changes in antibody titers. Complement fixation; viral neutralization; immunoprecipitation; enzyme-linked immunosorbent assay (ELISA); and, in a few instances, hemagglutination inhibition are the available techniques for assaying enterovirus antibodies. Neutralizing antibodies are type-specific, whereas complement fixation demonstrates group-reactive antibodies. In the course of a lifetime humans sustain multiple infections, occult or overt, with a variety of enteroviruses. IgM serology for coxsackievirus B has had some clinical use (McCartney et al., 1986). A specific infection elicits the production of antibody specific to that virus type but also may prompt an anamnestic response demonstrated by an increase in group-reactive antibody and by parallel rises in antibodies to serotypes of some of the other enteroviruses previously encountered. The concomitant serologic rises in heterologous antibody titer create problems with serologic surveys, rendering the complement fixation test inadequate to define a specific infection. In the absence of the recovery of a virus the problem of seeking specific antibody rises against the whole genus of enteroviruses remains. Thus the complexity of serology makes the serologic diagnosis of these infections impractical.

TREATMENT

Specific antiviral therapy for the EVs is not currently available for clinical use, although a number of drugs have been developed that have efficacy in vitro and in animal studies (O'Connell et al., 1995). One of these drugs, pleconaril, is in phase II clinical trials for aseptic meningitis and has recently been made available for compassionate use release to agammaglobulinemic patients with chronic enteroviral meningoencephalitis (Pevear et al., 1996). This drug, as well as several others of the same class in development, slips through a pore at the base of the receptor canyon (described earlier) and binds within a hydrophobic pocket beneath the canyon floor, preventing the steric change required by the EVs for uncoating.

As noted earlier, clearance of EVs by the host is antibody mediated, and, as might be expected, exogenously administered antibody has been useful in certain EV infections. Some patients with agammaglobulinemia and chronic EV meningitis or meningoencephalitis have shown stabilization and improvement during therapy with gamma globulin, often administered by multiple routes including directly into the CNS; other patients are less responsive to this therapy. Neonates with overwhelming EV sepsis, including meningitis, have received intravenous gamma globulin, maternal plasma, and exchange transfusions in attempts to reverse their otherwise bleak course, with occasional success. A single randomized trial of IV gamma globulin plus standard therapy versus standard therapy alone in neonates suspected of having EV infection in the first 2 weeks of life was undertaken; however, too few patients were enrolled for a definitive conclusion regarding clinical efficacy. A reduction in viral shedding was seen in the treatment group. For other EV infections in which antibody formation occurs endogenously, there is no evidence for a benefit of immune serum globulin administration once signs of the illness have already appeared. Treatment for these manifestations remains symptomatic.

PREVENTION

Because there currently is no widely available specific treatment for enterovirus infections, efforts have focused on means of prevention. The multiple antigenic types and the usual self-limited course of most echovirus and coxsackievirus infections have resulted in little stimulus to the development of vaccines. The story of the poliovirus vaccines, however, has been one of the most exciting and rewarding in microbiologic history.

Enders and colleagues' tissue culture techniques lent themselves to the propagation in vitro of sufficient amounts of relatively pure poliovirus, so that controlled formaldehyde inactivation could be used to produce a noninfectious virus that retained its antigenicity (Enders et al., 1949). Salk and his colleagues pursued this line of research and by 1954 were able to embark on a field trial that established the efficacy of an inactivated poliovirus vaccine in the prevention of paralytic disease. The vaccine was widely used in the United States during the 5 years from 1956 through 1960. The results were dramatic. With the widespread use of Salk vaccine, 10,000 to 20,000 cases of paralytic disease decreased to 2,000 to 3,000 reported annually.

By the early 1960s a second vaccine was available. Strains of poliovirus that Sabin had selected and studied in his laboratory were proven attenuated for monkey and man. Ingestion of these strains resulted in intestinal infection and viral excretion so that humoral and gastrointestinal tract immunity developed without any illness. This vaccine could be administered more readily (by the oral route) and the multiplication in the gastrointestinal tract more closely mimicked natural infection. These advantages led to its replacing the injectable Salk vaccine. Over the first 5 years of the 1960s more than 400 million doses of oral vaccine were distributed in the United States. At the same time, trials also were successfully conducted in European nations, Japan, and other countries. The use of oral vaccine in this country was accompanied by a further decrease in the annual reported polio cases (Fig. 7-2) so that, beginning in 1966, fewer than 100 cases have been reported each year. From 1980 through 1988 a total of 81 cases of paralytic polio have been reported. In less than 20 years a disease that had claimed thousands of victims annually and that had been the source of indescribable community anxiety was reduced to a rarity.

In the complex processes of development, commercial production, and widespread use of polio vaccines, a number of unexpected events transpired that merit consideration. After the highly successful field trials of 1954, commercial manufacture of the Salk type of vaccine was licensed. Within a few weeks of its use, paralytic disease was observed in April through June of 1955 among children in California and Idaho who had received some of the first lots of commercial vaccine manufactured by the Cutter Laboratories. By the time this occurrence had been fully investigated and resolved, it was learned that there were 204 cases of vaccine-associated disease. Seventy-nine were among children who had received the vaccine, 105 were among their family contacts, and 20 were in community contacts. Nearly three quarters of the cases were paralytic, and there were 11 deaths. The agent isolated from these patients was type 1 poliovirus. Laboratory tests on vaccine revealed viable virulent type 1 poliovirus in 7 of 17 lots (Nathanson and Langmuir, 1963). Revisions of the federal regulations governing the steps in vaccine manufacture were promulgated and implemented to prevent recurrence of such a tragic episode.

Manufacturers faced further difficulties in maintaining the fine balance between the complete elimination of the infectious live virus from the production process and the retention of effective antigenicity of the inactivated components. A number of lots of vaccine subsequently were proven to be poorly antigenic for type 3 poliovirus. As a result, when community polio outbreaks occurred among well-immunized groups, there were "breakthroughs" with paralytic disease, especially caused by type 3 virus, in previously immunized subjects. Such an outbreak was studied in 1959 in Massachusetts, where an analysis of polio cases revealed that 47% (62 of 137) of the patients had previously received three or more inoculations of inactivated vaccine (Berkovich et al., 1961).

In the United States almost all current immunization is performed with the oral attenuated product. A number of European countries, especially those in Scandinavia, have adhered to the use of in-

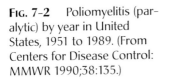

FIG. 7-2   Poliomyelitis (paralytic) by year in United States, 1951 to 1989. (From Centers for Disease Control: MMWR 1990;38:135.)

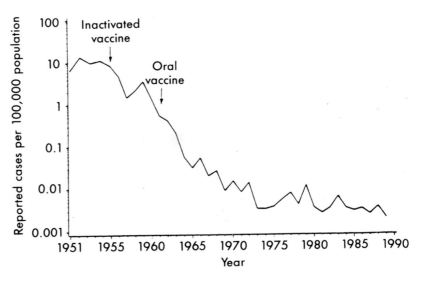

activated polio vaccine (IPV). Their record of achievement in the control of polio had been parallel to that of this country until 1984. From August 1984 through January 1985 nine cases of paralytic poliomyelitis and one case of aseptic meningitis caused by the wild type of virus occurred in Finland. Widespread poliovirus circulation was documented throughout the country by isolation of poliovirus type 3 from asymptomatic family members and sewage. Seven of the ten patients had received 3 to 5 doses of inactivated vaccine; one person received 1 dose; and two persons, ages 31 and 48 years, had not been immunized (Centers for Disease Control, 1986). The IPV vaccine in use in Finland produced lower levels of antibodies to poliovirus 3 than to types 1 and 2. As of 1987 more potent IPV became available and is now the standard IPV in use. However, persons immunized only with IPV can excrete polioviruses for longer periods and in larger quantities because of the absence of gastrointestinal tract immunity (Onorata et al., 1991). This may facilitate community circulation of polioviruses. An essential question is whether a person previously vaccinated with IPV with waning humoral immunity and lacking gastrointestinal immunity is again at risk of paralytic disease, because virulent virus can multiply in the gastrointestinal tract and produce viremia before an anamnestic humoral response to virus can occur.

The marked decrease in paralytic disease caused by "wild" polioviruses has disclosed a small but significant number of cases of oral vaccine recipients who have developed paralytic illness in temporal association with the ingestion of vaccine. Paralytic episodes have also been reported among susceptible family or community contacts of the vaccine recipients. Fewer than ten cases per year of paralytic disease are identified in the United States. A portion of these patients are immunodeficient children, particularly those with congenital hypogammaglobulinemia. Increased neurovirulence (i.e., reversion) has been documented after viral replication in the gastrointestinal tract. The overall figure of risk to recipients and their contacts is one case per 2.5 million doses of vaccine distributed. The calculated risk of paralysis is one case per 750,000 doses with the first dose of vaccine.

The small but disturbing risk of vaccine-associated paralytic poliomyelitis (VAPP) has prompted wide debate for many years regarding ideal immunization strategies in countries, such as the United States, where indigenous poliomyelitis has been eliminated. In countries with residual wild polio infections, there is universal agreement that strategies using live, attenuated, oral poliovirus vaccine are the most effective approaches toward ultimate eradication of the disease (see the following paragraphs). The concern over VAPP has very recently resulted in the first major change in nearly three decades in poliovirus vaccination recommendations in the United States. A total of 4 doses of poliovirus vaccine is still recommended. The Advisory Committee on Immunization Practices (of the Centers for Disease Control and Prevention) now recommends a sequential poliovirus immunization schedule in which IPV is given at the first two sittings (usually 2 and 4 months), followed by OPV for the final 2 doses (at 12 to 18 months and at 4 to 6 years). The use of initial IPV immunization is hoped to decrease the chances of VAPP associated with early OPV administration and still provide optimal intestinal immunity with the final 2 doses of OPV. The risk of VAPP is highest with the first dose of OPV, both to the vaccinee and to contacts of the vaccinee; IPV is expected to protect immunocompetent individuals from subsequent OPV and to decrease OPV shedding and subsequent exposure of contacts. The delay of several months in giving OPV is also envisioned as an opportunity to diagnose immunodeficiency in infants before they are inadvertently given live virus vaccine. The net effect is projected to prevent half or more cases of VAPP. Although it prefers the sequential IPV-OPV immunization schedule, the Advisory Committee on Immunization Practices continues to find traditional (4-dose) OPV-only or IPV-only regimens to be acceptable. The Committee on Infectious Diseases of the American Academy of Pediatrics has concluded that all three regimens are equally acceptable. The flexibility inherent in these guidelines acknowledges the difficulties anticipated in administering the sequential IPV-OPV series, including the need for additional injections and the potential for reduced compliance. Some have voiced concerns that the new recommendations will result in decreased overall vaccination rates because of the number of injections and additional physician visits required, with yet unproven capability of actually reducing the 6 to 8 annual cases of VAPP. Combination vaccines (polio with other childhood vaccines) are under development that should address compliance issues by resulting in fewer injections and physician visits. It is anticipated that the IPV-OPV sequential strategy is a transitional one only, with IPV-only recommended as global eradication nears reality.

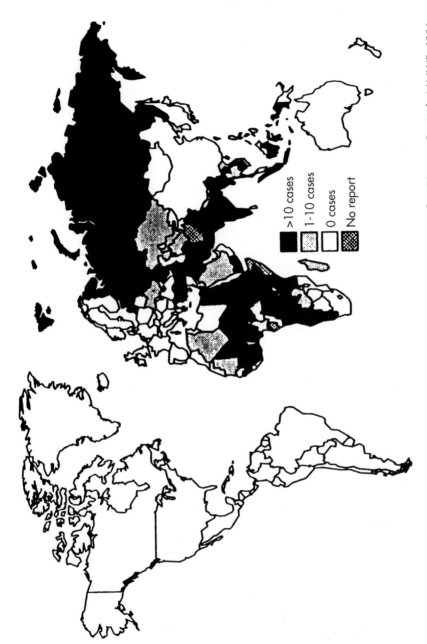

Fig. 7-3 Reported cases of poliomyelitis worldwide in 1995. (From Centers for Disease Control: MMWR 1996; 45:565–568.)

IPV-only schedules (i.e., 4 IPV doses) are still recommended for immunocompromised individuals and their household contacts and for infants of households where adults may be incompletely immunized against poliovirus. OPV-only schedules are recommended where accelerated immunization is required, such as for children who are beginning immunization after 6 months of age, and in populations where immunization is inadequate (as noted previously).

The achievements with poliovirus vaccination have been impressive in the United States, Canada, Latin America, and most of Europe, Australia, and some Asian and African nations. Wild paralytic poliomyelitis has been absent from the Western hemisphere since 1991. There have been no cases of the wild type of disease originating in the United States since 1979 (Fig. 7-3). In 1995 150 countries reported zero cases of poliomyelitis (see Fig. 7-3), compared to only 88 countries in 1988 (Centers for Disease Control, 1996). The total worldwide cases reported dropped 80% during this same period, and preliminary data for 1996 suggest a further decrease by greater than 50% from the 1995 incidence.

The global eradication strategy of the World Health Organization, which is responsible for much of this success, is founded in four principles: achievement and maintenance of high routine vaccination coverage levels among children, with at least 3 doses of oral poliovirus vaccine; development of sensitive systems of epidemiologic and laboratory surveillance (including molecular epidemiologic tools); administration of supplementary doses of oral poliovirus vaccine to all young children during National Immunization Days (NIDs) to rapidly interrupt poliovirus transmission; and "mopping up" vaccination campaigns targeted at high-risk areas. In 1995 all polio-endemic countries in Europe and Asia (with the exception of the Democratic People's Republic of Korea, Myanmar, Nepal, and Yemen) conducted NIDs; in 1996 each of the four countries that did not participate in 1995 conducted or had scheduled such NIDs to be conducted. More than 300 million children were immunized worldwide during NIDs in 1995. Approximately 60% of currently reported polio cases occur on the Indian subcontinent. Bangladesh, India, Nepal, Pakistan, and Sri Lanka have scheduled synchronized NIDs for December 1996 and January 1997; Myanmar and Thailand will also conduct NIDs in those months (Centers for Disease Control, 1996). Great challenges remain in the eradication of polio from the African continent, as well, because of infrastructure deficiencies in health, communications, and transportation. Nevertheless, NIDs have been scheduled for all countries in Africa by the end of 1997. A beneficial outgrowth of the WHO polio eradication program has been the mobilization of political and economic support for preventive medicine and public health, renewed focus on an infrastructure of child health programs, and enthusiasm for pursuing other diseases, such as measles. It is clearly premature to relax the use of poliovirus vaccination in those parts of the world where disease has been nearly eradicated. The possibility of the inadvertent introduction of virulent virus is omnipresent.

BIBLIOGRAPHY

Abzug MJ, Levin MJ, Rotbart HA. Profile of enterovirus disease in the first two weeks of life. Pediatr Infect Dis J 1993;12:820-824.

Aretz HT. Myocarditis: the Dallas Criteria. Hum Pathol 1987;18:619-624.

Berkovich S, Pickering JE, Kibrick S. Paralytic poliomyelitis in Massachusetts, 1959. A study of the disease in a well-vaccinated population. N Engl J Med 1961;264:1323.

Bodian D. Histopathologic basis of the clinical findings in poliomyelitis. Am J Med 1949;6:563.

Centers for Disease Control. MMWR update: poliomyelitis outbreak—Finland, 1984-85. MMWR 1986;35:82-86.

Centers for Disease Control. MMWR summary of notifiable disease, US 1989-1990. MMWR 1990;38:35.

Centers for Disease Control. MMWR update: Progress toward global eradication of poliomyelitis, 1995. MMWR 1996;45:565-568.

Cherry JD. Enteroviruses: polioviruses (poliomyelitis), coxsackieviruses, echoviruses, and enteroviruses. In Feigin RD, Cherry JD (eds). Textbook of pediatric infectious diseases, ed 3. Philadelphia: WB Saunders, 1992.

Cherry JD, Jahn CL. Herpangina: the etiologic spectrum. Pediatrics 1965;36:632-634.

Chonmaitree T, Mann L. Respiratory infections. In Rotbart HA (ed). Human enterovirus infections. Washington, D.C.: ASM Press, 1995.

Dalakas MC, Bartfield H, Kurland T (eds). The postpolio syndrome: advances in the pathogenesis and treatment. Annals of the New York Academy of Sciences, Vol. 753, 1995.

Dalldorf G, Sickless GM. An unidentified filtrable agent isolated from the faces of children with paralysis. Science 1948;108:61-62.

Enders JF, Weller TH, Robbins FC. Cultivation of the Lansing strain of poliomyelitis virus in cultures of various human embryonic tissues. Science 1949;109:85.

Hayward JC, Gillespie SM, Kaplan KM, et al. Outbreak of poliomyelitis like paralysis associated with enterovirus 71. Pediatr Infect Dis 1989;8:611-616.

Hellen CUT, Wimmer E. Enterovirus genetics. In Rotbart HA (ed). Human enterovirus infections. Washington, D.C.: ASM Press, 1995.

Hogle JM, Chow M, Filman DJ. Three-dimensional structure of poliovirus at 2.9Å resolution. Science 1985;229:1358-1365.

Jenista JA, Powell KR, Menegus MA. Epidemiology of neonatal enterovirus infection. J Pediatr 1984;104:685.

Kaplan MH, Klein SW, McPhee J, et al. Group B coxsackievirus infections in infants younger than three months of age: a serious childhood illness. Rev Infect Dis 1983;5:1019-1032.

Martino TA, Liu P, Petric M, Sole MJ. Enteroviral myocarditis and dilated cardiomyopathy: a review of clinical and experimental studies. In Rotbart HA (ed). Human enterovirus infections. Washington, D.C.: ASM Press, 1995.

McCartney RA, Banatvala JE, Bell EJ. Routine use of antibody capture ELISA for the serological diagnosis of coxsackie B virus infections. J Med Virol 1986;19:205-212.

McKinney RE, Katz SL, Wilfert CM. Chronic enteroviral meningoencephalitis in agammaglobulinemic patients. Rev Infect Dis 1987;2:334-356.

Melnick JL, Tagaya I, Von Magnus H. Enteroviruses 69, 70, and 71. Intervirology 1974;4:369-370.

Mendelsohn CL, Wimmer E, Racaniello VR. Cellular receptor for poliovirus: molecular cloning, nucleotide sequence, and expression of a new member of the immunoglobulin superfamily. Cell 1989;56:855-865.

Modlin JF. Perinatal echovirus infection: insights from a literature review of 61 cases of serious infection and 16 outbreaks in nurseries. Rev Infect Dis 8:918-926,1986.

Nathanson N, Langmuir AD. The Cutter incident, I, II, III. Am J Hyg 1963;78:16-81.

O'Connell J, Albin R, Blum D, et al. Development of antiviral agents for picornavirus infections. In Rotbart HA (ed). Human enterovirus infections. Washington, D.C.: ASM Press, 1995.

Onorata IM, Modlin JF, McBeam AM, et al. Mucosal immunity induced by enhanced potency inactivated and oral polio vaccines. J Infect Dis 1991;163:1-6.

Pevear DC, Seipel ME, Pallansch M, McKinlay MA. In vitro activity of VP 63843 against field isolates of nonpolio enteroviruses. Abstracts of the thirty-sixth ICAAC, New Orleans, 1996.

Racaniello VR. Early events in infection: receptor binding and cell entry. In Rotbart HA (ed). Human enterovirus infections. Washington, D.C.: ASM Press, 1995.

Ren R, Racaniello V. Human poliovirus receptor gene expression and poliovirus tissue tropism in transgenic mice. J Virol 1992;66:296-304.

Robinson CR, Doane FW, Rhodes AJ. Report of an outbreak of febrile illness with pharyngeal lesions and exanthem, Toronto summer 1957: isolation of group A coxsackievirus. Can Med Assoc J 1957;79:615.

Romero JR, Rotbart HA. Sequence analysis of the downstream 5′ nontranslated region of seven echoviruses with different neurovirulence phenotypes. J Virol 1995;69:1370-1375.

Rorabaugh ML, Berlin LE, Rosenberg L, et al. Absence of neurodevelopmental sequelae from aseptic meningitis. Pediatr Res 1992;30:177A.

Rotbart HA. Diagnosis of enteroviral meningitis with the polymerase chain reaction. J Pediatr 1990;117:85-89.

Rotbart HA, Kirkegaard K. Picornavirus pathogenesis: viral access, attachment, and entry into susceptible cells. Semin Virol 1992;3:483-499.

Sawyer MH, Holland D, Aintablian N, et al. Diagnosis of enteroviral central nervous system infection by polymerase chain reaction during a large community outbreak. Pediatr Infect Dis J 1994;13:177-182.

Strikas RA, Anderson LJ, Parker RA. Temporal and geographic patterns of isolates of nonpolio enterovirus in the United States, 1970-1983. J Infect Dis 1986;153:346-351.

van Creveld S, de Jager H. Myocarditis in newborns caused by coxsackievirus. Clinical and pathological data. Ann Pediatr 1956;187:100-112.

Wadia NH, Katrak SM, Misra VP, et al. Polio-like motor paralysis associated with acute hemorrhagic conjunctivitis in an outbreak in 1981 in Bombay, India: clinical and serologic studies. J Infect Dis 1983;147:660.

Webster ADB, Rotbart HA, Warner T, et al. Diagnosis of enterovirus brain disease in hypogammaglobulinemic patients by polymerase chain reaction. Clinical Infect Dis 1993; 17:657-661.

Weiner LS, Howell JT, Langford MP, et al. Effects of specific antibodies on chronic echovirus type 5 encephalitis in a patient with agammaglobulinemia. J Infect Dis 1979; 140:858.

Whitley RJ, Cobbs CG, Alford CA, et al. Diseases that mimic herpes simplex encephalitis. JAMA 1989;262:234-239.

Wilfert CM, Lehrman SN, Katz SL. Enteroviruses and meningitis. Pediatr Infect Dis 1983;2:333-341.

Yousef GE, Brown IN, Mowbray JF. Derivation and biochemical characterization of an enterovirus group–specific monoclonal antibody. Intervirology 1987;28:163-170.

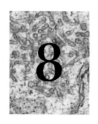

8   EPSTEIN-BARR VIRUS INFECTIONS

BEN Z. KATZ AND GEORGE MILLER

The Epstein-Barr virus (EBV) was discovered in the 1960s in cell lines derived from African Burkitt's lymphomas (Epstein et al., 1964). Today this virus is well recognized as the etiologic agent of infectious mononucleosis. Extensive virologic and serologic evidence also implicates EBV as the cause of various lymphoproliferative disorders such as large cell lymphomas and lymphocytic interstitial pneumonia in immunosuppressed patients (Andiman et al., 1985). EBV has also been regularly associated with two malignant conditions in patients who are not otherwise globally immunodeficient: (1) African (endemic) lymphoma, or Burkitt's lymphoma; and (2) nasopharyngeal carcinoma. Recently there has been increasing evidence of an association of EBV with Hodgkin's disease (Mueller et al., 1989; Weiss et al., 1989).

INFECTIOUS MONONUCLEOSIS

Infectious mononucleosis is the typical, symptomatic, primary EBV infection seen in the otherwise healthy host. Infectious mononucleosis is an acute infectious disease occurring predominantly in older children and young adults. It is characterized clinically by fever, exudative or membranous pharyngitis, generalized lymphadenopathy, and splenomegaly. Characteristically the peripheral blood shows an absolute increase in the number of atypical lymphocytes, and the serum has a high titer of heterophil antibody. Specific EBV antibodies are detected early in the illness and persist for years thereafter.

History

Infectious mononucleosis was first described as "glandular fever" by Pfeiffer in 1889. The term *infectious mononucleosis* was used by Sprunt and Evans (1920) in their description of hematologic changes in six young adults with a clinical syndrome characterized by a mononuclear leukocyto-sis. A diagnostic serologic test based on the association of heterophil antibody and mononucleosis was described by Paul and Bunnell (1932). This nonspecific test was made more specific by the development of differential absorption tests by Davidsohn (1937) (Table 8-1) and considerably simpler and more rapid (but occasionally less specific) by the more recent slide tests. The association of infectious mononucleosis with EBV was described by Henle et al. (1968) three decades later, 4 years after the virus was discovered.

Etiology

Although discovery of the causative agent of infectious mononucleosis eluded the efforts of competent investigators for many years, the assumption was that it was a virus. A report by Henle et al. (1968) provided evidence of a relationship between the herpesvirus now known as EBV and infectious mononucleosis.

In 1968 Niederman et al. detected antibodies against EBV in patients with infectious mononucleosis by means of an indirect immunofluorescence test. In twenty-four patients with infectious mononucleosis, antibodies that were absent in preillness specimens appeared early in the disease, rose to peak levels within a few weeks, and remained at high levels during convalescence. These antibodies were distinct from heterophil antibodies.

Subsequent studies by Niederman et al. in 1970 and Sawyer et al. in 1971 provided additional evidence indicating that EBV is the cause of infectious mononucleosis. The evidence that supports this concept is as follows: (1) EBV antibody is absent before onset of illness, appears during illness, and persists for many years thereafter; (2) clinical infectious mononucleosis occurs only in persons lacking antibody, and it fails to occur when antibody is present; (3) EBV has been isolated from the pharynx and saliva of patients with infectious

Table 8-1 Heterophil antibody reactions in normal and infectious mononucleosis (IM) sera

In the presence of:	Agglutination of sheep red blood cells after absorption with:	
	Guinea pig kidney cells	Beef red blood cells
Some normal human sera	−	+
Most IM sera	+	−

mononucleosis during their illness and for many months thereafter (Miller et al., 1973); and (4) cultured lymphocytes from patients who have had infectious mononucleosis will form continuous cell lines in vitro that contain the EBV genome and EBV antigens.

EBV is a member of the herpesvirus group. Mature infectious particles are 150 to 200 nm in diameter, with a lipid-containing envelope surrounding an icosahedral nucleocapsid. The genome is composed of approximately 172,000 base pairs of double-stranded DNA. The entire nucleotide sequence of one strain is known (Baer et al., 1984). Within the viral particle the genome is linear; within latently infected cells the genome is a circular extrachromosomal plasmid (Adams and Lindahl, 1975). In some cells EBV DNA also is integrated into the host cell chromosome (Matsuo et al., 1984).

In vitro the virus has a narrow host range, infecting B lymphocytes of human or other primate origin. However, in vivo the virus can be found in epithelial elements of the buccal mucosa, salivary glands, tongue, and ectocervix and in the epithelial cells of nasopharyngeal carcinoma. Within the mouth both parotid ductal epithelium and oropharyngeal squamous epithelial cells harbor EBV DNA and are sites of viral replication and release (Morgan et al., 1979; Sixbey et al., 1984; Wolf et al., 1984).

A number of viral antigen systems have been characterized, including viral capsid antigen (VCA), EB nuclear antigen (EBNA), membrane antigen (MA), and an early antigen (EA) complex of a diffuse component (D) and a restricted component (R). Each of these antigen systems is composed of a number of distinct viral gene products. For example, there are six different known EBNA genes. Antibodies to these different antigen systems can be demonstrated by a variety of techniques, including indirect immunofluorescence, immunoblotting, and enzyme-linked immunosorbent assay (ELISA).

Pathology

The generalized nature of infectious mononucleosis becomes apparent when the pathologic aspects of the disease are studied. Grossly, there may be diffuse enlargement of the lymphoid tissues, manifested by lymphadenopathy, splenomegaly, and pharyngeal lymphoid hyperplasia. Histologically, focal mononuclear infiltrations involve lymph nodes, spleen, tonsils, lungs, heart, liver, kidneys, adrenal glands, central nervous system (CNS), and skin. Bone marrow hyperplasia develops regularly, and in some instances small granulomas are present.

The lymphoid hyperplasia of infectious mononucleosis is not diagnostic; it can be seen in other conditions. Most of the hyperplasia involves T cells in the paracortical areas of the lymph node; however, in some instances there may be pronounced hyperplasia of B cells in the germinal follicle. The lymphoid hyperplasia is thought to consist of several distinct components. A few proliferating B cells are infected by EBV; they represent less than 0.1% of the circulating mononuclear cells in the acute phase of uncomplicated infectious mononucleosis. Other proliferating B cells may be "polyclonally activated" by the EBV infection but may not themselves contain EBV. The majority of the proliferating cells, represented by the atypical lymphocytes present in the blood, are reactive T cells (usually CD8-positive) and natural killer (NK) cells; they are not EBV-infected B lymphocytes (Pattengale et al., 1974). The proliferating T cells induce generalized lymph node hyperplasia and infiltrate many organs.

Thus it is the immune response against the virus that provides many of the pathologic conditions seen in acute infectious mononucleosis. Purtilo (1981) has called these atypical lymphocytes "combatants in an immune struggle." Some of these cells, cytotoxic T cells, have the specific ability to eliminate EBV-infected B cells (Svedmyr and Jondal, 1975). Others suppress activation of EBV-infected B cells (Tosato et al., 1979). There are also NK cells that nonspecifically eliminate EBV-infected cells (De Waele et al., 1981). Antibodies, especially neutralizing antibodies, may play a role in limiting acute infectious mononucleosis as well. These antibodies may limit the spread of extracellular virus and also participate in antibody-dependent cellular cytotoxicity (ADCC). It has been proposed that when this complex and finely tuned immunoregulatory mechanism fails, chronic or fatal EBV infection results. For example, if cytotoxic or suppressor T cells fail to eliminate infected B cells, excessive lymphoproliferation may occur. If, on the other hand, NK or cytotoxic T-cell activity is excessive, extensive B-cell death with resultant agammaglobulinemia may result (Andiman, 1984).

In the normal individual the extensive lymphoproliferation subsides, but the virus nevertheless persists in a latent state in the lymphoid compartment. Approximately one in a million peripheral blood mononuclear cells harbors EBV in the healthy EBV-seropositive individual (Rocchi et al., 1977).

Epidemiology

Although EBV infection is worldwide in distribution, clinical infectious mononucleosis is observed predominantly in developed countries, principally among adolescents and young adults. Seroepidemiologic surveys have revealed a gradual acquisition of antibody with age so that 50% to 90% of persons show a positive antibody reaction by young adult life. The overall incidence of clinical infectious mononucleosis is approximately 50 per 100,000 persons per year in the general population of the United States; however, the incidence of mononucleosis in susceptible college students is approximately 5,000 per 100,000 persons, 100 times higher than in the general population (Niederman et al., 1970). The total EBV infection rate in college students is estimated as at least twice as high (approximately 12,000 per 100,000 yearly), indicating that as many subclinical infections occur as overt infections. The so-called subclinical infections may be truly inapparent infections or atypical EBV-induced disease such as thrombocytopenia, hemolytic anemia, pneumonitis, or rash (Andiman, 1979; Andiman et al., 1981).

The epidemiologic factors that have a significant effect on the host response to EBV infection include age, socioeconomic status, and geographic location. In general, infection during infancy and childhood is usually clinically inapparent, perhaps because of the immaturity of the immunologic responses of children (Sumaya, 1977). Clinical infectious mononucleosis is generally seen only in adolescents and young adults (Evans et al., 1968). In developing countries of the world where sanitation is poor, exposure to EBV occurs at a very early age. In these countries most older children and adolescents are immune to the virus. Therefore infectious mononucleosis is rare. In the United States, infection generally occurs at an early age mainly in individuals in low socioeconomic groups who live in crowded conditions with poor hygiene.

Many seroepidemiologic studies have confirmed the well-known fact that infectious mononucleosis is not highly contagious, even in family settings. Henle and Henle (1970) found evidence of spread in three of eight families (37.5%), and Fleischer et al. (1981) found spread in seven of thirty-six susceptible contacts (19%). However, EBV infection appears to spread more efficiently under the conditions that exist in certain day-care nurseries (Pereira et al., 1969) and orphanages (Tischendorf et al., 1970).

The most likely modes of transmission are oral-salivary spread in children and close intimate contact (kissing) in young adults (Hoagland, 1955; Evans, 1960). Cell-free infectious virus is carried in saliva (Morgan et al., 1979). Prolonged pharyngeal excretion of EBV for periods up to several months after clinical infectious mononucleosis has been demonstrated (Miller et al., 1973; Niederman et al., 1976). Approximately 15% to 20% of immune individuals excrete EBV in saliva at any one point in time. Patients undergoing immunosuppression have an increased frequency ($>$50%) of oropharyngeal excretion (Strauch et al., 1974). If the saliva is concentrated, up to 100% of normal individuals may shed the virus (Yao et al., 1985). Thus the virus may never be truly "latent" in oropharyngeal elements but, instead, may produce a chronic, low-grade, productive infection. The infection can also be transmitted by transfusion of blood that is contaminated with EBV-infected lymphocytes (Gerber et al., 1969; Blacklow et al., 1971).

Clinical Manifestations

The incubation period has been estimated as 4 to 6 weeks on the basis of contact infections (Hoagland, 1984). After blood transfusion, heterophil-positive infectious mononucleosis has been shown to develop 5 weeks later (Blacklow et al., 1971; Turner et al., 1972).

The disease may begin abruptly or insidiously with headache, fever, chills, anorexia, and malaise, followed by lymphadenopathy and severe sore throat. The clinical picture is extremely variable in both severity and duration. The disease in children is generally mild; in adults it is more severe and has a more protracted course.

Fever. The temperature usually rises to 39.4° C (103° F) and gradually falls over a variable period, averaging 6 days. In a severe case it is not unusual for temperatures to hover between 40° and 40.6° C (104° and 105° F) and to persist for 3 weeks or more, after which low-grade fevers may persist for several more weeks. Children are more likely to have low-grade fever throughout the course or be afebrile.

Lymphadenopathy. Shortly after onset of illness, the lymph nodes rapidly enlarge to a variable size of approximately 1 to 4 cm. The nodes are typically tender, tense, discrete, and firm.

Any chain of lymph nodes may become enlarged, but the cervical group is most commonly involved. In addition, the following nodes are commonly affected: axillary, inguinal, epitrochlear, popliteal, mediastinal, and mesenteric. Massive mediastinal lymph node enlargement has been observed. Mesenteric lymphadenopathy frequently has been confused with acute appendicitis. Lymph node enlargement gradually subsides over a period of days or weeks, depending on the severity and extent of involvement.

Splenomegaly. Moderate enlargement of the spleen occurs in approximately 50% of cases. In rare instances enlargement may be followed by rupture, causing hemorrhage, shock, and death if it is not recognized. Rutkow (1978) reviewed 107 reports of splenic rupture in patients with infectious mononucleosis and concluded that only 18 ruptures were truly spontaneous; most followed trauma.

Tonsillopharyngitis. Sore throat is one of the cardinal symptoms of the disease. The tonsils are usually enlarged and reddened, and more than 50% develop exudate. Thick grayish-white, shaggy, membranous tonsillitis is a common finding and may persist for 7 to 10 days. During the first week, small petechiae are present on the palate in approximately one third of patients. In the past many patients referred to physicians with "diphtheria" because of the appearance of the throat proved to have infectious mononucleosis.

The triad of lymphadenopathy, splenomegaly, and exudative pharyngitis in a febrile patient is typical but not pathognomonic of infectious mononucleosis. Other manifestations of the disease include hepatitis, skin eruptions, pneumonitis, myocarditis, pericarditis, and CNS involvement.

Hepatitis. Liver involvement occurs relatively frequently in patients with infectious mononucleosis. Hepatomegaly is present in 10% to 15% of cases, but moderately abnormal hepatic isoenzymes are found in more than 80% of patients tested. Frank jaundice develops in less than 5% of cases and is usually mild; however, hyperbilirubinemia is reported in 25% of patients. Hepatitis may provoke such symptoms as anorexia, nausea, and vomiting.

Rash. In cases of infectious mononucleosis that are well documented clinically and serologically, the incidence of dermatitis is 3% to 19% (Bernstein, 1940; Contratto, 1944; Milne, 1945; Press et al., 1945; McCarthy and Hoagland, 1964). The rash, when present, is usually located on the trunk and arms; rarely, it may present solely as palmar dermatitis (Petrozzi, 1971). It appears during the first few days of illness, lasts 1 to 6 days, and is usually erythematous, macular, and papular or morbilliform. Sometimes, urticarial or scarlatiniform eruptions are seen (Press et al., 1945; McCarthy and Hoagland, 1964; Cowdrey and Reynolds, 1969). Occasionally, erythema multiforme, cold-induced urticaria, and acrocyanosis may be associated with infectious mononucleosis (Barth, 1981; Hughes and Burrows, 1993). Rarely, the rash may be petechial, vesicular, or hemorrhagic, but other more common and more serious causes of such rashes should be sought before they are ascribed to infectious mononucleosis.

In 1967 Pullen et al. and Patel nearly simultaneously observed an increased incidence of skin rashes in patients with infectious mononucleosis who were given ampicillin. The copper-colored rash begins 5 to 10 days after the drug is begun, mainly over the trunk. It then develops into an extensive, generalized (including the palms and soles), macular, and papular pruritic eruption. It can last up to a week, with desquamation persisting for several more days. At its peak the rash is confluent over exposed areas and pressure points and more marked extensor surfaces. A faint macular rash sometimes is seen on the palatal and buccal mucosae. This rash may also be seen with the administration of ampicillin derivatives, such as amoxicillin (Mulroy, 1973), and other penicillins, such as methicillin (Fields, 1980). This rash does not represent a long-lasting hypersensitivity to ampicillin; the drug may be used again once the infectious mononucleosis has subsided (Nazareth et al., 1972; Levene and Baker, 1968; McKenzie et al., 1976; Bjorg et al., 1975).

Pneumonitis. A small percentage of patients with infectious mononucleosis develop a cough that is paroxysmal in type, with a clinical picture and roentgenograms indistinguishable from those of atypical pneumonia. Pleural effusion also may develop. Hilar adenopathy is often observed in patients with extensive lymphoid hyperplasia in the course of infectious mononucleosis.

Central Nervous System Involvement. During the past three decades there have been increasing numbers of reports of CNS involvement in patients with infectious mononucleosis. These manifestations have been observed in the adult age group and also in children. The neurologic syndromes have included aseptic meningitis, encephalitis, the "Alice in Wonderland" syndrome, acute hemiplegia, infectious polyneuritis (Guillain-Barré syndrome), cranial nerve palsies, optic neuritis, peripheral neuropathy, transverse myelitis, acute cerebellar ataxia, and CNS lymphoma. Demyelinating disease may follow cases of acute infectious mononucleosis (Connelly and Demitt, 1994; Matoba, 1990; Bray 1992).

■ CASE 1 A 10-year-old black boy with generalized lymphadenopathy, splenomegaly, typical blood picture, and positive heterophil antibody titer developed encephalitis during the course of his infection. He had headache, vomiting, and drowsiness that progressed to stupor. The cerebrospinal fluid showed pleocytosis with a predominance of lymphocytes and an elevated protein level. His sensorium gradually improved, and he made an uneventful recovery.

■ CASE 2 A 12-year-old white girl with a classic picture of infectious mononucleosis developed weakness of both lower and upper extremities, with absent reflexes. Spinal fluid findings showed albuminocytological dissociation characteristic of the Guillain-Barré syndrome. There were no cells, and the protein value was 300 mg/dl. The paralysis cleared completely within 6 weeks. The diagnosis of infectious mononucleosis was confirmed by a typical blood smear and positive heterophil antibody test.

In general, the neurologic manifestations depend on the site of involvement, which may be anywhere in the CNS. The majority of patients recover completely, although fatalities have been associated with encephalitis.

Complications

Rupture of the Spleen. Rupture of the spleen is a serious but, fortunately, rare complication of infectious mononucleosis. It has been attributed to an extensive lymphocytic and mononuclear cell infiltrate that presumably causes stretching and weakening of the capsule and trabeculae. Consequently, minor trauma to the splenic area or sudden increases in intraabdominal pressure may precipitate rupture. In rare instances it may be a spontaneous development caused by progressive intrasplenic hyperplasia. The presence of this complication should be suspected in any patient who suddenly develops abdominal pain on the left side and signs of peritoneal irritation, hemorrhage, and shock (Rutkow, 1978).

Hematologic Complications. The development of epistaxis, petechial and ecchymotic skin lesions, and hematuria suggests a rare complication of infectious mononucleosis. Low platelet counts, prolonged bleeding time, and poor clot retraction confirm the diagnosis of thrombocytopenic purpura. Recovery is the rule (Clarke and Davies, 1964). Other rare hematologic complications include hemolytic anemia, aplastic anemia, agranulocytosis, and agammaglobulinemia (Grierson and Purtilo, 1987).

An acute hemophagocytic syndrome resembling malignant histiocytosis in infants and children has been linked to EBV infection (Wilson et al., 1981). Patients may present with fever, hepatosplenomegaly, pancytopenia, and disseminated intravascular coagulation; hemophagocytosis is found on examination of bone marrow. The mortality rate ranges from 30% to 40%. Overall the syndrome is poorly understood, except that it is associated with EBV and with many other infections. Some of these patients apparently are immunodeficient (McKenna et al., 1981). There is overlap between this syndrome and the X-linked lymphoproliferative syndrome, to be discussed later (Seemayer, 1995).

Cardiac Complications. Electrocardiographic changes during the course of infectious mononucleosis have been reported in adults. These are usually the only manifestations of cardiac involvement. However, there have been several reports of pericarditis and myocarditis characterized by severe chest pain and typical electrocardiographic findings (Hudgins, 1976; Butler et al., 1981).

Miscellaneous. Orchitis may occur rarely in association with infectious mononucleosis. In one case report (Ralston et al., 1960) the testicular involvement was bilateral; in another report (Wolnisty, 1962) it was unilateral. The orchitis subsided in 2 to 4 weeks. Renal failure, arthritis, rhabdomyolysis, pancreatitis, proctitis, and gall bladder hydrops have also been reported (Ray et al., 1982; Koutras, 1983; Dinulos et al., 1994; Mayer, 1996; Osamah, 1995).

Diagnosis

The diagnosis of infectious mononucleosis is usually made on the basis of (1) suggestive clinical features; (2) typical blood picture; (3) positive heterophil agglutination antibody test; and (4) ancillary laboratory findings, such as specific serologic findings to EBV antigens. Younger children especially may have EBV infection with symptoms not characteristic of infectious mononucleosis and with negative heterophil antibody titers. In such instances measurement of specific EBV serologic findings is required for diagnosis. The diagnosis can be confirmed by the specific tests for various antibodies against EBV antigens (Evans et al., 1975; Rapp and Hewetson, 1978). Examination and test results from a patient with mononucleosis seen early in the illness are illustrated in Fig. 8-1.

Clinical Features. A history of fever associated with the triad of lymphadenopathy, exudative

pharyngitis, and splenomegaly should suggest infectious mononucleosis as a diagnostic possibility. The following laboratory tests are not specific but are helpful in establishing the diagnosis.

Blood tests. An absolute increase in the number of atypical lymphocytes is a characteristic finding during some stages of the disease. In a blood smear these cells usually represent 10% or more of the field. These so-called Downey cells vary markedly in size and shape. With Wright's stain the cytoplasm is dark blue and vacuolated, presenting a foamy appearance; the nucleus is round, bean shaped, or lobulated and contains no nucleoli. The white blood cell count is variable. During the first week of the disease there may be leukopenia, but commonly there is leukocytosis with a predominance of lymphocytes. The white blood cell count may be so elevated that the presence of leukemia is suspected. In an occasional immunodeficient patient, infectious mononucleosis can progress to frank leukemia; in this instance all the primitive blasts in the circulation are EBV-transformed B cells (Robinson et al., 1980).

Atypical lymphocytes are not specific for infectious mononucleosis. They may be observed in a

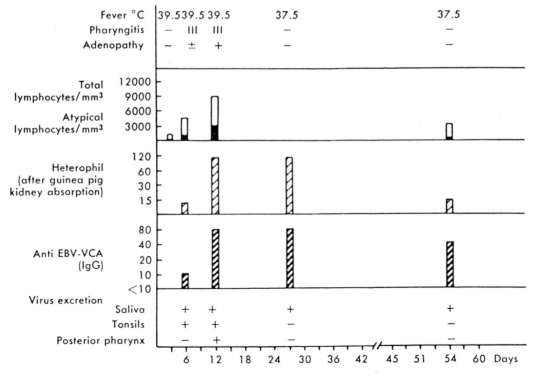

FIG. 8-1 Sequence of symptoms, atypical lymphocytosis, heterophil antibody, EBV antibody (anti-EBV–VCA), and EBV oral excretion in a patient with mononucleosis seen early in the illness. (From Niederman JC et al.: N Engl J Med 1976; 294:1355.)

variety of clinical entities, including infectious hepatitis, rubella, primary atypical pneumonia, allergic rhinitis, asthma, and other diseases. Morphologically, the atypical cells in these conditions are indistinguishable from those seen in infectious mononucleosis. However, there is a quantitative difference; in infectious mononucleosis there are usually more than 10% atypical cells, whereas these other conditions usually have a lower percentage of atypical cells.

Heterophil antibodies. The heterophil antibodies were the first serologic markers discovered that could reasonably confirm the diagnosis of infectious mononucleosis. Heterophil antibody tests are still used more frequently than any of the virus-specific assays. Most sera of patients with infectious mononucleosis cause sheep red blood cells to agglutinate after they have been absorbed with guinea pig kidney antigens but not after absorption with beef red blood cells. The reverse is often true of normal sera (see Table 8-1). The heterophil antibody responsible for this differential absorption in infectious mononucleosis is principally of the IgM class, appears during the first or second week of illness, and disappears gradually over 3 to 6 months. In a group of 166 patients studied by Niederman (1956) the heterophil antibody test was positive in 38% during the first week, in 60% during the second week, and in approximately 80% during the third week after onset of symptoms.

Sheep cell agglutinins are not specific for infectious mononucleosis. They occur in a number of other conditions, such as serum sickness, viral hepatitis, rubella, leukemia, and Hodgkin's disease. Low titers can also be demonstrated in the serum of some normal persons. Usually the absorption tests serve to distinguish these agglutinins from the heterophil antibodies of infectious mononucleosis. In general, the agglutinin titer is also higher in patients with infectious mononucleosis than in those with other conditions; an unabsorbed heterophil antibody titer above 1:128 and 1:40 or greater after absorption is considered significant.

A rapid slide test using equine red blood cells stabilized by formaldehyde has been evaluated as a diagnostic test for infectious mononucleosis. In 1965 Hoff and Bauer reported a high degree of correlation with the standard heterophil antibody test. They described the following advantages: (1) low incidence of false reactions; (2) high degree of specificity for infectious mononucleosis antibody; (3) great rapidity (2 minutes); and (4) ease of performance. This rapid test is a valuable diagnostic

aid in clinical practice. Other rapid slide tests have become available, using the same principle of the absorbed heterophil agglutination but using equine or bovine erythrocytes that are citrated or formalinized. All have shown a high index of positive correlation with the standard Paul-Bunnell test results (Rapp and Hewetson, 1978).

Antibody titers to specific EBV antigens. Although infectious mononucleosis occurs only in previously seronegative individuals, IgG antibody to the VCA may already be detectable early in the course of the illness. The acute illness may be diagnosed if VCA-specific IgM is present in serum, but this assay is difficult to perform and may yield false-positive reactions because of rheumatoid factors in blood. VCA-IgM responses disappear after several months, whereas VCA-IgG levels persist for life. Antibodies to the EA complex, associated with viral replication, are present in 70% to 80% of patients during acute disease and usually disappear after 6 months. Recent studies indicate that antibody to the component of the EA complex may be detectable in healthy individuals for years after having infectious mononucleosis (Horwitz et al., 1985). Antibody to the nuclear antigen (EBNA) appears more slowly, taking from 1 to 6 months to become detectable. The antibody response to EB nuclear antigen (EBNA-1) is more delayed (Niederman and Miller, 1986). Testing acute and convalescent sera for titer rises to EBNA-1 can be a useful diagnostic procedure. Thus a positive anti-VCA titer and a negative anti-EBNA titer are diagnostic of a primary EBV serologic response such as occurs in infectious mononucleosis. All late convalescent sera from healthy individuals contain EBNA antibodies. A diagram showing the sequence of development and persistence of these antibodies to EBV is shown in Fig. 8-2.

Detection of the virus. Biologically active virus can be isolated from saliva, peripheral blood, or lymphoid tissue by means of its ability to immortalize cultured human lymphocytes, usually from umbilical-cord blood. Occasionally, lymphoid cell lines can be grown directly from blood or lymph nodes. This assay is time-consuming (6 to 8 weeks) and requires specialized tissue-culture facilities that are not generally available.

Viral antigens representative of the latent life cycle of the virus can be found in lymphoid tissues, in nasopharyngeal carcinoma tumors, and occasionally in the peripheral blood if the level of leukoviremia is high enough. During the acute phase of mononucleosis, approximately 1% or less

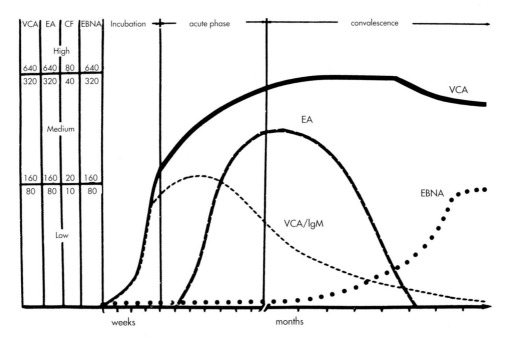

FIG. 8-2 EBV antibody response during the course of infectious mononucleosis. *EA,* Early antigen; *VCA,* viral capsid antigen; *EBNA,* EB nuclear antigen. (From de Thé G: In Klein G: Viral oncology, New York: Raven Press, 1980.)

of the circulating peripheral blood lymphocytes contain an EBNA.

The most specific method of demonstrating EBV in pathologic material is nucleic acid hybridization. Three general techniques have been used: (1) Southern hybridization, which is capable of distinguishing the specific portions of EBV DNA that are present in the lesions; (2) in situ hybridization, which identifies the cells that contain EBV DNA or RNA; and (3) polymerase chain reaction (PCR). Probes for nucleic acid detection methods are made from cloned EBV DNA fragments prepared by recombinant DNA techniques or from synthetic oligonucleotides. The probes are labeled by radioactive or nonisotopic methods.

The sensitivity of the Southern hybridization technique under the best conditions is approximately 10^5 EBV genomes, more often approximately 10^6 genomes. This sensitivity is sufficient to detect EBV DNA in nasopharyngeal carcinoma, Burkitt's lymphoma, and polyclonal lymphomas, all of which contain many copies of EBV DNA in each cell. However, it is not sensitive enough to detect EBV DNA regularly in peripheral blood of mononucleosis patients, in which only a few cells harbor EBV DNA. The PCR is highly sensitive; it can detect approximately 10^4 genomes or less; therefore in most cases of acute infectious mononu-

cleosis EBV DNA can be detected in the blood by PCR. Nucleic acid hybridization methods can be used as a rapid assay for salivary excretion of EBV.

Southern hybridization can determine whether patients are infected with the same or different viruses (Katz et al., 1988). Probes from regions of the genome near the termini provide additional information about whether the EBV is monoclonal or multiclonal (Raab-Traub and Flynn, 1986). Furthermore, the same probes can distinguish between latent and lytically replicating forms of EBV DNA. Using these techniques, it has been found that many EBV-associated lymphoproliferative diseases contain lytically replicating forms of EBV DNA (Katz et al., 1989).

In situ hybridization for the abundant EB virus–encoded small RNAs (EBERs) is a specific and sensitive technique for detection of EB viral gene expression in pathologic specimens (Howe and Steitz, 1986). EBER in situ hybridization permits the determination of the number and type of infected cells in paraffin-embedded tissues (Hamilton-Dutoit and Pallesen, 1994; Barletta et al. 1993).

Differential Diagnosis

Infectious mononucleosis is a notorious mimic of many other diseases. Lymphadenopathy, splenomegaly, and exudative tonsillitis are common manifestations of a number of entities. The following conditions are often confused with infectious mononucleosis.

Streptococcal Tonsillitis or Pharyngitis.
This condition is suggested by fever, sore throat, exudative tonsillitis, and cervical adenitis. An increase in the number of polymorphonuclear leukocytes, positive culture from a throat swab specimen, and prompt therapeutic response to penicillin all point to a streptococcal cause.

Diphtheria.
The membranous tonsillitis of infectious mononucleosis frequently resembles diphtheria. The diagnosis is confirmed by positive culture.

Blood Dyscrasias.
Blood dyscrasias, particularly leukemia, are suggested by the lymphadenopathy, splenomegaly, and increase in number of peripheral blood atypical lymphocytes. Laboratory tests, including bone marrow aspiration, establish the true diagnosis.

Rubella.
Rubella is commonly associated with a 2- to 4-day period of malaise and lymphadenopathy preceding the appearance of the rash. Rubella has a milder course, and frequently there is a history of exposure. A definite diagnosis of rubella can be established by evidence of a rise in the level of specific antibodies.

Measles.
Measles, which is less frequently confused with infectious mononucleosis, is easily identified by the pathognomonic Koplik's spots. In doubtful cases a diagnosis of measles can be confirmed by demonstration of a rise in the level of measles antibodies.

Viral Hepatitis.
This disease may be clinically indistinguishable from infectious mononucleosis with jaundice. Specific serologic tests can confirm a diagnosis of hepatitis A, B, or C.

Cytomegalovirus Infection.
A mononucleosis-like syndrome characterized by fever, splenomegaly, and atypical lymphocytes occurs in some patients with acute cytomegalovirus infection. These patients have a negative heterophil-agglutination determination and no evidence of recent EBV infection. Culture of urine or blood (buffy coat) or direct detection of antigen should be positive for cytomegalovirus.

Acquired Toxoplasmosis with Lymphadenopathy.
Toxoplasmosis infection may be clinically indistinguishable from infectious mononucleosis. It is characterized by generalized lymphadenopathy, chiefly of the cervical group, and occasionally by pharyngeal involvement and exanthem. These patients have a negative heterophil and a positive toxoplasma antibody determination.

In addition to simulating the diseases just described, infectious mononucleosis may simulate Hodgkin's disease, scarlet fever, secondary syphilis, typhoid fever, rickettsial diseases, and many others.

Prognosis

In general, the prognosis for patients with infectious mononucleosis is excellent. Severe cases may be followed by long periods (6 to 12 months) of asthenia. Spontaneous rupture of the spleen, which is very rare, is fatal if it is not recognized and treated promptly. Deaths reported in infectious mononucleosis have also resulted from CNS complications, secondary bacterial infection in neutropenic patients, myocarditis, disseminated lymphoproliferative disease, and hemophagocytic syndrome.

Treatment

Infectious mononucleosis is a self-limited disease, and treatment is chiefly supportive. Antimicrobial drugs are not effective and do not alter the course of the infection. Bed rest is indicated in the acute stage of the disease. Aspirin can usually control the pain or discomfort caused by the enlarged lymph nodes and pharyngeal involvement. In severe cases codeine or meperidine (Demerol) may be required.

Corticosteroid therapy has been reported to have a beneficial effect in certain situations. Severe symptoms referable to the throat and enlarged lymph nodes improve within 24 hours of corticosteroid therapy in many instances; if there is no response, tonsillectomy may be considered (Stevenson, 1992). In a well-controlled study of 132 patients with severe uncomplicated mononucleosis, Bender (1967) observed a significant decrease in the duration of fever; it persisted for an average of 1.4 days in the 66 corticosteroid-treated patients and an average of 5.6 days in the 66 matched control patients. Steroids may be considered for treatment of severe cases characterized by hematologic complications, marked toxemia, progressive tonsillar enlargement leading to airway encroachment, and evidence of neurologic or cardiac complications. Steroids are not recommended for treatment of mild cases of infectious mononucleosis because the long-term effects of intervention on the normal immune response to EBV are unknown. There are reports of neurologic or septicemic complications following steroid use (Waldo, 1981; Gold et al., 1995).

Contact sports should be avoided until the patient's spleen size has returned to normal. Spontaneous rupture of the spleen generally requires immediate surgery. Transfusions, treatment for shock, and splenectomy are lifesaving measures.

Acyclovir inhibits EBV DNA polymerase and thus blocks the lytic (but not the latent) phase of EBV replication. It inhibits viral DNA synthesis (represented by linear DNA) leading to virion production, but it has no effect on the number of latent (circular) genomes (Colby et al., 1980). The drug is preferentially incorporated into viral DNA through the action of the EBV thymidine kinase.

When given to patients with infectious mononucleosis, acyclovir given with or without steroids reduces the level of oropharyngeal viral replication during the period of administration (Ernberg and Andersson, 1986; Tynell et al., 1996). However, after cessation of treatment, replication returns to previously high levels. During acyclovir treatment there is little or no reduction in the number of EBV-infected B cells found in the peripheral circulation. Acyclovir has minimal effects on the symptoms of mononucleosis as well, and thus should not be routinely used in the treatment of patients with this disease.

OTHER EBV-ASSOCIATED DISEASES
X-Linked Lymphoproliferative Syndrome: Duncan's Disease

A spectrum of clinical manifestations of EBV infections in patients with recognized or presumed immunologic impairment has been reported. Severe and often fatal infectious mononucleosis, X-linked lymphoproliferative disease (XLP), with death occurring after 1 or 2 weeks from hemorrhage, hepatic failure, or bacterial superinfection, was described in kindred males by Bar et al. in 1974 and Purtilo et al. in 1977. This sex-linked recessive genetic disorder has variable phenotypic expression. Boys who survive EBV infection may subsequently develop a variety of hematologic complications, such as agammaglobulinemia, hypergammaglobulinemia, agranulocytosis, aplastic anemia, and malignancy. The mean age of 100 of these boys at death was approximately 6 years (Purtilo et al., 1982). The underlying problem appears to be an inappropriately regulated cytotoxic T-cell response to EBV under the control of a defective lymphoproliferative control locus (XLC) on the X chromosome (Xq24). In children who develop monoclonal B-cell neoplasms or fatal infectious mononucleosis, the cytotoxic T-cell response is probably ineffective. In contrast, agammaglobulinemia, agranulocytosis, and aplastic anemia may be secondary to an excescessive suppressor T-cell response (Seemayer, 1995). This disease may be difficult to diagnose because many patients have low or undetectable serologic responses to EBV despite infection. Many such patients experience lymphocytosis, hepatic necrosis and hemophagocytosis; EBV DNA or EBERs can be shown in liver or bone marrow by molecular hybridization techniques.

Rarely, cases of classic infectious mononucleosis in apparently normal girls have evolved into monoclonal or polyclonal lymphomas (Robinson et al., 1980; Abo et al., 1982). These patients presumably have undiagnosed immunoregulatory disorders with an abnormal immune response to EBV, which results in chronic or malignant disease following primary EBV infection.

EBV Infections in Transplant Patients

There is serologic and virologic evidence for reactivation of latent EBV in conjunction with immunosuppressive therapy (Strauch et al., 1974). Such reactivation, as well as primary EBV infection in this setting, may be associated with a spectrum of clinical manifestations, including benign or fatal lymphoproliferative disorders or non-Hodgkin's lymphomas (Ho et al., 1988). Thus it is not surprising that a variety of EBV-associated lymphoproliferative syndromes have been described in patients who have received kidney, heart, bone marrow, liver, or thymus transplants under cover of immunosuppressive therapy.

At least three factors are thought to contribute to the pathogenesis and timing of these lymphoproliferative syndromes: (1) the dosage, duration, and number of immunosuppressive drugs, particularly cyclosporin A or tacrolimus (FK506); (2) whether the patient is undergoing primary or reactivated EBV infection; and (3) the use of antibody to T cells (especially OKT3 antibody) as an immunosuppressive agent to maintain the graft or, in the case of bone marrow transplantation, to prevent graft-versus-host disease (Martin et al., 1984). Use of T cell–depleted allogeneic bone marrow and monoclonal anti–T cell antibodies to prevent graft-versus-host disease, are often associated with lymphomas arising in donor cells in bone marrow transplant recipients. The donor cells can be detected with markers such as a sex chromosome or mitochondrial DNA polymorphism (Schubach et al., 1982). Chronic antigenic stimulation caused by the engrafted cells was thought to play a role in pathogenesis of EBV-associated lymphomas in recipients of allogeneic transplants; however, EBV-associated B-cell lymphomas have been described in recipients of autologous marrow transplant as well (Ho et al., 1985, 1988).

The posttransplant lymphoproliferative lesions display the same latent EBV gene products observed in B cells immortalized in vitro. Thus they differ from those of Burkitt's lymphoma both in histologic conditions and in the spectrum of expression of EBV latent gene products.

Hanto et al. (1981) estimated an incidence of 1% (12 per 1,119) lymphomas and other lymphoproliferative disorders among recipients of renal transplants. The incidence of lymphomas among heart transplant patients in the Stanford series was 5% (9 per 182). The frequency of lymphomas in patients receiving transplantation of allogeneic T cell–depleted bone marrow may be as high as 15% to 20%. Nucleic acid hybridization is the principal technique used to demonstrate an association of EBV with these tumors. There is some evidence that discontinuation of cyclosporin A or tacrolimus therapy with or without concomitant acyclovir therapy is accompanied by remission of the lymphoproliferative disease. Chemotherapy and interferon-α have been used as well (Swinnen, 1992; Benkerrou et al., 1993). There is a recent report of a cure following bone marrow transplantation and treatment with etoposide (Pracher et al., 1994). A recent, highly encouraging therapeutic strategy involves the transfusion of EBV-specific cytotoxic T cells (Rooney, 1995). Anti–B cell antibodies have been used as well (Leblond, 1995).

EBV–Associated Diseases in AIDS Patients

Acquired immunodeficiency syndrome (AIDS) patients develop four different EBV-associated lesions: (1) lymphomas, (2) lymphocytic interstitial pneumonitis (LIP), (3) oral "hairy" leukoplakia of the tongue, and (4) leiomyosarcoma.

Lymphomas. AIDS predisposes to EBV-associated lymphomas of several histologic types, including classic Burkitt's lymphoma with its associated chromosome abnormality. However, many cases of Burkitt's lymphoma occurring in AIDS patients do not contain EBV (as is generally true of Burkitt's lymphoma outside the endemic regions) (Subar et al., 1988). Several other types of EBV-associated lymphomas, including CNS lymphoma and diffuse polyclonal or oligoclonal B-cell lymphoma found in extranodal sites such as the gut, are common complications of AIDS.

Lymphocytic Interstitial Pneumonitis. LIP is a polyclonal lymphoproliferative process (Joshi et al., 1987) seen mainly in children with AIDS. The occurrence of LIP correlates with lymphoproliferative activity (i.e., lymphadenopathy and parotitis) elsewhere in the body. It initially is seen as a subacute or chronic pulmonary process (e.g., with dyspnea on exertion and clubbing) rather than as acute pneumonitis. It is characterized by a reticulonodular pattern on chest radiography (Rubinstein et al., 1986). Histologically, lung biopsies of these lesions reveal mature lymphoid follicle formation in the lung, including germinal centers, and infiltration with plasmacytoid cells. Up to 80% of the lesions are associated with EBV DNA (Andiman et al., 1985), and patients, when compared to matched controls, often have evidence of a primary or reactivated EBV serologic response (Katz et al., 1992). LIP may regress with acyclovir treatment or a low dose of corticosteroids given every other day (Pahwa, 1988). The lesion tends to worsen concomitant with other pulmonary infections.

Oral Hairy Leukoplakia. Oral hairy leukoplakia, which resembles thrush, is seen principally on the lateral surface of the tongues of homosexual men with AIDS. Pathologically, the lesions resemble flat warts. Lytic EBV DNA replication and production of mature virions have been documented within the epithelial cells of these lesions, which regress with acyclovir treatment (Greenspan et al., 1985; Resnick et al., 1988).

CNS Lymphoma. One of the most serious CNS complications of EBV infection is the occurrence of CNS lymphoma. It is due to proliferation of EBV-infected B cells in an immunologically privileged site. It occurs infrequently in otherwise healthy individuals, but is more common in immunosuppressed patients with AIDS or organ transplants (Hochberg et al., 1983). EBV is invariably present in the CNS lymphoma (MacMahon, 1991).

Leiomyosarcoma. Leiomyosarcomas are malignant cancers of smooth muscle that are rare in childhood. Recently, five cases in children with AIDS and five cases in liver transplant recipients were found to be EBV associated. The tumors were monooligoclonal. There has been no report of an EBV-associated leiomyosarcoma in an immunocompetent host, thus strengthening the association between immunosuppression and EBV-associated malignancy (McClain, 1995; Lee, 1995).

Burkitt's Lymphoma

Epidemiology. Burkitt's lymphoma is a disease with striking epidemiologic features that first led to its recognition. In endemic areas Burkitt's lymphoma is the most common childhood cancer, and it may reach an incidence of 8 to 10 cases per 100,000 people per year. In Burkitt's original series of cases the mortality rate was high—approximately 80% within the first year after diagnosis. However, the tumor is sensitive to chemotherapy, and recent series have described a first-year mortality rate of 20%.

Burkitt's lymphoma occurs sporadically throughout the world. There are, however, high-incidence areas such as part of equatorial East Africa and New Guinea. Areas with extremely high incidences are in the hot, wet, rural lowlands. In these areas, malaria infection is universal, occurs very early in life, and is transmitted throughout the year; areas of Africa that are nearby but do not have holoendemic malaria as a result of malaria eradication campaigns do not have high rates of Burkitt's lymphoma. In areas such as Malaysia, Colombia, and Brazil the incidence is intermediate.

The median age of patients with Burkitt's lymphoma is remarkably constant within the endemic areas. For example, in Uganda, Nigeria, Ghana, and New Guinea the median age is from 7.7 to 9.2 years. Where the tumors occur in lower incidence, the patients are slightly older. In the United States the median age is 10½ years. However, Burkitt's lymphoma has been described in adults over the age of 30.

Association with EBV. The association of Burkitt's tumor with EBV is based on two types of findings: (1) demonstration of EBV genomes in the majority of tumors from endemic areas, and (2) serologic relationships. More than 90% of Burkitt's lymphoma biopsy specimens from Africa contain EBV DNA. A rare tumor in the endemic area that is histologically compatible with Burkitt's lymphoma fails to demonstrate the viral genome. In Burkitt's lymphoma occurring outside the endemic area, EBV DNA is associated with approximately 20% of the tumors.

Several seroepidemiologic findings indicate a relationship between Burkitt's lymphoma and EBV. In a prospective study of 42,000 children from the West Nile district of Uganda, it was determined that children who developed Burkitt's lymphoma were infected with the virus months to years before onset of the tumor (de Thé et al., 1978). Antibody titers to capsid antigen were approximately twofold higher in cases than in controls (matched for age) who did not develop Burkitt's lymphoma. Once the disease appears, Burkitt's lymphoma patients have considerably higher (approximately tenfold) antibody titers to capsid and early antigens than do children without the tumor. Seroepidemiologic studies show that, in the endemic area, EBV infections are acquired at a very early age and are readily transmitted. Elevated EBV antibody titers are not regularly seen in patients with other lymphomas, except for patients with Hodgkin's disease (see later discussion).

The association of elevated EBV antibody titers with Burkitt's lymphoma is most pronounced in the endemic areas. Outside the endemic areas patients with Burkitt's lymphoma seem to fall into two categories: (1) those whose tumors contain EBV DNA and who develop elevated EBV antibodies, and (2) those whose tumors are genome-negative and who may be infected with the virus but do not develop high antibody titers.

Clinical Features. In approximately 60% of children, Burkitt's lymphoma is seen initially as a unilateral swelling of the jaw. Characteristically, the jaw tumors are the presenting sign in younger children. Abdominal masses are usually the first sign in older children.

Jaw tumors are less frequently seen in patients with Burkitt's lymphoma outside the endemic areas of Africa. Only rarely does the tumor present as hepatosplenomegaly or enlargement of peripheral lymph nodes. Leukemic involvement of the bone marrow is also infrequent. Occasionally the tumor may become recognized because of signs of CNS involvement such as paraplegia, cranial nerve paralysis, or meningeal irritation.

Since the tumor grows rapidly, the clinical history is usually short. Some of the clinical features of the disease result from rapid tumor growth and the breakdown and release of intracellular metabolites. Thus complications include azotemia, hyperuricemia, hyperkalemia, and lactic acidosis.

Chromosome Abnormalities. Burkitt's lymphomas regularly contain abnormalities of those chromosomes that contain immunoglobulin genes and chromosome 8q24, which is the locus for the c-*myc* protooncogene (Leder et al., 1976). The cytogenetic abnormalities occur in both the endemic and sporadic forms of the tumor, independent of their geographical location and whether or not EBV is associated with the tumor. The chromosomal abnormalities are not detected in peripheral blood lymphocytes or hematopoietic stem cells of patients with Burkitt's lymphoma or in lymphoblastoid cells lines derived from Burkitt's lymphoma patients. They have been found only in the malignant cells. The most common abnormality, t(8;14), which is seen in approximately 75% of cases, is a reciprocal translocation between the long arm of chromosome 8 (24q) and the long arm of chromosome 14 (32q) bearing the heavy-chain locus. Variant translocations involve the c-*myc* gene on 8q24 and the genes for light chains on chromosome 2p11 (the kappa chain) and 22q11 (the lambda chain) (Lenoir et al., 1982).

Nasopharyngeal Carcinoma

Association with EBV. The association of EBV with nasopharyngeal carcinoma, an epithelial cell malignancy, is strong. EBV DNA is regularly found in all cases of undifferentiated nasopharyngeal carcinoma and also in differentiated forms of the carcinoma (Raab-Traub et al., 1987). Preinvasive lesions such as dysplasia and carcinoma in situ are also infected with EBV (Pathmanathan, 1995). On the basis of the structure of EBV episomes, which can vary in size as a result of different numbers of the EBV terminal repeats, it has been determined that a single clone of EBV is associated with each tumor (Raab-Traub and Flynn, 1986). This finding implies that EBV DNA has been associated with the progenitor of the tumor cell from the time of tumor initiation, although it does not prove that EBV induced the transformation event. There is, furthermore, a convincing serologic association between EBV and nasopharyngeal carcinoma: the sera of patients with the carcinoma have IgA antibodies to a variety of EBV latent and replicative antigens (Neel et al., 1983). Such antibodies rarely are found in the serum of healthy persons. A similar association has been found between EBV and several other carcinomas believed derived from embryonic branchial cleft remnants, such as carcinomas derived from the thymus, parotid, palatine tonsil, and supraglottic region of the larynx (Leyvraz et al., 1985; Brichacek et al., 1983, 1984).

In China, where there is a high incidence of nasopharyngeal carcinoma, mass serologic screening for serum IgA antibody to the EBV capsid antigen has been undertaken (Henle and Henle, 1976). The frequency of IgA antibody among 150,000 people studied was approximately 1%. Approximately 20% of those persons with elevated IgA anti-VCA who were biopsied had nasopharyngeal carcinoma. The use of serologic screening for IgA antibody accompanied by nasopharyngeal examination and radiological examination, including computerized tomography scans, has been useful in diagnosis of nasopharyngeal carcinoma at treatable stages of the disease.

Clinical Features. The presenting symptoms of nasopharyngeal carcinoma depend on the location of the primary tumor within the nasopharynx. In approximately half the cases the presenting sign is a cervical mass resulting from spread to regional lymph nodes. Other symptoms may include nasal obstruction, postnasal discharge, epistaxis or symptoms attributable to obstruction of the eustachian tube, such as impairment of hearing, tinnitus, or otitis media. If there has been local spread, the patient may present with cranial nerve involvement, headache, or trismus resulting from involvement of jaw muscles. Occasionally, initial symptoms result from obstruction of the paranasal sinuses. Nasopharyngeal carcinoma may metastasize to the skeleton, especially the spine, and to the liver, lung, skin, and peripheral lymph nodes.

Congenital Infection

Occasional infants with birth defects believed secondary to congenital EBV infection have been described. One infant manifested bilateral congenital cataracts, cryptorchidism, hypotonia, and mild micrognathia. A "celery stalk" appearance of long bones was noted radiologically, similar to the condition seen with congenital rubella (Goldberg et al., 1981). A report by Icart et al. (1981) described more than 700 pregnant women with serologic evidence of EBV infection during pregnancy. Their pregnancies were 3 times more likely to result in early fetal death, premature labor, or delivery of an infant who would become ill. Until further data are available, however, it is difficult to know whether these associations are real or coincidental. One prospective study of 4,063 pregnant women during 4,108 gestations failed to show any intrauterine EBV infections (Fleisher and Bologonese, 1984).

Hodgkin's Disease

EBERs and the EBV latent membrane protein 1 (LMP1) antigen have been detected in tissues of about 50% of patients with Hodgkin's disease (HD). The association of HD with EBV varies with age, being more frequent in young children and the elderly. It also differs with geography, occurring more frequently in children in economically underdeveloped countries than in those in developed countries (Weinreb et al., 1996). The EBERs are present predominantly in the Reed-Sternberg cells, but occasionally also in the Hodgkin's cells and in the infiltrating lymphoid cells of the tumor. The EBV DNA is often monoclonal. Patients with HD have slightly higher EBV titers than normal. The elevation is present before the diagnosis of Hodgkin's lymphoma (Mueller et al., 1989).

Chronic Active EBV Infections

Rarely, patients have a true chronic active infection with EBV. In these patients there are numerous objective clinical and laboratory findings, including pneumonitis, hepatitis, and uveitis, and a variety of hematologic abnormalities, such as neutropenia, eosinophilia, and thrombocytopenia (Schooley et al., 1986; Straus, 1988). These patients have prolonged, severe relapsing courses, occasionally with a fatal outcome. In some instances, death has been associated with respiratory failure caused by interstitial pneumonitis; in other instances it has been linked with diffuse T-cell lymphomas associated with EBV DNA (Jones et al., 1988). The pathogenesis of this syndrome is not clear, but it possibly is due to increased EBV replication, because patients often have extremely high levels of antibody to the EBV replicative antigens VCA and EA. Characteristically, these patients also have low or absent antibody to the EBNAs. Some of these patients have selective absence of antibody to EBNA-1 (Miller et al., 1987).

Several families have been described in which this syndrome has occurred in several members (Joncas et al., 1984). The pathogenesis of this familial form of chronic active EBV infection is also unclear. One hypothesis is that mechanisms involved in the restriction of viral replication are deficient, either at the cellular level or at the immune level. A deficiency of killer cells that participate in ADCC has been suggested. That it is difficult to identify transforming virus in the saliva of some of the patients has prompted the alternative hypothesis that they are infected with nontransforming, lytic EBV variants.

Chronic Fatigue Syndrome. Chronic active EBV infection should not be confused with a "neuromyasthenic," "polymyalgic," or "chronic fatigue" syndrome (Fukuda et al., 1994). In most patients EBV is not the causative agent of this syndrome, although some patients have elevations of antibody titers to EAs, and a few lack antibody to EBNA-1 (Jones et al., 1985; Katz et al., 1989). The symptoms of chronic fatigue syndrome include fatigue, chronic pharyngitis, tender lymph nodes, headaches, myalgia, and arthralgias. The symptoms are recurrent and prolonged, but no fatalities have been described. The natural history is variable.

BIBLIOGRAPHY

Abo W, Takada K, Kamada M, et al. Evolution of infectious mononucleosis into EVB carrying monoclonal malignant lymphoma. Lancet 1982;1:1272-1275.

Adams A, Lindahl T. Epstein-Barr virus genomes with properties of circular DNA molecules in carrier cells. Proc Natl Acad Sci USA 1975;72:1477-1481.

Anderson Lund BM, Bergen T. Temporary skin reactions to penicillins during the acute stage of infectious mononucleosis. Scand J Infect Dis 1975;7:21-28.

Andiman WA. The Epstein-Barr virus and EB virus infections in childhood. J Pediatr 1979;95:171-182.

Andiman WA. Epstein-Barr virus–associated syndromes: a critical reexamination. Pediatr Infect Dis 1984;3:198-203.

Andiman WA, Eastman R, Martin K, et al. Opportunistic lymphoproliferations associated with Epstein-Barr viral DNA in infants and children with AIDS. Lancet 1985;1390-1393.

Andiman WA, Markowitz RI, Horstmann DM. Clinical, virologic, and serologic evidence of Epstein-Barr virus infection in association with childhood pneumonia. J Pediatr 1981;99:880-886.

Baer R, Bankier AT, Biggin MD, et al. DNA sequence and expression of the B95-8 Epstein-Barr virus genome. Nature 1984;310:207-211.

Bar RS, DeLor CJ, Clauben KP, et al. Fatal infectious mononucleosis in a family. N Engl J Med 1974;290:363-367.

Barletta JM, Kingma DW, Ling Y, et al. Rapid in situ hybridization for the diagnosis of latent Epstein-Barr virus infection. Mol Cell Probes 1993;7:105-109.

Barth JH. Infectious mononucleosis (glandular fever) complicated by cold agglutinins, cold urticaria, and leg ulceration. Acta Dermatol Venereol (Stockh) 1981;61:451.

Bender CE. The value of corticosteroids in the treatment of infectious mononucleosis. JAMA 1967;199:97.

Benkerrou M, Durandy A, Fischer A. Therapy for transplant-related lymphoproliferative diseases. Hematol/Oncol Clin North Am 1993;7:467-475.

Bernstein A. Infectious mononucleosis. Medicine 1940;19:85-159.

Blacklow NR, Watson BK, Miller G, Jacobson BM. Mononucleosis with heterophile antibodies and EB virus infection.

Acquisition by an elderly patient in a hospital. Am J Med 1971;51:549-552.

Bray PF, Culp KW, McFarlin DE, et al. Demyelinating disease after neurologically complicated primary Epstein-Barr virus infection. Neurology 1992;42:278-282.

Brichacek B, Hirsch I, Sibl O, et al. Association of some supraglottic laryngeal carcinomas with EB virus. Int J Cancer 1983;32:193-197.

Brichacek B, Hirsch I, Sibl O, et al. Presence of Epstein-Barr virus DNA in carcinomas of the palatine tonsil. J Natl Cancer Inst 1984;72:809-815.

Butler T, Pastore J, Simon G, et al. Infectious mononucleosis myocarditis. J Infect 1981;3:172-175.

Clarke BF, Davies SH. Severe thrombocytopenia in infectious mononucleosis. Am J Med Sci 1964;248:703-708.

Colby BM, Shaw JE, Elion GB, Pagano JS. Effect of acyclovir [9-(2-hydroxyethoxymethyl)guanine] on Epstein-Barr virus DNA replication. J Virol 1980;34:560-568.

Conant MA. Hairy leukoplakia. A new disease of the oral mucosa. Arch Dermatol 1987;123:585-587.

Connelly KP, DeWitt D. Neurologic complications of infectious mononucleosis. Pediatr Neurol 1994;10:181-184.

Contratto AN. Infectious mononucleosis: a study of one-hundred and ninety-six cases. Arch Intern Med 1944;73:449-459.

Cowdrey SC, Reynolds JS. Acute urticaria in infectious mononucleosis. Ann Allergy 1969;27:182.

Davidsohn I. Serologic diagnosis of infectious mononucleosis. JAMA 1937;108:289.

de Thé G, Geser A, Day NE, et al. Epidemiological evidence for causal relationship between Epstein-Barr virus and Burkitt's lymphoma from Ugandan prospective study. Nature 1978;274:756-761.

De Waele M, Thielemans C, Van Camp BKG. Characterization of immunoregulatory T cells in EBV-induced infectious mononucleosis by monoclonal antibodies. N Engl J Med 1981;304:460-462.

Dinulos J, Mitchell DK, Egerton J, Pickering LK. Hydrops of the gall bladder associated with Epstein-Barr virus infection. Pediatr Infect Dis J 1994;13:924-929.

Epstein MA, Achong BG, Barr YM. Virus particles in cultural lymphoblasts from Burkitt's lymphoma. Lancet 1964;1:702-703.

Ernberg I, Andersson J. Acyclovir efficiently inhibits oropharyngeal excretion of Epstein-Barr virus in patients with acute infectious mononucleosis. J Gen Virol 1986;67:2267-2272.

Evans AS. Infectious mononucleosis in University of Wisconsin students. Report of five-year investigation. Am J Hyg 1960;71:342.

Evans AE, Niederman J, Cenabre LC, et al. A prospective evaluation of heterophile and Epstein-Barr virus-specific IgM antibody tests in clinical and subclinical infectious mononucleosis: specificity and sensitivity of the tests and persistence of antibody. J Infect Dis 1975;132:546.

Evans AS, Niederman JC, McCollum RW. Seroepidemiologic studies of infectious mononucleosis with EB virus. Engl J Med 1968;279:1121-1127.

Fields DA. Methicillin rash in infectious mononucleosis (letter). West J Med 1980;133:521.

Fleisher G, Bologonese R. Epstein-Barr virus infections in pregnancy: a prospective study. J Pediatr 1984;104:374-379.

Fleisher GR, Pasquariello PS, Warren WS, et al. Intrafamilial transmission of Epstein-Barr virus infections. J Pediatr 1981;98:16-19.

Fukuda K, Straus SE, Hickie I, et al. The chronic fatigue syndrome. Ann Intern Med 1994;121:953-959.

Gerber P, Walsh JN, Rosenblum EN, Purcell RH. Association of EB-virus infection with the post-perfusion syndrome. Lancet 1969;1:593-596.

Gold WL, Kapral MK, Witmer MR, et al. Postanginal septicemia as a life-threatening complication of infectious mononucleosis. Clin Infect Dis 1995;20:1439-1440.

Goldberg GN, Fulginiti VA, Ray CG, et al. In utero EBV (infectious mononucleosis) infection. JAMA 1981;246:1579-1581.

Greenspan D, Greenspan JS, Conant M, et al. Oral "hairy" leucoplakia in male homosexuals: evidence of association with both papillomavirus and a herpes-group virus. Lancet 1984;2:831-834.

Greenspan JS, Greenspan D, Lennette ET, et al. Replication of Epstein-Barr virus within the epithelial lesions of oral "hairy" leukoplakia, and AIDS-associated lesion. N Engl J Med 1985;313:1564-1571.

Grierson H, Purtilo DT. Epstein-Barr virus infections in males with X-linked lymphoproliferative syndrome. Ann Intern Med 1987;106:538-545.

Hamilton-Dutoit SJ, Pallesen G. Detection of Epstein-Barr virus small RNAs in routine paraffin sections using nonisotopic RNA/RNA in situ hybridization. Histopathol 1994;25:101-111.

Hanto DW, Frizzera G, Purtilo DT, et al. Clinical spectrum of lymphoproliferative disorders in renal transplant recipients and evidence for the role of the Epstein-Barr virus. Cancer Res 1981;41:4253-4261.

Henle G, Henle W. Observations on childhood infections with the Epstein-Barr virus. J Infect Dis 1970;121:303.

Henle G, Henle W. Epstein-Barr virus-specific IgA serum antibodies as an outstanding feature of nasopharyngeal carcinoma. Int J Cancer 1976;17:1-7.

Henle G, Henle W, Diehl V. Relation of Burkitt's tumor–associated herpes-type virus to infectious mononucleosis. Proc Natl Acad Sci USA 1968;59:94.

Ho M, Jaffe R, Miller G, et al. The frequency of Epstein-Barr virus infection and associated lymphoproliferative syndrome after transplantation and its manifestations in children. Transplantation 1988;45:719-727.

Ho M, Miller G, Atchison RW, et al. Epstein-Barr virus infections and DNA hybridization studies in posttransplantation lymphoma and lymphoproliferative lesions: the role of primary infection. J Infect Dis 1985;152:876-886.

Hoagland RJ. The transmission of infectious mononucleosis. Am J Med Sci 1955;229:262.

Hoagland RJ. The incubation period of infectious mononucleosis. Am J Public Health 1984;54:1699-1705.

Hochberg FH, Miller G, Schooley RJ, et al. Central-nervous system lymphoma related to Epstein-Barr virus. N Engl J Med 1983;309:745-748.

Hoff G, Bauer S. A new rapid slide test for infectious mononucleosis. JAMA 1965;194:351.

Horwitz CA et al. Long term serological follow-up of patients for Epstein-Barr virus after recovery from infectious mononucleosis. J Infect Dis 1985;151:1150-1153.

Howe JG, Steitz JA. Localization of Epstein-Barr virus–encoded small RNAs by in situ hybridization. Proc Natl Acad Sci USA 1986;83:9006-9010.

Hudgins JM. Infectious mononucleosis complicated by myocarditis and pericarditis. JAMA 1976;235:2626.

Hughes J, Burrows NP. Infectious mononucleosis presenting as erythema multiforme. Clin Experimen Dermatol 1993;18:373-374.

Icart J, Didier J, Dalens M, et al. Prospective study of Epstein-Barr virus (EBV) infection during pregnancy. Biomedicine 1981;34:160-163.

Joncas JH, Ghibu F, Blagdon M, et al. A familial syndrome of susceptibility to chronic active Epstein-Barr virus infection. Can Med Assoc J 1984;130:280-285.

Jones JF, Ray CG, Minnich LL, et al. Evidence for active Epstein-Barr virus infection in patients with persistent, unexplained illnesses: elevated anti–early antigen antibodies. Ann Intern Med 1985;102:1-7.

Jones JF, Shurin S, Abramowsky C, et al. T-cell lymphomas containing Epstein-Barr viral DNA in patients with chronic Epstein-Barr virus infections. N Engl J Med 1988;318:733-741.

Joshi VV, Kauffman S, Oleske JM, et al. Polyclonal polymorphic B-cell lymphoproliferative disorder with prominent pulmonary involvement in children with acquired immune deficiency syndrome. Cancer 1987;59:1455-1462.

Katz BZ, Andiman WA. Chronic fatigue syndrome. J Pediatr 1988;113:944-947.

Katz BZ, Berkman AB, Shapiro ED. Serologic evidence of active Epstein-Barr virus infection in Epstein-Barr virus–associated lymphoproliferative disorders in children with acquired immunodeficiency syndrome. J Pediatr 1992;120:228-232.

Katz BZ, Niederman JC, Olson BA, Miller G. Fragment length polymorphisms among independent isolates of Epstein-Barr virus from immunocompromised and normal hosts. J Infect Dis 1988;157:299-308.

Katz BZ, Raab-Traub N, Miller G. Latent and replicating forms of Epstein-Barr virus DNA in lymphomas and lymphoproliferative diseases. J Infect Dis 1989;160:589-598.

Koutras A. Epstein-Barr virus infection with pancreatitis, hepatitis, and proctitis. Pediatr Infect Dis J 1983;2:312-313.

Leblond V, Sutton L, Dorent R, et al. Lymphoproliferative disorders after organ transplantation. J Clin Oncol 1995;13:961-968.

Leder P, Battery J, Lenoir G, et al. Translocations among antibody genes in human cancer. Science 1976;222:765-771.

Lee ES, Locker J, Nalesnik M, et al. The association of Epstein-Barr virus with smooth muscle tumors occurring after organ transplantation. N Engl J Med 1995;332:19-25.

Lenoir G, Preud'homme JL, Bernheim A, Berger R. Correlation between immunoglobulin light chain expression and variant translocation in Burkitt's lymphoma. Nature 1982;298:474-476.

Levene G, Baker H. Drug reactions: ampicillin and infectious mononucleosis. Br J Dermatol 1968;80:417-421.

Leyvraz S, Henle W, Chahinian AP, et al. Association of Epstein-Barr virus with thymic carcinoma. N Engl J Med 1985;312:1296-1299.

MacMahon EME, Glass JD, Hayward SD, et al. Epstein-Barr virus in AIDS-related primary central nervous system lymphoma. Lancet 1991;338:969-973.

Martin PJ, Shulman HM, Schubach WH, et al. Fatal EBV-associated proliferation of donor B cells following treatment of acute graft-versus-host-disease with a murine monoclonal anti–T cell antibody. Ann Intern Med 1984;101:310.

Matoba AY. Ocular disease associated with Epstein-Barr virus infection. Arch Ophthalmol 1990;35:145.

Matsuo T, Heller M, Petti L, et al. Persistence of the entire Epstein-Barr virus genome integrated into human lymphocyte DNA. Science 1984;226:1322-1325.

Mayer HB, Wanke CA, Williams M, et al. Epstein-Barr virus–induced infectious mononucleosis is complicated by acute renal failure. Clin Infect Dis 1996;22:1009-1018.

McCarthy JT, Hoagland RJ. Cutaneous manifestations of infectious mononucleosis. JAMA 1964;187:153-154.

McClain KL, Leach CT, Jenson HB, et al. Association of Epstein-Barr virus with leiomyosarcomas in young people with AIDS. N Engl J Med 1995;332:12-18.

McKenna RW, Risdall RJ, Brunning RD. Virus associated with hemophagocytic syndrome. Hum Pathol 1981;12:395-398.

McKenzie H, Parratt D, White RO. IgM and IgG antibody levels to ampicillin in patients with infectious mononucleosis. Clin Exp Immunol 1976;26:214-221.

Miller G, Grogan E, Rowe D, et al. Selective lack of antibody to a component of EB nuclear antigen in patients with chronic active Epstein-Barr virus infection. J Infect Dis 1987;156:26-35.

Miller G, Niederman JC, Andrews LL. Prolonged oropharyngeal excretion of Epstein-Barr virus after infectious mononucleosis. N Engl J Med 1973;288:229.

Milne J. Infectious mononucleosis. N Engl J Med 1945; 233:727.

Morgan DG, Miller G, Neiderman JC, et al. Site of Epstein-Barr virus replication in the oropharynx. Lancet 1979;2:1154-1157.

Mueller N, Evans A, Harris NL, et al. Hodgkin's disease and Epstein-Barr virus: altered antibody pattern before diagnosis. N Engl J Med 1989;320:689-695.

Mulroy R: Amoxicillin rash in infectious mononucleosis (letter). Br Med J 1973;1:554.

Nazareth I, Mortimer P, McKendrick GD. Ampicillin sensitivity in infectious mononucleosis: temporary or permanent? Scand J Infect Dis 1972;4:229-230.

Neel HB, Pearson GR, Weiland LH, et al. Application of Epstein-Barr virus serology to the diagnosis of staging of North American patients with nasopharyngeal carcinoma. Otolaryngol Head Neck Surg 1983;91:255-262.

Niederman JC. Heterophil antibody determination in a series of 166 cases of infectious mononucleosis listed according to various stages of the disease. Yale J Biol Med 1956;28:629.

Niederman JC, Evans AS, Subrahmanyan MS, McCollum RW. Prevalence, incidence, and persistence of EB virus antibody in young adults. N Engl J Med 1970;282:361.

Niederman JC, McCollum RW, Henle G, Henle W. Infectious mononucleosis: clinical manifestations in relation to EB virus antibodies. JAMA 1968;203:205.

Niederman JC, Miller G. Kinetics of the antibody response to BamHI-K nuclear antigen in uncomplicated infectious mononucleosis. J Infect Dis 1986;154:346-349.

Niederman JC, Miller G, Pearson MA, et al. Infectious mononucleosis: Epstein-Barr virus shedding in saliva and oropharynx. N Engl J Med 1976;294:1355.

Osamah H, Finkelstein R, Brook JG. Rhabdomyolysis complicating acute Epstein-Barr virus infection. Infection 1995;23:119-120.

Pahwa S. Human immunodeficiency virus infection in children: nature of immunodeficiency, clinical spectrum, and management. Pediatr Infect Dis J 1988;7(suppl):61-71.

Pallesen G, Hamilton-Dutoit SJ, Zhou X. The association of Epstein-Barr virus (EBV) with T-cell lymphoproliferations and Hodgkin's disease. Adv Cancer Res 1993;62:179-239.

Patel BM. Skin rash with infectious mononucleosis and ampicillin. Pediatrics 1967;40:910-911.

Pathmanathan R, Prasad U, Sadler R, et al. Clonal proliferations of cells infected with Epstein-Barr virus in preinvasive lesions related to nasopharyngeal carcinoma. New Engl J Med 1995;333:693-698.

Pattengale PK, Smith RW, Perlin E. Atypical lymphocytes in acute infectious mononucleosis. Identification by multiple T and B lymphocyte markers. N Engl J Med 1974;291:1145.

Paul JR, Bunnell WW. The presence of heterophile antibodies in infectious mononucleosis. Am J Med Sci 1932;183:90.

Pereira MS, Blake JM, Macrae AD. EB virus antibody at different ages. Br Med J 1969;4:526.

Petrozzi JW. Infectious mononucleosis manifesting as a palmar dermatitis. Arch Dermatol 1971;104:207.

Pfeiffer E. Drüsenfieber. Jahrb Kinderheilkd 1889;29:257.

Pracher E, Panzer-Grumayer ER, Zoubeck A, et al. Successful bone marrow transplantation in a boy with X-linked lymphoproliferative syndrome and acute severe infectious mononucleosis. Bone Marrow Transplant 1994;13:655-658.

Press JH, et al. Infectious mononucleosis: a study of 96 cases. Ann Intern Med 1945;22:546.

Pullen H, Wright N, Murdock, JMcC: Hypersensitivity reactions to antimicrobial drugs in infectious mononucleosis. Lancet 1967;2:1176.

Purtilo DT. Malignant lymphoproliferative diseases induced by Epstein-Barr virus in immunodeficient patients, including X-linked, cytogenetic, and familial syndromes. Cancer Genet Cytogenet 1981;4:251-268.

Purtilo DT, DeFlorio D, Hutt LM, et al. Variable phenotypic expression of an X-linked recessive lymphoproliferative syndrome. N Engl J Med 1977;297:1077-1081.

Purtilo DT, Sakamoto K, Barnabei V, et al. Epstein-Barr virus–induced diseases in boys with the X-linked lymphoproliferative syndrome (XLP). Am J Med 1982;73:49-56.

Raab-Traub N, Flynn K. The structure of the termini of the Epstein-Barr virus as a marker of clonal cellular proliferation. Cell 1986;47:883-889.

Raab-Traub N, Flynn K, Pearson G, et al. The differentiated form of nasopharyngeal carcinoma contains Epstein-Barr virus DNA. Int J Cancer 1987;39:25-29.

Ralston LS, Saiki AK, Powers WT. Orchitis as a complication of infectious mononucleosis. JAMA 1960;173:1348.

Rapp CE Jr, Hewetson JF. Infectious mononucleosis and the Epstein-Barr virus. Am J Dis Child 1978;132:78.

Ray CG, Gall EP, Minnich LL, et al. Acute polyarthritis associated with active Epstein-Barr virus infection. JAMA 1982;248:2990-2993.

Resnick L, Herbst JS, Ablashi DV, et al. Regression of oral hairy leukoplakia after orally administered acyclovir therapy. JAMA 1988;259:384-388.

Robinson JE, Brown N, Andiman W, et al. Diffuse polyclonal B-cell lymphoma during primary infection with Epstein-Barr virus. N Engl J Med 1980;302:1293-1297.

Rocchi G, Felici A, Ragona G, Heinz A. Quantitative evaluation of Epstein-Barr virus–infected mononuclear peripheral blood leukocytes in infectious mononucleosis. N Engl J Med 1977;296:132.

Rooney CM, Smith CA, Ng CYC, et al. Use of gene-modified virus-specific T lymphocytes to control Epstein-Barr virus–related lymphoproliferation. Lancet 1995;345:9-13.

Rubinstein A, Morecki R, Silverman B, et al. Pulmonary disease in children with acquired immune deficiency syndrome and AIDS-related complex. J Pediatr 1986;108:498-503.

Rutkow IM. Rupture of the spleen in infectious mononucleosis. Arch Surg 1978;113:718.

Sawyer RN, Evans AS, Niederman JC, McCollum RW. Prospective studies of a group of Yale University freshmen: I. occurrence of infectious mononucleosis. J Infect Dis 1971;123:263.

Schooley RT, Carey RW, Miller G, et al. Chronic Epstein-Barr virus infection associated with fever and interstitial pneumonitis. Clinical and serologic features and response to antiviral chemotherapy. Ann Intern Med 1986;636-643.

Schubach WH, Hackman R, Neiman PE, et al. A monoclonal immunoblastic sarcoma in donor cells bearing Epstein-Barr virus genomes following allogeneic marrow grafting for acute lymphoblastic leukemia. Blood 1982;60:180-187.

Seemayer TA, Gross TG, Egeler RM, et al. X-linked lymphoproliferative disease. Pediatr Res 38:471-478, 1995.

Sixbey JW, Nedrud JG, Raab-Traub N, et al. Epstein-Barr virus replication in oropharyngeal epithelial cells. N Engl J Med 1984;310:1225-1230.

Sprunt TP, Evans FA. Mononuclear leukocytosis in reaction to acute infections ("infectious mononucleosis"). Bull Johns Hopkins Hosp 1920;31:410.

Stevenson SS, Webster G, Stewart IA. Acute tonsillitis in the management of infectious mononucleosis. J Laryngol Otol 1992;106:989-991.

Strauch B, Siegel N, Andrews LL, Miller G. Oropharyngeal excretion of Epstein-Barr virus by renal transplant recipients and other patients treated with immunosuppressive drugs. Lancet 1974;1:234.

Straus SE. The chronic mononucleosis syndrome. J Infect Dis 1988;157:405-412.

Subar M, Neri A, Inghirami G, et al: Frequent c-*myc* oncogene activation and infrequent presence of Epstein-Barr virus genome in AIDS-associated lymphoma. Blood 1988;72:667-671.

Sumaya CV. Primary Epstein-Barr virus infections in children. Pediatrics 1977;59:16.

Svedmyr E, Jondal M. Cytotoxic effector cells specific for B cell lines transformed by EBV are present in patients with infectious mononucleosis. Proc Natl Acad Sci USA 1975;7:1622-1626.

Swinnen LD. Posttransplant lymphoproliferative disorder. Leuk Lymphoma 1992;6:289-297.

Tischendorf P, Shramek GJ, Balagtas RC, et al. Development and persistence of immunity to Epstein-Barr virus in man. J Infect Dis 1970;122:401.

Tosato G, Magrath I, Koski I, et al. Activation of suppressor T cells during Epstein-Barr virus–induced infectious mononucleosis. 1979;301:1133-1137.

Turner AR, MacDonald RN, Cooper BA. Transmission of infectious mononucleosis by transfusion of preillness plasma. Ann Intern Med 1972;77:751-753.

Tynell E, Aurelius E, Brandell A, et al. Acyclovir and prednisilone treatment of acute infectious mononucleosis. J Infect Dis 1996;174:324-331. (Erratum in J Infect Dis 1996;174:678).

Waldo RT. Neurologic complications of infectious mononucleosis after steroid therapy. South Med J 1981;74:1159-1160.

Weinreb M, Day PJ, Niggli F, et al. The consistent association between Epstein-Barr virus and Hodgkin's disease in children in Kenya. Blood 1996;87:3828-3836.

Weiss LM, Movabhed LA, Warnke RA, Sklar J. Detection of Epstein-Barr viral genomes in Reed-Sternberg cells of Hodgkin's disease. N Engl J Med 1989;320:502-506.

Wilson ER, Malluh A, Stagno S, et al. Fatal Epstein-Barr virus–associated hemophagocytic syndrome. J Pediatr 1981;98:260-262.

Wolf H, Haus M, Wilmes E. Persistence of Epstein-Barr virus in the parotid gland. J Virol 1984;51:795-798.

Wolnisty C. Orchitis as a complication of infectious mononucleosis: report of a case. N Engl J Med 1962;266:88.

Yao QY, Rickinson AB, Epstein MA. A reexamination of the Epstein-Barr virus carrier state in healthy seropositive individuals. Int J Cancer 1985;35:35-42.

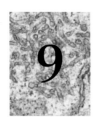

9   GASTROENTERITIS

DOUGLAS K. MITCHELL AND LARRY K. PICKERING

Acute infectious gastroenteritis is one of the most common infectious diseases of humans, ranking second to acute respiratory tract infections as a worldwide cause of morbidity. In developing areas of the world, diarrhea is a significant cause of death in infants. It is estimated that young children in developing countries experience 1.5 billion episodes of diarrhea and 4 million associated deaths each year (Bern et al., 1992; Claeson and Merson, 1990). Approximately 15% of children in developing nations die of diarrhea before 3 years of age. In the United States 20 to 35 million episodes of diarrhea occur every year, resulting in 2.1 to 3.7 million physician visits. In addition, an average of 220,000 children younger than 5 years of age with diarrhea are hospitalized in the United States, and approximately 125 deaths occur each year as a result of gastroenteritis (Cicerello and Glass, 1994). Hospitalization and outpatient care for pediatric diarrhea result in direct costs of more than $2 billion per year, with additional indirect costs to families (Avendano et al., 1993). The usual clinical syndrome is characterized by various combinations of nausea, vomiting, abdominal cramps, and diarrhea; fever and dehydration also may be present. Occasionally, systemic manifestations occur, including bacteremia and immune-mediated extraintestinal manifestations of enteric infections. The causative agents include bacteria, viruses, and parasites (Box 9-1). Bacterial and viral causes of diarrhea are reviewed in this chapter; parasitic causes of diarrhea are discussed in Chapter 21.

BACTERIAL GASTROENTERITIS

Bacterial agents associated with diarrhea that are discussed include *Aeromonas* species, *Campylobacter* species, *Clostridium difficile, Escherichia coli, Salmonella* species, *Shigella* species, *Vibrio cholerae,* and *Yersinia enterocolitica.* Some of these bacterial pathogens are identified routinely in

the microbiology laboratory, whereas others require specialized media or media environment. Fluid replacement is critical in all persons with diarrhea, and appropriate antimicrobial therapy may favorably alter the course of illness associated with some enteropathogens.

Etiology

Many bacteria are associated with diarrhea in humans (see Box 9-1) and vary in importance according to host factors, geography, epidemiologic considerations, and virulence mechanisms. Organisms are discussed here in alphabetic order.

Aeromonas. *Aeromonas* species are associated with several disease states in humans, including soft-tissue infections, bacteremia, and gastroenteritis. The association of *Aeromonas* species with gastroenteritis is controversial, but mounting evidence shows that *A. hydrophila, A. caviae,* and *A. sobria* are associated with gastroenteritis. These organisms are found in soil and in fresh and brackish water worldwide. *Aeromonas* species elaborate a large number of extracellular enzymes, including an enterotoxin (aerolysin) that causes fluid accumulation in rabbit intestinal loop models (Sears and Kaper, 1996; Utsalo et al., 1995; Wilcox et al., 1992).

Campylobacter. *Campylobacter* species are recognized as one of the most frequent causes of acute bacterial diarrhea throughout the world (Blaser and Reller, 1981; Karmali and Fleming, 1979; Pai et al., 1979). *C. jejuni* is the most commonly identified species, but other species— including *C. coli, C. concisus, C. fetus, C. lari, C. hyointestinalis, C. sputorum,* and *C. upsaliensis*— have also been associated with diarrhea and occasionally with invasive disease in humans. Animals, specifically poultry and cattle, are the reservoirs of *C. jejuni.* In most laboratories *C. coli* is identified humans that range in severity from asymptomatic colonization to severe diarrhea, pseudomembranous colitis, toxic megacolon, colonic perforation, and death (Bartlett, 1994; Gerding et al., 1995; Kelly et al., 1994). Toxin-producing *C. difficile* frequently is recovered from stools of asymptomatic infants during their first year of life, among whom 25% to 65% may be colonized; colonization rates decrease to 0% to 5% in older children and adults. Toxigenic *C. difficile* is a cause of antibiotic-associated diarrhea in adults, but the role of *C. difficile* in childhood illness, especially in infants, remains controversial (Cerquetti et al., 1995; Mitchell et al., 1995b). *C. difficile* can be isolated from soil and frequently is present in the hospital environment.

Escherichia coli. *E. coli* is a common inhabitant of the intestine and ordinarily causes no clinical symptoms. Although isolation of *E. coli* is not difficult, recognition of pathogenic strains is complex because of the multiple factors that enable this organism to cause disease. Specific recognition of pathogenic strains is accomplished readily in research or reference laboratories; therefore laboratory confirmation of gastrointestinal tract disease caused by *E. coli* generally is not available.

In 1951 *E. coli* organisms were shown as serologically heterogeneous by Kauffman, who divided the species into various somatic groups. *E. coli* possesses O (somatic) antigens, H (flagellar) antigens, and K (capsular) antigens. The serotype, which is a chromosomally determined characteristic, depends on these antigens.

E. coli strains that cause diarrhea currently are grouped according to their pathogenic phenotype(s) (Ulshen and Rollo, 1980). The provisional classification includes enterohemorrhagic *E. coli* (EHEC), which elaborates cytotoxins; enterotoxigenic *E. coli* (ETEC), which elaborates enterotoxins (Rudoy, 1975); enteroinvasive *E. coli* (EIEC), which invades the intestinal epithelium; enteropathogenic *E. coli* (EPEC), which demonstrates epithelial adherence and produces attaching and effacing lesions; and enteroaggregative *E. coli* (EAEC), which demonstrates a stacked-brick adherence to epithelial cells (Table 9-1). These categories of *E. coli* are associated with different epidemiologic patterns and clinical syndromes.

Enterohemorrhagic *E. coli*. In 1983 a previously unrecognized class of *E. coli* was described (Riley et al., 1983). The major virulence trait was production of cell-damaging toxins. The cytotoxins

as *C. jejuni*. *C. fetus* is an uncommon cause of disease in humans, but when infection occurs this organism produces fever, bacteremia, and meningitis, usually in immunocompromised hosts and neonates.

Clostridium difficile. *C. difficile* is the cause of pseudomembranous colitis and of a high percentage of cases of antimicrobial associated colitis. *C. difficile* is a spore-forming gram-positive anaerobic bacillus that produces two exotoxins: toxin A, an enterotoxin, and toxin B, a cytotoxin. The organism causes gastrointestinal tract infections in

Table 9-1 *E. coli* associated with diarrhea

Classification	Pathogenic mechanism	Common serogroups (somatic antigens)
Enterohemorrhagic *E. coli* (EHEC)	Protein synthesis inhibiting Shigatoxin I (VT1)* Shigatoxin II (VT2)* Shigatoxin II variants	157 (most common), 26, 111, others
Enterotoxigenic *E. coli* (ETEC)	Enterotoxins causing fluid loss Heat-stable (ST) Heat-labile (LT) (cholera-like) Adhesins Colonization factor antigens (CFA)	6, 8, 15, 20, 25, 27, 63, 78, 80, 85, 115, 128ac, 139, 148, 153, 159, 167
Enteroinvasive *E. coli* (EIEC)	Invasion of intestinal cells Invasion plasmid is closely related to invasion plasmid of Shigellae	28ac, 29, 124, 136, 143, 144, 152, 164, 167
Enteropathogenic *E. coli* (EPEC)	Adhesins Enteroadherent factor (EAF)† plasmid	Class I (EAF +): 55, 86, 111, 119, 125, 126, 127, 128ab, 142 Class II (EAF−): 18, 44, 112, 114
Enteroaggregative *E. coli* (EAEC)	Adhesins	Not determined

*VT, Verotoxin.
†EAF, EPEC adherence factor.

of EHEC are referred to as *verotoxins, verocytotoxins,* or *shigatoxins* (SLT). The most common EHEC serotype is *E. coli* 0157:H7, although approximately 50 EHEC serotypes have been recognized. Shortly after recognition of this class of *E. coli,* the distinctive hemorrhagic colitis associated with these organisms was shown to be complicated by development of hemolytic uremic syndrome (HUS) (Cleary, 1988; Karmali et al., 1983). Although other causes for HUS exist, the majority of HUS cases are associated with EHEC infection. Cattle are the reservoir of EHEC; humans also may serve as a reservoir for person-to-person transmission.

Enterotoxigenic *E. coli.* ETEC produce plasmid-encoded enterotoxins (Levine et al., 1978; Sack and Sack, 1975; Sears and Kaper, 1996; Shore et al., 1974; Thomas and Knoop, 1982, 1983). Although belonging to specific serogroups, these organisms are not identified routinely by serotyping. The heat-labile enterotoxin (LT) and heat-stable enterotoxin (ST) produced by ETEC are characterized in Table 9-2. LT, like cholera toxin, activates adenylate cyclase. ST activates guanylate cyclase, with a resulting increase in cyclic guanosine monophosphate (cGMP). Both LT and ST produce watery diarrhea without blood

or mucous. Many of the ETEC strains possess specific adhesion factors enabling them to colonize the small intestine. Such colonization factor antigens contribute to disease production by these toxigenic bacteria. Colonization factors appear in electron microscopy as filamentous structures that often resemble fimbriae. Humans constitute the reservoir for strains causing diarrhea in humans.

Enteroinvasive *E. coli.* EIECs produce intestinal tract disease by their ability to penetrate and multiply within the intestinal epithelial cells. These enteroinvasive *E. coli* organisms resemble shigella in this respect. Although these *E. coli* organisms tend to fall into certain serologic groups, serotyping to identify these organisms generally is not performed. Infections generally occur in adults; foodborne outbreaks have been reported.

Enteropathogenic *E. coli.* All *E. coli* strains that cause diarrhea were originally called enteropathogenic *E. coli* when certain serotypes were identified and associated with disease (Clausen and Christie, 1982; Goldschmidt and DuPont, 1976; Levine and Edelman, 1984). The terminology has evolved as the pathogenic mechanisms have been elucidated, so the term *enteropathogenic E. coli* currently refers only to those organisms that cause disease but do not produce LT or ST, do not have

Table 9-2 Diarrhea-associated toxins

Characteristics of organism toxin	V. cholerae Cholera toxin	E. coli Labile toxin (LT)	E. coli Stable toxin (ST)	Shiga toxin (SLT I,II,IIv)
Molecular weight (MW)	84,000	73,000	2,000	71,000
Immunogenic	Yes	Yes	No	Yes
Genetic control of toxin	Chromosomal Bacteriophage	Plasmid	Plasmid	Phage
Multimeric protein (A and B subunits)	Yes	Yes	No	Yes
A and B synthesized separately and then associated	Yes	Yes		Yes
B subunit binds to cell	Yes	Yes		Yes
Cell receptor	GM_1, ganglioside	GM_1, ganglioside	100,000 MW protein (not GM_1)	Galactose 1-4; galactose β1-4; glucose ceramide (Gb_3)
Internalization	By noncoated surface micro-invaginations	By noncoated surface micro-invaginations	Unknown	By receptor-mediated endocytosis through coated pits
Subunit with enzymatic activity	Yes	Yes		Yes
Intracellular target site	Inner-surface plasma membrane	Inner-surface plasma membrane	Inner-surface plasma membrane	Cytosol
Action	Modification of plasma membrane enzymes	Modification of plasma membrane enzymes	Modification of plasma membrane enzymes	Cleaves adenine residue from 28S ribosomal RNA
Enzyme affected	Activation of adenylate cyclase	Activation of adenylate cyclase	Activation of guanylate cyclase	Blocks attachment site for EF 1–dependent aminoacyl tRNA binding
Mode of action	NAD-dependent ADP ribosylation of GTP-binding compartment of adenylate cyclase		Unknown	A1-catalyzed inactivation of the 28S ribosomal subunit
Site of action	Small intestine epithelium	Small intestine epithelium	Small intestine epithelium	Small and large intestine
Physiologic action	Absorption	Absorption	Absorption	Probably causes fluid loss
	Secretion	Secretion	Secretion	Through injury to enterocytes with decreased absorption

the genes coding for these toxins, and are not enteroinvasive (Robins-Browne et al., 1982). EPEC has caused diarrhea in volunteers. Pathophysiologic studies have shown that some of these organisms adhere to the microvilli of the rabbit ileum. In vitro adherence to HEp-2 cells is a correlate of their ability to adhere in vivo. Biopsies of human intestine show that the brush border of the small intestine is effaced, and the organisms are densely adherent. This ability to adhere is apparently also associated with the presence of a enteroadherent factor (EAF) plasmid that is different from that necessary for the invasive qualities of EIEC mentioned previously. Two classes of EPEC can be distinguished by adherence patterns in tissue culture and by gene probe for this characteristic (EAF probe). The precise mechanism of adherence and diarrhea remains uncertain. Humans are the reservoir for strains that cause diarrhea in humans.

Enteroaggregative *E. coli*. This group of pathogens is not yet well characterized either mechanistically or clinically (Bhan et al., 1989; Mathewson et al., 1987). The major virulence trait thus far defined is the ability of these organisms to adhere to HEp-2 cells in tissue culture in a distinctive way. Some EAECs produce a distinct heat-stable enterotoxin named EAST1 (Savarino et al., 1996). Children infected with EAEC seem to be at particular risk for developing chronic diarrhea (Wanke et al., 1991).

Salmonellae. Salmonellae currently are classified into three species: *S. enteritidis, S. typhi,* and *S. choleraesuis.* There are more than 2,000 serotypes of *S. enteritidis,* which are typed by their O (somatic) antigens and H (flagellar) antigens. *S. typhi* and *S. choleraesuis* each have only one serotype. Salmonellae frequently are given names of locations (e.g., *S. newport*) in which outbreaks have occurred. Serogrouping may be useful epidemiologically and is generally performed by state health laboratories. Serotype *S. typhimurium,* one of the *S. enteritidis* group, is responsible for approximately 20% to 30% of all reported infections in the United States each year, and, although any serotype can cause human disease, in most areas a small number of serotypes account for the majority of confirmed cases. During the period from 1976 to 1994, rates of isolation of *S. enteritidis* increased in the United States from 0.5 to 3.9 per 100,000 population (Centers for Disease Control, 1996b; Mishu et al., 1994). Egg- and poultry-borne infections and reptile-associated infections are major problems. *S. typhi*

is a pathogen only of humans, and humans are the reservoir. For all other salmonella strains a wide range of domestic and wild animals serve as reservoirs.

Shigellae. There are four main serogroups that compose the genus *Shigella.* Each group includes a number of types that are distinguished by biochemical and serologic criteria: group A, *S. dysenteriae;* group B, *S. flexneri;* group C, *S. boydii;* and group D, *S. sonnei.* Group D accounts for 60% to 80% of the episodes of shigellosis in the United States.

The human intestinal tract is the natural habitat of shigellae. A specific virulence plasmid is necessary for the epithelial-cell invasiveness manifested by shigellae. *S. dysenteriae* type 1 (Shiga bacillus) produces a protein synthesis–inhibiting toxin (shigatoxin) (Bartlett et al., 1986). Other shigellae make little or no shigatoxin, although EHECs (described previously) produce a toxin either essentially identical to shigatoxin (SLT-I) or less closely related (SLT-II). Experimentally, shigatoxin causes hemorrhagic fluid secretion in the jejunum of animals and is a cytotoxin in cell culture. Shigatoxin recognizes a receptor, globotriaosylceramide (Gb3), in sensitive cells and is translocated by endocytosis to the cytoplasm, where it blocks protein synthesis. The presence of Gb3 is required but not sufficient for the action of shigatoxin (Jacewicz et al., 1994). The only significant reservoir of shigellae is humans, although primates may become infected.

Vibrio cholerae. In its severe form *Vibrio cholerae* causes sudden, profuse, watery diarrhea that can progress to rapid dehydration, acidosis, and death. The biotypes of *V. cholerae* O1 (classic and El Tor) each include organisms of Inaba, Ogawa, and (rarely) Hikojima serotypes. All clinical isolates of *V. cholerae* O1 from the United States have been biotype El Tor, serotype Inaba. These strains were isolated from people who had eaten contaminated raw and undercooked shellfish from the Gulf of Mexico or who had acquired the strain in South America, where an epidemic of cholera caused by El Tor biotype *V. cholerae* O1 has been occurring since 1991.

In 1992 large-scale epidemics of cholera were reported in India and Bangladesh. The causative agent was *V. cholerae* O139. This organism elaborates the same cholera toxin but differs from the O1 strains in the lipopolysaccharide structure. Cholera strains that are not classified as O1 or O139 are referred to as *non-O1 strains* (nonagglutinable vibrios or noncholera vibrios). These strains generally do not elaborate enterotoxin, are not associated with large outbreaks, and occasionally cause sporadic disease. The reservoirs of *V. cholerae* are humans and copepods and other zooplankton in brackish water or estuaries. *V. cholerae* O1 and O139 produce a heat-labile enterotoxin that activates adenylate cyclase and catalyzes the formation of cyclic AMP, which results in the secretion of fluid and electrolytes into the lumen of the intestine.

Other *Vibrio* species associated with acute diarrheal illness include *V. hollisae, V. parahaemolyticus, V. furnissii, V. flavialis,* and *V. mimicus. Vibrio vulnificus* has been associated with gastroenteritis following ingestion of raw oysters. This may be a severe and fatal illness in patients who are immunocompromised (Centers for Disease Control, 1993, 1996c).

Yersinia enterocolitica. The genus *Yersinia* includes *Y. pestis, Y. pseudotuberculosis,* and *Y. enterocolitica. Y. enterocolitica* can produce diarrhea, mesenteric adenitis, and extraintestinal infection. *Y. pseudotuberculosis* has been associated with abdominal pain. Five biotypes and fifty serotypes of *Y. enterocolitica* have been reported and inhabit the intestinal tract of many animals and birds and survive in fresh water. Strains pathogenic for humans include strains in serotypes 03, 05, 08, 09, and 027 and biotypes 1, 2, 3, and 4. Serotypes causing diseases may vary in different geographic areas; types 08 and 03 are responsible for most outbreaks in the United States. Laboratory personnel must be alerted to the possibility that this organism is being considered as a potential pathogen so that appropriate selective media can be used for isolation. Animals, especially pigs, are the principal reservoir of *Yersinia enterocolitica.*

Epidemiology

Bacterial enteropathogens are transmitted by the fecal-oral route, either through contaminated food or water or by person-to-person spread. The mode of transmission depends on the organism and the immune status of the host. In immunocompetent hosts a large inoculum is necessary for infection with virtually all bacteria, generally requiring ingestion of over 10^6 organisms. Shigellae (and perhaps EHEC) are the exceptions, with 10 to 100 organisms transmitting infection. *S. typhi* and shigellae are inhabitants of only the human intestinal tract, whereas the other bacterial enteric pathogens have animal hosts and can be transmitted to humans by contact with contaminated materials.

Major categories of diarrhea caused by enteric pathogens include illness acquired as a result of the following: (1) exposure to child-care settings or hospitals, (2) food-borne or water-borne disease, (3) antimicrobial agent exposure, (4) travel, or (5) immunosuppressed hosts. Children who attend day care have a significantly greater risk of diarrheal illness than age-matched children not in child care (Holmes et al., 1996; Reves et al., 1993). Diarrheal illnesses are increasing in less developed countries as a consequence of increased urbanization (crowding), decreasing incidence of breastfeeding, shifting agricultural patterns toward cash crops, and large numbers of refugees from wars.

Children less than 6 years of age are particularly at risk for diarrhea associated with *Aeromonas* spp. (Wilcox et al., 1992). Outbreaks of diarrhea caused by *Aeromonas* spp. in child-care centers also have been reported (de la Morena et al., 1993; Sempertegui et al., 1995), but volunteers who have been fed the organism have not become ill.

C. jejuni is an important cause of diarrhea worldwide. Disease occurs in all age groups, with the highest incidence in children under 5 years of age and young adults. Most farm animals; meat sources; poultry carcasses; and many pet dogs and cats, especially the young, harbor this organism. Transmission occurs from ingestion of undercooked chicken and pork, contaminated food and water, and unpasteurized milk. Transmission also can occur from contact with infected pets (puppies and kittens) and farm animals. Person-to-person spread appears to be uncommon; outbreaks have been reported, including outbreaks of *C. upsaliensis,* in child-care centers (Goossens et al., 1995). The incubation period is 2 to 5 days, with a range up to 10 days.

Spores of *C. difficile* are acquired from the environment or by fecal-oral transmission from colonized individuals. Colonization rates can reach 50% in asymptomatic neonates and infants but decline to less than 5% in children over 2 years of age and in adults. Risk factors for disease are administration of antimicrobial therapy, repeated enemas, prolonged nasogastric tube insertion, and intestinal tract surgery, all of which alter the normal intestinal flora and allow *C. difficile* to proliferate. Hospitals are reservoirs for *C. difficile,* and child-care centers may also be a source. The incubation period is unknown.

EHECs are recognized as a cause of sporadic diarrhea and have been associated with many outbreaks. EHEC outbreaks associated with undercooked beef, especially ground beef, are a major health problem. Outbreaks caused by contaminated water, unpasteurized milk, and apple cider have been reported (Centers for Disease Control, 1996a; Keene et al., 1994). Person-to-person transmission of *E. coli* O157:H7 has been described in child-care centers, custodial institutions, families, and hospitals (Belongia et al., 1993). The incubation period is 3 to 4 days, with a range up to 10 days. ETECs cause disease primarily in infants less than 18 months of age in developing nations and in adult travelers (Gorbach et al., 1975). Contaminated food, and less often water, are thought to be the major modes of transmission. Person-to-person transmission is uncommon. The incubation period is 1 to 3 days. EPECs cause outbreaks of disease, especially in infants in nurseries through contaminated instruments or other contaminated aspects of the environment or through health-care personnel. EPEC is uncommon in the United States but remains a major cause of diarrhea in many developing countries. EIECs are a rare cause of infantile diarrhea in the United States. EIECs are transmitted through contaminated food, and outbreaks have been described. EAECs have been recognized as a cause of diarrhea in infants in developing countries and in travelers to these locales. Some strains may cause chronic diarrhea in infants.

Disease resulting from salmonella is reported worldwide. Humans usually ingest salmonellae from contaminated food, including meat; raw milk; and poultry products, especially eggs. Organisms are present on the surface of meat; thus any conditions favoring multiplication enhance the possibility of disease production. Animals are infected and perpetuate the infection among themselves, easily contaminating other animals during transport. Selected salmonella serotypes frequently are associated with transmission from reptiles such as iguanas, snakes, lizards, and turtles (Ackman et al., 1995). A large U.S.-wide food-borne outbreak of *S. enteritidis* occurred in 1994 following national distribution of ice cream that had been contaminated by transport of ice cream mix in the same tanker trailers used for transport of unpasteurized eggs (Hennessy et al., 1996). Consumption of raw fruits and vegetables contaminated during slicing have been reported. An estimated 2 million cases of salmonella gastroenteritis occur per year in the United States, with the incidence rate of infection being highest in infants and young children. Nosocomial transmission within hospitals, nursing homes, and institutions results from cross-contamination involving personnel, equipment, and aerosol (Novak and Feldman, 1979). In regions where sewage disposal and water purification are inadequate, enteric infections are frequent and the likelihood of spread is enhanced. *S. typhi* is exclusively a human pathogen. The incubation period is 12 to 36 hours, with a range up to 72 hours.

Communicability of disease resulting from shigellae depends on human fecal material transmitting infection either through person-to-person contact or through food and water. The highest incidence of shigellae is in children 1 to 4 years of age, particularly during the warm season, with illness uncommon in infants under 6 months of age. In one study, 50% of children infected with shigellae were asymptomatic (Guerrero et al., 1994). Large outbreaks of infection are related to contaminated food or water or can occur in conditions of crowding where personal hygiene is poor, such as in jails, child-care centers, custodial institutions, and refugee camps. Infection can occur following ingestion of 10 to 100 organisms. The incubation period is 1 to 4 days, with a range up to 7 days.

Cholera has caused devastating worldwide pandemics, with perpetual endemic disease occurring in India and Bangladesh. An epidemic of cholera began in Peru in January of 1991 and subsequently has spread to several other countries in Latin America. Cases have been identified in the United States over the past decade and are related to eating shellfish from the Gulf of Mexico or from travel to South America. In 1995 most of the twenty-three reported cases of cholera in the United States were imported. Carriage and excretion of the organism usually last several weeks but may last longer. In endemic areas, cholera is a disease of childhood, although infants less than 1 year old are usually spared. When epidemics reach previously uninfected countries, all ages are infected. The *V. cholerae* O139 epidemics in Asia have occurred predominantly in adults. Presumably, *V. cholerae* O1 exposure during childhood does not protect against O139 exposure later in life. Because the cholera toxins of *V. cholerae* O1 and O139 are immunologically and genetically identical, this indicates that preexisting antitoxin antibody does not provide protection against *V. cholerae* O139 infections (Cholera Working Group, 1993; Nair et al., 1994). Transmission of cholera occurs following ingestion of food or water contaminated with feces or vomitus of infected persons. In the United States, most sporadic cases of infection follow ingestion of raw or inadequately cooked seafood from polluted waters. El Tor organisms can persist in water for long periods of time. The incubation period is 2 to 3 days, with a range up to 5 days.

Yersinia enterocolitica infection affects all age groups, but most episodes occur in infants and children in whom a spectrum of illness occurs, including gastroenteritis. Some geographic variation in recognized disease in the United States occurs for reasons that are not clear. The highest isolation rates have been reported during the cold season in temperate climates, including the United States, Canada, and Northern Europe. Outbreaks of disease have been traced to contaminated food, including milk, tofu, and pork chitterlings (Lee et al., 1990). Pathogenic strains most commonly are isolated from raw pork or pork products. Persons with excessive iron storage syndromes have increased susceptibility to *Yersinia* bacteremia.

Pathogenesis and Pathology

The intestinal tract has a number of nonimmunologic defense mechanisms that help form a barrier against infection (Grady and Keusch, 1971). The indigenous flora are present in numbers up to 10^{11} organisms per gram of stool in the large bowel. Competition for substrate plus other environmental alterations—such as decreased pH or production of antibacterial substances—probably contribute to which organisms succeed in causing disease. Antibiotics alter growth of indigenous flora and may contribute to colonization by enteric pathogens.

Secretions containing compounds such as mucin may diminish bacterial adherence to epithelial cells both mechanically and by competition at receptor sites. Normal peristalsis expels organisms that are not adherent. Gastric acid inhibits growth of many bacteria, and lysozyme and bile salts in the intestinal tract hinder growth of many bacteria. Immunologic defense mechanisms include secretory IgA, the production of which is dependent on antigen exposure to the local intestinal surface. The secretory piece of IgA increases resistance of these antibodies to protease; thus this class of antibody best withstands the environment of the lumen of the bowel. Antibody binds toxins and bacteria, thus preventing adsorption, and may be bactericidal in combination with complement and lysozyme.

Malabsorption or profuse watery isotonic diarrhea is caused by dysfunction of the small intestine. Some organisms (*V. cholerae* is the prototype) cause profuse malabsorption because of the effects of their enterotoxins on intestinal cells. In other instances, such as dysentery, the colon or the terminal ileum are invaded by bacteria. *Shigella* spp. constitute the prototype of invasive organisms causing dysentery. The mucosal invasion and disruption are visible as ulcerations and result in the presence of blood and mucus in stool.

Diarrhea can be categorized as inflammatory or noninflammatory, resulting from virulence mechanisms of enteropathogens. Inflammatory diarrhea occurs following adherence, invasion, or cytotoxin production by bacteria. Noninflammatory diarrhea occurs as a result of adherence, enterotoxin production by bacteria, or loss of villi cells caused by enteric viruses. Bacterial pathogens must be able to adhere in the intestinal mucosa to cause disease, establishing the adhesins of the bacteria as a critical part of virulence.

Bacteria produce one or more of four types of toxins: enterotoxin, cytoskeleton-altering toxin, cytotoxin, and toxins with neural activity (Sears and Kaper, 1996). Enterotoxins stimulate net intestinal secretion without histologic evidence of intestinal damage. Cytoskeleton-altering toxins produce an alteration in cell shape without inducing significant cell injury. Cytotoxins produce cellular damage, as documented by gross findings such as intestinal hemorrhage, light-microscopic evidence of intestinal damage, or cellular injury. Toxins with neural activity include those that involve release of one or more neurotransmitters from the enteric nervous system or alter smooth-muscle activity in the intestine.

The literature dealing with toxins produced by *Aeromonas* species is confusing. A definitive mechanism of secretion has not been identified for any of the *Aeromonas* toxins. An enterotoxin referred to as *aerolysin* causes secretion without histologic changes in perfused rat jejunum. At least four other noncytotoxic factors have been described to be produced by *Aeromonas* species, all of which have secretory activity.

Campylobacter jejuni has the potential to invade epithelial cells and produce dysentery. In addition, three major toxins have been reported to be produced by some *C. jejuni* strains associated with diarrheal disease. These toxins include a heat-labile enterotoxin, a cytoskeleton-altering toxin, and a cytotoxin. Consistent association between the toxins and clinical disease is lacking.

E. coli causes disease by several mechanisms, as described previously. The toxins of EHEC are referred to as *shigatoxin 1* (SLT-I), or verocytotoxin 1 (VT1), and *shigatoxin 2* (SLT-II), or verocytotoxin 2 (VT2). SLT-II is immunologically distinct from SLT-I but is genetically and mechanistically closely related. Other closely related variant toxins, some of which have been studied extensively, also exist. These toxins work like shigatoxin produced by *S. dysenteriae* type 1. The primary site of histopathologic conditions is the colon.

Approximately 40% to 50% of ETECs produce only ST, 30% to 40% produce ST and LT, and 20% to 30% produce only LT. Disease may be associated with production of either or both enterotoxins produced by ETEC. Stools are watery and often of large volume, as in a mild case of cholera.

The ability of EIEC to invade cells is due to virulence genes present on a 140-megadalton plasmid. This invasion contributes to the dysentery associated with infection by EIEC. Some EIECs produce an enterotoxin referred to as ShET2 (shigella enterotoxin 2 or EIEC enterotoxin), which may play a role in the watery diarrhea associated with EIEC infections.

The adherent but noninvasive EPECs colonize the small intestine and produce a distinctive histopathologic lesion, which involves destruction of microvilli and close adherence of the bacteria to the membrane of the enterocyte, which results in a cuplike pedestal formation, on which each bacterium rests. This classic lesion is referred to as the *attaching-effacing* (AE) *lesion* and requires the presence of several virulence genes. EAEC strains have been reported to produce three toxins that potentially are able to stimulate intestinal secretion, the best characterized of which is EAEC heat-stable enterotoxin 1 (EAST 1).

Salmonellae produce disease by adhering to and then penetrating intestinal mucosal cells by endocytosis (mucosal translocation) before reaching the lamina propria. Bacterial proliferation occurs in the lamina propria and mesenteric nodes. Penetration is rapid, and macrophage engulfment without killing has been demonstrated. The terminal ileum and cecum are maximally involved, and neutrophilic inflammation is apparent in these locations. Peyer's patches and the mesenteric nodes may be enlarged. Salmonellae seem to survive in an intracellular location and gain access to the reticuloendothelial system, and are thus protected from antibody and some antibiotics. This intracellular location may contribute to prolonged carriage and excretion of the organism. *S. typhi* elicits a mononuclear cell response in the lamina propria. *S. typhi* traverses the mucosa and is more likely to cause bacteremia than other *Salmonella* species.

Nontyphoidal salmonella serotypes, including *S. typhimurium*, usually cause watery diarrhea. The pathogenesis of the secretory response to salmonella infection is uncertain. Although several enterotoxins are produced by various salmonella strains, their role in disease is not well defined. Water and electrolyte transport abnormalities accompany experimental salmonella infections.

Shigella species are recognized primarily for causing dysentery, although watery diarrhea more characteristic of small bowel involvement is a frequent occurrence. The molecular mechanisms by which shigella organisms invade epithelial cells have been studied extensively. In addition to invasion, *Shigella* species produce several toxins. *S. dysenteriae* type 1 produces a cytotoxin referred to as *shigatoxin*. The other *Shigella* species do not produce shigatoxin. Two distinct enterotoxins have been reported to be produced by *S. flexneri* and are referred to as *shigella enterotoxins 1* and 2 (ShET1 and ShET2).

The severe diarrhea caused by *V. cholerae* is produced by the O1 and O139 serogroups. The rapidly dehydrating noninflammatory diarrhea is due to its ability to produce a heat-labile enterotoxin referred to as *cholera toxin*. The toxin production of this organism is coded by chromosomal DNA (see Table 9-2) (Holmgren, 1981). Nontoxigenic *V. cholerae* can acquire the cholera toxin gene by infection by a filamentous bacteriophage that carries the cholera toxin gene. The bacteriophage gains entry to the *V. cholerae* cell by way of pili, which also function as adhesion molecules in the intestine. Once the bacteriophage gains entry to the *V. cholerae* cell, the cholera toxin gene is incorporated into the bacterial chromosome, and the cell can produce cholera toxin (Waldor and Mekalanos, 1996). This toxin has provided a wealth of information about the structure and function of enterotoxins and about the pathogenesis of diarrheal diseases. This protein exotoxin activates adenylate cyclase and catalyzes the formation of cyclic AMP, resulting in the secretion of fluid into the lumen of the intestinal tract. The toxin has two component parts. The B subunit binds to a receptor, GM_1 ganglioside, present on the surface of intestinal cells. The A subunit of the toxin penetrates the cell and must gain access to the interior to catalyze the adenosine diphosphate (ADP) ribosylation of guanosine triphosphate

(GTP)–binding protein. This results in activation of adenylate cyclase and conversion of adenosine triphosphate (ATP) to cAMP. The increased concentration of intracellular cAMP activates electrolyte transport isosmotically with water from the extracellular fluid to the lumen of the intestinal tract. Secretion then exceeds fluid absorption.

Increased cAMP also inhibits the transport of sodium and chloride from the lumen of the gut across the brush border and into the cell, with decreased absorption as membrane permeability in the villus cell is diminished. Glucose-coupled sodium and water transport into cells occurs by an independent mechanism that is unaltered. Thus oral electrolyte solution can still be absorbed from the intestine.

Y. enterocolitica produces several disease syndromes, including watery diarrhea, ulcerative enterocolitis, and mesenteric adenitis not associated with diarrhea. *Y. enterocolitica* infection mimics the mucosal translocation and bacterial proliferation in nodes and lamina propria described for *Salmonella* species. Strains of *Y. enterocolitica* produce a heat-stable enterotoxin thought to be important in the pathogenesis of the watery diarrhea syndrome.

Clinical Manifestations

Clinical manifestations that occur following infection with an enteropathogen include signs and symptoms related to the gastrointestinal tract, systemic manifestations, and complications that may be intestinal or extraintestinal in origin.

Aeromonas Species. *Aeromonas* spp. have been associated with a variety of intestinal and extraintestinal infections. A wide spectrum of gastrointestinal tract symptoms have been associated with *Aeromonas* infections, but the most common presentation is an acute, self-limited, watery diarrhea. A dysenteric illness is less common.

Campylobacter jejuni. *C. jejuni* may produce enteric disease ranging from watery diarrhea to dysentery; it is often excreted without producing symptoms. Infected individuals may manifest diarrhea, abdominal pain, chills, and fever. Abdominal pain can mimic that associated with appendicitis. Blood, mucus, and fecal leukocytes may be present in stool, resembling the illness produced by shigellae. Organisms may be excreted for two to three weeks in untreated persons. *Campylobacter jejuni* have caused bacteremia in children with immunodeficiency, in malnourished children, and in neonates (Reed et al., 1996). Immunoreactive complications include reactive arthritis, Guillain-Barré syndrome, Reiter's syndrome, and erythema nodosum.

Escherichia coli. EHEC produce a variety of clinical syndromes that begin with nausea, vomiting, significant abdominal pain, and watery diarrhea that may progress to bloody diarrhea and hemorrhagic colitis over several days. Only 20% of patients have fever as part of this syndrome. Although bloody diarrhea is the most distinctive presentation for EHEC, nonspecific watery diarrhea and asymptomatic infections also occur. Hemolytic uremic syndrome (HUS) follows EHEC enteritis in approximately 10% of patients, and thrombotic thrombocytopenia purpura is a postdiarrheal complication in adults (Pickering et al., 1994).

ETEC strains are an important cause of traveler's diarrhea and diarrheal illness in children in developing countries. ETEC strains produce watery diarrhea without blood or mucus. The severity of illness following ETEC infection varies from mild to severe, with up to ten to twenty stools per day. Disease is self-limited, lasting 3 to 5 days in an immunocompetent host, but severe dehydration may occur in infants. The disease is a malabsorptive diarrhea with watery stools without blood or white blood cells, and low-grade fever may be present.

EIEC can produce either dysentery with blood and mucus in the stools or watery diarrhea. Onset of fever, nausea, cramps, and tenesmus may be rapid. The clinical manifestations of dysentery are similar to those produced by shigellae. EIEC disease is uncommon in infants.

EPEC characteristically infects infants, particularly in developing countries, and has caused numerous outbreaks of acute and chronic infantile diarrhea. These organisms are of particular importance in tropical countries and developing nations where crowding and poor hygiene occur. EPEC-associated diarrheal illness is uncommon in older children and adults. Frequent, green, slimy stools are produced, usually without blood or fecal leukocytes. Diarrhea may be severe and can result in dehydration. Infections occur during the rainy season and warm-weather months.

EAEC has been recognized, primarily in children in the developing world, as a cause of both acute and chronic diarrhea. Data suggest that these organisms may be common enteropathogens of early childhood.

Salmonella Species. Infection with salmonellae have been associated with several clinical syndromes: (1) acute gastroenteritis, which is most common; (2) enteric fever; (3) septicemia with or without localized infections; and (4) inapparent infection and carrier state (Saphra and Winter, 1957). The clinical manifestations of these syndromes often overlap.

Gastroenteritis. Salmonella infection varies in severity from mild to severe. Nausea, vomiting, and diarrhea are associated with severe abdominal cramps and tenderness. Fever and prostration may be pronounced. Chills and weakness are common. Stools are numerous and may contain mucus and blood. Bloody diarrhea is observed often in young children but is rare in adults. In approximately 50% of the patients, the temperature falls to normal within 1 or 2 days, and recovery is uneventful. In others the disease may last 1 week or more. Protracted or recurrent diarrhea occurs and may represent secondary consequences of mucosal invasion and destruction of the epithelium. In severe infections, shock with cyanosis, hypothermia, and circulatory collapse, which precedes death, may occur. In some patients, gastroenteritis is followed by septicemia or by signs of localization. Metastatic foci are more likely to occur in patients with sickle cell disease, infants less than 6 months of age, and in immunocompromised persons such as those with AIDS (Centers for Disease Control, 1992).

Enteric fever. Although infections caused by *Salmonella* spp. constitute a serious public health problem, those caused by *S. typhi* have become relatively infrequent in the United States. The number of cases of typhoid fever reported in the United States during the last two decades rarely has exceeded 500 per year.

The onset of symptoms of typhoid fever in most cases is gradual, with fever, headache, malaise, and loss of appetite. The typical course in an adult is illustrated in Fig. 9-1. The temperature rises in a steplike manner for 2 to 7 days to an average of approximately 40° C (104° F) and characteristically remains at this level for 3 to 4 weeks in the absence of specific antimicrobial therapy. The pulse rate is slow relative to the fever. Diarrhea is present in some patients, although constipation may persist throughout infection. Either manifestation may be accompanied by abdominal tenderness, distention, and pain. In the early stages of illness, discrete rose-colored spots may be scattered over the trunk, especially the abdomen. The spleen is enlarged in most patients. Severely ill patients may become delirious or stuporous. The white blood cell count, as a rule, shows leukopenia.

Typhoid fever in children in the first 2 years of life exhibits certain differences from the clinical course in adults (Hornick et al., 1970). The diagnosis in infancy is often made by the chance isolation of *S. typhi* from stools or blood in infants in whom the onset is often abrupt, with high fever, vomiting, convulsions, and meningeal signs. The slow pulse rate is not a frequent finding. Rose spots occur less commonly than in adults. Leukocytosis is the rule, and the white blood cell count may be as high as 20,000 to 25,000 cells/µl, but neutrophils rarely

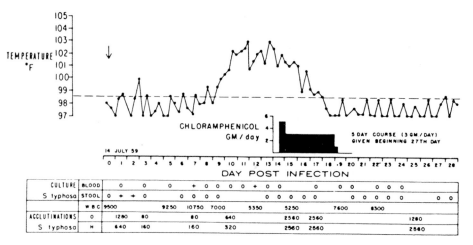

Fig. 9-1   Summary of the clinical course of induced typhoid fever in an adult volunteer. Therapy consisted of two 5-day courses of chloramphenicol separated by a 1-week interval. (From Hornick RB, et al: N Engl J Med 1970;283:686.)

exceed 60% to 70%. The spleen usually is palpable. The course of the disease is short, rarely persisting more than 2 weeks. The mortality rate in infancy is low when appropriate therapy is administered.

Salmonella spp. other than *S. typhi* may produce a disease with all the manifestations of typhoid fever, including persistent fever; intestinal tract symptoms; rose spots; leukopenia; and positive cultures of blood, stool, and urine.

Septicemia with or without localized infection. *Salmonella* spp. are also responsible for a disease characterized by intermittent fever, chills (in adults), anorexia, and loss of weight. The characteristic features of typhoid fever are absent. Stool cultures usually are negative, although blood cultures yield the causative organism. A focus of infection is identified in approximately one fourth of patients with bacteremia. The acute focal process may be directly or indirectly connected with the intestinal tract and may cause appendicitis, cholecystitis, peritonitis, or salpingitis. Hematogenous spread of organisms may result in foci of infection in the brain, skin, lungs, spleen, middle ear, bone, or joints. Meningitis is caused by a variety of salmonella types and occurs principally in young infants, with a high morbidity rate. The urinary tract also can be infected. Osteomyelitis and pyarthrosis, caused by many serotypes, can occur in any bone, but the long bones, spine, and ribs are affected most commonly. Pneumonia usually is accompanied by a high temperature and often terminates fatally. This manifestation occurs almost exclusively in elderly patients, many of whom suffer from unrelated medical problems.

Inapparent infection and the carrier state. Asymptomatic infection with salmonellae occurs in an estimated 0.2% of people, as documented by positive stool cultures in the absence of clinical illness. Some of these persons have had known contact with symptomatic persons or are being investigated because of a recognized source of contaminated food. Persons who have been infected usually excrete organisms for weeks to months. Carriers of *S. typhi,* especially those with abnormal gall bladders, may excrete organisms for years.

Shigella Species. Mild illness with transient diarrhea is a common manifestation of shigella infection. Persons with mild infection have watery diarrhea or loose stools for a few days, with mild or absent constitutional symptoms. The classic clinical picture of bacillary dysentery is characterized by severe abdominal pain, tenesmus, and constitutional symptoms with frequently passed stools containing mucus and blood (Scragg et al., 1978). Patients with moderately severe disease may have an abrupt onset with fever, abdominal pain, vomiting, and then diarrhea. Stools occur seven to twelve times daily, are watery, green, or yellow, and contain mucus and undigested food. Disease may progress with development of all of the features of dysentery. Acute symptoms may persist for 7 to 10 days, and meningismus, delirium, and convulsions may accompany dysentery caused by shigella infection. Morbidity and mortality usually result from severe dehydration. Bacteremia is uncommon but may occur in persons who are immunocompromised or malnourished. The most severe illness occurs most frequently in young infants, in the elderly, and in debilitated persons. Sequelae of shigella infection include toxic megacolon; hemolytic uremic syndrome associated only with *S. dysenteriae* type 1; reactive arthropathy (Reiter's syndrome) following infection with *S. flexneri* in persons genetically predisposed; and fulminant toxic encephalopathy.

Vibrio cholerae. Infection with *V. cholerae* results in a spectrum ranging from asymptomatic excretion to mild to moderate diarrhea to severe, dehydrating illness. Asymptomatic infection is much more common than clinical illness. Severe illness in adults may be characterized by rapid fluid loss in excess of 20 L per 24 hours. Profound shock and death can occur within a day if fluid replacement is not instituted. The acutely ill patient usually appears in a shocklike state, with soiling of clothes by excessive fecal discharge. The feces usually are clear and without odor, contain flecks of mucus that impart a "rice-water" appearance, and have high concentrations of sodium and bicarbonate. Vomiting without nausea, described as effortless, usually follows the onset of diarrhea. The skin of the hands may have a characteristic appearance resembling wrinkled "washer woman hands" in persons with severe dehydration. Fever, if present, is low grade, or the patient may develop hypothermia.

Yersinia enterocolitica. Clinical manifestations of infection with *Y. enterocolitica* depend on the age and immune status of the host. Watery diarrhea is a common manifestation of *Y. enterocolitica.* Infection with this organism also can produce a dysentery syndrome, most often occurring in young children. Older children and adolescents may develop acute mesenteric adenitis or ileitis with diarrhea, fever, right lower quadrant tenderness, abdominal pain, and leukocytosis. Acute bacteremia with metastatic foci, including involvement of the liver and spleen, occurs in elderly adults or immunocompromised hosts. Postinfectious sequelae include erythema nodosum and reactive arthritis, most often in adults.

Diagnosis and Differential Diagnosis

Demographic data, epidemiologic information, clinical manifestations, and knowledge of virulence mechanisms of enteropathogens provide the framework for establishing the cause of enteric infection using microscopy, culture, rapid diagnostic tests, and specialized laboratory tests (Box 9-2). Examination of stool for the presence of leukocytes and blood provides insight into whether the organism is invasive. Culture of stool can detect *Campylobacter* spp., *V. cholerae*, salmonella, shigella, and *Y. enterocolitica*. Laboratory confirmation of *E. coli*–associated disease generally is not available in

most diagnostic laboratories because detection of toxins or invasive properties requires cell cultures, animal models, or other specific assays. Serotyping of *E. coli* in diarrheal outbreaks in infants is potentially helpful for recognition of EPEC but is more helpful in outbreak evaluation than in the diagnostic evaluation of a single infant. *E. coli* O157:H7 should be suspected if non–sorbitol fermenting *E. coli* are present; confirmation in a reference laboratory is necessary. All laboratories should include a sorbitol-MacConkey agar plate as part of routine stool culture to screen for non–sorbitol fermenting *E. coli* O157:H7. If present, these organisms should be confirmed by serologic testing.

S. typhi frequently is detected in blood cultures during the first 2 weeks of illness. When enteric fever is suspected, blood and bone marrow must be obtained for culture. In patients not from endemic areas serologic tests may be helpful if they are positive but generally are not useful. The leukocyte count is usually 10,000 to 15,000 cells/μl, with a slight increase in number of polymorphonuclear

---

BOX 9-2

DIAGNOSTIC METHODS FOR BACTERIAL ENTERIC PATHOGENS

Nonspecific Tests

Microscopy
Fecal lactoferrin assay
Fecal leukocytes
Stool occult blood
Complete blood count

Routine Screening Culture

Enteric agar media
    Differential media (e.g., MAC, EMB)
    Moderately selective media (e.g., Hektoen enteric [HE],
        xylose-lysine-desoxycholate [XLD], *Salmonella-Shigella* [SS])
Enrichment broth
Sorbitol-MAC agar

Organism-Specific Identification

Organism	*Media or method*
Salmonella	Brilliant green or bismuth sulfite agar
Campylobacter	Skirrow's formula, Campy-BAP, Butzler's formula, Preston's formula
Aeromonas	BAP, MAC, EMB
Vibrio	TCBS agar, *V. cholerae* 01 antisera
Yersinia	Cefsulodin-irgasan-novobiocin (CIN) agar
Clostridium difficile	Cycloserine–cefoxitin–fructose–egg yolk (CCFA) anaerobically, *C. difficile* toxin EIA
Enterohemorrhagic *E. coli*	Sorbitol MAC, 0157 antisera, H7 antisera

cells. Leukopenia found in the enteric fever type of infection is seldom seen in the gastroenteric form. Positive blood cultures are more frequent in infants less than 6 months of age and occasionally occur in older persons, especially in the presence of severe infections. Stool cultures usually yield salmonellae during the acute phase of the disease and often for weeks to months thereafter. Symptoms subside despite continued colonization with the organism.

Most clinical microbiology laboratories now include Campy BAP and Butzler's media, or Skirrow's medium for culture of stool at 42° C in a reduced-oxygen, high–carbon dioxide environment for *C. jejuni*. However, since this practice is not universal, the physician must be aware of available laboratory practices and procedures. In addition, other *Campylobacter* species require specialized media and conditions not generally used in most diagnostic laboratories.

V. cholerae presents diagnostic problems in the United States, where it is an uncommon pathogen. The unprepared laboratory may miss the diagnosis, so it is essential that the clinician suspect the diagnosis, alert the laboratory personnel, and thus increase the likelihood of a correct diagnosis. *V. cholerae* grows rapidly on certain alkaline-enrichment media, such as thiosulfate citrate bile salts sucrose (TCBS) agar, which has a pH greater than 6.0. The organisms can be distinguished from other enteric bacteria on TCBS agar by the fact that they form characteristic opaque yellow colonies.

Suspect colonies are confirmed serologically by agglutination with specific antisera. Isolated specimens of *V. cholerae* O1 and O139 should be confirmed and tested for production of cholera toxin. Similarly, to culture *Y. enterocolitica*, laboratory personnel must be alerted to use specific conditions or media to facilitate growth and recognition of this organism.

Complications

The severity of acute bacterial gastroenteritis is correlated best with fluid and electrolyte loss and the extent of dehydration. Most infections are self-limited and localized to the gastrointestinal tract. The availability of fluid replacement has altered the morbidity and mortality rates of cholera. Extracellular volume depletion secondary to intestinal loss of isotonic fluid, acidosis secondary to bicarbonate loss in stool, and hypokalemia secondary to fecal potassium loss are the major abnormalities that occur during cholera. Abnormalities in renal function occur secondary to the initial deficits, and renal failure has occurred as a result of hypovolemia and shock. Replacement fluids have diminished the morbidity rate for all diarrheal illnesses, and specific antibiotics have contributed to effective therapy of several of these entities. In developing nations in which nutrition is poor, diarrheal illnesses often contribute to protein-calorie malnutrition, growth failure, and susceptibility to additional pathogens.

Salmonella suppurative foci such as meningitis, pyarthrosis, and osteomyelitis occur infrequently. The patient may have an altered mental status, with a spectrum of effects including delirium, stupor, and aphasia. It is important to ascertain if direct invasion of the central nervous system (CNS) has occurred in the presence of such signs and symptoms. Fortunately, intestinal tract perforation and hemorrhage are rare in the United States even with *S. typhi,* primarily because infections are treated. These complications characteristically occur after 2 weeks of untreated disease. Relapse may occur in 15% to 20% of persons treated for *S. typhi* and does so usually within 10 to 18 days of withdrawal from antibiotics. Chronic carriage of *S. typhi* has been attributed to chronic infection of the gallbladder.

Campylobacter jejuni enteritis complications include reports of Reiter's syndrome, reactive arthritis, Guillain-Barré syndrome and erythema nodosum (Rees et al., 1995; Walker et al., 1986). Reiter's syndrome also has been associated with *Salmonella, Shigella,* and *Yersinia* infections. *Y. enterocolitica* rarely can cause chronic and recurrent enteric symptoms, which respond to antibiotic therapy. Septicemic illness is potentially severe and has occurred in immunocompromised hosts. The nonsuppurative arthritis usually is self-limited and usually lasts a few months.

Prognosis

Prognosis generally is dependent on the age and nutritional status of the patient and the presence of an underlying disease. The vast majority of intestinal tract infections are self-limited, with no complications and complete recovery. The very young, the aged, and those with protein-calorie malnutrition or underlying disease are at risk for complications or prolonged illness (Centers for Disease Control, 1992). Overall, fatality from any of these agents seldom exceeds 1% when health-care delivery is adequate. Patients with meningitis or endocarditis caused by salmonellae have a higher mortality rate than do individuals with compromised immune systems (Centers for Disease Control, 1992).

Treatment

Therapy of children with gastroenteritis includes fluid and electrolyte replacement and maintenance; maintenance of dietary intake; specific therapy with antimicrobial agents; and infrequent use of nonspecific therapy, including antidiarrheal compounds.

Infants, children, and adults with gastroenteritis require fluid replacement. Oral hydration with fluid containing carbohydrates and electrolytes has significantly reduced the morbidity and mortality from diarrheal disease. The American Academy of Pediatrics and the CDC have made similar recommendations for management of acute diarrhea in children (Duggan et al., 1992; Provisional Committee on Quality Improvement, 1996). Oral rehydration therapy is the preferred treatment of fluid and electrolyte losses caused by diarrhea in children with mild to moderate dehydration. Children who have diarrhea and who are not dehydrated should continue to be fed age-appropriate diets (Brown et al., 1994; Snyder, 1994). Children who require rehydration should be fed age-appropriate diets as soon as they have been rehydrated. Antimotility agents, opiates, bismuth subsalicylate, and adsorbents are not recommended for treatment of diarrhea in children 1 month to 5 years of age (Provisional Committee on Quality Improvement, 1996).

Hospitalization usually is not necessary unless a fluid deficit of ≥5% has occurred and rehydration cannot be provided through oral solutions. *V. cholerae* causes the most rapid losses, and replacement may be an emergency. Since glucose-coupled electrolyte and water transport across the epithelium are unaltered by the various toxins, it is possible to replace fluids orally. Replacement fluids should not be prepared by parents without medical supervision, since hypernatremia is a risk of inappropriately prepared fluid and electrolyte solutions. Fluid replacement using the World Health Organization formulation, mixed and used as recommended, is preferred (Fekety, 1983; Hayani et al., 1992), but premixed fluid and electrolyte replacement solutions also are available.

Specific antimicrobial therapy (Table 9-3) alters the course of typhoid and shigella infections (Pickering, 1996). Additionally, the period of time shigellae are excreted is shortened; therefore communicability is lessened. In contrast, the course of infections of salmonellae, other than *S. typhi,* is not altered by antibiotics, and excretion of the organisms may be prolonged by their use. Routine antibiotic therapy is not of benefit for most children with salmonella gastroenteritis, with possible exceptions being infants, immunocompromised patients, and persons with severe episodes. Patients with salmonella infections in sites other than the intestinal tract also should be treated with antimicrobial agents (Pickering, 1991; Pickering and Matson, 1995).

V. cholerae, ETEC, and *C. jejuni* infections are all treated with antibiotics when the patient is symptomatic and the organism has been identified. Excretion of the organism is shortened, and therapy may alter the disease. At present it is unclear whether antibiotics decrease the severity of illness or complications with *Y. enterocolitica.*

Preventive Measures

Preventive measures include handwashing, education, proper food preparation and hygiene, knowledge of risks of animal exposure and travel, immu-

Table 9-3   Antimicrobial therapy for bacterial organisms causing gastroenteritis

Organism	Antimicrobial agent
*Campylobacter jejuni**	Erythromycin
Escherichia coli	
EPEC, ETEC, EIEC	Trimethoprim-sulfamethoxazole (TMP/SMX)
EHEC, EAEC	Uncertain
Salmonella gastroenteritis*	None (ampicillin, TMP/SMX, chloramphenicol, cefotaxime, or ceftriaxone for other sites of infection)
*Salmonella typhi** (typhoid fever)	Chloramphenicol, TMP/SMX, ampicillin, ceftraxione, or cefotaxime
Shigella species*	TMP/SMX and cefixime; ceftriaxone or cefotaxime for resistant strains
Vibrio cholerae	Doxycycline or tetracycline or TMP/SMX
Yersinia enterocolitica	
Gastroenteritis	None
Bacteremia*	TMP/SMX, tetracycline, aminoglycoside, cefotaxime, or chloramphenicol

*Ciprofloxacin or ofloxacin can be used for nonpregnant persons over 17 years old.

nization, and interaction with public health officials when illness occurs. Interruption of fecal-oral spread is essential for diminishing transmission of enteric pathogens. Individual patients should be isolated during the illness. Strict handwashing should be initiated, as should appropriate processing or disposal of contaminated materials. Guidelines for prevention of enteric infections in persons infected with human immunodeficiency virus are applicable to all children (Kaplan et al., 1995).

To prevent *S. typhi* and *Shigella* species that are exclusively human pathogens, as well as other enteropathogens, the incidence of disease can be diminished by (1) sanitary disposal of human feces; (2) purification and protection of water supplies; (3) pasteurization of milk and milk products; (4) strict sanitary supervision of preparation and serving of all foods; (5) proper refrigeration of food and milk; (6) exclusion of persons with diarrhea from handling food; (7) avoidance of eating raw or undercooked food, including eggs, meat, and poultry; (8) avoiding contact with reptiles and ill animals; (9) use of appropriate precautions when traveling to developing countries; and (10) stressing the importance of handwashing.

Reducing the spread of enteric pathogens where animal reservoirs play an important role is more complex. Animal reservoirs are probably responsible for the majority of human salmonella infections in the United States. Poultry and milk products often are implicated, either directly or indirectly, with contamination of meat-processing areas, markets, or kitchens. By-products of the meat-packing industry (e.g., fertilizer or bone meal) perpetuate infection in animals. Prevention of salmonella infections in humans depends on interrupting transmission. The task of controlling salmonellosis among animals and preventing the spread of infection to people is enormous. The consumption of raw or undercooked eggs should be avoided and all egg products must be stored and prepared as recommended. Households with young children or immunosuppressed individuals should not keep reptiles as pets because of the risk of zoonotic salmonellosis. Continued surveillance is needed to identify and eliminate the multiple sources of infection.

Immunization

Vibrio Cholerae. Parenterally inoculated, killed, whole-cell vaccine has been available for years, but it is of little value in epidemic control or management of contacts of cases. This vaccine stimulates high titers of serum vibriocidal antibodies, but it does not induce antibodies to toxin. In an individual previously primed by intestinal tract contact with *V. cholerae,* the vaccine also produces an anamnestic response of intestinal tract secretory IgA directed against the O antigen. In field trials, homologous protection by vaccine has been induced for approximately 1 year with vaccine efficacy approximately 70%. These vaccines provide partial protection (50%) of short duration (3 to 6 months) in highly endemic areas and do not prevent asymptomatic infection. They are not recommended.

Local intestinal tract immunity against the organism and against the toxin by oral vaccines should provide a better, less reactogenic immunogen. Using recombinant DNA technology, an "attenuated" *V. cholerae* organism that lacks the genes for production of the A subunit of toxin was created. This live attenuated *V. cholerae* O1 oral vaccine, CVD103-HgR—containing all the cell wall antigens necessary for adherence and the capacity to produce only the B subunit of toxin—has been engineered (Levine and Kaper, 1993). In theory it could provide ideal local immunity without toxicity. Initial trials have demonstrated a vaccine efficacy of 90% to rechallenge with virulent organisms. Another strategy is to create a hybrid organism by the insertion of the cholera O antigen genes into *S. typhi* vaccine strain Ty21a. These trials are underway.

Salmonella Typhi. Typhoid immunization is not recommended routinely in the United States but is recommended for persons with occupational exposure, those traveling to endemic areas, persons living in areas of high endemicity, and household members of known carriers. Three vaccines are available to U.S. civilians: (1) an orally administered, live, attenuated vaccine using *S. typhi* strain Ty21a is given in 3 to 4 doses, 2 days apart, and is not recommended for children younger than 6 years of age; (2) a parenteral vaccine containing the capsular polysaccharide Vi antigen is given in a single dose and is not recommended for children younger than 2 years of age; and (3) a whole-cell parenteral bacterial vaccine, which is not recommended because of higher incidence of side effects and is not given to children younger than 6 months of age (Levine and Noriega, 1994).

VIRAL GASTROENTERITIS
Etiology

Acute viral gastroenteritis affects all age groups, may occur in either sporadic or epidemic form, and is responsible for a large proportion of diarrhea for which an etiologic agent can be defined. Most illnesses are self-limited, and in healthy hosts recovery is complete. If severe dehydration occurs, morbidity and mortality may be substantial. The viral agents discussed in this chapter are outlined in Box 9-1 and shown in Fig. 9-2.

Enteric Adenoviruses. Adenoviruses are DNA viruses that include 47 distinct serotypes that cause disease in humans. Types 40 and 41, and rarely 31, have been associated with gastroenteritis (Brandt et al., 1985). The enteric adenoviruses are 70 to 90 nm in diameter, nonenveloped, and contain double-stranded DNA. The enteric adenoviruses are sec-

ond to rotavirus among recognized causes of viral gastroenteritis in children.

Astroviruses. Astroviruses, which were first described in 1975, are nonenveloped, single-stranded RNA viruses 28 to 30 nm in diameter, with a characteristic five- or six-pointed star appearance when seen by electron microscopy. The single-stranded RNA genome encodes three structural proteins and is approximately 7.2 Kb long. Eight antigenic types have been described.

Caliciviruses. Caliciviruses are 28 to 34 nm in diameter with a distinct "star of David" appearance when seen by electron microscopy (Fig. 9-2, *C*).

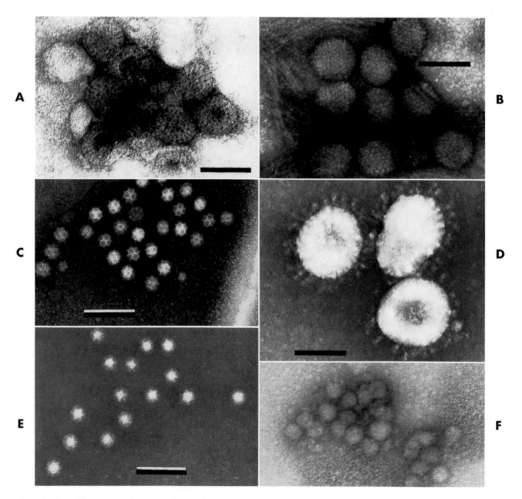

FIG. 9-2   Electron microscopic appearance of viruses visualized in stool. All micrographs are printed with a bar representing 100 nm to illustrate differences in size. **A**, Rotavirus; **B**, adenovirus; **C**, calicivirus; **D**, coronavirus; **E**, astrovirus; **F**, small round virus. (A, B, and F, courtesy of Miller SE, Duke University, Durham, North Carolina; C and E, courtesy of Szymanski MT, Hospital for Sick Children, Toronto; D, courtesy of Bradley DW, Centers for Disease Control and Prevention, Atlanta.)

Caliciviruses were recognized as pathogens in animals in 1932 and in humans in 1976. The caliciviruses now include human and animal strains that have been separated phylogenetically into genogroups: (1) Norwalk-like; (2) Snow Mountain–like; (3) Sapporo-like human calicivirus; (4) enterically transmitted non-A, non-B hepatitis virus or hepatitis E virus (HEV); (5) rabbit caliciviruses; and (6) feline caliciviruses-like animal caliciviruses. All are associated with diarrhea except hepatitis E virus, which causes hepatitis. Each genogroup has a unique genomic organization of the protein-encoding region. The relatedness of these viruses was confirmed by similar physical properties such as a single structural protein of approximately 60 kDa and by molecular characteristics. The genome of human caliciviruses has been cloned and is a positive-sense, single-stranded RNA approximately 7.5 Kb long.

Norwalk virus was first described from an outbreak of gastroenteritis that occurred in Norwalk, Ohio, in 1969. A bacteria-free filtrate from a stool specimen produced gastroenteritis in several volunteers, and stools from the infected individuals could be serially passed in additional volunteers. In 1972 immune electron microscopic examination using serum from a symptomatic patient demonstrated 27-nm particles in an infectious stool filtrate (Fig. 9-2) (Dolin et al., 1972; Kapikian et al., 1972). Several other morphologically similar but antigenically unrelated or partially related small, round enteric viruses have been described (Okada et al., 1990). Many of these viruses are known from a single outbreak and have been named after the site in which the outbreak occurred. The antigenic relatedness of these viruses is not yet clear. These viruses cannot be cultivated in cell culture, thus hindering acquisition of information about the epidemiology and properties of these viruses. Each virus was initially detected by electron microscopy or immune electron microscopy.

Rotaviruses. In 1973 rotavirus particles were visualized in a duodenal biopsy by electron microscopy (Bishop et al., 1973; Kapikian et al., 1974). Rotaviruses currently are recognized as the single most common agent causing diarrhea in infants from 6 to 24 months of age in the United States. Rotaviruses also cause diarrhea in foals, lambs, piglets, rabbits, deer, monkeys, and other species.

Rotaviruses consist of an eleven-segment genome of double-stranded RNA. The genome of this 70- to 75-nm virus is located within the inner core, and each gene segment codes for a separate viral protein (Estes and Cohen, 1989; Prasad et al., 1990). Rotavirus groups A through F have been described, but only groups A, B, and C have been identified in humans. Group A rotaviruses are common causes of gastroenteritis in children, but the significance of groups B and C has not been fully defined. The group designation of rotavirus is determined by VP6. Group A rotaviruses can be classified further into serotypes, which are determined by VP7 glycoprotein (G type) and VP4 protease-cleaved hemagglutinin (P type). There are 14 serotypes of group A rotaviruses, six of which (G types 1, 2, 3, 4, 8, 9, and 12) have been identified in humans. Serotypes 1 through 4 are the major causes of human disease.

Coronaviruses. Coronaviruses are 180 to 200 nm in diameter and have characteristic petal-shaped surface projections that, when visualized by electron microscopy, give the appearance of a corona. These viruses are a well-documented cause of gastroenteritis in animals and the common cold in humans. Coronaviruses have been identified in stools of children with diarrhea, but their role as a cause of diarrhea is unknown.

Parvoviruses. Parvoviruses appear as 20- to 30-nm round particles when visualized in stools. They have no detectable surface structure and do not grow in vitro in routine cell culture systems. These particles have been visualized in stools from patients with diarrhea and in persons who have no clinical symptoms; more information is needed to establish their causative role in gastroenteritis.

Other Viruses. Pestiviruses appear as 40- to 60-nm particles when visualized by electron microscopy. They have been implicated as a cause of diarrhea in children. A virus resembling the Breda virus of calf diarrhea has been detected in stool specimens from children with diarrhea.

Epidemiology

Enteric adenovirus types 40 and 41 are widespread and cause endemic diarrhea and outbreaks of diarrhea in hospitals, orphanages, and child-care centers (Van et al., 1992). These viruses infect all age groups (Kotloff et al., 1989), with antibody prevalence studies showing that more than 50% of children are seropositive by the third or fourth year of life. Infection appears to occur all year. The mode of transmission is fecal-oral and the incubation period lasts from 3 to 10 days. Enteric adenoviruses cause 2% to 22% of pediatric diarrhea in inpatients or outpatients. Enteric adenoviruses are a more important cause of viral gastroenteritis in infants less than 6 months of age than in older children (Bates et al., 1993). Children admitted with enteric adenovirus infection are more likely to have diarrhea for more than 5 days but less likely to be febrile or dehydrated than children with rotavirus infection (Grimwood et al., 1995). Asymptomatic infection is common and asymptomatic excretion after illness may last for several weeks (Van et al., 1992).

Astrovirus has been associated with diarrhea worldwide and has been linked to outbreaks of diarrhea in schools, pediatric wards, nursing homes, and child care centers (Mitchell et al., 1993, 1995a). Illness occurs mainly in children less than 4 years of age and in the elderly. More than 80% of adults have antibodies against the virus. Astrovirus accounts for 3% of hospital admissions for diarrhea. Asymptomatic infection is common and asymptomatic excretion after an illness may last for several weeks. The incubation period is 3 to 4 days.

Antibodies to calicivirus have been demonstrated in virtually all children by the age of 5 years. By 2 years of age, 85% of children have antibody to Norwalk virus, as found by antibody EIA (Jiang et al., 1995). Studies in child-care centers showed that calicivirus-associated diarrhea and asymptomatic infection are both widespread (Matson et al., 1990). Human calicivirus accounts for at least 3% of diarrhea episodes in child-care centers. Human calicivirus infections occur year-round as a result of fecal-oral transmission. This virus also may be a cause of food-borne and water-borne outbreaks of gastroenteritis (Kaplan et al., 1995). Roughly one third of identified outbreaks of gastroenteritis can be attributed to a human calicivirus. The outbreaks have occurred in schools, recreation camps, cruise ships, nursing homes, and after ingestion of inadequately cooked contaminated shellfish or contaminated water. The incubation period ranges from 1 to 4 days.

Epidemic gastroenteritis caused by the Norwalk group of caliciviruses may affect an entire community. Outbreaks have involved school-age children, family contacts, and adults. Roughly one third of the identified outbreaks of gastroenteritis may be attributed to a Norwalk-like agent. Outbreaks have occurred at all times of the year, and antibody surveys suggest that the agent is worldwide in distribution. Transmission of Norwalk virus occurs as a result of ingestion of contaminated food (shellfish, salads, and cake frosting), ingestion of water or ice, and by person-to-person spread. In less developed nations, antibody to Norwalk virus is detected in early childhood, but, in the United States, antibody to Norwalk virus usually develops during late adolescence and early adulthood.

Rotavirus infection occurs most frequently during the cooler months of the year in temperate climates, but in tropical areas, infection occurs throughout the year. Rotavirus appears first in the Southwestern United States in November and moves to the Northeast by March or April of each year. Infection with group A rotaviruses most frequently occurs in children 6 to 24 months of age. Infections in neonates are often asymptomatic, and both asymptomatic and symptomatic reinfections are common (Velazquez et al., 1996). Incidence rates in community-based and child-care center studies in this age group range from 0.2 to 0.8 episodes per child/year (Brandt et al., 1979; Kapikian et al., 1976). Rotaviruses cause up to 50% of the episodes of diarrhea requiring hospitalization in infants and children and are common causes of outbreaks in children in child-care centers (O'Ryan and Matson, 1990; O'Ryan et al., 1990) and hospitals (Bartlett et al., 1988). Rotavirus results in 55,000 hospitalizations per year, 20 to 40 deaths per year, and over $1 billion per year in health-care costs in the United States (Glass et al., 1996). According to some estimates, rotavirus is the fifth leading cause of death among children living in less developed countries. Serotypes 1 and 3 are the most frequently isolated serotypes from children with rotavirus diarrhea in the United States (Matson et al., 1990). Rotaviruses can be excreted for several days before and for up to 10 days after diarrhea occurs, with the quantity of virus highest early in the course of illness (Pickering et al., 1988). Transmission occurs through the fecal-oral route. The incubation period ranges from 1 to 3 days.

Pathogenesis and Pathology

Caliciviruses are transmitted by the fecal-oral route. Infected volunteers have had detectable virus in their stools during the first 72 hours after the onset of illness. Infection with these agents results in delayed gastric emptying, although the gastric mucosa is morphologically normal. Microscopic broadening and blunting of the villi in the jejunum are apparent. The mucosa remains histologically intact, but there is a mononuclear cell infiltration. Viruses have not yet been detected in involved mucosal cells. Small-intestinal enzyme studies showed decreased amounts of the enzymes measured.

Rotavirus is excreted in extraordinarily high concentrations early in the course of the illness, with as many as 10^{11} particles per gram of feces. Rotavirus particles have been visualized by electron microscopy in intestinal epithelial cells, aspirated duodenal secretions, and feces of infected persons. In addition, rotavirus has been detected in the liver and kidneys of children with immunodeficiencies (Gilger et al., 1992). Morphologically, shortening and blunting of the villi of the duodenum and upper small intestine accompany acute illness (Schreiber et al., 1973). The microvilli of the absorptive cells are distorted, and other cells have swollen mitochondria. Rotavirus particles infect the mature enterocytes located in the middle and upper villous epithelium. This destruction of the mature enterocyte is associated with a decrease in the surface area of the intestine and decreased production of one or more mucosal disaccharidases. The destroyed infected cells are replaced by immature cells, resulting in a deficit in glucose-facilitated sodium transport. Diarrhea then results from decreased absorption secondary to the altered ion transport. Complete recovery has been confirmed by biopsy as early as 4 weeks after the episode of diarrhea.

Clinical Manifestations

Enteric adenoviruses cause diarrhea that lasts 6 to 9 days and may be associated with emesis and fever. Diarrhea is watery without blood or fecal leukocytes. Persistent lactose intolerance has been reported. Enteric adenovirus diarrhea can last longer than other types of viral gastroenteritis. Asymptomatic infection is common.

Diarrhea caused by astroviruses usually occurs in children and in the elderly. Symptoms include low-grade fever, malaise, nausea, vomiting, and watery diarrhea that usually lasts 4 days. Vomiting is less common than with other viruses. Cow's milk intolerance has been reported following infection. Asymptomatic infection is common.

Most patients who sustain calicivirus infections have nausea, vomiting, headache, malaise, and abdominal cramps, and approximately half of them have associated diarrhea. Fever and chills are less common. The symptoms last from 12 to 24 hours. Stools usually are not bloody and do not contain mucus or lymphocytes. Transient lymphopenia has

been observed in volunteers challenged with these agents.

Acute infections caused by rotavirus are characterized by an abrupt onset of watery diarrhea that characteristically is not associated with blood or mucus in the stool. The mean duration of illness in immunocompetent hosts is 5 to 7 days, but chronic infection can occur in immunodeficient children, and disease can be more severe in malnourished hosts. Vomiting is often present before or after onset of diarrhea. Dehydration and metabolic acidosis are common and may necessitate hospitalization. Rotaviruses are responsible for at least one half of the cases of infantile diarrhea requiring hospitalization. Rotaviruses have been associated with liver damage in immunodeficient hosts. In children in child-care centers asymptomatic infections represent up to 50% of all rotavirus infections (O'Ryan and Matson, 1990; O'Ryan et al., 1990). Recurrent infections are common in children in child care and in other settings in which exposure is frequent (Velazquez et al., 1996).

Diagnosis and Differential Diagnosis

The clinical differentiation of viral gastroenteritis from bacterial gastroenteritis is often difficult. Various epidemiologic factors such as season and age, as well as clinical manifestations, may be helpful. Viral gastroenteritis rarely is associated with bloody diarrhea. Laboratory support is needed to substantiate a clinical diagnosis. The most widely used assays for detection of a viral enteropathogen are electron microscopy, immune electron microscopy, enzyme immunosorbent assay (EIA), latex agglutination, gel electrophoresis, culture of the virus, polymerase chain reaction (PCR), and reverse transcriptase–PCR (RT-PCR). Different assays currently are used for each virus (Table 9-4). Commercial EIAs are available for detection of rotavirus and enteric adenoviruses. Commercial assays for other viral enteropathogens may be available soon.

Electron microscopy initially was used to detect enteric adenoviruses, but commercially available assays that use monoclonal antibodies in EIA techniques are now available (Van et al., 1992). Enteric adenoviruses can be cultivated in special cell lines. Restriction enzyme analysis is the definitive method used for classifying individual isolates.

Astroviruses grow in human colonic carcinoma cells in the presence of trypsin. Electron microscopy, immune electron microscopy, immunofluorescence of cell culture, EIA (Herrmann et al., 1990), and RT-PCR (Mitchell et al., 1993, 1995a)

Table 9-4   Diagnostic methods for enteric viral pathogens

Organism	Routine identification	Research or reference methods
Enteric adenovirus	EM, EIA*	PCR, culture, restriction enzyme analysis
Astrovirus	EM	EIA, RT-PCR, culture
Caliciviruses	EM	EIA, RT-PCR
Rotavirus	EM, EIA*	RT-PCR, electropherotyping

EM, Electron microscopy; *EIA*, enzyme immunoassay; *RT-PCR*, reverse transcriptase–polymerase chain reaction.
*Assays are available commercially.

can be used as detection methods. These methods currently are available in research laboratories. RT-PCR and genome sequencing have been used for epidemiologic studies.

Caliciviruses can be detected in stool specimens by electron microscopy or EIA. The current EIA tests are strain specific. Little is known about antigenic variation of the caliciviruses. RT-PCR and EIA tests using monoclonal antibodies are used in research laboratories.

For detection of rotavirus in stool specimens the original diagnostic technique of electron microscopy is still used as the single method available to identify all of the viral pathogens, including group A and non–group A rotavirus. EIA and latex agglutination assays are more readily available and detect group A rotaviruses (Yolken et al., 1978). As a general rule, latex agglutination tests have shown as high a specificity but a lower sensitivity when compared to EIA (Dennehy et al., 1988). Electropherotyping is a valuable means of studying the epidemiology of rotavirus infection, but it is not used as a diagnostic test. Oligonucleotide probes and polymerase chain reaction (PCR) tests have been used in research settings (Gouvea et al., 1990). Serologic assays for total antibody to rotavirus or serotype-specific response are useful to substantiate an infection but are currently not useful diagnostic tests during the acute course of an infection.

Complications

Severe dehydration as a consequence of vomiting and diarrhea is the major complication of viral gastroenteritis, especially in young infants and elderly debilitated adults. Immunocompromised patients may have prolonged viral shedding and symptoms of diarrhea caused by viral enteropathogens.

Prognosis

In general, the prognosis with any of these viral infections of the intestinal tract is excellent. The illness is self-limited and usually lasts for 1 to 4 days.

Treatment

The general principles of rehydration therapy are the same as those described for bacterial gastroenteritis (Provisional Committee on Quality Improvement, 1996). There is no specific antiviral therapy for any of the viral enteropathogens. Oral rehydration should be used for most children, except those who are severely dehydrated and cannot tolerate oral feedings. For the mildly dehydrated patient (3% to 5% fluid deficit), oral rehydration should commence with a fluid containing 50 to 90 mEq/L of sodium. The amount of fluid administered should be 50 ml/kg over a period of 2 to 4 hours. After 2 to 4 hours, hydration status should be reassessed. After the patient is rehydrated, treatment should progress to the maintenance phase of therapy. During rehydration and maintenance therapy, ongoing stool and vomit fluid losses must be replaced. Stool losses can be approximated by administering 10 ml/kg for each watery or loose stool passed, and 2 ml/kg of fluid should be administered for each episode of emesis (Duggan et al., 1992).

Preventive Measures

Appropriate hygiene and frequent handwashing are necessary for interruption of the fecal-oral spread of these agents. Careful food preparation measures must be enforced to reduce spread by contaminated food and water (Hedberg and Osterholm, 1993; Kramer et al., 1996).

Hospital isolation measures must be followed to prevent nosocomial diarrhea. Hospitalized patients with diarrhea should be isolated using "enteric precautions" (using the old CDC guidelines) or "contact precautions" (using the newest 1994 CDC isolation guidelines) (Garner, 1996). The prevention of rotavirus infection would be a major contribution to reducing the morbidity and mortality of acute infectious gastroenteritis. Therefore it is expected that immunization will make a major contribution toward this goal.

Immunizations

Various approaches to immunization are being considered. Rotavirus reassortant viruses containing the gene from the human rotavirus–encoding VP7 and the remaining ten genes from an animal rotavirus are being studied. These vaccines include three or four of the major G serotypes commonly found in the United States. The vaccines are safe and nonreactogenic. They give 50% to 60% protection against all rotavirus disease and ≥80% protection against severe dehydrating diarrhea (Rennels et al., 1996). Based on this partial protection, rotavirus vaccine is estimated to be cost-effective in the United States (Smith et al., 1995). The reassortant vaccines induce similar seroresponses and protection in breast-fed and non–breast fed children in the United States (Rennels et al., 1995). Based on the finding of antirotavirus secretory IgA in human milk (Pickering et al., 1995), there is interest in immunizing women immediately postpartum to provide protection to the infant through breast-feeding.

BIBLIOGRAPHY

Ackman DM, Drabkin P, Birkhead G, Cieslak P. Reptile-associated salmonellosis in New York state. Pediatr Infect Dis J 1995;14:955-959.

Avendano P, Matson DO, Long J, et al. Costs associated with office visits for diarrhea in infants and toddlers. Pediatr Infect Dis J 1993;12:897-902.

Bartlett AV, Prado D, Cleary TG, Pickering LK. Production of shigatoxin and other enterotoxins by serogroups of *Shigella*. J Infect Dis 1986;154:996-1002.

Bartlett AV, Reves RR, Pickering LK. Rotavirus in infant-toddler day-care centers: epidemiology relevant to disease control strategies. J Pediatr 1988;113:435-441.

Bartlett JG. *Clostridium difficile:* history of its role as an enteric pathogen and the current state of knowledge about the organism. Clin Infect Dis 1994;18:S265-S272.

Bates PR, Bailey AS, Wood DJ, et al. Comparative epidemiology of rotavirus, subgenus F (types 40 and 41) adenovirus, and astrovirus gastroenteritis in children. J Med Virol 1993;39:224-228.

Belongia EA, Osterholm MT, Soler JT, et al. Transmission of *Escherichia coli* O157:H7 infection in Minnesota child day-care facilities. JAMA 1993;269:883-888.

Bern C, Martines J, de Zoysa I, Glass RI. The magnitude of the global problem of diarrhoeal disease: a 10-year update. Bull World Health Organ 1992;70:705-714.

Bhan MK, Raj P, Levine MM, et al. Enteroaggregative *E. coli* associated with persistent diarrhea in a cohort of rural children in India. J Infect Dis 1989;159:1061-1064.

Bishop RF, Davidson GP, Holmes IH, Ruck BJ. Evidence for viral gastroenteritis. N Engl J Med 1973;289:1096-1097.

Blaser MJ, Reller LB. Campylobacter enteritis. N Engl J Med 1981;305:1444-1452.

Brandt CD, Kim HW, Rodriguez WJ, et al. Adenovirus and pediatric gastroenteritis. J Infect Dis 1985;151:437-443.

Brandt CD, Kim HW, Yolken RH, et al. Comparative epidemiology of two rotavirus serotypes and other viral agents associated with pediatric gastroenteritis. Am J Epidemiol 1979;110:243-254.

Brown KH, Peerson JM, Fontaine O. Use of nonhuman milks in the dietary management of young children with acute diarrhea: a meta-analysis of clinical trials. Pediatrics 1994;93:17-27.

Centers for Disease Control. 1993 Revised classification system for HIV infection and expanded AIDS surveillance case definition for AIDS among adolescents and adults. MMWR 1992;41:1-19.

Centers for Disease Control. *Vibrio vulnificus* infections associated with raw oyster consumption: Florida, 1981-1992. MMWR 1993;42:405-407.

Centers for Disease Control. Lake-associated outbreak of *Escherichia coli* O157:H7-Illinois, 1995. MMWR 1996a;45:437-439.

Centers for Disease Control. Outbreaks of Salmonella serotype Enteritidis infection associated with consumption of raw shell eggs: United States, 1994-1995. MMWR 1996b;45:737-742.

Centers for Disease Control. *Vibrio vulnificus* infections associated with eating raw oysters: Los Angeles, 1996. MMWR 1996c;45:621-624.

Cerquetti M, Luzzi I, Caprioli A, et al. Role of *Clostridium difficile* in childhood diarrhea. Pediatr Infect Dis J 1995;14:598-603.

Cholera Working Group, International Centre for Diarrhoeal Diseases Research, Bangladesh. Large epidemic of cholera-like disease in Bangladesh caused by *Vibrio cholerae* O139 synonym Bengal. Lancet 1993;342:387-390.

Cicirello HG, Glass RI. Current concepts of the epidemiology of diarrheal diseases. Semin Pediatr Infect Dis 1994;5:163-167.

Claeson M, Merson MH. Global progress in the control of diarrheal diseases. Pediatr Infect Dis J 1990;9:345-355.

Clausen CR, Christie DL. Chronic diarrhea in infants caused by adherent enteropathogenic *E. coli.* J Pediatr 1982;100:358-361.

Cleary TG. Cytotoxin producing *E. coli* and the hemolytic uremic syndrome. Pediatr Clin North Am 1988;30:485-501.

de la Morena ML, Van R, Singh K, et al. Diarrhea associated with *Aeromonas* species in children in day-care centers. J Infect Dis 1993;168:215-218.

Dennehy PH, Gauntlett DR, Tente WE. Comparison of nine commercial immunoassays for the detection of rotavirus in fecal specimens. J Clin Microbiol 1988;26:1630-1634.

Dolin R, Blacklow NR, DuPont H, et al. Biological properties of Norwalk agent of acute infectious nonbacterial gastroenteritis. Proc Soc Exp Biol Med 1972;140:578-583.

Duggan C, Santosham M, Glass RI. The management of acute diarrhea in children: oral rehydration, maintenance, and nutritional therapy: Centers for Disease Control and Prevention. MMWR 1992;41:1-20.

Estes MK, Cohen J. Rotavirus gene structure and function. Microbiol Rev 1989;53:410-449.

Fekety R. Recent advances in management of bacterial diarrhea. Rev Infect Dis 1983;5:246-257.

Garner JS. Guideline for isolation precautions in hospitals. Infect Control Hosp Epidemiol 1996;17:53-80.

Gerding DN, Johnson S, Peterson LR, et al. *Clostridium difficile*–associated diarrhea and colitis. Infect Control Hosp Epidemiol 1995;16:459-477.

Gilger MA, Matson DO, Conner ME, et al. Extraintestinal rotavirus infections in children with immunodeficiency. J Pediatr 1992;120:912-917.

Glass RI, Kilgore PE, Holman RC, et al. The epidemiology of rotavirus diarrhea in the United States: surveillance and estimates of disease burden. J Infect Dis 1996;174(suppl 1): S5-S11.

Goldschmidt MC, DuPont HL. Enteropathogenic *Escherichia coli:* lack of correlation of serotype with pathogenicity. J Infect Dis 1976;133:153-156.

Goossens H, Giesendorf AJ, Vandamme P, et al. Investigation of an outbreak of *Campylobacter upsaliensis* in day-care centers in Brussels: analysis of relationships among isolates by phenotypic and genotypic typing methods. J Infect Dis 1995; 172:1298-1303.

Gorbach SL, Kean BH, Evans DG, et al. Travelers' diarrhea and toxigenic *Escherichia coli.* N Engl J Med 1975;292:933-936.

Gouvea V, Glass RI, Woods P, et al. Polymerase chain reaction amplification and typing of rotavirus nucleic acid from stool specimens. J Clin Microbiol 1990;28:276-282.

Grady GF, Keusch GT. Pathogenesis of bacterial diarrheas. N Engl J Med 1971;285:831-900.

Grimwood K, Carzino R, Barnes GL, Bishop RF. Patients with enteric adenovirus gastroenteritis admitted to an Australian pediatric teaching hospital from 1981 to 1992. J Clin Microbiol 1995;33:131-136.

Guerrero L, Calva JJ, Morrow AL, et al. Asymptomatic Shigella infections in a cohort of Mexican children younger than two years of age. Pediatr Infect Dis J 1994;13:597-602.

Hayani KC, Ericsson CD, Pickering LK. Prevention and treatment of diarrhea in the traveling child. Semin Pediatr Infect Dis 1992;3:22-32.

Hedberg CW, Osterholm MT. Outbreaks of food-borne and water-borne viral gastroenteritis. Clin Microbiol Rev 1993; 6:199-210.

Hennessy TW, Hedberg CW, Slutsker L, et al. A national outbreak of *Salmonella enteritidis* infections from ice cream. N Engl J Med 1996;334:1281-1286.

Herrmann JE, Nowak NA, Perron-Henry DM, et al. Diagnosis of astrovirus gastroenteritis by antigen detection with monoclonal antibodies. J Infect Dis 1990;161:226-229.

Holmes SJ, Morrow AL, Pickering LK. Child care practices: effects of social changes on epidemiology of infectious diseases and antibiotic resistance. Epidem Rev 1996;18:10-28.

Holmgren J. Actions of cholera toxin and the prevention and treatment of cholera. Nature 1981;292:413-417.

Hornick RB, Greisman SE, Woodward TE, et al. Typhoid fever: pathogenesis and immunologic control. N Engl J Med 1970;283:739-746.

Jacewicz MS, Mobassaleh M, Gross SK, et al. Pathogenesis of *Shigella* diarrhea: XVII. a mammalian cell membrane glycolipid, Gb3, is required but not sufficient to confer sensitivity to Shiga toxin. J Infect Dis 1994;169:538-546.

Jiang X, Matson DO, Velazquez FR, et al. Study of Norwalk-related viruses in Mexican children. J Med Virol 1995; 47:309-316.

Kapikian AZ, Kim HW, Wyatt RG, et al. Reovirus-like agent in stools: association with infantile diarrhea and development of serologic tests. Science 1974;185:1049-1053.

Kapikian AZ, Kim HW, Wyatt RG, et al. Human reovirus-like agent as the major pathogen associated with "winter" gastroenteritis in hospitalized infants, young children, and their contacts. N Engl J Med 1976;294:965-972.

Kapikian AZ, Wyatt RG, Dolin R, et al. Visualization by immune electron microscopy of a 27-nm particle associated with acute infectious nonbacterial gastroenteritis. J Virol 1972;10:1075-1081.

Kaplan JE, Masur H, Holmes KK. USPHS/IDSA guidelines for the prevention of opportunistic infections in person infected with human immunodeficiency virus: a summary. MMWR 1995;44:1-34.

Karmali MA, Fleming PC. Campylobacter enteritis in children. J Pediatr 1979;94:527-533.

Karmali MA, Petric M, Steele BT, Lin C. Sporadic cases of hemolytic uremic syndrome associated with faecal cytotoxin and cytotoxin producing *E. coli* in stools. Lancet 1983;1:619-620.

Keene WE, McAnulty JM, Hoesly FC, et al. A swimming-associated outbreak of hemorrhagic colitis caused by *Escherichia coli* O157:H7 and *Shigella sonnei.* N Engl J Med 1994; 331:579-584.

Kelly CP, Pothoulakis C, LaMont JT. *Clostridium difficile* colitis. N Engl J Med 1994;380:256-261.

Kotloff KL, Losonsky GA, Morris JG, et al. Enteric adenovirus infection and childhood diarrhea: an epidemiologic study in three clinical settings. Pediatrics 1989;84:219-225.

Kramer MH, Herwaldt BL, Craun GF. Surveillance for waterborne disease outbreaks: United States, 1993-1994. MMWR 1996;459(SS-1):1-30.

Lee LA, Gerber AR, Lonsway DR, Smith JD. *Yersinia enterocolitica* O:3 infections in infants and children, associated with the household preparation of chitterlings. N Engl J Med 1990;322:984-987.

Levine MM, Berquist EJ, Nalin DR, et al. *Escherichia coli* strains that cause diarrhea but do not produce heat-labile or heat-stable enterotoxins are noninvasive. Lancet 1978; 1:1119-1122.

Levine MM, Edelman R. Enteropathogenic *E. coli* of classic serotypes associated with infant diarrhea: epidemiology and pathogenesis. Epidemiol Rev 1984;6:31-51.

Levine MM, Kaper JB. Live vaccines against cholera: an update. Vaccine 1993;11:207-212.

Levine MM, Noriega F. Current status of vaccine development for enteric diseases. Semin Pediatr Infect Dis 1994;5:245-250.

Mathewson JJ, Oberhelman RA, DuPont HL, et al. Enteroadherent *E. coli* as a cause of diarrhea among children in Mexico. J Clin Microbiol 1987;25:1917-1919.

Matson DO, Estes MK, Burns JW, et al. Serotype variation of human group A rotaviruses in two regions of the United States. J Infect Dis 1990;162:605-614.

Matson DO, Estes MK, Tanaka T, et al. Asymptomatic human calicivirus infection in a day-care center outbreak. Pediatr Infect Dis J 1990;9:190-196.

Mishu B, Koehler J, Lee LA, et al. Outbreaks of *Salmonella enteritidis* infections in the United States, 1985-1991. J Infect Dis 1994;169:547-552.

Mitchell DK, Monroe SS, Jiang X, et al. Virologic features of an astrovirus diarrhea outbreak in a day-care center revealed by reverse transcriptase-polymerase chain reaction. J Infect Dis 1995a;172:1437-1444.

Mitchell DK, Van R, Mason EH, et al. Prospective study of infection with *Clostridium difficile* in children given amoxicillin/clavulanate for otitis media. Pediatr Infect Dis J 1995b;15:514-519.

Mitchell DK, Van R, Morrow AL, et al. Outbreaks of astrovirus gastroenteritis in day-care centers. J Pediatr 1993;123:725-732.

Nair GB, Ramamurthy T, Bhattacharya SK, et al. Spread of *Vibrio cholerae* 0139 Bengal in India. J Infect Dis 1994; 169:1029-1034.

Novak R, Feldman S. Salmonellosis in children with cancer: review of 42 cases. Am J Dis Child 1979;133:298-300.

Okada S, Sekine S, Ando T, et al. Antigenic characterization of small, round-structured viruses by immune electron microscopy. J Clin Microbiol 1990;28:1244-1248.

O'Ryan ML, Matson DO. Viral gastroenteritis pathogens in the day-care center setting. Semin Pediatr Infect Dis 1990;1:252-262.

O'Ryan ML, Matson DO, Estes MK, et al. Molecular epidemiology of rotavirus in children attending day-care centers in Houston. J Infect Dis 1990;162:810-816.

Pai CH, Sorger S, Lackman L. Campylobacter gastroenteritis in children. J Pediatr 1979;94:589-591.

Pickering LK. Therapy for acute infectious diarrhea in children. J Pediatr 1991;118:S118-S128.

Pickering LK. Emerging antibiotic resistance in enteric bacterial pathogens. Semin Pediatr Infect Dis 1996;7:272-280.

Pickering LK, Bartlett AV, Reves RR, Morrow AL. Asymptomatic excretion of rotavirus before and after rotavirus diarrhea in children in day-care centers. J Pediatr 1988;112:361-365.

Pickering LK, Matson DO. Therapy for diarrheal disease in children. In Blaser MJ, Smith PD, Ravdin JI, et al. (eds). Infections of the gastrointestinal tract. New York: Raven Press; 1995.

Pickering LK, Morrow AL, Herrera I, et al. Effect of maternal rotavirus immunization on milk and serum antibody titers. J Infect Dis 1995;172:723-728.

Pickering LK, Obrig TG, Stapleton FB. Hemolytic uremic syndrome and enterohemorrhagic *Escherichia coli*. Pediatr Infect Dis J 1994;13:459-475.

Prasad BVV, Burns JW, Mariette E, et al. Localization of VP4 neutralization sites in rotavirus by three-dimensional cryo-electron microscopy. Nature 1990;343:476-479.

Provisional Committee on Quality Improvement, Subcommittee on Acute Gastroenteritis, American Academy of Pediatrics. Practice parameter: the management of acute gastroenteritis in young children. Pediatrics 1996;97:424-433.

Reed RP, Friedland IR, Wegerhoff FO, et al. *Campylobacter* bacteremia in children. Pediatr Infect Dis J 1996;15:345-348.

Rees JH, Soudain SE, Gregson NA, Hughes RAC. *Campylobacter jejuni* infection and Guillain-Barré syndrome. N Engl J Med 1995;333:1374-1379.

Rennels MB, Glass RI, Dennehy PH, et al. Safety and efficacy of high-dose rhesus-human reassortant rotavirus vaccines: report of the national multicenter trial. Pediatrics 1996;97:7-13.

Rennels MB, Wasserman SS, Glass RI, Keane VA. Comparison of immunogenicity and efficacy of rhesus rotavirus reassortant vaccines in breast-fed and non–breast fed children. Pediatrics 1995;96:1132-1136.

Reves RR, Morrow AL, Bartlett AV, et al. Child day-care increases the risk of clinic visits for acute diarrhea and diarrhea due to rotavirus. Am J Epidemiol 1993;137:97-107.

Riley LW, Remis RS, Helgerson SD, et al. Hemorrhagic colitis associated with a rare *Escherichia coli* serotype. N Engl J Med 1983;308:681-685.

Robins-Browne RM, Levine MM, Rowe B, Gabriel EM. Failure to detect conventional enterotoxins in classical enteropathogenic (serotyped) *E. coli* strains of proven pathogenicity. Infect Immun 1982;138:798-801.

Rudoy RC. Enteroinvasive and enterotoxigenic *Escherichia coli:* occurrence in acute diarrhea of infants and children. Am J Dis Child 1975;129:688-672.

Sack DA, Sack RB. A test for enterotoxigenic *Escherichia coli*. Infect Immun 1975;11:334-336.

Saphra I, Winter JW. Clinical manifestations of salmonellosis in man. An evaluation of 7,779 human infections identified at the New York Salmonella Center. N Engl J Med 1957; 256:1128.

Savarino SJ, McVeigh A, Watson J, et al. Enteroaggregative *Escherichia coli* heat-stable enterotoxin is not restricted to enteroaggregative *E. coli*. J Infect Dis 1996;173:1019-1022.

Schreiber DS, Blacklow NR, Trier JS. The mucosal lesion of the proximal small intestine in acute infections nonbacterial gastroenteritis. N Engl J Med 1973;288:1318-1323.

Scragg JN, Rubidge CJ, Applebaum PC. Shigella infection in African and Indian children with special reference to septicemia. J Pediatr 1978;93:796-797.

Sears CL, Kaper JB. Enteric bacterial toxins: mechanisms of action and linkage to intestinal secretion. Microbiol Rev 1996;60:167-215.

Sempertegui F, Estrella B, Egas J, et al. Risk of diarrheal disease in Ecuadorian day-care centers. Pediatr Infect Dis J 1995; 14:606-612.

Shore EG, Dean AG, Holik KJ, Davis BR. Enterotoxin-producing *Escherichia coli* and diarrheal disease in adult travelers: a prospective study. J Infect Dis 1974;129:577-582.

Smith JC, Haddix AC, Teutsch SM, Glass RI. Cost-effectiveness analysis of a rotavirus immunization program for the United States. Pediatrics 1995;96:609-615.

Snyder J. The continuing evolution of oral therapy for diarrhea. Semin Pediatr Infect Dis 1994;5:231-235.

Thomas DD, Knoop FC. The effect of calcium and prostaglandin inhibitors on the intestinal fluid response to heat-stable enterotoxin of *E. coli*. J Infect Dis 1982;145: 141-147.

Thomas DD, Knoop FC. Effect of heat-stable enterotoxin of *E. coli* on cultured mammalian cells. J Infect Dis 1983; 147:450-459.

Ulshen MH, Rollo JL. Pathogenesis of *E. coli* gastroenteritis in man: another mechanism. N Engl J Med 1980; 302:99-101.

Utsalo SJ, Eko FO, Antia Obong OE, Nwaigwe CU. Aeromonads in acute diarrhoea and asymptomatic infections in Nigerian children. Eur J Epidemiol 1995;11:171-175.

Van R, Wun C, O'Ryan MC, et al. Outbreaks of human enteric adenovirus types 40 and 41 in Houston day-care centers. J Pediatr 1992;120:516-521.

Velazquez FR, Matson DO, Calva JJ, et al. Rotavirus infection in infants as protection against subsequent infections. N Engl J Med 1996;335:1022-1028.

Waldor MK, Mekalanos JJ. Lysogenic conversion by a filamentous phage encoding cholera toxin. Science 1996;272:1910-1914.

Walker RI, Caldwell MB, Lee EC, et al. Pathophysiology of *Campylobacter* enteritis. Microbiol Rev 1986;50:81-94.

Wanke CA, Schorling JB, Barrett LJ, et al. Potential role of adherence traits of *Escherichia coli* in persistent diarrhea in an urban Brazilian slum. Pediatr Infect Dis J 1991;10:746-751.

Wilcox MH, Cook AM, Eley A, Spencer RC. *Aeromonas* spp. as a potential cause of diarrhea in children. J Clin Pathol 1992;45:959-963.

Yolken RH, Wyatt RG, Zissis G, et al. Epidemiology of human rotavirus types 1 and 2 as studied by enzyme-linked immunosorbent assay. N Engl J Med 1978;229:1156-1161.

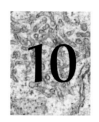

10 *HAEMOPHILUS INFLUENZAE* TYPE B

DENNIS A. CLEMENTS

Haemophilus influenzae type b (HIB) is a small, pleomorphic, nonmotile gram-negative bacterium that is naturally a parasite only of humans. Its name derives from the mistaken identification by Pfeiffer in 1892 that it was responsible for the influenza pandemic and from the fact that it requires two factors from blood for growth. *Haemophilus influenzae* is easily divided into encapsulated forms, which cause invasive disease (discussed in this chapter), and unencapsulated forms, which Pfeiffer had identified in the airways of those dying from influenza. The unencapsulated forms typically cause mucosal disease (otitis media, bronchitis, and conjunctivitis), except in aged, immunosuppressed, malnourished, or premature individuals, in whom may cause invasive disease.

HIB was once the most common bacterial pathogen to cause meningitis in children in countries where nationwide reporting of diseases is established (Box 10-1). In 1978 *Haemophilus influenzae* type b was estimated to have caused 46% of all bacterial meningitis (10,000 cases) in the United States, regardless of age. In addition, it caused an equal number of other invasive diseases, such as buccal and periorbital cellulitis, pneumonia, arthritis, epiglottitis and pericarditis. This disease burden is equivalent to that caused by paralytic polio in the United States in the 1950s (Cochi et al., 1988).

Since the introduction of HIB vaccine in 1987 the incidence of HIB disease in the United States has decreased 95% among children <5 years of age. The disease incidence in persons > 5 years of age has not changed and remains about 0.5 per 100,000. Non–type b *Haemophilus influenzae* disease in children <5 years of age has decreased slightly but is now more common than type b disease (Centers for Disease Control, 1996).

ETIOLOGY

HIB organisms are gram-negative coccobacilli or filamentous rods, hence the descriptive term *pleomorphic*. They grow on chocolate agar, where they have a glistening, semitransparent appearance. They are further identified by the requirement for X (hemin or other porphyrins) and V (coenzyme nicotinamide adenine dinucleotide) factors for growth on blood agar. (A more sensitive test for the X factor requirement is to test the ability of *Haemophilus influenzae* to convert delta aminolevulinic acid to porphyrin.) Other tests such as the production of indole from tryptophan and detection of β-galactosidase (ONPG test) activity are also useful in discriminating *Haemophilus influenzae* from other *Haemophilus* species.

A more rapid method of identifying type b organisms is to use type b antiserum on a slide with the unidentified organism. If agglutination does not occur, one can be sure that the organism is not a type b. However, if agglutination does occur, it is possible that the organism is a type b. False positives are frequent because of cross-reactivity of antigens and because of autoagglutination by nontypable strains.

Another method for selective identification of type b organisms is to use antiserum agar as described by Michaels and Stonebraker (1975). A suitable clear nutrient agar is prepared containing hyperimmune *Haemophilus influenzae* type b antiserum (produced in burros). When this selective medium is inoculated with appropriate specimens, a halo of agglutination is observed around each HIB colony after 24 to 48 hours. This is a very sensitive method for detecting colonization and also allows for a quantitative assay.

Typable and nontypable *Haemophilus influenzae* can be divided into biotypes by the presence or absence of three enzyme activities: urease, ornithine

---

BOX 10-1

A BRIEF HISTORY

1892: Pfeiffer erroneously identified *Haemophilus influenzae* as the causative agent in the lungs of patients dying during the influenza pandemic.

1930: Margaret Pittman described 6 serotypes (a through f) of encapsulated *Haemophilus influenzae* based on antigenic differences in their capsular polysaccharides.

1935: Fothergill and Wright described an inverse relationship between the age of HIB disease and the serum level of bactericidal antibody against *Haemophilus influenzae* type b.

1944: Alexander demonstrated that hyperimmune sera protected rabbits against developing meningitis when inoculated with HIB.

1950: The use of chloramphenicol markedly decreased the mortality from infection resulting from HIB.

1970: Schneerson purified the HIB polysaccharide capsule component polyribosyl-ribotyl phosphate (PRP), to be used as a vaccine immunogen.

1974: Peltola demonstrated that PRP was immunogenic in children over 18 months of age in a vaccine trial of 100,000 children in Finland.

1984: Kayhty reported a 90% protective vaccine efficacy in children older than 18 months in the 1974 Finnish HIB trial.

1985: PRP vaccine was licensed in the United States to be given to children >2 years of age.

1980s: PRP was conjugated with various proteins to increase its immunogenicity in children less than 18 months of age.

1985 to 1987: A controlled trial of PRP-D given in the first 6 to 12 months of life in Finland was shown to be protective.

1987: PRP-D was licensed for use in the United States in children who had reached 18 months of age.

1990: HboC and PRP-OMP were licensed for use in children as young as 2 months in the United States.

1993: PRP-T and DTP-HbOC combination vaccines licensed in the United States.

1995: Multiple reports of decreased HIB disease to 5% to 10% of previous levels in the United States.

---

decarboxylase, and production of indole from tryptophan (Kilian, 1976). This system divides *Haemophilus influenzae* organisms into eight (I to VIII) groups, but 90% of type b organisms are biotype I. Hence this has proved to be of little epidemiologic use for type b organisms. Unencapsulated *Haemophilus influenzae,* however, show a much wider distribution of biotypes, and this technique is more useful in epidemiologic studies of nontypable disease.

The polysaccharide capsule of *Haemophilus influenzae* is an important virulence factor. The type b capsule consists of a repeating polymer of five carbon sugar units, ribose, and ribitol phosphate. The cell envelope includes lipo-oligosaccharide (LOS) and outer-membrane proteins (OMP). Pili or fimbriae extend from the outer membrane, but their presence appears to be variable. They apparently mediate the attachment of HIB to epithelial cells, which is essential to establish colonization but perhaps disadvantageous in the blood.

Haemophilus influenzae was invariably sensitive to ampicillin until the early 1970s, when resistance resulting from the production of a plasmid-mediated β-lactamase was first described. At present 15% to 50% of HIB isolates are β-lactamase producers, depending on geographical location (Wenger et al., 1990). Resistance to chloramphenicol because of plasmid-mediated chloramphenicol acetyltransferase production has also been described.

There has been keen interest in determining which subtypes of *Haemophilus influenzae* type b cause invasive disease. This was explored in the United States by Barenkamp et al. (1983). They reported that a high proportion of cases (84%) of invasive HIB disease is caused by only a few OMP subtypes (1H, 44%; 3L, 28%; and 1L, 12%), but there was no specificity of disease by subtype. They also reported that subtype prevalence varies over time. Subtype 2L accounted for 22% of CSF and blood isolates during the years 1977 through 1980 but only 4% in 1981 and 1982. In Holland, van Alphen et al. (1987) documented that 80% to 90% of HIB organisms causing invasive disease in Europe are OMP subtype 3L (van Alphen subtype 1) and that 83% of the isolates from Iceland are subtype 2L (van Alphen subtype 2). Takala et al.

(1989) reported that one subtype (van Alphen 1c), which has been rarely isolated elsewhere, causes very little epiglottitis, compared to meningitis, in Finland. Thus there is suggestive evidence that virulence may vary with OMP subtype.

Attempts have also been made to categorize HIB isolates by LOS (lipo-oligosaccharide) typing because LOS subtypes are more varied, which could increase their value as an epidemiologic tool. Unfortunately, LOS patterns of individual isolates appear to be unstable during storage, and, in the animal model, LOS expression by an individual clone may vary according to environmental conditions.

Newer techniques such as multilocus enzyme electrophoresis (ET) and clonotyping attempt to identify HIB isolates by differences in single enzyme loci or DNA sequence changes, respectively. Most isolates with the same ET pattern belong to the same OMP subtype and LOS subtypes, suggesting homogeneity of isolates. Musser et al. (1988) showed that HIB strains could be separated into three genetic groups or "clonotypes," each of which is associated with a restricted group of OMP subtypes, suggesting limited clonal ancestry of HIB. One clonotype was predominant in Europe, but all three were found in the United States.

PATHOGENESIS

HIB, a natural infection only in humans, is spread by respiratory secretions. However, most colonized children do not become ill, and carriage alone does not necessarily induce an antibody response. Type b strains may persist in the airway for prolonged periods, thus increasing the opportunity for transmission. Animal models indicate that, in the minority in whom disease occurs, invasion through the mucosa into the blood is facilitated by mucosal damage (viral infection, trauma, etc.) or increased numbers of mucosal organisms. After penetration into the bloodstream they are protected from phagocytosis by their capsules and multiply while disseminating to the meninges, epiglottis, or synovial surfaces. The patient may become symptomatic at any time after bacteremia occurs. The predilection of HIB for the epiglottis is not understood, but it is known that blood colony counts in patients with epiglottitis are considerably lower than those in patients with meningitis.

CLINICAL MANIFESTATIONS
Meningitis

The pathology of meningitis is discussed in Chapter 17. HIB appears to have associated subdural ef-fusions more than other causes of bacterial meningitis. The slow resolution of these effusions, some of which may be empyemas, has led to debate about the length of time these patients should be treated and whether surgical intervention is necessary. The persistance of bacterial cell products (particularly LOS) in the subdural space is thought to be responsible for prolonged fever in some of these patients.

Cellulitis

Buccal cellulitis occurs principally in children less than 18 months of age and may be related to bottle feeding. It can appear overnight in an otherwise healthy child. It often has a violaceous hue or it can appear erysipeloid. HIB can often be cultured from the blood or a saline aspirate of the cheek. Due consideration should be given to whether the child might have another focus of infection, particularly if blood cultures are positive. Other bacterial causes need to be considered, particularly in the older child or if there is an associated facial abrasion.

Orbital cellulitis (Fig. 10-1) can be a medical emergency. It is usually an extension of an ethmoid sinusitis, and, if there is proptosis of the eye or paralysis of eye movement, decompression of the orbit is mandatory. This disease needs to be distinguished from "preseptal," or periorbital, cellulitis (Fig. 10-2), which is a cellulitis of the eyelid and contiguous structures but which does not compromise the blood supply or the movement of the eye (Goldberg et al., 1978).

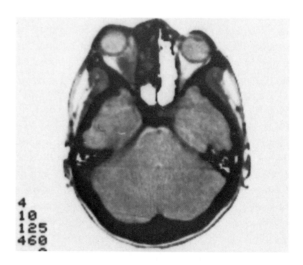

FIG. 10-1   CT scan of a child with orbital cellulitis. Proptosis of the eye and involvement of deeper structures is evident.

Epiglottitis

In epiglottitis manifestation the epiglottis is acutely edematous and erythematous. HIB can often be cultured from the surface of the pharynx, as well as from the blood. Some investigators feel that there may be an allergic component to this disease, which accounts for the extremely rapid course (as few as 4 to 6 hours) with which this disease often manifests. Children appear toxic, but more strikingly they hold their heads forward trying to keep their airway patent. A short period of intubation with appropriate antibiotic treatment reverses this process quickly.

Septic Arthritis

HIB may cause septic arthritis in the young child. It is clinically indistinguishable from the disease caused by *Staphylococcus aureus.* Large joints—the hip in particular—are involved. It is important to have adequate drainage when large joints are affected, both for organism identification and for healing. Latex agglutination tests may be positive from fluid from the joint space. If the child is very young, it is important to consider whether there is a contiguous osteomyelitis.

Pneumonia

The incidence of this infection is truly unknown. Many children are probably inadvertently treated when they are given antibiotics for other upper-respiratory illnesses, such as otitis media or sinusitis. Children with documented meningitis, pericarditis, or epiglottitis may have pneumonia as well. A definitive diagnosis is hampered in many cases because of the inability to obtain a positive diagnosis. One British study has suggested that a positive HIB latex agglutination test in children with pneumonia

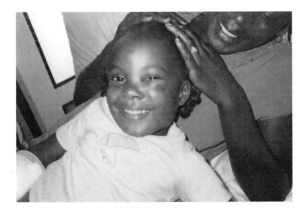

FIG. 10-2   Child recovering from a case of HIB preseptal (periorbital) cellulitis.

may not be accurate (Isaacs, 1989). Thus many children in the past may have been falsely assumed to have HIB pneumonia. HIB cultured from the blood in a patient with clinical or roentgenographic pneumonia can be considered confirmatory. It has been reported that as many as 90% of patients with HIB pneumonias will have a pleural reaction and effusion.

Pericarditis

Although infrequent, this disease manifestation is frightening for its rapidity of onset and lack of clinical symptoms. Respiratory distress in a child who is toxic and has a normal chest roentgenogram are often the only symptoms. The child may have an underlying pneumonia or meningitis, and this disease process has been reported to occur in children who are on antibiotic treatment. Echocardiography followed by pericardiocentesis and appropriate antibiotic therapy are indicated. Copious pericardial exudate often persists for several days after therapy is initiated.

Bacteremia

Children who appear toxic but have no focus of infection may have HIB bacteremia, which is diagnosed with a positive blood culture.

DIAGNOSIS

The isolation of HIB from a normally sterile body site is the diagnosis of choice in all diseases. HIB bacteremia, for instance, is always diagnosed with the isolation of HIB from the blood. However, there are limitations to this otherwise optimal standard. Occasionally a child may be given an antibiotic for treatment of a less severe disease before manifesting clinical meningitis. If the clinical history is compatible with meningitis and there are CSF changes (low sugar, high protein, and increased number of neutrophils) and a positive CSF latex agglutination test for HIB, most would agree that the child should be assumed to have HIB meningitis. If the CSF latex agglutination test is negative however, even if the urine antigen test is positive, it is unlikely that this patient should be considered to have HIB meningitis if HIB does not grow from the CSF. If HIB grows from the CSF culture and the CSF is otherwise benign, it should be assumed that the child has HIB meningitis and that the disease was detected at an early stage.

A positive diagnosis for HIB is often difficult in a patient with cellulitis because clinicians are often reluctant to aspirate from the inflamed tissue. If blood cultures are positive for HIB or if the clinical picture is compatible and the urine latex test is positive, the diagnosis can be assumed to be correct. Where there are no positive results, it is prudent to treat with an antibiotic that would also treat *S. aureus* infections.

If an aspirate is performed in septic arthritis, it will often confirm the bacterial cause of the infection, but if it is not performed then the physician must rely on positive blood cultures and/or positive urine latex tests. If the child is already receiving an oral antibiotic, all the same difficulties with negative cultures just mentioned prevail. It is extremely important, however, that if there is doubt about the cause of the arthritis the patient be treated with antibiotics (and surgical drainage, if indicated) that would be suitable for *S. aureus* infections, as well as for *Haemophilus influenzae* type b.

Pericarditis always requires drainage, and, if the drainage is performed early in the course of disease, a positive culture for HIB from the fluid or blood is likely. If, however, the child has been on antibiotics and cultures are negative, a positive latex agglutination for HIB from the pericardial fluid or urine would be useful.

Pneumonia remains the most difficult of all the infections to document, because there is question about the meaning of positive latex agglutination tests in these patients (see the previous discussion). A positive blood culture or positive latex agglutination test from pleural fluid may be confirmatory, but these tests may not be positive even if performed.

Laboratory Tests

Gram stain and culture are the tests of choice to document infection. However, prior antibiotic treatment often makes blood cultures sterile. CSF cultures are less critically affected, particularly by the prior use of oral antibiotics, and thus may still be positive. Additionally, diseases with localized infection (arthritis and epiglottitis) have a lower level of bacteremia, and positive cultures may be missed if an inadequate volume of blood is taken for culture.

Several methods of antigen detection are useful even when the organisms have been made nonviable by antibiotics. The most popular and sensitive is the latex particle agglutination test, which uses anti-PRP antibody on latex particles that agglutinate in the presence of PRP antigen. This test may be negative, however, if there is an overabundance or, alternately, a shortage of PRP antigen. It is also occasionally falsely positive as a result of cross-reactivity with some *E. coli, S. pneumoniae, S. aureus,* and *N. meningitidis* strains. Nevertheless, a positive latex test, in the presence of a strongly suggestive clinical course, is useful.

DIFFERENTIAL DIAGNOSIS
Meningitis

In the developed world the most common cause of meningitis in children between the ages of 3 months and 3 years was once HIB. The disease is indistinguishable from other causes of meningitis by clinical signs and symptoms alone. Chapter 17 deals with clinical symptoms so they are not discussed here. With the advent of HIB immunization in children as young as 2 months old in the United States it is expected that HIB as a cause of meningitis in this age group should diminish. *Neisseria meningitidis* and *Streptococcus pneumoniae* would then be the leading causes of meningitis in this age group (Wenger et al., 1990). HIB meningitis can be differentiated from the previously mentioned causes of bacterial meningitis preferably by the results of CSF culture or by positive blood culture with a compatible CSF picture. A positive urine latex test for HIB with a compatible clinical course and CSF analysis would also be acceptable. Other possible diagnoses include *Streptococcus agalactia* (group B streptococcus) or *Listeria monocytogenes* in infants, and TB meningitis or aseptic meningitis in a child of any age. TB meningitis typically has a CSF lymphocytosis, increased protein, and decreased glucose. Aseptic meningitis may have a CSF pleocytosis and slightly elevated protein, but the glucose is usually within normal limits.

Epiglottitis

The presenting symptoms for epiglottitis include upper-airway obstruction and a toxic appearance. Symptoms often appear rapidly, frequently in just a few hours. In areas where epiglottitis is common, it is customary to visualize the epiglottis with an anesthesiologist or intensivist present so that the child can be immediately intubated if necessary. At the time of intubation the epiglottis is cherry red and swollen, and it is useful to swab the epiglottis for bacterial culture. If the epiglottis is not typical in appearance (for epiglottitis) but the child requires intubation, it is useful to send the swab for viral culture. Most viral causes of a similar clinical-appearing syndrome have other symptoms of a respiratory infection (e.g., cough, coryza, conjunctivitis) and have a longer period of recovery. Children who present with drooling and with their head placed forward to facilitate air entry occasionally have other pharyngeal structures red and swollen (uvula or posterior pharynx); these children often grow HIB from their blood or mucosal surface culture.

There is evidence that virtually all cases of epiglottitis in young children, as determined by inspection of the epiglottis during intubation, are caused by HIB. HIB was isolated from 114 of 123 (93%) blood cultures collected from epiglottitis patients in the study in Melbourne, Australia, and no other pathogens were isolated (Gilbert et al., 1990). When the diagnosis is not bacteriologically confirmed, it is usually because appropriate specimens are not taken.

Pneumonia

The diagnosis of HIB pneumonia is difficult because blood cultures may not be positive, as a result of prior antibiotic therapy or an associated low level of bacteremia. If there is a pleural effusion, aspiration of fluid for culture or latex agglutination may provide a positive result. However, the value of only a positive urine latex for HIB is debatable, as previously mentioned. The presence of a significant effusion is suggestive that the pneumonia may be caused by HIB: up to 90% of HIB pneumonias have effusions (compared to only 10% for *S. pneumoniae*) in some reports. Drainage of a large effusion may not be required for recovery, unless there is an empyema, but usually speeds the healing process.

Septic Arthritis

This disease manifestation is assumed to be secondary to seeding synovial surfaces subsequent to bacteremia. Large joints, particularly the hip, are most commonly affected and should be surgically drained to avoid permanent damage. If the child was febrile and/or irritable before diagnosis, he or she may already be taking an antibiotic, and thus blood cultures may be negative. If there is a small antigen load in the blood or if the urine is dilute, then the urine latex test may be negative as well. In this case only an aspirate of the joint for culture and latex agglutination may provide a diagnosis. In the absence of a positive culture it is prudent to treat for a possible *S. aureus* septic arthritis as well because it is common in the same age group and the symptoms are identical. If the child is very young it is important to determine whether there is a contiguous osteomyelitis.

Cellulitis

Cellulitis of the face or around the orbit (periorbital) often develops rapidly. There is some suggestion that facial cellulitis may be associated with maxillary sinusitis or bottle feeding. These superficial skin infections are markedly different from the deep orbital tissue infection, "orbital" cellulitis, that commonly has an associated ipsilateral ethmoid sinusitis. CT imaging may be required to distinguish the difference, since the eyelid is often too swollen to allow inspection of eye movement. The inability to move the eye suggests "orbital" infection, and decompression of the orbit is often required to avoid permanent sequelae. A positive microbiologic diagnosis can only be made in these infections if there is a positive blood culture or aspirate from the infected tissue. A positive urine latex alone is suggestive and, some would believe, sufficient. However, if the diagnosis is uncertain, treatment to cover *Staphylococcus aureus, Streptococcus pneumoniae,* and *Streptococcus pyogenes* would be prudent.

COMPLICATIONS

Most of the complications of HIB disease are found in the youngest patients who have meningitis. This is not unexpected. The youngest children often have the most fulminant disease and the fewest focal symptoms to alert parents and physicians of their diagnosis before the disease progresses to meningitis, the consequences of which necessarily affect the brain.

Subdural Fluid

Subdural effusions are frequently associated with HIB meningitis. Some of these effusions probably represent subdural empyemas, and there is debate about which of these require surgical drainage. It would seem appropriate to treat with antibiotics and perform serial CT scans, or other appropriate imaging procedures, to document whether the effusion/empyemas will resolve on their own. Children with these fluid collections often have persistent fever, which is compatible with the presence of persistent HIB antigen (particularly LOS) in the subdural space, causing the febrile reaction. Subdural fluid HIB antigen tests in some patients are positive for as long as a month after initial treatment, although cultures of the fluid are sterile.

Hearing Loss

The most common sequealae of HIB disease is hearing loss, which has been reported in 5% to

15% of cases. It appears that prior treatment of the child with oral antibiotics may actually increase the incidence of hearing loss—probably by decreasing bacteremia and hence symptoms but masking a smoldering CNS infection. There is also evidence that the early treatment of meningitis with steroids decreases the incidence of hearing loss in some patients. If this finding is verified, it will be useful in preventing significant morbidity in these children.

Intellectual Functioning

A sizable minority of children (5% to 20%) will have significant intellectual impairment after HIB meningitis. In the United States, as compared to other developed nations, there are more sequelae after HIB disease, but the median and mean age of patients with meningitis is younger in the United States, which may predispose patients to more complications. In addition, there have been studies that look at more subtle measurements of intellectual functioning in the United States. It has been reported that a disturbingly high percentage (up to 40%) of patients have "soft" intellectual problems, such as the inability to concentrate or specific learning disabilities when compared to their siblings or peers (Sell, 1987). With the advent of preventive immunization the incidence of all of these sequelae should decrease.

PROGNOSIS

In the United States the death rate from HIB disease is approximately 3% of those known to be infected (Wenger et al., 1990). Meningitis carries the highest death rate, since it occurs in the youngest children and affects the brain. Mental retardation, hearing loss, and mild neurologic abnormalities have also been described; the rates of each are dependent on the population examined and the intensity of investigation.

IMMUNITY

The protective role of PRP antibodies was first demonstrated by Fothergill and Wright in 1933. They noted an increased incidence of HIB disease when maternal antibody began to wane at 4 to 6 months of age. Like other polysaccharide antigens, PRP is T-cell independent and thus does not induce immunologic memory; the ability to respond to PRP with production of antibody (particularly IgG_2) is not acquired until about 18 to 24 months old. Thus the greatest period of susceptibility to disease is between 4 and 24 months old, which is the peak incidence of disease in the United States.

This lack of response to polysaccharide antigen is also responsible for the susceptibility of these children to *Neisseria meningitidis* and *Streptococcus pneumoniae* infections. Immunization for the prevention of these diseases has necessitated the conjugation of the polysaccharide to a protein moiety to induce the infant immune system to make antibody to the polysaccharide and thus protect itself. This is discussed at the end of the chapter.

It is therefore apparent that children who acquire HIB infection at an early age may not mount an immunologic response. Therefore even children who have had HIB disease should be vaccinated with the conjugate vaccine.

EPIDEMIOLOGIC FACTORS

The HIB nasopharyngeal carriage rate is generally less than 5%, but most children have acquired antibody to PRP by the age of 5 years without becoming ill, suggesting that they have been exposed to HIB or cross-reacting polysaccharides of other organisms. Disease is more common in children living under crowded conditions such as in day-care centers or inner-city areas. Although there is seasonal variation in disease, clear-cut epidemics have not been described.

Before the advent of conjugate HIB vaccine, the incidence and type of disease varied by country, but approximately 90% to 95% of disease occurred before the age of 5, regardless of location. The case attack rate per 100,000 children less than 5 years of age was 50 to 60 in Australia and Scandinavia and 60 to 130 in the United States. In certain ethnic groups such as Alaskan Eskimos, American Indians, and Australian aboriginals, the case attack rate was as high as 400 per 100,000 children less than 5 years old (1% to 2% of all children). When the incidence was high (e.g., in Alaskan Eskimos), the median age of disease was low (6 months), and epiglottitis was rare. In Australia and Finland, where the incidence of disease was lower, the median age was higher (27 months) and 30% to 40% of the disease was epiglottitis.

The differences in incidence of disease in different locations may be a result of genetic, as well as environmental, factors. Alaskan Eskimos in the same environment as non-Eskimos had a higher incidence of HIB disease, despite apparently adequate antibody levels. In addition, black Americans without the Km1 allotype had a higher incidence of disease than did black Americans with this allotype.

Population-based epidemiologic studies in Australia, Finland, and the United States before widespread use of conjugate vaccine demonstrated differences in the case attack rates for all invasive HIB disease and, in particular, in the relative frequency of the major clinical manifestations, namely, meningitis and epiglottitis (Table 10-1). A comprehensive study from Australia showed that the annual case attack rate of invasive HIB infections was 58.5 per 100,000 in children less than 5 years old and almost two thirds (64%) of cases occurred in children over 18 months old (Gilbert et al., 1990). Meningitis (mean age, 20 months) and epiglottitis (mean age, 36 months) each accounted for approximately 40% of infections (attack rates of 23 per 100,000 each). Interestingly, attack rates for *Haemophilus influenzae* disease in Australian aboriginal children were reported to be 450 per 100,000, which is similar to that found in Alaskan natives. Population-based studies from Finland showed that the HIB case attack rate (52 per 100,000) and proportion of cases of meningitis (46%) and epiglottitis (29%) were similar to those in Australia (Takala, 1989). The attack rate for HIB disease was higher in the United States, even in populations that are primarily white. Studies from the United States estimated that the overall HIB attack rate was 60 to 100 per 100,000, of which approximately 60% were meningitis and 5% to 15% were epiglottitis.

In general, meningitis occurs at an earlier age than epiglottitis, so populations with a higher proportion of cases of meningitis have a lower mean age overall of HIB disease. In addition, populations with higher HIB attack rates also have a lower mean age of meningitis relative to those populations with lower attack rates. Thus a lower mean age of disease is relative to HIB disease incidence and disease manifestations (Fig. 10-3). One could hypothesize that there is a pool of susceptible young children that gradually diminishes over time, coincident with the maturation of the immune system. If the environment provides for early exposure to the HIB organism, then there is an increased frequency of meningitis. If exposed later, they are less likely to become diseased even if infected, and their diseases are more likely to be localized. However, this hypothesis is still unproven.

Sex Distribution

Generally, the sex distribution for HIB disease manifestations—except pneumonia and epiglottitis—is equal. There is perhaps a small predominance of males when all studies are considered, but it is small. The distribution for epiglottitis is however unequivocally dominated by males. Most studies show a 1.5 to 2.0:1 male/female ratio. In studies of HIB pneumonia there is a predominance of males (2:1), but, as previously mentioned, complete case ascertainment for pneumonia is questionable, which may (or may not) bias this finding.

Age Distribution

HIB disease is primarily a disease of children between 3 months and 5 years old. Most disease manifestations, except epiglottitis, are concentrated in the younger ages. Epiglottitis, although varying in incidence in different populations, seems to have a median age of disease between 2 and 3 years (compared to 12 to 18 months for most other disease manifestations). The reason for this difference in age distribution is not known. Except for epiglottitis, the incidence of HIB disease is inversely proportional to the level of anti-PRP antibody measured in children's serum.

The age distribution of HIB disease is best demonstrated by data from Australia, where the in-

Table 10-1   Estimated incidence of invasive *Haemophilus influenzae* type b disease

| Population/place | Annual rate/100,000 children <5 years of age | | |
	Meningitis	Epiglottitis	Mean age (mo)
Alaskan natives	601	5	10
Australia (aboriginal)	450	0	7
Navajo Indians	152	0	8
United States (average)	19-69	5-15	8-15
Sweden	27	28[*]	30
Finland	26	13	28
Australia	25	23[*]	27
England	18	9	24

Adapted from Clements, 1990 and Broome, 1987.

[*]Includes patients with clinically, but not bacteriologically, confirmed epiglottitis (of which >95% probably result from HIB).

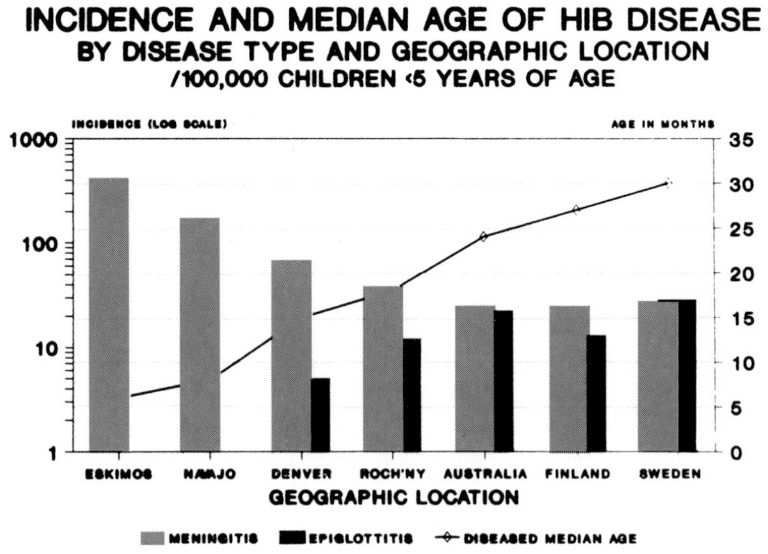

INCIDENCE AND MEDIAN AGE OF HIB DISEASE
BY DISEASE TYPE AND GEOGRAPHIC LOCATION
/100,000 CHILDREN <5 YEARS OF AGE

FIG. 10-3 Median age by country by disease type. (Modified from Clements DA, Gilbert GL: Aust NZ J Med 1990; 20:828-834.)

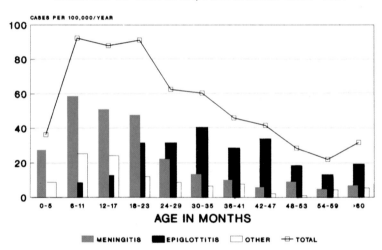

AGE SPECIFIC INCIDENCE OF INVASIVE HIB
DISEASE IN VICTORIA, AUSTRALIA 1985-1987

FIG. 10-4 Australia age distribution of disease. (Modified from Ward JI, Cochi S: In Plotkin SA, Mortimer EA [eds]. Vaccines, ed 1. Philadelphia: WB Saunders, 1988.)

AGE SPECIFIC INCIDENCE OF INVASIVE HIB
DISEASE IN USA 1976-1984

FIG. 10-5 United States age distribution of disease. (Modified from Gilbert GL, et al. Pediatr Infect Dis 1990; 9:252-257.)

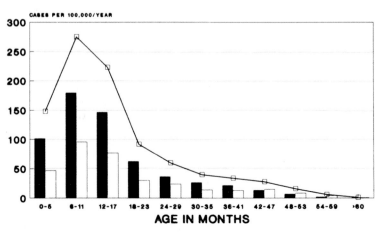

cidence of epiglottitis is common. Data from the United States gives similar age distributions, except the meningitis cases tend to occur even earlier in life. It is instructive to see that the overall distribution of disease is dependent on the predominant disease manifestations. Most other causes of HIB disease have an age distribution similar to that of meningitis (Figs. 10-4 and 10-5).

Seasonal Incidence and Year-to-Year Variation

There appears to be very little year-to-year variation in HIB disease incidence in countries where HIB disease has been systematically followed (Finland and Australia). There is, however, a seasonal variation. HIB is least common in the summer months; the disease clusters around the winter months. Some investigators have shown a bimodal fall-spring distribution, but others have shown that winter is the most common time.

RISK FACTORS

Infection rates depend on host susceptibility and exposure to the infectious agent. Protection from HIB disease in the first few months of life is provided by maternal antibody; thereafter the risk is relatively high until the child can mount an antibody response to HIB polysaccharide antigen, which develops gradually over the first few years of life.

Two studies from the United States have reported that crowded conditions increase the risk of HIB disease (Cochi et al., 1986; Istre et al., 1985). Crowding can result from smaller or fewer rooms per family unit or an increased number of persons per family. Attendance at day-care centers also appears to increase the risk of HIB disease, and children with HIB infection are more likely to have siblings who attend day care or school. Breast-feeding appears to be protective, but children who breast feed may be less likely to be exposed to environments where there is a large number of other children. After controlling for number of siblings and residence size, family income does not seem to be a risk factor for disease.

Family members of children with HIB disease are often HIB carriers, particularly siblings aged 3 to 6 years. In an Australian study in which day-care exposure and siblings were risk factors for HIB disease, the risk of disease by attending day care was modified by whether the child had siblings, suggesting that day care has an effect similar to an increased number of siblings. Both of these measures

are probably related to crowding or the potential for organism transmission.

Some unknown genetic factors may increase the risk of HIB disease. Aboriginals, Eskimos, and American Indians have a particularly high incidence of HIB disease. The environmental exposure may be the predominant determinant in the setting of a homogeneous genetic background. Black Americans who lack the Km1 immunoglobulin allotype have an increased incidence of HIB disease. Reasons for this increase in disease rate are unknown.

TREATMENT

Until 1974 *Haemophilus influenzae* type b was universally susceptible to ampicillin. Beginning in that year, sporadic reports of resistance to ampicillin began to appear. Chloramphenicol, which had not been routinely used except in children known to be allergic to ampicillin, became commonly used. The advent of second-generation cephalosporins, such as cefuroxime, provided another possible treatment for HIB disease in the subsequent years, but variable CNS penetration and treatment failures precluded their use. At present, with 15% to 50% of HIB producing β-lactamase, the antibiotics of choice are the third-generation cephaloporins cefotaxime (100 to 150 mg/kg/day divided q6h) and ceftriaxone (50 to 75 mg/kg/day divided q12h). These two antibiotics have very low MICs against all HIB, regardless of whether they produce β-lactamase. Some clinicians have concluded that ampicillin can be used if the HIB organism isolated does not produce β-lactamase, but HIB isolates both sensitive and resistant to ampicillin have been recovered from the same patient on occasion.

Although chloramphencol is infrequently used at present, it is important to note that there are recent reports of resistance to this antibiotic as a result of the ability of some HIB organisms to produce chloramphenicol acetyltransferase.

PREVENTIVE MEASURES
Immunization

PRP Alone. In 1974 100,000 Finnish children were immunized with unconjugated PRP or with meningococcal group A vaccine in a trial to prevent an outbreak of meningococcal A disease. In the 4 years after vaccination there were twenty cases of HIB disease in children over 18 months of age in the group that received meningococcal vaccine and only two cases in the PRP vaccine group—90% vaccine efficacy (Peltola et al., 1984). Protective efficacy for the polysaccharide antigen was not demonstrated in children less than 18 months of age. In an attempt to overcome the inability of the polysaccharide antigen alone to protect the youngest children, PRP was subsequently conjugated to several proteins to better stimulate antibody production and convert the immunogen to a T-cell–dependent antigen.

In spite of the limitations of the use of PRP alone as an immunogen to children over 2 years of age, it was judged to be cost effective and was licensed for use in the United States in 1985. Because PRP is at least partially effective in children between 18 and 24 months, it was also recommended at that time that high-risk children (those attending daycare centers and close contacts of cases) in the 18- to 24-month age group be vaccinated, with the proviso that they be vaccinated again at 24 months of age.

Replacement immunoglobulin therapy and the 1974 vaccine trials suggested that an anti-PRP antibody level above 0.15 µg/ml would be protective. However, because antibody levels fall over time, a higher level (>1.0 µg/ml) after immunization was postulated to be required for sustained protection. In addition, in children less than 6 months of age, levels of anti-PRP antibody acquired prenatally from the mother are falling, which complicates the assessment of vaccine immunogenicity.

Complicating these findings is the fact that, in Finnish children over 18 months of age, PRP immunization was 90% protective against HIB disease in 1974. However, when licensed in the United States for children over 2 years of age, vaccine efficacy averaged only 60%, estimated by several retrospective case-control studies (Ward et al., 1988a). This may have been a result of differences in populations or possibly the differences in use of vaccine under controlled versus uncontrolled conditions. Nevertheless, it gives reason to be cautious when extrapolating results of vaccine trials from one population to another.

PRP Conjugate Vaccines. After unsuccessful attempts to enhance PRP immunogenicity by changing the PRP polymer length and mixing PRP with DTP or pertussis vaccine, PRP was conjugated (covalently linked) to one of several protein carriers, including a mutant diptheria toxin (PRP-CRM—Lederle-Praxis), diphtheria toxoid (PRP-D—Connaught), an outer membrane protein of *Neisseria meningitidis* (PRP-OMP—Merck,

Sharp, and Dohme), and tetanus toxoid (PRP-T—Merieux). The amount of specific antibody produced (IgG_1, IgG_2, and IgM) after immunization depends on the method of conjugation and the age of the child. It is not clear whether a level of 1.0 µg/ml of anti-PRP antibody is required in response to T-cell–dependent vaccines in order to maintain protection. A lower antibody level may be protective if there is a prompt anamnestic response to a second PRP exposure as a result of vaccine or natural infection.

PRP-D. PRP-D contains PRP conjugated to diphtheria toxoid with a 6-carbon spacer (Connaught Laboratories). In children over 14 months of age, one 20-µg (PRP) dose gives antibody levels >1 µg/ml in 67% of children. For children between 9 and 15 months 2 doses were required to give the same levels. In younger children, antibody produced is primarily IgM and thus relatively short-lived, whereas proportionally higher levels of IgG are produced in older children. Nevertheless, the antibody levels achieved are considerably higher than those with PRP alone, even in the youngest age groups. In children less than 6 months of age, even 3 injections may fail to achieve levels greater than 1 µg/ml, and levels decline rapidly in the subsequent year. A booster dose of the conjugate or PRP vaccine alone at 18 months produces a good response. These data encouraged the use of this vaccine in two efficacy trials; one in Alaska and the other in Finland.

In 1985 the PRP-D vaccine was given to Finnish children in a 3-dose schedule of 3, 5, and 7 months of age. The protective efficacy was 83% for 1 injection, 90% for 2 injections, and 100% for 3 injections. However, the antibody response was relatively poor in children less than 7 months of life; invasive disease occurs less often in this age group in Finnish children. The same vaccine was also used in a trial in Alaskan children but was not protective. A genetic or environmental factor may contribute to the early mean age of disease in Alaskan children and, because of the poor antibody response in the youngest children, may have been responsible for the difference in vaccine efficacy reported. Until recently, PRP-D was still the most commonly commercially available conjugate HIB vaccine in Europe. It has never been widely used in the United States.

HbOC. Low–molecular-weight oligosaccharides of PRP are coupled to a mutant variant of diphtheria toxin in this Lederle-Praxis vaccine. This was the first conjugate vaccine to be licensed for use in children at 2 months of age in the United States. There is little antibody response to the initial dose of vaccine at 2 months of age, but there is a brisk and sustained antibody response to subsequent doses of vaccine. As in all conjugate vaccines, there are almost no side effects to vaccination. The present recommendation for vaccination includes 3 doses of vaccine (preferably 2 months apart) by 6 months of age and a booster at 15 months of age.

PRP-OMP. Merck, Sharp, and Dohme have conjugated PRP to a protein from group B *Neisseria meningitidis*. This vaccine is immunogenic with the first dose given. Its demonstrated efficacy in the Navajo population (even after 1 dose), where there is a very early median age of HIB disease, was particularly impressive. The only case of disease (arthritis) in the immunized group was in a child who was over a year of age and who had failed to receive her booster immunization. It was subsequently licensed for use in children as young as 2 months of age. It requires 2 immunizations (preferably 2 months apart) in the first 6 months of life and a booster at 12 months.

Response to subsequent doses of vaccine is less than to HbOC and, although it appears to be T-cell dependent, it does not boost to the same level as the other licensed product. However, there is an extremely good antibody response to the first dose of vaccine. There are no significant side effects to receiving this vaccine.

PRP-T. PRP-T is composed of high–molecular-weight PRP covalently linked to a formalin-detoxified tetanus toxin. Active surveillance for adverse events after immunization shows some mild local and systemic reactions, similar to those of the other conjugate HIB vaccines. Of 107,000 infants who received vaccine in Finland, only forty-three adverse events were noted; thirty-three were reported after the first dose, eight after the second, and two after the booster dose. Most reactions occurred in children who received the DTP vaccine at the same time. Immunogenicity from the vaccine is high, with 90% to 95% of recipients having anti-PRP antibody levels above 1 μg/ml after the third dose. This vaccine (compared to other conjugate PRP vaccines) reportedly yields the highest percentage of children with anti-PRP antibodies above 1 μg/ml after the primary series (Fritzell and Plotkin, 1992).

Mixed-Conjugate Vaccine Administration. Although each conjugate HIB vaccine is tested before approval in many children, children in clinical trials all receive the same manufacturer's vaccine for the series. In the real world, families move, or health providers change vaccine brands because of supply problems or price differences. Several studies have looked at whether there is a difference in anti-PRP antibody production if different conjugate vaccines are used during the third and fourth series of immunizations. To date, none have shown any decreased immunogenicity because of changing vaccine sources during the series; in fact, there is a subtle suggestion that some mixed-brand strategies actually enhance anti-PRP antibody production. It is obviously not feasible to design a mixed strategy to be routinely given to children, so researchers must accept at least that there are no untoward effects if patients receive mixed-brand conjugate HIB vaccines during the series.

Neonatal Immunization. Studies assessing the preterm and newborn's response to conjugate HIB vaccines are few but support that infants with a gestational age of at least 28 weeks respond adequately (although not optimally) to vaccination at 2, 4, and 6 months of chronologic age. Children less than 28 weeks have less response and may need a different strategy (such as delay to 3, 5, and 7 months of age). The number of studies is small, however, and each study has only used one vaccine brand, so further analysis is needed. But, to date, it is preferable to immunize infants of 28 weeks or greater gestation with conjugate HIB vaccination on the regularly suggested schedule.

Prenatal Maternal Immunization. One study of approximately 100 mothers, half of whom received HIB vaccine in the last trimester (one-third PRP, two-thirds conjugate PRP) demonstrated significant increase in the infant's anti-PRP level in cord blood (17 to 29 μg/ml versus 0.29 μg/ml). This may be a reasonable strategy in populations that have very early HIB disease (Alaskan Eskimos) or where vaccination of infants is problematic. The effect of this increased antibody level on subsequent infant HIB immunization is unclear at this time.

CHEMOPROPHYLAXIS

There has been considerable controversy about the use of rifampin to prevent secondary cases of HIB. There is sufficient evidence that rifampin, taken orally, will markedly decrease the carrier rate of

HIB in the pharynx (estimates are as high as 95%) and thereby reduce secondary or coprimary cases if it is administered soon after the discovery of the primary case. What is not clear is the advantage this has in stopping the spread of disease. Several studies show that family members or close contacts often carry the organism in the throat, which is presumably where the diseased child obtains the infection. But unless there is another susceptible child in the environment, rifampin treatment may be of little use. At present the recommendations are to treat all members of a family, including the patient, with rifampin (20 mg/kg per day, max. 600 mg) once daily for 4 days if there is another child less than 48 months of age in the home. Treatment of contacts at day-care centers should be individualized, but, in general, prophylaxis at day care is no longer routinely recommended. In fact, HIB immunization is an admission requirement for entry to day care, so the need for prophylaxis should not be a concern.

Two approaches other than immunization have been taken to decrease disease incidence in populations where the median age of patients with HIB disease is very low. Maternal immunization with HIB before delivery has been performed in Navajo Indians, a measure that boosts the mother's anti-PRP IgG levels. In addition, newborns of Navajo mothers have received repeated doses of intramuscular immunoglobulin to boost IgG levels. Both of these strategies have had some effect on increasing anti-PRP antibody in the newborn, but the advent of conjugated HIB vaccines that can be given at 2 months of age may have obviated the use of these therapies.

HIB Disease Epidemiology Since the Inception of HIB Vaccine

HIB disease has decreased markedly since the licensure of the HIB vaccine. Interestingly, there was a decrease in the disease incidence in children less than 18 months of age (in addition to the expected decrease in children over 18 months of age) when the vaccine was first given to 18-month-old children. This was in spite of the fact that there did not seem to be a decreased oral-pharyngeal HIB colonization rate after vaccination. Subsequently, when the conjugate HIB vaccines were licensed and given, there was a further decrease in the HIB disease rate and concomitant decrease in the oral HIB colonization rate (suggesting less ability to spread infection). At present the HIB disease rate in the United States has been reduced between 70% and 90%, depending on the population measured (Fig. 10-6) (Adams et al., 1993; Michaels and Ali, 1993;

Murphy 1993). Even in Alaskan Eskimos the disease incidence has decreased 90% (but this has included passive immunoglobulin therapy also) (Singleton et al., 1994). In addition, since the inception of HIB vaccination, acute epiglottitis has also decreased significantly in many locations (85% in Quebec).

A new concern is that the welcome decrease in HIB disease has made it unusual for those training in pediatrics to have experience with what was once a common disease. This is similar to the decreased experience and awareness with measles, mumps, and rubella. But this is not such a high price to pay for what has been a great cause of morbidity and mortality in young children.

• • •

The recommendations of the Advisory Committee on Immunization Practices (ACIP) for the use of HIB vaccines are as follows (MMWR 1993;42 [RR-13]:8-12).

RECOMMENDATIONS FOR HIB VACCINATION
General

All infants should receive a conjugate Hib vaccine (separate or in combination with DTP [TETRAMUNE™]), beginning at age 2 months (but not earlier than 6 weeks). If the first vaccination is delayed beyond age 6 months, the schedule of vaccination for previously unimmunized children should be followed (Table 10-2). When possible, the Hib conjugate vaccine used at the first vaccination should be used for all subsequent vaccinations in the primary series. When either Hib vaccines or TETRA-MUNE™ is used, the vaccine should be administered intramuscularly using a separate syringe and administered at a separate site from any other concurrent vaccinations.

HbOC or PRP-T

Previously unvaccinated infants aged 2-6 months should receive three doses of vaccine administered 2 months apart, followed by a booster dose at age 12-15 months, at least 2 months after the last vaccination. Unvaccinated children ages 7-11 months should receive two doses of vaccine, 2 months apart, followed by a booster dose at age 12-18 months, at least 2 months after the last vaccination. Unvaccinated children ages 12-14 months should receive two doses of vaccine, at least 2 months apart. Any previously unvaccinated child aged 15-59 months should receive a single dose of vaccine.

PRP-OMP

Previously unvaccinated infants ages 2-6 months should receive two doses of vaccine administered at least 2 months apart. Although PRP-OMP induces a substantial antibody response after one dose, all children should receive all recommended doses of PRP-OMP. Because

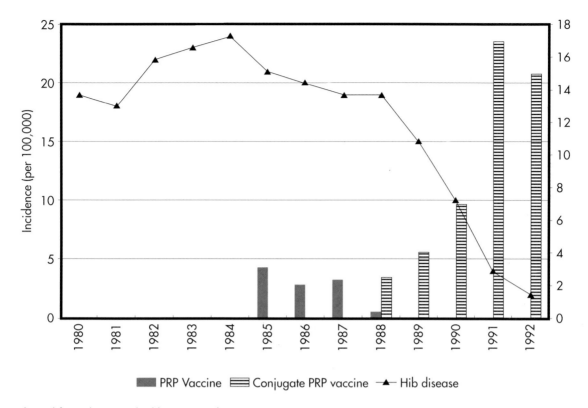

FIG. 10-6 *Haemophilus influenza* type b meningitis incidence in children <5 years of age and (PRP) vaccine doses distributed by year in the United States.

of the substantial antibody response after one dose, it may be advantageous to use PRP-OMP vaccine in populations that are known to be at increased risk for disease during early infancy (e.g., Alaskan Natives). A booster dose should be administered to al children at 12-15 months of age at least 2 months after the last vaccination. Unvaccinated children ages 7-11 months should receive two doses of vaccine, 2 months apart, followed by a booster dose at 12-18 months of age, at least 2 months after the last dose. Unvaccinated children ages 12-14 months should receive two doses of vaccine, 2 months apart. Any previously unvaccinated child 15-59 months of age should receive a single dose of vaccine.

PRP-D

One dose of PRP-D may be administered to unvaccinated children aged 15-59 months. This vaccine may be used as a booster dose at 12-18 months of age following a two- or three-dose primary series, regardless of the vaccine used in the primary series. This vaccine is not licensed for use among infants because of its limited immunogenicity and variable protective efficacy in this age group.

TETRAMUNE™

This combination vaccine TETRAMUNE™ may be used for routine vaccination of infants, beginning at age 2 months, to prevent diphtheria, tetanus, pertussis, and invasive Hib disease. Previously unvaccinated infants aged 2-6 months should receive three doses administered at least 2 months apart. An additional dose should be administered at 12-15 months of age, after at least a 6-month interval following the third dose. Alternatively, acellular DTP and Hib vaccine can be administered as separate injections at 12-15 months of age. Acellular DTP is preferred for doses four and five of the five-dose DTP series. For infants who begin both Hib an DTP vaccinations late (after 2 months of age), TETRAMUNE™ may be used for the first and second doses of the vaccine series. However, because delay in initiation of the DTP series does not reduce the number of required doses of DTP, additional doses of DTP without Hib are necessary to ensure that all four doses are administered. Infants ages 7-11 months who have not previously been vaccinated with DTP or Hib vaccines should receive two doses of TETRAMUNE™, administered at least 2 months apart, followed by a dose of DTP vaccine 4-8 weeks after the second dose of TETRAMUNE™. An additional dose of DTP and Hib vaccines should then be administered: DTP vaccine at least 6 months after the third

Table 10-2 Schedule for Hib conjugate vaccine administration among previously vaccinated children

Vaccine	Age at first vaccination (mos)	Primary series	Booster
HbOC/PRP-T*	2-6	3 doses, 2 mos apart	12-15 mos
	7-11	2 doses, 2 mos apart	12-18 mos
	12-14	1 dose	2 mos later
	15-59	1 dose	—
PRP-OMP	2-6	2 doses, 2 mos apart	12-15 mos
	7-11	2 doses, 2 mos apart	12-18 mos
	12-14	1 dose	2 mos later
	15-59	1 dose	—
PRP-D	15-59	1 dose	—

*TETRAMUNE™ may be administered by the same schedule for primary immunization as HbOC/PRP-T (when the series begins at 2 to 6 months of age). A booster dose of DTP or DTaP should be administered at 4 to 6 years of age, before kindergarten or elementary school. This booster is not necessary if the fourth vaccinating dose was administered after the fourth birthday. See ACIP statement for information on use of DTP and contraindications for use of pertussis vaccine (44).
—Not applicable.

immunizing dose against diphtheria, tetanus, and pertussis; and Hib vaccine at 12-18 months of age, at least 2 months after the last Hib dose.

TETRAMUNE™ may be used to complete an infant immunization series started with any Hib vaccine (licensed for use in this age group) and with any DTP vaccine if both vaccines are to be administered simultaneously. Completion of the primary series using the same Hib vaccine, however, is preferable. Conversely, any DTP vaccine may be used to complete a series initiated with TETRAMUNE™ (see the general ACIP statement on Diphtheria, Tetanus and Pertussis: Recommendations for Vaccine Use and Other Preventive Measures [44] for further information).

Other considerations for Hib vaccination
Other considerations for Hib vaccination are discussed in the following section:

1) Although an interval of 2 months between doses of Hib vaccine in the primary series is recommended, an interval of 1 month is acceptable, if necessary.
2) Unvaccinated children aged 15-59 months may be administered a single dose of any one of the four Hib conjugate vaccines or TETRAMUNE™ (if both Hib and DTP vaccines are indicated).
3) After the primary infant vaccination series is completed, any of the four licensed Hib conjugate vaccines (or TETRAMUNE™ if both Hib vaccine and DTP vaccine are indicated) may be used as a booster dose at age 12-15 months.
4) The primary vaccine series should preferably be completed with the same Hib conjugate vaccine. If, however, different vaccines are administered, a total of three doses of Hib conjugate vaccine is adequate. Any combination of Hib conjugate vaccines that is licensed for use among infants may be used to complete the primary series.

5) Infants born prematurely should be vaccinated according to the schedule recommended for other infants, beginning at age 2 months.
6) Hib conjugate vaccines may be administered simultaneously with DTP (or DTaP) vaccine, OPV, IPV, MMR, influenza, and hepatitis B vaccines. TETRAMUNE™ may be administered simultaneously with OPV, IPV, MMR, influenza, and hepatitis B vaccines.
7) Because natural infection does not always result in the development of protective anti-PRP antibody levels (45), children <24 months of age who develop invasive Hib disease should receive Hib vaccine as recommended in the schedule. These children should be considered unimmunized, and vaccination should start as soon as possible during the convalescent phase of the illness.
8) Hib vaccine is immunogenic in patients with increased risk for invasive disease, such as those with sickle-cell disease (46), leukemia (47), human immunodeficiency virus (HIV) infection (48,49), and in those who have had splenectomies (50). However, in persons with HIV infection, immunogenicity varies with stage of infection and degree of immunocompromise. Efficacy studies have not been performed in populations with increased risk of invasive disease (see the general ACIP statement on Use of Vaccines and Immune Globulins in Persons with Altered Immunocompetence [51]).
9) Children who attend day care are at increased risk for Hib disease. Therefore, efforts should be made to ensure that all day care attendance <5 years of age are fully vaccinated.
10) Rifampin chemoprophylaxis for household contacts of a person with invasive Hib disease is no longer indicated if all contacts ages <4 years are fully vaccinated against Hib disease. A child is considered fully

immunized against Hib disease following a) at least one dose of conjugate vaccine at ≥15 months of age, b) two doses of conjugate vaccine at 12-14 months of age, or c) two or more doses of conjugate vaccine at <12 months of age, followed by a booster dose at ≥12 months of age. In households with one or more infants <12 months of age (regardless of vaccination status) or with a child aged 1-3 years who is inadequately vaccinated, all household contacts should receive rifampin prophylaxis following a case of invasive Hib disease that occurs in any family member. The recommended dose is 20 mg/kg as a single daily dose (maximal daily dose 600 mg) for 4 days. Neonates (<1 month of age) should receive 10 mg/kg once daily for 4 days.

Adverse reactions

Adverse reactions to each of the four Hib conjugate vaccines are generally uncommon. Swelling, redness, and/or pain have been reported in 5%-30% of recipients and usually resolve within 12-24 hours. Systemic reactions such as fever and irritability are infrequent. Available information on side effects and adverse reactions suggests that the risks for local and systemic events following TETRAMUNE™ administration are similar to those following concurrent administration of its individual component vaccines (i.e., DTP and Hib vaccines), and may be due largely to the pertussis component of the DTP vaccine (*52*).

Surveillance regarding the safety of TETRAMUNE™, PRP-T, and other Hib vaccines in large-scale use aids in the assessment of vaccine safety by identifying potential events that may warrant further study. The Vaccine Adverse Events Reporting System (VAERS) of the U.S. Department of Health and Human Services encourages reports of all serious adverse events that occur after receipt of any vaccine.* Invasive Hib disease is a reportable condition in 43 states. All health-care workers should report any case of invasive Hib disease to local and state health departments.

Contraindications and precautions

Vaccination with a specific Hib conjugate vaccine is contraindicated in persons known to have experienced anaphylaxis following a prior dose of that vaccine. Vaccination should be delayed in children with moderate or severe illnesses. Minor illnesses (e.g., mild upper-respiratory infection) are not contraindications to vaccination.

Contraindications and precautions of the use of TETRAMUNE™ are the same as those for its individual component vaccines (i.e., DTP or Hib) (see the general ACIP statement on Diphtheria, Tetanus, and Pertussis: Recommendations for Vaccine Use and Other Preventive Measures [*44*] for more details on the use of vaccines containing DTP).

---

*Questions about reporting requirements, completion of report forms, or requests for reporting forms should be directed to VAERS at 1-800-822-7967.

BIBLIOGRAPHY

Adams WG, Deaver KA, Cochi SL, et al. Decline of childhood *Haemophilus influenzae* type b (Hib) disease in the HIB vaccine era. JAMA 1993;269:221-226.

Barenkamp SJ, Granoff DM, Pittman M. Outer membrane protein subtypes and biotypes of *Haemophilus influenzae* type b: relation between strains isolated in 1934-1954 and 1977-1980. J Infect Dis 1983;148:1127.

Broome CV. Epidemiology of *Haemophilus influenzae* type b infections in the United States. Pediatr Infect Dis J 1987;6:779-782.

Centers for Disease Control. Recommendations of the Advisory Committee on Immunization Practices (ACIP) for the use of HIB vaccines. MMWR 1993;42:1-15.

Centers for Disease Control. Progress toward elimination of *Haemophilus influenzae* type b disease among infants and children: United States 1987-1995. MMWR 1996;45:901-905.

Clements DA, Gilbert GL. Immunization for the prevention of *Haemophilus influenzae* type b infections: a review. Aust NZ J Med 1990;20:828-834.

Cochi SL, Fleming DW, Hightower AW, et al. Primary invasive *Haemophilus influenzae* type b disease: a population-based assessment of risk factors. J Pediatr 1986;108:887-896.

Cochi SL, O'Mara D, Preblud SR. Progress in *Haemophilus* type b polysaccharide vaccine use in the United States. Pediatrics 1988;81:166-168.

Fritzell B, Plotkin S. Efficacy and safety of a *Haemophilus influenzae* type b capsular polysaccharide-tetanus protein conjugate vaccine. J Pediatr 1992;121:355-362.

Gilbert GL, Clements DA, Broughton S. *Haemophilus influenzae* type b infections in Victoria, Australia 1985-87: A population based study to determine the need for immunization. Pediatr Infect Dis J 1990;9:252-257.

Goldberg F, Berne AS, Oski FA. Differentiation of orbital cellulitis from preseptal cellulitis by computed tomography. Pediatrics 1978;62:1000-1005.

Isaacs D. Problems in determining the etiology of community-acquired childhood pneumonia. Pediatr Infect Dis J 1989;8:143-148.

Istre CR, Conner JS, Broome CV, et al. Risk factors for primary invasive *Haemophilus influenzae* disease: increased risk from day-care attendance and school-age household members. J Pediatr. 1985;106:190-195.

Kilian M. A taxonomic study of the genus *Haemophilus* with the proposal of a new species. J Clin Micro 1976;93:9-62.

Michaels RH, Ali O. A decline in *Haemophilus influenzae* type b meningitis. J Pediatr 1993;122:407-409.

Michaels RH, Stonebraker FE, Robbins JB. Use of antiserum agar for detection of *Haemophilus influenzae* type b in the pharynx. Pediat Res 1975;9:513-516.

Moxon ER. Virulence genes and prevention of *Haemophilus influenzae* infections. Arch Dis Child 1985;60:1193-1196.

Murphy TV, White KE, Pastor P, et al. Declining incidence of *Haemophilus influenzae* type b disease since introduction of vaccination. JAMA 1993;269:246-248.

Musser JM, Granoff DM, Pattison PE, Selander RK. A population genetic framework for the study of invasive diseases caused by serotype b strains of *Haemophilus influenzae*. Proc Natl Acad Sci 1985;82:5078-5082.

Musser JM, Kroll JS, Moxon ER, Selander RK. Clonal populations structure of encapsulated *Haemophilus influenzae*. Infect Immun 1988;56:1837-1845.

Peltola H, Kayhty H, Virtanen M, Makela PH. Prevention of *Haemophilus influenzae* type b bacteremic infections with the capsular polysaccharide vaccine. N Engl J Med 1984; 310:1566-1569.

Sell SH. *Haemophilus influenzae* type b meningitis: manifestations and long-term sequelae. Pediatr Infect Dis J 1987; 6:775-778.

Singleton RJ, Davidson NM, Desmet IJ, et al. Decline of *Haemophilus influenzae* type b disease in a region of high risk: impact of passive and active immunization. Pediatr Infect Dis J 1994;13:362-367.

Takala AK, Eskola J, Peltola H, Mäkelä PH. Epidemiology of invasive *Haemophilus influenzae* type b disease among children in Finland before vaccination with *Haemophilus influenzae* type b conjugate vaccine. Pediatr Infect Dis J 1989; 8:297-302.

Takala AK, van Alphen L, Eskola J, et al. *Haemophilus influenzae* type b strains of outer membrane subtypes 1 and 1c cause different types of invasive disease. Lancet 1987;2:647-650.

van Alphen L, Geelen L, Jonsdottir K, et al. Distinct geographical distribution of HIB subtypes in Western Europe. J Infect Dis 1987;156:216-218.

Ward JI, Broome CV, Harrison LH, et al. *Haemophilus influenzae* type b vaccines: lessons for the future. Pediatrics 1988a;81:886-892.

Ward JI, Cochi S. *Haemophilus influenzae* vaccines. In Plotkin SA, Mortimer EA (eds). Vaccines, ed 1. Philadelphia: WB Saunders, 1988b.

Wenger JD, Hightower AW, Facklam RR, et al. Bacterial meningitis in the United States, 1986: report of a multistate surveillance study. J Infect Dis 1990;162:1316-1323.

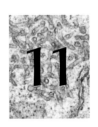

11 VIRAL HEPATITIS: A, B, C, D, E, AND NEWER HEPATITIS AGENTS

WILLIAM BORKOWSKY AND SAUL KRUGMAN

The term *viral hepatitis* refers to a primary infection of the liver caused by at least five etiologically and immunologically distinct viruses: hepatitis A (HAV), hepatitis B (HBV), hepatitis C (HCV), hepatitis D (HDV), and hepatitis E (HEV). Hepatitis may occur also during the course of disease caused by the following viruses: adenovirus, cytomegalovirus (CMV), Epstein-Barr virus (EBV), herpes simplex virus (HSV), human herpes virus 6 (HHV-6), human immunodeficiency virus (HIV), and varicella-zoster virus (VZV).

Hepatitis A is synonymous with infectious hepatitis, an ancient disease described by Hippocrates and formerly known as epidemic jaundice, acute catarrhal jaundice, and other designations. The fulminant form of the disease was called acute yellow atrophy of the liver.

Hepatitis B is synonymous with serum hepatitis, a disease with a more recent history. The first known outbreak occurred in 1883 among a group of shipyard workers who were vaccinated against smallpox with glycerinated lymph of human origin (Lürman, 1885). Later an increased incidence of the disease was observed among patients attending venereal disease clinics, diabetic clinics, and other facilities in which multiple injections were given with inadequately sterilized syringes and needles contaminated with the blood of a carrier. The most extensive outbreak occurred in 1942, when yellow fever vaccine containing human serum caused 28,585 cases of hepatitis B infection with jaundice among U.S. military personnel. It was unknown at the time of vaccination that the human serum component of the vaccine was contaminated with HBV. The additional aliases of hepatitis B recorded in the literature include homologous serum jaundice, transfusion jaundice, syringe jaundice, and postvaccinal jaundice.

Hepatitis C was formerly designated *parenterally transmitted non-A, non-B hepatitis* (PT-

NANB). Non-A, non-B (NANB) hepatitis was recognized as a clinical entity in the 1970s, when specific tests for the identification of HAV and HBV infections became available. The identification of HCV as the most common cause of PT-NANB hepatitis was reported in 1989 (Choo et al., 1989; Kuo et al., 1989).

Hepatitis delta virus is a "defective" RNA virus that can replicate only in the presence of acute or chronic HBV infection. The genome of HDV codes for an internal antigen (HDAg), but the virus is encapsulated by hepatitis B surface antigen (HBsAg) of the helper HBV. The delta antigen was discovered by Rizzetto et al. in 1977.

Hepatitis E was previously called *enterically transmitted NANB* (ET-NANB). Serologic studies of various outbreaks of ET-NANB hepatitis revealed no evidence of HAV or HBV infection (Khuroo, 1980). In retrospect it is clear that these outbreaks were caused by HEV, an agent that was cloned by Reyes et al. in 1990.

Several new hepatitis agents, genetically related to HCV, have been identified and sequenced. These have been designated GB virus A (GBV-A), GB virus B (GBV-B), and GB virus C (GB-C). The first two were obtained from primates and the last isolated from human serum. In addition, a transfusion transmissible hepatitis virus closely related to GBV-C, termed *hepatitis G virus*, has also been cloned.

ETIOLOGY
Hepatitis A

Before the mid-1960s knowledge of the properties of HAV was derived from human volunteer studies. The agent survived a temperature of 56° C for 30 minutes (Havens et al., 1944) and was inactivated by heating at 98° C for 1 minute (Krugman et al., 1970). It retained its infectivity after storage at −18° to −70° C for several years. HAV was more resistant to chlorine than many bacteria found in drinking water.

Oral or parenteral administration of the virus caused hepatitis after an incubation period ranging from 15 to 40 days, averaging approximately 30 days. Extensive studies with the MS-1 strain of HAV and the MS-2 strain of HBV confirmed observations by Havens et al. (1944) and Neefe et al. (1946) that hepatitis A and B viruses were immunologically distinct (Krugman et al., 1967).

In 1966 Deinhardt et al. reported the successful transmission of hepatitis A to marmoset monkeys. Later, additional studies by his group (Holmes et al., 1969), Mascoli et al. (1973), Provost et al. (1973), and Maynard (1974) confirmed the successful transmission of human HAV to marmosets. In addition, Dienstag et al. (1975b) successfully transmitted HAV to susceptible chimpanzees.

In 1973 Feinstone et al. reported the identification of 27-nm viruslike particles in the stools of adults who had been infected with the MS-1 strain of HAV. These particles were identified by immune electron microscopy (IEM). These findings were confirmed by Maynard (1974), who induced hepatitis in marmosets by inoculating them with stool filtrates containing the 27-nm particles.

Human HAV was further characterized by Provost et al. (1975b), who reported that the 27-nm particles appeared to have the physical, chemical, and biologic characteristics of an enterovirus. It has been designated enterovirus type 27 (Melnick, 1982). Electron micrographs comparing HAV with HBV are shown in Fig. 11-1. Unlike HBV, HAV is a simple, nonenveloped RNA virus with a nucleocapsid that has been designated hepatitis A antigen (HA Ag). The HAV capsid consists of thirty-two capsomeres arranged in icosahedral conformation; it is composed of four virion polypeptides (VP1, VP2, VP3, and VP4). A single-stranded molecule of RNA is present inside the capsid.

Purified HAV is inactivated by formalin, ultraviolet irradiation, heating at 100° C for 5 minutes, or treatment with chlorine (Provost et al., 1975b; Peterson et al., 1982). The purified virus was shown

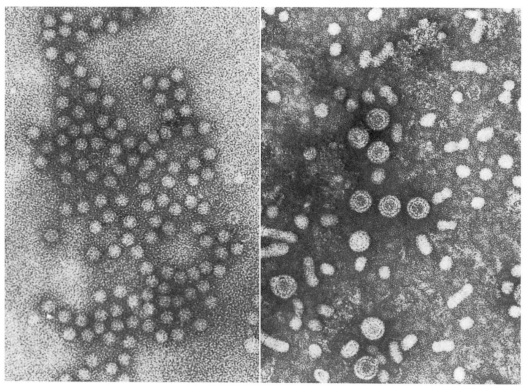

Type A   Type B

FIG. 11-1 Electron micrographs of type A and type B hepatitis viruses. Type A: Note 27-nm particles, uniform in size. Type B: Note 43-nm Dane particles (hepatitis B virus) and spherical and filamentous particles 20 nm in diameter (hepatitis B surface antigen). (From Provost PJ, et al.: Am J Med Sci 1975b;270:87.)

by IEM as specifically aggregated by hepatitis A antibody (anti-HAV).

Miller et al. (1975) prepared HA Ag from infected marmoset liver for use in an immune adherence hemagglutination antibody (IAHA) test. Both HA Ag and anti-HAV can be detected by various established serologic methods, including IEM (Feinstone et al., 1973), radioimmunoassay (RIA) (Hollinger et al., 1975), enzyme immunoassay (EIA) (Duermeyer et al., 1978), and immunofluorescence (IF) (Murphy et al., 1978). The RIA and EIA tests are the most practical for serodiagnosis of acute hepatitis A.

In 1979 Provost and Hilleman reported the propagation of human HAV in primary explant cell cultures of marmoset livers and in the normal fetal rhesus kidney cell line (FRhK6). Provost et al. (1981) subsequently isolated HAV directly from acute-phase human stool specimens by in vitro propagation in an FRhK6 line. Other workers demonstrated that HAV could be cultivated in human diploid fibroblasts (Gauss-Muller et al., 1981), in human amniotic (FL) and Vero cells (Kojima et al., 1981), and in African green monkey kidney (AGMK) cell cultures (Daemer et al., 1981). HAV propagates in the cytoplasm and is noncytopathic.

The HAV genome has been cloned by various investigators (Ticehurst et al., 1983; Baroudy et al., 1985). Modern molecular biologic techniques have provided insight into the structure and organization of the virus, thereby revealing similarities to and differences from other enteroviruses.

Hepatitis B

The human volunteer studies of the 1940s indicated that hepatitis B was highly infectious by inoculation. These studies suggested that HBV caused a parenteral infection characterized by a long incubation period of 50 to 180 days and, unlike HAV, was not infectious by mouth. Studies in the 1960s provided evidence for the existence of two types of viral hepatitis with distinctive clinical, epidemiologic, and immunologic features (Krugman et al., 1967). One type, MS-1, resembled hepatitis A; it was characterized by an incubation period of 30 to 38 days and a high degree of contagion by contact. The other type, MS-2, resembled hepatitis B; it had an incubation period of 41 to 108 days. Contrary to the prevailing concept, the MS-2 strain of HBV was infectious both by mouth and parenterally. The discovery of Australia antigen by Blumberg et al. (1965), and its subsequent association with hepatitis B, had a major impact on the un-

derstanding of the etiology and natural history of the disease.

The successful transmission of HBV to chimpanzees was achieved in the early 1970s (Maynard et al., 1972; Barker et al., 1973). The chimpanzee has proved to be a highly sensitive animal model for the study of hepatitis B infection.

By the early 1970s the agent responsible for hepatitis B had been identified and characterized. Electron microscopic examination of serum obtained from patients with acute or chronic type B hepatitis revealed the following types of viruslike particles: (1) spherical particles, 20 nm in diameter (Bayer et al., 1968); (2) filamentous particles, 100 nm or more in length and 20 nm in diameter (Hirschman et al., 1969); and (3) "Dane particles," approximately 42 nm in diameter (Dane et al., 1970) (see Fig. 11-1). The available evidence indicates that the Dane particle is the complete hepatitis B virion and that the 20-nm spherical particles represent excess virus-coat (HBsAg) material. The HbsAg and Dane particles occur free in serum.

Hepatitis B Virus (Dane Particle). The HBV, a complex 42-nm virion, is a member of a new class of viruses designated *hepadna.* The precise nomenclature of HBV is hepadna virus type 1 (Melnick, 1982). Unlike HAV, it has not been propagated successfully in cell culture. Nevertheless, its biophysical and biochemical properties have been well characterized, and the HBV genome has been cloned and sequenced.

A schematic illustration of the structure of HBV and its antigens is shown in Fig. 11-2. The virus is a double-shelled particle; its outer surface component, the hepatitis B surface antigen (HBsAg), is immunologically distinct from the inner core component, the hepatitis B core antigen (HBcAg). The core contains the genome of HBV, a single molecule of partially double-stranded DNA. One of the strands is incomplete, leaving a single-stranded or gap region. Additional components of the core include DNA-dependent DNA polymerase and hepatitis B e antigen (HbeAg).

A simple, direct molecular hybridization test has been developed to detect HBV DNA in serum. Studies by various investigators have revealed that most HbeAg-positive sera have detectable HBV DNA (Lieberman et al., 1983; Scotto et al., 1983).

Hepatitis B Surface Antigen. The HBsAg particle contains approximately seven polypeptides. Multiple antigenic specificities of HBsAg are

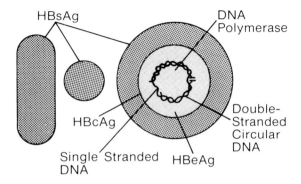

HBsAg

DNA Polymerase

HBcAg

Double-Stranded Circular DNA

Single Stranded DNA

HBeAg

Fig. 11-2 Schematic illustration of the hepatitis B virus and its antigens: hepatitis B surface antigen *(HBsAg)*, hepatitis B core antigen *(HBcAg)*, and hepatitis B e antigen *(HBeAg)*.

associated with these polypeptides. Serologic analysis of HBsAg particles indicates that (1) they share a common group-specific determinant, a; and (2) they usually carry at least two mutually exclusive subdeterminants, d or y and w or r (LeBouvier, 1972). The subtypes are the phenotypic expressions of distinct genotype variants of HBV. Four principal phenotypes have been recognized: adw, adr, ayw, and ayr. Other complex permutations of these subdeterminants and new variants are listed in Table 11-1. The subtypes are valuable epidemiologic markers of infection. Protection against infection apparently is conferred by antibody against the a specificity.

Various tests for the detection of HBsAg and anti-HBs have been developed. These techniques have proved very useful for various studies involving (1) the testing of blood donors and blood products, (2) the diagnosis of acute and chronic hepatitis and the hepatitis B carrier state, (3) the epidemiology of hepatitis B infections, (4) various investigations designed to enhance knowledge of the pathogenesis and immunologic aspects of the disease, and (5) the evaluation of active and passive immunization procedures for the prevention of HBV infections.

Hepatitis C

Studies in chimpanzees by Bradley et al. (1987) revealed the presence of a transmissible agent in blood products that caused NANB hepatitis. The agent was sensitive to organic solvents, and it was less than 80 nm in diameter as assessed by filtration. Using large quantities of Bradley's well-characterized highly infectious plasma as a source of virus, Choo et al. (1989) cloned the genome of

Table 11-1 Nomenclature of hepatitis B antigens and antibodies

HBV	Hepatitis B virus; a 42-nm double-shelled virus, originally known as the Dane particle
HBsAg	Hepatitis B surface antigen; the hepatitis B antigen found on the surface of the virus and on the accompanying unattached spherical (22 nm) and tubular particles
HBcAg	Hepatitis B core antigen; the hepatitis B antigen found within the core of the virus
HBeAg	The e antigen, which is closely associated with hepatitis B infection
anti-HBs	Antibody to hepatitis B surface antigen
anti-HBc	Antibody to hepatitis B core antigen
anti-HBc	Antibody to the e antigen

Subdeterminants of hepatitis B surface antigen:

ayw1	(a_1y2)	*adw$_2$*	(a_2^1dw)
ayw2	(a_2^1yw)	*adw$_4$*	(a_3dw)
ayw3	(a_2^3yw)	*adr*	
ayw4	(a_3yw)	*adyw*	
ayr			

From World Health Organization Expert Committee on Viral Hepatitis: Advances in viral hepatitis, WHO Tech Rep Ser No. 602, 1977.

this NANB agent, HCV. It contains a positive single-stranded RNA molecule and consists of about 9,400 bases coding for about 3,100 amino acids. There is about a 40% sequence homology with the family of *Flavivirus* in the conserved 5' region and HCV is now considered a member of this family, most closely resembling pestiviruses. The 5' untranslated region (UTR) extends from the N terminal and probably plays a regulatory role in transcription or translation. Downstream from the UTR are structural sequences encoding the nucleocapsid core and structural regions, called *E1* and *E2/NS1*, that code for the glycosylated envelope protein. Further downstream are nonstructural genes, designated sequentially *NS-2* to *NS-5*, that code for a polymerase, replicase, and helicase. There is only one open reading frame with splicing performed by viral and cellular enzymes.

Variation in the envelope region is considerable and results in more than 4 strains now classified as genotypes based on genetic relatedness (Okamoto et al., 1992). A recent change in nomenclature (Simmonds et al., 1993, 1994) classifies HCV into "type" (corresponding to major phylogenetic branches for genomic and subgenomic regions) and "subtypes" (divided into more closely related sequences among major groups). The known types are numbered from 1 and the subtypes as a, b, and c. HCV in the United States and Europe is classified as 1a, 1b, 2a, 2b, and 3a. In Japan and China 1b, 2, and 2b predominate. Individuals may be infected with more than one type and subtype, indicating that there is little cross-protection between types. Type 1 HCV appears to be overrepresented among patients with cirrhosis, although all types are capable of producing cirrhosis. Patients with type 1 are also less likely to respond to interferon therapy. Although HCV viral load is inversely correlated with potential clearance after interferon therapy, there appears to be no inherent difference in the ability of HCV to replicate and produce unique levels of virus, indicating that viral type and load are independent variables for clinical outcomes.

In addition to infection by HCV types, individuals are usually infected by multiple "quasispecies" within a given classification. These viral swarms represent unique viruses that differ minimally from each other in genetic sequences, produced by both viral mutation and immunologic selection.

HCV can now be quantified using a polymerase chain reaction–based (PCR-based) assay (Hoffman laRoche) or by a branched chain oligonucleotide technique (Chiron). Although virtually all types can be measured by these two techniques, there may be selective differences in the relative sensitivity of assays for different HCV types, resulting in different measurements.

Hepatitis D

The 35-nm HDV double-shelled particle resembles HBV on electron microscopy. It has an external coat antigen of HBsAg provided by the genome of HBV (the helper virus) and an internal delta antigen (HDAg) provided by the HDV genome. A small, circular RNA molecule is associated with the HDAg; it is single stranded. HDV RNA isolated from infected liver is present in linear or circular forms. The structure and replicative cycle of HDV place it outside of any known family of animal viruses. Three genotypes (I, II, and III) have been described.

Hepatitis E

Viruslike particles, 27 to 30 nm in diameter, were detected by Balayan et al. (1981) in fecal samples from a volunteer who ingested an aqueous extract of feces obtained from patients with enterically transmitted NANB hepatitis. A similar agent was transmitted to marmosets and chimpanzees by Bradley et al. (1987). This cause of ET-NANB hepatitis is the HEV. The genome is a single-stranded positive-sense RNA molecule about 7.5 kilobases long. Three open reading frames (ORF) are present. ORF1 codes for nonstructural regulatory proteins; ORF2 codes for structural protein; ORF3 codes for a protein of undetermined function. The virus is very labile. Its biophysical properties indicate that it is a calicivirus-like agent, although genomic sequences more closely resemble rubella virus.

PATHOLOGY
Acute Viral Hepatitis

The histologic features of acute viral hepatitis caused by various hepatitis viruses (A, B, C, D, and E) may be indistinguishable. The characteristic findings on liver biopsy include necrosis and inflammation of the lobule, architectural consequences of the necrosis, and proliferation of the mesenchymal and bile duct elements. Anicteric hepatitis shows the same histologic appearance as icteric but usually with less severity.

The fully developed stage of hepatitis is characterized by degeneration and death of liver cells, proliferation of the Kupffer's cells, mononuclear cell infiltration, and bile duct proliferation. The hepatic cell changes involve the entire lobule, with a concentration of lesions in the centrolobular areas. The cells are usually swollen, but occasionally they are shrunken. As the lesions progress, there may be a variable degree of collapse, condensation of reticulin fibers, and accumulation of ceroid pigment and large phagocytic cells, first within the lobules and later in the portal tracts. In HEV infection the typical changes are focal necrosis with little infiltration and no lobular predilection. The focal lesions resemble those seen in drug-associated toxic hepatitis, with evidence of cholestasis.

During the recovery period the following residual changes may be seen: pleomorphic liver cells around central veins, focal inflammatory infiltration of portal tracts, and a mild degree of fibrosis extending from the portal tracts. Liver cell necrosis is slight or absent, but ceroid pigment may be found in the portal tracts.

Complete resolution is the usual course of all types of viral hepatitis. In most cases complete regeneration of the liver cells is observed after 2 or 3 months. However, other possible consequences include chronic persistent or chronic active hepatitis, resolution of hepatitis with postnecrotic scarring, cirrhosis, or fatal massive necrosis.

Chronic Active Hepatitis

Chronic active hepatitis caused by HBV, HCV, and HDV is characterized histologically by accumulations of lymphocytes and plasma cells that are located in the portal tracts and in foci of necrosis scattered throughout the hepatic lobules. Other findings include disruption of the limiting plate of the hepatic lobule adjacent to the portal tract and extension of the inflammatory reaction out of the portal tract into the hepatic parenchyma. The hepatocytes undergoing necrosis in these areas apparently are entrapped by the inflammatory infiltrate (known as "piecemeal necrosis"). Small clusters of hepatocytes may be surrounded by the inflammatory process, thereby creating a "rosette" appearance. The inflammation may vary in severity and distribution. A predominance of plasma cells may be found in patients with lupoid hepatitis. The pattern of lobular collapse and necrosis bridging portal areas and central veins has been termed *submassive necrosis* or *bridging necrosis* (Boyer and Klatskin, 1970). These findings during a biopsy indicate a poor prognosis.

The presence of portal fibrosis is variable. In more severe cases there is a marked deposition of fibrous tissue in the portal areas, accompanied by collapse of the hepatic lobular architecture and formation of fibrous tissue "bridges" between adjacent portal areas and central veins. In advanced stages the extensive cirrhosis may mask the chronic inflammatory process, resulting in histologic evidence of cryptogenic or macronodular cirrhosis.

Chronic Persistent Hepatitis

In patients with chronic persistent hepatitis the lymphocytic inflammatory infiltration is confined chiefly to the portal tracts. The lobular architecture of the liver is preserved, evidence of hepatocellular damage is minimal or absent, and fibrosis is only slight or absent. Piecemeal necrosis, very typical with chronic active hepatitis, is lacking in chronic persistent hepatitis.

Fulminant Hepatitis

In patients with fulminant hepatitis with death occurring within 10 days, the size of the liver is reduced, and its color is yellow or mottled (acute yellow atrophy). Histologic findings include extensive, diffuse necrosis and loss of hepatocytes, which are replaced by an inflammatory infiltrate composed of both polymorphonuclear and monocytic cells. Since the virus is usually not directly cytotoxic to liver cells, it has been suggested that an exaggerated immune response to a viral antigen is responsible for the cell death. The lobular structure of the liver may be collapsed. Occasionally, however, the architecture of the liver may be well preserved. Kupffer's cells and histiocytes contain phagocytized material from disintegrated liver cells. Bile thrombi may be seen in the canaliculi. Portal triads that usually are retained are filled with monocytes, lymphocytes, and polymorphonuclear cells. Occasionally, surviving liver tissue may be seen in the periphery of the lobules.

Regeneration of liver tissue may begin if patients survive for several days. The regeneration appears as clusters of cells scattered randomly throughout the liver. As regeneration advances, these "pseudolobules" of liver parenchyma appear to form adenoma-like groups of liver cells unrelated to the normal lobular architecture and lacking central veins. Patients who survive fulminant hepatitis usually have a remarkable recovery of liver function. Little or no residual liver damage is seen in biopsy specimens, although occasionally a coarse lobular type of cirrhosis is noted (Karvountzis et al., 1974).

IMMUNOPATHOLOGY
Hepatitis A

Hepatitis A antigen is detected in the cytoplasm of hepatocytes shortly before onset of acute hepatitis. Viral expression decreases rapidly after the appearance of clinical and histologic manifestations and IgM-specific anti-HAV. These findings indicate that hepatocellular damage is caused chiefly by immunologic rather than cytotoxic factors. Propagation of HAV in tissue culture is not associated with a cytopathic effect.

Hepatitis B

The pathologic and clinical consequences of hepatitis B infection is related to at least two factors: (1) HBV is not cytopathogenic, and (2) liver cell necrosis is in great part the result of host defenses. Cell necrosis may be the result of a cellular and immune response to HBV. Acute hepatitis with recovery may be associated with an efficient immune response that eliminates virus-infected cells by means of spotty necrosis. Viral antigens (HBsAg and HBcAg) that may be present in the liver before elicitation of the immune response are eliminated at the height of the acute disease. In contrast, chronic forms of hepatitis B may be the result of a quantitatively or qualitatively ineffective immune response. Under the conditions of high-grade immunosuppression such as occurs in kidney transplant recipients, HBV may persist in the liver without any substantial liver cell damage. On the other hand, in patients with chronic active hepatitis the occurrence of piecemeal necrosis may be a consequence of a partially deficient immune state. The available evidence indicates that an immune defect resulting in the incomplete elimination of infected hepatocytes is a cause of chronic HBV infection.

Hepatitis C

Once infection occurs, apoptosis—as well as ballooning degeneration of hepatocytes, damage of bile duct epithelium, microsteatosis and macrosteatosis, and fibrosis—are typical but not pathognomonic of HCV. It remains debatable whether HCV is directly cytopathic. Evidence to support this comes from the rare cases of unusually fulminant hepatitis in immunocompromised liver transplant recipients. It is also unclear whether the exuberance of the immune response or the lack thereof is the principal process resulting in chronic HCV hepatonecrosis. Portal changes (including lymphoid follicular aggregates) are mild and may be due to immunologic mechanisms, including potential autoimmune ones. Histologic events do not appear to reflect simultaneous measurements of serum transaminases. There is also no correlation between histologic activity and the presence of HCV RNA in the liver tissue. It may be difficult to differentiate acute from chronic hepatitis, and it is also difficult to predict clinical outcome based on a single biopsy. HCV RNA sequences may also be found in the lymphocytes of patients with chronic HCV (Zignego et al., 1995). These cells may serve as a source for reinfection of previously infected liver transplant recipients.

CLINICAL MANIFESTATIONS

The similarities and differences between the clinical manifestations of viral hepatitis types A, B, C, D, and E are listed in Table 11-2. The incubation period of hepatitis A ranges between 15 and 40 days, and the onset of symptoms is usually acute. In contrast, the incubation period of hepatitis B is longer (50 to 180 days), and the onset more commonly is insidious. The incubation period of hepatitis C may be the same as that of both type A and type B hepatitis; it may range between 1 and 5 months. In general, the clinical features of hepatitis C resemble type B infection more than type A.

The clinical picture shows great variation. In children the acute disease is generally milder and its course is shorter than in adults. In children or adults, jaundice may be inapparent or evanescent, or it may persist for many weeks. The course of the disease often may be separated into two phases: preicteric and icteric. However, occasionally jaundice may be the initial symptom.

Preicteric Phase

Fever, when present, appears during the preicteric phase of the disease; often it is absent or fleeting in young children, but in adolescents and adults it may last for 5 days. The temperature ranges from 37.8° to 40° C (100° to 104° F) and generally is accompanied by headache, lassitude, anorexia, nausea, vomiting, and abdominal pain. Urticaria and arthralgia or arthritis occurring during the preicteric phase usually are manifestations of hepatitis B. The liver may be enlarged and tender, and splenomegaly and lymphadenopathy may be present in some patients.

Icteric Phase

Jaundice begins to emerge as the fever subsides; it usually is preceded by the appearance of dark urine (biliuria). In young children the transition to the icteric phase is most often marked by disappearance of symptoms. On the other hand, in adults and older children the icteric phase may be accompanied by an exacerbation of some of the original symptoms, such as anorexia, nausea, vomiting, and abdominal pain. Mental depression, bradycardia, and pruritus—all frequently occurring in adults—are uncommon in children. The stools may be clay colored, but this is an inconstant finding. The icteric phase persists from a few days to as long as a month, with an average duration of 8 to 11 days in children and 3 to 4 weeks in adults. As jaundice fades, the patient's symptoms subside. As a rule, convalescence is rapid and uneventful. Excessive weight loss is more common in adults than in children. In small infants and children less than 3 years of age, hepatitis is usually anicteric. Jaundice is a very rare manifestation of neonatal hepatitis B infection. Most HBV-infected infants born to mothers who are HBV carriers have a chronic asymptomatic infection.

Table 11-2 Viral hepatitis types A, B, D, C, and E: comparison of clinical, epidemiologic, and immunologic features

Features	A	B	D	C	E
Virus	HAV	HBV	HDV	HCV	HEV
Family	Picornavirus	Hepadnavirus	Satellite	Flavivirus	Calicivirus
Genome	RNA	DNA	RNA	RNA	RNA
Incubation period	15-40 days	50-180 days	21-90 days	1-5 months	2-9 weeks
Type of onset	Usually acute	Usually insidious	Usually acute	Usually insidious	Usually acute
Prodrome: arthritis and rash	Not present	May be present	Unknown	May be present	Not present
Mode of transmission					
Oral (fecal)	Usual	No	No	No	Usual
Parenteral	Rare	Usual	Usual	Usual	No
Other	Food- or water-borne	Intimate (sexual) contact, perinatal	Intimate (sexual) contact less common	Intimate (sexual) contact less common	Water-borne transmission in developing countries
Sequelae					
Carrier	No	Yes	Yes	Yes	No
Chronic hepatitis	No cases reported	Yes	Yes	Yes	No cases reported
Mortality	0.1%-0.2%	0.5%-2.0% in uncomplicated cases; may be higher in complicated cases	2%-20%	1%-2% in uncomplicated cases; may be higher in complicated cases	20% in pregnant women; 1%-2% in general population
Immunity					
Homologous	Yes	Yes	Yes	Yes	Yes
Heterologous	No	No	No	No	No

Hepatitis A (HAV)

The course of hepatitis A is shown in Fig. 11-3. After an incubation period of approximately 30 days, there is a spiking rise in serum alanine aminotransferase (ALT) levels. The duration of abnormal ALT levels in children is brief, rarely exceeding 2 to 3 weeks. The serum bilirubin value usually becomes abnormal when ALT reaches peak levels. The increased level of serum bilirubin may be transient, and the duration may be as short as 1 day or may persist for more than 1 month. In general, jaundice is transient in children and more prolonged in adults.

The following tests are available for the detection of hepatitis A antibody: IAHA, RIA, and EIA. As indicated in Fig. 11-3, RIA anti-HAV is detected very early—at the time of onset of disease. Initially, RIA anti-HAV is predominantly IgM; later it is exclusively IgG. The time of appearance of EIA anti-HAV is the same for RIA, and the test apparently is equally sensitive.

The duration of illness caused by HAV is variable, ranging from several weeks to several months. The degree of morbidity and the duration of jaundice correlate directly with the patient's age. Even with prolonged acute illness lasting several months, complete resolution of hepatitis usually occurs. Unlike hepatitis B, C, and D, HAV infection does not cause chronic liver disease. Viremia is transient; it is not characterized by a chronic carrier state. Although the outcome of HAV infection is usually favorable, fulminant hepatitis may occur. McNeil et al. (1984) reported three deaths (0.14%) in a series of 2,174 consecutive virologically or

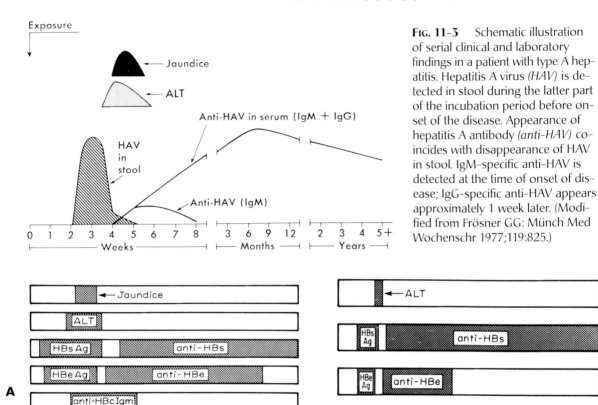

FIG. 11-3 Schematic illustration of serial clinical and laboratory findings in a patient with type A hepatitis. Hepatitis A virus *(HAV)* is detected in stool during the latter part of the incubation period before onset of the disease. Appearance of hepatitis A antibody *(anti-HAV)* coincides with disappearance of HAV in stool. IgM-specific anti-HAV is detected at the time of onset of disease; IgG-specific anti-HAV appears approximately 1 week later. (Modified from Frösner GG: Münch Med Wochenschr 1977;119:825.)

FIG. 11-4 **A,** Acute hepatitis B followed by recovery, showing results of serial tests for serum alanine aminotransferase *(ALT)*, hepatitis B surface antigen *(HBsAg)* and its antibody *(anti-HBs)*, hepatitis B e antigen *(HBeAg)* and its antibody *(anti-HBe)*, hepatitis B core antibody *(anti-HBc)*, and anti-HBc IgM. **B,** Subclinical hepatitis B infection followed by an immune response. Shaded areas denote "abnormal" or "detectable," and white areas denote "normal" or "not detectable." (From Krugman S: Pediatr Rev 1985;7:3-11.)

serologically confirmed hospitalized cases. Thus the death rate among all hepatitis A cases must be negligible.

Hepatitis B (HBV)

The course of HBV infection is shown in Figs. 11-4 and 11-5. The incubation period may range from 2 to 6 months. The detection of HBsAg in the blood of a patient with acute hepatitis is indicative of HBV infection. The characteristic laboratory findings and the profile of abnormal liver function are shown in Table 11-3 and Fig. 11-4.

HbsAg may be detected by RIA 6 to 30 days after a parenteral exposure and 56 to 60 days after an oral exposure (Krugman, 1979; Krugman et al.,

1979). The antigen may be detected approximately 1 week to 2 months before the appearance of abnormal levels of ALT and jaundice. In most patients with acute hepatitis B, HBsAg is consistently present during the latter part of the incubation period and during the preicteric phase of the disease. The antigen may become undetectable shortly after onset of jaundice.

The pattern of serum ALT activity is illustrated in Fig. 11-4, *A*. After an incubation period of approximately 50 days, the serum ALT values become abnormal, rising gradually over a period of several weeks. The duration of abnormal ALT activity may be prolonged, usually exceeding 30 to 60 days.

As indicated in Fig. 11-4, *A*, the first antibody that is detectable is anti-HBc. It appears approximately 1 week or more after the onset of hepatitis. The anti-HBc titers, predominantly IgM, are usually high for several months. Thereafter IgM values decline to low or undetectable levels, but anti-HBc persists for many years (Chau et al., 1983). The commercially available test for anti-HBc IgM is a solid-phase immunoassay; its cut-off assay value was established to differentiate high levels of antibody (positive) from low or undetectable levels (negative). The test is negative in healthy HBsAg carriers and in patients with cirrhosis. It may be positive in those with chronic hepatitis characterized by marked inflammatory changes without cirrhosis.

The anti-HBc IgM assay should be useful for differentiating recent from past HBV infections and identifying acute hepatitis B in patients whose HBsAg has declined to undetectable levels before the appearance of anti-HBs (window phase). Antibody to the HBsAg usually appears late, approximately 2 weeks to 2 months after HbsAg is no longer detectable. Anti-HBs is detected in approximately 80% of patients with hepatitis B who eventually become HBsAg-negative. In the remainder the antibody levels are too low for detection. Anti-HBs may be detected in approximately 5% to 10% of HBsAg carriers. Up to one third of Chinese and half of Japanese patients with serologic evidence of past HBV infection have detectable HBV DNA in their blood when tested with sensitive detection techniques such as PCR; the loss of HbsAg followed by the emergence of anti-HBsAg antibody does not necessarily indicate the absence of viremia.

The results of tests for HBsAg, HBeAg, anti-HBs, and anti-HBc during the course of hepatitis B are shown in Table 11-3 and in Figs. 11-4 and 11-5.

Table 11-3 Detection of hepatitis B surface antigen (HBsAg), antibody to HBsAg (anti-HBs), antibody to hepatitis B core antigen (anti-HBc), hepatitis B e antigen (HBeAg), and antibody to HBeAg (anti-HBe) during the course of type B hepatitis infection

Time of hepatitis B infection	HBsAg	Anti-HBs	Anti-HBc	HBeAg	Anti-HBe
Late incubation period	0	0	0	+	0
Early in course of acute hepatitis (<1 week)	+	0	+	+	0
Late in course of acute hepatitis (1 to 4 weeks)	+ or 0	+ or 0	+	+ or 0	0 or +
Convalescence from acute hepatitis					
Early (4 to 8 weeks)	0	+ or 0	+	0	+ or 0
Late (>8 weeks)	0	+	+	0	+ or 0

+, Present; 0, not present.

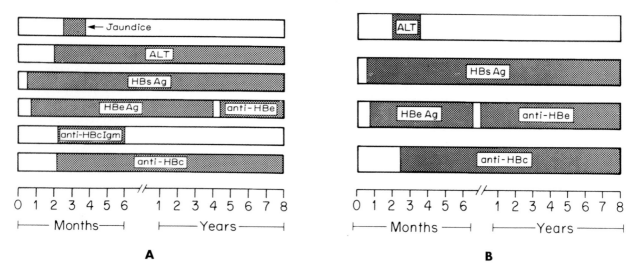

FIG. 11-5 **A,** Chronic hepatitis B infection. **B,** Subclinical hepatitis B followed by an asymptomatic chronic carrier state. See Fig. 11-4 for key. (From Krugman S: Pediatr Rev 1985;7:3-11.)

Most patients with hepatitis B infection recover completely. However, progression to chronic hepatitis with persistence of HBsAg has been reported in 3% of Taiwanese university students (Beasley et al., 1983), in 8% of homosexual men (Szmuness et al., 1981), and in 13% of Eskimos (McMahon et al., 1985). The risk of chronic hepatitis B infection in infants born to mothers who are HbsAg- and HBeAg-positive carriers may exceed 60%. Other serious consequences of acute HBV infection include fulminant hepatitis, cirrhosis, and hepatocellular carcinoma.

Hepatitis C (HCV)

Most patients with HCV infection are anicteric, especially those who have the contact-acquired sporadic form. The incubation period ranges from 1 to 5 months. The clinical signs and symptoms of the acute illness are milder than those with HAV and HBV infections. However, biochemical evidence of chronic liver disease develops in approximately 50% of patients with posttransfusion hepatitis C (Alter, 1985). HCV infection is found in 0.5% to 8% of blood donors worldwide. As indicated in Fig. 11-6, the ALT elevations fluctuate over prolonged periods of time. The interval between exposure to HCV or onset of illness and detection of anti-HCV may be prolonged. In recipients of transfusions the mean interval from onset of hepatitis to anti-HCV detection may be 15 weeks (range, 4 to 32 weeks). In general, anti-HCV persists in patients with chronic disease; it may disappear in those with acute resolving hepatitis C (Alter et al., 1989; Farci et al., 1991).

The course of a typical case of posttransfusion hepatitis C is shown in Fig. 11-6. Evidence of viremia was detected by the use of PCR technology 2 weeks after a transfusion of HCV-contaminated blood. The first increase in ALT values was de-tected at 8 weeks, and anti-HCV was detectable at 11 weeks. A 6-year follow-up revealed persistence of positive PCR, detectable anti-HCV, and biopsy evidence of chronic active hepatitis. Long-term prospective studies of patients with posttransfusion (NANB) hepatitis (HCV disease) have revealed evidence of progression to cirrhosis and to hepatocellular carcinoma. In most blood centers, units of blood are screened for antibody to HCV and for elevations of liver transaminases. This should reduce but not completely eliminate HCV transmission, since antibody responses to HCV may be absent for a long time after HCV infection, and liver transaminases may continue to be normal. In the future, HCV RNA screening may be added to decrease the likelihood of HCV infection.

Hepatitis D (HDV)

The clinical manifestations and course of type D hepatitis resemble those of acute or chronic hepatitis B. In general, however, hepatitis D is a more severe disease. The mortality rate of acute HDV hepatitis has ranged from 2% to 20%, compared to less than 1% for acute hepatitis B. In addition, cirrhosis and complications of portal hypertension occur more often and progress more rapidly in patients with hepatitis D. Acute delta hepatitis occurs as either a coinfection or superinfection of hepatitis B (see Table 11-2). Coinfection entails a simultaneous onset of acute HBV and HDV infection. In superinfection a chronic HBV carrier is infected with HDV.

The course of acute delta coinfection is shown in Fig. 11-7. During the latter part of the incubation period, HBsAg—followed by HDV RNA—appears. Thereafter serum ALT levels begin to rise, followed by the development of clinical symptoms and jaundice. Serum ALT activity is often biphasic. Resolution of acute liver disease follows clearance

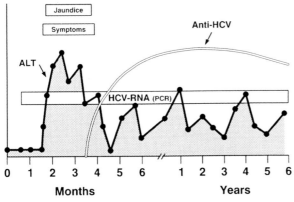

FIG. 11-6   Typical course of a case of acute hepatitis C that progresses to chronic infection and disease. *ALT,* alanine aminotransferase; *HCV-RNA,* hepatitis C virus ribonucleic acid; *PCR,* polymerase chain reaction; *anti-HCV,* antibody to hepatitis C virus. (From Hoofnagle JH, DiBisceglie AM: Semin Liver Dis 1991;11:78.)

FIG. 11-7 Typical course of a case of acute delta hepatitis coinfection. *ALT*, alanine aminotransferase; *HBsAg*, hepatitis B surface antigen; *HDV-RNA*, hepatitis delta virus ribonucleic acid; *anti-HDV*, antibody to HDV; *anti-HBs*, antibody to HBsAg. (From Hoofnagle JH, DiBisceglie AM: Semin Liver Dis 1991;11:79.)

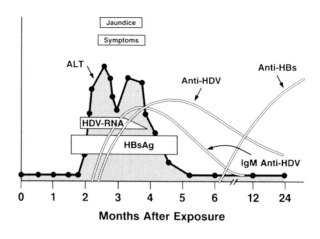

FIG. 11-8 Typical course of a case of acute delta hepatitis superinfection. See Fig. 11-7 for key. (From Hoofnagle JH, DiBisceglie AM: Semin Liver Dis 1991;11:80.)

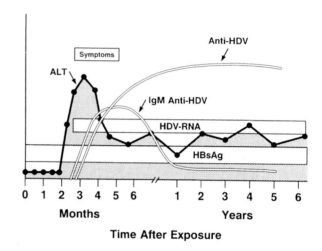

of HBsAg and cessation of HDV replication. The antibody to HDV (anti-HDV) that appears shortly after onset of clinical disease is transient. The course of acute delta superinfection followed by the development of chronic delta hepatitis is shown in Fig. 11-8. At the time of exposure to HDV this patient was an asymptomatic chronic HBsAg carrier with normal ALT values. At the end of the incubation period there are (1) a rise in serum ALT values; (2) appearance and persistence of HDV RNA; followed by (3) appearance of IgM anti-HDV, which is transient; and (4) a rise of IgG anti-HDV to high levels that persist.

Hepatitis E (HEV)

The clinical manifestations and course of hepatitis E are essentially the same as those for hepatitis A. However, there are several striking differences. During various epidemics the disease has been rare in children and common in adolescents and young

adults. The typical clinical and immunologic correlates of infection are seen in Fig. 11-9.

HEV, like HAV, does not cause chronic liver disease. In most patients the illness is self-limiting, and there is no evidence of a chronic carrier state. However, unlike hepatitis A, hepatitis E can be a devastating disease in pregnant women. Whereas the mortality rate from hepatitis A in pregnant women is less than 1%, the rate has ranged from 10% to 20% in outbreaks of hepatitis E. The deaths are caused by fulminant hepatitis and disseminated intravascular coagulation. Mortality is highest during the third trimester and lowest during the first trimester. The mortality rate in nonpregnant women is the same as that among men, less than 1%. Transmission from mother to infant has been reported, with most of the infected infants recovering from their hepatitis. However, one of the infants developed massive hepatic necrosis and died (Khuroo et al., 1995).

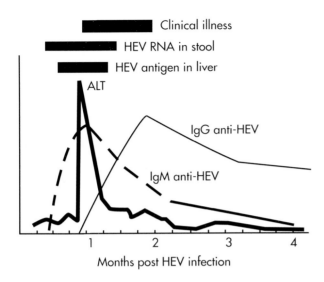

FIG. 11-9 Typical clinical and immunologic correlates of infection.

At the present time a practical serologic test to confirm a diagnosis of hepatitis E is not available. Immune electron microscopy was the first-generation test used by investigators. Second-generation tests using recombinant proteins in ELISA or Western blot format have an 80% to 100% sensitivity. Comparative sensitivity and specificity data are unavailable. Diagnostic tests can also detect HEV antigens using immunofluorescent probes, as well as RNA by PCR.

NEONATAL HEPATITIS B INFECTION

HBV is the most common and most important cause of neonatal hepatitis infection. To date, perinatal transmission of HAV, HCV, HDV, and HEV has not been well documented. It is unlikely that HAV and HEV will prove to be problems, since these infections are not characterized by a carrier state. The risk of perinatal transmission of HCV (ranging from 5% to 50%, depending on the population studied) is controversial at the present time (Thaler et al., 1991; Nagata et al., 1992; Ohto et al., 1994; Giacchinno et al., 1995; Palomba et al., 1996).

Perinatal transmission of HBV from mother to infant during the course of pregnancy or at the time of birth was first reported by Stokes et al. (1954). They observed an infant born by cesarean section to a mother who was a hepatitis B carrier. The infant, who developed hepatitis with jaundice at 2 months of age, later died at age 18 months with advanced fibrosis of the liver.

The availability of tests to detect HBsAg has enabled various investigators to study infants whose mothers had acute hepatitis B or an asymptomatic chronic carrier state during pregnancy (Schweitzer et al., 1972; Stevens et al., 1975). Signs of neonatal hepatitis B infection (antigenemia) are usually not present at the time of birth but may be detected between 2 weeks and 5 months of age. Approximately 5% of infants are infected in utero and approximately 95% at the time of birth. Certain infants escape infection completely; others develop only persistent antigenemia with no liver disease; others may develop severe chronic active hepatitis; and still others may develop fulminant hepatitis (Fawaz et al., 1975).

Perinatal transmission of hepatitis B infection from mother to infant depends in great part on the presence of HbeAg (an indirect marker of viral load that exceeds a million particles per ml of plasma). Infection is most likely to occur if the mother is HBeAg-positive (Stevens et al., 1975). Infants born to HbeAg-positive carrier mothers have a 60% to 90% chance of contracting chronic hepatitis B infection and of possible subsequent progression to cirrhosis and hepatocellular carcinoma. In contrast, the attack rate of hepatitis B in infants whose HbsAg-positive mothers are HbeAg-negative is less than 20%. These infants usually recover completely, and chronic hepatitis is rare, but occasionally the infection may be fulminant with a fatal outcome (Delaplane et al., 1983). The viruses associated with this rare fulminant course have often been HBV variants with precore mutations (Bahn et al., 1995).

Possible routes of transmission from mother to baby include (1) leakage of virus across the placenta late in pregnancy or during labor; (2) ingestion of amniotic fluid or maternal blood; and (3) breast-feeding, especially if the mother has cracked nipples. Studies by Alter (1980) with HBsAg-positive and HbeAg-positive pregnant chimpanzees revealed that cesarean section and postdelivery isolation did not prevent infection of newborn chimpanzees. They became HBsAg-positive in spite of these precautions.

Infants who inadvertently receive contaminated blood or blood products during the neonatal period may subsequently develop severe hepatitis B. Dupuy et al. (1975) described their experience with fourteen infants 2 to 5 months of age who were admitted to the hospital with severe or fulminant hepatitis. Of the fourteen infants, eleven had serologic evidence of hepatitis B infection. Of the eleven infants with hepatitis B, seven received blood derivatives during the neonatal period, and four were exposed to their mothers who were chronic HBsAg carriers. The case fatality rate was very high; eight of the fourteen infants died.

COURSE AND COMPLICATIONS

Various factors can affect the course of hepatitis infection: age, type of virus, and immunocompetence. In general, hepatitis A and E are mild or inapparent infections in infants and children. However, they are generally more severe in adults. In contrast, infants infected with HBV are more likely to develop chronic hepatitis B than older children and adults. Compared to hepatitis A infections, hepatitis B, C, and D infections are more likely to progress to chronic liver disease.

Acute Hepatitis

The duration of illness caused by HAV is variable, ranging from several weeks to several months. The degree of morbidity and duration of jaundice correlate directly with age. Even with prolonged acute illness lasting several months, complete resolution of hepatitis usually occurs. Most patients with hepatitis A recover completely. Hepatitis B, C, and D, on the other hand, are associated with more debility and a substantial risk of chronic liver disease. In rare instances, acute hepatitis may progress to a fulminant fatal outcome.

Chronic Persistent Hepatitis

Chronic persistent hepatitis is a pathologic diagnosis based on a liver biopsy. It is an inflammatory process involving only the portal areas. This form of hepatitis usually lasts longer than 6 months, and it is more common and less severe than chronic active hepatitis. In general, the patient is asymptom-atic and usually has mild hepatomegaly and moderate elevation of serum aminotransferases without jaundice. Chronic persistent hepatitis may resolve after several years or may progress to chronic active hepatitis. These patients may be HBsAg carriers.

Chronic Active Hepatitis

Chronic active hepatitis, also referred to as *chronic aggressive hepatitis,* is more likely to progress to cirrhosis. The disease is characterized by chronic and recurrent episodes of jaundice, abnormal levels of serum aspartate aminotransferase (AST) and ALT, and evidence of portal hypertension with ascites if the disease progresses to cirrhosis. Severe episodes of hepatic necrosis may terminate in hepatic failure. Most patients with chronic hepatitis (persistent or active) have not had a past history of acute illness with jaundice. The disease usually follows mild, anicteric forms of hepatitis.

Fulminant Hepatitis

The occurrence of hepatic failure within the first few days or within 4 weeks after onset of acute hepatitis indicates a fulminant course. When the course is more prolonged and hepatic failure occurs after 1 to 3 months of illness, the term *subacute hepatitis* is used; it is associated with portal hypertension, ascites, and submassive hepatic necrosis. Fulminant hepatitis usually is characterized by mental confusion, emotional instability, restlessness, bleeding manifestations, and coma. The progressive jaundice and coma are associated with a shrinking liver. The Fulminant Hepatic Failure Surveillance Study (Trey, 1972) included 142 patients with fulminant viral hepatitis. The survival rate was influenced by the age of the patient. Of 27 patients less than 15 years of age, 10 (37%) survived; of 73 patients 15 to 44 years of age, 12 (16%) survived; and of 42 patients 45 to more than 75 years of age, 3 (7%) survived. The overall survival rate was 18%.

Each of the hepatitis viruses can cause fulminant hepatitis with similar courses and prognoses, and there are no clinical or prognostic differences between these different forms of fulminant viral hepatitis (Gimson et al., 1983). Fulminant hepatitis B probably occurs more frequently than recognized because HbsAg may be cleared faster in this form of hepatitis than in regular hepatitis B (Tabor et al., 1981). HBV with precore mutations resulting in variants unable to express HbeAg can be associated with fulminant hepatitis (Hasegawa et al., 1991; Liang et al., 1991; Shafritz, 1991).

Simultaneous infection with HBV and HDV seems to increase liver necrosis and to favor the development of fulminant hepatitis B. In a report by Smedile et al. (1982) HDV markers were more common in patients with fulminant (39%) than with ordinary acute hepatitis B (19%), and serologic markers for acute HDV infection (anti-HDV IgM) were positive among 33.8% of patients with fulminant hepatitis B, compared to 4.2% of patients with acute hepatitis B (Govindarajan et al., 1984).

Hepatoma

The striking association between chronic hepatitis B infection and primary hepatocellular carcinoma (PHC) has been well established. The relationship is supported by the following factors: (1) geographic distribution of PHC, (2) presence of HBsAg in serum of patients with PHC, (3) detection of HBV markers in tumor tissue and PHC cell lines, (4) occurrence of PHC in certain animals infected with hepadnaviruses, and (5) integration of the HBV genome in the tumor cell genome.

Worldwide seroepidemiologic studies have revealed a remarkable correlation between the prevalence of HBsAg carriers and the incidence of PHC (Szmuness, 1978). The highest frequency of carrier and PHC rates has been observed in Southeast Asia and sub-Saharan Africa. Various studies have revealed that the prevalence of HBsAg is significantly higher in patients with PHC than in comparable controls (Szmuness, 1978).

Histochemical and immunochemical methods have revealed the presence of HBsAg and HBcAg in the livers of patients with PHC. HBsAg has been detected in both the tumor and the surrounding liver tissue. In addition, cultured cell lines derived from human PHC secrete enormous quantities of HBsAg into supernatant culture media (MacNab et al., 1976). Integration of HBV genome has been demonstrated by molecular hybridization analysis of DNA extracted from human PHC. These studies revealed HBV DNA sequences integrated into the tumor cell genome (Shafritz and Kew, 1981).

The occurrence of PHC in certain animals has provided additional evidence of an association with chronic hepatitis infection. The tumors have been observed in woodchucks infected with woodchuck hepatitis virus (WHV), a member of the hepadnavirus group. The inflammatory hepatic lesion caused by active viral infection is associated with a high frequency of hepatoma formation (Popper et al., 1981).

EXTRAHEPATIC MANIFESTATIONS OF VIRAL HEPATITIS

HBV infections may be associated with a variety of extrahepatic manifestations. The following sites may be affected: skin, joints, small arteries and arterioles, and renal glomeruli. The underlying pathology is usually a diffuse and widespread immune complex type of vasculitis. The following syndromes have been identified: (1) serum sicknesslike prodrome, (2) polyarteritis nodosa, (3) glomerulonephritis, (4) "essential" mixed cryoglobulinemia, (5) polymyalgia rheumatica, and (6) infantile papular acrodermatitis (Gianotti-Crosti syndrome) (Gocke, 1975).

Serum Sicknesslike Prodrome

Serum sicknesslike prodrome is characterized by a transient erythematous maculopapular eruption, polyarthralgia, and occasionally actual arthritis and urticaria. These symptoms and signs usually occur during the latter part of the incubation period or early acute phase of the disease, and they last just a few days. During the early phase of the skin and joint manifestations the complement titer and C3 and C4 levels may be transiently suppressed (Alpert et al., 1971). The critical role that the composition of the immune complex plays in the causation of tissue injury has been demonstrated in studies by Wands et al. (1974) on the pathogenesis of arthritis associated with type B (HBsAg-positive) hepatitis.

Polyarteritis Nodosa

The association of polyarteritis nodosa with persistent hepatitis B antigenemia initially was described by Gocke et al. (1970) and Trepo and Thiyolet (1970). The illness usually begins with fever, polyarthralgia, myalgia, rash, and urticaria. The syndrome may evolve over a period of months, and it is characterized by various manifestations of acute vasculitis, including peripheral neuropathies, hypertension, and evidence of renal damage. Biopsy reveals lesions in small arteries characterized by typical fibrinoid necrosis and perivascular infiltration associated with polyarteritis nodosa. Approximately 30% to 40% of patients with polyarteritis nodosa have high titers of HBsAg, but the liver involvement that is present is not the primary problem. Circulating immune complexes composed of HBsAg and anti-HBs are present during the acute phase of the disease. At this time the whole complement titer and C3 levels are decreased. Immunofluorescent studies of biopsy specimens reveal deposition of HBsAg, IgM, IgG, and C3 in a nodular pattern along the elastic membrane of damaged vessels (Gocke et al., 1971). A study of HBsAg-positive and HBsAg-negative polyarteritis nodosa revealed that the fatality rate was essentially equal (42% and 44%, respectively) in the two groups after a 3-year follow-up period (Sergent et al., 1976).

Glomerulonephritis

The association of glomerulonephritis with chronic hepatitis B has been studied by various investigators (Combes et al., 1971; Brzosko et al., 1974; Kohler et al., 1974). They observed typical immune complex deposits along the subepithelial surface of the glomerular basement membrane by electron microscopy. Fluorescent antibody studies showed nodular deposition of HbsAg, immunoglobulin, and C3 in the glomeruli. The glomerulonephritis is usually of the membranous or membranoproliferative type. Most cases of glomerulonephritis in adults have occurred in patients with existing evidence of chronic active hepatitis and a persistent HBsAg carrier state. However, studies by Brzosko et al. (1974) revealed the presence of HBsAg-antibody complex deposits in renal glomeruli in approximately 35% of children with clinical nephrosis or glomerulonephritis. Glomerulonephritis has also been associated with chronic HCV infection.

Other Possible Extrahepatic Syndromes

Mixed Cryoglobulinemia. Mixed cryoglobulinemia is an immune complex disease characterized by arthralgias, purpura, weakness, vasculitis, and diffuse glomerulonephritis (Meltzer et al., 1966). Levo et al. (1977) described this syndrome in patients who had evidence of HBV infection and circulating immune complexes composed of HBsAg and anti-HBs. In a recent study, cryoglobulinemia was found in 36% of patients with chronic HCV infection, and rheumatoid factor was found in the serum of 71% of patients (Pawlotsky et al., 1995).

Autoimmune Manifestation. Various autoantibodies have been found in the sera of 40% to 50% of patients with HCV infection, including ANA, antismooth muscle, and antithyroid antibodies (Pawlotsky et al., 1994). In addition, salivary gland lesions with lymphocytic capillaritis, resembling Sjögren's syndrome, were seen in half of patients with chronic HCV. Autoimmune hepatitis because of HCV appears to be rare in the United States but a possible entity in Europe (Krawitt, 1996).

Polymyalgia Rheumatica. Polymyalgia rheumatica is another distinct connective tissue disorder that has been associated with hepatitis B infection (Bacon et al., 1975; Plouvier et al., 1978).

Papular Acrodermatitis. The association of infantile papular acrodermatitis with hepatitis B infection was first described by Gianotti (1973). A striking epidemic of this disease occurred in Japan, involving 153 patients in a pediatric clinic from 1974 to 1977 (Ishimaru et al., 1976; Toda et al., 1978). Of these cases 89% were associated with HBsAg. During the outbreak all of the index cases were 1 year old or younger, but the age ranged from 3 months to 10 years. In approximately 40% of the patients with infantile papular acrodermatitis who were 1 year of age or younger, HBsAg persisted for 1 year.

DIAGNOSIS

The diagnosis of viral hepatitis usually is based on clinical and epidemiologic grounds. The occurrence of jaundice in association with a prior febrile episode and anorexia, nausea, and abdominal pain suggests viral hepatitis. The presence of an elevated serum AST or ALT value provides additional evidence. The diagnostic features of viral hepatitis types A, B, C, D, and E are listed in Table 11-2. The value of specific serologic tests for the diagnosis of various types of hepatitis is dependent on the time the blood is obtained during the course of the disease. The presence of IgM-specific anti-HAV indicates hepatitis A infection. The detection of HBsAg in the serum is indicative of hepatitis B infection. The interpretation of various serologic tests for the diagnosis of hepatitis B infection is shown in Table 11-3. Diagnosis of HCV infection is most easily made serologically using second- and third-generation assays. The first-generation ELISA used a recombinant antigen derived from the NS-4 region but had limited sensitivity. The newer assays include additional antigens derived from the core and NS-3 regions (second generation) and the NS-5 region (third generation). A confirmatory recombinant immunoblot assay (RIBA) is also available for the purpose of determining the specificity of the ELISA. The sensitivity of the later-generation assays is greater than 90%. Since antibodies may appear months after infection or not at all, the use of PCR to detect RNA remains the standard for HCV detection.

DIFFERENTIAL DIAGNOSIS

Before jaundice emerges, the following diseases may be considered in the differential diagnosis: infectious mononucleosis; acute appendicitis; gastroenteritis; influenza; and, in some parts of the world, malaria, dengue, and sandfly fever. The diagnosis of these diseases may be established by the detection of specific etiologic agents, by serologic tests, or by the subsequent course.

In the presence of jaundice the diseases that may be confused with viral hepatitis are congenital or acquired hemolytic jaundice or obstructive jaundice caused by blockage of the bile ducts by stone or tumor or, in infants, congenital atresia; hepatocellular jaundice resulting from chemical poisons, cirrhosis, or neoplasm of the liver (primary or metastatic); spirochetal jaundice (Weil's disease); yellow fever; acute cholangitis; and jaundice associated with various other infections such as infectious mononucleosis, brucellosis, amebiasis, malaria, and syphilis. Before considering these diseases in the differential diagnosis, it would be important to rule out a diagnosis of hepatitis A (absence of IgM anti-HAV) and hepatitis B (absence of HBsAg and IgM anti-HBc). At the present time the test for anti-HVC is not useful for the diagnosis of acute HCV infection. A negative test does not rule out HCV infection; it may not be detectable for several months after onset of disease. A positive test may be indicative of a past unrelated infection.

Hemolytic Jaundice

Hemolytic jaundice can be differentiated from obstructive jaundice by the history, the presence of anemia, positive Coombs' test, presence of urobilin in the stools, and absence of bilirubinuria.

Extrahepatic Obstructive Jaundice

Calculi and neoplasms are rare in children. In infancy, congenital obliteration of the bile ducts may present difficulties at first. The distinction should become clear in the course of the illness, since the jaundice progressively deepens and the stools remain chalky or gray. Serum aminotransferase levels are lower than those found in viral hepatitis.

Hepatocellular Jaundice

Hepatocellular jaundice or parenchymal jaundice caused by chemical poisons may be difficult to diagnose in the absence of a history of ingestion of toxic agents. The history is also important in the recognition of cirrhosis or neoplasm, both of which are uncommon in children in the United States.

Drug-Associated Hepatitis

Hepatitis induced by the following drugs may be clinically, biochemically, and morphologically indistinguishable from viral hepatitis: pyrazinamide, isoniazid, zoxazolamine, gold, and cinchophen. A clinical picture similar to the cholestatic form of the disease may be produced by the phenothiazine derivatives (e.g., chlorpromazine), methyltestosterone, and contraceptive drugs. Fatal toxic hepatitis has been described in a child receiving indomethacin for rheumatoid arthritis.

Jaundice Associated with Infection

In patients with jaundice associated with infection the diagnosis is established by demonstrating the specific etiologic agent or a rise in the specific antibody in convalescence. Jaundice in the neonatal period should suggest bacterial sepsis, syphilis, CMV infection, toxoplasmosis, congenital rubella, HSV, or coxsackie B infections. Neonatal hepatitis associated with these infections is present at the time of birth or several days thereafter. In contrast, hepatitis B is usually detected several weeks to as long as 5 months after birth. The diagnosis is established by detection of HBsAg in the blood.

TREATMENT
Acute Viral Hepatitis

The management of patients with acute hepatitis involves decisions about (1) the duration of bed rest, (2) the choice of a diet, and (3) the value of various nonspecific drugs. At the present time there is no antiviral agent that has been shown to alter the course of either type A or type B hepatitis consistently. Bed rest is recommended for patients who are symptomatic during the acute stage of the disease. Studies by Chalmers et al. (1955) provided the basis for a more liberal attitude toward bed rest during the convalescent period. They observed that ad-lib activity was preferable to rigidly enforced bed rest for prolonged periods of time. The liberal attitude toward bed rest described by Chalmers et al. in the 1950s is just as pertinent in the 1990s. Resumption of normal activity is usually gradual.

Progressively decreasing serum aminotransferase and bilirubin levels are helpful guides to increasing activity. It is not necessary to restrict the activity of an asymptomatic patient for the many weeks and months that the transaminase levels may be elevated. Generally, children return to normal activity much sooner than adults.

Diet is best regulated by the patient's appetite. When the child shows signs of anorexia, liquids such as chicken soup and fruit juices should be given. It is recommended that, with the return of appetite, a normal diet be given that is nutritious, properly balanced, and palatable. There is no contraindication to ingesting fats in moderate amounts.

Corticosteroids and antiviral agents are not recommended for the treatment of acute hepatitis infections caused by HAV, HBV, HCV, HDV, and HEV.

Chronic Persistent Hepatitis

Since chronic persistent hepatitis is usually a benign, self-limited disorder, normal activity is advised, and dietary restrictions are unnecessary. Corticosteroid or other immunosuppressive forms of therapy are not indicated.

Chronic Active Hepatitis

Patients with chronic active hepatitis may be permitted to carry out normal activities on an ad-lib basis. There is no evidence that bed rest and limitation of activity are of benefit. Alcohol should be avoided. A normal, well-balanced diet is recommended. The effect of various antiviral and immunomodulatory agents has been evaluated for the treatment of chronic hepatitis B, C, and D infections. Several studies have revealed that the use of corticosteroids may be detrimental in treating chronic hepatitis B (Hoofnagle, 1987). Adenine arabinoside (Ara-A) and its monophosphate derivative have not been shown effective. To date, the most promising agent has been leukocyte interferon, or IFN-α. Various controlled studies in adults have revealed that it is possible to eliminate HBV replication and to ameliorate liver disease in approximately 40% of patients treated with IFN-α (Hoofnagle et al., 1988). However, it should be noted that (1) the therapy involved a 3- to 6-month course of daily or three-times-per-week subcutaneous inoculations; (2) relapses occurred in approximately 50% of responders after therapy was discontinued; and (3) potential side effects included fever, chills, myalgia, anorexia, irritability, weight loss, and hair loss. In one small trial in Hong Kong the effect of IFN-α on chronic hepatitis B in Asian children was not encouraging (Lai et al., 1987). A more recent American study suggested that IFN-α therapy was more successful when given to younger children than it was when given to older children (Narkewicz et al., 1995).

A very promising preliminary study of the effects of 12 weeks of lamivudine (3TC), a nucleoside analog, found a dose-related clearance of HBV DNA in chronically infected adults. Fifteen percent of treated patients, most of whom had already failed interferon therapy, permanently cleared HBV (Dienstag et al., 1995). Additional studies are eagerly awaited.

Chronic Hepatitis C

Corticosteroid therapy has not been effective against chronic hepatitis C. Recombinant IFN-α therapy was evaluated in a double-blind, placebo-controlled trial (DiBisceglie et al., 1989). Approximately 50% of patients treated with 2 million units of IFN-α three times weekly for 6 months responded with a fall of ALT values to normal and an improvement in liver histologic conditions. However, in about half of responding patients, relapses occurred after cessation of interferon therapy. In fact, the response rate in patients with HCV type 1b is only 40%, whereas those with type 2 have a response rate of almost 80%. A recent report has described an interferon response gene, located in the NS5A region, that may cause these differences (Enomoto et al., 1995). In addition, the presence of preexisting cirrhosis decreases the likelihood of successful interferon therapy.

Several studies have revealed that adding ribavirin as additional primary therapy to interferon or for reinduction of patients who relapse results in diminished liver transaminases and often lower viral RNA levels. Ribavirin itself will lower liver transaminases, but the effects are lost when therapy is continued. Its sole effects on HCV RNA levels are controversial but certainly unimpressive.

Chronic Hepatitis D

Corticosteroid therapy has not been beneficial in treating chronic hepatitis D; it is not recommended. A controlled trial with IFN-α revealed transient improvement. Cessation of interferon therapy was followed by a return of viral replication and liver disease (Rizzetto et al., 1986).

Fulminant Hepatitis

Sudden onset of mental confusion, emotional instability, restlessness, coma, and hemorrhagic manifestations in a patient with hepatitis require prompt therapy. The rationale for the treatment is to combat the deleterious systemic effects of liver failure. The major objective of treatment of fulminant hepatitis is to reduce the load of nitrogenous products entering the portal circulation. Failure of the compromised liver to remove and detoxify these products is probably responsible for the cerebral dysfunction. The following measures are used: (1) restriction of protein intake, (2) removal of protein already in the gastrointestinal tract (use of a laxative and high-colonic irrigations), and (3) suppression of the bacterial population of the bowel (use of neomycin sulfate by mouth or nasogastric tube). The following therapeutic procedures of unproved benefit have been used: (1) corticosteroids; (2) exchange transfusion; (3) cross-perfusion with human, baboon, or pig liver; and (4) total body perfusion. Studies by the Acute Hepatic Failure Study Group (1977) failed to show any difference in survival rates between groups treated with hepatitis B immune serum globulin (HBIG) and those treated with standard immune globulin (IG). There have been isolated reports of dramatic improvement after liver transplantation.

PROGNOSIS

The prognosis of various types of viral hepatitis has been discussed in the sections of this chapter devoted to clinical manifestations and to course and complications. Hepatitis A is a relatively benign disease. Occasionally the illness may be prolonged, but eventually there is complete recovery with no evidence of chronic liver disease. Fatal fulminant hepatitis A may occur, but it is an extraordinarily rare phenomenon.

Most patients with hepatitis B recover completely. However, the risk of chronic infection is extremely variable; it may be low in young healthy adults (approximately 3%) or very high in infants born to HBsAg- and HbeAg-carrier mothers (60% to 90%). The overall risk is near 10%. Chronic hepatitis B infection may progress to cirrhosis of the liver and primary hepatocellular carcinoma. The risk of fatal fulminant hepatitis B is low (<2%), except when there is superinfection with HDV. Under these circumstances the mortality rate may be as high as 30% (Hadler et al., 1984).

Observations of patients with posttransfusion and community-acquired hepatitis C have revealed a relatively high incidence of chronic liver disease—approximately 50% (Alter, 1985; Sampliner et al., 1984). Fulminant hepatitis is an occasional outcome. The overall mortality rate is 1% to 2%. Studies in Japan have revealed that HCV infection is associated with the development of hepatocellular carcinoma (Saito et al., 1990).

Hepatitis E is a relatively benign disease that does not progress to chronic hepatitis. However, it is a highly fatal disease in pregnant women (Kane et al., 1984).

EPIDEMIOLOGIC FACTORS
Hepatitis A

The geographic distribution of hepatitis A is worldwide. It is endemic in parts of the world such as the Mediterranean littoral and parts of Africa, South America, Central America, and the Far East, where its presence creates a danger to susceptible military and civilian persons working or traveling in such areas.

Although no age group is immune, the highest incidence in civilian populations occurs among persons less than 15 years of age. In military groups the youngest persons are the ones chiefly affected. Persons of either sex are equally susceptible to infection.

The well-defined autumn-winter seasonal incidence has changed; no consistent seasonal patterns have been observed. In general, at the present time the incidence of hepatitis is fairly constant throughout the year.

Abundant evidence favors transmission through intestinal-oral pathways. HAV is found in the stools of both naturally and experimentally infected persons. Various studies have revealed that HAV is detectable in blood and stools during the latter part of the incubation period. Viremia is no longer detectable after onset of jaundice when anti-HAV appears. Fecal shedding of HAV persists for approximately 1 week after onset of jaundice (Krugman et al., 1962; Dienstag et al., 1975a). These findings indicate that the infection is usually spread during the preicteric phase of the disease and that it is generally not communicable after the first week of jaundice.

Epidemics have long been known to occur in association with poor sanitation in military camps. Explosive water-, milk-, and food-borne epidemics have been reported. Ingestion of raw shellfish from polluted waters has caused many epidemics. For example, an epidemic of hepatitis A in Shanghai, China, in 1988 involved more than 300,000 persons who had eaten raw hairy clams. HAV was isolated from the gills and digestive tracts of the contaminated clams.

There is evidence also for human association as the principal mode of spread. HAV may be transmitted through the use of blood and blood products or contaminated needles, syringes, and stylets. However, this potential mode of transmission is very rare, chiefly because viremia is transient in hepatitis A infection, and a carrier state does not exist.

When hepatitis A occurs in circumscribed situations—such as in households, day-care centers, orphanages, institutions for mentally handicapped children, military installations, and children's camps—it may smolder for months or years, or it may strike in explosive outbreaks. In families, secondary cases may occur in approximately 20 to 30 days.

Seroepidemiologic surveys by various investigators have provided valuable information about the distribution of anti-HAV in various population groups (Miller et al., 1975; Szmuness et al., 1976; Villarejos et al., 1976). The investigators observed a striking correlation between the presence of anti-HAV and socioeconomic status. Persons from lower socioeconomic groups were more likely to have detectable anti-HAV (past hepatitis A infection) than those from middle and upper socioeconomic groups. The detection of anti-HAV was strongly correlated with age. In New York City the prevalence increased gradually in adults, reaching peak levels in persons 50 years of age or older. In Costa Rica, however, peak levels were reached by 10 years of age. It is clear that the prevalence of anti-HAV (1) varies among different population groups, (2) increases with age, and (3) is independent of sex and race.

It is likely that the continued improvement of environmental and socioeconomic conditions will decrease the probability of exposure to hepatitis A, thereby changing a predominantly childhood infection to one that is more apt to occur in adults. This changing epidemiologic pattern was typical for poliomyelitis during the first half of the twentieth century in the United States. Poliomyelitis, like hepatitis A, is currently a more severe and more disabling disease in adults than in children.

Hepatitis B

Early epidemiologic concepts indicated that HBV was transmitted exclusively by the parenteral route. It is now clear, however, that other modes of transmission play an important role in the dissemination of the HBV. The experimental demonstration of oral transmission and the demonstration that contact-associated transmission is common have altered previous epidemiologic concepts. The term *contact-associated hepatitis* denotes one or more of the following possible modes of transmission: (1) oral-oral, (2) sexual, (3) perinatal, and (4) intimate physical contact of any type. Hepatitis B antigen has been detected in saliva (Ward et al., 1972), in semen (Heathcote et al., 1974), and in many other body fluids.

The major reservoirs of HBV are healthy chronic carriers and patients with acute hepatitis. The infection is transmitted to susceptible persons by transfusion of blood, plasma, or other blood products or by the use of inadequately sterilized needles and syringes. Medical and paramedical personnel may be infected by accidental inoculation or ingestion of contaminated materials. Outbreaks have occurred among drug addicts using unsterilized equipment. Tattooing and acupuncture have been responsible for transmitting the infection. Patients and personnel in the following areas are at high risk: renal dialysis, intensive care, oncology units, and various laboratories in which potentially contaminated blood and tissues are examined.

Seroepidemiologic surveys to detect the presence of HBsAg and anti-HBs have confirmed the worldwide distribution of the disease. The antigen has been detected in all populations, even in those living in the most remote areas devoid of parenteral modes of transmission. The antigen is most prevalent among persons living under crowded conditions and with poor hygienic standards, thus accounting for the endemicity of the disease in institutions for mentally retarded persons and in certain developing countries of the world. The HbsAg carrier rate may range from 0.1% to more than 10%; it is dependent on such factors as geographic location, age, and sex. The carrier rate is higher in tropical, underdeveloped areas than in temperate, developed countries; it is higher in urban communities than in rural communities and higher among males than among females. As indicated in Table 11-4, the prevalence of anti-HBs in various populations ranges from 3.1% in Switzerland to 78% in Taiwan.

The period of infectivity of patients with hepatitis B is dependent on the presence or absence of a carrier state. HBsAg is detectable in the blood during the latter part of the incubation period and for a variable period after onset of jaundice. Infectivity has also been associated with the presence of HbeAg and a high titer of HBsAg. For example, perinatal transmission of hepatitis B infection from HbsAg-positive mothers to their infants is highly likely if they are HBeAg-positive. On the other hand, HBsAg-positive and anti-HBe–positive mothers are much less likely to transmit infection.

Hepatitis C

The availability of a specific serologic test to detect anti-HCV has clarified the epidemiology of parenterally transmitted and sporadic HCV infection. The distribution of the disease is worldwide, with

Table 11-4 Prevalence of antibody to hepatitis B surface antigen (anti-HBs) in the populations surveyed for HAV infections

Country	Number tested	Number anti-HBs–positive	Percent positive
United States	1,000	108	10.8
Switzerland	98	3	3.1
Belgium	133	7	5.3
Yugoslavia	97	33	34.0
Israel	112	17	15.2
Taiwan	123	96	78.0
Senegal	96	60	62.5

From Szmuness W et al. Am J Epidemiol 1977;106:392.

an estimated 100 million HCV carriers. In the United States, hepatitis C may be the cause of 20% to 40% of all acute hepatitis cases. The largest group of HCV-infected adults has no known risk factor. Persons at high risk of contracting HCV infection include transfusion recipients, intravenous drug users, hemodialysis patients, and health-care workers with frequent blood contact. The risk of transmission from an individual needle stick incident from a known HCV infected person is about 5% to 10% (Mitsui et al., 1992). Promiscuous homosexual and heterosexual persons have a low risk of contracting HCV infection, which is not true for HBV. Perinatal transmission of HCV has been well documented and appears to occur at frequencies ranging from 5% to 10%. This rate may rise to levels in excess of 25% in children born to mothers who are HIV infected and may approach 50% if the child also acquires HIV (Papaevangelou et al., unpublished).

Hepatitis D

The epidemiology of hepatitis D is characterized by striking similarities to and certain differences from hepatitis B (see Table 11-2). The modes of transmission are the same, except that HDV perinatal infection is rare. In general, the prevalence of HDV correlates with the prevalence of HBV in the following high-risk groups: intravenous drug users, hemophiliacs, and institutionalized mentally retarded patients. In contrast, HDV has not been reported as prevalent in the following HBV high-risk groups: homosexual men and chronic carriers in such highly endemic areas as Southeast Asia, Southern Africa, and Alaska.

Superinfection of chronic HBV carriers has been responsible for epidemics of HDV-associated fulminant hepatitis in Venezuela, Colombia, and Brazil (Hadler et al., 1984; Buitrago et al., 1986).

In the United States and in Northern Europe HDV is most common in drug abusers.

Hepatitis E

The epidemiology of hepatitis E is characterized by certain similarities to and many differences from hepatitis A (see Table 11-2). Both hepatitis E and hepatitis A are enterically transmitted diseases that are spread through the fecal-oral route.

Hepatitis A is worldwide in distribution; it is predominantly an infection of children, and the secondary attack rate in household contacts is in excess of 20%. In contrast, hepatitis E has occurred predominantly in certain developing areas of the world during the course of water-borne outbreaks. Hepatitis E is most common in adults but rare in children, and the secondary attack rate in household contacts has been relatively low: less than 3% (Kane et al., 1984).

Hepatitis E epidemics have occurred in China, Southeast and Central Asia, Northern and Western Africa, Mexico, and Central America with periodicity of 5 to 10 years. The epidemics have either been extensive, involving thousands of persons, or smaller focal outbreaks. In endemic areas, HEV accounts for over 50% of acute sporadic hepatitis in adults and children. Seroprevalence studies performed on blood donors from nonendemic countries have found evidence of infection in 1% to 5%. With the exception of a few imported cases, hepatitis E has not occurred in the United States (DeCock et al., 1987). Hepatitis E, unlike hepatitis A, is a highly fatal disease in infected pregnant women, in whom the mortality rate may be 10% to 20%. Few studies have evaluated the efficacy of preexposure and postexposure prophylaxis with immune globulin for the prevention of HEV. In studies that compared disease rates of those who received immunoglobulin prepared from individuals (presumably hyperimmune) in endemic areas, no statistical differences were seen when compared to those who received no immunoglobulin.

A detailed discussion of recommendations for prevention of viral hepatitis follows. These recommendations of the Immunization Practices Advisory Committee (ACIP) were reported in the February 9, 1990, issue of the Public Health Service, Centers for Disease Control Morbidity and Mortality Weekly Report.

IMMUNE GLOBULINS

Immune globulins are important tools for preventing infection and disease before or after exposure to hepatitis viruses. Immune globulins used in medical practice are sterile solutions of antibodies (immunoglobulins) from human plasma. They are prepared by cold ethanol fractionation of large plasma pools and contain 10% to 18% protein. In the United States, plasma is primarily obtained from paid donors. Only plasma shown to be free of hepatitis B surface antigen (HBsAg) and antibody to human immunodeficiency virus (HIV) is used to prepare immune globulins.

Immune globulin (IG) (formerly called *immune serum globulin, ISG,* or *gamma globulin*) produced in the United States contains antibodies against the hepatitis A virus (anti-HAV) and the HBsAg (anti-HBs). Hepatitis B immune globulin (HBIG) is an IG prepared from plasma containing high titers of anti-HBs.

There is no evidence that hepatitis B virus (HBV), HIV (the causative agent of acquired immunodeficiency syndrome [AIDS]), or other viruses have ever been transmitted by IG or HBIG commercially available in the United States. Since late April 1985 all plasma units for preparation of IGs have been screened for antibody to HIV, and reactive units are discarded. No instances of HIV infection or clinical illness have occurred that can be attributed to receiving IG or HBIG, including lots prepared before April 1985. Laboratory studies have shown that the margin of safety based on the removal of HIV infectivity by the fractionation process is extremely high. Some HBIG lots prepared before April 1985 have detectable HIV antibody. Shortly after being given HBIG, recipients have occasionally been noted to have low levels of passively acquired HIV antibody, but this reactivity does not persist.

Serious adverse effects from IGs administered as recommended have been rare. Igs prepared for intramuscular administration should be used for hepatitis prophylaxis. IGs prepared for intravenous administration to immunodeficient and other selected patients are not intended for hepatitis prophylaxis. IG and HBIG are not contraindicated for pregnant or lactating women. Preparations of intravenous gamma globulin (IVIG) have been associated with the transmission of HCV (Bjoro et al., 1994). Manufacturers of IVIG are currently modifying production routines and screening lots by PCR for HCV RNA to virtually eliminate future HCV transmissions by this route.

HEPATITIS A
Preexposure Prophylaxis

The major group for whom preexposure prophylaxis is recommended is international travelers. The risk of hepatitis A for U.S. citizens traveling abroad varies with living conditions, length of stay, and the incidence of hepatitis A infection in areas visited. In general, travelers to developed areas of North America, western Europe, Japan, Australia, and New Zealand are at no greater risk of infection than they would be in the United States. For travelers to developing countries, risk of infection increases with duration of travel and is highest for those who live in or visit rural areas, trek in back country, or frequently eat or drink in settings of poor sanitation. Nevertheless, recent studies have shown that many cases of travel-related hepatitis A occur in travelers with "standard" tourist itineraries, accommodations, and food and beverage consumption behaviors. In developing countries, travelers should minimize their exposure to hepatitis A and other enteric diseases by avoiding potentially contaminated water or food. Travelers should avoid drinking water (or beverages with ice) of unknown purity and eating uncooked shellfish or uncooked fruits or vegetables that they did not prepare.

It should be noted that studies with inactivated hepatitis A vaccine have confirmed its safety, immunogenicity, and efficacy. Hepatitis A vaccines were licensed for use in 1993 and are currently the agent of choice for prophylaxis. Persons should be vaccinated before departure. Immunity is assumed to be protected by 18 to 28 days after vaccination, but a second dose 6 to 12 months later may be necessary for long-term immunity. The dosage of Havrix (manufactured by SmithKline Beecham Pharmaceuticals) for adults is 1,440 ELISA units per dose. Children and adolescents are given a smaller dose (360 ELISA units per dose) at 0, 1, and 6-12 months. Vaqta (manufactured by Merck and Co., Inc) is another inactivated HIV vaccine that has been licensed.

Those allergic to a vaccine component in both vaccines should receive IG, which is 80% to 90% effective in preventing clinical hepatitis A and is recommended as preexposure prophylaxis for all susceptible travelers, who have no access to the vaccine, going to developing countries. For travelers a single dose of IG of 0.02 ml/kg of body weight is recommended if travel is for less than 3 months. For those who anticipate a longer stay, 0.06 ml/kg should be used every 5 months.

Postexposure Prophylaxis

Hepatitis A cannot be reliably diagnosed on clinical presentation alone, and serologic confirmation of index patients is recommended before contacts are treated. Serologic screening of contacts for anti-HAV before they are given IG is not recommended because screening is more costly than IG and would delay its administration. For postexposure IG prophylaxis a single intramuscular dose of 0.02 ml/kg is recommended. IG should be given as soon as possible after last exposure; giving IG more than 2 weeks after exposure is not indicated.

Specific recommendations for IG prophylaxis for hepatitis A depend on the nature of the HAV exposure. Candidates for prophylaxis include the following individuals:

1. All household and sexual contacts of persons with hepatitis A.
2. All staff and attendees of day-care centers or homes if (a) one or more children or employees are diagnosed as having hepatitis A, or (b) cases are recognized in two or more households of center attendees.
3. Persons who have close contact with a school- or classroom-centered outbreak.
4. Residents and staff in some institutions, such as prisons and facilities for the developmentally disabled, who have close contact with patients with hepatitis A.
5. Persons exposed to feces of infected patients usually in association with an unsuspected index patient who is fecally incontinent.

IG use might be effective in preventing food-borne or water-borne hepatitis A if exposure is recognized in time. However, IG is not recommended for persons exposed to a common source of hepatitis infection after cases have begun to occur, since the 2-week period during which IG is effective will have been exceeded. If a food handler is diagnosed as having hepatitis A, common-source transmis-sion is possible but uncommon. IG should be administered to other food handlers but is usually not recommended for patrons. However, IG administration to patrons may be considered if all of the following conditions exist: (1) the infected person is directly involved in handling, without gloves, foods that will not be cooked before they are eaten; (2) the hygienic practices of the food handler are deficient, or the food handler has had diarrhea; and (3) patrons can be identified and treated within 2 weeks of exposure. Situations in which repeated exposures may have occurred, such as in institutional cafeterias, may warrant stronger consideration of IG use.

Hepatitis B Prevention Strategies in the United States

The incidence of reported acute hepatitis B cases increased steadily over the past decade and reached a peak in 1985 (11.50 cases/105/year), despite the introduction of hepatitis B vaccine 3 years previously. Incidence decreased modestly (18%) by 1988 but still remains higher than a decade ago. This minimal impact of hepatitis B vaccine on disease incidence is attributable to several factors. The sources of infection for most cases include intravenous drug abuse (28%), heterosexual contact with infected persons or multiple partners (22%), and homosexual activity (9%). In addition, 30% of patients with hepatitis B deny any of the recognized risk factors for infection.

The present strategy for hepatitis B prevention is to vaccinate all babies, as well as those individuals at high risk of infection. Most persons receiving vaccine as a result of this strategy are persons at risk of acquiring HBV infection through occupational exposure, a group that accounts for approximately 4% of cases. The major deterrents to vaccinating the other high-risk groups include the lack of knowledge about the risk of disease and its consequences, the lack of public-sector programs, the cost of vaccine, and the inability to access most of the high-risk populations.

For vaccine to have an impact on the incidence of hepatitis B, a comprehensive strategy must be developed that will provide hepatitis B vaccination to persons before they engage in behaviors or occupations that place them at risk of infection. Universal HBsAg screening of pregnant women was recently recommended to prevent perinatal HBV transmission. The previous recommendations for selective screening failed to identify most HBsAg-positive pregnant women. Universal immunization of neonates and adolescents would be expected to successfully prevent infection before entering into a high-risk group. Immunization between infancy and adolescence is suggested only for those children who were not immunized as infants, particularly in those who are in groups where person-to-person transmission has been documented to be significant. This group includes Alaskan natives, Pacific Islanders, and children of immigrants from countries that experience high rates of HBV infection.

Hepatitis B Prophylaxis

Two types of products are available for prophylaxis against hepatitis B. Hepatitis B vaccines, first licensed in 1981, provide active immunization against HBV infection, and their use is recommended for both preexposure and postexposure prophylaxis. HBIG provides temporary, passive protection and is indicated only in certain postexposure settings.

HBIG

HBIG is prepared from plasma preselected to contain a high titer of anti-HBs. In the United States, HBIG has an anti-HBs titer of >100,000 by radioimmunoassay (RIA). Human plasma from which HBIG is prepared is screened for antibodies to HIV; in addition, the Cohn fractionation process used to prepare this product inactivates and eliminates HIV from the final product. There is no evidence that the causative agent of AIDS (HIV) has been transmitted by HBIG.

Hepatitis B Vaccine

Two types of hepatitis B vaccines are currently licensed in the United States. Plasma-derived vaccine consists of a suspension of inactivated, alum-adsorbed, 22-nm HBsAg particles that have been purified from human plasma by a combination of biophysical (ultracentrifugation) and biochemical procedures. Inactivation is a threefold process using 8 M urea; pepsin at pH 2; and 1:4,000 formalin. These treatment steps have been shown to inactivate representatives of all classes of viruses found in human blood, including HIV. Plasma-derived vaccine is no longer being produced in the United States, and use is now limited to hemodialysis patients, other immunocompromised hosts, and persons with known allergy to yeast.

Currently licensed recombinant hepatitis B vaccines are produced by *Saccharomyces cerevisiae* (common baker's yeast), into which a plasmid con-

taining the gene for the HBsAg has been inserted. Purified HBsAg is obtained by lysing the yeast cells and separating HBsAg from yeast components by biochemical and biophysical techniques. These vaccines contain more than 95% HBsAg protein. Yeast-derived protein constitutes no more than 5% of the final product.

The recommended series of 3 intramuscular doses of hepatitis B vaccine induces an adequate antibody response in >90% of healthy adults and in >95% of infants, children, and adolescents from birth through 19 years of age. The deltoid (arm) is the recommended site for hepatitis B vaccination of adults and children; immunogenicity of vaccine for adults is substantially lower when injections are given in the buttock. Larger vaccine doses (2 or 4 times normal adult dose) or an increased number of doses (4 doses) are required to induce protective antibody in a high proportion of hemodialysis patients and may also be necessary for other immunocompromised persons (such as those on immunosuppressive drugs or with HIV infection). An adequate antibody response is 10 milli–International Units (mIU)/ml, approximately equivalent to 10 sample ratio units (SRU) by RIA or positive by enzyme immunoassay (EIA), measured 1 to 6 months after completion of the vaccine series.

Field trials of the vaccines licensed in the United States have shown 80% to 95% efficacy in preventing infection or clinical hepatitis among susceptible persons. Protection against illness is virtually complete for persons who develop an adequate antibody response after vaccination. The duration of protection and need for booster doses are not yet fully defined. Between 30% and 50% of persons who develop adequate antibody after three doses of vaccine will lose detectable antibody within 7 years, but protection against viremic infection and clinical disease appears to persist. Immunogenicity and efficacy of the licensed vaccines for hemodialysis patients are much lower than in normal adults. Protection in this group may last only as long as adequate antibody levels persist.

Vaccine Usage

Primary vaccination comprises 3 intramuscular doses of vaccine, with the second and third doses given 1 and 6 months, respectively, after the first. Adults and older children should be given a full 1.0 ml/dose, whereas children <11 years of age should usually receive half (0.5 ml) this dose. See Table 11-5 for complete information on age-specific dosages of currently available vaccines.

An alternative schedule of four doses of vaccine given at 0, 1, 2, and 12 months has been approved for one vaccine for postexposure prophylaxis or for more rapid induction of immunity. However, there is no clear evidence that this regimen provides greater protection than the standard 3-dose series. Hepatitis B vaccine should be given only in the deltoid muscle for adults and children or in the anterolateral thigh muscle for infants and neonates. For patients undergoing hemodialysis and for other immunosuppressed patients, higher-vaccine doses or increased numbers of doses are required. A special formulation of one vaccine is available for such persons (see Table 11-5). Persons with HIV infection have an impaired response to hepatitis B vaccine. The immunogenicity of higher doses of vaccine is unknown for this group, and firm recommendations on dosage cannot be made at this time.

Vaccine doses administered at longer intervals provide equally satisfactory protection, but optimal protection is not conferred until after the third dose. If the vaccine series is interrupted after the first dose, the second and third doses should be given separated by an interval of 3 to 5 months. Persons who are late for the third dose should be given this dose when convenient. Postvaccination testing is not considered necessary in either situation.

In one study the response to vaccination by the standard schedule using 1 or 2 doses of one vaccine, followed by the remaining doses of a different vaccine, was comparable to the response to vaccination with a single vaccine. Moreover, because the immunogenicities of the available vaccines are similar, it is likely that responses in such situations will be comparable to those induced by any of the vaccines alone.

The immunogenicity of a series of 3 low doses (0.1 standard dose) of plasma-derived hepatitis B vaccine administered by the intradermal route has been assessed in several studies. The largest studies of adults show lower rates of developing adequate antibody (80% to 90%) and twofold to fourfold lower antibody titers than with intramuscular vaccination with recommended doses. Data on immunogenicity of low doses of recombinant vaccines given intradermally are limited. The principal advantage is the lower cost of vaccination with lower concentrations of vaccine antigen, which is a factor in some countries, and the possible enhanced immunogenicity in dialysis patients when it is given repeatedly for many doses. At this time, intradermal vaccination of adults using low doses of vaccine should be done only under research protocol, with appropriate informed consent and with postvaccination testing to identify persons with inadequate response who would be eligible for revaccination. Intradermal vaccination is not recommended for infants or children.

All hepatitis B vaccines are noninfective products, and there is no evidence of interference with other simultaneously administered vaccines.

Table 11-5 Recommended doses and schedules of currently licensed HB vaccines

| | Vaccine | | | | | |
| | Heptavax-B*,† | | Recombivax HB* | | Engerix-B*,‡ | |
Group	Dose (μg)	(ml)	Dose (μg)	(ml)	Dose (μg)	(ml)
Infants of HBV-carrier mothers	10	(0.5)	5	(0.5)	10	(0.5)
Other infants and children <11 years	10	(0.5)	2.5	(0.25)	10	(0.5)
Children and adolescents 11-19 years	20	(1.0)	5	(0.5)	20	(1.0)
Adults >19 years	20	(1.0)	10	(1.0)	20	(1.0)
Dialysis patients and other immunocompromised persons	40	(2.0)§	40	(1.0)‖	40	(2.0)§,¶

*Usual schedule: 3 doses at 0, 1, 6 months.
†Available only for hemodialysis and other immunocompromised patients and for persons with known allergy to yeast.
‡Alternative schedule: 4 doses at 0, 1, 2, 12 months.
§Two 1.0-ml doses given at different sites.
‖Special formulation for dialysis patients.
¶Four-dose schedule recommended at 0, 1, 2, 6 months.

Data are not available on the safety of hepatitis B vaccines for the developing fetus. Because the vaccines contain only noninfectious HBsAg particles, there should be no risk to the fetus. In contrast, HBV infection of a pregnant woman may result in severe disease for the mother and chronic infection of the newborn. Therefore pregnancy or lactation should not be considered a contraindication to the use of this vaccine for persons who are otherwise eligible.

Vaccine Storage and Shipment

Vaccine should be shipped and stored at 2° C to 8° C but not frozen. Freezing destroys the potency of the vaccine.

Side Effects and Adverse Reactions

The most common side effect observed following vaccination with each of the available vaccines has been soreness at the injection site. Postvaccination surveillance for 3 years after licensure of the plasma-derived vaccine showed an association of borderline significance between Guillain-Barré syndrome and receipt of the first vaccine dose. The rate of this occurrence was very low (0.5 per 100,000 vaccinees) and was more than compensated for by disease prevented by the vaccine, even if Guillain-Barré syndrome is a true side effect. Such postvaccination surveillance information is not available for the recombinant hepatitis B vaccines. Early concerns about safety of plasma-derived vaccine have proven to be unfounded, particularly the concern that infectious agents such as HIV present in the donor plasma pools might contaminate the final product.

Effect of Vaccination on Carriers and Immune Persons

Hepatitis B vaccine produces neither therapeutic nor adverse effects for HBV carriers. Vaccination of individuals who possess antibodies against HBV from a previous infection is not necessary, but it will not cause adverse effects. Such individuals will have a postvaccination increase in their anti-HBs levels. Passively acquired antibody, whether acquired from HBIG or IG administration or from the transplacental route, will not interfere with active immunization.

Prevaccination Serologic Testing for Susceptibility. The decision to test potential vaccine recipients for prior infection is primarily a cost-effectiveness issue and should be based on whether the costs of testing balance the costs of vaccine saved by not vaccinating individuals who have already been infected. Estimation of cost-effectiveness of testing depends on three variables: the cost of vaccination, the cost of testing for susceptibility, and the expected prevalence of immune individuals in the group. Testing in groups with the highest risk of HBV infection (HBV marker prevalence of >20%) is usually cost-effective unless testing costs are extremely high. Cost-effectiveness of screening may be marginal for groups at intermediate risk. For groups with a low expected prevalence of HBV serologic markers, such as health professionals in their training years, prevaccination testing is not cost-effective. For routine testing, only one antibody test is necessary (either anti-HBc or anti-HBs). Anti-HBc identifies all previously infected persons, both carriers and noncarriers, but does not differentiate members of the two groups. Anti-HBs identifies persons previously infected, except for carriers. Neither test has a particular advantage for groups expected to have carrier rates of <2%, such as health-care workers. Anti-HBc may be preferred to avoid unnecessary vaccination of carriers for groups with higher carrier rates. If RIA is used to test for anti-HBs, a minimum of 10 sample ratio units should be used to designate immunity (2.1 is the usual designation of a positive test). If EIA is used, the positive level recommended by manufacturers is appropriate.

Postvaccination Testing for Serologic Response and Revaccination of Nonresponders. Hepatitis B vaccine, when given in the deltoid, produces protective antibody (anti-HBs) in >90% of healthy persons. Testing for immunity after vaccination is not recommended routinely but is advised for persons whose subsequent management depends on knowing their immune status (such as dialysis patients and staff). Testing for immunity is also advised for persons for whom a suboptimal response may be anticipated, such as those who have received vaccine in the buttock, persons >50 years of age, and persons known to have HIV infection. Postvaccination testing should also be considered for persons at occupational risk who may have needle-stick exposures necessitating post-exposure prophylaxis. When necessary, postvaccination testing should be done between 1 and 6 months after completion of the vaccine series to provide definitive information on response to the vaccine.

Revaccination of persons who do not respond to the primary series (nonresponders) produces adequate antibody in 15% to 25% after 1 additional dose and in 30% to 50% after 3 additional doses when the primary vaccination has been given in the deltoid. Some individuals appear to be nonresponders by virtue of their HLA-DR type (Hsu et al., 1993; Watanabe et al., 1988). Such individuals are not likely to respond when vaccinated with the same antigen. In the future, immunization with a DNA-based vaccine may prove useful in this situation, since studies performed in "nonresponder" mice suggest that such an approach may extend the spectrum of immunogenic epitopes (Schirmbeck et al., 1995).

For persons who do not respond to a primary vaccine series given in the buttock, data suggest that revaccination in the arm induces adequate antibody in >75%. Revaccination with 1 or more additional doses should be considered for persons who fail to respond to vaccination in the deltoid and is recommended for those who have failed to respond to vaccination in the buttock.

Need for Vaccine Booster Doses

Available data show that vaccine-induced antibody levels decline steadily with time and that up to 50% of adult vaccinees who respond adequately to vaccine may have low or undetectable antibody levels by 7 years after vaccination. Nevertheless, both adults and children with declining antibody levels are still protected against hepatitis B disease. Current data also suggest excellent protection against disease for 5 years after vaccination among infants born to hepatitis B–carrier mothers. For adults and children with normal immune status, booster doses are not routinely recommended within 7 years after vaccination, nor is routine serologic testing to assess antibody levels necessary for vaccine recipients during this period. For infants born to hepatitis B–carrier mothers, booster doses are not necessary within 5 years after vaccination. The possible need for booster doses after longer intervals will be assessed as additional information becomes available.

For hemodialysis patients, for whom vaccine-induced protection is less complete and may persist only as long as antibody levels remain above 10 mIU/ml, the need for booster doses should be assessed by annual antibody testing, and booster doses should be given when antibody levels decline to <10 mIU/ml.

Groups Recommended for Preexposure Vaccination

Persons at substantial risk of HBV infection who are demonstrated or judged likely to be susceptible should be vaccinated. They include the following:

1. Persons with occupational risk (i.e., health-care and public-safety workers).
2. Clients and staff of institutions for the developmentally disabled.
3. Staff of nonresidential day-care programs (e.g., schools, sheltered workshops for the developmentally disabled) attended by known HBV carriers.
4. Susceptible hemodialysis patients.
5. Sexually active homosexual men.
6. Users of illicit injectable drugs who are susceptible to HBV.
7. Household and sexual contacts of HBV carriers.
8. Families accepting orphans or unaccompanied minors from countries of high or intermediate HBV endemicity who prove to be chronic carriers.
9. Populations with high endemicity of HBV infection (e.g., Alaskan natives, Pacific Islanders, and refugees from HBV-endemic areas).
10. Inmates (and possibly workers) of long-term correctional facilities.
11. Sexually active heterosexual persons with multiple sexual partners.
12. Persons who plan to reside for more than 6 months in areas with high levels of endemic HBV and who will have close contact with the local population.

Ideally, hepatitis B vaccination of travelers should begin at least 6 months before travel to allow for completion of the full vaccine series. Nevertheless, a partial series will offer some protection from HBV infection. The alternative 4-dose schedule may provide better protection during travel if the first 3 doses can be delivered before travel (second and third doses given 1 and 2 months, respectively, after the first).

Postexposure Prophylaxis for Hepatitis B

Prophylactic treatment to prevent hepatitis B infection after exposure to HBV should be considered in the following situations: perinatal exposure of an infant born to an HBsAg-positive mother, accidental percutaneous or permucosal exposure to HBsAg-positive blood, sexual exposure to an HBsAg-positive person, and household exposure of an infant <12 months of age to a primary caregiver who has acute hepatitis B.

Various studies have established the relative efficacies of HBIG and hepatitis B vaccine in different exposure situations. For an infant with perinatal exposure to an HBsAg-positive and HBeAg-positive mother, a regimen combining 1 dose of HBIG at birth with the hepatitis B vaccine series started soon after birth is 85% to 95% effective in preventing development of the HBV carrier state. Regimens involving either multiple doses of HBIG alone or the vaccine series alone have 70% to 85% efficacy.

For accidental percutaneous exposure only regimens including HBIG or IG have been studied. A regimen of 2 doses of HBIG, 1 given after exposure and 1 a month later, is about 75% effective in preventing hepatitis B in this setting. For sexual exposure a single dose of HBIG is 75% effective if given within 2 weeks of last sexual exposure. The efficacy of IG for postexposure prophylaxis is uncertain. Because of the availability of HBIG and the wider use of hepatitis B vaccine, IG no longer has a role in postexposure prophylaxis of hepatitis B.

Recommendations on postexposure prophylaxis are based on available efficacy data and on the likelihood of future HBV exposure of the person requiring treatment. In all exposures a regimen combining HBIG with hepatitis B vaccine will provide both short- and long-term protection, will be less costly than the 2-dose HBIG treatment alone, and is the treatment of choice.

Perinatal Exposure and Recommendations

Transmission of HBV from mother to infant during the perinatal period represents one of the most efficient modes of HBV infection and often leads to severe long-term sequelae. Infants born to HBsAg-positive and HBeAg-positive mothers have a 70% to 90% chance of acquiring perinatal HBV infection, and 85% to 90% of infected infants will become chronic HBV carriers. Estimates are that >25% of these carriers will die from primary hepatocellular carcinoma (PHC) or cirrhosis of the liver. Infants born to HBsAg-positive and HbeAg-negative mothers have a lower risk of acquiring perinatal infection; however, such infants have had acute disease, and fatal fulminant hepatitis has been reported. Based on 1987 data in the United States, an estimated 18,000 births occur to HBsAg-positive women each year, resulting in approximately 4,000 infants who become chronic HBV carriers. Prena-

tal screening of all pregnant women identifies those who are HBsAg-positive and allows treatment of their newborns with HBIG and hepatitis B vaccine, a regimen that is 85% to 95% effective in preventing the development of the HBV chronic carrier state.

On February 26, 1991, the ACIP recommended that universal vaccination of infants be incorporated in the routine immunization schedule for infants and children in the United States. The two options proposed by the ACIP committee and the Committee on Infectious Diseases of the American Academy of Pediatrics are as follows:

Option 1. First dose at birth, second dose at 1 to 2 months, and third dose at 6 to 18 months.

Option 2. First dose at 1 to 2 months, second dose at 4 months, and third dose at 6 to 18 months.

The optimal time for immunization of preterm infants has not been determined, but it is suggested that immunization be delayed until the child has achieved a weight of 2 kg or until 2 months of age, when other immunizations are offered.

The ACIP recommendations describing a comprehensive strategy for eliminating transmission of HBV in the United States through universal childhood vaccination are given in the following CDC Morbidity and Mortality Weekly Report (1991).

Postexposure Prophylaxis for HCV

The ACIP has offered the following recommendations: "Recent studies indicate that IG does not protect against infection with HCV. Thus, available data do not support the use of IG for prophylaxis of HCV."

Preexposure Prophylaxis of HDV

Prevention of HDV currently depends on preventing chronic HBV infection as HDV requires HBV for its replication. No products exist which can prevent HDV infection in HBV chronic carriers.

Preexposure Prophylaxis of HEV

No products are available to prevent HEV. IG prepared from plasma of individuals residing in non–HEV endemic areas is not effective. The efficacy of an IG prepared from plasma of individuals in an endemic area is unclear.

BIBLIOGRAPHY

Acute Hepatic Failure Study Group. Failure of specific immunotherapy in fulminant type B hepatitis. Ann Intern Med 1977;86:272.

Alpert E, Isselbacher KJ, Schur PH: The pathogenesis of arthritis associated with viral hepatitis. N Engl J Med 1971; 285:185.

Alter HJ: The infectivity of the healthy hepatitis B surface antigen carrier. In Bianchi L, Gerok W, Sickinger K, Stalder GA (eds). Virus and the liver. Lancaster, England: M.T.P. Press, Ltd, 1980.

Alter HJ: Posttransfusion hepatitis: clinical features, risk, and donor testing. In Dodd RY, Barker LF (eds). Infection, immunity, and blood transfusion. New York: Alan R Liss, 1985.

Alter JH, Purcell RH, Shih JW, et al. Detection of antibody to hepatitis C virus in prospectively followed transfusion recipients with acute and chronic non-A, non-B hepatitis. N Engl J Med 1989;321:1494-1500.

Alter MS, Margolis H, Krawczynski K, et al. The natural history of community-acquired hepatitis C in the United States. N Engl J Med 1992;327:1899-1905.

Bacon PA, Doherty SM, Zuckerman AJ. Hepatitis B antibody in polymyalgia rheumatics. Lancet 1975;2:476.

Bahn A, Hilbert K, Matine U, et al. Selection of a precore mutant after vertical transmission of different hepatitis B virus mutants is correlated with fulminant hepatitis in infants. J Med Virol 1995;47:336-341.

Balayan MS, Anlzhaparidze AG, Savinskaya SS, et al. Evidence for a virus in non-A, non-B hepatitis transmitted via the fecal-oral route. Intervirology 1981;20:23.

Barker LF, Chisari FV, McGrath PP, et al. Transmission of type B viral hepatitis to chimpanzees. J Infect Dis 1973; 127:648.

Baroudy BM, Ticehurse JR, Miele TA, et al. Sequence analysis of hepatitis A virus cDNA coding for capsed proteins and RNA polymerase. Proc Natl Acad Sci USA 1985; 82:2143-2147.

Bayer ME, Blumberg BS, Werner B: Particles associated with Australia antigen in the sera of patients with leukemia, Down's syndrome, and hepatitis. Nature 1968;218:1057.

Beasley RP, Hwang L-Y, Lin C-C, et al. Incidence of hepatitis among students at a university in Taiwan. Am J Epidemiol 1983;117:213-222.

Bjoro K, Froland S, Yun Z, et al. Hepatitis C infection in patients with primary hypogammaglobulinemia after treatment with contaminated immuno globulin. N Engl J Med 1994; 331:1607-1611.

Blumberg BS, Alter HJ, Visnich S. A "new" antigen in leukemia sera. JAMA 1965;191:541.

Boyer JL, Klatskin G. Pattern of necrosis in acute viral hepatitis: prognostic value of bridging (subacute hepatic necrosis). N Engl J Med 1970;283:1063.

Bradley DW, Krawczynski K, Cook EH, et al. Enterically transmitted non-A, non-B hepatitis: serial passage of disease in cynomologous macaques and tumorous and recovery of disease-associated 27-34 nm viruslike particles. Proc Natl Acad Sci 1987;84:6277-6281.

Brzosko WJ, Krawczynski K, Nazarewicz T, et al. Glomerulonephritis associated with hepatitis B surface antigen immune complexes in children. Lancet 1974;2:477.

Buitrago B, Popper H, Hadler SC, et al. Specific histologic features of Santa Marta hepatitis: a severe form of hepatitis D virus infection in northern South America. Hepatology 1986;6:1285-1291.

Centers for Disease Control. Protection against viral hepatitis. MMWR 1990;39/52:1-26.

Centers for Disease Control. Hepatitis B Virus: A comprehensive strategy for eliminating transmission in the United States through universal childhood vaccination. MMWR 1991;40(RR-13):1–25.

Chalmers TG, et al. Treatment of acute infectious hepatitis. Controlled studies of the effects of diet, rest, and physical reconditioning on the acute course of the disease and on the incidence of relapses and residual abnormalities. J Clin Invest 1955;34:1163.

Chau KH, Hargie MP, Decker RH, et al. Serodiagnosis of recent hepatitis B infection by IgM class anti-HBc. Hepatology 1983;3:141.

Choo QL, Kuo G, Weiner AJ, et al. Isolation of a cDNA derived from blood-borne non-A, non-B viral hepatitis genome. Science 1989;244:359-361.

Combes B, Shorey J, Barrera et al. Glomerulonephritis with deposition of Australia antigen-antibody complexes in glomerular basement membrane. Lancet 1971;2:234.

Daemer RJ, Feinstone SM, Gust ID, et al. Propagation of human hepatitis A virus in African green monkey kidney cell culture: primary isolation and serial passage. Infect Immunol 1981: 32:388.

Dane DS, Cameron CH, Briggs M. Viruslike particles in serum of patients with Australia-antigen–associated hepatitis. Lancet 1970;1:695.

DeCock, KMD, Bradley DW, Sanford NL, et al. Epidemic non-A, non-B hepatitis in patients from Pakistan. Ann Intern Med 1987;106:227.

Deinhardt F, Holmes AW, Capps RB, Popper H. Studies on the transmission of human viral hepatitis to marmoset monkeys: I. transmission of disease, serial passages, and description of liver lesions. J Exp Med 1966;125:673.

Delaplane D, Yogev R, Crussi G, Schulman ST. Fatal hepatitis in early infancy. Pediatrics 1983;72:176.

Desmyter J, DeGoote J, Desmet VJ, et al. Administration of human fibroblast interferon in chronic hepatitis-B infection. Lancet 1976;2:645.

DiBisceglie AM, Hoofnagle JH. Antiviral therapy of chronic viral hepatitis. Am J Gastroenterol 1990;85:650-654.

DiBisceglie AM, Martin P, Kassianides C, et al. Recombinant interferon alpha therapy for chronic hepatitis C: a randomized, double-blind, placebo-controlled trial. N Engl J Med 1989;321:1506-1510.

Dienstag JL, Feinstone SM, Kapikian AZ, Purcell RH. Fecal shedding of hepatitis-A antigen. Lancet 1975a;1:765.

Dienstag JL, et al. Experimental infection of chimpanzees with hepatitis A virus. J Infect Dis 1975b;132:532.

Duermeyer W, van der Veen J, Koster B. ELISA in hepatitis A. Lancet 1978;1:823.

Dupuy JW, Frommel D, Alagille D. Severe viral hepatitis type B in infants. Lancet 1975;1:191.

Edmondson HA. Needle biopsy in differential diagnosis of acute liver disease. JAMA 1965;191:136.

Enomoto N, Sakuma I, Asahina Y, et al. Comparison of full-length sequences of interferon-sensitive and resistant hepatitis C virus 1b: sensitivity to interferon is conferred by amino acid substitutions in the NS5A region. J Clin Invest 1995;96:224-230.

Farci P, Alter HJ, Wong D, et al. A long-term study of hepatitis C virus replication in non-A, non-B hepatitis. N Engl J Med 1991;325:98-104.

Fawaz KA, Grady GF, Kaplan MM, Gellis SS. Repetitive maternal-fetal transmission of fatal hepatitis B. N Engl J Med 1975;293:1357.

Feinstone SM, Kapikian AZ, Purcell RH. Hepatitis A: detection by immune electron microscopy of a viruslike antigen associated with acute illness. Science 1973;182:1026.

Gauss-Muller V, Frosner GG, Deinhardt F. Propagation of hepatitis A virus in human embryo fibroblasts. J Med Virol 1981;7:233.

Gerber MA, Thung SN. The diagnostic value of immunohistochemical demonstration of hepatitis viral antigens in the liver. Hum Pathol 1987;18:771-774.

Giacchinno R, Picciotto A, Tasso L, et al. Vertical transmission of hepatitis C. Lancet 1995;345:1122-1123.

Gianotti F. Papular acrodermatitis of childhood: an Australia antigen disease. Arch Dis Child 1973;48:794.

Gimson AE, Tedder RS, White YS, et al. Serological markers in fulminant hepatitis. B Gut 1983;24:615-617.

Gocke DJ. Extrahepatic manifestations of viral hepatitis. Am J Med Sci 1975;270:49.

Gocke DJ, Hsv K, Morgan C, et al. Association between polyarteritis and Australia antigen. Lancet 1970;3:1149.

Gocke DJ, et al. Vasculitis in association with Australia antigen. J Exp Med 1971;134:330.

Govindarajan S, Chin KP, Redeker AG, et al. Fulminant B viral hepatitis: role of delta agent. Gastroenterology 1984; 86:1417-1420.

Hadler SC, DeMonzon M, Ponzetto A, et al. Delta virus infection and severe hepatitis: an epidemic in Yuepa Indians of Venezuela. Ann Intern Med 1984;100:339-344.

Hasewaga K, Hvang JK, Wands JR, et al. Association of hepatitis B viral precore mutations with fulminant hepatitis B in Japan. Virology 1991;185(1):460-463.

Havens WP Jr, Ward R, Drill VA, Paul JR. Experimental production of hepatitis by feeding icterogenic materials. Proc Soc Exp Biol Med 1944;53:206.

Heathcote J, Cameron CH, Dane DS. Hepatitis-B antigen in saliva and semen. Lancet 1974;1:71.

Hirschman RJ et al. Viruslike particles in sera of patients with infectious and serum hepatitis. JAMA 1969;208:1667.

Hollinger FB, Bradley DW, Dreesman GR, et al. Detection of hepatitis A viral antigen by radioimmunoassay. J Immunol 1975;115:1464.

Holmes AW, Wolfe L, Rosenblate H, et al. Hepatitis in marmosets: induction of disease with coded specimens from a human volunteer study. Science 1969;165:816.

Hoofnagle JH. Antiviral treatment of chronic type B hepatitis. Ann Intern Med 1987;107:413-415.

Hoofnagle JH, DiBisceglie AM. Serologic diagnosis of acute and chronic viral hepatitis. Sem Liver Dis 1991.

Hoofnagle JH, Peters M, Mullen KD, et al. Randomized, controlled trial of recombinant human alpha interferon in patients with chronic hepatitis B. Gastroenterology 1988; 95:1318-1325.

Hsu HY, Chang MH, Ho HN, et al. Association of HLA-DR14-DR52 with low responsiveness to hepatitis B vaccine in Chinese residents in Taiwan. Vaccine 1993;11:1437-1440.

Ishimaru Y, Ishimaru H, Toda G, et al. An epidemic of infantile papular acrodermatitic (Gianotti's disease) in Japan associated with hepatitis B surface antigen subtype ayw. Lancet 1976;1:707.

Kane MA, Bradley DW, Shrestha SM, et al. Epidemic non-A, non-B hepatitis in Nepal. JAMA 1984;252:3140-3145.

Karvountzis GD, Redeker AG, Peters RL. Long-term follow-up studies of patients surviving fulminant viral hepatitis. Gastroenterology 1974;67:870.

Khuroo MS. Study of an epidemic of non-A, non-B hepatitis. Am J Med 1980;68:818-824.

Khuroo MS, Kamili S, Jameel S. Vertical transmission of hepatitis E virus. Lancet 1995;345:1025-1026.

Kohler PF, Cronin RE, Hammond WS, et al. Chronic membranous glomerulonephritis caused by hepatitis B antigen-antibody immune complexes. Ann Intern Med 1974;81:488.

Kojima S, Shibayoma T, Sato A, et al. Propagation of human hepa-titis A virus in conventional cell lines. J Med Virol 1981; 7:273.

Krawitt E. Autoimmune hepatitis. N Engl J Med 1996;334:897-903.

Krugman S. Viral hepatitis, type B: prospects for active immunization. Am J Med Sci 1975;270:391.

Krugman S. Incubation period of type B hepatitis. N Engl J Med 1979;300:625.

Krugman S, Friedman H, Lattimer C. Viral hepatitis, type A: identification by specific complement fixation and immune adherence tests. N Engl J Med 1975;292:1141.

Krugman S, Giles JP. Viral hepatitis: new light on an old disease. JAMA 1970;212:1019.

Krugman S, Giles JP. Viral hepatitis type B (MS-2 strain): further observations on natural history and prevention. N Engl J Med 1973;288:755.

Krugman S, Giles JP, Hammond J. Infectious hepatitis: evidence for two distinctive clinical, epidemiological, and immunological types of infection. JAMA 1967;200:365.

Krugman S, Giles JP, Hammond J. Hepatitis virus: effect of heat on the infectivity and antigenicity of the MS-1 and MS-2 strains. J Infect Dis 1970;122:432.

Krugman S, Giles JP, Hammond J. Viral hepatitis, type B (MS-2 strain): prevention with specific hepatitis B immune serum globulin. JAMA 1971a;218:1665.

Krugman S, Giles JP, Hammond J. Viral hepatitis, type B (MS-2 strain): studies on active immunization. JAMA 1971b;217:41.

Krugman S, Ward R. Infectious hepatitis: current status of prevention with gamma globulin. Yale J Biol Med 1962;34:329.

Krugman S, Ward R, Giles JP. The natural history of infectious hepatitis. Am J Med 1962;32:717.

Krugman S, Ward R, Giles JP, Jacobs AM. Infectious hepatitis: studies on the effect of gamma globulin and on the incidence of inapparent infection. JAMA 1960;174:825.

Krugman S, Hoofnagle JH, Gerety RI, et al: Viral hepatitis, type B: DNA polymerase activity and antibody to hepatitis B core antigen. N Engl J Med 1974;290:1331.

Krugman S et al. Viral hepatitis, type B: studies on natural history and prevention reexamined. N Engl J Med 1979; 300:101.

Kuo G, Choo QL, Alter HJ, et al. An assay for circulating antibodies to a major ecologic virus of human non-A, non-B hepatitis. Science 1989;244:362-364.

Lai CL, Lok ASF, Lin HJ, et al. Placebo-controlled trial of recombinant alpha-2 interferon in Chinese patients with chronic hepatitis B infection. Lancet 1987;2:877-880.

LeBouvier GL. Subspecificities of the Australia antigen complex. Am J Dis Child 1972;123:420.

Levo Y, Gorevic PD, Kassab HJ, et al. Association between hepatitis B virus and essential mixed cryoglobulinemia. N Engl J Med 1977; 296:1501.

Liang TJ, Hasegawa K, Rimon N et al. A hepatitis B virus mutant associated with an epidemic of fulminant hepatitis. New Engl;324(24):1705-1709.

Lieberman HM, La Breeque DR, Kew MC, et al. Detection of hepatitis B virus DNA directly in human serum by a simplified molecular hybridization tests: comparison to HBeAg/anti-HBe status in BhsAg carriers. Hepatology 1983;3:285.

Linnen J, Wages J, Zhang-Kack ZY, et al. Molecular cloning and disease association of hepatitis G virus: a transfusion-transmissible agent. Science 1996;271:505-508.

Lorenz D, et al. Hepatitis in the marmoset: *Saguinus mystax,* Proc Soc Exp Biol Med 1970;135:348.

Lürman A. Eine Icterusepidemie. Berl Klin Wochenschr 1885;22:20.

MacNab GM, Alexander JJ. Lecatsas G, et al. Hepatitis B surface antigen produced by a human hepatoma cell line. Br J Cancer 1976;34:509.

Martell M, Esteban JI, Quer J, et al. Hepatitis C virus (HCV) circulates as a population of different but closely related genomes: quasispecies nature of HCV genome distribution. J Virol 1992;66:3225-3229.

Mascoli CC, Ittensohn OL, Villarejos VM, et al. Recovery of hepatitis agents in the marmoset from human cases occurring in Costa Rica. Proc Soc Exp Biol Med 1973;143:276.

Maynard JE. Infectivity studies of hepatitis A and B in nonhuman primates. Proc Int Assoc Biol Stand symposium on viral hepatitis, Milan, Italy, December 16-19, 1974.

Maynard JE, Berquist KR, Krushak DH, Purcell RH. Experimental infection of chimpanzees with the virus of hepatitis B. Nature 1972;237:514.

McMahon BJ, Alward WLM, Hall DB, et al. Acute hepatitis B virus infection: relation of age to the clinical expression of disease and subsequent development of the carrier state. J Infect Dis 151:1985;599-603.

McNeil M, Hoy JF, Richards MJ, et al. Etiology of fatal hepatitis in Melbourne. Med J Aust 1984;2:637-640.

Melnick JL. Classification of hepatitis A virus as enterovirus type 72 and of hepatitis B virus as hepadna virus, type 1. Intervirology 1982;18:105.

Meltzer M, Franklin EC, Elias K, et al. Cryoglobulinemia—a clinical and laboratory study: II. cryoglobulins with rheumatoid factor activity. Am J Med 1966;40:837.

Miller WJ, Prorost PJ, McAleer WJ, et al. Specific immune adherence assay for human hepatitis A antibody. Application of diagnostic and epidemiologic investigations. Proc Soc Exp Biol Med 1975;149:254.

Mitsui T, Iwano K, Masuko K, et al. Hepatitis C infection in medical personnel after needle stick accident. Hepatology 1992;16:1109-1114.

Morrow RH Jr, Smetana HF, Sai FT, et al. Unusual features of viral hepatitis in Accra, Ghana. Ann Intern Med 1968; 68:1250-1264.

Murphy BL, Maynard JE, Bradley DW, et al. Immunofluorescence of hepatitis A virus antigen in chimpanzees. Infect Immunol 1978;21:663.

Nagata I, Shiraki K, Tanimoto K, et al. Mother-to-infant transmission of hepatitis C virus. J Pediatr 1992;120:432-434.

Narkewicz, MR, Smith D, Silverman A, et al. Clearance of chronic hepatitis B virus infection in young children after alpha interferon treatment. J Pediatr 1995;127:815-818.

Neefe JR, Gellis SS, Stokes J Jr. Homologous serum hepatitis and infectious (epidemic) hepatitis. Studies in volunteers bearing on immunological and other characteristics of the etiological agents. Am J Med 1946;1:3.

Ohto H, Terazawa S, Sasaki N, et al. Transmission of hepatitis C virus from mother to infants. N Engl J Med 1994; 330:744-750.

Okamoto H, Sugiyama Y, Okada S, et al. Typing hepatitis C virus by polymerase chain reaction with type-specific primers: application to clinical surveys and tracing infectious sources. J Gen Virol 1992;73:673-679.

Palomba E, Manzini P, Flammengo P, et al. Natural history of perinatal hepatitis C virus infection. Clin Infect Dis 1996;23:47-50.

Papaevangelou V, Pollack H, Borkowsky W. (Unpublished.)

Pawlotsky JM, Ben Yahia M, Andre C, et al. Immunologic disorders in C virus chronic active hepatitis: a prospective case-control serotypes. Hepatology 1994;19:841-848.

Pawlotsky JM, Roudot-Thoraval F, Simmonds P, et al. Extrahepatic immunologic manifestations in chronic hepatitis C and hepatitis C serotypes. Ann Int Med 1995;122:169-175.

Perillo RP, Schiff ER, Davis GL, et al. A randomized controlled trial of interferon alpha-2b alone and after prednisone withdrawal for the treatment of chronic hepatitis B. N Engl J Med 1990;323:295-301.

Peterson DA, Hurley TR, Hoff JC, et al. Hepatitis A virus infectivity and chlorine treatment. In Szmuness W, Alter HJ, Maynard JE (eds). Proceedings of the 1981 international symposium on viral hepatitis. Philadelphia: Franklin Institute Press, 1982.

Plouvier B, Wattre P, Devulder B. HBsAg in superficial artery of a patient with polymyalgia rheumatica. Lancet 1978;2:932.

Popper H, Shih JW-K, Gerin JL, et al. Woodchuck hepatitis and hepatocellular carcinoma: correlation of histologic with virologic observations. Hepatology 1981;1:91.

Provost PJ, Giesa PA, McAleer WJ, et al. Isolation of hepatitis A virus in vitro in cell culture directly from human specimens. Proc Soc Exp Biol Med 1981;167:201.

Provost PJ, Hilleman MR. Propagation of human hepatitis A virus in cell culture in vitro. Proc Soc Exp Biol Med 1979;160:213.

Provost PJ, Ittensohn OL, Villarejos VM, Hilleman MR. A specific complement fixation test for human hepatitis A employing CR326 virus antigen: diagnosis and epidemiology. Proc Soc Exp Biol Med 1975a;148:961.

Provost PJ, Wolanski BS, Miller WJ, Ittensohn OL. Biophysical and biochemical properties of CR326 human hepatitis virus. Am J Med Sci 1975b;270:87.

Provost PF, Ittensohn OL, Villarejos VM, et al. Etiologic relationship of marmoset-propagated CR326 hepatitis A virus to hepatitis in man. Proc Soc Exp Biol Med 1973;142(4):1257-1267.

Reyes GR, Purdy MA, Kim JP. Isolation of cDNA from virus responsible for enterically transmitted non-A, non-B hepatitis. Science 1990;247:1335-1339.

Rizzetto M, Canese MG, Arico S, et al. Immunofluorescence detection of new antigen-antibody system associated to hepatitis B virus in liver and serum of HBsAg carriers. Gut 1977;18:997-1003.

Rizzetto M, Ponzetto A, Borino A. Hepatitis delta virus infection: clinical and epidemiological aspects. In (ed). Viral hepatitis and liver disease. New York: Alan R Liss, 1988.

Rizzetto M, Rosina F, Saracco G, et al. Treatment of chronic delta hepatitis with alpha 2 recombinant interferon. J Hepatol 1986;3:S229-S233.

Saito I, Miyamura T, Ohbayashi A, et al. Hepatitis C virus infection is associated with the development of hepatocellular carcinoma. Proc Natl Acad Sci USA 1990;87:6547-6549.

Sampliner RE, Woronow DI, Alter HJ, et al: Community-acquired non-A, non-B hepatitis. J Med Virol 1984;13:125-130.

Schirmbeck R, Bohm W, Ando K, et al. Nucleic acid vaccination primes hepatitis B surface antigen-specific cytotoxic T lymphocytes in nonresponder mice. J Virol 1995; 69:5929-5934.

Schweitzer IL, Wing A, McPeak C, Spears RL. Hepatitis and hepatitis-associated antigen in 56 mother-infant pairs. JAMA 1972;220:1092.

Scotto J, Hadchouel M, Herej C, et al. Detection of hepatitis B virus DNA in serum by a simple spot hybridization technique. Comparison with results for other viral markers. Hepatology 1983;3:279.

Sergent I, Lockshin MD, Christian CL, et al. Vasculitis with hepatis B antigenemia. Long-term observations in nine patients. Medicine 1976;55:1.

Shafritz DA, Kew MC. Identification of integrated hepatitis B virus DNA sequences in human hepatocellular carcinoma. Hepatology 1981;1:1.

Shafritz DA. Variants of hepatitis B virus associated with fulminant liver disease. New Eng J Med 1991;324(24):1737-1739.

Shrestha SM, Kane MA. Preliminary report of non-A, non-B hepatitis in Kathmandu Valley. J Inst Med 1983;5:1-10.

Simmonds P, Alberti A, Alter HJ, et al. A proposed system for nomenclature of hepatitis C virus genotypes. Hepatology 1994;19:1321-1324.

Simmonds P, Holmes EC, Cha TA, et al. Classification of hepatitis C virus into 6 major genotypes and a series of subtypes by phylogenetic analysis of the NS-5 region. J Gen Virol 1993;74:2391-2399.

Smedile A, Farci P, Verme G, et al. Influence of delta infection on severity of hepatitis B. Lancet 1982;2:945.

Stevens CE, Beasley RP, Tsui J, Lee WC. Vertical transmission of hepatitis B antigen in Taiwan. N Engl J Med 1975;292:771.

Stokes J Jr, et al. The carrier-state in viral hepatitis. JAMA 1954;154:1059.

Szmuness W. Hepatocellular carcinoma and hepatitis B virus: evidence for a causal association. Prog Med Virol 1978;24:40.

Szmuness W, Stevens CE, Zang EA, et al. A controlled clinical trial of the efficacy of the hepatitis B vaccine (Heptavax B): a final report. Hepatology 1981;1:377-385.

Szmuness W, et al. Distribution of antibody to hepatitis A antigen in urban adult population. N Engl J Med 1976;295:755.

Szmuness W, Dienstag JL, Purcell RH, et al. The prevalence of antibody to hepatitis A antigen in various parts of the world: a pilot study. Am J Epidemiol 1977;106:392.

Tabor E, Krugman S, Weiss EC, et al. Disappearance of hepatitis B surface antigen during an unusual case of fulminant hepatitis B. J Med Virol 1981;8:277-282.

Thaler MM, Park C-K, Landers DV, et al. Vertical transmission of hepatitis C virus. Lancet 1991;338:17-18.

Ticehurst JR, Recaniello VR, Baroudy BM, et al. Molecular cloning and characterization of hepatitis A virus with DNA. Proc Natl Acad Sci USA 1983;80:5885.

Toda G, Ishimaru Y, Mayumi M, Oda T. Infantile papular acrodermatitis (Gianotti's disease) and intrafamilial occurrence of acute hepatitis B with jaundice: age dependency of clinical manifestations of hepatitis B virus infection. J Infect Dis 1978;138:211.

Trepo CH, Thiyolet J. Hepatitis-associated antigen and periarteritis nodosa (PAN). Vox Sang 1970;19:410.

Trey C. The fulminant hepatic surveillance study. CMA J 1972;106:525.

Villarejos VM, Provost PJ, Ittensohn OL, et al. Seroepidemiologic investigations of human hepatitis caused by A, B, and a possible third virus. Proc Soc Exp Biol Med 1976;152:524.

Wands JR, Mann E, Alpert E, Issel Bacher KJ. The pathogenesis of arthritis associated with acute HB, Ag-positive hepatitis: complement activation and characterization of circulating immune complexes. J Cun Invest 1975;55:930-936.

Ward R, Borchert B, Wright A, Kline E. Hepatitis B antigen in saliva and mouth washing. Lancet 1972;2:726.

Watanabe H, Matsushita S, Kamikawaji N, et al. Immune suppression gene on HLA-Bw54-DR4-DRw53 haplotype controls nonresponsiveness in humans to hepatitis B surface antigen via CD8+ suppressor T-cells. Hum Immunol 1988; 22:9-17.

World Health Organization Expert Committee on Viral Hepatitis. Advances in viral hepatitis. Who Tech Rep Ser No 602, 1977.

Wu JC, Cho KD, Chen CM, et al. Genotyping of hepatitis D virus by restriction fragment length polymorphism and relation to outcome of hepatitis D. Lancet 1995;346:939-941.

Zignego AL, DeCarli M, Monti M, et al. Hepatitis C virus infection of mononuclear cells from peripheral blood and liver infiltrates in chronically infected patients. J Med Virol 1995;47(1):58-64.

12 HERPES SIMPLEX VIRUS

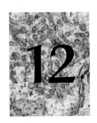

Paula Winter Annunziato

Herpes simplex viruses (HSV) are among the most widely disseminated infectious agents of humans. The ubiquity of these viruses is not generally appreciated because they often do not produce overt disease. However, the various clinical syndromes caused by HSV in infants and children—particularly, neonatal infections, gingivostomatitis, encephalitis, and infections in the immunocompromised—are clinically significant problems.

ETIOLOGY

A member of the herpesvirus group, HSV is composed of an inner core containing linear double-stranded DNA, surrounded concentrically by an icosahedral capsid of approximately 100 nm, an amorphous material termed the *tegument,* and an outer envelope composed of lipids and glycoproteins. Enveloped HSV particles range in size from 150 to 200 nm. HSV usually is considered the prototype of the human herpesviruses, and cytomegalovirus (CMV), varicella-zoster virus (VZV), and Epstein-Barr virus (EBV) resemble it in morphological appearance. The two antigenic types of HSV, types 1 (HSV-1, recently designated human herpes virus 1) and 2 (HSV-2, recently designated human herpes virus 2), show 50% homology of their DNA (Nahmias and Dowdle, 1968). The two types can be distinguished by the following means: (1) restriction enzyme analysis of the DNA (Buchman et al., 1978; Buchman et al., 1979), (2) antigenic structure determined by Western blotting (Growdon et al., 1987), and (3) certain antibody determinations (see the following paragraphs). Subtypes of HSV-1 and HSV-2 can be further distinguished by analysis of viral DNA with restriction enzymes (Buchman et al., 1978; Buchman et al., 1979; Corey, 1982). Subtypes differ in less than 10% of their DNA, and they do not show significant antigenic variation, so they can only be distinguished from one another by DNA analysis.

HSV DNA encodes for a number of structural and nonstructural viral proteins and glycoproteins (g). As with all of the herpesviruses, replication occurs in a regulated cascading sequence, with immediate early alpha genes controlling subsequent transcription and translation of early beta and late γ gene products (Whitley, 1996). Certain alpha genes initiate viral transcription, beta genes control synthesis of proteins and enzymes such as thymidine kinase necessary for viral replication, and γ genes encode structural proteins of HSV, including the glycoproteins. There are at least ten envelope glycoproteins of HSV: gB, gC, gD, gE, gG, gH, gI, gK, gL, and gM. These glycoproteins are antigenic and therefore play an important role in generating immune responses by the infected host. They also play important roles in viral infectivity. Some glycoproteins (gB, gC, gD, and gH) mediate viral attachment to and penetration of host cells; gC binds to the C3b component of complement, and gE binds to the Fc portion of IgG.

The relative importance of immune responses to each of the glycoproteins and to nonstructural proteins (alpha gene products) for protection of the host is the subject of much investigation. Infection with one HSV does not result in immunity to the other type, but there is some indication that partial protection is induced against HSV-2 infection when there is preexisting immunity to HSV-1 (Boucher et al., 1990; Breinig et al., 1990).

Antibody responses to each type of HSV cannot be distinguished by commercially available antibody assays, but they may be detected by Western blot, using known strains of HSV-1 and HSV-2 as antigens. Antibodies to types 1 and 2 can also be distinguished by using gG as the antigen in an immunologic antibody assay such as enzyme-linked immunosorbent assay (ELISA), since gG is distinct for each type of HSV (Whitley, 1996).

189

HSV is readily transmitted to a variety of animals. Animal models are useful for studying viral latency and the effects of antiviral drugs.

Tissue cultures infected with HSV show cytopathic effects characterized by degeneration and clumping of the cells and the presence of typical intranuclear inclusion bodies and giant cells. Infection in tissue cultures is at first focal, reflecting cell-to-cell viral spread, and then generalized throughout a culture, reflecting release of infectious virus into supernatant media.

HSV-1 has been associated chiefly with nongenital infections of the mucous membranes of the mouth, lips, eyes, and of the central nervous system (CNS). HSV-2 most commonly has been associated with genital and neonatal infections. There are no strict anatomic barriers; however, HSV-1 can cause genital and neonatal infection, and HSV-2 can infect the oral mucosa.

Latency

All of the herpesviruses share the characteristic of becoming latent after primary infection; the virus may subsequently reactivate periodically and produce clinical symptoms in certain individuals. The phenomenon of latent infection permits long-term persistence of the virus within the host and potential future transmissibility to others. Presumably, HSV reaches the ganglia during primary infection when the sensory nerve endings, as well as the skin or mucous membranes, are invaded by the virus. Based on studies in animals, HSV is thought to reach the ganglia by retrograde axonal transport. Various factors such as fever, sunlight, stress, and trauma may trigger a recurrent infection, but at times no stimulus is apparent. Sites and, possibly, mechanisms of latent infection vary for different herpesviruses; for both HSV-1 and HSV-2, however, the site of latency is the sensory ganglia. Surgical transection of the trigeminal nerve frequently results in the appearance of herpetic vesicles in the facial skin. In studies of ganglia obtained at autopsy from patients with no clinical evidence of HSV infection at death, it was found that HSV-1 or HSV-2 can be isolated in tissue culture by cocultivation techniques from approximately 50% of trigeminal ganglia and 15% of sacral ganglia (Baringer, 1974; Baringer and Swoveland, 1973).

There is no morphologic or antigenic evidence of the presence of HSV in latently infected ganglia; however, limited amounts of viral RNA are detectable. During latent infection there is consistent expression of RNA that is transcribed in the oppo-

site orientation to and overlapping the part of the alpha gene encoding a viral protein termed the *infected cell protein 0* (ICP0). This RNA is referred to as the *latency-associated transcript* (LAT); it is hypothesized to play a major role in regulating whether an infection will remain latent or reactivate (Stevens et al., 1988; Croen et al., 1987, 1991). The presence of LAT markedly reduces ICP0 expression (Farrell et al., 1991). The role of this transcript in latency, however, has been seriously questioned, since latent HSV infection in animals can be established in its absence (Steiner et al., 1989). It is more likely that LAT has a role in reactivation, since reactivation is limited in guinea pigs and rabbits infected with LAT-deficient HSV (Bloom et al., 1996; Krause et al., 1995; Perng et al., 1994).

Immunologic factors have long been hypothesized to control reactivation of HSV, since immunocompromised patients are at high risk to develop reactivation syndromes, but no specific abnormal or absent immunologic reactions have been consistently implicated. In general, HSV can reactivate despite specific humoral and cell-mediated immunity. The following cells or cell-mediated immune reactions may play roles in host defense against HSV: macrophages, cytotoxic T cells, natural killer (NK) cells, antibody-dependent cellular cytotoxicity (ADCC), and cytokines released as a result of antigenic stimulation of lymphocytes and macrophages (Corey and Spear, 1986). Antibody may play a role by neutralization of virus and participation in ADCC. It seems most likely that specific immune reactions in the host determine the extent to which reactivated HSV is able to multiply and cause disease. The phenomena of viral latency and reactivation, however, probably are regulated by the latently infected cell rather than controlled by the immune system.

PATHOLOGY

The characteristic lesion caused by HSV on the skin is a vesicle and on the mucous membranes is an ulcer. The epidermis but not the dermis is usually involved so that healing followed by scarring is uncommon. Invaded epithelial cells are destroyed by the virus and the associated inflammatory response of the host, sparing an intact superficial cornified layer that covers the vesicle; in the ulcer this upper layer is not present. Cells invaded by HSV demonstrate the following characteristics: coalescence to form multinucleated giant cells, nuclear degeneration, ballooning, and intranuclear inclusions. Cells in deeper tissues characteristically exhibit hemorrhagic necrosis. A biopsy specimen of a herpetic vesicle showing eosinophilic intranuclear inclusions and giant cells is shown in Plate 2, *E*.

CLINICAL MANIFESTATIONS OF PRIMARY INFECTIONS

Primary infections are defined as those that occur in individuals with no preexisting antibody to HSV. The clinical manifestations of primary herpetic infections are determined by a variety of factors including (1) the portal of entry of the virus and (2) host factors such as age, immune competence, and integrity of the cutaneous barrier. The various clinical entities that may be encountered are listed in Fig. 12-1. The most common recognized HSV infection in children is acute gingivostomatitis. The other diseases are relatively uncommon or rare. The incubation period for primary infection is approximately 6 days, with a range of 2 to 20 days. The host-parasite relationship for HSV is shown in Fig. 12-1. Primary infection of a sus-

ceptible host is frequently inapparent for both HSV-1 and HSV-2 (Boucher et al., 1990; Breinig et al., 1990; Brock et al., 1990; Langenberg et al., 1989; Strand et al., 1986). Clinically apparent primary infections may be characterized by a vesicular eruption, fever, and other constitutional symptoms. Recurrent clinical infections usually are characterized by a localized vesicular eruption and absence of constitutional symptoms. The primary infection can be asymptomatic, and recurrent infections can be symptomatic. The primary infection, however, may be symptomatic with asymptomatic recurrences, or there may be any other combination of symptomatic and asymptomatic infections (Corey and Spear, 1986; Langenberg et al., 1989; Strand et al., 1986). Because of this phenomenon, it is impossible to differentiate between primary and recurrent HSV infections on clinical grounds alone.

Acute Herpetic Gingivostomatitis

Acute herpetic gingivostomatitis almost always is caused by HSV-1. Most children have no symptoms during their primary infection with the virus;

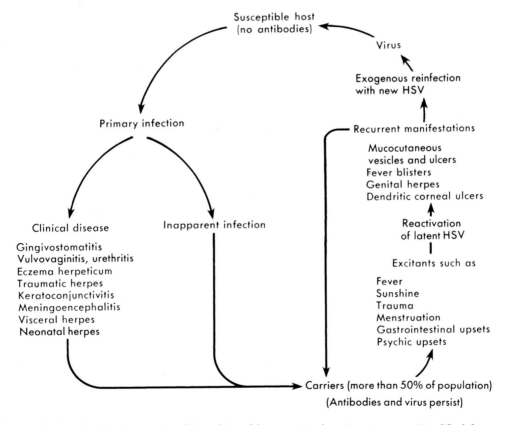

FIG. 12-1 The host-parasite relationship of herpes simplex virus in man. (Modified from Blank H, Rake G: Viral and rickettsial diseases of the skin, eye, and mucous membranes of man, Boston: Little, Brown, 1955.)

an estimated 5% develop clinically apparent gingivostomatitis. Primary infection of the mucous membranes of the mouth occurs most often in the 1- to 4-year age group and occasionally in adolescents and adults. The illness begins with the abrupt onset of fever (39.4° to 40.6° C; 103° to 105° F), irritability, anorexia, and sore mouth. Along with these constitutional symptoms, striking lesions appear on the mucous membranes of the oropharynx. The gums are swollen, reddened, and friable and bleed very easily (Plate 2, A and B). White 2- to 3-mm plaques or shallow ulcers with red areolae develop on the buccal mucosa, tongue, palate, and fauces. The lesions usually appear in the mouth first. Occasionally, however, they may develop first on the tonsils and subsequently progress forward. The regional anterior cervical lymph nodes become enlarged and tender. Satellite vesicular lesions around the mouth are not uncommon. Infants with gingivostomatitis who are thumbsuckers can also infect the thumb (or other fingers) by self-inoculation.

The disease varies considerably in severity and duration. It may be extremely mild, with a paucity of lesions, low-grade fever, and minimal constitutional symptoms. Under these circumstances, the patient improves within 5 to 7 days. On the other hand, an occasional infant is desperately ill with high fever, extensive hemorrhagic mouth lesions, evidence of dehydration and acidosis, and a course that does not abate until the tenth to fourteenth day.

Acute Herpetic Vulvovaginitis

Acute herpetic vulvovaginitis is usually a sexually transmitted infection. An exception is vulvovaginitis that is an unusual manifestation of HSV-1 infection in children secondary to autoinoculation from gingivostomatitis (Krugman, 1952). Vulvovaginitis caused by HSV-2 is not uncommon in sexually active adolescents and adults. The counterpart of this disease in sexually active males is development of penile ulcers and vesicles caused by HSV. The spectrum of disease is similar to that of herpetic gingivostomatitis, with a high percentage of subclinical infections (Brock et al., 1990; Corey and Spear, 1986; Johnson et al., 1989; Strand et al., 1986). In infants and children who develop isolated vulvovaginitis caused by HSV, the virus should be typed, since the possibility of child abuse must be considered if HSV-2 is implicated.

Symptomatic patients often complain of dysuria, and children may refuse to void. The perineal area is usually reddened, edematous, and studded with painful, shallow, white ulcers 2 to 4 mm in diameter. Many of these lesions coalesce to form larger ulcers (Plate 2, C). The regional inguinal lymph nodes are enlarged and tender. Fever and constitutional symptoms subside within 5 to 7 days, and nonmucosal lesions become crusted by the tenth to fourteenth day. Healing is complete without scarring by the end of the third week.

Eczema Herpeticum (Kaposi's Varicelliform Eruption)

Eczema herpeticum, a manifestation of herpetic infection of the skin, was first described by Kaposi in 1887. It is characterized by vesicular and crusting eruptions superimposed on atopic eczema or chronic dermatitis (Lynch et al., 1945). Primary infection usually is more severe than secondary infection. This disease starts abruptly with high fever (40° to 40.6° C; 104° to 105° F), irritability, and restlessness, followed by the appearance of crops of vesicles concentrated chiefly on the eczematous skin. In areas of broken skin there may be ulcers and weeping, with a hemorrhagic component. A smaller number of lesions may involve the normal skin. The lesions may appear in crops over a period of 7 to 9 days, then rupture and become crusted within a few days. Thus, as the disease progresses in some children, it may resemble varicella.

Like other herpetic infections, this disease varies considerably in severity from extremely mild to potentially rapidly fatal, especially if it is primary. Severe cases have been related to deficient cell-mediated immunity to HSV (Vestey et al., 1990). Extensive areas of weeping, oozing skin may be associated with severe fluid loss and with bacterial superinfection.

Traumatic Herpetic Infections

Traumatic herpetic infections of the skin are similar to eczema herpeticum except that they are localized rather than generalized. The site of an abrasion, burn, or break in the skin may be infected with HSV. The source of the virus may be a sympathetic parent or caretaker who "kissed to make well" the injured site for reassurance. HSV also may be transmitted during athletic activities, such as wrestling, in which there are both skin trauma and close physical contact with others. Vesicular lesions that develop at the site of inoculation may be associated with fever, constitutional symptoms, and regional lymphadenopathy. Another form is due to trauma to a nerve that is latently infected with HSV, with resultant reactivation of the virus.

These syndromes may be difficult to differentiate clinically.

Acute Herpetic Keratoconjunctivitis

Primary herpetic infections of the eye are relatively rare. Fever and constitutional symptoms are associated with keratoconjunctivitis and preauricular adenopathy. Usually the infection is unilateral. The cornea has a hazy appearance, and the patient may be unable to close the eyelid (Plate 2, *D*). A purulent and membranelike exudate is present. The skin around the eye may exhibit discrete vesicles. The eye usually clears completely in 2 weeks if the infection is confined chiefly to the conjunctiva. Superficial corneal involvement is characterized by the formation of typical dendritic ulcers. These infections may cause a serious impairment of sight. Deep infections such as keratitis disciformis, hypopyon keratitis, and iridocyclitis are almost always accompanied by significant scarring.

Acute Herpetic Encephalitis and Meningoencephalitis

Primary infection of the CNS is an unusual manifestation of HSV infection in children. Infection of the CNS with HSV-2 beyond the neonatal period (often in conjunction with genital HSV) in an otherwise healthy individual is almost always associated with a self-limited form of meningitis rather than encephalitis, although it may occasionally cause a serious illness (Boucquey et al., 1990). An estimated 15% of patients with primary genital HSV infection will have mild concomitant meningitis (Kohl, 1988).

In contrast, HSV-1 typically causes a rapidly progressive, fatal type of encephalitis, with death after 1 to 2 weeks in approximately 70% of patients who are untreated. There are few reports of cases of benign HSV-1 meningitis (Rathore et al., 1996). The clinical manifestations of 113 biopsy-proved cases of HSV encephalitis are listed in Table 12-1. The encephalitis frequently may be localized in the frontotemporal area, simulating a mass lesion, or it may be widespread, involving both cerebral hemispheres. The cerebrospinal fluid (CSF) usually shows pleocytosis with a predominance of lymphocytes. Computed tomography (CT) and magnetic resonance imaging (MRI) often can be used to localize the area of affected brain (Kohl, 1988; Schroth et al., 1987).

Approximately one third of patients with herpes encephalitis experience a primary infection, but there is no known clinical difference between pri-

Table 12-1 Historical findings and signs at presentation of 113 patients with biopsy-proved herpes simplex encephalitis

Characteristics	Number/total	Percent
Historical findings		
Altered consciousness	109/112	97
Fever	101/112	90
Personality change	62/87	71
Headache	89/110	81
Vomiting	51/111	46
Recurrent herpes labialis	24/108	22
Memory loss	14/59	24
Signs and presentation		
Dysphasia	58/76	76
Autonomic nervous system dysfunction	53/88	60
Ataxia	22/55	40
Seizures	43/112	38
Hemiparesis	41/107	38

Modified from Whitley RJ et al: JAMA 1982b; 247:318.

mary and secondary HSV infection in this instance (Whitley and Lakeman, 1995). The virus is believed to reach the brain either by the hematogenous route, from olfactory neurons of the respiratory mucosa, or from infected ganglia. No immunologic component has been identified, and immunocompromised patients are not at increased risk to develop this form of HSV infection (Kohl, 1988).

Neonatal HSV Infections

HSV infections in premature and newborn infants are usually caused by HSV-2, most often the consequence of primary maternal genital HSV-2 infection at term. Characteristically, the mother's genital infection is asymptomatic, she delivers vaginally, and the infant is unwittingly exposed to the virus during delivery. Less commonly, the infant is infected by HSV-1 secondary to primary maternal gingivostomatitis at term (Amortegui et al., 1984) or exposure to someone else with HSV infection, such as a father or grandparent. The reported incidence of neonatal herpes is 1 in 2,500 to 5,000 live births (Whitley, 1994).

The inability to distinguish accurately between type-specific antibodies of HSV has led to confusion and controversy about whether antibodies could protect an infant from the virus (Nahmias et al., 1971; Yeager et al., 1980). It is now becoming apparent, based on a small number of reported cases, that the presence of specific antibodies in an infant is likely to play at least some role in protection after exposure (Sullender et al., 1988). To a large extent, this may account for the observation in prospective studies that the rate of infection during primary maternal HSV-2 infection is approximately 50%, whereas during recurrent infection it is less than 8%. In this report none of the thirty-four infants born vaginally to women with recurrent HSV at delivery were later found infected; all had detectable neutralizing antibodies to HSV-2 (Prober et al., 1987). Similarly, high titers of ADCC antibodies at presentation in HSV-infected neonates have not been associated with disseminated infections, but high titers are seen in babies who have been exposed to HSV but have not been infected or have had only localized infections (Kohl, 1991; Kohl et al., 1989).

Rarely, infants may be infected in utero with either HSV-1 or HSV-2 during an episode of maternal viremia that may or may not have been clinically apparent (Florman et al., 1973; Hutto et al., 1987; Rabalais et al., 1990). The spectrum of congenital disease varies from chronic to fulminant; some infants have died within days of birth, and others have survived with severe neurologic sequelae. Most have evidence of acute, chronic, or recurrent skin infections with HSV. Infants with zosteriform rashes present at birth may have had HSV infection (Music et al., 1971; Rabalais et al., 1990).

The clinical picture of full-blown neonatal herpes is well recognized. At the end of the first week of life the infant develops fever or hypothermia, progressively increasing icterus, hepatosplenomegaly, and vesicular skin lesions. Anorexia, vomiting, lethargy, respiratory distress, cyanosis, and circulatory collapse may follow. Untreated, the outcome is frequently fatal. The presence of skin vesicles is helpful in distinguishing neonatal herpes from other infections; however, they may be absent in approximately 20% of affected babies. In infants without rash, neonatal HSV infection should be considered when there are signs and symptoms of bacterial meningitis but no bacterial cause can be identified (Arvin et al., 1982) and when there is an interstitial pneumonic process beginning at approximately 4 days of age. Infected infants are usually also febrile and thrombocytopenic and have evidence of liver involvement (Anderson, 1987; Hubbell et al., 1988). Fulminant hepatitis has also been described as the initial symptom of neonatal HSV (Benador et al., 1990). One study has reported HSV infection of the CNS in an infant who did not develop symptoms until he was 2 months old, when he developed a skin lesion caused by HSV-2 (Thomas et al., 1989).

Whitley et al. (1980) have classified neonatal HSV into three presenting groups on the basis of their experience with ninety-five proven cases. These groups include (1) disseminated disease (hepatitis, pneumonia, or disseminated intravascular coagulation, with or without CNS involvement) in 51%; (2) isolated CNS involvement in 32%; and (3) disease localized to the eye, skin, or mouth in 17%. Untreated, the mortality rates were 85%, 50%, and 0%, respectively (Whitley et al., 1980).

HSV in Immunocompromised Hosts

In the immunocompromised host, HSV infections may show two unusual courses: (1) disseminated disease may occur with widespread dermal, mucosal, and visceral involvement; or (2) disease may remain localized but with a greatly prolonged course, persisting for periods as long as 9 months with indolent, often painful ulcerative lesions (Schneidman et al., 1979). These two forms of the infection appear more likely in patients whose T-lymphocyte function is depressed. In immunocompromised patients both primary and recurrent HSV infections may be severe.

Other Illnesses Associated with HSV

Other illnesses associated with HSV include infection of the fingers (herpetic whitlow) (Gill et al., 1988); respiratory infection, including epiglottitis (Bogger-Goren, 1987; Schwenzfeier and Fechner, 1976); lymphadenitis with lymphangitis (Sands and Brown, 1988; Tamaru et al., 1990); parotitis (Arditi et al., 1988); and erythema multiforme (Arditi et al., 1988; Brown et al., 1987a), which may result from hypersensitivity of the host to HSV. All are either unusual or rare in children. Although it once was thought that HSV played at least some causal role in cervical cancer, this is now considered unlikely, based on current evidence (Meigner et al., 1986).

RECURRENT INFECTIONS

Recurrent herpetic infections are more common than clinically apparent primary infections. The most common type is herpes labialis, the well-known fever sore that is manifested by vesicular lesions at the corner of the mouth. Other recurrent lesions may appear on any part of the skin or mucous membranes. As indicated before, these are generally mild and not associated with constitutional symptoms. Two exceptions to this general rule are

HSV encephalitis, which may be a primary or secondary infection, and severe HSV in the immunocompromised patient, which may be recurrent and yet severe (Corey and Spear, 1986).

DIAGNOSIS

Infection with HSV should be suspected in a patient who develops fever, constitutional symptoms, and a vesicular exanthem or enanthem. The diagnosis can be confirmed by (1) isolation of virus from local lesions, (2) demonstration of viral antigens or DNA in skin lesions or CSF, (3) serologic tests showing a significant rise in the level of antibodies during convalescence from a primary infection, and (4) histologic evidence of type A intranuclear inclusion bodies and multinucleated giant cells in infected tissue.

Isolation of Virus and Viral Antigen Tests

HSV can be cultivated in a variety of cell cultures; inoculation of these cultures produces cytopathic changes that are usually evident within 24 to 48 hours. Cultures with suspected infection can be stained with fluorescein-labeled monoclonal antibodies so that identification and simultaneous typing of HSV can be performed rapidly and the results made available to the clinician. Cultures are now available in many hospital laboratories, since HSV is rather easy to propagate and grows rapidly. Culture is superior to Papanicolaou and Tzanck smears, since the latter tests are nonspecific and may yield false-positive and false-negative reactions.

Smears from skin or mucous membrane lesions for direct staining with fluorescein-tagged monoclonal antibodies are very useful for rapid diagnosis. For preparing smears, vigorous swabbing of an open ulcer or ruptured vesicle should be performed to include epithelial cells that harbor the virus in the specimen. An ELISA that identifies HSV antigens in samples from lesions with sensitivity equal to that of culture may be used for rapid identification of HSV, although it will not distinguish between types 1 and 2 (Baker et al., 1989; Dascal et al., 1989). Diagnosis is often difficult when HSV encephalitis or pneumonia is suspected. In the latter case, smears of tracheal or bronchial secretions may be submitted to the diagnostic laboratory, but positive results may reflect asymptomatic shedding of virus from the respiratory tract rather than true infection. When CNS infection is suspected, skin lesions may or may not be present; in any case they offer no specific diagnostic clues. To make a certain diagnosis of herpes encephalitis, a brain biopsy may be required. At present, performing a brain biopsy for diagnosis of HSV encephalitis is controversial. Proponents cite its diagnostic sensitivity and specificity, low rate of complications, and ability to limit the use of the antiviral acyclovir (ACV) to patients with proven disease (Hanley et al., 1987; Whitley et al., 1982b, 1986). Opponents cite the risk of complications of the procedure, delay in ACV therapy, potential for false-negative results, and lack of serious toxicity of ACV (Fishman, 1987; Wasiewski and Fishman, 1988). When a brain biopsy can be performed readily and safely, it may be worth the small risk of complications (approximately 2%), although polymerase chain reaction (PCR) detection of HSV DNA in CSF may eventually supplant it (Rozenberg and Lebon, 1991; Troendle-Atkins et al., 1993; Lakeman and Whitley, 1995; Guffond et al., 1994). The reported incidence of false-negative results for biopsied brain specimens is approximately 4% (Kohl, 1988). CT scan and MRI can be used to localize the affected area of the brain, and an electroencephalogram (EEG) may provide nonspecific clues, such as periodic slow and sharp waves that suggest HSV encephalitis. The abnormalities of the CT scan in neonates with HSV probably will not be localized to the temporal or frontal lobes of the brain, as in herpes encephalitis in an older child, but more likely will be generalized. In patients with neonatal HSV of the CNS the CT scan is at times normal (Noorbehesht et al., 1987). Brain biopsy material can be examined by culture for virus or viral antigens or by electron microscopy. Demonstration of HSV by in situ hybridization in brain biopsy specimens has been reported (Bamborschke et al., 1990).

It is rare to isolate HSV from CSF in patients with either neonatal or postnatal HSV encephalitis, although it is more common to isolate the virus from the CSF of neonates. The presence of antibodies to HSV in CSF, if significantly greater in titer than the serum titer, is considered diagnostic of HSV encephalitis (Kahlon et al., 1987). These antibodies are not always detected early enough in the illness, however, to make this test useful in providing guidance about whether or not to institute antiviral therapy (Van Loon et al., 1989). An especially promising technique for diagnosis of HSV encephalitis is PCR (Rowley et al., 1990; Lakeman and Whitley, 1995). In PCR, DNA is amplified and detected with a molecular probe; this technique has been successful diagnostically in a number of patients early in the illness. It is specific, accurate, and rapidly performed, but experience with this technique in the clinical setting is limited.

The interest in diagnosing maternal HSV in pregnant women at term, especially in those with asymptomatic infections, has been great. It is now recognized, based on studies of over 6,000 pregnant women cultured before and at delivery, that performing maternal genital cultures from those women who have a history of genital HSV is not only expensive but yields little useful information. Women who have had positive cultures during pregnancy are not likely to have positive cultures at delivery, and only a minority of infants at risk are identified if asymptomatic viral shedding is looked for only in women with a past history of genital herpes (Arvin et al., 1986; Prober et al., 1988). PCR is a sensitive and specific procedure for identifying women with genital HSV at delivery (Hardy et al., 1990). However, PCR detects virus DNA rather than infectious virus particles, and studies have not yet addressed whether this is a useful procedure for predicting which infants will be infected with HSV.

Serologic Tests

Although neither as rapid nor as specific as demonstration of virus in lesions, paired samples of sera from the acute and convalescent phases of an illness may be tested for HSV antibodies for diagnostic purposes in a variety of suspected herpetic infections. The levels of these antibodies begin to rise by the end of the first week of illness after a primary infection. Often, however, there is no rise in antibody titer with recurrent HSV infection, and these tests may yield false-positive results, since rising levels of antibodies to HSV may also be seen with VZV infections.

An ELISA method in which gG of HSV-1 and HSV-2 is used for the antigen is an important newly developed antibody test. With this assay, antibodies specific to either type of HSV can be measured; therefore it is possible to determine if an individual has been infected with either or both types of HSV (Corey and Spear, 1986; Johnson et al., 1989). This test is not yet available commercially.

Histologic Studies

The demonstration of acidophilic intranuclear inclusion bodies, multinucleated giant cells, and ballooning degeneration of the epithelial cells of a lesion from biopsy material reinforces the diagnosis of HSV. Immunofluorescence with specific antiserum or monoclonal antibodies is important to confirm a tissue diagnosis.

DIFFERENTIAL DIAGNOSIS
Acute Herpetic Gingivostomatitis

Acute herpetic gingivostomatitis can usually be recognized clinically without laboratory confirmation. The following diseases may be confused with it:

1. *Herpangina.* The lesions of herpangina, caused by group A coxsackievirus, are clinically indistinguishable in appearance from those of HSV (Plate 2, *F*). However, the distribution of the lesions makes it possible to separate these two conditions. With herpangina, they usually are confined to the anterior fauces and soft palate, and gingivitis does not occur, whereas, with herpetic infection, gingivitis is a typical manifestation.

2. *Acute membranous tonsillitis.* Acute membranous tonsillitis secondary to streptococcal infection, EBV infection, diphtheria, and other infectious agents may simulate herpetic involvement of the tonsillar area. Invariably, herpetic lesions appear on the tongue, buccal mucosa, palate, and gingival tissues. Cultures and blood smears are the most helpful diagnostic laboratory procedures.

3. *Thrush.* Thrush is generally not associated with fever and constitutional symptoms. Lesions are polymorphous elevated white plaques without ulceration.

Acute Herpetic Vulvovaginitis

Acute involvement of the skin of the perineal area may simulate herpetic vulvovaginitis. The following conditions are most commonly confused:

1. *Ammoniacal dermatitis with secondary infection.* Fever and systemic symptoms are absent as a rule with this condition. The lesions extend onto the thighs and diaper area.

2. *Gonorrheal and monilial vulvovaginitis.* Lesions can be identified by appropriate cultures.

3. *Impetigo.* Lesions are usually present elsewhere, particularly on the nares and other sites readily scratched. Viral diagnostic procedures (see section on diagnosis) and bacterial cultures may provide helpful diagnostic information.

Eczema Herpeticum

Herpetic infection of eczematous skin lesions must be differentiated from the following conditions:

1. *Eczema with secondary bacterial infection.* These lesions may resemble eczema herpeticum, but fever and constitutional symptoms are usually not present.

2. *Varicella.* Varicella is not an unusually severe infection in children with eczema, and the rash does not become disseminated or confluent.

3. *Eczema vaccinatum.* This disease may be almost impossible to distinguish clinically from eczema herpeticum, and the diagnosis requires the performance of laboratory procedures. Fortunately, however, eczema vaccinatum has become a disease of the past, since routine vaccination of children for smallpox is no longer performed.

Traumatic Herpes Infections

Traumatic herpetic infections may be confused with herpes zoster or with secondary bacterial infection of the site that has been traumatized. Performing methods of viral diagnosis of HSV may be necessary to make a certain diagnosis.

Acute Herpetic Keratoconjunctivitis

A variety of bacteria—including *Haemophilus* species, pneumococci, and staphylococci—and viruses such as picornaviruses, influenza viruses, rubeola, and adenoviruses may cause conjunctivitis. Adenovirus infection with enlargement of the preauricular lymph nodes may be an isolated phenomenon or may be accompanied by respiratory symptoms. Differentiation requires assessment of the history and accompanying symptoms and physical findings of the patient. Cultures and scrapings are often required to make the correct diagnosis.

Neonatal HSV

In infants with vesicular skin lesions HSV may be confused with varicella. Historical information concerning exposure to varicella or VZV is helpful. It may be necessary either to identify the viral antigen in the vesicular lesion or to perform a culture. In infants without skin lesions, neonatal HSV infection may be confused with bacterial sepsis, enteroviral infections, pneumonia, or meningitis. The average length of time until onset of pneumonia caused by group B beta-hemolytic streptococcus is 20 hours, whereas HSV pneumonia begins on average at 5 days (Hubbell et al., 1988). Rapid diagnosis is important because early treatment with either appropriate antimicrobials or antivirals improves the outcome. If skin lesions are not present, the diagnosis may be made by isolation of HSV from the mouth or conjunctiva or, more rarely, from the urine or CSF (Hammerberg et al., 1983). Occasionally it may be possible to isolate HSV from buffy coat cells if the infant has viremia (Golden, 1988).

On rare occasions it is necessary to obtain a biopsy of the brain to diagnose infants with obvious CNS involvement and no skin lesions (Arvin et al., 1982; Koskiniemi et al., 1989). Infants with positive throat cultures only in the first 24 hours of life born vaginally to women with genital herpes have been reported (Arvin et al., 1986). These infants appear to "carry" HSV briefly but are not actually infected.

HSV Encephalitis

Many other conditions mimic HSV encephalitis. These include vascular disease, brain abscess, other forms of viral encephalitis (enterovirus, mumps, EBV, measles, influenza, arbovirus), cryptococcal infection, tumor, toxic encephalopathy, Reye's syndrome, toxoplasmosis, tuberculosis, and lymphocytic choriomeningitis.

COMPLICATIONS

Bacterial complications rarely occur in a patient with acute gingivostomatitis. Dehydration and acidosis may result from the patient's refusal of fluids because of extensive and painful lesions in the mouth. Eczema herpeticum occasionally may become secondarily infected with bacteria, which may be a potential focus for the development of septicemia.

PROGNOSIS

The prognosis of patients with acute herpetic gingivostomatitis is excellent. Extensive eczema herpeticum, neonatal HSV, and herpes simplex encephalitis are highly fatal if not treated with an antiviral drug. Early therapy of eczema herpeticum is associated with a good prognosis. The prognosis of neonatal HSV and herpes encephalitis has improved since the development of antiviral drugs, particularly ACV.

As is true for many HSV infections, the prognosis for patients with neonatal herpes depends on the extent of the infection at the time antiviral therapy is begun. Early therapy improves the outcome, but progression of the disease (e.g., development of chorioretinitis) has been reported despite antiviral treatment. Poor prognosis has been associated with acute primary maternal disease at delivery, prematurity, visceral involvement, and EEG abnormalities (Koskiniemi et al., 1989). Collaborative studies of Whitley et al. (1991a,b) on 202 infants infected with HSV-1 or HSV-2 have revealed the following information. The death rate for patients who have been treated for disseminated HSV infection is approximately 60%, and for those treated for encephalitis it is approximately 15%. Approximately 60% of survivors of disseminated disease and 30% to 40% of those surviving encephalitis are developing normally at 1 year of age (Whitley et al., 1991a, 1991b; Whitley and Hutto, 1985). The mortality after neonatal HSV infection limited to the skin, eye, or mouth is essentially nil, with approximately 10% having sequelae. Among infants with skin, eye, or mouth disease, those who experienced three or more recurrences of skin lesions during the first 6 months of life were at greater risk of neurologic impairment (Whitley et al., 1991b). The prognosis has been reported as better after HSV-1 than after HSV-2 neonatal encephalitis (Corey et al., 1988; Whitley et al., 1991b). For example, of fifteen infants with HSV-2 encephalitis, only 23% were normal at 18 months of age, whereas, of nine who had encephalitis caused by HSV-1, all were normal at the same age. These infants had all been treated appropriately with vidarabine or ACV (Corey et al., 1988).

Treatment with ACV has also decreased the mortality and morbidity of herpes encephalitis beyond the neonatal period, and ACV therapy has proved to offer a better prognosis than vidarabine (Whitley et al., 1986). The mortality rate for thirty-two patients treated with ACV was approximately 30%, as compared to 54% in thirty-seven who received vidarabine. Roughly 40% of ACV-treated patients were free of sequelae 6 months later, compared to only 14% of vidarabine-treated patients. The better the patient's condition is before initiation of therapy, particularly with regard to neurological status, the better the outcome (Whitley et al., 1986).

IMMUNITY

Many infants are born with HSV antibodies passively acquired from the mother. This passive immunity is somewhat protective, but it disappears by approximately 6 months of age. Active immunity in the form of long-lasting humoral and cellular immune responses develops after an apparent or inapparent primary infection with HSV. This immunity to HSV, however, is incomplete and does not necessarily protect against future exogenous herpetic infections or against recurrent endogenous herpetic infections, although the infection may be modified (Buchman et al., 1979). The virus may reactivate after latent infection, and reinfection may also occur. In addition, patients may have latent infection with more than one type of HSV (Whitley et al.,

1982a). A prior infection with HSV-1 appears to attenuate the severity of subsequent infection with HSV-2 (Corey and Spear, 1986; Johnson et al., 1989).

Host factors important in defense have been analyzed best in infants. Although the presence of neutralizing antibodies in infants does not necessarily prevent disseminated infection, they may attenuate the illness considerably (Arvin et al., 1986; Sullender et al., 1987; Yeager et al., 1980). The functions of NK cells and T lymphocytes—including production of cytokines such as interleukin-2 and interferon—are all immature in infants, which appears to predispose infants to serious infection with HSV (Kohl, 1989; Kohl et al., 1988, 1989; Sullender et al., 1987). In all probability, in the healthy child and adult, antibodies and cellular immunity act in concert in host defense against HSV.

EPIDEMIOLOGIC FACTORS

In lower socioeconomic groups most individuals have been infected with HSV-1 before 6 years of age. In contrast, in upper socioeconomic groups much of the population may escape primary HSV-1 infection in the first decade of life; in these groups young adults are therefore more likely to experience primary HSV-1 gingivostomatitis. For HSV-2 infections, as with other sexually transmitted diseases, the highest rate of infection is during the second and third decades. Herpetic infections are worldwide in distribution.

Not all of the details about the spread of HSV are known, but it appears that one means of transmission is by intimate contact. Infectious virus may be recovered from saliva, skin and mucosal lesions, and urine, all of which are potential sources. Patients with recurrent lesions are infectious to others for a shorter period of time than those with primary infections.

An extensive study of the natural history of herpetic infection in 4,191 Yugoslavian children has been reported (Juretic, 1966). The incidence of clinically apparent infection, primary herpetic gingivostomatitis, was 12%. The peak incidence according to age was in the second year of life, and there was no seasonal variation. Adults with herpetic lesions were the chief source of infection. Nine minor epidemics were observed. The incubation period was 2 to 12 days, with a mean of 6 days.

A seroepidemiologic study of HSV-2 infection in 4,201 participants in which a type-specific (gG) antibody assay was used revealed the following. Between 1976 and 1980, 16.4% of the U.S. population between 15 and 74 years of age had detectable antibodies to HSV-2. The prevalence of antibodies increased from less than 1% positive in children less than 15 years old to 20.2% in young adults. The highest prevalence of positive titers in elderly individuals was 19.7% in whites and 64.7% in blacks (Johnson et al., 1989).

Neonatal HSV is usually acquired from a maternal genital source. Maternally transmitted HSV infections in the perinatal period apparently are increasing in incidence (Sullivan-Bolyai et al., 1983b). Intrauterine infection has been reported but seems rare (Florman et al., 1973; Hutto et al., 1987; Stone et al., 1989). Delivery of an infant by cesarean section usually prevents neonatal infection if the fetal membranes remain intact or have been ruptured for less than 4 hours before delivery. Most infants who develop neonatal HSV are born vaginally to mothers with no history or knowledge of genital HSV infection. Although an infant may be infected with HSV after exposure to a woman with recurrent HSV (Growdon et al., 1987), the high-risk situation for transmission is not in women with a history of recurrent genital HSV but in those with no history of this disease. Transmission to an infant is far greater after maternal primary infection than after maternal recurrent genital HSV.

The effects on the fetus of a first episode of genital herpes during pregnancy have been analyzed prospectively in a report of twenty-nine women infected in various trimesters and their offspring (Brown et al., 1987b). This study confirmed the serious nature of primary, in contrast to secondary, infection during pregnancy, since there were three of fifteen infected offspring in the first group and zero of fourteen infected in the second. In addition, the incidence of premature birth and intrauterine growth retardation increased in the babies whose mothers had a primary infection during pregnancy, especially if the infection occurred in the third trimester.

Infants may on occasion be inadvertently infected through scalp monitors during delivery (Parvey and Ch'ien, 1980), during breast-feeding (Sullivan-Bolyai et al., 1983a), in intensive-care nurseries (Hammerberg et al., 1983), and from family members besides the mother (Yeager et al., 1983). The availability of molecular biologic techniques for viral "fingerprinting," using restriction endonucleases to evaluate the DNA of HSV isolates, has been invaluable in proving many of these transmissions.

TREATMENT

The treatment of mucocutaneous HSV beyond the neonatal period is chiefly supportive. Infants require careful observation for possible dehydration. Fluids should be given intravenously if necessary. Citrus fruit juices and other irritating liquids should be avoided. Cold drinks such as apple, pear, and peach juices often seem well tolerated. Only those children with extensive oral involvement should be treated with specific antiviral chemotherapy; intravenous ACV (10 mg/kg every 8 hours) should usually be given. Some pediatricians may first try administration of oral ACV; however, the dosage for infants with primary HSV gingivostomatitis is not known (Arvin, 1987). In a study of 174 nonimmunocompromised adults with oral herpes, many of whom probably had secondary HSV, a dose of 400 mg 5 times a day by mouth for 5 days hastened the healing if therapy was begun in the very early stages of the illness (Spruance et al., 1990). ACV is relatively nontoxic; the main associated adverse effects include rash, gastrointestinal discomfort, and mild azotemia, which can be avoided by maintenance of good hydration. ACV is both an inhibitor of and a faulty substrate for viral DNA polymerase; because ACV requires phosphorylation by a viral enzyme to exert its antiviral effects, it is relatively nontoxic to uninfected cells that lack the enzyme. Approximately 20% of the oral formulation is absorbed by the gastrointestinal tract. ACV is marketed in topical, oral, and intravenous formulations. Topical ACV has very little use; it shortens the course of primary genital HSV from an average of 14 to 11 days. This interval is shortened significantly further by administration of oral ACV (200 mg 5 times a day for an adult), which is the treatment of choice for primary genital herpes. Frequently, recurring genital HSV can be suppressed by long-term oral administration of ACV (400 to 800 mg per day [two to four 200-mg capsules in divided doses]) (Gold and Corey, 1987; Guinan, 1986; Merz et al., 1988; Straus et al., 1989).

Children with herpetic keratoconjunctivitis should be treated with topical trifluridine; topical ophthalmic ACV ointment is not a licensed product in the United States. Children with conjunctivitis and mucosal or cutaneous lesions should also be treated with oral ACV. The care of children with this disease should be supervised by an ophthalmologist. However, some infants with neonatal HSV present with conjunctivitis; special consideration should be taken with infants less than 1 month old. They should receive intravenous ACV and topical ophthalmic ointment (Liesegang, 1988) and should be evaluated for systemic HSV infection.

Serious HSV infections such as encephalitis and neonatal HSV should be treated with intravenous ACV (10 to 20 mg/kg every 8 hours) for 2 to 3 weeks. Immunocompromised children with severe mucocutaneous involvement should be given 5 to 10 mg/kg every 8 hours, usually for 5 to 7 days. Lower dosages should be used for children with renal compromise (Balfour and Englund, 1989).

For both neonatal HSV and HSV encephalitis it is often necessary to begin therapy before a proven diagnosis, since the earlier treatment is begun, the better the outcome (Sullivan-Bolyai et al., 1986; Whitley et al., 1986; Whitley and Hutto, 1985). Treatment with ACV for 1 to 2 days before obtaining a diagnostic culture usually will not interfere with obtaining a positive result (Balfour and Englund, 1989). All babies under 1 month of age who have HSV infection must be treated intravenously, even if their symptoms are mild, since the incidence of progression to CNS or disseminated disease is more than 50% in babies presenting with infection localized to the skin, mouth, or eye.

The increased awareness of neonatal HSV and the use of antiviral therapy appear to have made a significant impact on the presentation of the disease. For example, during the 1970s approximately 50% of infants presented with disseminated disease, but now the rate has been reduced to less than 25%. Moreover, the frequency of skin, eye, and mouth infections has increased to approximately 40% from approximately 20% (Whitley et al., 1988).

Close follow-up of patients after treatment of neonatal HSV and HSV encephalitis is also critical, since relapses in both diseases have been reported (Brown et al., 1987a; Gutman et al., 1986; Kohl, 1988). In most instances of relapse, retreatment with ACV for several weeks is believed helpful, but it is not known whether additional therapy with orally administered ACV on a long-term basis adds any additional benefit. Some experts in the field advocate treating infants with HSV infection with oral acyclovir until they are 6 to 12 months old, but clinical data supporting this strategy are lacking. Relapse of HSV encephalitis caused by hypersensitivity to HSV, a form of postinfectious encephalitis, has been reported (Koenig et al., 1979). Relapse has also been reported after treatment for only 10 days (VanLandingham et al., 1988).

Resistance of HSV to ACV is an emerging problem (Hirsch and Schooley, 1989). HSV may become resistant in three ways. Most commonly, it may cease producing thymidine kinase, the enzyme that phosphorylates ACV into an active antiviral compound. It may also produce either an altered form of thymidine kinase or an altered form of DNA polymerase (Balfour and Englund, 1989). Strains of HSV resistant to ACV have been found in immunocompromised patients (Englund et al., 1990) and, less commonly, in immunocompetent patients (Kost et al., 1993). These strains have limited ability to spread to others because they are also less invasive than ACV-sensitive strains of HSV. Resistance to ACV may arise rapidly in immunocompromised patients, and, although the ability to detect these strains remains a research tool, clinically useful methods to detect them are being developed (Englund et al., 1990). Since the ACV-resistance of HSV is increasing, the wisdom of using prophylactic therapy in patients with non–life-threatening herpetic illnesses must be carefully considered in every instance.

Currently the therapy of choice for serious HSV infections that do not respond to acyclovir is foscarnet (Safrin et al., 1991). Foscarnet inhibits HSV replication by acting directly on the virus DNA polymerase and does not require phosphorylation by the virus thimidine kinase. The dose of foscarnet for the treatment of HSV infections is 40 mg/kg/dose IV every 8 hours. Adverse effects associated with its administration include renal toxicity, electrolyte disturbances, and CNS toxicity. HSV strains with altered DNA polymerase may be resistant to foscarnet, acyclovir, or both drugs. In some cases, therapy with both foscarnet and acyclovir may be successful (Safrin et al., 1994).

Valaciclovir and famciclovir are both prodrugs with good oral bioavailability. Valaciclovir is an ester of acyclovir; the recommended dosage for treatment of genital HSV infection is 1,000 mg orally twice a day for 5 days. Famciclovir is metabolized to its active form, pencyclovir. The dosage of famciclovir for the treatment of first episodes of genital HSV infection is 250 mg orally every 8 hours for 5 days and for recurrent episodes is 125 mg twice a day for 5 days. Neither of these drugs is approved for use in children, and there are no pediatric suspensions available. They may be useful for the treatment of HSV infections in adolescents.

PREVENTIVE MEASURES

Most herpetic infections are difficult to prevent. Children with eczema should avoid contact with others with HSV infections if possible. Infants whose mothers have active genital HSV during labor should be delivered by cesarean section, particularly if the membranes are intact or have been ruptured for less than 4 hours. Newborn infants should not have contact with persons with active herpes labialis.

The advantages of a successful herpes simplex vaccine are apparent; attempts to develop one are in progress, including efforts with subunit vaccines and with a live attenuated vaccine (Whitley, 1996; Straus et al., 1994). Recombinant gD and combination gD and gB vaccines are well tolerated and immunogenic in people without prior HSV-2 infection (Straus et al., 1993; Adria et al., 1995). The gD vaccine also decreases the frequency of recurrences in people with genital HSV infections (Straus et al. 1994). It is hoped that these vaccines will decrease HSV-2 transmission.

The risk/benefit ratio of administration of ACV to pregnant women who develop primary HSV to prevent infection of the infant or to prevent infection of an infant delivered vaginally to a woman with known genital HSV is unknown. Therefore neither of these possible preventive strategies is encouraged at this time.

BIBLIOGRAPHY

Adria GM, Langenberg MD, Burke RL, et al. A recombinant glycoprotein vaccine for herpes simplex type 2: safety and efficacy. Ann Intern Med 1995;122:889-898.

Amortegui AJ, Macpherson TA, Harger JH. A cluster of neonatal herpes simplex infections without mucocutaneous manifestations. Pediatrics 1984;73:194-198.

Anderson RD. Herpes simplex virus infection of the neonatal respiratory tract. Am J Dis Child 1987;141:274-276.

Arditi M, Shulman S, Langman CB, et al. Probable herpes simplex type 1–related acute parotitis, nephritis, and erythema multiforme. Pediatr Infect Dis J 1988;7:427-428.

Arvin AM. Oral therapy with acyclovir in infants and children. Pediatr Infect Dis J 1987;6:56-58.

Arvin AM, Hensleigh PA, Prober C, et al. Failure of antepartum maternal cultures to predict the infant's risk of exposure to herpes simplex virus at delivery. N Engl J Med 1986; 315:796-800.

Arvin AM, Yeager AS, Bruhn FW, Grossman M. Neonatal herpes simplex infection in the absence of mucocutaneous lesions. J Pediatr 1982;100:715-721.

Baker DA, Gonik B, Milch PO, et al. Clinical evaluation of a new virus ELISA: a rapid diagnostic test for herpes simplex virus. Obstet Gynecol 1989;73:322-325.

Balfour HH, Englund JA. Antiviral drugs in pediatrics. Am J Dis Child 1989;143:1307-1316.

Bamborschke S, Porr A, Huber M, Heiss WD. Demonstration of herpes simplex virus DNA in CSF cells by in situ hybridization for early diagnosis of herpes encephalitis. J Neurol 1990;237:73-76.

Baringer JR. Recovery of herpes simplex virus from human sacral ganglions. N Engl J Med 1974;291:828.

Baringer JR, Swoveland R. Recovery of herpes simplex virus from human trigeminal ganglions. N Engl J Med 1973; 288:648-650.

Benador N, Mannhardt W, Schranz D, et al. Three cases of neonatal herpes simplex virus infection presenting as fulminant hepatitis. Eur J Pediatr 1990;149:555-559.

Bloom DC, Hill JM, Devi-Rao G, et al. A 348-pair region in the latency-associated transcript facilitates herpes simplex virus type 1 reactivation. J Virol 1996;70:2449-2459.

Bogger-Goren S. Acute epiglottitis caused by herpes simplex virus. Pediatr Infect Dis J 1987;6:1133-1134.

Boucher FD, Yasukawa LL, Bronzan RN, et al. A prospective evaluation of primary genital herpes simplex virus type 2 infections acquired during pregnancy. Pediatr Infect Dis J 1990;9:499-504.

Boucquey D, Chalon M-P, Sindic CJM, et al. Herpes simplex virus type 2 meningitis without genital lesions: an immunoblot study. J Neurol 1990;237:285-289.

Breinig MK, Kingsley LA, Armstrong JA, et al. Epidemiology of genital herpes in Pittsburgh: serologic, sexual, and racial correlates of apparent and inapparent herpes simplex infections. J Infect Dis 1990;162:299-305.

Brock BV, Selke MA, Benedetti J, et al. Frequency of asymptomatic shedding of herpes simplex virus in women with genital herpes. JAMA 1990;263:418-420.

Brown ZA, Ashley R, Douglas J, et al. Neonatal herpes simplex virus infection: relapse after initial therapy and transmission from a mother with an asymptomatic genital herpes infection and erythema multiforme. Pediatr Infect Dis J 1987a; 6:1057-1061.

Brown ZA, Vontver LA, Benedetti J, et al. Effects on infants of a first episode of genital herpes during pregnancy. N Engl J Med 1987b;317:1246-1251.

Buchman TG, Roizman B, Adams G, Stover BH. Restriction endonuclease fingerprinting of herpes simplex virus DNA: a novel epidemiologic tool applied to a nosocomial outbreak. J Infect Dis 1978;138:488-498.

Buchman TG, Roizman B, Nahmias AJ. Demonstration of exogenous genital reinfection with herpes simplex virus type 2 by restriction endonuclease fingerprinting of viral DNA. J Infect Dis 1979;140:295-304.

Corey L. The diagnosis and treatment of genital herpes. JAMA 1982;248:1041-1049.

Corey L, Spear P. Infections with herpes simplex viruses. N Engl J Med 1986;314:686-691, 749-757.

Corey L, Stone EF, Whitley RJ, Mohan K. Difference between herpes simplex virus type 1 and type 2 neonatal encephalitis in neurological outcome. Lancet 1988;1:1-4.

Croen KD, Ostrove JM, Dragovic LJ, et al. Latent herpes simplex virus in human trigeminal ganglia. N Engl J Med 1987;317:1427-1432.

Croen KD, Ostrove JM, Dragovic LJ, et al. Characterization of herpes simplex virus type 2 latency-associated transcription in human sacral ganglia and in cell culture. J Infect Dis 1991;163:23-28.

Dascal A, Chan-Thim J, Morahan M, et al. Diagnosis of herpes simplex virus infection in a clinical setting by a direct antigen detection enzyme immunoassay. J Clin Microbiol 1989; 27:700-704.

Englund JA, Zimmerman ME, Swierkosz EM, et al. Herpes simplex virus resistant to acyclovir: a study in a tertiary care center. Ann Intern Med 1990;112:416-422.

Farrell MJ, Dobson AT, Feldman L. Herpes simplex virus latency-associated transcript is a stable intron. Proc Natl Acad Sci USA 1991;88:790-794.

Fishman RA. No, brain biopsy need not be done in every patient suspected of having herpes simplex encephalitis. Arch Neurol 1987;44:1291-1292.

Florman AL, Gershon AA, Blackett PR, Nahmias AJ. Intrauterine infection with herpes simplex virus: resultant congenital malformations. JAMA 1973;225:129-132.

Gill MJ, Arlett J, Buchan K. Herpes simplex virus infection of the hand. Am J Med 1988;84:89-93.

Gold D, Corey L. Acyclovir prophylaxis for herpes simplex infection. Antimicrob Ag Chemo 1987;31:361-367.

Golden SE. Neonatal herpes simplex viremia. Pediatr Infect Dis 1988;7:425-426.

Growdon WA, Apodaca L, Cragun J, et al. Neonatal herpes simplex virus infection occurring in second twin of an asymptomatic mother. JAMA 1987;257:508-511.

Guffond T, Dewilde A, Lobert PE, et al. Significance and clinical relevance of the detection of herpes simplex virus DNA by the polymerase chain reaction in cerebrospinal fluid from patients with presumed encephalitis. Clin Infect Dis 1994; 18:744-749.

Guinan ME. Oral acyclovir for treatment and suppression of genital herpes simplex virus infection. JAMA 1986; 255:1747-1749.

Gutman LT, Wilfert CM, Eppes S. Herpes simplex virus encephalitis in children: analysis of cerebrospinal fluid and progressive neurodevelopmental deterioration. J Infect Dis 1986;154:415-421.

Hammerberg O, Watts J, Chernesky M, et al. An outbreak of herpes simplex virus type 1 in an intensive care nursery. Pediatr Infect Dis J 1983;2:290-294.

Hanley DF, Johnson RT, Whitley RJ. Yes, brain biopsy should be a prerequisite for herpes simplex encephalitis treatment. Arch Neurol 1987;44:1289-1290.

Hardy DA, Arvin AM, Yasukawa LL, et al. Use of polymerase chain reaction for successful identification of asymptomatic genital infection with herpes simplex virus in pregnant women at delivery. J Infect Dis 1990;162:1031-1035.

Hirsch MS, Schooley RT. Resistance to antiviral drugs: the end of innocence. N Engl J Med 1989;320:313-314.

Hubbell C, Dominguez R, Kohl S. Neonatal herpes simplex pneumonitis. Rev Infect Dis 1988;10:431-438.

Hutto C, Arvin AM, Jacobs R, et al. Intrauterine herpes simplex infections. Ann Intern Med 1987;110:97-101.

Johnson RE, Nahmias AJ, Magder LS, et al. A seroepidemiologic survey of the prevalence of herpes simplex virus type 2 infection in the United States. N Engl J Med 1989; 321:7-12.

Juretic M. Natural history of herpetic infection. Helv Pediatr Acta 1966;21:356.

Kahlon J, Chatterjee S, Lakeman F, et al. Detection of antibody to herpes simplex virus in the cerebrospinal fluid of patients with herpes simplex encephalitis. J Infect Dis 1987; 155:38-44.

Koenig H, Rabinowitz SG, Day E, Miller V. Post-infectious encephalomyelitis after successful treatment of herpes simplex encephalitis with adenine arabinoside. N Engl J Med 1979; 300:1089-1093.

Kohl S. Herpes simplex virus encephalitis in children. Pediatr Clin N Am 1988;35:465-483.

Kohl S. The neonatal human's immune response to herpes simplex virus infection: a critical review. Pediatr Infect Dis J 1989;8:67-74.

Kohl S. Role of antibody-dependent cellular cytotoxicity in defense against herpes simplex virus infections. J Infect Dis 1991;13:108-114.

Kohl S, West MS, Loo LS. Defects in interleukin-2 stimulation of neonatal natural killer cytotoxicity to herpes simplex virus–infected cells. J Pediatr 1988;112:976-981.

Kohl S, West MS, Prober CG, et al. Neonatal antibody–dependent cellular cytotoxicity antibody levels are associated with the clinical presentation of neonatal herpes simplex virus infection. J Infect Dis 1989;160:770-776.

Koskiniemi M, Happonen M-M, Jarvenpaa A-L, et al. Neonatal herpes simplex virus infection: a report of 43 patients. Pediatr Infect Dis J 1989;8:30-35.

Kost RG, Hill EL, Tigges M, et al. Recurrent acyclovir-resistant genital herpes in an immunocompetent patient. N Engl J Med 1993:1777-1782.

Krause PR, Stanberry N, Bourne B, et al. Expression of the herpes simplex virus type 2 latency-associated transcript enhances spontaneous reactivation of genital herpes in latently infected guinea pigs. J Exp Med 1995;181:297-306.

Krugman S. Primary herpetic vulvovaginitis: report of a case; isolation and identification of herpes simplex virus. Pediatrics 1952;9:585.

Lakeman FD, Whitley RJ. Diagnosis of herpes simplex encephalitis: application of polymerase chain reaction to cerebrospinal fluid from brain-biopsied patients and correlation with disease. J Infect Dis 1995;171:857-863.

Langenberg A, Benedetti J, Jenkins J, et al. Development of clinically recognizable genital lesions among women previously identified as having "asymptomatic" herpes simplex virus type 2 infection. Ann Intern Med 1989;110:882-887.

Liesegang TJ. Ocular herpes simplex infection: pathogenesis and current therapy. Mayo Clin Proc 1988;63:1092-1105.

Lynch FW, Evans CA, Bolin VS, Steves RJ. Kaposi's varicelliform eruption: extensive herpes simplex as a complication of eczema. Arch Dermatol Syph 1945;51:129.

Meigner B, Norrild B, Thunning C, et al. Failure to induce cervical cancer in mice by long-term frequent vaginal exposure to live or inactivated herpes simplex virus. Int J Cancer 1986;38:387-394.

Merz GJ, Jones CC, Mills J, et al. Long-term acyclovir suppression of frequently recurring genital herpes simplex virus infection. JAMA 1988;260:201-206.

Music SI, Fine EM, Togo Y. Zoster-like disease in the newborn caused by herpes simplex virus. N Engl J Med 1971;284:24-26.

Nahmias AJ, Dowdle WR. Antigenic and biologic differences in herpesvirus hominis. Prog Med Virol 1968;10:110.

Nahmias AJ, Josey WE, Naib ZM, et al. Perinatal risk associated with maternal genital herpes simplex virus infection. Am J Obstet Gynecol 1971;110:825.

Noorbehesht B, Enzmann DR, Sullender W, et al. Neonatal herpes simplex encephalitis: correlation of clinical and CT findings. Radiology 1987;162:813-819.

Parvey LS, Ch'ien LT. Neonatal herpes simplex virus infection introduced by fetal-monitor scalp electrodes. Pediatrics 1980;65:1150-1153.

Perng GC, Dunkel EC, Geary PA, et al. The latency-associated transcript gene of herpes simplex virus type 1 (HSV-1) is required for efficient in vivo spontaneous reactivation of HSV-1 from latency. J Virol 1994; 68:8045-8055.

Prober G, Hensleigh PA, Boucher FD, et al. Use of routine viral cultures at delivery to identify neonates exposed to herpes simplex virus. N Engl J Med 1988;318:887-891.

Prober CG, Sullender WM, Yasukawa LL, et al. Low risk of herpes simplex virus infections in neonates exposed to the virus at the time of vaginal delivery to mothers with recurrent genital herpes simplex virus infections. N Engl J Med 1987; 316:240-244.

Rabalais GP, Yusk JW, Wilkerson SA. Zosteriform denuded skin caused by intrauterine herpes simplex virus infection. Pediatr Infect Dis J 1990;10:79-81.

Rathore MH, Mercurio K, Halstead D. Herpes simplex type 1 meningitis. Pediatr Infect Dis J 1996;15:824-828.

Rowley AH, Whitley RJ, Lakeman FD, Wolinsky SM. Rapid detection of herpes-simplex-virus DNA in cerebrospinal fluid of patients with herpes simplex encephalitis. Lancet 1990; 1:440-441.

Rozenberg F, Lebon P. Amplification and characterization of herpesvirus DNA in cerebrospinal fluid from patients with acute encephalitis. J Clin Micro 1991;29:2412-2417.

Safrin S, Crumpacker C, Chatic P, et al. A controlled trial comparing foscarnet with vidarabine for acyclovir-resistant mucocutaneous herpes simplex in the acquired immunodeficiency syndrome. N Engl J Med 1991;325:551-555.

Safrin S, Kemmerly S, Plotkin B, et al. Foscarnet-resistant herpes simplex virus infections in patients with AIDS. J Infect Dis 1994;169:193-196.

Sands M, Brown R. Herpes simplex lymphangitis. Arch Intern Med 1988;148:2066-2067.

Schneidman DW, Barr RJ, Graham JH. Chronic cutaneous herpes simplex. JAMA 1979;241:592.

Schroth G, Gawehn J, Thron A, et al. Early diagnosis of herpes simplex encephalitis by MRI. Neurology 1987;37:179-183.

Schwenzfeier CW, Fechner RE. Herpes simplex of the epiglottis. Arch Otolaryngol 1976;102:374-375.

Spruance SL, Stewart JCB, Rowe N, et al. Treatment of recurrent herpes simplex labialis with oral acyclovir. J Infect Dis 1990;161:185-190.

Steiner I, Spivack JG, Lirette R, et al. Herpes simplex virus type 1 latency-associated transcripts are evidently not essential for latent infection. EMBO J 1989;8:505-511.

Stevens JG, Haarr L, Porter DD, et al. Prominence of the herpes simplex virus latency-associated transcript in trigeminal ganglia from seropositive humans. J Infect Dis 1988; 158:117-123.

Stone KM, Brooks CA, Guinan ME, Alexander ER. National surveillance for neonatal herpes simplex virus infections. Sex Trans Dis 1989;16:152-156.

Strand A, Vahlne A, Svennerholm B, et al. Asymptomatic virus shedding in men with genital herpes infection. Scand J Infect Dis 1986;18:195-197.

Straus S, Corey L, Burke RL, et al. Placebo-controlled trial of vaccination with recombinant glycoprotein D of herpes simplex virus type 2 for immunotherapy of genital herpes. Lancet 1994;343:1460-1463.

Straus SE, Savarese B, Tigges M, et al. Induction and enhancement of immune responses to herpes simplex virus type 2 in humans by use of a recombinant glycoprotein D vaccine. J Infect Dis 1993;167:1045-1052.

Straus S, Seidlin M, Takiff H, et al. Effect of oral acyclovir treatment on symptomatic and asymptomatic virus shedding in recurrent genital herpes. Sex Trans Dis 1989;16:107-113.

Sullender WM, Miller JL, Yasukawa LL, et al. Humoral and cell-mediated immunity in neonates with herpes simplex virus infection. J Infect Dis 1987;155:28-37.

Sullender WM, Yasukawa LL, Schwartz M, et al. Type-specific antibodies to herpes simplex virus type 2 (HSV-2) glycoprotein G in pregnant women, infants exposed to maternal HSV-2 infection at delivery, and infants with neonatal herpes. J Infect Dis 1988;157:164-171.

Sullivan-Bolyai J, Fife KH, Jacobs RF, et al. Disseminated neonatal herpes simplex type 1 from a maternal breast lesion. Pediatrics 1983a;71:455-457.

Sullivan-Bolyai J, Hull HF, Wilson C, et al. Herpes simplex virus infection in King County, Washington. JAMA 1983b; 250:3059-3062.

Sullivan-Bolyai JZ, Hull HF, Wilson C, et al. Presentation of neonatal herpes simplex virus infections: implications for a change in therapeutic strategy. Pediatr Infect Dis J 1986; 5:309-314.

Tamaru J, Mikata A, Horie H, et al. Herpes simplex lymphadenitis. Am J Surg Pathol 1990;14:571-577.

Thomas EE, Scheifele DW, MacLean BS, Ashley R. Herpes simplex type 2 aseptic meningitis in a two-month-old infant. Pediatr Infect Dis J 1989;8:184-186.

Troendle-Atkins J, Demmler GJ, Buffone GJ. Rapid diagnosis of herpes simplex virus encephalitis by using the polymerase chain reaction. J Pediatr 1993;123:376-380.

VanLandingham KE, Marsteller HB, Ross GW, Hayden FG. Relapse of herpes simplex encephalitis after conventional acyclovir therapy. JAMA 1988;259:1051-1053.

Van Loon AM, Van der Logt JTM, Heessen FWA, et al. Diagnosis of herpes simplex virus encephalitis by detection of virus-specific immunoglobulins A and G in serum and cerebrospinal fluid by using an antibody-capture enzyme-linked immunosorbent assay. J Clin Microbiol 1989;27:1983-1987.

Vestey JP, Howie SEM, Norval M, et al. Severe eczema herpeticum is associated with prolonged depression of cell-mediated immunity to herpes simplex virus. Curr Probl Dermatol 1989;18:158-161.

Wasiewski WW, Fishman MA. Herpes simplex encephalitis: the brain biopsy controversy. J Pediatr 1988;113:575-578.

Whitley RJ. Herpes simplex virus infections of women and their offspring: implications for a developed society. Proc Nat Acad Sci USA 1994;91:2441-2447.

Whitley R. Herpes simplex viruses. In Fields B (ed). Virology, ed 3. New York: Raven Press, 1996.

Whitley RJ, Alford CA, Hirsch MS, et al. Vidarabine versus acyclovir therapy in herpes simplex encephalitis. N Engl J Med 1986;314:144-149.

Whitley R, Arvin A, Prober C, et al. Predictors of morbidity and mortality in neonates with herpes simplex virus infections. N Engl J Med 1991a;324:450-454.

Whitley R, Arvin A, Prober C, et al. A controlled trial comparing vidarabine with acyclovir in neonatal herpes simplex virus infection. N Engl J Med 1991b;324:444-454.

Whitley RJ, Corey L, Arvin AM, et al. Changing presentation of herpes simplex viral infection in neonates. J Infect Dis 1988;158:109-116.

Whitley RJ, Hutto C. Neonatal herpes simplex virus infections. Pediatr Rev 1985;7:119-126.

Whitley RJ, Lakeman FD. Herpes simplex virus infection of the central nervous system: therapeutic and diagnostic considerations. Clin Infect Dis 1995;20:414-420.

Whitley RJ, Lakeman FD, Nahmias AJ, Roizman B. DNA restriction-enzyme analysis of herpes simplex virus isolates obtained from patients with encephalitis. N Engl J Med 1982a;307:1060-1062.

Whitley RJ, Nahmias AJ, Visintine AM, et al. The natural history of herpes simplex virus infection of mother and child. Pediatrics 1980;66:489-494.

Whitley RJ, Soong S, Linneman C Jr, et al. Herpes simplex encephalitis. JAMA 1982b;247:317-320.

Yeager A, Arvin AM, Urbani LJ, Kemp JA. Relationship of antibody to outcome in neonatal herpes simplex virus infections. Infect Immunol 1980;29:532-538.

Yeager A, Ashley R, Corey L. Transmission of herpes simplex virus from father to neonate. J Pediatr 1983;103:905-907.

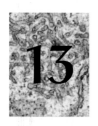

13   HUMAN HERPESVIRUS 6, 7, AND 8

CAROLINE BREESE HALL

Unmasked within its cellular cache
a microbe minuscule unknown;
Creator of the rose-like rash
described by sages ages past.

Molecular techniques unfold
its programmed, dark genomic soul,
Revealing its recondite hold
on newly born to those now old.

CBH

The sixth exanthematous disease of childhood, long of unknown ancestry, has now been recognized to be one of the manifestations of the sixth member of the human herpes family, HHV-6. With this has come the recognition that this virus responsible for roseola, like other members of its family, has multiple personalities and potential import at all ages.

HISTORY

The first description of roseola may have been in Meigs and Pepper's *A Practical Treatise of the Diseases of Children* of 1870, wherein it is referred to as *roseola aestiva* or *roseola autumnalis*. In this textbook the exanthematous disease was described as "chilliness alternating with heat, with loss of strength and spirits, headache, restlessness, sometimes mild delirium and slight convulsive phenomena," and the rash of roses as "irregularly circular with rather large patches, at first of red, but soon changing to a deep rose color."

In 1910 Zahorsky described the first clear cases of roseola, and in 1941 Breese conducted the first prospective study of roseola cases. The epidemiologic and clinical description of these roseola cases from Breese's practice closely mimics those subsequently described for HHV-6. A decade later Kempe et al. (1950) described the transmission of

the agent of roseola via blood from one infant to another and to monkeys via both blood and nasal secretions. Although a viral etiology was suspected, the attempts at identification and isolation by Breese and subsequently by Kempe were unsuccessful.

HHV-6 was initially discovered by Salahuddin et al. in 1986 in adult patients with lymphoreticular diseases and HIV infection. Two years later Yamanishi et al. (1988) isolated the same virus from the blood of four infants with roseola infantum. Although this novel virus was found initially in the B-lymphocytes of adult immunocompromised patients, it was subsequently noted to have primary affinity for T-lymphocytes, and its original appellation, human B lymphotrophic virus (HBLV), was changed to HHV-6.

HHV-6 is a member of the *Roseolovirus* genus of the Betaherpesvirus subfamily. Like other herpesviruses, HHV-6 possesses the characteristic electron-dense core and an icosahedral capsid, surrounded by a tegument and outer envelope, the location of the important glycoproteins and membrane proteins. HHV-6's capsid, with a diameter of 90 to 110 nm, is assembled initially in the nucleus, where the tegument is acquired. Fully tegumented capsids of a diameter of 165 nm are subsequently released into the cytoplasm; the capsids then become enveloped by budding into cytoplasmic vesicles. The extruded virions have a diameter of about 200 nm.

HHV-6 is composed of two variants, HHV-6A and HHV-6B (Pellett et al., 1992). These two variants are closely related, but distinct in terms of their cellular tropism, molecular biologic characteristics, epidemiology, and clinical associations. The genomic identity between strains from the two variants is generally high, sometimes 95%. The double-stranded DNA genomes of HHV-6 are approximately 162 to 170 kb, with a unique long (UL) segment of about 141 to 143 kb bracketed by direct repeats (D_{RL} and D_{RR}) of variable length.

HHV-6A and HHV-6B are closely related to HHV-7 but share some amino acid similarities with human cytomegalovirus (HCMV). Currently no serologic tests can distinguish between HHV-6A and HHV-6B; HHV-6 shares some serologic cross-reactivity with HHV-7, but not with other herpesviruses (Black et al., 1993).

EPIDEMIOLOGY

Recent serologic studies of HHV-6 have highlighted the ubiquitous occurrence of HHV-6 infection in every country in which it has been studied. Acquisition of infection is usually in the first year or two of life, and in adults ≥95% possess antibody. In the United States, Japan, and other countries, HHV-6 infection is acquired during infancy, primarily at 6 to 18 months of age, with the mean age about 9 months (Fig. 13-1). Infection occurs with amazing alacrity within a few months and correlates with the decline of maternal antibody (see Fig. 13-1). In a prospective study of approximately 4,000 children in Rochester, New York, essentially all infants at birth possessed passive maternal antibody, which declined over the next several months, reaching a nadir by 4 months, with a subsequent rapid increase in the proportion of seropositive infants to 18 months of age (Hall et al., 1994). Detection of the HHV-6 genome by polymerase chain re-

action assays (PCR) in the peripheral blood mononuclear cells of these same infants, indicating the acquisition of infection and persistence of the viral DNA, mimicked the same curve as that for seroprevalence but preceded it by about 2 months (Hall et al., 1994).

The major modes of transmission of HHV-6 are incompletely defined. HHV-6 persists after primary infection in the blood, respiratory secretions, and other anatomic sites. Presumably, the source of the rapid and complete acquisition of infection by the infant, therefore, is the asymptomatic shedding of HHV-6 in secretions of the caretakers and close contacts of the infant. Other modes of transmission also may be possible, including perinatal transmission. This possibility has been suggested by the detection of the HHV-6 genome in the peripheral blood mononuclear cells of asymptomatic neonates (Hall et al., 1994). HHV-6 DNA has been detected in the cervical secretions of pregnant women, but not in breast milk (Leach et al., 1994; Okuno et al., 1995).

The impact of HHV-6 infection, not suspected by the long-held general clinical conceptions of roseola, is indicated by the proportion of acute emergency room visits for young children that HHV-6 engenders because of high fevers, toxicity, and seizures (Hall et al., 1994). Approximately

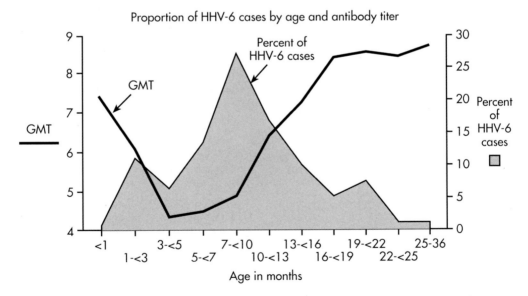

FIG. 13-1   The proportion of 335 cases of HHV-6B primary infection occurring according to age in months and in relation to their mean titer (GMT) (log$_2$) of IgG antibody to HHV-6. The 335 cases of primary HHV-6 infection were identified by isolation of HHV-6 from the blood and by seroconversion from a prospective study of children less than 3 years of age with febrile illnesses presenting to outpatient facilities at the University of Rochester Medical Center, Rochester, N.Y. (Some cases reported in Hall CB et al.: N Engl J Med 1994;331:432–438.)

20% of the visits for acute infection evaluated in Rochester, New York, for infants 6 to 12 months of age were identified as primary HHV-6 infection, and for children in the first 2 years of life 10% of such visits were from HHV-6 infection. The cost of evaluating these children places an appreciable burden on the health-care system.

IMMUNITY

The relative protection of infants against primary infection until maternal antibody declines indicates that serum antibody does provide protection, though not complete. Primary infection is characterized by viremia, which results in the production of neutralizing antibody. Specific IgM antibodies are the first to appear, 1 week from the onset of clinical symptoms. Within the subsequent 2 months, IgM declines and is no longer detectable. Specific IgG antibody rises in the second week, with a subsequent increase in the avidity, and generally persists for life. Specific IgA antibodies have been identified in a few adult patients. Antibody levels may fluctuate subsequent to primary infection, possibly as a result of reactivation of latent virus, and significant increases in antibody levels have been noted with the occurrence of other infections, such as cytomegalovirus (Pellett et al., 1992). Specific IgM antibodies may also be present in reactivated disease and are present in a small proportion of normal individuals (Suga et al., 1992). Fourfold rises in IgG antibody to HHV-6 have been documented in normal children during the 2 years after their primary infection (Hall et al., 1994). Although some of these significant antibody rises occurred during an acute infection with another agent, many remain unexplained. Reinfection with HHV-6 of a different variant or strain is possible. Two different HHV-6B infections have been documented by genomic analysis in one infant (Dewhurst et al., 1992). Roseola and other primary infections with HHV-6 appear to be almost exclusively from variant B. The occurrence and circumstances of primary infection from variant A alone have yet to be determined.

Little is known about the role of cellular immunity in HHV-6 infection. The importance of cellular immunity, however, is evident from the appearance of reactivated HHV-6 infection with clinical findings, sometimes dissemination, in patients who are immunosuppressed. HHV-6 infection is associated with increased NK cellular activity and the induction of IFN-α; in vitro replication is diminished with exogenous IFN-α.

CLINICAL MANIFESTATION
Primary HHV-6 Infection

Contact cases or the source for primary HHV-6 infection that occurs in an infant is almost always unknown, but the incubation period may be estimated from Kempe's studies (Kempe et al., 1950) to be approximately 10 days. Although roseola is the major manifestation of primary HHV-6 infection in Japan, in the large prospective studies of U.S. children the classical manifestations of roseola are present only in about 15% to 20% of primary cases evaluated in clinics and the emergency room. Clinical manifestations are varied (Hall et al., 1994; Kusuhara et al., 1992). Most striking and characteristic is the abrupt onset of high fever, which tends to persist for 3 to 6 days. The peak fever over the first several days usually reaches 39° to 40° C, and approximately half of the patients have fevers above 40° C. This febrile period generally correlates with the occurrence of viremia. The fever may only be accompanied by nonspecific signs and symptoms, including lethargy, anorexia, and toxicity, although many children appear relatively well considering the height of the fever. Such children are often diagnosed as having nonspecific or "viral" febrile illness, frequently with otitis. The latter diagnosis appears to be based mostly on the erythematous condition of the tympanic membranes, which frequently occurs in these young children. On follow-up, however, many of these children do not have the typical signs of otitis media and sequelae, such as middle-ear effusions. The most frequent diagnosis on the initial presentation of children with primary HHV-6 infection usually is a febrile illness of unknown etiology with otitis. Approximately 20% to 25% have the primary diagnosis of gastroenteritis or respiratory illness (Table 13-1).

The physical findings accompanying primary HHV-6 infection may also be varied. Lymphadenopathy commonly is present in the cervical region and particularly in the posterior occipital area. The lymphadenopathy it usually becomes most prominent on the third or fourth day of the illness. The pharynx may be mildly injected, and sometimes an enanthema of small red maculopapular spots on the soft plate and uvula (Nagayama's spots) may be present. The palpebral conjunctivae also may be mildly inflamed and slightly edematous. As mentioned earlier, the tympanic membranes are frequently inflamed, in part because of the fever and mild catarrhal otitis.

Table 13-1 Clinical manifestations of primary HHV-6 infection in 335 children ≤25 months of age*

Sign of symptom	Proportion of HHV-6 patients with sign or symptom
Fever	100%
Fever >39°C	88%
Irritability	76%
Lethargy	77%
Lymphadenopathy (cervical, occipital)	74%
Toxic appearance	68%
Palpebral erythema	62%
Inflamed tympanic membranes	55%
Upper respiratory tract signs	41%
Gastrointestinal signs (vomiting, diarrhea)	38%
Rash	
During fever	11%
At defervescence	21%
Seizures	13%

*From prospective study of children presenting to outpatient facilities at the University of Rochester, New York, with primary HHV-6 infection identified by isolation of HHV-6 from blood and seroconversion.

Roseola. All of the aforementioned findings may be present in children with roseola. The typical course of roseola is similar to that just outlined, with the abrupt onset of high fever; nonspecific signs, especially irritability; cervical and posterior occipital lymphadenopathy; and the appearance of a rash with defervescence. Occasionally the rash appears before the fever has subsided completely and sometimes not until after one afebrile day. The rash may be varied in appearance and is not distinctive for roseola. It may be evanescent, lasting only a few hours or remaining for 1 to 3 days. Characteristically the lesions are rose colored, as noted by Meigs and Pepper (1870); macular or maculopapular; and approximately 2 to 3 mm in diameter. The lesions fade on pressure, rarely coalesce, and may be rubelliform or morbilliform. The rash usually is first noted on the trunk, with subsequent spread to the neck, upper extremities, face, and lower extremities. The rash, however, may be more limited in distribution, occurring primarily on the trunk, neck, and face. The exanthem clears completely leaving no pigmentation or desquamation.

Neonatal Infection. Despite the general conception and observations for roseola, HHV-6 infection may occur in very young infants, including

neonates. In Rochester approximately 15% of the primary HHV-6 infections studied were in infants in the first 8 weeks of life. The clinical manifestations of symptomatic primary HHV-6 infection in these young infants generally are similar to that of older infants. A febrile illness with no localizing signs is the most frequent presentation, but the fever tends to be lower than that of older infants.

Newborns may have asymptomatic infection, as indicated by the detection of HHV-6 DNA in their peripheral blood mononuclear cells at birth or in the subsequent neonatal period (Hall et al., 1994). The import of this remains unclear. In some but not all of these infants the HHV-6 DNA persists in their peripheral blood cells for variable periods, and some subsequently develop clinical primary HHV-6 infection. This may suggest perinatal transmission of HHV-6 without durable immunity.

Laboratory Findings. The most distinctive laboratory finding to accompany primary HHV-6 infection is the course of the peripheral white blood cell (WBC) count. On initial presentation the total WBC count is diminished for age, usually about 8,000 cells/mm^3 (Hall et al., 1994) (Fig. 13-2). Subsequently, the total WBC count falls, reaching its nadir on days 3 and 4, and then rises toward normal, thus correlating with the febrile course. The peripheral lymphocyte count is most diminished, but the proportion of neutrophils also falls below the normal for age. Most other laboratory findings remain within normal limits. Occasionally the erythrocyte sedimentation rate (ESR) is slightly elevated, but in most children it remains within the normal range.

DIAGNOSIS
Differential Diagnosis

The clinical diagnosis of primary HHV-6 infection is difficult because of its varied manifestations, which may mimic many other infections. The abrupt onset of high fever and toxicity often suggests the diagnosis of sepsis or meningitis in the initial evaluation. Other viral infections, such as enteroviral infections, appear similar. The distinctive features of HHV-6 infection are the abrupt and initially persistent high fever, commonly 40° C or more, in an infant with the characteristic demographics, primarily age, between 6 and 18 months, without known contact. HHV-6 is also not seasonal, as are such viruses as enteroviruses and influenza. The subsequent characteristic pattern of development of lymphadenopathy, particularly posterior occipital nodes, and the pattern of the

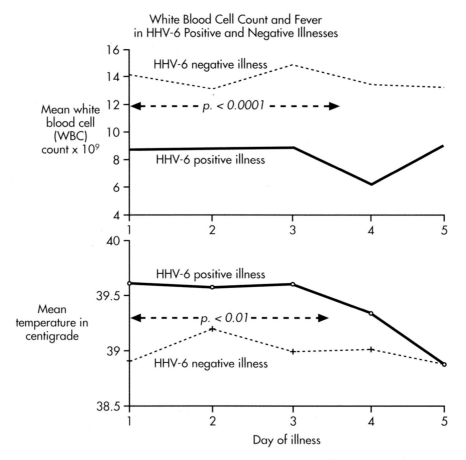

White Blood Cell Count and Fever
in HHV-6 Positive and Negative Illnesses

FIG. 13-2   Mean peripheral white blood cell count (WBC) ($\times 10^9$) and temperature in 2,005 children under 3 years of age presenting with acute febrile illness to outpatient facilities at University of Rochester Medical Center. Compared are 285 children with primary HHV-6 illness to 1,720 children with illness resulting from other causes according to day of illness. (Unpublished data plus data adapted from Hall CB: Contemporary pediatrics 1996;13(1):45–57 and Hall CB: In Long SS, Prober CG, Pickering LK [eds]. Principles and practice of pediatric infectious diseases, 1997;1176–1181.)

WBC count are not likely to be helpful initially. Roseola often may be diagnosed retrospectively once the typical course has been observed and the rash has appeared at defervescence. Other viral diseases, such as echovirus 16 infection, may produce similar rubelliform or morbilliform rashes, occasionally on defervescence. Recently HHV-7 has been identified as causing some cases of roseola and other febrile illnesses, which may be indistinguishable clinically. HHV-7, however, tends to occur slightly later in life (Caserta et al., 1996; Tanaka et al., 1994).

Laboratory Diagnosis

The laboratory diagnosis of primary HHV-6 infection currently remains problematic, requiring diffi-cult or laboratory research techniques. The diffi-culty of diagnosis is further compounded by the persistent or latent nature of HHV-6. Detection of HHV-6 DNA in peripheral blood lymphocytes or in other sites does not necessarily indicate primary infection; most frequently it is persistent virus from previous infection. Serologic diagnosis has similar drawbacks, in that fourfold rises may be detected with reactivation and sometimes in association with other infections (Black et al., 1996). In normal children the definitive diagnosis of primary HHV-6 infection therefore requires the detection of viremia (i.e., isolation of HHV-6 from the peripheral blood mononuclear cells) and significant serologic rises. In normal children HHV-6 viremia occurs rarely other than with primary infection. Isolation of HHV-6, however, requires cocultivation with stimulated cord blood cells and subsequent identification techniques that are currently available only in research laboratories. Rapid diagnostic techniques, such as polymerase chain reaction, are available for detection of HHV-6 DNA, but are not yet available to differentiate between persistent virus and primary viremic infection.

Serologic diagnosis may be accomplished by several assays, including the indirect immunofluorescent assay, anticomplement immunofluorescent assay, neutralization assay, competitive radioimmune assays, and enzyme immunoassays (Black et al., 1996; Pellett et al., 1992). However, all serologic assays currently available have several drawbacks. First, HHV-6 and HHV-7 are so closely related that cross-reactive antibodies may be present in some individuals, thus requiring that sera be absorbed for both viruses before performance of the assay (Black et al., 1996). Second, the serologic assay cannot differentiate between HHV-6A and HHV-6B infections. Third, the ubiquity of HHV-6 infection results in the seropositivity of almost all individuals. Young infants have passive maternal antibody for the first several months of life, and the subsequent acquisition of antibody via infection is so rapid and complete that essentially all are seropositive by 2 years of age.

Detection of IgM antibodies to HHV-6 is also not a reliable sign of primary HHV-6 infection, since not all infants with culture-positive primary infection develop detectable IgM responses, and since previously infected individuals may possess IgM antibody at any time or during reactivation (Suga et al., 1992).

COMPLICATIONS

The major complications of primary HHV-6 infection involve the central nervous system. Roseola has long been observed to have occasional central nervous system complications such as seizures, bulging of the anterior fontanelle, meningoencephalitis or encephalitis, and hemiplegia, as noted in past case reports.* In most instances these complicating manifestations resolve, but long-term sequelae occasionally have been reported (Yanagihara et al., 1995). The most frequent complication of acute infection, however, is febrile seizures (Barone et al., 1995; Hall et al., 1994). In a prospective study of over 200 children with pri-

---

*Berenberg et al., 1949; Burnstine and Paine, 1959; Holliday, 1950; Huang et al., 1991; Möller, 1956; Posson, 1949.

mary HHV-6 infection, seizures occurred in 13%, with the highest rate in children 12 to 15 months of age, in whom 36% developed seizures, compared to only 13% of matched children with acute febrile illnesses not caused by HHV-6 (Hall et al., 1994). The seizures associated with primary HHV-6 infection are characteristic of febrile seizures in terms of age, occurring primarily after 6 months of age, but also have differentiating characteristics. In this study approximately half of the febrile seizures occurred after the first day of fever and tended to be prolonged or recurrent.

HHV-6 DNA has been detected in the CSF of children with acute primary HHV-6 infection with or without CNS complications and subsequently in normal children with past HHV-6 infection. The significance of this is unclear, but some studies suggest that the presence of HHV-6 DNA in the CSF is associated with acute and long-term CNS sequelae (Caserta et al., 1994; Kondo et al., 1993; Suga et al., 1992). Recent studies have shown that HHV-6 DNA frequently may be detected in brains of individuals dying of multiple causes (Luppi et al., 1994a, 1994b). Whether HHV-6 invades the brain during primary infection—with subsequent persistence and development of sequelae—is unknown. In cases of encephalitis associated with HHV-6 in children and adults, HHV-6 DNA in the CSF has been detected (Jones et al., 1994; McCullers et al., 1995; Yoshikawa et al., 1992). Case reports have noted a variety of other complications associated with HHV-6 infection, including idiopathic thrombocytopenic purpura, granulocytopenia, hepatitis, and myocarditis (Kitamura et al., 1994; Tajiri et al., 1990).

HHV-6's frequent persistence in multiple sites—including peripheral white blood cells, brain, lymph nodes, secretions, and skin—portend the possibility of reactivation and complications at later times. In normal children, little information currently exists about this possibility. In immunocompromised patients, however, reactivation with the detection and isolation of HHV-6 from multiple sites is frequent. The role that HHV-6 plays in the subsequent course of such patients is incompletely defined, but in organ transplant recipients some studies have suggested that HHV-6 reactivation is associated with rejection, bone marrow suppression, and pneumonitis (Carrigan, 1995; Yalcin et al., 1994). HHV-6 DNA particularly has been detected in the brains of children with HIV infection and associated with reactivation in adult HIV patients. Whether HHV-6 is a cofactor in the course of HIV infection is not clear.

THERAPY

Currently no therapy, other than symptomatic, is available for the treatment of HHV-6 infection. Several antiviral agents, including ganciclovir and foscarnet, have been examined in vitro and show some antiviral effect (Burns and Sandford, 1990). No studies of antiviral agents for normal children with HHV-6 have been conducted, but a few uncontrolled studies have been reported for immunocompromised patients with disease associated with HHV-6 reactivation (Drobyski et al., 1993).

Summary

With discovery of its etiology, the sixth exanthematous disease of old has assumed a new mien as the sixth member of the herpesvirus family. HHV-6 primary infection presents in varied, and not always benign, ways and causes an appreciable burden on the healthcare of children in the first 2 years of life. The ubiquity of the agent, the high proportion of acute ambulatory visits it engenders, and the cost of the evaluations for these infants who may appear toxic or septic indicate the need for rapid, specific, and feasible diagnostic assays. The tendency of the virus to persist and potentially to reactivate requires much further investigation. The import of such latency—as well as strain variation, reinfection, and its role as a potential cofactor for other diseases of later life—has yet to be delineated.

HUMAN HERPESVIRUS 7 (HHV-7) AND HUMAN HERPESVIRUS 8 (HHV-8)

The younger siblings of the now infamously expanding family of herpesviruses, HHV-7 and HHV-8, also owe their discovery to the advancing technology stemming from investigation of HIV infection. Indeed, perhaps more is known currently about the internal structure of these viruses than about their clinical implications, a reversal of the classic investigative process of infectious agents. Rather than looking from the outside eventually to the inside, the view in these cases appears to have begun within the capsid.

HHV-7 bears the closest familial resemblance to HHV-6 morphologically, antigenically, and genomically, and is thus also classified as a β-herpesvirus (Frenkel and Roffman, 1996). Amino acid sequencing shows variable but appreciable homology with HHV-6 and some degree of serologic cross-reactivity may exist in some sera, especially of older individuals (Black and Pellett, 1993). Like HHV-6, HHV-7 is a ubiquitous agent, occurring in early childhood, usually after HHV-6, and it is most capable of persistence or latency. HHV-7 DNA may be detected in three fourths of salivas from healthy adults, which is likely to be the source of the early and widespread acquisition of infection in children.

No clear clinical personality yet has emerged for HHV-7. Case reports from Japan indicate that initial infection with HHV-7 may present as typical roseola and may account for second or recurrent cases of roseola (Asano et al., 1994; Tanaka et al., 1994; Torigoe et al., 1995). A large prospective study of children under 3 years of age in Rochester, New York, suggests that primary infection manifest as marked acute clinical illness may be relatively uncommon, but when it does present with illness requiring medical attention (as with HHV-6) the signs and symptoms may be varied, evoking diagnoses other than roseola (Caserta et al., 1996). Of eight children with primary HHV-7 infection confirmed by viral isolation from the blood and by serology, 75% had febrile seizures (Caserta et al., 1996).

Proving a direct causal relationship between HHV-7 infection and clinical disease is confounded by the few cases yet described of primary infection confirmed by both viral isolation from peripheral blood lymphocytes and serologic tests; by its ability to persist asymptomatically after primary infection; and also by its interaction with other viruses, especially HHV-6. HHV-7 infection may reactivate latent HHV-6 genomes, and latent HHV-7 could possibly be reactivated by primary HHV-6 infection (Frenkel and Roffman, 1996; Caserta et al., 1996). Of particular interest is the in vitro evidence suggesting that HHV-7 infection could influence the course of HIV infection. Both use the cellular receptor of CD 4 cells, and coinfection results in diminished HIV replication (Frenkel and Roffman, 1996; Lusso et al., 1994).

The clinical implications for children of the newly discovered γ-herpesvirus, the eighth member of the herpesvirus family, is even less clear. In adults, however, HHV-8 has been associated closely with the development of Kaposi's sarcoma (Chang et al., 1994; Voevodin, 1996). The agent was first discovered by Chang et al. (1994) in Kaposi's sarcoma lesions of patients with AIDS and thus also bears the name *Kaposi's sarcoma–associated herpesvirus* (KSHV). The oncogenic potential of HHV-8 is an area of major interest and investigation, since two cellular homologues to protooncogenes, human cyclin D and bcl-2, have been identified in HHV-8 (Voevodin, 1996). HHV-8 is detected most commonly by PCR, and limited studies thus far indicate that it is uncommon in healthy individuals not at risk of developing AIDS or becoming immunocompromised (Voevodin, 1996). Antibodies against HHV-8 are found in people with AIDS who develop Kaposi's sarcoma, but not in HIV-seronegative blood donors (Gas et al., 1996). Information in children is lacking. Detection of HHV-8 is most frequent in patients with Karposi's sarcoma, but it also has been identified in patients with other HIV-associated, body cavity–based B-cell lymphomas; with transplants; and with multicentric Castleman's disease (Voevodin, 1996).

BIBLIOGRAPHY

Asano Y, Yoshikawa T, Suga S, et al. Clinical features of infants with primary human herpesvirus 6 infections (exanthem subitum, roseola infantum). Pediatrics 1994;93:104-108.

Barone SR, Kaplan MH, Krilov LR. Human herpesvirus–6 infection in children with first febrile seizures. J Pediatr 1995; 127:95-97.

Berenberg W, Wright S, Janeway CA. Roseola infantum (exanthem subitum). N Engl J Med 1949;241:253-259.

Black JB, Inoue N, Kite-Powell K, et al. Frequent isolation of human herpesvirus 7 from saliva. Virus Res 1993;29:91-98.

Black JB, Pellett PE, Human herpesvirus 7. Rev Med Virol 1993;3:217-223.

Black JB, Schwarz TF, Patton JL, et al. Evaluation of immunoassays for detection of antibodies to human herpesvirus 7. Clin Diagn Lab Immunol. 1996;3:79-83.

Breese BB Jr. Roseola infantum (exanthem subitum). NY State J Med 1941;41:1854-1859.

Burns WH, Sandford GR. Susceptibility of human herpesvirus 6 to antivirals in vitro. J Infect Dis 1990;162:634-637.

Burnstine RC, Paine RS. Residual encephalopathy following roseola infantum. Am J Dis Child 1959;98:144-152.

Carrigan DR. Human herpesvirus 6 and bone marrow transplantation. Blood 1995;85(1):294-295.

Caserta M, Hall CB, Schnabel K, O'Heron N, Human herpesvirus 7 in U.S. children, Pediatric Res 1996;39:168.

Caserta MT, Hall CB, Schnabel K, et al. Neuroinvasion and persistence of human herpesvirus 6 in children. J Infect Dis 1994;170:1586-1589.

Chang Y, Cesarman E, Pessin MS, et al. Identification of herpesvirus-like DNA sequences in AIDS-associated Kaposi's sarcoma. Science 1994;266:1865-1869.

Dewhurst S, Chandran B, McIntyre K, et al. Phenotypic and genetic polymorphisms among human herpesvirus–6 isolates from North American infants. Virology 1992;190:490-493.

Drobyski WR, Dunne WM, Burd EM, et al. Human herpesvirus–6 (HHV-6) infection in allogeneic bone marrow transplant recipients: evidence of a marrow-suppressive role for HHV-6 in vivo. J Infect Dis 1993;167:735-739.

Frenkel N, Roffman E. Human herpesvirus 7. In Fields BN, Knipe DM, Howley PM, et al. (eds). Fields virology, ed 3. Philadelphia: Lippincott-Raven, 1996.

Gao SJ, Kingsley L, Hoover DR, et al. Seroconversion to antibodies against Kaposi's sarcoma–associated herpesvirus-related latent nuclear antigens before the development of Kaposi's sarcoma. N Engl J Med 1996;335:233-241.

Hall CB. Herpesvirus 6: new light on an old childhood exanthem. Contemp Pediatr 1996;13(1):45-57.

Hall CB. Human herpesviruses 6 (roseola, exanthem subitum). In Long SS, Prober CG, Pickering LK (eds). Principles and Practice of Pediatric Infectious Diseases. New York: Churchill Livingstone, 1997.

Hall CB, Long CE, Schnabel KC, et al. Human herpesvirus–6 infection in children: prospective evaluation for compli-cations and reactivation. N Engl J Med 1994;331(7):432-438.

Holliday PB Jr. Pre-eruptive neurological complications of the common contagious diseases: rubella, rubeola, roseola, and varicella. J Pediatr 1950;36:185-198.

Huang LM, Lee CY, Chen JY, et al. Roseola infantum caused by human herpesvirus 6: report of 7 cases with emphasis on complications. J Formos Med Assoc 1991;90:579-582.

Jones CMV, Dunn HG, Thomas EE, et al. Acute encephalopathy and status epilepticus associated with human herpesvirus–6 infection. Dev Med Child Neurol 1994;36:646-650.

Kempe HC, Shaw EB, Jackson JR, Silver HK. Studies on the etiology of exanthema subitum (Roseola infantum). J Pediatr 1950;37:561-568.

Kitamura K, Ohta H, Ihara T, et al. Idiopathic thrombocytopenic purpura after human herpesvirus–6 infection. Lancet 1994; 344:830.

Kondo K, Nagafuji H, Hata A, et al. Association of human herpesvirus–6 infection of the central nervous system with recurrence of febrile convulsions. J Infect Dis 1993; 167:1197-1200.

Kusuhara K, Ueda K, Miyazaki C, et al. Attack rate of exanthem subitum in Japan. Lancet 1992;340:482.

Leach CT, Newton ER, McParlin S, Jenson HB. Human herpesvirus–6 infection on the female genital tract. J Infect Dis 1994;169:1281-1283.

Luppi M, Barozzi P, Maiorana A, et al. HHV-6 in normal brain tissue. J Infect Dis 1994a;169:943-944.

Luppi MP, Barozzi P, Maiorana A, et al. Detection of human herpesvirus–6 sequences in normal human brains and in neurological tumors. Proc Ann Meet Assoc Cancer Res 1994b; 35:A3518.

Lusso P, Secchiero P, Crowley RW, et al. CD4 is a critical component of the receptor for human immunodeficiency virus. Proc Nat Acad Sci USA 1994;266:1865-1869.

McCullers JA, Lakeman FD, Whitley RJ. Human herpesvirus 6 is associated with focal encephalitis. Clin Infect Dis 1995; 21:571-576.

Meigs JF, Pepper W. A practical treatise of the diseases of children. In Philadelphia: Lindsay and Blakiston, 1870.

Möller KL. Exanthema subitum and febrile convulsions. Acta Paediatr 1956;45:534-540.

Okuno T, Oishi H, Hayashi K, et al. Human herpesvirus 6 and 7 in cervixes of pregnant women. J Clin Microbiol 1995; 33(7):1968-1970.

Pellett PE, Black JB, Yamamoto M. Human herpesvirus 6: the virus and the search for its role as a human pathogen. Adv Virus Res 1992;41:1-52.

Posson DD. Exanthem subitum (roseola infantum) complicated by prolonged convulsions and hemiplegia. J Pediatr 1949;35:235-236.

Salahuddin SZ, Ablashi DV, Marleham PD, et al. Isolation of a new virus, HBLV, in patients with lymphoproliferative disorders. Science 1986;234:596-601.

Suga A, Yoshikawa T, Asano Y, et al. Clinical and virological analyses of 21 infants with exanthem subitum (roseola infantum) and central nervous system complications. Ann Neurol 1993;33(6):597-603.

Suga S, Yoshikawa T, Asano Y, et al. IgM neutralizing antibody responses to human herpesvirus 6 in patients with exanthem subitum or organ transplantation. Microbiol Immunol 1992; 36(5):495-506.

Tajiri H, Nose O, Baba K, Okada S. Human herpesvirus–6 infection with liver injury in neonatal hepatitis. Lancet 1990; 335:863.

Tanaka K, Kondo T, Torigoe S, et al. Human herpesvirus 7: another causal agent for roseola (exanthem subitum). J Pediatr 1994;125:1-5.

Torigoe S, Kumamoto T, Koide W, et al. Clinical manifestations associated with human herpesvirus–7 infection. Arch Dis Child 1995;72:518-519.

Voevodin AF. Human herpesvirus, type 8, early days. Rev Med Virol 6:173-178.

Yalcin S, Karpuzoglu T, Suleymanlar G, et al. Human herpesvirus–6 and human herpesvirus–7 infections in renal transplant recipients and healthy adults in Turkey. Arch Virol 1994;136:183-190.

Yamanishi K, Okuno T, Shiraki K, et al. Identification of human herpesvirus 6 as a causal agent for exanthem subitum. Lancet 1988;1:1065-1067.

Yanagihara K, Tanaka-Taya K, Itagaki Y, et al. Human herpesvirus–6 meningoencephalitis with sequelae. Pediatr Infect Dis J 1995;14(3):240-241.

Yoshikawa T, Nakashima T, Suga S, et al. Human herpesvirus–6 DNA in cerebrospinal fluid of a child with exanthem subitum and meningoencephalitis. Pediatrics 1992;89:888-890.

Zahorsky J. Roseola infantilis. Pediatrics 1910;22:60-64.

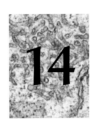

14 INFECTIONS IN THE HOSPITALIZED AND IMMUNOINCOMPETENT CHILD

LINDA L. LEWIS AND PHILIP A. PIZZO

The risk of infectious complications in children undergoing intensive cytotoxic therapy for cancer has been investigated extensively over the last 25 years, resulting in advances in their diagnosis and treatment and decreases in their morbidity and mortality. This chapter reviews the alterations of host defense that heighten the risk for infection, the current diagnostic considerations, and the principles of treatment and prevention of these complications.

HOST DEFENSE DISTURBANCES ASSOCIATED WITH INCREASED RISK OF INFECTION

Alterations in host defense mechanisms increase the risk for viral, bacterial, fungal, and protozoan pathogens (Table 14-1). Although specific defects in host defense can increase susceptibility to particular types of organisms (e.g., with splenectomy and the increased risk for bacteremia with encapsulated bacteria), only the immunocompromised child frequently has deficiencies of multiple components of the immune network, rendering him or her at risk for a wide variety of infectious complications.

Anatomic abnormalities resulting in breaks in skin or mucosal integrity or mechanical obstruction of a usually patent body cavity or lumen provide an environment conducive to the rapid multiplication of potential pathogens. Oral and gastrointestinal (GI) mucosal surfaces may be disrupted by chemotherapeutic regimens, allowing normal or hospital-acquired flora to have access to the bloodstream. Enlarged lymph nodes, tumor mass, or scar tissue from previous surgical procedures or radiation therapy may also obstruct body passages, allowing overgrowth of microorganisms in usually sterile sites, with consequent transmigration of bacteria across mucosal surfaces or proximal perforation.

Bacteremias with organisms such as fastidious streptococci, *Peptococcus* spp., or *Capnocy-*

tophaga spp. can also implicate certain body sites (e.g., the oral cavity) as the potential source of infection. Similarly, bacteremia with gram-negative aerobes, anaerobes, enterococci, or other enteric pathogens (e.g., *Streptococcus bovis*) should prompt investigation of the GI tract as the source of infection. Frequent hospitalization and frequent use of antibiotics or chemotherapeutic agents can alter the "normal" flora of many patients with chronic illnesses and provide an endogenous microflora more likely to result in infectious complications.

Asplenia, whether surgical, congenital, or functional, predisposes to serious infections with encapsulated bacteria such as *Streptococcus pneumoniae, Haemophilus influenzae, Klebsiella* spp., and *Neisseria meningiditis*. The increased risk of salmonella infections in patients with sickle cell disease has been attributed to both splenic dysfunction and humoral immune deficits. Patients who underwent splenectomy following trauma are less likely to develop overwhelming infections than those asplenic for other reasons, presumably because of the presence of residual splenic rests that provide functional activity (Rubin et al., 1991).

The ability of granulocytes to respond appropriately to infection requires migration of the cells to the site of infection (chemotaxis), phagocytosis, and killing of the organism. Defects in all of these steps have been described in hereditary disorders, with hematologic malignancies, and as the result of certain medications. Chronic granulomatous disease of childhood (CGD), perhaps the best understood inherited leukocyte disorder, most commonly is due to an X-linked recessive disorder. Because of faulty metabolism of hydrogen peroxide, superoxide, and oxygen radicals, intracellular killing of bacteria by neutrophils is deficient. Patients with this disease are most susceptible to recurrent infections with catalase-producing bacteria such as

Table 14-1 Predominant pathogens in compromised patients: association with selected defects in host defenses

Host defense impairment	Bacteria	Fungi	Viruses	Other

Neutropenia	Gram-negative
	  Enteric organisms
	    (*E. coli, K. pneumoniae,*
	    Enterobacter spp.,
	    Citrobacter spp.)
	  Pseudomonas aeruginosa
	Gram-positive
	  Staphylococci
	    (coagulase-negative,
	    coagulase-positive)
	  Streptococci
	    (group D, a-hemolytic)
	Anaerobes
	  (anaerobic streptococci,
	  Clostridia spp.,
	  Bacteroides spp.)
		Candida spp.
		  (*C. albicans, C.*
		  tropicalis, other
		  species)
		Aspergillus spp.
		  (*A. fumigatus, A. flavus*)		

Abnormal cell-mediated immunity	*Legionella* spp.
	Nocardia asteroides
	Salmonella spp.
	Mycobacteria
	  (*M. tuberculosis* and
	  atypical mycobacteria)
	Disseminated infection from live
	  mycobacterial vaccine (BCG)
		Cryptococcus neoformans
		Histoplasma capsulatum
		Coccidioides immitis
		Candida spp.
			Varicella-zoster virus
			Herpes simplex virus
			Cytomegalovirus
			Epstein-Barr virus
			Herpesvirus B
			Disseminated infection from live
			  virus vaccines (vaccinia,
			  measles, rubella, mumps,
			  yellow fever, live polio)
				Pneumocystis carinii
				Toxoplasma gondii
				Cryptosporidium spp.
				Strongyloides stercoralis

	Bacteria	Fungi	Viruses	Parasites
Immunoglobulin abnormalities	Gram-positive Streptococcus pneumoniae Staphylococcus aureus Gram-negative Haemophilus influenzae Neisseria spp. Enteric organisms		Enteroviruses (including polio)	Giardia lamblia
Complement abnormalities C3, C5	Gram-positive S. pneumoniae Staphylococci Gram-negative H. influenzae Neisseria spp. Enteric organisms			
C5 through C9	Neisseria spp. (N. gonorrhea, N. meningitides)			
Anatomic disruption Oral cavity	α-Hemolytic streptococci, oral anaerobes (Peptococcus, Peptostreptococcus)	Candida spp.	Herpes simplex virus	
Esophagus	Staphylococci, other colonizing organisms	Candida spp.	Herpes simplex virus Cytomegalovirus	
Lower gastrointestinal tract	Gram-positive Group D streptococci Gram-negative Enteric organisms Anaerobel (bacteroidel) etc Anaerobes (Bacteroides fragilus, Clostridium spp.)	Candida spp.		S. stercoralis

Continued

Table 14-1 Predominant pathogens in compromised patients: association with selected defects in host defenses—cont'd

Host defense impairment	Bacteria	Fungi	Viruses	Other
Skin (intravenous catheter)	Gram-positive Staphylococci Streptococci Corynebacteria *Bacillus* spp. Gram-negative *P. aeruginosa* Enteric organisms Mycobacteria *M. fortuitum, M. chelonei*	*Candida* spp. *Aspergillus* spp. *Malassezia furfur*		
Urinary tract	Gram-positive Enterococci Gram-negative Enteric organisms *P. aeruginosa*	*Candida* spp.		
Splenectomy	Gram-positive *S. pneumoniae* Gram-negative *H. influenzae* *Salmonella* spp. DF-2 bacillus (*Capnocytophaga* spp.)			*Babesia* spp.

Staphylococcus aureus, Serratia spp., *Escherichia coli, Pseudomonas* spp., and *Candida* spp. Recent advances in understanding the disease have lead to therapy for some patients with interferon-γ, resulting in a significant decrease in infections and in the need for hospitalization (Esekowitz et al., 1988; Sechler et al., 1988; International Chronic Granulomatous Disease Cooperative Study Group, 1991). Other disorders—including myeloperoxidase deficiency, deficiency of the synthesis of β-2 integrin chain, CD18, Chédiak-Higashi syndrome, and glucose-6-phosphate dehydrogenase (G6PD) deficiency—affect granulocytic microbicidal functions, predisposing patients to bacterial infections, particularly soft-tissue abscesses, dermatitis, adenitis, and sinopulmonary infections.

Abnormal neutrophil function also has been documented in a number of hematologic diseases, including acute myelogenous leukemia, preleukemia, and myelodysplastic syndromes. Neutrophils from some of these patients have decreased myeloperoxidase, elastase, and other granule constituents (Davey et al., 1988). Cytotoxic agents and radiation therapy may also result in abnormalities of granulocyte functioning. These deficits may relate to an increased risk of infectious complications.

Defects in cell-mediated immunity can result from congenital disorders or acquired deficits secondary to lymphoid malignancies; certain immunosuppressive drugs; some chronic illnesses; and viral infections, including human immunodeficiency virus (HIV) infection. Abnormal cellular immunity arises when the normal T lymphocyte–macrophage interactions fail, predisposing the patient to infections with intracellular organisms such as *Salmonella* spp., *Listeria* spp., mycobacteria, cytomegalovirus (CMV), herpes simplex virus (HSV), varicella-zoster virus (VZV), Epstein-Barr virus (EBV), *Histoplasma* spp., *Cryptococcus* spp., *Coccidioides* spp., *Toxoplasma* spp., and *Pneumocystis carinii*. Several congenital disorders affect cellular immunity, either as isolated T-lymphocyte dysfunction (as in Nezelof's syndrome) or in combination with defects of humoral immunity (as in severe combined immune deficiency) (Van Der Meer, 1988).

For many years the use of corticosteroids also has been implicated in increased risk of infection. Although steroids adversely affect several host defense mechanisms—such as wound healing, lymphocyte function, and lymphokine production—they are also notorious as agents that decrease granulocyte chemotaxis to sites of infection, thus

"masking" the usual signs and symptoms of inflammation (Cupps and Fauci, 1982).

Immunosuppressive drugs may interfere with cellular immunity by different mechanisms. The cytotoxic agents have profound effects on cell proliferation. Corticosteroids decrease production of and response to cytokines by macrophages and induce lymphopenia through a redistribution of these cells (Cupps and Fauci, 1982). Cyclosporin A, a potent immunosuppressive agent used to prevent rejection in solid organ transplant patients, is associated with disturbances of T–helper cell population, inhibits production of interleukin-2 (IL-2) and interferon-γ, and can alter the risk for infectious complications.

The group of immunocompromised children at risk for serious infectious complications that increased most rapidly in the past decade were those with HIV infection. A detailed discussion of HIV-related risks of infection and immunosuppression is presented in Chapter 1.

Nevertheless, the most frequent reason for host compromise in children remains cancer and its treatment. Indeed, infection is a major cause of morbidity in children with cancer, especially in association with neutropenia. The relationship between falling neutrophil numbers, absolute neutrophil count, and risk of infection was first reported in 1966 by investigators at the National Cancer Institute. This group followed fifty-two leukemia patients through the course of their illness and treatment, charting white blood cell counts, absolute numbers of neutrophils and lymphocytes, clinically and microbiologically diagnosed infections, fevers without proven infections, and relapses and remissions of the underlying malignancy. These investigators concluded the following: (1) the risk of infection was related directly to the number of circulating neutrophils, with an increased incidence of infection when the absolute neutrophil count fell below 1,000 cells/mm^3 and especially when the absolute neutrophil count reached levels below 100 cells/mm^3; (2) the risk of infection was greater for all absolute neutrophil count levels during relapse; (3) the most important factor in predicting risk of infection was the duration of neutropenia with episodes longer than 3 weeks leading to the highest rates of infection and highest mortality; and (4) the degree of fall in the absolute neutrophil count was not as important as the final level that was observed (Bodey et al., 1966). Since the time of this sentinel report the relationship between cancer, neutropenia, and infection has been clearly established, and advances in management have focused attention on this high-risk group of patients. Studies performed during the last three decades confirm that patients with an absolute neutrophil count less than 500 cells/mm^3 constitute a population that requires urgent empirical therapy when those patients become febrile. More recently it has been identified that intensive chemotherapy also has significant effects on the number and distribution of T-cell subsets, leading to depletion of CD4+ and CD8+ cells that may persist for months after completion of chemotherapy. These changes may contribute to increasing the risk for opportunistic infections in these children (Mackall et al., 1994). The considerations that surround the diagnosis, treatment, and prevention of infections in these neutropenic patients offer a paradigm for the management of any immunocompromised child and is the focus of this chapter.

INFECTIONS ENCOUNTERED IN IMMUNOCOMPROMISED PATIENTS
Bacterial Infections

By far the majority of organisms infecting compromised children arise from endogenous flora of the respiratory or GI tracts or the skin. With hospitalizations and treatment there is a shift in the endogenous flora, manifested by colonization with gram-negative organisms and, at some institutions, more resistant bacteria.

During the past 30 years there has been a shift in the cause of the bacterial infections in neutropenic patients. In the 1950s and early 1960s, gram-positive organisms (especially *Staphylococcus aureus*) predominated. With more intensive chemotherapy in the late 1960s and 1970s, gram-negative bacteria, especially *Enterobacteriaceae* species (Van der Waaij et al., 1977) and *Pseudomonas aeruginosa* emerged as the predominant pathogens. Because infections with gram-negative bacilli, especially *P. aeruginosa.* spp., were associated with the rapid onset of overwhelming sepsis and a high mortality rate (Bodey et al., 1985), guidelines for empiric therapy emerged as the standard of practice. Although gram-negative organisms continue to be important, certain of these organisms, *P. aeruginosa* in particular, inexplicably declined as pathogens during the 1980s. Currently, gram-positive organisms—including the staphylococci (both coagulase-positive and coagulase-negative), α-hemolytic streptococci, and enterococci—now predominate at most large medical centers (Pizzo et al., 1978; Wade et al., 1982). Such shifts have an impact on the management and outcome of patients with neutropenia.

Recently infections with some of the gram-positive organisms have attracted increased notice because of changes in the previously expected antibiotic susceptibility patterns. Alpha-hemolytic or viridans streptococci, especially *Streptococcus mitis* and *Streptococcus sanguis,* have increasingly been recognized in neutropenic patients as a cause of bacteremia, with conditions often accompanied by fever and hypotension, and occasionally by circulatory collapse, acute respiratory failure, renal failure, and encephalopathy (Sotiropoulos et al., 1989; Elting et al., 1992; Bochud, 1994). A substantial proportion of these isolates are penicillin-resistant and, to a lesser degree, cephalosporin-resistant, although they have remained susceptible to vancomycin to date. Predisposing factors for the α-streptococcal sepsis syndrome include chemotherapeutic regimens that include high-dose cytosine arabinoside, presence of mucositis, prophylactic use of trimethoprim-sulfamethoxazole or quinolones, profound neutropenia, and administration of antacids or H2-blockers (Elting, 1992; Bochud et al., 1994).

Similarly, the enterococcal species, both *Enterococcus faecalis* and *Enterococcus faecium,* have emerged as pathogens with extremely worrisome susceptibility profiles. Over the last several years these organisms have acquired antibiotic resistance plasmids that render them resistant to multiple antibiotics, including ampicillin, the aminoglycosides, and vancomycin. From 1989 to 1993 the National Nosocomial Infections Surveillance system established by the Centers for Disease Control documented a twentyfold increase in the percentage of nosocomial infections resulting from enterococci that were associated with vancomycin-resistant enterococci (VRE). Among ICU patients with nosocomial infections, the proportion of infections caused by VRE increased from 0.4% in 1989 to 13.6% in 1993 (CDC, 1993). Outbreaks of infections and colonization with these organisms have been reported in oncology units, and morbidity and mortality have been significant (Rubin et al., 1992; Montecalvo et al., 1994). Risk factors associated with colonization with VRE include prior use of antibiotic, especially vancomycin, and length of hospitalization in the period preceding colonization (Rubin et al., 1992). In a recent review of cases in a pediatric oncology ward, risk factors associated with progression of VRE colonization to VRE infection included greater number of days of neutropenia. This report also identified prolonged periods of fecal shedding (median, 112 days) in over 40% of those colonized and found that some children excreted VRE intermittently for up to 1 year of follow-up (Henning et al., 1996).

In spite of their numerical preponderance, anaerobic bacteria are less commonly associated with bacteremia in immunocompromised hosts, accounting for only approximately 5% of episodes. Anaerobes have, however, been associated with specific clinical syndromes, including intraabdominal abscesses, peritonitis, mucositis, or perianal cellulitis. Most anaerobes isolated under these circumstances are *Bacteroides* or *Clostridium* species (Fainstein et al., 1989). *C. difficile* toxin-mediated gastrointestinal disease may also cause a variety of symptoms, from mild gastroenteritis to severe pseudomembranous colitis, but rarely results in bacteremia.

Fungal Infections

During recent years the increased use of intensive chemotherapy for almost all varieties of pediatric cancers has resulted in more regimens that lead to prolonged neutropenia. Under these circumstances fungi have emerged as a major cause of infectious complications. The duration of neutropenia after initiation of antibiotics was the significant risk factor for an invasive mycosis in a recent multivariate analysis (Wiley et al., 1990). Moreover, invasive mycoses are most likely to occur as secondary infections during periods of prolonged neutropenia. The majority of fungal infections in children with cancer are caused by *Candida* spp., with *Aspergillus* spp. the second most frequent cause of invasive mycoses. Depending on the patient's underlying cancer, treatment regimen, and geographic location, a variety of other fungal organisms— including *Cryptococcus, Histoplasma, Coccidioides, Fusarium,* and *Trichosporon* spp.; the Zygomycetes; and the dematiaceous molds—may also result in serious infection. Although some of these fungi, particularly *Candida albicans,* compose part of the normal gastrointestinal or skin flora, most invasive mycoses in immunocompromised hosts represent nosocomial infections. Alterations of mucosal surfaces by chemotherapy, surgery, or tumor invasion may increase the risk of invasive disease, and it has been noted that certain species, such as *Candida tropicalis* and *Torulopsis glabrata,* may be intrinsically more invasive (Wingard et al., 1979; Aisner et al., 1976). Other

fungi such as *Aspergillus* and *Mucor* spp. are not part of the normal microbial flora and are most often acquired from environmental sources. Yeasts such as *Cryptococcus neoformans* and *Histoplasma capsulatum* more commonly produce infection in patients with impaired cell-mediated immunity and, although rarely considered nosocomial processes, they can result from either primary or secondary infection.

Viral Infections

Viruses also have emerged as important pathogens in neutropenic or otherwise immunocompromised children. Early epidemiologic studies probably underestimated the importance of viruses as pathogens, since techniques for viral detection or isolation were less reliable in the 1960s and 1970s. It has been well documented that the herpes group viruses may cause severe and even life-threatening infections in this population. Herpes simplex virus (HSV) and varicella-zoster virus (VZV) were clearly identified as the most common viral pathogens in a comprehensive, prospective study of 150 pediatric leukemia patients, but significant morbidity was associated with isolation of a wide variety of other community-acquired viruses, including the influenza viruses, parainfluenza viruses, cytomegalovirus (CMV), measles, adenovirus, enteroviruses, respiratory syncytial virus (RSV), and rhinoviruses. Because of difficulties in obtaining specimens from some sites (e.g., lower respiratory tract, central nervous system, or liver), this study was unable to make conclusions about the cause-and-effect relationship of virus detection and most clinical syndromes. The investigators were able to document an increased incidence of virus infections during induction or relapse, compared to patients who were in remission. Furthermore, there was an increased rate of virus isolation from patients with acute myeloblastic leukemia, compared to acute lymphoblastic leukemia (Wood and Corbitt, 1985).

Like fungal infections, viral infections may represent either primary or secondary processes. HSV, VZV, and CMV commonly affect large numbers of children early in life and may become latent for long periods, only to recur as reactivation disease when the immune system fails during cancer, chemotherapy (including administration of steroids), organ transplantation, or HIV infection. Untreated primary VZV in leukemic children carries with it the potential for serious pneumonitis, encephalitis, hepatitis, Reye's syndrome, purpura fulminans, and a mortality rate of 7% to 14% (Feldman et al., 1975). Zoster, which represents recrudescent VZV, has a low mortality rate when it occurs as localized cutaneous disease, but it can disseminate cutaneously and potentially viscerally in up to 26% of compromised patients (Strauss et al., 1988). CMV infection in compromised patients may be manifested as a spectrum of involvement ranging from asymptomatic viral shedding to life-threatening pneumonitis. Among bone marrow transplant patients, the incidence of CMV infection is greater in patients already seropositive (Meyers et al., 1986), but there is some evidence that, although it occurs more frequently, reactivation CMV disease results in less morbidity than primary infection (Chou, 1986). Those at highest risk for serious morbidity and mortality are seronegative individuals who receive seropositive organs or leukocyte-containing blood products (Rubin, 1990). It has also been documented that CMV infection may cause further immunosuppression and lead to a higher incidence of secondary bacterial infections (Rand et al., 1978). Prophylactic strategies using acyclovir for HSV infections and preemptive use of ganciclovir in bone marrow transplant patients at risk for CMV disease have reduced the incidence of these infections in susceptible hosts and decreased morbidity and mortality.

Infections caused by common respiratory viruses were documented in 25% of the febrile episodes encountered in one series of neutropenic patients followed at the National Cancer Institute. Unfortunately, the role of these viruses in illness could not be predicted on the basis of presenting symptoms, chest radiograph, degree of fever, or the duration of neutropenia, so this information did not have much impact on patient management (Cotton et al., 1984). Recent studies have documented that adult oncology patients are at increased risk for severe disease resulting from RSV, with significant mortality in bone marrow transplant populations (Whimbey et al., 1995b). Outbreaks on oncology wards have been described that result from nosocomial spread of the infection (Englund et al., 1991; Harrington et al., 1992; Whimbey et al., 1995a), emphasizing the need for careful attention to infection control procedures during periods when respiratory viruses are known to be circulating in the community. Improvement in rapid diagnostic assays and increased treatment options for viral infections make this one of the most rapidly changing areas in the care of febrile, immunosuppressed patients.

Parasites

Pneumocystis carinii has been the major pathogenic parasite in immunocompromised children, although there have always been arguments over its exact taxonomic position (Bartlett and Smith, 1991), and ribosomal RNA sequencing places it among the fungi (Edman et al., 1988). In children with cancer, *P. carinii* is most often a reactivation infection, in contrast to its presumptive role as a primary infection in young infants with HIV infection. In cancer patients, *P. carinii* causes a more rapidly progressive, severe infection characterized by lower numbers of cysts than seen in HIV patients, though there is no difference in overall mortality (Kovacs et al., 1984). A variety of other protozoan pathogens are seen in HIV-infected adults, but since they frequently occur as reactivations of latent infections, organisms such as *Toxoplasma gondii* and *Cryptosporidium* spp. are relatively unusual in children. Infections with *Strongyloides stercoralis,* frequently seen in patients with adult T-cell leukemia and human T-lymphotropic virus 1 (HTLV-1) infection, are rare complications in children living in the United States.

DIAGNOSTIC EVALUATION

In nonneutropenic cancer patients, infection is the presumed cause of fever in less than 20% of the episodes. More often, fever is a consequence of the use of chemotherapeutic agents or of the underlying malignancy. Although "tumor fever" occurs in less than 5% of children with leukemia or lymphoma, it may be present in up to 25% of children with those solid tumors that are associated with necrosis. Unless these children are neutropenic or have rapidly falling neutrophil counts after receiving chemotherapy, empiric therapy is unnecessary, and treatment can be based on whether an infectious etiology can be demonstrated. An exception to this approach pertains to nonneutropenic children who have central venous catheters. Because these patients are at increased risk of bacteremia (Hiemenz et al., 1986), it has been the current practice to treat these children with intravenous antibiotics while blood cultures are in progress (see Central Venous Catheter-Associated Infection).

In a neutropenic child the occurrence of a single oral temperature greater than 38.5° C or three episodes of temperature greater than 38.0° C within a 24-hour period mandates hospital admission for evaluation and empiric antibiotic therapy. The importance of empiric therapy has been underscored by the fact that, among the 1,001 febrile episodes that occurred in 324 pediatric and young adult patients followed at the National Cancer Institute, there were no clearly definable signs, symptoms, treatment modalities, or invasive procedures that were predictive of bacteremia (Pizzo et al., 1982b). In fact, the classic signs of inflammation may be notably absent in neutropenic patients. At the same time, the patient's clinical status may change over time, making serial (at least daily) examinations of critical importance. Each patient should have at least two sets of blood cultures obtained before the institution of antibiotics and, if a central venous catheter is present, blood cultures should be obtained both from peripheral venipuncture and from all lumens of the indwelling device. Urine analysis and urine culture should also be done before antibiotics are given, although this is sometimes more difficult to obtain in young children. Cultures of any other potentially infected sites revealed by the history or initial examination should be aggressively pursued for the source of fever. A chest radiograph at the onset of illness not only provides information regarding infiltrates that may be present at the time of presentation, but also provides a baseline by which to monitor the evolution of infiltrates as neutrophils recover or as secondary infections arise. Routine serum electrolyte profiles, including liver and kidney function tests, allow monitoring of organ system dysfunction or antibiotic toxicities and should be part of the initial evaluation. Special diagnostic procedures such as thoracentesis, paracentesis, lumbar puncture, sinus radiographs or other imaging studies, or surgical biopsy should be pursued as indicated by the patient's presentation and clinical course.

Although colonization with a particular organism usually precedes infection, the use of routine surveillance cultures has not proved useful. In a series of 652 episodes of neutropenia with fever, serial surveillance cultures of nose, throat, urine, and stool were evaluated. The clinical value of this information was limited, however, because no single body site was predictive of bacteremia, multiple organisms were frequently isolated from the same site, the organisms responsible for sepsis were often known before the results of the surveillance cultures, and the results of the cultures rarely influenced initial patient management. Additionally, the cost of such a surveillance program is tremendous and not justified on the basis of available data (Kramer et al., 1982).

ASSESSMENT OF RISK IN FEBRILE NEUTROPENIC CHILDREN

Although the degree and duration of neutropenia have been shown to be the most important factors affecting the risk of the infectious complications just stated, it is becoming increasingly clear that febrile, neutropenic patients can be further stratified, and empiric therapy may be tailored to the level of risk for some patients. Often patients presenting for medical evaluation of fever may be categorized as being at relatively high risk or relatively low risk for serious infectious complications.

In reviewing 261 episodes of fever and neutropenia in adult oncology patients followed at the Dana Farber Cancer Institute, Talcott et al. (1988) identified three groups of patients at higher risk for serious complications, whereas the remaining patients were at lower risk. Serious morbidity or mortality occurred significantly more often in (1) patients who were already hospitalized at the time of fever and neutropenia (this group included all of the patients receiving bone marrow transplantations); (2) patients who presented with serious comorbid conditions requiring hospitalization (e.g., uncontrolled pain or vomiting, hypotension, respiratory distress, significant localized infection, etc.); and (3) patients whose cancer was uncontrolled. Patients found to be free of these conditions were determined to have a low (2%) risk of serious medical complications during febrile, neutropenic periods.

Using these criteria, the same group performed a pilot study in which thirty low-risk patients were observed in hospital for a short period then discharged home to receive outpatient intravenous antibiotics and be reevaluated by a visiting nurse. Five of these patients were readmitted for prolonged or recurrent fever and four others had significant medical complications, a higher rate than seen in the earlier study. None died or had irreversible complications during the study. Interestingly, however, treatment costs were not different for those patients enrolled in the study receiving outpatient antibiotics and those who were eligible but refused enrollment, and the duration of therapy was longer for those treated at home (Talcott et al., 1994).

In a similar series of studies conducted with pediatric patients in Dallas, investigators identified groups of children at lower risk for serious complications during hospitalization (Mullen and Buchanan, 1990; Griffin and Buchanan, 1992; Bash et al., 1994). Children were felt to be at low risk for infection and therefore eligible for early discharge while still neutropenic if they (1) exhibited some evidence of bone marrow recovery (e.g., increasing monocytes); (2) had negative blood cultures; (3) defervesced promptly; (4) had improvement of any localized site of infection; (5) had no other reason for intravenous antibiotics; and (6) could return to the hospital immediately if complications occurred (Buchanan, 1993). A separate analysis was undertaken to stratify children at low risk for bacteremia at the time of initial evaluation (Pappo and Buchanan, 1991). This study identified the following criteria for low risk of infectious complications: (1) some evidence of bone marrow recovery (e.g., ANC > 100 cells/mm^3; platelet count > 75,000/mm^3); (2) underlying malignancy in remission; (3) age over 1 year; (4) ≥10 days since the start of last course of chemotherapy; (5) well-appearing child; (6) no measure of comorbidity; and (7) no evidence of significant localized infection. These criteria have now been tested in a small pilot study of outpatient management of children with fever and neutropenia, which found that eighteen of nineteen children enrolled were successfully managed with daily administration of intravenous ceftriaxone and outpatient follow-up (Mustafa et al., 1996). None of the children in this study were found to be bacteremic. Although the results of these studies are encouraging and indicate that a subset of children with fever and neutropenia can be cared for in the outpatient setting, additional studies involving larger numbers are required to establish the optimal guidelines for assessing the risks and benefits of outpatient therapy.

PRINCIPLES OF EMPIRIC THERAPY

The morbidity and mortality associated with fever in neutropenic children have been greatly reduced by the rapid initiation of empiric antibiotics. This policy evolved during the 1960s and 1970s, when it became clear that a delay in starting antibiotics of even 24 to 48 hours while waiting for results of cultures could have disastrous consequences, particularly when gram-negative organisms ultimately were identified. Not surprisingly, the earliest empiric regimens were directed against gram-negative pathogens, particularly *P. aeruginosa*. To optimize the benefits of empiric antibiotic therapy, the regimen should have a broad spectrum of activity that includes *P. aeruginosa* spp., antibiotic effectiveness in the absence of neutrophils, ability to achieve high serum bactericidal concentrations

quickly, an acceptable incidence of adverse side effects, and a low potential for the emergence of resistant pathogens (Rubin et al., 1991).

MONOTHERAPY VERSUS COMBINATION ANTIBIOTICS

Numerous antibiotic regimens have been proposed and used for the initial management of the febrile neutropenic child over the last 25 years. To provide broad coverage against the many potential pathogens, the use of combinations of antibiotics has been the standard practice at most institutions. Although both the carboxypenicillins (carbenicillin and ticarcillin) and the more recent ureidopenicillins and piperazyl penicillins (azlocillin and piperacillin) have excellent activity against gram-negative bacteria, including *P. aeruginosa*, resistant organisms can emerge when these are used alone. Thus an aminoglycoside or another β-lactam antibiotic should be combined with an extended-spectrum penicillin. Similarly, in the neutropenic patient, aminoglycosides cannot be used alone, since clinical and microbiologic failures frequently occur. Nonetheless, combinations of a penicillin and an aminoglycoside have proven highly effective, although the use of aminoglycosides requires careful monitoring of serum levels to ensure adequate therapy and reduce the likelihood of toxicity. The selection of a particular aminoglycoside should be based on local antibiotic resistance patterns.

During the late 1970s and early 1980s two major developments introduced the possibility that single-agent therapy could be an effective empiric regimen: (1) the availability of new β-lactam antibiotics with extended gram-negative activity and (2) the gradual decrease in the prevalence of gram-negative organisms, especially *Pseudomonas* spp., at many centers. The third-generation cephalosporins (such as ceftazidime and cefoperazone) and the carbapenems (imipenem-cilastatin and meropenem) represent significant advances in activity that make them attractive for use in febrile immunocompromised patients. These third-generation cephalosporins have been studied as monotherapy in a number of trials and, although a variety of combination regimens were used in comparison, the investigators concluded that monotherapy was equivalent to combination therapy in nine of thirteen studies reviewed in one report (Pizzo et al., 1985). A comparison of ceftazidime alone versus "standard" combination therapy (in this case cephalothin, gentamicin, and carbenicillin) conducted at the National Cancer

Institute encompassed 550 consecutive admissions for fever and neutropenia. For both initial regimens the outcome was successful in 98% of the patients who presented with unexplained fever. Success was also similar for the two regimens in patients who had documented infections (89% and 91%), but many of these patients required modification of their initial antibiotics. Patients who required more frequent modifications in therapy usually were those with documented infections and those who remained neutropenic for longer than 1 week. This study also confirmed a shift toward a higher percentage of unexplained febrile episodes (72%) than of documented infections and assumed that this phenomenon was related to the early initiation of antibiotics with any defined fever (Pizzo et al., 1986).

A subsequent trial at the National Cancer Institute explored the use of imipenem-cilastatin, the first in the carbapenem class of antibiotics, as monotherapy for initial empiric antibiotic therapy. In this study, patients were randomized to receive either imipenem or ceftazidime as initial therapy for neutropenia-associated fever. No clear difference in overall outcome in the two treatment groups was identified. A higher number of patients than expected in the imipenem group required modification of antibiotics secondary to nausea, but fewer modifications were made in order to provide coverage for anaerobic infections (Freifeld et al., 1995). Although the antibacterial coverage provided by imipenem is broad and rapid development of resistance has not been a problem in clinical trials, its use as empiric monotherapy in febrile neutropenic patients has been limited by its GI side effects and its potential to lower the seizure threshold in patients with CNS disease. The newer carbapenem, meropenem, may have similar efficacy as monotherapy in this setting and lower incidence of adverse effects (Boogaerts et al., 1995).

A number of studies have also investigated the use of intravenous ciprofloxacin, a fluoroquinolone antibiotic with broad-spectrum activity, as initial treatment in febrile neutropenic adults. Although the studies included relatively small numbers of patients, it appears that this agent achieved a successful outcome in a majority of patients (Rolston et al., 1989), despite some indication that a higher incidence of secondary streptococcal infections occurred (Bayston et al., 1989). At present the quinolone antibiotics are not approved for use in children because of concern for potential age-related arthropathy; however, emerging data suggests that ciprofloxacin may be safe in pediatric patients (Schaad et al., 1995).

Although the third-generation cephalosporins and the carbapenems have excellent gram-negative activity, as well as coverage of a number of gram-positive organisms, none are active against the methicillin-resistant staphylococci. This factor, together with the increased frequency of gram-positive infections (particularly those caused by coagulase-negative staphylococci and α-streptococci), has led several investigators to evaluate the inclusion of vancomycin as part of initial empiric therapy. Although these studies have suggested that the early use of vancomycin reduces the incidence of secondary infections or even the need for empiric amphotericin B, there was no difference in mortality in patients randomized to receive initial vancomycin or not (Karp et al., 1986). The experience at the National Cancer Institute has suggested that patients could be successfully treated with pathogen-directed vancomycin and that there was no adverse effect on outcome when vancomycin was not included as part of the initial empiric regimen. Importantly, this pathogen-directed use of vancomycin appeared to be much more cost-effective than if vancomycin were simply given to every patient with fever and neutropenia (Rubin et al., 1988). The emergence of more virulent and more resistant gram-positive organisms (such as methicillin-resistant *S. aureus* and penicillin- and cephalosporin-resistant α-streptococci) in some institutions may necessitate the use of vancomycin in initial empiric regimens. At present, recommendations for the addition of vancomycin to empiric regimens for the treatment of fever during neutropenia should be based on local experience, institutional antibiotic resistance patterns, and susceptible host populations. The Working Committee of the Infectious Diseases Society of America established guidelines in 1990 for the use of antimicrobial agents in neutropenic patients; these recommendations, which outline all acceptable regimens (Hughes et al., 1990), are currently being updated.

A number of new antimicrobial agents are currently in development for use against resistant organisms, especially the resistant enterococci. Quinupristin-dalfopristin (Synercid), an antibiotic in the new class Streptogramin, has been shown to have good activity against a variety of gram-positive organisms, including vancomycin-resistant enterococci, methicillin-resistant staphylococci, and penicillin-resistant streptococci (Finch, 1996). The antibiotic shows some variability in susceptibility to enterococci, however, and it has limited activity against gram-negative organisms. Recent studies have shown Synercid to be synergistic with other antibiotics against some strains of resistant organisms (Vouillamoz et al., 1996). There is also optimism that some of the newer quinolone antibiotics, such as clinafloxacin and trovafloxacin (Zaman et al., 1996; Coque et al., 1996; Cohen et al., 1996), may prove to be useful against the resistant enterococci. Whether these agents will prove efficacious in immunosuppressed children with serious infections remains to be determined.

MODIFICATIONS AND LENGTH OF THERAPY

The question of how long to continue therapy or when to modify the empiric treatment regimen frequently arises in the management of the febrile neutropenic patient. Indeed, empiric therapy really relates to the management of patients until the results of the pretreatment cultures become available. Even when a pathogen is isolated in a febrile neutropenic child, there is evidence to suggest that, during the period of neutropenia, broad-spectrum antibiotic coverage should be continued (Pizzo et al., 1980). Specific clinical settings that develop during an episode may also warrant a change in therapy. Table 14-2 lists some common events for which modifications of the empiric regimen are warranted.

The appropriate length of antibiotic therapy in a febrile neutropenic patient depends on the clinical setting and the length of neutropenia. Minimal data exist to support specific recommendations regarding length of therapy, especially in those patients with no defined site of infection. In patients with fever of unexplained origin who become afebrile and have resolution of neutropenia in less than 7 days, it is probably reasonable to discontinue antibiotics and observe them carefully. Those who become afebrile but remain neutropenic may benefit from continuing antibiotics for a full 14 days or until the resolution of neutropenia (Pizzo et al., 1984). Limited evidence supports either of these positions, but it has been demonstrated that discontinuing antibiotics after 7 days of empiric therapy in patients who remain neutropenic may result in recurrent fever and hypotensive events (Pizzo et al., 1979). Any neutropenic patient in whom antibiotic treatment is discontinued must be observed closely, since evidence of recurrent fever mandates reinstitution of antibiotic therapy.

As stated earlier there are increasing data to support simplification of intravenous antibiotic regimens or discontinue intravenous antibiotics and discharge patients before full bone marrow recovery in selected groups of children who are thought to be at low risk of serious infectious complications. Data from Europe suggest that single daily doses of amikacin and ceftriaxone may be as effec-

Table 14-2 Modifications of therapy during fever and neutropenia

Clinical event	Possible modifications in therapy
Breakthrough bacteremia	If gram-positive isolate, add vancomycin.
	If gram-negative isolate (presumably resistant), change regimen.
Catheter-associated soft tissue infections*	Add vancomycin (and gram-negative coverage, if not already being given).
Severe oral mucositis or necrotizing gingivitis	Add specific anaerobic agent (clindamycin, metronidazole); may need trial of acyclovir.
Esophagitis	Trial of clotrimazole, ketoconazole, fluconazole, or amphotericin B; may need trial of acyclovir.
Diffuse or interstitial pneumonitis	Trial of trimethoprim-sulfamethoxazole and erythromycin in addition to broad-spectrum antibiotics if the patient remains neutropenic.
New infiltrate in neutropenic patient on antibiotics	If neutrophil count rising, may observe
	If neutrophil count not recovering, pursue biopsy; if biopsy not possible, add amphotericin B.
Perianal cellulitis	If patient already on broad-spectrum antibiotics, add a specific anaerobic agent.
	If patient not on antibiotics, begin broad-spectrum regimen with anaerobic coverage.
Prolonged fever and neutropenia	After 1 week of antibiotics, add amphotericin B.

*No specific modification necessary for catheter present without soft tissue infection.

tive as a multidose ceftazidime plus amikacin regimen; the former regimen had a toxicity profile similar to that of the latter (EORTC, International Antimicrobial Therapy Cooperative Group, 1993). In this study, *P. aeruginosa* accounted for 10 episodes and gram-positive organisms for 104 episodes among 205 microbiologically proven infections; outcomes were similar in the two treatment groups. This type of daily regimen would certainly be more amenable to outpatient administration. In another study, investigators in Dallas evaluated the safety of early discharge of children with fever and neutropenia before complete marrow recovery in those who defervesced promptly, appeared clinically well, had negative cultures and control of any local infection, and had some evidence of bone marrow recovery even though still neutropenic (Bash et al., 1994). Sixty-nine of seventy children who met all these criteria did well clinically after discharge, but six of eight children who were inadvertently discharged without any signs of bone marrow recovery required readmission for recurrent fever.

In patients with a defined site of infection who have resolution of both fever and neutropenia and show a good response to antibiotics, the length of therapy can be based on usual standards of treatment. For those patients who remain neutropenic, antibiotics should be continued until there is microbiologic and clinical resolution of the infection and the patient has been afebrile for at least 7 days. Under those circumstances the patient should also be free of mucosal or skin lesions and must again be observed closely for evidence of recurrent infection at the same or another site (Hughes et al., 1990).

EMPIRIC ANTIFUNGAL THERAPY

Standard practice is to begin empiric antifungal therapy if a patient remains febrile and neutropenic without an obvious source after 4 to 7 days of receiving broad-spectrum antibiotics. This policy is based on an accumulating body of knowledge and experience in caring for both pediatric and adult cancer patients. Studies from different groups have documented the rate of serious fungal infection in this patient population to be from 9% to 31% (Pizzo et al., 1982a; EORTC, International Antimicrobial Therapy Cooperative Group, 1989; Wiley et al., 1990). These rates include cases diagnosed at autopsy, emphasizing the difficulty in making a diagnosis of fungal infection even in some cases of disseminated disease. Empiric amphotericin B

(usually 0.5 mg/kg/day) has appeared to decrease the rates of documented fungal infection. However, doses of amphotericin B used in empiric therapy may be less effective with some fungi (e.g., *Aspergillus* spp. and *C. tropicalis*); infection with these organisms may benefit from higher doses of antifungals.

In spite of its potential benefit, amphotericin B has considerable toxicity, making the search for newer and less toxic antifungal agents an important priority. Among the most promising are the imidazoles (such as ketoconazole) and thiazoles (such as fluconazole and itraconazole). Ketoconazole has been compared to amphotericin B in two trials of neutropenic patients already on antibiotic therapy, with reported equivalent efficacy (Hathorn et al., 1985; Fainstein et al., 1987). Unfortunately, because of its lack of activity against *Aspergillus* spp. and *C. tropicalis* and the lack of a parenteral form, ketoconazole cannot be recommended for routine use in this setting (Walsh, 1990). Fluconazole has been investigated as a potential agent for empiric antifungal therapy in a prospective randomized trial coordinated through the National Cancer Institute. This study evaluated the addition of fluconazole to empiric antibiotic regimens early in febrile episodes in patients who were anticipated to have longer than 7 days of neutropenia in an effort to prevent fungal infection and avoid the use of amphotericin B. Results of this multicenter study are currently being analyzed. Lipid formulations of amphotericin B are also being investigated at a number of centers and appear to have greatly decreased toxicity over the currently available preparation. Recently one of these products containing amphotericin B incorporated into lipid complexes (ABeLCet) has been approved for use in the United States.

CLINICAL SYNDROMES OF INFECTION IN COMPROMISED CHILDREN

More than half of children with fever and neutropenia have no definable site of infection. Of those with clinically or microbiologically documented infections, 10% to 15% may have bacteremia with any of a wide variety of organisms, and a small percentage may have fungemia. The range of infections seen in three different large series of febrile neutropenic patients followed at the National Cancer Institute is compiled in Table 14-3. Some of these clinical syndromes and their management in neutropenic or immunocompromised children are discussed in more detail.

Table 14-3   Documented sites of infection in febrile neutropenic cancer patients during three studies conducted at the National Cancer Institute

Site of infection	Study A*	Study B†	Study C‡	Total
Sepsis/bacteremia	81[§]	109	48	238
Pulmonary	28	88	11	127
Cutaneous/cellulitis	42	43	31	116
HEENT	11	69	21	101
GI	4	35	9	48
Urinary tract	22	29	15	66
Other	2	38	15	55
Total documented infections	156[§]	411	135	702 (40%)
No documented source	394	382	264	1040 (60%)

*Data from Pizzo PA et al.: N Engl J Med 1986;315:552-558
†Data from Pizzo PA et al.: Medicine 1982b;61:153-165
‡Data from Freifeld AG et al.: J Clin Oncol 1995;13:165-176
§Some patients with bacteremia had other sites of infection as well, but these were counted as only one infection in this study.

PULMONARY INFILTRATES

Pulmonary infections are the most common localized infection seen in neutropenic hosts and initially can have a wide range of symptoms and radiographic appearances. In children who are severely neutropenic, there may be no obvious infiltrate at the time of the initial evaluation. Use of invasive diagnostic procedures such as bronchoalveolar lavage must be considered for a child with respiratory symptoms and a "normal" chest roentgenogram if the initial evaluation provides no etiology for the clinical manifestations.

A localized pulmonary infiltrate at the onset of fever in a neutropenic child should be considered bacterial and should be treated with broad-spectrum antibiotics while the initial assessment proceeds. Routine childhood pathogens such as *S. pneumoniae, H. influenzae, Chlamydia* spp., and *Mycoplasma* spp. must be considered in addition to the pathogens associated with immunocompromised hosts, such as the gram-negative enteric bacteria (including *E. coli, Klebsiella pneumoniae,* and *Pseudomonas* spp). *Legionella* pneumonia should be considered, especially if the patient also has diarrhea and headache. Localized infiltrates that fail to improve with broad-spectrum antibiotics usually represent infection with mycobacteria, fungi (especially *Aspergillus* spp.), *Nocardia* spp., or multiply resistant bacteria.

Interstitial infiltrates in immunocompromised patients are more likely to represent a nonbacterial process. *Pneumocystis carinii* is the entity most frequently diagnosed in interstitial pneumonitis in children who do not receive prophylactic trimetho-

prim-sulfamethosoxazole. A high index of suspicion should be maintained for any compromised patient, but especially for those receiving steroid therapy or those with significant defects in cellular immunity. Common symptoms include fever, dry cough, and significant hypoxemia. An arterial blood gas and an induced sputum examination to look for cysts should be performed when *P. carinii* is being considered. The incidence of *P. carinii* in this patient population has been decreased dramatically by the routine use of trimethoprim-sulfamethoxazole for prophylaxis in high-risk patients (Hughes et al., 1977). In nonneutropenic hosts with diffuse infiltrates who are unable to undergo biopsy, an empiric trial of trimethoprim-sulfamethoxazole and erythromycin is reasonable (Browne et al., 1990). *Legionella, Mycoplasma,* and viral infections may also cause diffuse or interstitial infiltrates. Of the viral pathogens, CMV has been most frequently linked to serious pneumonias, especially in allogeneic bone marrow transplant patients (Meyers, 1986). CMV pneumonitis is suspected when CMV is found by culture or hybridization in bronchoalveolar lavage fluid, but confirmation requires lung or transbronchial biopsy. Therapeutic options for CMV pneumonitis are limited, although a regimen of ganciclovir and intravenous immune globulin appears successful in some patients (Emmanuel et al., 1988; Reed et al., 1988).

Whether localized or diffuse, infiltrates that develop during antibiotic therapy present a more complex problem. A review of thirty-four patients who developed infiltrates while receiving broad-

Table 14-4 Approach to empiric antibiotic use in immunocompromised patients with extensive pulmonary infiltrates

Empiric regimen	Pathogens likely to be treated
Patient with deficient cell-mediated immunity (HIV−)	
Trimethoprim-sulfamethoxazole	*Pneumocystis* and *Nocardia* spp.
and	
Erythromycin	*Legionella, Mycoplasma,* and *Chlamydia* spp.
with or without	
Nafcillin or vancomycin	Aerobic gram-positive cocci
and	
Aminoglycoside	Aerobic gram-negative bacilli
Neutropenic patient	
Trimethoprim-sulfamethoxazole	*Pneumocystis* and *Nocardia* spp.
and	
Erythromycin	*Legionella, Mycoplasma,* and *Chlamydia*
and	
Nafcillin or vancomycin	Aerobic gram-positive cocci
and	
Aminoglycoside	Aerobic gram-negative bacilli
and	
Third-generation cephalosporin or extended spectrum penicillin	*Pseudomonas aeruginosa*
(In many cases bacterial etiologies can be covered by third-generation cephalosporin alone.)	
HIV-infected patient	
Trimethoprim-sulfamethoxazole	*Pneumocystis* spp.
and	
Erythromycin	*Legionella* and *Mycoplasma* spp.

Modified from Masur H, Shelhamer J, Parrillo JE: J Am Med Assoc 1985;253:1769.

spectrum antibiotics during a granulocytopenic period revealed that those whose infiltrates were diagnosed at the time of bone marrow recovery were more likely to have no etiologic factors determined. Moreover, 92% of these cases recovered. On the other hand, those whose infiltrates were detected during continued neutropenia were more likely to have a fungal pathogen ultimately isolated and had a much lower survival rate (32%) (Commers et al., 1984). Thus a new infiltrate occurring during recovery of the neutrophils may represent localization of the inflammatory response in an area of previously unrecognized pneumonia, whereas a similar infiltrate not concomitant with recovering neutrophil counts has a much more ominous prognosis and strongly argues for the need for lung biopsy and antifungal therapy. One approach to empiric antibiotics in immunocompromised patients with severe or extensive infiltrates is shown in Table 14-4.

The presentation of a progressive infiltrate during neutropenia that is accompanied by fever, dry cough or hemoptysis, and pleuritic chest pain strongly suggests the diagnosis of invasive *Aspergillus* pneumonia. Computed tomography studies of the chest may be useful in showing multiple nodular infiltrates, sometimes with cavitation, that may not have been readily apparent on routine radiographs (Walsh, 1990). Isolation of *Aspergillus flavus* from the anterior nares of neutropenic patients was shown to be highly predictive of invasive infection in one study (Aisner et al., 1979). A more recent study confirms that identification of *Aspergillus* in lower–respiratory tract specimens (sputa, tracheal aspirations, bronchoalveolar lavage fluid, etc.) from patients with neutropenia, hematologic malignancies, bone marrow transplantation, or corticosteroid use was associated with invasive pulmonary aspergillosis in almost two thirds of the episodes (Horvath and Dummer, 1996). Children rarely have other risk factors for colonization of the airway with *Aspergillus* spp. (e.g., cigarette smoking or chronic obstructive pulmonary disease), so recovery of this organism from the respiratory tract in neutropenic patients with persistent fever should be considered as strong evidence for infection and the need for higher doses of amphotericin B (1.5 mg/kg/day). In contrast, recovery of *Aspergillus* spp. from the respiratory tree in nonneutropenic patients may only represent evidence of colonization (Yu et al., 1986).

CENTRAL VENOUS CATHETER–ASSOCIATED INFECTION

The use of indwelling central venous catheters (Hickman-Broviac catheters or subcutaneously implanted access devices) has in many ways simplified the administration of chemotherapeutic agents and blood products and has allowed monitoring and repeated blood sampling in children who have poor venous access. Catheter use, however, is accompanied by an intrinsic risk of infection, since the devices breach the body's first line of defense, skin integrity. Rates of catheter-related infections and noninfectious complications vary considerably from one institution to another, probably because of differences in patient populations, insertion techniques, frequency of catheter access, and routine care.

The gram-positive cocci, particularly the coagulase-negative staphylococci, have emerged as the most frequent causes of bacteremias associated with these catheters, although many other organisms have been associated with catheter infections. At the National Cancer Institute the frequency of bacteremia was compared in patients with and without catheters: 39% of patients with catheters developed an episode of bacteremia, with 60% of the episodes occurring during periods of neutropenia. A fourfold increase in incidence of bacteremia was found in neutropenic patients with catheters compared to those without catheters, and a forty-fold increase was found in nonneutropenic patients with catheters compared to those without catheters (Hiemenz et al., 1986). Although unusual, infections with mixed flora (multiple organisms) have occurred in patients whose only risk for bacteremia was the catheter. This type of infection should provoke questions about catheter maintenance and unusual occurrences (i.e., bathing habits or swimming, close contact with family pets, and even young infants chewing on catheter tubing).

Bacteremia may exist as a consequence of localized infection at the exit site of the catheter or along the subcutaneously tunneled portion of the tubing, or these soft-tissue infections may occur without evidence of dissemination. Although a mi-

nor exit site infection in a nonneutropenic child may respond to oral antibiotics, intravenous antibiotics are required when there is evidence of significant erythema, tenderness, or purulent discharge. Similarly, any evidence of infection at the catheter site in a neutropenic patient warrants hospitalization and initiation of broad-spectrum intravenous therapy. The presence of erythema, tenderness, and induration or fluctuance along the tunnel tract of the catheter necessitates parenteral antibiotics and removal of the catheter to resolve the infection. Although staphylococcal infections represent a growing percentage of catheter-related complications, it has been shown that empiric vancomycin may not be necessary in a stable patient receiving broad-spectrum antibiotics unless there are signs of an exit site or tunnel infection or if cultures suggest a β-lactam–resistent organism (Rubin et al., 1988).

The vast majority of patients with catheter-related bacteremia who do not have a tunnel infection can be successfully treated without removing the catheter (Hiemenz et al., 1986). Specific settings that may warrant catheter removal include persistent, severe clinical findings (i.e., hypotension); persistently positive blood cultures after 48 hours of appropriate antibiotics; infection with *Candida* spp. (Eppes et al., 1989); infections with *Bacillus* spp. (Cotton et al., 1987); and infections along the subcutaneous tract of the catheter. Standard practice at many centers is to deliver antibiotics on a rotating schedule through all lumens or ports of the device.

MUCOSITIS

Children receiving chemotherapeutic agents often develop mucositis that may range in severity from a few small oral ulcers to extensive sloughing of the oral and gastrointestinal mucosa. The most recognizable manifestation of this process is marginal or necrotizing gingivitis, characterized by a periapical line of erythema and tenderness. These lesions can become colonized with the normal oral flora and can provide a portal of entry for organisms including anaerobic streptococci, lactobacilli, and other usually nonpathogenic bacteria. In addition, patients who have been hospitalized or have been on antibiotics for extended periods of time may become colonized with gram-negative organisms or fungi. The lesions of oral candidiasis (thrush) and herpetic stomatitis may sometimes be confused with chemotherapy-induced mucositis or may cause superinfection. Candidal lesions usually respond to oral therapy with clotrimazole troches, but in severe cases—or those accompanied by esophagitis—ketoconazole, fluconazole, or intravenous amphotericin B may be necessary. The oral lesions of HSV usually respond to oral or intravenous acyclovir. Preventive measures such as mouth rinses with chlorhexidine and fastidious oral hygiene may reduce the incidence and severity of mucositis.

INTRAABDOMINAL INFECTIONS

Invasion or obstruction of the bowel by tumor predisposes to bowel perforation that can result in peritonitis or intraabdominal abscesses. Extension of mucosal ulcerations and sloughing into the intestinal tract secondary to chemotherapy also predispose to intraabdominal infections. A necrotic, agranulocytic enteropathy may result when leukemic infiltrates in the bowel wall or mesentery necrose after chemotherapy. When this process involves the terminal ileum, cecum, and appendix, it is termed *typhlitis,* and it may present with many of the classic findings of appendicitis (Wagner et al., 1970; Skibber et al., 1987). Most commonly this syndrome is caused by the infiltration of the bowel wall by gram-negative aerobic bacilli. A review of typhlitis spanning 30 years at St. Jude Children's Research Hospital identified twenty-four children with this process, only eight of whom were bacteremic. Abdominal CT was remarkable for thickening of the bowel wall in seventeen of the twenty patients evaluated (Sloas et al., 1993). Surgical resection may be necessary if necrosis of the bowel results in perforation, uncontrolled bleeding, abscess formation, or septic shock, but most patients respond to conservative medical management including broad-spectrum antibiotics (Shamberger et al., 1986; Skibber et al., 1987). Therefore the timing and extent of surgical procedures must be carefully considered.

Antibiotic-associated pseudomembranous colitis results from a toxin produced by *Clostridium difficile.* The spectrum of illness caused by this syndrome ranges from mild abdominal pain to severe bloody diarrhea or toxic megacolon. Almost all classes of antibiotics and some chemotherapeutic agents have been reported to cause pseudomembranous colitis, and recurrent episodes are not unusual. Most cases of *C. difficile*–associated diarrhea occurring in hospitalized patients represent nosocomial spread of the organism, though there is evidence that many patients colonized with the organism never have symptoms (McFarland et al., 1989). Asymptomatic colonization rates may be very high in young infants and decrease with age. This infection can usually be effectively treated with either oral vancomycin or metronidazole, and relapses may be treated successfully with repeated courses of the same agents.

PERIANAL CELLULITIS

Although children in general have fewer problems with perianal disorders than adults, pediatric patients receiving chemotherapy are prone to develop lesions of the rectal mucosa similar to those seen in the oral cavity. These lesions not only provide access to the bloodstream to whatever organisms are colonizing the intestinal tract, but also may be the focal point for cellulitis and perirectal abscesses. Anorectal infections commonly involve multiple organisms, with the enterococci, gram-negative bacilli, and anaerobes the most frequently isolated. Broad-spectrum antibiotic regimens that included both an aminoglycoside and a specific anaerobic agent showed increased efficacy in treatment. In general, surgical drainage should be avoided, if possible, while patients are neutropenic, since there is a high incidence of postoperative complications in this setting (Glenn et al., 1988).

CENTRAL NERVOUS SYSTEM INFECTIONS

Fortunately, infections of the central nervous system (CNS) are rare causes of fever in neutropenic children. They must be considered, however, whenever there is a history of neurosurgical procedures, especially placement of an indwelling intraventricular device (ventriculoperitoneal shunt or Ommaya reservoir). A review of the infectious complications of Ommaya reservoirs in children with cancer documented that 75% of these children had never had an infection of the device, and there were no Ommaya infection-related deaths in the series. *Proprionibacterium acnes* was the most common organism isolated in children with reservoir infections in this review (Browne et al., 1987). As with intravascular devices most of these infections can be resolved without removing the reservoir. Patients with impaired cellular immunity are susceptible to a variety of nonbacterial CNS infections, such cryptococcal meningitis or toxoplasmosis, although these are much more common in adults than in children.

PREVENTIVE MEASURES

Techniques for the prevention of infections in immunocompromised patients have been extensively investigated. These methods include isolation measures, preventive antibiotic regimens, active and passive immunizations, and the use of immune modulating agents. Since the majority of infections in compromised children are caused by organisms that are part of the patient's own flora, simple reverse isolation per se provides no benefit. A totally protective environment using a laminar airflow room, specially prepared food, sterilization of all items entering the chamber, and a regimen of oral antibiotics offers some protection from infection in profoundly neutropenic children such as those undergoing bone marrow transplantation or those with severe combined immune deficiency syndrome, but the cost of this kind of program is enormous and the setting quickly becomes intolerable for the patient. Although the number of infections decreased in one study comparing patients treated in a total protected environment to a standard hospital room, the mortality rate was not significantly different and almost half of the patients in the protected environment were unwilling to continue the oral antibiotics required (Pizzo, 1989).

PROPHYLACTIC ANTIMICROBIAL REGIMENS

Many centers have attempted to decrease the incidence of infection in immunosuppressed patients by using oral antibiotics to "decontaminate" the gastrointestinal tract or to prevent specific infections. Oral nonabsorbable antimicrobials such as vancomycin, gentamicin, and nystatin have been used in an attempt to decrease the number of potential pathogens in the GI tract. However, this approach has offered little benefit and is frequently poorly tolerated. Also, the use of these agents in some centers was associated with increased emergence of resistant bacteria. Recently the use of fluoroquinolone antibiotics as prophylaxis for bacterial infections in neutropenic patients has been evaluated. Both norfloxacin and ciprofloxacin have reduced the number of infections caused by gram-negative bacteria in neutropenic patients, although the incidence of fever with neutropenia and the need for intravenous antibiotics have not been consistently changed (Karp et al., 1987; Dekker et al., 1987). Additionally, the emergence of resistant organisms must be considered as a potential long-term liability of the use of these agents. Patients receiving long courses of the fluoroquinolone antibiotics may be more at risk for the development of infections with gram-positive organisms

such as *Staphylococci* and α-hemolytic streptococci. It is our opinion that the quinolones should not be used routinely for prophylaxis in neutropenic patients, but they may have some value in patients at high risk for developing gram-negative bacterial infections.

In some specific settings, preventive antimicrobial agents have a well-defined role. Trimethoprim-sulfamethoxazole is clearly effective in preventing *P. carinii* pneumonia in pediatric cancer patients (Hughes et al., 1977), and its use has become part of standard care in areas where *P. carinii* is a common pathogen in this population. Further studies have revealed that intermittent dosing is as effective and less toxic for prophylaxis as daily therapy for cancer patients (Hughes et al., 1987), and its use has also been recommended in pediatric patients whose immunosuppression is caused by HIV infection (Centers for Disease Control, 1991, 1995). Trimethoprim-sulfamethoxazole has also been used in the prevention of infections in children with CGD (Hill, 1988).

Similarly, it has been shown that acyclovir can reduce the incidence of recurrent HSV disease in patients undergoing intensive chemotherapy or bone marrow transplant (Saral et al., 1981). There is also some evidence that intravenous acyclovir given early in the course of bone marrow transplantation (Meyers et al., 1988) or kidney transplantation (Balfour et al., 1989) may reduce serious CMV infections in these high-risk populations. However, use of ganciclovir has been shown to be effective in preventing CMV disease in patients undergoing bone marrow transplantation (Schmidt et al., 1991; Goodrich et al., 1994) and has become part of the standard management of patients known to be seropositive for CMV antibody or to have received marrow from a seropositive donor.

The increasing concern for invasive fungal infections in immunocompromised patients has led to the investigation of the oral antifungal agents in prophylactic regimens. Large randomized studies evaluating fluconazole as prophylaxis in severely compromised adults have demonstrated a decrease in fungal colonization and infections in patients who undergo bone marrow transplantation (Goodman et al., 1992; Winston et al., 1993). Unfortunately, although fluconazole may eliminate *C. albicans* from the normal flora, fungi such as *Torulopsis glabrata, Candida krusei,* and *Aspergillus* spp. that are less susceptible may proliferate and become invasive (Wingard et al., 1991) and can cause significant morbidity.

IMMUNIZATIONS

Many children have already received their routine childhood immunizations before becoming immunosuppressed. For those who have not completed the immunization schedule at the time they become immunocompromised, the American Academy of Pediatrics provides some guidelines in administering immunizations (American Academy of Pediatrics, 1994). In general, nonreplicating vaccines should be given because the immune response to these agents seems to be adequate (although not optimal) even in immunosuppressed children. Booster doses may be needed when or if children are no longer immunocompromised. Live virus vaccines are generally contraindicated in all immunosuppressed children, and, in the case of the polio vaccine, the affected child and all siblings should receive the inactivated vaccine. The live attenuated varicella vaccine may be an exception to this rule, since it has proven to be safe and effective for up to 3 years in children with cancer who receive maintainance therapy (Gershon et al., 1989). This vaccine has recently been approved for use in children in the United States, but not for immunocompromised children, in spite of extensive investigation in this patient population. Another exception includes HIV-infected children who should receive live measles vaccine. Children recovering from allogeneic bone marrow transplantation are considered unimmunized and should be reimmunized with inactivated vaccines. Live virus vaccines (such as measles vaccine or MMR) may be given in leukemia patients in remission whose chemotherapy has been completed for at least 3 months and in bone marrow transplant patients with no evidence of graft-versus-host disease 2 years following transplantation.

ROLE FOR IMMUNE GLOBULIN

The use of immune globulins in passive immunization can be divided into those hyperimmune globulins specific for a certain type of infection and pooled serum immune globulin. Administration of varicella-zoster immune globulin (VZIG) significantly reduces the incidence of pneumonia and encephalitis and decreases mortality in seronegative immunocompromised patients exposed to varicella if given within the first 72 hours of exposure. Protection lasts only 3 to 4 weeks, however, so during a community outbreak of varicella it may be necessary for a child to receive more than 1 dose of VZIG if there are multiple exposures at home or school. During community epidemics of measles, unimmunized children may benefit from administration of pooled human immune globulin, since these preparations usually have protective titers of measles antibody. A number of studies have investigated the use of CMV-immune globulin in bone marrow transplant patients to prevent severe CMV disease, but, to date, this approach appears to have no clear advantage over careful monitoring of CMV serologic status and use of CMV-seronegative blood products in susceptible patients (Bowden et al., 1986). Clearly, children with congenital deficiencies of immunoglobulin G production benefit from replacement therapy with IVIG. However, a randomized trial performed at the National Cancer Institute failed to demonstrate any significant benefit from intravenous immune globulin in reducing the incidence of fever or infection in children and adults undergoing prolonged neutropenia. A new approach in the treatment of sepsis, although not specific to immunocompromised patients, involves the use of specific antiserum or monoclonal antibodies directed against different components of bacteria or the host response (i.e., tumor necrosis factor or interleukin-1).

ROLE OF CYTOKINES AND BIOLOGICALS

One of the most exciting areas of research in the field of infectious diseases is the discovery, characterization, and clinical application of various biologic substances capable of boosting a compromised immune system. The hematopoietic growth factors, such as granulocyte-macrophage colony-stimulating factor (GM-CSF) and granulocyte colony-stimulating factor (G-CSF), have been evaluated in clinical trials involving cancer and bone marrow transplant patients in an attempt to reconstitute the granulocyte line and decrease the incidence of infectious complications during periods of neutropenia. Primary use of G-CSF has been shown to decrease the incidence of febrile neutropenic episodes by about half in three studies in which the incidence of fever and neutropenia was about 40% in the control group. In some studies, although not all, this resulted in decreased hospitalizations and use of antibiotics. G-CSF has generally been well tolerated; GM-CSF has had more reported side effects, ranging from fever and myalgias to polyserositis with capillary leak syndrome. No survival advantage or improved tumor response rate has been identified with use of these agents. Many of these studies and recommendations for the use of hematopoietic growth factors are summarized in a consensus paper published by the American Society of Clinical Oncology (American Society of Clinical Oncology, 1994). Increasingly, data suggest that these agents may enhance the bactericidal activity of neutrophils (Groopman et al., 1989; Laver and Moore, 1989), whether they have normal or abnormal function (Roilides et al., 1991).

SUMMARY

Although the number of children with immunodeficiencies has increased with the expansion of cancer chemotherapeutic options and improved transplantation techniques expectant management of infectious complications in these patients have dramatically decreased morbidity and mortality. The principles outlined here, based on the experience with children with chemotherapy-induced neutropenia, provide a framework for evaluation and management of infections in any population of immunocompromised children. The goal of basic science and clinical research in this field is to decrease the duration and intensity of immune dysfunction during more intensive chemotherapy, hasten immune reconstitution, decrease the risk of significant infectious complications, and thereby decrease morbidity and mortality.

BIBLIOGRAPHY

Aisner J, Schimpff SC, Sutherland JC, et al. *Torulopsis glabrata* infections in patients with cancer: increasing incidence and relationship to colonization, Am J Med 1976;61:23.

Aisner J, Murillo J, Schimpff SC, et al. Invasive *Aspergillus* in acute leukemia: correlation with nose cultures and antibiotic use. Ann Intern Med 1979;90:4.

American Academy of Pediatrics. Immunization in special clinical circumstances. In Peter G (ed). 1994 Red Book: Report of the Committee on Infectious Diseases, ed 23. Elk Grove Village, Ill.: American Academy of Pediatrics, 1994.

American Society of Clinical Oncology. American Society of Clinical Oncology recommendations for the use of hematopoietic colony–stimulating factors: evidence-based, clinical practice guidelines. J Clin Oncol 1994;12:2471.

Balfour HH, Chase BA, Stapleton JJ, et al. A randomized, placebo-controlled trial of acyclovir for the prevention of cytomegalovirus disease in recipients of renal allografts. N Engl J Med 1989;320:1381.

Bartlett MS, Smith JW. *Pneumocystis carinii,* an opportunist in immunocompromised patients. Clin Microbiol Rev 1991; 4:137.

Bash RO, Katz JA, Cash JV, Buchanan GR. Safety and cost effectiveness of early hospital discharge of lower risk children with cancer admitted for fever and neutropenia. Cancer 1994;74:189.

Bayston KF, Want S, Cohen J. A prospective, randomized comparison of ceftazidime and ciprofloxacin as initial empirical therapy in neutropenic patients with fever. Am J Med 1989; 87(suppl 5A):269.

Bochud P-Y, Calandra R, Francioli P. Bacteremia due to viridans streptococci in neutropenic patients: a review. Am J Med 1994;97:256.

Bodey GP, Buckley M, Sathe YS, Freireich EJ. Quantitative relationships between circulating leukocytes and infection in patients with acute leukemia. Ann Intern Med 1966;64: 328.

Bodey GP, Jadeja L, Elting L. *Pseudomonas* bacteremia: a retrospective analysis of 410 episodes. Arch Intern Med 1985; 145:1621.

Boogaerts MA, Demuynck H, Mestdagh N, et al. (Meropenem Study Group of Leuven, London, and Nijmegen). Equivalent efficacies of meropenem and ceftazidime as empirical monotherapy of febrile neutropenic patients. J Antimicrobiol Chemother 1995;36:185.

Bowden RA, Sayers M, Flournoy N, et al. Cytomegalovirus immune globulin and seronegative blood products to prevent primary cytomegalovirus infection after marrow transplantation. N Engl J Med 1986;314:1006.

Browne MJ, Perek D, Dinndorf PA, et al. Infectious complications of intraventricular reservoirs in cancer patients. Pediatr Infect Dis 1987;6:182.

Browne MJ, Potter D, Gress J, et al. A randomized trial of open lung biopsy versus empirical antimicrobial therapy in cancer patients with diffuse pulmonary infiltrates. J Clin Oncol 1990;8:222.

Buchanan GR. Approach to treatment of the febrile cancer patient with low-risk neutropenia. Hematol Oncol Clin N Amer 1993;7:919.

Centers for Disease Control. Guidelines for prophylaxis against *Pneumocystis carinii* pneumonia for children infected with human immunodeficiency virus. MMWR 1991;40:1.

Centers for Disease Control. Nosocomial enterococci resistant to vancomycin: United States, 1989-1993. MMWR 1993; 42:597.

Centers for Disease Control. 1995 revised guidelines for prophylaxis against *Pneumocystis carinii* pneumonia for children infected with or perinatally exposed to human immunodeficiency virus. MMWR 1995;44(RR-4):1.

Chou S. Acquisition of donor strains of cytomegalovirus by renal-transplant recipients. N Engl J Med 1986;314:1418.

Cohen MA, Huband MD, Gage JW, et al. In vitro activity of clinafloxacin, trovafloxacin, and ciprofloxacin, Abstract E85. Abstracts of the thirty-sixth Interscience Conference on Antimicrobrial Agents and Chemotherapy, New Orleans, September 15-18, 1996.

Commers JR, Robichaud KJ, Pizzo PA. New pulmonary infiltrates in granulocytopenic cancer patients being treated with antibiotics. Pediatr Infect Dis 1984;3:423.

Coque TM, Singh KV, Murray BE. Assessment of the bactericidal activity of trovafloxacin, CP(99,129) against multiresistant strains of enterococci, Abstract E77. Abstracts of the thirty-sixth Interscience Conference on Antimicrobial Agents and chemotherapy. New Orleans, September 15-18, 1996.

Cotton DJ, Gill V, Hiemenz J. Bacillus bacteremia in an immunocompromised patient population: clinical features, therapeutic interventions, and relationship to chronic intravascular catheters. J Clin Micro 1987;25:672.

Cotton DJ, Yolken RH, Hiemenz JW. Role of respiratory viruses in the etiology of fever occurring during chemotherapy-induced granulocytopenia. Pediatr Res 1984;18:272A.

Cupps TR, Fauci AS. Corticosteroid-mediated immunoregulation in man. Immunol Rev 1982;65:133.

Davey FR, Erber WN, Gatter KC, Mason DY. Abnormal neutrophils in acute myeloid leukemia and myelodysplastic syndrome. Hum Pathol 1988;19:454.

Dekker AO, Rozenberg-Arska M, Verhoef J. Infection prophylaxis in acute leukemia: a comparison of ciprofloxacin with trimethoprim-sulfamethoxazole and colistin. Ann Intern Med 1987;106:7.

Edman JC, Kovacs JA, Masur H, et al. Ribosomal RNA sequence shows *Pneumocystis carinii* to be a member of the fungi. Nature 1988;334:519.

Elting LS, Bodey GP, Keefe BH. Septicemia and shock syndrome due to viridans streptococci: a case-control study of predisposing factors. Clin Infect Dis 1992;14:1201.

Emmanuel D, Cunningham I, Jules-Elysee K, et al. Cytomegalovirus pneumonia after bone marrow transplantation successfully treated with the combination of ganciclovir and high-dose intravenous immune globulin. Ann Intern Med 1988;109:777.

Englund JA, Anderson LJ, Rhame FS. Nosocomial transmission of respiratory syncytial virus in immunocompromised adults. J Clin Microbiol 1991;29:115.

EORTC, International Antimicrobial Therapy Cooperative Group. Efficacy and toxicity of single daily doses of amikacin and ceftriaxone versus multiple daily doses of amikacin and ceftazidime for infection in patients with cancer and granulocytopenia. Ann Intern Med 1993;119:584.

EORTC, International Antimicrobial Therapy Cooperative Group. Empiric antifungal therapy in febrile granulocytopenic patients. Am J Med 1989;86:668.

Eppes SC, Troutman JL, Gutman LT. Outcome of treatment of candidemia in children whose central catheters were removed or retained. Pediatr Infect Dis 1989;8:99.

Esekowitz RAB, Dinaur MC, Jaffe HS, et al. Partial correction of the phagocytic defect in patients with X-linked chronic granulomatous disease by subcutaneous interferon gamma. N Engl J Med 1988;319:146.

Fainstein V, Bodey GP, Elting L, et al. Amphotericin B or ketoconazole therapy of fungal infections in neutropenic cancer patients. Antimicrob Agents Chemother 1987;31:11.

Fainstein V, Elting LS, Bodey GP. Bacteremia caused by nonsporulating anaerobes in cancer patients: a 12-year experience. Medicine 1989;68:151.

Feldman S, Hughes WT, Daniel CB. Varicella in children with cancer: seventy-seven cases. Pediatrics 1975;56:388.

Finch RG. Antibacterial activity of quinopristin/dalfopristin: rationale for clinical use. Drugs 1996;51(suppl 1):31.

Freifeld AG, Walsh T, Marshall D, et al. Monotherapy for fever and neutropenia in cancer patients: a randomized comparison of ceftazidime versus imipenem. J Clin Oncol 1995; 13:165.

Gershon AA, Steinberg SP, the Varicella Vaccine Collaborative Study Group of the National Institute of Allergy and Infectious Diseases. Persistence of immunity to varicella in children with leukemia immunized with live attenuated varicella vaccine. N Engl J Med 1989;320:892.

Glenn J, Cotton D, Wesley R, Pizzo P. Anorectal infections in patients with malignant diseases. Rev Infect Dis 1988; 10:42.

Goodman JL, Winston DJ, Greenfield RA, et al. A controlled trial of fluconazole to prevent fungal infections in patients undergoing bone marrow transplantation. N Engl J Med 1992;326:845.

Goodrich JM, Boeckh M, Bowden R. Strategies for the prevention of cytomegalovirus disease after marrow transplantation. Clin Infect Dis 1994;19:287.

Griffin TC, Buchanan GR. Hematologic predictors of bone marrow recovery in neutropenic patients hospitalized for fever: implications for discontinuation of antibiotics and early hospital discharge. J Pediatr 1992;121:28.

Groopman JE, Molina J-M, Scadden DT. Hematopoietic growth factors: biology and clinical applications. N Engl J Med 1989;321:1449.

Harrington RD, Hooton RD, Hackman RC, et al. An outbreak of respiratory syncytial virus in a bone marrow transplant center. J Infect Dis 1992;165:987.

Hathorn J, Thaler M, Skelton J, et al. Empiric amphotericin B versus ketoconazole in febrile granulocytopenic cancer patients, Abstract 248. Programs and abstracts of the twenty-fifth Interscience Conference on Antimicrobial Agents and Chemotherapy, Minneapolis, 1985.

Henning KJ, Delencastre H, Eagan J, et al. Vancomycin-resistant *Enterococcus faecium* on a pediatric oncology ward: duration of stool shedding and incidence of clinical infection. Pediatr Infect Dis J 1996;15:848.

Hiemenz J, Skelton J, Pizzo PA. Perspective on the management of catheter-related infections in cancer patients. Pediatr Infect Dis 1986;5:6.

Hill H. Infections complicating congenital immunodeficiency syndromes. In Rubin RH, Young LS (eds). Clinical approach to infection in the compromised host. New York: Plenum Medical Book Co, 1988.

Horvath JA, Dummer S. The use of respiratory-tract cultures in the diagnosis of invasive pulmonary aspergillosis. Amer J Med 1996;100:171.

Hughes WT, Armstrong D, Bodey GP, et al. Guidelines for the use of antimicrobial agents in neutropenic patients with unexplained fever. J Infect Dis 1990;161:381.

Hughes WT, Kuhn S, Chaudhary S, et al. Successful chemoprophylaxis for *Pneumocystis carinii* pneumonitis. N Engl J Med 1977;297:1419.

Hughes WT, Rivera GK, Schell MJ, et al. Successful intermittent chemoprophylaxis for *Pneumocystis carinii* pneumonitis. N Engl J Med 1987;316:1627.

International Chronic Granulomatous Disease Cooperative Study Group. A controlled trial of interferon-γ to prevent infection in chronic granulomatous disease. N Engl J Med 1991;324:509.

Karp JE, Dick JD, Angelopulos C, et al. Empiric use of vancomycin during prolonged treatment-induced granulocytopenia: randomized, double-blind, placebo-controlled clinical trial in patients with acute leukemia. Am J Med 1986; 81:237.

Karp JE, Merz WG, Hendricksen C, et al. Oral norfloxacin for prevention of gram-negative bacterial infections in patients with acute leukemia and granulocytopenia: a randomized, double-blind, placebo-controlled trial. Ann Intern Med 1987;106:1.

Kovacs JA, Hiemenz JW, Macher AM, et al. *Pneumocystis carinii* pneumonia: a comparison between patients with the acquired immunodeficiency syndrome and patients with other immunodeficiencies. Ann Intern Med 1984;100:663.

Kramer BK, Pizzo PA, Robichaud DJ, et al. Role of serial microbiological surveillance and clinical evaluation in the management of cancer patients with fever and granulocytopenia. Am J Med 1982;72:561.

Laver J, Moore MAS. Clinical use of recombinant human hematopoietic growth factors. J Natl Cancer Inst 1989; 81:1370.

Mackall CL, Fleisher TA, Brown MR, et al. Lymphocyte depletion during treatment with intensive chemotherapy for cancer. Blood 1994;84:2221.

Masur H, Shelhamer J, Parrillo JE. The management of pneumonias in immunocompromised patients. J Amer Med Assoc 1985;253:1769.

McFarland LV, Mulligan ME, Kwok RYY, Stamm WE. Nosocomial acquisition of *Clostridium difficile* infection. N Engl J Med 1989;320:204.

Meyers JD. Infection in bone marrow transplant recipients. Am J Med 1986;81(suppl 1A):27.

Meyers JD, Flournoy N, Thomas ED. Risk factors for cytomegalovirus infection after human marrow transplantation. J Infect Dis 1986;153:478.

Meyers JD, Reed EC, Shepp DH, et al. Acyclovir for prevention of cytomegalovirus infection and disease after allogeneic marrow transplantation. N Engl J Med 1988;318:70.

Montecalvo MA, Horowitz H, Gedris C, et al. Outbreak of vancomycin-, ampicillin-, and aminoglycoside-resistant *Enterococcus faecium* bacteremia in an adult oncology unit. Antimicrob Agents Chemother 1994;38:1363.

Mullen CA, Buchanan GR. Early hospital discharge of children with cancer treated for fever and neutropenia. Identification and management of the low-risk patient. J Clin Oncol 1990;8:1998.

Mustafa MM, Aquino VM, Pappo A, et al. A pilot study of outpatient management of febrile neutropenic children with cancer at low risk of bacteremia. J Pediatr 1996;128:847.

Pappo AS, Buchanan GR. Predictors of bacteremia in febrile neutropenic children with cancer. Proc Am Soc Clin Oncol 1991;10:331.

Pizzo PA. Considerations for the prevention of infectious complications in patients with cancer. Rev Infect Dis 1989; 11(suppl 7):S1551.

Pizzo PA, Commers J, Cotton D, et al. Approaching the controversies in the antibacterial management of cancer patients. Am J Med 1984;76:436.

Pizzo PA, Hathorn JW, Hiemenz J, et al. A randomized trial comparing ceftazidime alone with combination antibiotic therapy in cancer patients with fever and neutropenia. N Engl J Med 1986;315:552.

Pizzo PA, Ladisch S, Robichaud K. Treatment of gram-positive septicemia in cancer patients. Cancer 1980;45:206.

Pizzo PA, Ladisch S, Simon RM, et al. Increasing incidence of gram-positive sepsis in cancer patients. Med Pediatr Oncol 1978;5:241.

Pizzo PA, Robichaud KJ, Gill FA, Witebsky FG. Empiric antibiotic and antifungal therapy of cancer patients with prolonged fever and granulocytopenia. Am J Med 1982a; 72:101.

Pizzo PA, Robichaud KJ, Gill FA, et al. Duration of empirical antibiotic therapy in granulocytopenic cancer patients. Am J Med 1979;67:194.

Pizzo PA, Robichaud KJ, Wesley R, Commers JR. Fever in the pediatric and young adult patient with cancer: a prospective study of 1,001 episodes. Medicine 1982b;61:153.

Pizzo PA, Thaler M, Hathorn J, et al. New β-lactam antibiotics in granulocytopenic patients: new options and new questions. Am J Med 1985;79(suppl 2A):75.

Rand KH, Pollard RB, Merigan TC. Increased pulmonary superinfections in cardiac transplant patients undergoing primary cytomegalovirus infection. N Engl J Med 1978; 298:951.

Reed EC, Bowden RA, Dandliker PS, et al. Treatment of cytomegalovirus pneumonia with ganciclovir and intravenous cytomegalovirus immunoglobulin in patients with bone marrow transplants. Ann Intern Med 1988;109:783.

Roilides E, Walsh TJ, Pizzo PA, Rubin M. Granulocyte colony–stimulating factor enhances the phagocytic and bactericidal activity of normal and defective human neutrophils. J Infect Dis 1991;163:579.

Rolston KVI, Haron E, Cunningham C, Bodey GP. Intravenous ciprofloxacin for infections in cancer patients. Am J Med 1989;87(suppl 5A):261.

Rubin LG, Tucci V, Cercenado E, et al. Vancomycin-resistant *Enterococcus faecium* in hospitalized children. Infect Control Hosp Epidemiol 1992;13:700.

Rubin M, Hathorn JW, Marshall D, et al. Gram-positive infections and the use of vancomycin in 550 episodes of fever and neutropenia. Ann Intern Med 1988;108:30.

Rubin M, Walsh TJ, Pizzo PA. Clinical approach to infections in the compromised host. In Benz E, Cohen H, Furip B, et al. (eds). Hematology: basic principles and practice, 1991.

Rubin RH. Impact of cytomegalovirus infection on organ transplant recipients. Rev Infect Dis 1990;12(suppl 7):S754.

Saral R, Burns WH, Laskin OL, et al. Acyclovir prophylaxis of herpes simplex virus infections: a randomized, double-blind, controlled trial in bone-marrow-transplant recipients. N Engl J Med 1981;305:63.

Schaad UB, Salam MA, Aujard Y, et al. Use of fluoroquinolones in pediatrics consensus report of an International Society of Chemotherapy commission. Pediatr Infect Dis J 1995; 14:1.

Schmidt GM, Horak DA, Niland JC, et al. A randomized, controlled trial of prophylactic ganciclovir for cytomegalovirus pulmonary infection in recipients of allogeneic bone marrow transplants. N Engl J Med 1991;324:1005.

Sechler JMF, Malech HL, White CJ, Ballin JI. Recombinant human interferon-γ reconstitutes defective phagocyte function in patients with chronic granulomatous disease of childhood. Proc Natl Acad Sci USA 1988;85:4874.

Shamberger RC, Weinstein HJ, Delorey MJ, Levey RH. The medical and surgical management of typhlitis in children with acute nonlymphocytic (myelogenous) leukemia. Cancer 1986;57:603.

Skibber JM, Matter GJ, Pizzo PA, Lotze MT. Right lower quadrant pain in young patients with leukemia: a surgical perspective. Ann Surg 1987;206:711.

Sloas MM, Flynn PM, Kaste SC, Patrick CC. Typhlitis in children with cancer: a 30-year experience. Clin Infect Dis 1993;17:484.

Sotiropoulos SV, Jackson MA, Woods GM, et al. Alpha-streptococcal septicemia in leukemic children treated with continuous or large dosage intermittent cytosine arabinoside. Pediatr Infect Dis J 1989;8:755.

Straus SE, Ostrove JM, Inchauspe G, et al. Varicella-zoster virus infections: biology, natural history, treatment, and prevention. Ann Intern Med 1988; 108:221.

Talcott JA, Finberg R, Mayer RJ, Goldman L. The medical course of cancer patients with fever and neutropenia: clinical identification of a low-risk subgroup at presentation. Arch Intern Med 1988;148:2561.

Talcott JA, Whalen A, Clark J, et al. Home antibiotic therapy for low-risk cancer patients with fever and neutropenia: a pilot study of thirty patients based on a validated prediction rule. J Clin Oncol 1994;12:107.

Van Der Meer JWM. Defects in host-defense mechanisms. In Rubin RH, Young LS (eds). Clinical approach to infection in the compromised host. New York: Plenum Medical Book, 1988.

Van der Waaij D, Tielemans-Speltie TM, Roeck-Houben AMJ. Infection by and distribution of biotyped of *Enterobacteriaceae* species in leukaemic patients treated under ward conditions and in units for protective isolation in seven hospitals in Europe. Infection 1977;5:188.

Vouillamoz J, Entenza JM, Giddey M, et al. In vitro activity of Synercid (quinopristin-dalfopristin)(SYN) combined with other classes of antibiotics against vancomycin-susceptible (VS) *E. faecalis* and vancomycin-susceptible or -resistant (VR) *E. faecium* (VSEF and VREF), Abstract E8. Abstracts of the thirty-sixth Interscience Conference on Antimicrobial Agents and Chemotherapy. New Orleans, September 15-18, 1996.

Wade JC, Schimpff SC, Newman KA, Wiernik PH. *Staphylococcus epidermidis:* an increasing cause of infection in patients with granulocytopenia. Ann Intern Med 1982;97:503.

Wagner ML, Rosenberg HS, Fernbach DJ, Singleton EB. Typhlitis: a complication of leukemia in childhood. Am J Roentgenol Rad Therapy and Nuclear Med 1970;109:341.

Walsh TJ. Invasive pulmonary aspergillosis in patients with neoplastic diseases. Sem Resp Infect 1990;5:111.

Whimbey E, Champlin RE, Englund JA, et al. Combination therapy with aerosolized ribavirin and intravenous immunoglobulin for respiratory syncytial virus disease in adult bone marrow transplant recipients. Bone Marrow Transplantation 1995;16:393.

Whimbey E, Couch RB, Englund JA, et al. Respiratory syncytial virus pneumonia in hospitalized adult patients with leukemia. Clin Infect Dis 1995b;21:376.

Wiley JM, Smith N, Leventhal BG, et al. Invasive fungal disease in pediatric acute leukemia patients with fever and neutropenia during induction chemotherapy: a multivariate analysis of risk factors. J Clin Oncol 1990;8:280.

Wingard JR, Merz WG, Rinaldi MG, et al. Increase in *Candida krusei* infection among patients with bone marrow transplantation and neutropenia treated prophylactically with fluconazole. N Engl J Med 1991;325:1274.

Wingard JR, Merz WG, Saral RR. *Candida tropicalis:* a major pathogen in immunocompromised patients. Ann Intern Med 1979;91:539.

Winston DJ, Chandrasekar PH, Lazarus HM, et al. Fluconazole prophylaxis of fungal infection in patients with acute leukemia: results of a randomized, placebo-controlled, double-blind, multicenter trial. Ann Intern Med 1993;118:495.

Wood DJ, Corbitt G. Viral infections in childhood leukemia. J Infect Dis 1985;152:266.

Yu VL, Muder RR, Poorsattar A. Significance of isolation of aspergillus from the respiratory tract in diagnosis of invasive pulmonary aspergillosis: results from a 3-year prospective study. Am J Med 1986;81:249.

Zaman MM, Landman D, Burney S, et al. Treatment of experimental endocarditis due to multidrug-resistant *Enterococcus faecium* with clinafloxacin and penicillin. J Antimicrob Chemo 1996;37:127.

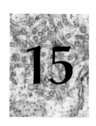

15   KAWASAKI SYNDROME

MARIAN E. MELISH AND PETER HOTEZ

Kawasaki syndrome, or mucocutaneous lymph node syndrome, is an acute febrile multisystem vasculitis affecting children. It was first described by Dr. Tomisaku Kawasaki in Japan in 1967 (Kawasaki, 1967; Kawasaki et al., 1974). Dr. Kawasaki's particular genius was the clear description of the disease and the identification of six clinical criteria, which remain the foundation of diagnosis 25 years later. Originally termed "benign" mucocutaneous lymph node syndrome, it is no longer considered necessarily benign. It was recognized in the early 1970s that death caused by myocardial infarction occurred in approximately 2% of cases; subsequently, it has been appreciated that approximately 30% of patients develop clinical evidence of cardiac disease, 20% develop coronary artery abnormalities large enough for detection by echocardiogram, and 30% develop inflammatory arthritis. In North America Kawasaki syndrome currently is a more common cause of acquired heart disease and inflammatory arthritis than acute poststreptococcal rheumatic fever. No longer confined to the Orient, Kawasaki syndrome has been recognized on all continents in children of all racial groups. Although the cause of this disorder remains unexplained, therapy is available. Intravenous gamma globulin given during the first week of illness has a dramatic effect on the clinical illness and reduces the likelihood of coronary abnormalities from greater than 20% to less than 5% (Furusho et al., 1984; Newburger et al., 1986; Newburger et al., 1991).

ETIOLOGY

Because of its febrile, exanthematous, and self-limited clinical characteristics, Kawasaki syndrome is widely believed to have a microbial cause. Despite intensive investigation, the causative agent had not been discovered by 1992. Studies (Shulman and Rowley, 1986; Burns et al., 1987) reporting the detection of reverse transcriptase, possibly indicating a retroviral cause, have not been confirmed by others (Melish et al., 1989; Marchette et al., 1990) or in subsequent experiments in one of the original laboratories (Shulman and Rowley, 1986). Although the human herpesvirus family, especially Epstein-Barr virus, has come under suspicion, all, including the newest member (human herpes virus 6), have been exonerated (Marchette et al., 1990).

Although some studies show a provocative link between toxin-producing strains of *Staphylococcus aureus* to Kawasaki syndrome, they have not been replicated (Melish et al., 1994). Of interest in this regard is a case report in which a 13 year old simultaneously presented with both Kawasaki syndrome and toxic syndrome in association with *S. aureus* colonization (Davies et al., 1996).

PATHOLOGY AND PATHOGENESIS

By the mid-1970s it became evident that approximately 2% of children affected with Kawasaki syndrome, originally considered a benign condition, died suddenly, generally between 10 and 40 days from onset in the subacute or convalescent stage of illness (Kawasaki et al., 1974).

At autopsy, the major findings are multisystem vasculitis with special predilection for the coronary arteries (Landing and Larson, 1977; Fujiwara and Hamashima, 1978). The immediate cause of death is acute thrombosis of inflamed coronary arteries in more than 80% of fatal cases. In some deaths occurring early (within the first 2 weeks after onset), pancarditis with inflammation in the atrioventricular conduction system is thought to result in death from fatal arrhythmias or intractable congestive heart failure, whereas some late deaths (months to years after acute disease) apparently are secondary to coronary stenosis with chronic myocardial ischemia. Rupture of a coronary aneurysm is rare. Involvement of other arteries, particularly large and medium-sized muscular arteries, is variable and scattered. The history of the vascular lesion is directly related to the stage of illness at the time of death, demonstrating that the insult in Kawasaki syndrome is episodic and has a self-limited relationship to the acute illness rather than being chronic or progressive.

Early lesions (<10 days from onset of fever) are characterized by acute inflammation involving the intima of the coronary arteries. There is also an intense perivascular infiltration in the adventitia, with evidence of acute inflammation in the microvessels or vasa vasorum supplying the arterial wall. The media is spared, and aneurysmal dilation is absent. The clinical correlation is that the first evidence of coronary dilation by serial echocardiography appears at a mean of 10 days in those children ultimately developing coronary aneurysms. At this early stage carditis with an acute polymorphonuclear infiltrate in the pericardium, in the perivascular spaces of the myocardium, and in the endothelium—especially the mitral, tricuspid, and aortic valves—is present. Polymorphonuclear leukocyte infiltration is notable in the atrioventricular conduction system.

By the second week of illness through the sixth week, the intensity and nature of the inflammatory infiltrate progressively change, maturing from a dominant polymorphonuclear cell infiltrate to a less intense infiltrate composed predominantly of plasma cells and lymphocytes. The inflammation of the pericardium, myocardium, and endocardium gradually subsides. In the blood vessel wall destruction of the media appears, with multiple fractures of the internal elastic lamina and the development of aneurysmal dilation. The cause of death at this stage almost invariably involves coronary thrombosis close to the origin of the vessel, with massive myocardial infarction. Deaths occurring during this stage represent the most commonly encountered cardiac pathology of Kawasaki syndrome and are indistinguishable from a previously described pathologic entity, infantile periarteritis nodosa. Infantile periarteritis nodosa was encountered rarely from the late nineteenth century to 1975; it was characterized by a fatal 2- to 6-week illness compatible with what is now recognized as Kawasaki syndrome. Both Kawasaki syndrome and infantile periarteritis nodosa have major differences from classic periarteritis nodosa, which is generally a chronic progressive illness of older children and adults, resulting in hypertension and renal and pulmonary disease and involving most

often small and medium-sized muscular arteries, especially in the lung, kidney, and intestines.

Patients whose deaths occur more than 2 months from onset generally show little or no evidence of inflammation in the vessel walls or the heart. There is evidence of stenosis and myocardial infarction, both recent and remote, and the cause of death is generally acute infarction or chronic myocardial ischemia.

Although changes in multiple arteries, especially axillary, iliac, and femoral arteries and extraparenchymal portions of arteries supplying the stomach, spleen, and intestines, are seen, the intensity of involvement of other vessels in fatal cases is nearly always less than that found in the heart. Nonspecific changes in the lymph nodes, including focal necrosis with microthrombi, T-zone hyperplasia, macrophage infiltration of B zones, immunoblast proliferation, and mononuclear cell infiltration, have been described.

Recently, considerable progress has been made in elucidating aspects of the immunopathogenesis of vasculitis in Kawasaki syndrome. An acute rise and a convalescent fall of all classes of immunoglobulins occur during the illness so that 50% of IgE values and 80% of IgM values exceed 2 standard deviations for age-matched norms (Eluthesen et al., 1985). Immunoregulatory abnormalities resulting in a dramatic increase in the numbers of circulatory B cells spontaneously secreting immunoglobulin have been reported. The increase in immunoglobulin is polyclonal, with a very high proportion of activated B cells, apparently the result of a relative and absolute depression of suppressor T cells, which results in an elevated T-helper–T-suppressor ratio in the acute stage. T cells from patients with early Kawasaki syndrome stimulate normal, control B cells to produce immunoglobulins. The relative and absolute T-suppressor deficiency resolves rapidly with time, with normalization at 2 to 3 weeks of illness (Leung et al., 1983; Mason et al., 1985).

Immune complexes can be detected in more than 50% of patients by either C1q or Raji cell assays. These immune complexes are present very early in the illness, tend to peak approximately 4 weeks after onset, and become undetectable in late convalescence. The quantity of immune complexes in patients with Kawasaki syndrome is lower than that found in those with systemic lupus erythematosus but higher than that found in normal, afebrile children (Levin et al., 1985; Ono et al., 1985). Concentrations of complement are of special interest because of the increased levels of immune complexes in Kawasaki syndrome. C3 is universally elevated in weeks 1 through 3 of illness and then becomes normal, whereas C4 remains normal throughout the illness (Eluthesen et al., 1985). The coexistence of immune complexes with normal or high complement values in Kawasaki syndrome is markedly different from the classic immune complex disorders in which there is complement consumption, generally with renal involvement. Renal involvement is extremely unusual in Kawasaki syndrome. With Kawasaki syndrome, immune complexes may aggregate platelets, resulting in release of vasoactive factors. It is possible that the immune complexes bind directly to the vascular endothelium and induce an inflammatory reaction.

Increased elaboration of cytokines from peripheral blood mononuclear cells and high levels of serum interleukin-1 (IL-1), tumor necrosis factor (TNF), and interferon-gamma (IFN-γ) have been documented (Leung, 1989; Leung et al., 1989; Maury et al., 1989). In contrast, levels of interferon-alpha (IFN-α) in acute or convalescent sera of patients with Kawasaki syndrome were undetectable (Ogle et al., 1991). Serum-soluble interleukin-2 (IL-2) receptor levels are increased in the acute phase and early subacute phase (up to 14 days), becoming normal thereafter (Lang et al., 1990). This provides another marker of lymphocyte activation that is associated with increased production of the cytokine IL-2.

Endothelial injury with Kawasaki syndrome may be related both to increased cytokine production, which may induce novel endothelial cell antigens, and to the generation of harmful autoantibodies to these new antigens. IgG and IgM antibodies, which are cytotoxic to cultured human umbilical vein endothelial cells that have been exposed to IFN-γ, IL-1, or TNF, can be detected in early illness. These novel cytokine-induced antigens might also make the endothelial cell surface more thrombogenic and induce adhesion antigens that could attract inflammatory cells (Leung et al., 1986). Some investigators believe that vigorous cytokine production occurs in a genetically predisposed individual who becomes infected with an as yet unidentified infectious pathogen. As noted previously, although the epidemiologic and clinical features of Kawasaki syndrome appear to suggest an infectious etiology, no consensus for its identification has emerged.

In all of these studies the period of most intense cytokine elaboration and immune activation occurs during the acute and early subacute phase, coinciding with the period of most intense vascular inflammation through aneurysm formation. Leukotriene B$_4$ production by polymorphonuclear cells is increased in the subacute phase 13 to 29 days from onset. This powerful endogenous chemoattractant released from polymorphonuclear cells at an inflammatory site may play a role in attracting more inflammatory cells to the site, thus prolonging the period of intense inflammation (Hamasaki et al., 1989).

The strongest evidence of the importance of immunologic factors in the pathogenesis of vasculitis in Kawasaki syndrome is provided by the remarkable beneficial effect of large-dose intravenous gamma globulin (IVIG) on both the acute febrile illness and the prevalence of coronary aneurysms. After IVIG therapy, B-cell activation and cytokine secretion are reduced, and T-suppressor cells return more rapidly to normal. Endothelial cell activation antigens disappeared after treatment in four of six patients in whom skin biopsies were performed before and while being given IVIG (Leung, 1989). The possible importance of endothelial cell antigens is demonstrated by a necropsy study that showed that endothelial cells of coronary arteries from Kawasaki syndrome patients, but not from normal individuals, expressed the major histocompatibility class II activation antigen (Terai et al., 1990). Prompt reversal of cytokine elaboration and other aspects of immune activation affecting endothelial cell function and antigen expression provide an attractive explanation of the still unknown mechanism of action of high-dose IVIG. Other theories attempting to explain the beneficial action of IVIG in this disease include down regulation of immunoglobulin production by a negative-feedback mechanism, specific immunoglobulin neutralization of the elusive causative agent or toxin, and nonspecific blockade of attachment sites for immune complexes or harmful autoantibodies on the vascular endothelium.

EPIDEMIOLOGY

The epidemiology of Kawasaki syndrome demonstrates that the disease virtually is restricted to young children: 50% are less than 2 years of age, 80% are less than 4 years, and cases are rare in individuals over the age of 12 years. Males outnumber females by a ratio of 1.4 to 1.6:1. Race-specific incidence rates developed from active surveillance in diverse locations such as Japan, Hawaii, Los Angeles, Chicago, and Heilbronn, Germany, demonstrate that Japanese and Korean children have an annual incidence of 40 to 150 cases per 100,000 children less than 5 years old, whereas Caucasian children in the diverse areas outside of Japan have rates of 6 to 10 cases per 100,000 children less than 5 years old. Intermediate rates have been recorded for children of black, Hispanic, Chinese, Filipino, and Polynesian ancestry. These rates are higher than those obtained from a nationwide passive surveillance in the United States and Britain (1.1 and 1.5 per 100,000 children <5 years old, respectively) but undoubtedly more accurately represent the true incidence. Projecting these figures to the United States as a whole, an estimated 3,000 to 5,000 cases occur per year, a figure close to that reported for Lyme disease. Community-wide epidemics generally occurring in the winter and spring with a 2- to 4-year interepidemic frequency have been recorded in several well-studied communities in Japan and North America. In these outbreaks no point-source exposure or direct person-to-person spread is apparent. In Japan, large cyclic epidemics of Kawasaki syndrome have been reported in 1979, 1982, and 1985 (Yanagawa et al., 1995). Such spread has not been reported in North America, where outbreaks to date have been limited to single communities. Epidemiologic and case-control investigations have demonstrated no striking climatic or urban-rural differences, no evidence of association with drugs or immunizations, no evidence to suggest insect vector or animal contact transmission, and no evidence of parenteral spread, contact with specific environmental toxins, or diets unusual for age. Two intriguing associations—exposure to freshly shampooed carpets and residence near a body of standing water—have been found in some investigations but not in others (Patriarca et al., 1982; Klein et al., 1986; Rogers, 1986; Rauch, 1987; Burns et al., 1991).

The clinical and epidemiologic features of sudden onset, the febrile exanthematous and self-limited character of the disease, and the regular occurrence of epidemics at 2- to 4-year intervals suggest a microbial cause. The widespread nature of the community-wide outbreaks with little evidence of direct person-to-person spread, the epidemic periodicity, and the restriction to young children further suggest that the elusive causative agent probably is highly transmissible and human associated, spreading widely through the community, producing infection and immunity in nearly all individuals by the age of 12 years, but resulting in clinically apparent disease in only a few, particularly those

with a race-related genetic predisposition to disease. The 2- to 4-year interepidemic frequency, superimposed on endemic occurrence, coincides with the age at greatest occurrence and suggests that outbreaks can be generated when a sufficient number of new susceptibles have been added to the population by birth. No evidence has yet been found supporting a bacterial cause, for no bacterial agent has been isolated regularly from a normally sterile site. The possibility that an agent constituting the normal flora of the respiratory tract or the gut might have pathologic potential, perhaps through elaboration of a toxin, has been suggested. A novel, difficult to cultivate virus would be equally likely.

CLINICAL MANIFESTATIONS

In its fully developed form Kawasaki syndrome is a distinctive clinical entity with a predictable clinical course. Because no single pathognomonic laboratory test or clinical sign has yet emerged, the diagnosis must be made by careful adherence to clinical criteria (Box 15-1 and Plate 3). These criteria were described by Dr. Kawasaki and are discussed in detail in the following sections.

Fever

The fever usually begins abruptly and is of a remittent, high-spiking nature, with two to four peaks

---

BOX 15-1

PRINCIPAL DIAGNOSTIC CRITERIA FOR KAWASAKI SYNDROME

Five of the six criteria are necessary to make a secure diagnosis.
- Fever
- Conjunctival injection
- Changes in the mouth
    Erythema, fissuring, and crusting of the lips
    Diffuse oropharyngeal erythema
    Strawberry tongue
- Changes in the peripheral extremities
    Induration of hands and feet
    Erythema of palms and soles
    Desquamation of fingertips and toetips approximately 2 weeks after onset
    Transverse grooves across fingernails 2 to 3 months after onset
- Erythematous rash
- Enlarged lymph node mass measuring more than 1.5 cm in diameter

per day. The temperature usually ranges from 38.5° to more than 40° C. Unless the patient is treated with a combination of aspirin and IVIG, the mean duration of fever exceeds 10 days but ranges from 5 to 35 days. The fever drops dramatically to the normal range in more than 80% of patients within 24 hours of single-dose IVIG treatment.

Conjunctival Changes

In patients with Kawasaki syndrome there is discrete vascular injection of the bulbar conjunctiva, which is more severe than injection in the tarsal or palpebral conjunctiva. Finding a zone of decreased infection around the iris (limbal sparing) is characteristic. Some patients also have follicular palpebral conjunctivitis. These findings develop in the first week of illness. There is no associated exudate, and edema of the conjunctiva and corneal ulceration do not occur, thus distinguishing the conjunctivitis of Kawasaki syndrome from the purulent conjunctivitis of Stevens-Johnson syndrome. Mild acute iridocyclitis or anterior uveitis also occurs early in the acute phase and is diagnosed by visualization of cells or "flare" during office slit-lamp examination. The finding rapidly resolves and rarely is associated with photophobia or eye pain.

Mouth Changes

Any or all of the following mouth changes can occur in patients with Kawasaki syndrome: lip involvement, strawberry tongue, and oropharyngeal erythema. Lip changes first appear 2 to 5 days after onset of fever, starting as generalized erythema with mild edema. Erythema and edema progressively increase over the next several days, with cracking and bleeding. The development of fissures coincides with lip changes. A strawberry tongue develops, with prominent hypertrophied papillae. The tongue is usually reddened; the white strawberry tongue characteristic of early scarlet fever is encountered less often. Patients may have diffuse oropharyngeal erythema, but exudates on the tonsils and vesicles and ulcers within the mouth are rarely encountered; therefore their appearance should prompt consideration of an alternate diagnosis.

Hand and Foot Lesions

Changes in the hands and feet are among the most distinctive features of Kawasaki syndrome. The first and most constant finding is the development of diffuse red-purple discoloration of the palms and soles 2 to 5 days after onset of fever. This erythema may wrap partially around the fingers and soles and extend a few centimeters up the wrists. Discrete macules on the palms and soles as seen in measles and other viral illnesses are not part of Kawasaki syndrome and constitute strong evidence against the diagnosis. The hands and feet may be edematous or firmly indurated. Patients often refuse to stand or walk because of discomfort from edema, and older children find that edema of their hands prevents using crayons and scissors. In the subacute phase of illness, days 10 to 20 from onset of fever, a characteristic desquamation begins at the fingertips just under the nailbed. It is followed by toe desquamation a few days later. Extensive desquamation of the entire palm and sole, with the shedding of large, thick sheets of skin, usually is present. This desquamation differs considerably from the fine, branny flakes that begin at the sides of the fingernails as a characteristic of the convalescent stage of scarlet fever. A transverse groove across the fingernails and toenails (Beau's lines) becomes apparent 6 to 8 weeks after onset and grows out with the nail.

Rash

The rash of Kawasaki syndrome is deeply erythematous, nonvesicular, and nonbullous, but it is polymorphic in both its nature and distribution. The most common type of rash consists of raised, deeply erythematous pruritic plaques of varying sizes ranging from 2 to more than 10 mm in diameter. These lesions resemble intensely erythematous urticaria or incompletely developed target lesions of the erythema multiforme type. The second most frequently encountered type of rash is maculopapular. It may be widely scattered or coalescent. This type of rash strongly resembles that of measles, but it rarely has the same distribution and does not progress from the face and trunk to the extremities in a centripetal fashion. A generalized or blotchy scarlatiniform erythroderma occurs in approximately 10% of cases. Rarely have we encountered a flat erythema marginatum rash in small infants. The distribution of rash is quite variable; in some patients it is truly generalized, and in others it is more prominent on the trunk or on the extremities. Occasionally, the rash is most prominent on or even limited to the lower abdomen and perineal area.

Lymph Nodes

An enlarged lymph node mass is seen in approximately 50% of cases. When present, it is virtually always unilateral and cervical, with considerable firm induration measuring from 1.5 to 7 cm in diameter. It may be extremely tender and have overlying erythema. At times it may result in acute torticollis or swallowing difficulty.

Once present, rash, hand and foot erythema, edema, and lymph node swelling persist throughout the febrile phase and disappear dramatically when the fever resolves. Conjunctival infection and mouth changes resolve more gradually.

Associated Features

The associated features of Kawasaki syndrome attest to its multisystemic nature (Box 15-2). Sterile pyuria reflecting urethritis is found in three quarters of patients. Arthritis developing in the first week of illness tends to involve multiple joints, including the small interphalangeal joints and large weight-bearing joints. Arthrocentesis during this phase reveals copious, thick purulent fluid, with a mean white blood cell (WBC) count of 125,000/mm^3 up to 300,000/mm^3. Glucose determinations are within normal limits; gram stain results and cultures are invariably negative. Approximately one third of patients with arthritis have the onset in the first 10 days of illness. Arthritis developing after 10 days has a predilection for large weight-bearing joints, especially the knees and ankles. It is associated with slightly less intense inflammation as measured by the WBC count of the joint fluid. Gastrointestinal complaints, including abdominal pain, severe diarrhea, and nausea, occur in approximately one third of children during the early stages of the disease. Central nervous system (CNS) involvement, with severe lethargy, semicoma, and aseptic meningitis, occurs in one quarter

of the patients. Obstructive jaundice and acute gallbladder hydrops are seen in approximately 5% of patients. Vomiting, diarrhea, and other gastrointestinal symptoms have been described in patients with Kawasaki syndrome. Pancreatitis has also been reported (Lanting et al., 1992).

The most important associated feature of Kawasaki syndrome is involvement of the heart. Clinical cardiac disease occurs in approximately 20% of patients and most often is manifested as pericardial effusion, transient myocardiopathy with congestive heart failure, and/or arrhythmias. Angiographic and two-dimensional echocardiographic studies performed on a routine basis 4 to 8 weeks after onset demonstrate coronary artery aneurysms in approximately 20% of patients.

Clinical Course

The clinical course of Kawasaki syndrome is triphasic. The acute febrile phase of the disease is marked by rash, conjunctival injection, strawberry tongue, edema and erythema of the hands and feet, lymphadenitis, aseptic meningitis, and hepatic dysfunction. Without aspirin or IVIG treatment, this phase generally lasts 8 to 15 days (mean, 11). After defervescence, the physical findings disappear rapidly, but the child remains irritable and anorectic. Arthritis and cardiac disease may develop in the subacute phase of the illness, which is marked also by desquamation and thrombocytosis. The subacute phase persists until the child's behavior returns to normal, approximately 3 weeks after onset. The subacute and early convalescent periods (3 to 4 weeks from onset) constitute the time of greatest risk of sudden death from acute coronary artery thrombosis.

Laboratory abnormalities with Kawasaki syndrome are quite nonspecific. In the acute phase most patients have leukocytosis with abundant band-form neutrophils. Increased acute phase reactants, with elevated sedimentation rate, C-reactive protein, or alpha$_1$-antitrypsin, are universally found during the acute and subacute stages; they return to normal 8 to 12 weeks after onset. The platelet count shows a gradual rise from normal levels, becoming elevated above 450,000 between days 7 and 10 and peaking between days 15 and 25. Virtually all patients ultimately have elevated platelet counts, which may persist for 3 months after onset.

DIAGNOSIS

Management of Kawasaki syndrome starts with diagnosis. Kawasaki syndrome should be considered

---

BOX 15-2

ASSOCIATED FEATURES (IN ORDER OF FREQUENCY)

Pyuria and urethritis
Arthralgia and arthritis
Aseptic meningitis
Diarrhea
Abdominal pain
Myocardiopathy
Pericardial effusion
Obstructive jaundice
Hydrops of gallbladder
Acute mitral insufficiency
Myocardial infarction

in the differential diagnosis of patients with fever and any of the following: generalized polymorphous erythematous rash, conjunctival injection, characteristic changes in the mouth, characteristic changes in the hands and feet, or unilateral cervical lymph node swelling measuring greater than 1.5 cm. A secure diagnosis of Kawasaki syndrome is made in patients who fulfill five of the six criteria and for whom other illnesses that may mimic Kawasaki syndrome have been excluded. The most commonly encountered diseases to exclude are (1) nonspecific exanthems, presumably viral; (2) measles; (3) streptococcal and staphylococcal infections with scarlatiniform eruptions; (4) infectious mononucleosis; and (5) hypersensitivity reactions. If all clinical features of Kawasaki syndrome are present, it is not necessary to wait until the fifth day from onset before making the diagnosis and beginning therapy (Levy and Koren, 1990).

Some "incomplete" cases of Kawasaki syndrome do not fulfill the diagnostic criteria but are at risk for the development of coronary artery aneurysms. Children under the age of 6 months are particularly likely to develop coronary abnormalities while not expressing complete diagnostic criteria (Burns et al., 1986). Most young infants with Kawasaki syndrome fulfill diagnostic criteria, but many of the manifestations are milder or more subtle than those usually seen in older children. Therefore Kawasaki syndrome should be considered even if the diagnostic criteria are not fulfilled; in some cases patients with incomplete forms should receive care just as patients who fulfill all the clinical criteria.

The laboratory tests provide modest diagnostic support. An elevated C-reactive protein result or elevated sedimentation rate is almost universal in pa-

tients with Kawasaki syndrome and is not commonly found in patients with viral exanthems, hypersensitivity reactions, or measles. Platelet count elevation greater than $450,000/mm^3$ is usually seen in patients presenting after the seventh day of illness, but the platelet count is usually normal for the first week. An analysis of reported cases of atypical Kawasaki syndrome with coronary abnormalities demonstrated that platelet elevation and elevated sedimentation rate were universal in these cases. Our experience in Hawaii and with the 900 patients in the U.S. Multicenter Study Group experience corroborates that finding to the point that a diagnosis of Kawasaki syndrome is extremely unlikely if the platelet count and a full panel of acute phase inflammatory reactants (sedimentation rate, C-reactive protein, alpha$_1$-antitrypsin) are normal after day 7.

TREATMENT
Intravenous Immune Globulin

As soon as the disease can be diagnosed, patients should have a baseline echocardiogram and receive IVIG, 2 gm/kg given in a 10- to 12-hour infusion (Fig. 15-1). This dosage has recently been demonstrated as equally efficacious in reducing the risk of coronary disease as a schedule of 400 mg/kg/day given for 4 consecutive days. The single-dose schedule is superior to the four-dose schedule in rapidity of return of fever and acute phase reactants to normal (Newburger, 1990; Newburger et al., 1991). Single-dose infusion is safe, having been given to 273 children in a controlled trial with no significant adverse effects. Pulse, heart rate, and blood pressure should be monitored at the beginning of infusion, at 30 minutes, at 1 hour, and then at 2 hours during infusion. Although this dose does provide a substantial fluid and protein load, it does

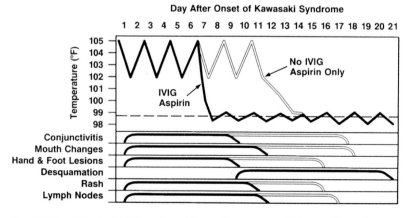

FIG. 15-1 Effect of IVIG and aspirin on the course of Kawasaki syndrome.

not increase the risk of congestive heart failure, even in patients with decreased myocardial function. A recent report suggests that different formulations of IVIG may differ markedly in their efficacy (Silverman et al., 1995), although this was not confirmed with respect to worsening coronary artery disease (Burns et al., 1995).

No large clinical experience is available demonstrating efficacy of lower-dose single-infusion therapy. Multiple studies in Japan have also demonstrated efficacy for multiple-dose regimens of more than 1 gm/kg. Total doses at or below 1 gm/kg have been ineffective in reducing the incidence of coronary abnormalities.

Limited data are available to guide therapy of patients encountered later than 10 days from onset. If patients are still febrile or have other signs of active disease, including progressive coronary dilation, IVIG therapy should be instituted, because it may result in prompt clinical improvement (Marasini et al., 1991). Patients who have become afebrile and have normal coronary arteries by day 21 of illness are unlikely to benefit from receiving IVIG but should receive aspirin 3 to 5 mg/kg once daily. Currently, no evidence suggests any beneficial effect of IVIG in patients who have already developed coronary aneurysms once active inflammation has subsided.

Aspirin

On the same day that IVIG is administered, the patient should start to receive aspirin. The dose of aspirin best studied in the United States is 100 mg/kg/day until the fever is controlled or until day 14 of illness, followed by a dose of 5 to 10 mg/kg/day (40 to 80 mg by mouth once daily) until the sedimentation rate and platelet count are normal, approximately 3 months from onset of illness. The appropriate dose of aspirin in Kawasaki syndrome has been controversial. Theoretically, high-dose aspirin (>80 mg/kg/day) adjusted to produce a serum total salicylate level of 18 to 28 mg/dl might decrease the intensity of the vasculitis, whereas much lower doses (3 to 10 mg/kg/day) would provide optimal inhibition of platelet aggregation. Both regimens have supporters in North America. Japanese clinicians generally have received an intermediate antipyretic dose of 30 to 50 mg/kg/day. To date there is no conclusive evidence favoring any of these dosages.

Difficulty in obtaining therapeutic antiinflammatory serum salicylate levels during the acute phase of illness has been reported. Koren et al. (1985) found this difficulty related to both impaired bioavailability and enhanced clearance of salicylate. Because IVIG appears to have potent antiinflammatory effects, a lower dose of aspirin throughout the illness may be more appropriate. A study to answer this important question is currently under way. Salicylate levels should be obtained if symptoms of vomiting, hyperpnea, lethargy, or liver function abnormalities develop while the patient is receiving high-dose aspirin. To decrease the risk of Reye's syndrome, aspirin administration can be interrupted for a few days if patients develop varicella or influenza during the follow-up phase.

Monitoring

All patients with Kawasaki syndrome should be admitted to the hospital for administration of IVIG and for observation until the fever is controlled. Cardiovascular function should be monitored carefully. Once a child's fever has subsided, it is unlikely that significant congestive heart failure or myocardial dysfunction will occur. The patient should be evaluated within a week after discharge and should have an echocardiogram between 21 and 28 days after onset of fever. If baseline and 3- to 4-week echocardiograms reveal normal results with no evidence of coronary abnormality, further echocardiograms are unnecessary. The peak period to demonstrate coronary abnormalities detectable by echocardiogram is 3 to 4 weeks after onset. In a recent study of more than 800 patients, we found no new abnormalities at 8 weeks if the 3- to 4-week echocardiogram was normal. Patients with no evidence of coronary abnormalities should receive 80 mg of aspirin per day for approximately 3 months, the period required for both the platelet count and the sedimentation rate to return to normal.

Myocardial Infarction

Myocardial infarction occurs most commonly in patients with giant coronary aneurysms, 8 mm or greater, in the first year after onset of Kawasaki syndrome. Patients with a history of giant aneurysms are also at higher risk for later coronary thrombosis than those with smaller lesions. Parents of all children with coronary abnormalities should be instructed to contact a physician and alert the emergency medical system if chest pain, dyspnea, extreme lethargy, or syncope develop. Prompt fibrinolytic therapy with streptokinase, urokinase, or tissue plasminogen activator should be attempted at a tertiary care center if acute coronary thrombosis is diagnosed.

Noncardiac Complications

Kawasaki syndrome is a multisystem disease, but, except for cardiac complications, other systemic involvement is generally self-limited. In most patients with arthritis, joint inflammation occurs in the acute stage and is intense and painful but self-limited, usually lasting less than 2 weeks. Although we have treated patients with both high-dose aspirin (100 mg/kg/day) and other nonsteroidal anti-inflammatory drugs, particularly tolmetin sodium (20 mg/kg/day in three divided doses), we have not been impressed with prompt temporal response to antiinflammatory therapy. Many patients with effusions appear to benefit most from arthrocentesis, which usually must be done only once. Abdominal pain–diarrhea complex, also a feature of the early acute stage, usually responds to intravenous hydration and supportive care. Gallbladder hydrops, presenting clinically as a right upper-quadrant mass, sometimes in association with obstructive jaundice, can be confirmed by diagnostic ultrasonography and can be monitored until resolution occurs. Surgical removal of the dilated gallbladder is not necessary, because this complication is self-limited. A rare complication seen in the acute febrile stage is peripheral vasoconstriction threatening distal extremities. It is usually seen only in patients with severe systemic illness and widespread vascular involvement. This complication has been managed either with prostaglandin E_1 infusion (0.007 to 0.03 mg/kg/minute), maintained over several days in an intensive care unit with constant hemodynamic monitoring (Westphalen et al., 1988), or with systemic heparin therapy and corticosteroid pulse therapy (methylprednisolone, 25 mg/kg intravenous push). There are anecdotal reports of success with both approaches but no controlled experience. Telephone consultation with a center treating large numbers of Kawasaki syndrome patients should be sought by the physician faced with rare or serious complications.

LONG-TERM MANAGEMENT

Patients with No History of Coronary Artery Abnormalities. There is no need for administration of aspirin or other antiplatelet medications beyond 3 months or for restriction of physical activities. Cardiac evaluation and electrocardiograms obtained every 2 to 3 years may be warranted.

Patients with Transient or Small Coronary Aneurysms. These patients should receive long-term antiplatelet therapy with aspirin (3 to 5 mg/kg/day) at least until resolution of abnormalities, preferably indefinitely. Restricting physical activities is not necessary unless there are cardiac stress test abnormalities. Patients should be followed with yearly cardiac evaluations and have periodic stress testing when they are over the age of 5 years. Echocardiograms should be performed yearly or more often until stable regression has been demonstrated. Angiography is indicated if electrocardiographic or stress test abnormalities develop.

Patients with Giant Aneurysms, 8 mm or Greater. Indefinite therapy with aspirin (3 to 5 mg/kg once daily, with or without dipyridamole, 3 to 4 mg/kg/day in three doses) is advised. Anticoagulant therapy with warfarin (Coumadin) and/or subcutaneous heparin may be added, especially during the first 2 years after onset. Cardiac evaluation should be performed every 6 months along with periodic stress testing, and yearly or more frequent echocardiograms should be performed to monitor aneurysm size. Angiography should be performed to define the extent of disease at least once and whenever symptoms or stress tests indicate myocardial ischemia. Physical activity is regulated on the basis of stress test results and the level of anticoagulation. Patients with obstructive lesions or signs of ischemia may need evaluation for possible surgical intervention. These patients require consultation with a pediatric cardiologist with extensive experience managing Kawasaki syndrome patients. Some Japanese children with severe coronary artery aneurysms have had successful outcomes after bypass surgery or even cardiac transplantation (Kitamura et al., 1994).

PROGNOSIS

Kawasaki syndrome is primarily an acute and self-limited disease; however, cardiac damage sustained when the disease is active may be permanent and progressive. This damage may manifest soon after onset or may not become apparent until years later. From multiple studies it is clear that approximately 20% of all patients untreated with IVIG develop coronary artery aneurysms that are detectable by angiography or two-dimensional echocardiography. These abnormalities may appear as early as 7 days and as late as 4 weeks after onset of the syndrome. The risk of coronary aneurysms is lowered to 4% by 8 weeks overall if IVIG is given in the first 10 days of illness. For infants less than 1 year of age, even with IVIG treatment, the risk of coronary abnormalities at 8 weeks is 12% (Newburger et al., 1991). Patients with coronary artery abnormalities are at risk for myocardial infarction, sudden death, and myocardial ischemia for a period of at least 5 years after onset of illness (Kato et al., 1986). Regression of aneurysms is known to occur. Approximately two thirds of patients with coronary aneurysms at 8 weeks after onset have regression within 1 year to apparently normal vessels by angiography or echocardiography. Approximately one third continue to have coronary dilation. Among patients whose aneurysms regress, stenosis, tortuosity, and thrombosis of coronary vessels may occur (Kato et al., 1988). Patients with giant aneurysms (coronary lumen >8 mm in diameter) are at risk for the development of significant stenosis with resultant myocardial ischemia (Tatara and Kusakawa, 1987). The risk of giant aneurysm, originally found in 3% to 7% of all patients, has also been dramatically lowered by the use of IVIG (Rowley et al., 1988). Chung and the United States Multicenter Kawasaki Study Group (1989) administered IVIG to more than 800 patients. Six of these patients developed giant aneurysms; three had coronary dilation at the time IVIG was begun.

A mortality rate of approximately 2% was reported in the mid-1970s. In Japan the mortality rate is approximately 0.1% in 1989 (Kawasaki, 1989). This improvement in mortality came during a decade in which there was (1) widespread use of aspirin; (2) awareness of the possibility of cardiac disease, with more intensive follow-up and supportive care; and (3) increased recognition of Kawasaki syndrome, possibly leading to the inclusion of milder cases in the total. The true long-term prognosis for patients with Kawasaki syndrome is not well understood, because long-term follow-up studies into the second and third decade after disease have not been performed. Inoue et al. (1989) have surveyed cardiologists in Japan and found adults with newly detected coronary aneurysms discovered by angiography performed to evaluate myocardial infarction or ischemia. One quarter of these patients had a history of Kawasaki syndrome or compatible childhood illness 19 to 60 years before discovery of coronary aneurysms.

Other complications of Kawasaki syndrome such as arthritis and hepatic disease apparently are entirely self-limited, last for less than 3 months, and are not associated with chronic or progressive disability or recurrent attacks.

Recurrence of Kawasaki syndrome is uncommon, with approximately 3% of patients suffering one or more episodes. Recurrences may occur as long as 8 years after the first attack.

PREVENTION

Without knowledge about its cause, no effective preventive strategies for Kawasaki syndrome have been determined.

ISOLATION AND QUARANTINE

To date there has been no evidence of point-source exposure or direct person-to-person spread. Therefore isolation and quarantine are not indicated.

BIBLIOGRAPHY

Burns JC, Geha RS, Schneeberger EE, et al. Polymerase activity in lymphocyte culture supernatants from patients with Kawasaki disease. Nature 1987;323:814-816.

Burns JC, Glode MP, Capparelli E, et al. Intravenous gamma globulin (IVIG) in the treatment of Kawasaki syndrome (KS): are all brands equal? Abstract presented at 5th International Kawasaki Disease Symposium, May 22-25, 1995, Fukuoka, Japan.

Burns JC, Wiggins JW, Toews WH, Glode M. Clinical spectrum of Kawasaki syndrome in infants younger than 6 months of age. J Pediatr 1986;109:759-763.

Burns JC, Wilbert MH, Mary GP, et al. Clinical and epidemiologic characteristics of patients referred for evaluation of possible Kawasaki disease. J Pediatr 1991;118:680-686.

Chung KJ, U.S. Multicenter Kawasaki Study Group. Incidence and prognosis of giant coronary artery aneurysms in Kawasaki disease (Abstract 1123). Circulation 1989;80: II-282.

Davies HD, Kirk V, Jadavji T, Kotzin BL. Simultaneous presentation of Kawasaki disease and toxic shock syndrome in an adolescent male. Pediatr Infect Dis J 1996;15:1136-1138.

Eluthesen K, Marchette N, Melish ME. Immunoglobulins, complimental circulating immune complexes in Kawasaki syndrome. Presented at the 21st Interscience Conference on Antimicrobial Agents and Chemotherapeutics, November 1985.

Fujiwara H, Hamashima Y. Pathology of the heart in Kawasaki disease. J Pediatr 1978;61:100-107.

Furusho K, Kamiya T, Nakano H, et al. High-dose intravenous gamma globulin for Kawasaki disease. Lancet 1984;2:1055-1058.

Hamasaki Y, Ichimaru T, Koga H, et al. Increased in-vitro leukotriene B4 production by stimulated polymorphonuclear cells in Kawasaki disease. Acta Pediatr Jpn Overseas Ed 1989;31:346-348.

Inoue O, Akagi T, Kato H. Fate of giant coronary artery aneurysms in Kawasaki disease: long term follow-up study (Abstract 1046). Circulation 1989;80:II-262.

Kato H, Ichinose E, Kawasaki T. Myocardial infarction in Kawasaki disease. J Pediatr 1986;108:923-928.

Kato H, Inoue O, Akagi T. Kawasaki disease: cardiac problems and management. Pediatr Rev 1988;9:209-217.

Kawasaki T. Acute febrile mucocutaneous syndrome with lymphoid involvement with specific desquamation of the fingers and toes in children [Japanese]. Jpn J Allerg 1967;16: 178-222.

Kawasaki T. Kawasaki disease. Asian Med J 1989; 32:497-506.

Kawasaki T, Kosaki F, Okawa S, et al. A new infantile acute febrile mucocutaneous lymph node syndrome (MLNS) prevailing in Japan. Pediatrics 1974;54:271-276.

Kitamura S, Kameda Y, Seki T, et al. Long-term outcome of myocardial revascularization in patients with Kawasaki coronary artery disease—a multicenter cooperative study. J Thorac Cardiovasc Surg 1994;107:663.

Klein BS, Rogers MF, Patrican LA, et al. Kawasaki syndrome: a controlled study of an outbreak in Wisconsin. Am J Epidemiol 1986;124:306-316.

Koren G, Rose V, Levi S. Probable efficacy of high dose salicylates in reducing coronary involvement in Kawasaki disease. JAMA 1985;254:767.

Landing BH, Larson EJ. Are infantile periarteritis nodosa with coronary artery involvement and fatal mucocutaneous lymph node syndrome the same? Comparison of 20 patients from North America with patients from Hawaii and Japan. J Pediatr 1977;59:651-662.

Lang BA, Silverman ED, Laxer RM, et al. Serum soluble interleukin-2 receptor levels in Kawasaki disease. J Pediatr 1990;116:592-596.

Lanting WA, Muinos WI, Kamani NR. Pancreatitis heralding Kawasaki disease. J Pediatr 1992;121:743.

Leung DYM. Immunomodulation by intravenous immune globulin in Kawasaki disease. J Allergy Clin Immunol 1989;84:588-894.

Leung DYM, Chu ET, Wood N, et al. Immunoregulatory T cell abnormalities in mucocutaneous lymph node syndrome. J Immunol 1983;130:2002-2004.

Leung DYM, Collins T, LaPierre LA, et al. IgM antibodies present in the acute phase of Kawasaki syndrome lyse cultured vascular endothelial cells stimulated by gamma interferon. J Clin Invest 1986;77:1428-1435.

Leung DYM, Kurt-Jones E, Newberger JW, et al. Endothelial cell activation and high interleukin-1 secretion in the pathogenesis of acute Kawasaki disease. Lancet 1989;2:1298-1302.

Levin M, Holland PC, Nokes TJC, et al. Platelet immune complex interaction in pathogenesis of Kawasaki disease and childhood polyarteritis. Br Med J 1985;290:1456-1460.

Levy M, Koren G. Atypical Kawasaki disease: analysis of clinical presentation and diagnostic clues. Pediatr Infect Dis 1990;9:122-126.

Marasini M, Pongiglione G, Gazzolo D, et al. Late intravenous gamma globulin treatment in infants and children with Kawasaki disease and coronary artery abnormalities. Am J Cardiol 1991;68:796.

Marchette NJ, Melish ME, Hicks R, et al. Epstein-Barr virus and other herpes virus infections in Kawasaki syndrome. J Infect Dis 1990;161:680-684.

Mason WH, Jordan SC, Sakai R, et al. Circulating immune complexes in Kawasaki syndrome. Pediatr Infect Dis 1985;4:48-51.

Maury CPJ, Sal E, Pelkemen P. Elevated circulating tumor necrosis factor in patients with Kawasaki disease. J Lab Clin Med 1989;113:651.

Melish ME, Marchette NJ, Kaplan JC, et al. Absence of significant RNA-dependent DNA polymerase activity in lymphocytes from patients with Kawasaki syndrome. Nature 1989;337:288-290.

Melish ME, Parsonnett J, Nyven M. Kawasaki syndrome is not caused by toxic shock syndrome toxin-1 (TSST-1) and staphylococci. Presented at the Society for Pediatric Research, May 1994, Seattle, Washington.

Newberger JW, Takahashi M, Beiser AS, et al. A single infusion of intravenous gamma globulin compared to four daily doses in the treatment of acute Kawasaki syndrome. N Engl J Med 1991;324:1633-1637.

Newburger JW, Takahashi M, Burns JC, et al. The treatment of Kawasaki syndrome with intravenous gamma globulin. N Engl J Med 1986;315:341-347.

Newberger JW, United States Multicenter Kawasaki Study Group. Preliminary results of multicenter trial on IVIG treatment of Kawasaki disease with single infusion vs four-infusion regimen (abstract). Pediatr Res 1990;27:22A.

Ogle JW, Waner JL, Joffe LS, et al. Absence of interferon in sera of patients with Kawasaki syndrome. Pediatr Infect Dis J 1991;10:25.

Ono S, Onimaru T, Kawakami K, et al. Impaired granulocyte chemotaxis and increased circulating immune complexes in Kawasaki disease. J Pediatr 1985;106:567-570.

Patriarca PA, Rogers MF, Morens DM, et al. Kawasaki syndrome: association with the application of rug shampoo. Lancet 1982;2:578-580.

Rauch AM. Kawasaki syndrome: critical review of U.S. epidemiology. Progr Clin Biol Res 1987;250:33-44.

Rogers MF. Kawasaki syndrome. Am J Dis Child 1986;140:191.

Rowley DH, Duffy E, Shulman ST. Prevention of giant aneurysms in Kawasaki disease by intravenous gamma globulin therapy. J Pediatr 1988;113:290-294.

Shulman ST, Rowley AH. Does Kawasaki disease have a retroviral aetiology? Lancet 1986;2:545-546.

Silverman ED, Huang C, Rose V, et al. IVGG treatment of Kawasaki disease: are all brands equal? Abstract presented at 5th International Kawasaki Disease Symposium, May 22-25, 1995, Fukuoka, Japan.

Tatara K, Kusakawa S. Long-term prognosis of giant coronary aneurysms in Kawasaki disease: an angiographic study. J Pediatr 1987;111:705-710.

Terai M, Kohno Y, Koichiro N, Nakajima H. Class II antigen expression in the coronary artery endothelium in Kawasaki disease. Hum Pathol 1990;21:231-234.

Westphalen MA, McGrath MA, Kelly W, et al. Kawasaki disease with severe peripheral ischemia: treatment with prostaglandin E_1 infusion. J Pediatr 1988;112:431-433.

Yanagawa H, Yashiro M, Nakamura Y, et al. Nationwide surveillance of Kawasaki disease in Japan, 1984 to 1993. Pediatr Infect Dis J 1995;14:69.

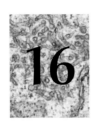

16 MEASLES (RUBEOLA)

Measles is an acute, highly contagious viral disease characterized by fever, coryza, conjunctivitis, cough, and a specific enanthem (Koplik's spots) followed by a generalized maculopapular eruption, which usually appears on the fourth day of the disease. The rash and accompanying illness reach a climax on approximately the sixth day, followed by subsidence in a few days and, in most cases, complete recovery. Serious complications involving the gastrointestinal and respiratory tracts and central nervous system occur in 5% to 15% of patients in highly developed countries. In other parts of the world, however, the high mortality and morbidity associated with measles present serious problems. The widespread use of live attenuated measles virus vaccine has been followed by a sharp decline in the incidence of the disease in the United States, as well as other nations, where immunization has been established as a cornerstone of child health practices.

ETIOLOGY

Although measles had been demonstrated to be a transmissible infection of viral etiology early in the twentieth century, it was not until 1954 that Enders and Peebles reported the successful isolation of measles virus in human and rhesus monkey kidney tissue cultures. The characteristic cytopathic changes in tissue culture included (1) formation of multinucleated giant cells, (2) vacuolization in the syncytial cytoplasm, and (3) presence of eosinophilic intranuclear and intracytoplasmic inclusion bodies. Measles virus has been adapted to a number of tissue cultures, including human amnion, human embryonic lung, a variety of cell lines, and chick embryo cells. The cytopathic effects in tissue culture have provided a basis for virus isolation procedures, for assay of infectivity, and for determination of neutralizing antibody. The property of hemagglutination of simian erythrocytes by in-fected tissue culture fluids has been utilized as the basis for a convenient serologic test.

Measles is the sole human member of the genus *Morbillivirus,* family Paramyxoviridae. Other viruses of that genus are the agents of canine distemper; rinderpest of cattle; peste des petits ruminants and morbilliviruses of dolphins, seals, and porpoises. Recently a fatal respiratory illness of horses in Australia resulting from an apparent new member of the genus, equine morbillivirus (EMV), has been reported by Murray et al. (1995). Of special note was its spread to human contacts, with one death resulting from respiratory involvement and another from a progressive encephalitis (O'-Sullivan et al., 1997). If proven correct, this would be the first example of the spread of a morbillivirus from one to another mammalian order. The natural host of EMV may be the Australian fruit bat (Young et al., 1996).

Measles virions are spherical, pleomorphic, lipid-enveloped particles, ranging from 100 to 250 nm in diameter, with a helical nucleocapsid. They are morphologically identical to the other paramyxoviruses. Two transmembrane glycoproteins, H (hemagglutinin) and F (fusion), project from the surface of the virus envelope, a lipid bilayer derived from the plasma membrane of infected cells. The M (matrix) protein is in the inner surface of the membrane. The helical nucleocapsid within the envelope contains the nucleoprotein (N) bound to the genomic RNA, along with the phosphoprotein (P) and the large polymerase protein (L). The genome is linear, single stranded, of negative polarity, and nonsegmented and contains approximately 15,900 nucleotides. The genome has been fully sequenced, and there is a surprising degree of stability and homogeneity among various strains and isolates, with some changes in the N and H genes (Bellini et al., 1994; Rota et al., 1992, 1994). These observations coincide with the apparent clinical and immunologic stability of measles over the centuries of observation and decades of laboratory investigations. Naniche et al. (1993) identified a member of the regulators of complement activation, CD46, as the cell receptor for measles virus permitting binding of virus to the host cell. It is a 57-67 kDa protein expressed on nearly all human cell types except erythrocytes. A monoclonal antibody to CD46 inhibits measles virus binding, syncytium formation, and subsequent viral replication.

Measles virus is very sensitive to heat and cold and is rapidly inactivated at 37° C and at 20° C. It is also inactivated by ultraviolet light, ether, trypsin, and β-propiolactone. Formalin destroys infectivity, but it does not alter complement-fixing activity. The virus in the presence of protein is well preserved at low temperature, surviving storage at −15° to −70° C for 5 years and at 4° C for 5 months. In the lyophilized state with a protein stabilizer it is preserved at 4° C for 18 months.

PATHOLOGY

Because measles is a generalized infection, the pathologic lesions are widespread. During the prodromal period there is hyperplasia of the lymphoid tissue in the tonsils, adenoids, lymph nodes, spleen, and appendix. Large (100 μm) multinucleated giant cells can be demonstrated in these tissues and in the pharyngeal and bronchial mucosa.

Suringa et al. (1970) found that Koplik's spots and the skin lesions of measles share the following histologic features: foci of syncytial epithelial giant cells with pale-staining cytoplasm, intercellular and intracellular edema, and parakeratosis and dyskeratosis. Many of the giant cell nuclei contain pink-staining inclusion bodies. Electron microscopy reveals aggregates of "viral" microtubules within the nuclei and cytoplasm of syncytial giant cells. These tubules are indistinguishable from those seen in tissue cultures infected with measles virus.

The lungs show evidence of a peribronchiolar inflammatory reaction with a mononuclear cell infiltrate in the interstitial tissues. The large giant cells are occasionally identified there.

The brain and spinal cord in measles encephalomyelitis show gross evidence of edema, congestion, and scattered petechial hemorrhages. Microscopically, the early stage is characterized by perivascular hemorrhages and lymphocytic cell infiltration. Later there is evidence of demyelination throughout the central nervous system (CNS). His-

tologically, these lesions are very similar to those encountered in postvaccinal encephalitis.

CLINICAL MANIFESTATIONS

The clinical course of a typical case of measles is illustrated in Fig. 16-1. After an incubation period of 10 to 11 days the illness is ushered in by fever and malaise. Within 24 hours there is onset of coryza, conjunctivitis, and cough. These symptoms gradually increase in severity, reaching a peak with the appearance of the eruption on the fourth day. Approximately 2 days before the development of the rash, Koplik's spots appear on the buccal mucous membranes opposite the molars. Over a 3-day period these lesions increase in number and spread to involve the entire mucous membrane. The fever subsides and Koplik's spots disappear by the end of the second day of the rash. The coryza and conjunctivitis clear considerably by the third day of the rash. The duration of the exanthem rarely exceeds 5 to 6 days.

Fever

The temperature curve illustrated in Fig. 16-1 is the one most commonly observed. There is a stepwise increase until the fifth or sixth day of illness at the height of the eruption. Occasionally, however, the temperature curve may be biphasic; an initial elevation for the first 24 to 48 hours is followed by a normal period for 1 day and then by a rapid rise to 39.4° to 40.6° C (103° to 105° F) when the rash is in full bloom. At times the temperature may reach its peak by the end of the first day and remain ele-

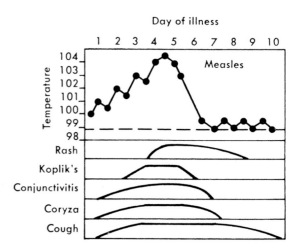

Fig. 16-1 Schematic diagram of clinical course of typical case of measles. The rash appears 3 to 4 days after onset of fever, conjunctivitis, coryza, and cough. Koplik's spots usually develop 2 days before the rash.

vated at levels of 39.4° to 40.6° C (103° to 105° F) for the remaining prodromal and early rash period. In uncomplicated measles the temperature falls by crisis or rapid lysis between the second and third days after the onset of the exanthem.

Coryza

The coryza of measles is indistinguishable from that of a severe common cold. The early sneezing is followed by nasal congestion and a mucopurulent discharge that becomes most profuse at the height of the eruption. It clears very rapidly after the patient becomes afebrile.

Conjunctivitis and Keratitis

A transverse marginal line of conjunctival injection across the lower lids may be observed in the early prodromal period. Subsequently, it is obscured by an extensive conjunctival inflammation associated with edema of the lids and the caruncles. There is evidence of increased lacrimation, and occasionally the patient complains of photophobia. In severe cases, Koplik's spots may be observed on the caruncle. The conjunctivitis, like the coryza, disappears shortly after the fever has subsided. Among children with malnutrition accompanied by vitamin A deficiency, a more severe conjunctivitis with accompanying keratitis and corneal ulcerations may leave damage sufficient to impair vision permanently.

Cough

The cough is caused by the inflammatory reaction of the respiratory tract. Like the other catarrhal manifestations, it increases in frequency and intensity, reaching its climax at the height of the eruption. However, it persists much longer, gradually subsiding over the next several weeks.

Koplik's Spots

Approximately 2 days before the rash appears, the pathognomonic Koplik's spots may be detected. These lesions were described by Koplik (1896) as

small irregular spots of bright red color[;] in the center of each red spot is seen a minute bluish-white speck. There may at first be only two or three or six such rose-red spots, with a bluish-white speck in the center. The combination of a bluish-white speck with a rose-red background on the buccal and labial mucous membrane is absolutely pathognomonic of the invasion of measles. Sometimes the bluish-white speck is so small and delicately colored that only in a very direct and strong day-

light is it possible to bring out the above effect, but the combination is always present.

Koplik's spots increase to uncountable numbers so that by the end of the first day of rash they usually involve the entire buccal and labial mucosa. The rose-red areas coalesce to form a diffuse erythematous background that is peppered with many pinpoint blue-white elevations. At this stage, Koplik's spots resemble grains of salt sprinkled on a red background (Plate 4). By the end of the second day of the rash the spots already begin to slough, and by the third day of rash the mucous membranes look perfectly normal.

Rash

As indicated in Fig. 16-1, the rash of unmodified measles first makes its appearance 3 to 4 days after the onset of catarrhal symptoms. Occasionally the prodromal period may be as short as 1 day or as long as 7 days.

The exanthem begins as an erythematous maculopapular eruption (Fig. 16-2). It appears first at the hairline and involves the forehead, the area behind the earlobes, and the upper part of the neck. It then spreads downward to involve the face, neck, upper

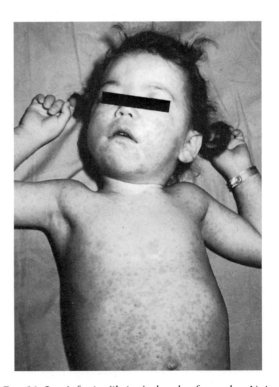

FIG. 16-2   Infant with typical rash of measles. Note confluent maculopapular lesions on face.

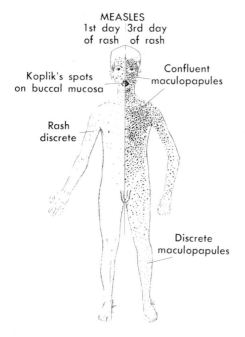

MEASLES
1st day   3rd day
of rash   of rash

Koplik's spots
on buccal mucosa

Confluent
maculopapules

Rash
discrete

Discrete
maculopapules

FIG. 16-3 Development and distribution of measles rash.

extremities, and trunk. It continues downward until it reaches the feet by the third day. The earlier sites contain many more lesions than those that are affected later. Consequently, the lesions high up on the face and neck tend to become confluent, whereas those more peripheral on the extremities tend to remain discrete (Fig. 16-3).

The rash begins to fade by the third day in order of appearance. Therefore, although the face and upper trunk may be clear by the fourth day, an eruption may still be apparent on the lower extremities. The early erythematous lesions blanch on pressure. After 3 or 4 days they assume a brownish appearance. This staining of the skin, which is probably the result of capillary hemorrhages, does not fade on pressure. With the disappearance of the rash, a fine branny desquamation may be noted over the sites of most extensive involvement. In contrast to the extensive peeling seen in scarlet fever, the skin of the hands and feet does not desquamate. Morley (1962) observed extensive desquamation after severe measles in West African children who were protein deficient.

Other Manifestations

Anorexia and malaise are usually present during the febrile period. Gastroenteritis with both vomiting and diarrhea is commonly present and in malnourished children may be especially severe, often

accompanied by painful stomatitis (Makhene and Diaz, 1993). Generalized lymphadenopathy is noted in moderate to severe cases. Like rubella, measles may be associated with enlarged postauricular, cervical, and occipital lymph nodes. Occasionally a transient prodromal rash may be observed. This eruption may be scarlatiniform or morbilliform and usually disappears within 24 hours. Laryngotracheitis, sometimes of severity sufficient to require intubation in patients under 2 years of age (Fortenberry et al., 1992), bronchitis, bronchiolitis, and pneumonitis caused by the primary viral infection are present in various degrees in most patients.

Convalescence

The illness reaches its climax between the second and third days of the rash. At this time, the temperature is at its peak, Koplik's spots have covered the entire buccal mucous membrane and are beginning to slough, the eyes are puffy and red, the coryza is profuse, and the cough is most distressing. The child looks "measly" and feels miserable. Within the next 24 to 36 hours the temperature falls by crisis or rapid lysis, the coryza and conjunctivitis clear, and the cough decreases in severity. Within a few days the child feels normal. Fever persisting beyond the third day of rash is usually caused by a complication. The convalescent period of measles is of short duration, although cough often persists for longer periods.

ATYPICAL MEASLES IN CHILDREN PREVIOUSLY IMMUNIZED WITH INACTIVATED MEASLES VIRUS VACCINE

A severe, atypical type of measles was first reported by Rauh and Schmidt in 1965, by Nader et al. in 1968, and by Fulginiti et al. in 1967 in children who had received inactivated measles virus vaccine 2 to 4 years previously. The following clinical manifestations have been observed: fever, pneumonitis, pneumonia with pulmonary consolidation and pleural effusion, and an unusual rash. The eruption has been urticarial, maculopapular, petechial, purpuric, and occasionally vesicular with a predilection for the extremities. Edema of the hands and feet, myalgia, and severe hyperesthesia of the skin also have been observed. The appearance and distribution of the exanthem resemble Rocky Mountain spotted fever.

Patients with atypical measles may have extraordinarily high measles hemagglutination-inhibition (HI) antibody titers (1:25,000 to 1:200,000). These levels are sixfold or more higher than those observed following typical measles infection.

It has been estimated that 600,000 to 900,000 children were immunized with inactivated measles vaccine between the time of licensure in 1963 and 1967, when it was removed from the market. Consequently, this disease now is seen exclusively in adults (Cherry et al., 1990). It was appropriate for Martin et al. (1979) and Hall and Hall (1979) to describe this problem in detail in the adult medical literature.

The pathogenesis of the atypical measles syndrome is based on the failure of formalin-inactivated measles vaccine to induce antibody to the F protein. Immunity to the F protein is necessary to prevent cell-to-cell spread of infection. In addition, hypersensitivity develops to other viral antigens to which immunity had been stimulated previously by the inactivated measles vaccine. Studies of six patients with atypical measles syndrome by Annunziato et al. (1982) revealed that five of six acute-phase sera lacked antibody to F antigen but contained antibody to H antigen.

SEVERE HEMORRHAGIC MEASLES

Severe hemorrhagic measles (black measles) was not uncommon several decades ago. Recently, however, cases of this type have become rare. The illness may begin with a sudden onset of hyperpyrexia (40.6° to 41.1° C; 105° to 106° F), convulsions, delirium, or stupor that may progress to coma. This is followed by marked respiratory distress and an extensive confluent hemorrhagic eruption of the skin and mucous membranes. Bleeding from the mouth, nose, and bowel may be severe and uncontrollable. This type of measles is often fatal, probably because it involves disseminated intravascular coagulation (DIC).

Severe hemorrhagic measles should not be confused with the purpuric type of eruption that may occur in fair-skinned children with severe ordinary measles. This type of hemorrhagic eruption is not associated with excessive toxicity, and the illness pursues a more favorable course.

MODIFIED MEASLES

Modified measles most commonly develops in children who have been passively immunized with immune globulin (IG) after exposure to the disease. Occasionally it may also occur in infants whose transplacental passive immunity has only partially waned. The incubation period may be prolonged to 14 or even to 20 days. The illness is an abbreviated, milder version of ordinary measles.

The usual prodromal period of 3 to 4 days may be decreased to 1 or 2 days, or it may even be absent. The fever is generally low grade, but the temperature may be normal. The coryza, conjunctivitis, and cough are usually minimal and may even be absent. Koplik's spots may not be present; if they do appear, they are few in number and disappear within a day or less. The rash is generally sparse and discrete and in some cases is so mild that it may be missed.

Modification of measles converts a severe 6- to 9-day illness to one that is very mild and of much shorter duration. In contrast to the unmodified disease, modified measles are rarely followed by complications. Nevertheless, the patient with modified illness is a potential source of infection to susceptible contacts.

DIAGNOSIS
Confirmatory Clinical Factors

The development of a generalized maculopapular eruption preceded by a 3- to 4-day period of fever, cough, coryza, and conjunctivitis associated with the pathognomonic Koplik's spots points to a clear-cut diagnosis of measles. During the prevaccine era, confirmatory laboratory procedures were usually unnecessary.

Identification of Causative Agent

Measles virus may be isolated from the blood, urine, or nasopharyngeal secretions during the febrile period of the illness. However, these are costly, time-consuming, and technically demanding cell culture procedures that are infrequently available or utilized for purposes other than investigation. A sensitive and specific RT-nested PCR (polymerase chain reaction with reverse transcription) has been employed successfully by Matsuzono et al. (1994).

Serologic Tests

A significant titer of antibodies may be detected in serum collected 2 weeks after the onset of illness. Antibodies usually appear within 1 to 3 days after onset of rash. Peak titers are reached 2 to 4 weeks later. Measles neutralizing and HI antibodies may be detected for many years. The pattern of development and persistence of measles HI antibody is illustrated in Fig. 16-4. A fourfold or greater increase in antibody titer during convalescence is strongly indicative of measles infection. The enzyme immunoassay (EIA), because of its increased sensitivity and rapidity and its relative

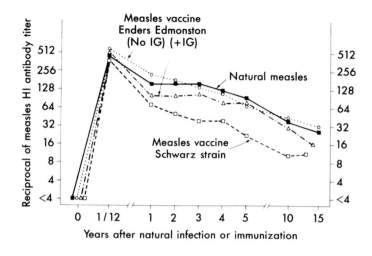

Fig. 16-4   Measles hemagglutination-inhibition (HI) antibody response and persistence. Fifteen-year follow-up. (From Krugman S: J Pediatr 1977;90:1.)

simplicity, is the test currently used most often to assay measles-specific antibodies. A single determination of IgM antibody to measles in an acute-phase serum specimen confirms the diagnosis. Helfand et al. (1996) have demonstrated the reliability of an antibody-capture IgM EIA for detection of measles-specific IgM in oral fluids obtained from a cotton-fiber pad rubbed between the cheek and gum of infants. Their results correlated well (91% with positives, 95% with negatives) when compared to serum specimens of the same infants. The most sensitive assay for measles is a plaque reduction neutralization test (PRN), which has detected antiviral activity at levels below those obtained by ELISA, HI, or CF. It has been used in evaluating persistence of transplacental antibodies in infants and duration of immunity in vaccine recipients who have become seronegative by the usual, more convenient methods of measurement (Albrecht et al., 1977).

Other Laboratory Findings

Uncomplicated measles typically is associated with leukopenia. A characteristic multinucleated giant cell has been identified in sputum and nasal secretions of patients during the prodromal period and in urinary sediment throughout the course of the disease (Scheifele and Forbes, 1972; Tompkins and Macaulay, 1985).

DIFFERENTIAL DIAGNOSIS

Differential diagnosis of measles is discussed in Chapter 40.

COMPLICATIONS

The virus of measles is responsible for an inflammatory reaction that extends from the nasopharynx down the respiratory tract to the bronchi. Thus nasopharyngitis with coryza and tracheobronchitis with cough are both manifestations of the natural disease. The more common complications are usually caused by (1) an extension of the inflammation caused by the virus, (2) an invasion of damaged tissues by bacteria, or (3) a combination of both. The sites of involvement of complications of measles include the middle ear, the respiratory tract, the CNS, the eyes, and the skin.

Otitis Media

Infection of the middle ear is one of the most common complications of measles. Early in the course of measles the tympanic membranes should be examined frequently for signs such as redness, bulging, and obliteration of the light reflex and landmarks. Particularly in infants, the first sign of otitis media may be a purulent discharge from the middle ear. Complicating otitis media is usually responsible for persistence of pyrexia beyond the normal course.

The incidence of otitis media as a complication of measles is affected by factors related to the disease, the host, and the environment. Severe measles more likely will be complicated than mild forms. Susceptibility is increased in infants as compared with older children and in patients of any age with a history of previous ear infections. In the 1990 U.S. outbreak nearly 7% of reported cases of measles were complicated by otitis media (Centers for Disease Control, 1991).

Mastoiditis

Mastoiditis formerly was a common sequela of otitis media. Prompt antibacterial therapy has virtually eliminated this complication.

Pneumonia

Pulmonary complications are as frequent as otitis media but more common as a cause of death. The pneumonia may result from (1) an extension of the viral infection, (2) a superimposed bacterial infection, or (3) a combination of both. It is manifested clinically as bronchiolitis (in infants), bronchopneumonia, or lobar pneumonia. The presence of a pneumonic complication should be suspected when any child with measles develops respiratory distress associated with persistence or recrudescence of fever. Examination of the chest may reveal dullness to percussion, suppression of breath sounds, bronchial breathing, and localized or generalized rales. A chest roentgenogram should clarify the diagnosis.

In some adults and especially in immunocompromised individuals of any age lacking normal cellular immune functions, a persisting giant cell pneumonia may occur as a result of chronic replication of measles virus in the lower respiratory tract. This has usually been a fatal complication, sometimes occurring without any rash or dermal manifestations of measles (Enders et al., 1959).

Obstructive Laryngitis and Laryngotracheitis

Transient mild laryngitis and tracheitis are both part of the normal course of measles. Occasionally, however, the inflammatory process progresses and causes obstruction of the airway. The increased hoarseness, barking cough, and inspiratory stridor associated with suprasternal retractions indicate the development of this complication. These symptoms usually subside when the rash begins to fade. The development of increasing restlessness, dyspnea, and tachycardia points to increasing obstruction, which may necessitate intubation and maintenance of airway support until the subsidence of the acute inflammation.

Cervical Adenitis

Mild generalized lymphadenopathy is associated with most cases of measles. In most cases this represents lymphoid hyperplasia caused by the virus itself. Bacterial cervical adenitis may occur as an extension of pharyngitis secondary to upper respiratory flora.

Acute Encephalomyelitis

Acute encephalomyelitis is a serious, potentially crippling, and fatal complication that occurs in approximately 0.1% of measles cases. It begins most commonly between the second and sixth days after onset of the rash. However, it rarely develops during the preeruptive period.

Fever, headache, vomiting, drowsiness, convulsions, coma, or personality changes may usher in this complication. Frequently, there are signs of meningeal irritation such as a stiff neck and Brudzinski's and Kernig's signs. The cerebrospinal fluid (CSF) shows a modest pleocytosis with a predominance of lymphocytes. The protein level is generally elevated; the glucose level is either normal or elevated. In rare instances the CSF may be normal.

The course of encephalomyelitis may be extremely variable. It may be very mild, clearing completely within several days, or it may be a rapidly progressive and fulminating disease, terminating fatally within 24 hours. Between these two extremes are many variations. In general, approximately 60% of patients recover completely; 15% die; and 25% subsequently show manifestations of brain damage such as mental retardation, recurrent seizures, severe behavior disorders, nerve deafness, hemiplegia, and paraplegia. The course is unpredictable. It is not unusual for a child to be in a coma for several weeks and subsequently to recover completely without sequelae.

Other CNS complications of measles include cerebellar ataxia, retrobulbar neuritis, and hemiplegia caused by infarctions in the distribution of major arteries (Tyler, 1957). Although the pathogenesis of measles encephalomyelitis remains uncertain, it does not seem to involve viral replication in the CNS; rather, it more closely resembles the neuropathologic findings of experimental allergic encephalomyelitis, suggesting an autoimmune-mediated process (Johnson et al., 1984).

Infants with dehydration and hyperelectrolytemia may present a neurologic picture that closely resembles that of measles encephalomyelitis. Correction of the water and electrolyte disturbance is usually followed by rapid improvement.

Subacute Sclerosing Panencephalitis

The rare condition of subacute sclerosing panencephalitis (SSPE) is a late complication of measles, with an incidence of approximately 1 per 100,000 cases. It has clinical and pathologic features that are characteristic of a slowly progressing viral infection. The syndrome, first described by Dawson in 1934 and by van Bogaert in 1945, has also been called *subacute inclusion-body encephalitis*.

The early clinical manifestations are characterized by insidious and progressive behavioral and intellectual deterioration, possibly initially manifested by declining school performance. These symptoms are associated with awkwardness, stumbling, and falling. Later, the course may be characterized by involuntary myoclonic seizures and increasing mental deterioration that frequently are followed by death within a 6-month period. The confirmatory laboratory findings include (1) an electroencephalogram with paroxysmal spiking at regular intervals and depressed activity between spikes; (2) elevation of the CSF globulin, predominantly the IgG fraction; (3) an exceptionally high serum measles antibody titer; and (4) detectable oligoclonal measles antibody in the CSF.

Pathologic and clinical differences have been observed between SSPE and acute encephalomyelitis. The early neuropathologic features of SSPE include perivascular round cell infiltration, neuronal degeneration, and intranuclear and intracytoplasmic inclusion bodies. Later, extensive gliosis and demyelination occur. The demonstration of measles-virus antigen in the brain and the serologic findings incriminate the virus itself as the causative agent or, more probably, a defective variant of the virus. Further confirmation of the role of measles virus in SSPE has been provided by electron microscopic demonstration of paramyxovirus nucleocapsids in the inclusion bodies, immunofluorescence with specific measles antiserum of affected cells, and recovery in the laboratory by cocultivation techniques of infectious measles–like virus from brain biopsy or autopsy specimens.

Using immunoprecipitation methods, Hall and Choppin (1981) found a relative lack of antibodies to M protein in serum and CSF of patients with SSPE. However, there were high levels of antibody to other viral proteins. The onset of SSPE occurs many months or many years after an attack of measles. Epidemiologic studies have shown a possible relationship to age of the person. It is usually the youngest male child in the family who develops SSPE, even though older siblings had measles at the same time. Moreover, the initial measles infection is usually very mild. It has been postulated that during the course of a relatively mild or inapparent infection, the virus may survive and persist as a defective virion. The defects are apparently in expression of the M, H, and F genes of the measles virus.

There is a spectrum of gene defects in virus recovered from brains of SSPE patients, but most frequently the virus demonstrates absent or defective synthesis of M protein. By a method combining in situ reverse transcriptase–PCR amplification with labeled-probe hybridization (in situ RT-PCR-LPH) Isaacson et al. (1996) have detected measles virus RNA in neurons, astrocytes, oligodendrocytes, and vascular endothelial cells of SSPE patients, suggesting a far wider spread of the virus in the brain than had been appreciated by previous neuropathologic and virus culture studies. Since the advent of measles immunization programs, SSPE has nearly disappeared from countries with high rates of vaccination. However, it persists in those nations where measles vaccines are not yet widely utilized.

Subacute Measles Encephalitis

In addition to acute measles encephalitis and SSPE, a third CNS syndrome has been described—subacute measles encephalitis (SME). This occurs primarily in immunodeficient patients, most commonly children under treatment for acute leukemia but more recently in HIV-infected patients. Whereas SSPE patients have a latency period of years between measles and the onset of SSPE, patients with SME have undergone measles within the past six months. Focal or generalized seizures, altered level of consciousness, and a variety of other CNS dysfunctions are observed. The mortality rate is 85%, with death a few weeks to several months after onset. Mustafa et al. (1993) reviewed the past literature and reported two additional patients studied during the outbreaks of measles in Dallas from 1989 to 1991. Confirmatory findings include the characteristic intranuclear or intracytoplasmic inclusions on neurohistologic staining, paramyxovirus nucleocapsids on electron microscopy, measles virus RNA by PCR, and isolation of measles virus from affected brain cells.

Other Complications

Purpura, thrombocytopenic and nonthrombocytopenic, rarely may complicate measles. The deleterious effect of measles on pregnancy and on tuberculosis was clearly demonstrated in the southern Greenland epidemic (Christensen et al., 1953). Of twenty-six pregnant women with measles, half either aborted or gave birth to premature infants; there were no congenital malformations. There apparently were a reactivation of previously arrested cases, a striking increase of new cases of tuberculosis, and an increased mortality rate with this disease.

A positive tuberculin test may temporarily revert to negative during the course of measles. This anergy may persist for as long as 6 weeks. In the majority of cases the tuberculin test becomes positive again within 2 weeks.

Pneumomediastinum and subcutaneous emphysema may occur in rare instances. Bloch and Vardy (1968) described four cases that occurred during an epidemic in a small town in the northern Negev in Israel.

Corneal ulceration is a potentially serious complication that fortunately is uncommon. However, nearly all patients have a mild superficial keratoconjunctivitis.

Among children with nutritional deficiencies, particularly of vitamin A, the combination of infection and epithelial cell vulnerability has resulted in a more extensive involvement frequently ending in blindness (Morley, 1962).

Appendicitis may develop, perhaps as a result of lymphoid hyperplasia in the appendix, and may be so extensive it obliterates the lumen. In most instances perforation occurs before the complication is recognized.

In certain areas of the world (sub-Saharan Africa and India) where measles remains a severe and often fatal disease, the following complications are frequently observed: severe diarrhea and dehydration, kwashiorkor, pyogenic infections of the skin, cancrum oris, and septicemia.

Among children infected with human immunodeficiency virus (HIV), measles has an enhanced severity, with a higher incidence of pneumonia, hospitalization, and death (Krasinski and Borkowsky, 1989; Kaplan et al., 1992) (see also Chapter 1).

An association between either intrapartum exposure to measles virus (Ekbom et al., 1996) or childhood receipt of measles vaccine (Thompson et al., 1995) and inflammatory bowel disease has been suggested but questioned by a number of critical reviewers (Patriarca and Beeler, 1995). Resolution of the issue awaits more specific and definitive virologic investigation.

PROGNOSIS

The prognosis of measles has improved significantly during the past three decades. Many of the serious bacterial complications are easily controlled by antimicrobial therapy. In general, the prognosis is better in older children than in infants. A preexisting tuberculous infection may be aggravated. The majority of deaths is the result of severe bronchopneumonia or encephalitis. In 1989 and 1990 in outbreaks in the United States the reported case fatality rates were from 3 to 4 per 1,000 (Centers for Disease Control, 1991).

Modified measles, which is rarely complicated, has an excellent prognosis.

IMMUNITY
Active Immunity

One attack of measles is generally followed by permanent immunity. Most so-called recurrent attacks reflect errors in diagnosis. The available evidence suggests that in most cases lasting immunity follows an attack of modified measles also. Contemporary studies indicate that comparable lasting immunity will follow immunization with live attenuated measles virus vaccine. Markowitz et al. (1990a) reviewed extensively the literature on duration and quality of measles vaccine–induced immunity in the 27 years since licensure of vaccine. Although a number of issues remain unresolved, waning immunity has been demonstrated in only a very small proportion of vaccinees (Edmonson et al., 1990; Anders et al., 1996).

A number of studies have explored the causes of the suppression of cell-mediated immune responses observed during and following measles for weeks or months. These same alterations have been detected after live measles virus vaccination (Hussey et al., 1996). Reported factors include a down-regulation of IL-12 production by infected monocyte-macrophages and a suppression of TH-1 type cytokines, including IL-4, which inhibits CD4 and CD8 cell-mediated responses. The effects on the monocyte-macrophages resulted from binding of measles virus to the cells (Karp et al., 1996) with or without the initiation of productive virus infection. This binding occurs at the CD 46 receptor on the cell membrane, suggesting an interaction with the complement system, since C3b binds to the same site.

Passive Immunity

Neutralizing antibodies for measles virus are present in convalescent-phase serum and in pooled adult serum. These antibodies are contained in the immune globulin (IG) fraction that has been used for passive immunization. Passively acquired measles antibody is detected in cord blood and is usually not measurable after the infant reaches 12 months of age.

Studies by Albrecht et al. (1977) revealed the presence of passively acquired measles-neutralizing antibody in serum specimens obtained from 12-month-old infants who had no detectable HI antibody. In those populations where measles vaccines have been widely used since the mid-1960s, most pregnant women have vaccine-induced antibodies rather than those resultant from the natural infection. Because these are of lower titer, they are catabolized earlier in the first year of life by their infants, who then may lack detectable antibody by 9 to 12 months of age (Markowitz et al., 1996).

EPIDEMIOLOGIC FACTORS

Patients with measles harbor the virus in their nasopharyngeal secretions during the acute stage of the disease. Epidemiologic evidence suggests that the patients are contagious for at least 7 days after the onset of the first symptom. Contacts may acquire the infection (1) *directly,* by being sprayed with droplets emanating from a cough or sneeze; (2) *indirectly,* by a third person; or (3) by airborne spread. The most common mode of spread is by direct contact. Indirect contact within a house or a hospital ward is also possible but is an unlikely mode of transmission. In crowded settings such as classrooms, residential institutions, day-care centers, and homes, the spread of large respiratory droplets accounts for the major amount of communicability. Airborne spread by viruses persisting in fine droplets for several hours has also been demonstrated in physicians' waiting rooms.

An extraordinary study of an epidemic in Greenland in 1962 may contribute to a better understanding of the *communicability* of measles (Littauer and Sørenson, 1965). A correlation between time of exposure and communicability was observed during this epidemic. It was obvious that the available health facilities would be inadequate to cope with the problems associated with a major outbreak. Accordingly, it was decided that a "guided epidemic" would be the best solution for a potentially critical situation. The area was divided into three quarantinable units: the 800 inhabitants of the town of Umanak, the 500 inhabitants of the four most remote settlements, and the 700 inhabitants of the five nearest settlements. The plan involved the deliberate exposure of large groups of susceptible individuals to a person or persons with measles; half the adults and half the children in each household were asked to volunteer for "artificial infection."

The results of this unique plan were very interesting. Approximately 400 persons visited a patient named Josef on the first day of his measles rash. Josef coughed twice in the face of each person. In spite of this exposure, not a single contact acquired measles. Consequently, the procedure was repeated 3½ weeks later, but this time patients in the catarrhal, prerash stage of measles were chosen as

the source of infection. Under these circumstances the disease was successfully transmitted to the susceptible contacts.

Measles virus is present in the nasopharynx during the first day of rash and during the catarrhal period of the disease. The failure to transmit the infection on the first day of the rash was due to the minimal quantity of virus present at that time. The larger quantities of virus present during the catarrhal period are undoubtedly responsible for the communicability of the disease.

During the prevaccine era (before 1963) the *age incidence* varied with the particular environment. In general, measles was a disease of childhood. In congested urban areas the highest incidence occurred in the infant and preschool age groups. In rural and less crowded urban areas the highest incidence was in children 5 to 10 years of age. In epidemics that occurred in isolated communities, children of all ages were equally affected. In developing countries, measles is most common in infants 1 to 2 years of age and is frequently seen in those less than 9 months old. Because of this early occurrence among small infants, for whom morbidity and mortality are often very marked, a number of programs were initiated to evaluate the immunogenicity, safety, and efficacy of several higher-titered live virus measles vaccines administered early (Aaby et al., 1988; Markowitz et al., 1990b; Tidjani et al., 1989; Whittle et al., 1988a, 1988b).

Vaccines containing 10 to 50 times more virus than usual were administered to 4- to 6-month-old infants in an attempt to overcome maternal transplacental immunity and "close the window of susceptibility" that exists between catabolism of maternal antibody and ability to immunize successfully with conventional attenuated live measles virus vaccines. The success of these studies in a number of nations (Senegal, Guinea-Bissau, Gambia, Haiti, Togo, Sudan, Mexico, and Peru) led to a 1989 World Health Organization recommendation that high-titered vaccines be administered at 6 months of age, instead of waiting until 9 months with conventional vaccines, in those areas where measles below age 9 months caused significant mortality (World Health Organization, 1990). In subsequent years, surveillance revealed that, despite the successful prevention of measles, there was an unexplained increase in deaths from other infections in female recipients (Aaby et al., 1993, 1996). This was an inconsistent finding among the study populations, but its occurrence in Senegal, Guinea-Bissau and Haiti was of sufficient concern to call a halt to further use of high-titered vaccines (World Health Organization, 1992).

The disease is extremely rare in infants less than 3 to 4 months of age because of passively acquired maternal antibodies. If the mother, however, has never had measles, the newborn infant is susceptible.

Seasonal incidence in the temperate zones is fairly consistent. Measles is essentially a winter-spring disease, with the peak of the outbreak occurring during March and April. In heavily populated areas, epidemics usually occurred at intervals of 2 to 3 years during the prevaccine era. This periodicity was in part caused by the accumulation of a new crop of susceptible children during this interval. The extensive use of live attenuated measles virus vaccine since licensure in 1963 has had a profound effect on the incidence of measles (Fig. 16-5).

Following the initiation in 1966 of major federal funding for measles vaccine programs, a precipitous drop in the reported cases of disease resulted so that by 1981 a reduction of greater than 99% from prevaccine years had occurred. In 1983 an all-time low was reached, with fewer than 1,500 cases, in contrast to the half million or more reported annually before 1963. In 1989 and 1990 a striking in-

crease in measles cases was observed, especially among inner-city, poor, unimmunized preschool children (see inset of Fig. 16-6). This resulted in great part from a failure to reach these infants and children with recommended health care measures, including basic immunizations (Katz, 1991). With enhanced efforts to reach these unimmunized children and with the introduction of second doses of vaccine, measles has been reduced to fewer than 1,000 reported cases annually in the years 1993 through 1996 (Centers for Disease Control, 1996a). Using genomic analysis (Rota et al., 1992, 1994) as a technique for molecular epidemiology, it has been demonstrated that measles virus isolates in the United States have all been of international origin, with no United States strain of virus identified since late in 1993 (Centers for Disease Control, 1996a).

Geographic distribution is worldwide. Modern air transportation can carry an infected individual to all parts of the world within the incubation period. Through the Pan American Health Organization's leadership, measles control and elimination have been initiated and have progressed rapidly in much of Latin America and the Caribbean countries (de Quadros et al., 1996). The English-

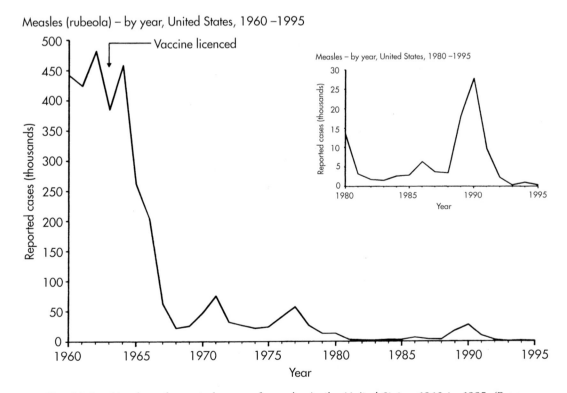

FIG. 16-5   Number of reported cases of measles in the United States, 1960 to 1995. (From CDC: Measles: United States, 1995. MMWR 1996a;45:305-307.)

speaking Caribbean countries have reported no cases of measles since 1991 despite careful surveillance and laboratory investigation of suspect patients with febrile rash illnesses (Pan American Health Organization, 1996a).

Measles is one of the most highly contagious diseases. The secondary attack rate after an intimate household exposure is greater than 90%. The reduced intimacy and duration of exposure in a school, bus, or hospital ward are followed by a lower attack rate in susceptible persons—less than 25%.

TREATMENT

Measles is a self-limited disease. The course of uncomplicated infection is not altered by antimicrobial therapy. Treatment is chiefly supportive.

Studies in Africa by Barclay et al. (1987) and by Hussey and Klein (1990) have demonstrated the striking beneficial effects of giving vitamin A to children with severe measles. Hussey and Klein—in a randomized, double-blind trial of hospitalized children (median age, 10 months)—found that those who received 400,000 IU of vitamin A within 5 days of onset of rash had less croup, recovered more rapidly from pneumonia and diarrhea, spent fewer days in the hospital, and had a much lower mortality rate than those given a placebo. Only 2 of 92 patients died among the vitamin A recipients; 10 of 97 placebo patients died. The World Health Organization has recommended vitamin A supplementation for all children in regions where vitamin A deficiency exists or where the measles mortality rate is 1% or higher. To take advantage of the 9-month health visit at which measles vaccine is administered in the Expanded Programme Immunization (EPI), vitamin A was recommended to be given simultaneously. Unfortunately, there has been a recent study reporting reduced vaccine immunogenicity when both were given at the same time (Semba et al., 1995).

Supportive Therapy

Bed rest is advisable and not difficult to enforce during the febrile period. The diet should be either liquid or soft as tolerated. When the child becomes afebrile and the anorexia subsides, regular indoor activity and diet may be resumed.

The measles *cough* is difficult to control. Most cough medicines are not very effective.

The *coryza,* too, is unaffected by treatment and runs a self-limited course. Generally, nose drops are ineffective and unnecessary. The skin around

the nares, however, should be protected with petrolatum.

The *conjunctivitis* usually requires no medication. The eyelids should be cleansed with warm water to remove any secretions or crusts. The cornea should be examined for possible ulceration. Corneal complications should be treated by an ophthalmologist. If photophobia is present, bright lights should be avoided; it is depressing and unnecessary to darken the room completely.

Infants with very high fever and children with headache should be treated with appropriate doses of antipyretic drugs.

Prevention of Bacterial Complications

Antibiotics should not be routinely administered to children with measles for the purpose of preventing bacterial complications. These agents not only may fail to achieve this goal but also may have the adverse effect of encouraging overgrowth by antibiotic-resistant bacteria or fungi that later may be responsible for complicating secondary infections (pneumonia, otitis, mastoiditis, sinusitis). This was demonstrated clearly by Weinstein (1955) in his studies of measles and its complications in the prevaccine era. Consequently, each case of measles should be carefully evaluated before antimicrobial agents are prescribed. The following factors pertaining to the host, the environment, and the disease may influence the decision to administer or withhold these drugs.

Host Factors. Age and past experience influence the development of complications. Infants are more prone to develop complications than are older children. Children with a past history of recurrent otitis media are particularly susceptible.

Environmental Factors. Patients at home are less likely to acquire a secondary infection than those in hospital wards.

Disease Factors. A mild case of measles is usually uncomplicated and need not be treated. A severe case, however, more likely will be complicated by otitis media or pneumonia.

Treatment of Complications

The complications of measles may be treated as follows.

Otitis Media. The pathogenesis and the treatment of otitis media complicating measles are no different than those following other respiratory virus infections. For a complete discussion, see Chapter 20.

Pneumonia. Bacterial pneumonia may be caused by *Streptococcus pneumoniae,* hemolytic streptococci, *Staphylococcus* species, or *Haemophilus influenzae.* These infections are discussed in Chapters 10, 25, 30, and 31.

Bronchiolitis. The treatment of infants who develop complicating bronchiolitis is difficult. The details are discussed in Chapter 25.

Obstructive Laryngitis and Laryngotracheitis. The development of a severe measles croup requires emergency treatment. The child should be hospitalized and placed in an intensive care unit. Treatment of this complication is discussed in detail in Chapter 25.

Encephalitis. Treatment is primarily symptomatic. There is no measles-specific antiviral drug currently available. Most patients require the detailed monitoring and supportive interventions available in a critical care unit. These may include stabilization of circulatory function, maintenance of respiration and ventilation, anticonvulsant therapy, lowering of increased intracranial pressure, and management of fluid and electrolyte balance (Chapter 38).

The use of corticosteroids remains controversial. The very favorable clinical experience reported by Applebaum and Abler in 1956 with seventeen treated cases and by Allen in 1957 with ten treated cases appeared impressive. Although the number of cases was small (twenty-seven), the reported incidence of twenty-six complete recoveries was striking. On the other hand, in 1959 Meade reported comparable results without corticosteroid therapy. He cited a personal observation of more than fifty patients, many with respiratory paralysis and status epilepticus, who recovered without sequelae. The evidence for the efficacy of corticosteroids in the treatment of measles encephalitis is not convincing.

An important aspect of the treatment of encephalitis is the supportive medical and nursing care necessary to tide over a comatose child for a period of days and sometimes weeks. This includes careful attention to hydration and nutrition and the prevention and treatment of intercurrent infections.

PREVENTIVE MEASURES
Immune Globulin

Measles can be modified or prevented by human IG, which induces passive immunity of variable duration. IG is given intramuscularly. The dose for prevention is 0.25 ml/kg of body weight.

With the increasing use of human immune globulin preparations for a variety of conditions, especially intravenous immune globulin (IVIG), measles and measles vaccine virus infections are inadvertently modified or prevented in a number of scenarios dependent on the product used and the dose administered (Halsey, 1995). Although the Food and Drug Administration has established a minimum concentration of measles antibody for IG preparations, there is no such standard for IVIG. Because of the resultant uncertainty regarding duration of protection from such globulin administration, measles vaccine should be given to recipients promptly after a known exposure in hopes of providing active protection if the exogenous antibody has been catabolized to an extent unlikely to prevent illness.

MEASLES VIRUS VACCINES

Within a decade of the first report of successful isolation and replication of measles virus in cell culture systems (Enders and Peebles, 1954), an attenuated live measles virus vaccine was licensed in the United States and subsequently in a number of other nations (Markowitz and Katz, 1994). With rare exceptions (Japan, China, Russia) these products are all descendents of the prototype Edmonston virus. Widespread administration of these vaccines in developed nations and through the Expanded Programme on Immunization of the World Health Organization (WHO) has resulted in a marked decrease in both morbidity and mortality resulting from measles. Previously in the United States, 500,000 to 800,000 cases were reported annually, but this was gross underreporting since nearly an entire birth cohort (3.5 to 4.0 million children) was infected each year. From a global perspective the WHO estimates that, before initiation of the EPI in 1977, there were 6 to 8 million deaths annually from measles; by 1995 there were fewer than 1 million. After a brief resurgence of measles in the United States, mainly among unimmunized inner-city children 1989 through 1991 (Katz, 1991; Hutchin et al., 1996), increased efforts to immunize all children shortly after their first birthday and to administer second doses at elementary or middle school entry have resulted in 4 successive years with fewer than 1,000 cases reported—this at a time when surveillance and reporting are more complete and precise than ever in the past. With optimism regarding the possibility of measles elimination (following the examples of smallpox and of current progress in the global polio eradication program), participants at a July 1996 meeting sponsored by PAHO, CDC, and WHO agreed that progress to date in measles control justified the establishment of a target date between 2005 and 2010 for global measles eradication, following shortly on the polio target year of 2000 (Pan American Health Organization, 1996b). Currently the EPI schedule calls for administration of measles vaccine at age 9 months. In the United States, vaccine is given between 12 and 15 months of age and a second dose before school entry. In the United States, measles vaccine is ordinarily administered as a combination with measles, mumps, and rubella (MMR). EPI uses monovalent measles vaccine without mumps or rubella.

Measles vaccine is produced in cell cultures of chick embryo fibroblasts and is stabilized with human albumin, sorbitol, and hydrolyzed gelatin to yield a final concentration of at least 1,000 tissue culture infectious doses of virus. There is also a small amount of neomycin in the final solution. The only measles vaccine currently licensed in the United States is Moraten (an Enders-Edmonston descendant) by Merck. Although the complete genome of measles virus has been sequenced (Kobune et al., 1995), and it is thereby possible to differentiate vaccine strain from circulating wild virus, the molecular basis for attenuation or virulence has not been identified. Past epidemiologic history and current laboratory observations confirm the overall antigenic stability of the virus, but there are sufficient variations in the F and H gene products to permit the discrimination of vaccine from wild strains. Immunologically, it is reassuring to note that sera from vaccine recipients are capable in vitro of neutralizing wild viruses isolated more than 40 years ago. Likewise, sera from individuals infected many years ago neutralize current measles virus isolates.

In the United States, two committees are responsible for recommendations governing the use of measles virus vaccines. The Advisory Committee on Immunization Practices (ACIP) of the U.S. Public Health Service publishes its recommendations as supplements to the Morbidity and Mortality Weekly Reports (MMWR), and the Committee on Infectious Diseases (COID—"Redbook Commit-

tee") of the American Academy of Pediatrics publishes its recommendations in the journal *Pediatrics* and in its *Redbook* publication, which is issued approximately every 3 years, most recently in May 1997.

In susceptible children, measles vaccine produces febrile response ($\geq 39.4°$ C) in 5% to 15% of recipients 7 to 12 days after vaccination, and rash in approximately 5% 7 to 10 days after vaccine administration. More than 95% of susceptible recipients show seroconversion with a measles-specific antibody response first detectable 12 to 15 days after vaccination and achieving peak titers 21 to 28 days thereafter. Serum antibodies are of the IgM, IgG, and IgA isotypes, and there is also detectable measles-specific secretory IgA at the respiratory mucosal surfaces. In general, these antibodies are enduring but may fall to undetectable levels in a variable number of recipients over lengthy periods of observation. Reexposure to vaccine results in a rapid anamnestic response, indicating persistence of immunity. Undoubtedly, a significant aspect of this memory resides in T-cell function, an essential component of the measles immune response. Concern regarding secondary vaccine failures (that is, those individuals who initially responded to vaccine but subsequently lost their immunity) has challenged full resolution over the years. Recent observations suggest that, if they occur, they are extremely unusual, probably less than 0.2% (Watson et al., 1996; Anders et al., 1996).

As noted, fever and rash are the most common reactions observed after primary immunization of susceptible children. From an exhaustive review by a committee of the Institute of Medicine (Stratton et al., 1994) available evidence pointed to febrile seizures, thrombocytopenia, and anaphylaxis as the only adverse events for which sufficient evidence existed to establish a causal relationship. Anaphylaxis has been reported in less than 1 per 1 million doses of MMR vaccine in the United States. Although children may have febrile seizures after MMR vaccination, especially among those with a prior history of seizures, there is no evidence for the production of a residual seizure disorder or chronic neurologic disability. Suspected encephalopathies following a nonrandom distribution cluster between days 5 and 14 after vaccine administration. If measles vaccine is the cause, the frequency may be 1 per 500,000, significantly fewer than the 1 per 1,000 rate observed following natural measles. Thrombocytopenia, which may be an unusual complication of natural measles, has also been reported after vaccine at an estimated rate of 1 per 1 million doses (Beeler et al., 1996). This may be a more frequent complication for patients who have previously had an immune thrombocytopenic purpura.

Because vaccine is derived from chick embryo cell cultures, there has been a concern regarding its administration to children with egg allergy. James et al. (1995) studied fifty-four children with severe allergies to egg, twenty-six of whom had anaphylaxis after ingestion of eggs. None of the fifty-four had either an immediate or a delayed adverse reaction on receipt of a standard dose of MMR subcutaneously.

Because vaccine is a live, replicating virus, it's administration to immunocompromised patients has received careful scrutiny. In early studies with the first (less attenuated) Edmonston vaccine, two children under chemotherapy for acute leukemia developed giant cell pneumonia after vaccination (Mitus et al., 1962). After subsequent further attenuation of the vaccine virus and extensive experience over a 33-year period, only six severely immunocompromised patients have been reported who suffered fatal complications attributable to vaccine virus. This occurs in a background denominator of more than 100 million doses administered. In the current era of HIV and AIDS, increased attention has been focused on the possible risks associated with measles immunization of HIV-infected children. Because wild measles has resulted in such a high mortality rate among these patients (Kaplan et al., 1992), the hypothetical risk of vaccine-induced disease has been an acceptable one, so until 1996 MMR was recommended for asymptomatic HIV-infected persons and considered for symptomatic ones. The publication in 1996 (CDCb 1996) of a single, highly unique exception initiated a reconsideration of this policy. One year after receipt of his second dose of MMR, given to fulfill a college prematriculation requirement, this young man developed a progressive illness with pneumonia, shown later to be giant cell pneumonia resulting from measles virus, which was identified as vaccine strain by its sequence analysis. As a result, recommendations were reformulated, advising the withholding of measles vaccine from HIV-infected individuals with severe immunosuppression (for children age 1 to 5 years, CD4 counts of less than 200 or percentages less than 15). Among those infants and children who have received measles vaccine, there has been a spectrum of response with lower antibody titers,

fewer seroconversions, and shortened persistence of detectable antibodies (Walter et al., 1994; Palumbo et al., 1992).

Despite the impressive success of current vaccines in controlling measles and eliminating transmission in some countries, the challenge of immunizing infants at an even younger age (when transplacentally acquired maternal antibody aborts the infection with attenuated virus) has stimulated attempts to develop other forms of vaccine that would immunize successfully despite circulating measles-specific antibody. These have included the use of recombinant vaccinia virus or canarypox virus expressing measles F and H proteins, immune-stimulating complexes containing these same proteins, (Hsu et al., 1996) and chimeras of measles and other viruses.

Other modifications of current measles vaccine include the incorporation of live attenuated varicella vaccine in a tetravalent preparation (measles-mumps-rubella-varicella vaccine [MMRV]), which has been immunogenic and safe in initial studies (Watson et al., 1996; also see Chapter 37).

Whether global elimination of measles can be achieved is an enormous challenge, given the marked communicability of the infection, the susceptibility of infants once maternal antibody has been catabolized, the need to immunize close to 100% of susceptibles, and the lack of public health infrastructure in those countries where it remains endemic (Katz and Gellin, 1994).

ISOLATION AND QUARANTINE

In general, isolation and quarantine procedures are of limited value in the prophylaxis of measles. Exposure usually occurs before the diagnosis is obvious. Attempts to isolate siblings from each other are useless. The availability of IG and live attenuated measles virus vaccine for household and other susceptible contacts has obviated the need for quarantine.

Isolation of Patient

Epidemiologic evidence has indicated that measles is no longer contagious after the fourth day of rash. Consequently, children may return to school or other group activities after this time.

Quarantine of Contact

The susceptible contact is a potential source of infection from the eighth day after exposure to as long as the twenty-first day if IG has been administered. Consequently, if quarantine were to be instituted, a child would have to be isolated for almost 2 weeks. Experience has shown that quarantine rarely affects the course of an epidemic. On the contrary, it usually disrupts household and school activities unnecessarily. Once the outbreak has occurred, it is best to continue normal school and group activities and to rely chiefly on IG and live attenuated measles virus vaccine as prophylactic agents.

BIBLIOGRAPHY

Aaby P, Jensen TG, Hansen HL, et al. Trial of high-dose Edmonston-Zagreb measles vaccine in Guinea-Bissau: protective efficacy. Lancet 1988;2:809-811.

Aaby P, Knudsen K, Whittle H, et al. Child mortality after Edmonston-Zagreb measles vaccination in Guinea-Bissau increased female mortality rate. J Pediatr 1993;122:904-908.

Aaby P, Samb B, Simondon F, et al. Five-year follow-up of morbidity and mortality among recipients of high-titer measles vaccines in Senegal. Vaccine 1996;14:226-229.

Albrecht P, Ennis FA, Saltzmann EJ, Krugman S. Persistence of maternal antibody in infants beyond 12 months: mechanism of measles vaccine failure. J Pediatr 1977;91:715.

Allen JE. Treatment of measles encephalitis with adrenal steroids. Pediatrics 1957;20:87.

Anders JF, Jacobson RM, Poland GA, et al. Secondary failure rates of measles vaccines: a metaanalysis of published studies. Pediatr Infect Dis J 1996;15:62-66.

Annunziato D, Kaplan MH, Hall WW, et al. Atypical measles syndrome: pathologic and serologic findings. Pediatrics 1982;70:203-209.

Applebaum E, Abler C. Treatment of measles encephalitis with corticotropin. Am J Dis Child 1956;92:47.

Barclay AJG, Foster A, Sommer A. Vitamin A supplements and mortality related to measles: a randomized clinical trial. Br Med J 1987;294:294-296.

Beeler J, Varrichio F, Wise R. Thrombocytopenia after immunization with measles vaccines: review of the vaccine adverse events reporting system (1990 to 1994). Pediatr Infect Dis J 1996;15:88-90.

Bellini WJ, Rota JS, Rota PA. Virology of measles virus. J Infect Dis 1994;170(suppl 1):S15-S23.

Bloch A, Vardy P. Pneumomediastinum and subcutaneous emphysema in measles. Clin Pediatr 1968;7:7.

Centers for Disease Control: Measles: United States, 1990. MMWR 1991;40:369:372.

Centers for Disease Control. Measles: United States, 1995. MMWR 1996a; 45:305-307.

Centers for Disease Control. Measles pneumonitis following M-M-R vaccination of a patient with HIV infection, 1993. MMWR 1996b;45:603-606.

Chen RT, Markowitz LE, Albrecht P, et al. Measles antibody: reevaluation of protective titers. J Infect Dis 1990; 162:1036-1042.

Cherry JD, Cohen LM, Panosian CB. Diarrhea, fever, hypoxia, and rash in a house officer. Rev Infect Dis 1990; 12:1044-1051.

Christensen PO, Schmidt H, Bang HO, et al. An epidemic of measles in Southern Greenland in 1951. Acta Med Scand 1953;144:430,450.

Dawson JR Jr. Cellular inclusions in cerebral lesions of epidemic encephalitis. Arch Neurol Psychiatr 1934;31:685.

Degen JA Jr. Visceral pathology in measles: a clinicopathological study of 100 fatal cases. Am J Med Sci 1937;194: 104.

de Quadros C, Olive J, Hersh B, et al. Measles elimination in the Americas: evolving strategies. JAMA 1996;275:224-229.

Edmunson MB, Addiss DG, McPherson JT, et al. Mild measles and secondary vaccine failure during a sustained outbreak in a highly vaccinated population. JAMA 1990;263:2467-2471.

Ekbom A, Daszak P, Kraaz W, et al. Crohn's disease after in utero measles virus exposure. Lancet 1996;348;515-517.

Enders JF, Katz SL, Milovanovic MJ, Holloway A. Studies on an attenuated measles virus vaccine. I. Development and preparation of the vaccine: techniques for assay of effects of vaccination. N Engl J Med 1960;263:153.

Enders JF, McCarthy K, Mitus A, Cheatham WJ. Isolation of measles virus at autopsy in cases of giant-cell pneumonia without rash. N Engl J Med 1959;261:875.

Enders JF, Peebles TC. Propagation in tissue cultures of cytopathogenic agents from patients with measles. Proc Soc Exp Biol Med 1954;86:277.

Fortenberry J, Mariscalco M, Louis P, et al. Severe laryngotracheobronchitis complicating measles. Amer J Dis Child 1992;146:1040-1043.

Fulginiti VA, Eller JJ, Downie AW, Kempe CH. Altered reactivity to measles virus: atypical measles in children previously immunized with inactivated measles virus vaccine. JAMA 1967;202:1075.

Griffin DE, Ward BJ, Esolen LM. Pathogenesis of measles virus infection: an hypothesis for altered immune responses. J Infect Dis 1994;170(suppl):S24-S31.

Guris D, McCready J, Watson JC, et al. Measles vaccine effectiveness and duration of vaccine-induced immunity in the absence of boosting from exposure to measles virus. Pediatr Infect Dis J 1996;15:1082-1086.

Hall WJ, Hall CB. Atypical measles in adolescents: evaluation of clinical and pulmonary function. Ann Intern Med 1979;90:882.

Hall WW, Choppin PW. Measles-virus proteins in the brain tissue of patients with subacute sclerosing panencephalitis: absence of M protein. N Engl J Med 1981;304:1152-1155.

Halsey N. Dose-adjusted timing of measles vaccine after administration of Ig. Rep Pediatr Infect Dis 1995;5(6):21-22.

Helfand R, Kebede S, Alexander J, et al. Comparative detection of measles-specific IgM in oral fluid and serum from children by an antibody-capture IgM EIA. J Infect Dis 1996; 173:1470-74.

Holt EA, Boulos R, Halsey NA, et al. Childhood survival in Haiti: protective effect of measles vaccination. Pediatrics 1990;85:188-194.

Hsu S, Schadeck E, Delmas A, et al. Linkage of a fusion peptide to a CTL epitope from the nucleoprotein of measles virus enables incorporation into ISCOMs and induction of CTL responses following intranasal immunization. Vaccine 1996; 14:1159-1166.

Hussey G, Goddard E, Hughes J, et al. The effect of Edmonston-Zagreb and Schwarz measles vaccines on immune responses in infants. J Infect Dis 1996;173:1320-1326.

Hussey GD, Klein M. A randomized controlled trial of vitamin A in children with severe measles. N Engl J Med 1990; 323:160-164.

Hutchin S, Markowitz L, Atkinson W, et al. Measles outbreaks in the United States, 1987 through 1990. Pediatr Infect Dis J 1996;15:31-38.

Isaacson S, Asher D, Godec M, et al. Widespread, restricted low-level measles virus infection of brain in a case of suba-cute sclerosing panencephalitis. Acta Neuropathol 1996; 91:135-139.

James J, Burks A, Roberson P, et al. Safe administration of the measles vaccine to children allergic to eggs. N Engl J Med 1995;332:1262-1266.

Johnson RT, Griffin DE, Hirsch RL, et al. Measles en-cephalomyelitis: clinical and immunologic studies. N Engl J Med 1984;310:137-141.

Kaplan LJ, Daum RS, Smaron M, McCarthy CA. Severe measles in immunocompromised patients. JAMA 1992; 267:1237-1241.

Karp C, Wysocka M, Wahl L, et al. Mechanism of suppression of cell-mediated immunity by measles virus. Science 1996; 273:228-231.

Katz SL. Measles in the United States: 1989 and 1990. In Arnoff SC (ed). Advances in pediatric infectious diseases, vol 6. St. Louis: Mosby, 1991.

Katz SL, Gellin BG. Measles vaccine: do we need new vaccines or new programs? Science 1994;265:1391-1392.

Kobune F, Funatu M, Takahashi H, et al. Characterization of measles viruses isolated after measles vaccination. Vaccine 1995;13:370-372.

Koplik H. The diagnosis of the invasion of measles from a study of the exanthema as it appears on the buccal mucous mem-brane. Arch Pediatr 1896;13:918.

Krasinski K, Borkowsky W. Measles and measles immunity in children infected with human immunodeficiency virus. JAMA 1989;261:2512-2516.

Krugman S. Present status of measles and rubella immunization in the United States: a medical progress report. J Pediatr 1977;90:1.

Krugman S, Giles JP, Jacobs AM, Friedman H. Studies with a further attenuated live measles-virus vaccine. Pediatrics 1963;31:919.

Littauer J, Sørensen K. The measles epidemic at Umanak in Greenland in 1962. Dan Med Bull 1965;12:43.

Makhene M, Diaz P. Clinical presentations and complications of suspected measles in hospitalized children. Pediatric Infect Dis J 1993;12:836-840.

Mallory FB, Medlar EM. Skin lesions in measles. J Med Res 1920;41:327.

Markowitz L, Albrecht P, Rhodes P et al. Changing levels of measles antibody titers in women and children in the United States: impact on response to vaccination. Pediatrics 1996; 97:53-58.

Markowitz LE, Katz SL. Measles vaccine. In Plotkin SA, Mor-timer EA Jr. (eds). Vaccines. Philadelphia: WB Saunders, 1994.

Markowitz LE, Preblud SR, Fine PEM, et al. Duration of live measles vaccine-induced immunity. Pediatr Infect Dis 1990a; 9:101-110.

Markowitz LE, Sepulveda J, Diaz-Ortega JL, et al. Immuniza-tion of six-months-old infants with different doses of Edmon-ston-Zagreb and Schwarz measles vaccines. N Engl J Med 1990b;322:580-587.

Martin DB, Werher LB, Nieburg PI, et al. Atypical measles in adolescents and young adults. Ann Intern Med 1979;90: 977.

Matsuzono Y, Narita M, Ishiguro N, et al. Detection of measles virus from clinical samples using the polymerase chain reac-tion. Arch Pediatr Adolesc Med 1994;148:289-293.

Meade RH III. Common viral infections in childhood: a discus-sion of measles, German measles, mumps, chickenpox, vac-cinia, and smallpox. Med Clin North Am 1959;43:1355.

Mitus A, Holloway A, Evans AE, Enders JF. Attenuated measles vaccine in children with acute leukemia. Amer J Dis Cli H 1962;103:243-248.

Morley DC. Measles in Nigeria. Am J Dis Child 1962;103:230.

Murray K, Selleck P, Hooper P, et al. A morbillivirus that caused fatal disease in horses and humans. Science 1995;268:94-97.

Mustafa M, Weitman S, Winick N, et al. Subacute measles en-cephalitis in the young immunocompromised host: report of two cases diagnosed by polymerase chain reaction and treated with ribavirin and review of the literature. Clin Infect Dis 1993;16:654-660.

Nader PR, Horwitz MS, Rousseau J. Atypical exanthem follow-ing exposure to natural measles: 11 cases in children previ-ously inoculated with killed vaccine. J Pediatr 1968;72:22.

Naniche D, Varior G, Cervoni F, et al. Human membrane cofac-tor protein (CD46) acts as a cellular receptor for measles virus. J Virol 1993;67:6025-6032.

O'Sullivan JD, Allworth AM, Paterson DL, et al. Fatal en-cephalitis due to novel paramyxovirus transmitted from horses. Lancet 1997;349:93-95.

Pan American Health Organization. Record five years measles-free! EPI Newsletter 1996a;18:1-3.

Pan American Health Organization. Global measles eradication: target 2010? EPI Newsletter 1996b;18(4):1-3.

Palumbo P, Hoyt L, Demasio K, et al. Population-based study of measles and measles immunization in human immunodefi-ciency virus–infected children. Pediatr Infect Dis J 1992; 11:1008-1014.

Patriarca PA, Beeler JA. Measles vaccination and inflammatory bowel disease. Lancet 1995;345:1062-1063.

Rauh LW, Schmidt R. Measles immunization with killed virus vaccine. Am J Dis Child 1965;109:232.

Rota J, Hummel K, Rota P, et al. Genetic variability of the gly-coprotein genes of current wild-type measles isolates. Virol 1992;188:135-142.

Rota PA, Bloom AE, Vanchiere JA, Bellini WJ. Evolution of the nucleoprotein and matrix genes of wild-type strains of measles virus isolated from recent epidemics. Virology 1994;198:724-730.

Scheifele DW, Forbes CE. Prolonged giant cell excretion in se-vere African measles. Pediatrics 1972;50:867.

Semba R, Munasir Z, Beeler J, et al. Reduced seroconversion to measles in infants given vitamin A with measles vaccination. Lancet 1995;345:1330-1332.

Stratton K, Howe C, Johnson R (eds). Adverse events associated with childhood vaccines: evidence bearing on causality. Washington, D.C.: National Academy Press, 1994.

Suringa DWR, Bank LJ, Ackerman AB. Role of measles virus in skin lesions and Koplik's spots. N Engl J Med 1970;283:1139.

Thompson N, Montgomery S, Pounder R, et al. Is measles vac-cination a risk factor for inflammatory bowel disease? Lancet 1995;345:1071-1074.

Tidjani O, Grunitsky G, Guerin N, et al. Serological effects of Edmonston-Zagreb, Schwarz, and AIK-C measles vaccine strains given at 4-5 or 8-10 months. Lancet 1989;2:1357-1360.

Tompkins V, Macaulay JC. A characteristic cell in nasal secretions during prodromal measles. JAMA 1955;157:711.

Tyler HR. Neurological complications of rubeola (measles). Medicine 1957;25:147-167.

van Bogaert L. Une Leuco-encephalite sclerosante subaiguë. J Neurol Neurosurg Psychiatry 1945;8:101.

Walter EB, Katz SL, Bellini WJ. Measles immunity in HIV-infected children. Pediatr AIDS HIV Infect 1994;5:300-304.

Ward B, Boulianne N, Ratnam S, et al. Cellular immunity in measles vaccine failure: demonstration of measles antigen–specific lymphoproliferative responses despite limited serum antibody production after revaccination. J Infect Dis 1995; 172:1591-1595.

Watson B, Laufer D, Kuter B, et al. Safety and immunogenicity of a combined live attenuated measles, mumps, rubella, and varicella vaccine (MMRV) in healthy children. J Infect Dis 1996a;173:731-734.

Watson J, Pearson J, Markowitz L, et al. An evaluation of measles revaccination among school-entry-aged children. Pediatr 1996b;97:613-618.

Weinstein L. Failure of chemotherapy to prevent the bacterial complications of measles. N Engl J Med 1955;253:679.

Whittle HC, Hanlon P, O'Neill K, et al. Trial of high-dose Edmonson-Zagreb measles vaccine in the Gambia: antibody response and side effects. Lancet 1988a;2:811-814.

Whittle HC, Mann G, Eccles M, et al. Effects of dose and strain of vaccine on success of measles vaccination of infants aged 4-5 months. Lancet 1988b;1:963-966.

World Health Organization, Expanded Programme on Immunization, Global Advisory Group. Measles immunization before 9 months of age (part 1). Wkly Epidemiol Rec 1990; 65:5-12.

World Health Organization, Expanded Programme on Immunization. Safety of high titer measles vaccines. Wkly Epidemiol Rec 1992;67:357-361.

Young PL, Halpin K, Selleck PW, et al. Serological evidence for the presence in pteropus bats of a paramyxovirus related to equine morbillivirus. Emerg Infect Dis 1996;2:239-240.

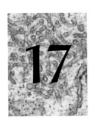

17 MENINGITIS

XAVIER SÁEZ-LLORENS AND GEORGE H. MCCRACKEN, JR.

Bacterial meningitis is a potentially fatal acute infectious disease caused by a variety of microorganisms. Current case fatality rates associated with this entity can be as low as 2% in infants and children and as high as 30% in neonates. Deafness or other long-term neurologic sequelae are present in up to one third of survivors. Antimicrobial agents have had a profound effect on the clinical course and prognosis of meningitis. Sophisticated medical intensive care technology and the availability of newer, extraordinarily active β-lactam antibiotics, however, have resulted in only a slight improvement in outcome from this disease.

In the last decade there has been an increasing recognition that further improvements in the treatment of bacterial meningitis can result only from a better understanding of the pathophysiologic events that occur after activation of the host's inflammatory pathways by either the bacteria or their products (Sande et al., 1989).

With the recent introduction of effective conjugated vaccines against *Haemophilus influenzae* type b organisms, the incidence of bacterial meningitis has declined dramatically. This enthusiasm has been neutralized, however, by the worldwide spread of pneumococcal strains exhibiting resistance to multiple, commonly used, antimicrobial agents and the continued widespread epidemics of meningococcal disease in many areas of the developing world.

ETIOLOGY

A wide range of pathogenic and nonpathogenic bacteria has been incriminated as causative agents of purulent meningitis. The most commonly implicated organisms are listed for the various pediatric age-groups.

Newborn Infants

Group B streptococci *(Streptococcus agalactiae)*
Escherichia coli K1 and other gram-negative enteric bacilli
Listeria monocytogenes
Enterococci

Infants and Children

Streptococcus pneumoniae
Neisseria meningitidis
H. influenzae type b (rare in areas with routine *Haemophilus* vaccination)

Children Older than 5 Years

S. pneumoniae
N. meningitidis

In immunocompromised hosts and in patients undergoing neurosurgical procedures, meningitis can be caused by a variety of different bacteria such as *Staphylococcus* species, gram-negative enteric bacilli, or *Pseudomonas aeruginosa.*

In the neonatal period group B streptococci are the most common organisms causing bacterial meningitis in many developed countries. Most cases of meningitis are caused by subtype III strains, and the disease usually occurs after the first week of life. Coliform bacilli are the second most common meningeal pathogens, particularly strains of *E. coli* possessing K1 antigen. In many developing countries *E. coli* and other gram-negative enteric bacilli such as species of *Klebsiella, Enterobacter,* and *Salmonella* are the leading cause of meningitis in newborns. *L. monocytogenes* can be recovered in 1% to 10% of all cases of bacterial meningitis in this age-group. As with group B streptococcal infections, meningeal infection caused by *L. monocytogenes* usually occurs after the first week of life. *Listeria* serotype IVb has been implicated in most cases.

In infants and children *H. influenzae* type b, *N. meningitidis,* and *S. pneumoniae* are responsible for the vast majority of bacterial meningitis cases. Young infants 1 to 3 months of age, however, are in a special category because pathogens found both in neonates and in older infants and children can cause meningitis.

Encapsulated strains of *H. influenzae* are classified by capsular polysaccharide types a through f; however, more than 95% of invasive diseases are caused by type b strains. With the routine use of conjugated vaccines against the type b strain in many countries, disease caused by this organism has almost disappeared. The capsule of the type b strain (polylribosyl ribitol phosphate [PRP]) is believed to play an important role in the ability of these pathogens to evade immunologic recognition by the host, whereas the lipopolysaccharide (LOS) or endotoxin component of the bacterial outer cell membrane constitutes the main virulence factor (Syrogiannopoulos et al., 1988).

Although more than 80 serotypes of pneumococci have been identified on the basis of their capsular polysaccharides, only relatively few have commonly been associated with invasive disease and with meningitis. Almost all penicillin-resistant pneumococcal strains causing meningitis belong to serotypes 6, 14, 19, and 23. The capsule of these organisms aids the bacteria to resist phagocytosis, whereas the teichoic acid polymers of the pneumococcal cell wall are important in determining virulence and eliciting the host's inflammatory responses (Tuomanen et al., 1985).

Meningococci have been divided into sero-groups on the basis of antigenic differences in their capsular polysaccharides (A, B, C, D, X, Y, Z, W-135, and 29-E). Groups B, C, Y, and W-135 are the predominant serogroups associated with severe clinical disease in the United States, whereas the group A strain accounts for epidemic disease in many other countries; group B strains are the most common isolates in Latin America (Riedo et al., 1995). Meningococcal serotypes are defined on the basis of antigenic differences in the class 2 and 3 outer membrane proteins (OMPs), whereas differences in the class 1 OMPs determine subtypes. There are currently more than twenty serotypes and at least ten class 1 subtypes. As with the pathogenesis of *H. influenzae* disease, the presence of the meningococcal capsule is important in avoiding the host's clearance mechanisms, whereas its endotoxin contributes to virulence.

PATHOGENESIS

Meningitis most commonly follows invasion of the bloodstream by organisms that have colonized mu-

cosal areas. In the neonatal period pathogens are acquired primarily, although not exclusively, during birth by contact and aspiration of intestinal and genital tract secretions at the time of delivery. Neonates with longer nursery stays can also be exposed to multiple nosocomial pathogens. Colonization of babies with potential meningeal organisms can result in bacteremia and subsequent cerebrospinal fluid (CSF) invasion in a small percentage of cases, especially in very low birth weight infants.

In infants and children meningitis usually develops after hematogenous dissemination with encapsulated bacteria that have colonized the nasopharynx. It is believed that mild upper respiratory viral infections commonly precede bloodstream bacterial invasion (Feldman, 1966). Consequently, organisms penetrate vulnerable sites of the blood-brain barrier (e.g., choroid plexus and cerebral capillaries) and reach the subarachnoid space.

In some cases meningitis may also develop by direct extension from a paranasal sinus or from the middle ear to the mastoid and finally to the meninges. Severe head trauma with a skull fracture and/or CSF rhinorrhea may lead to meningitis, usually caused by *S. pneumoniae*. Direct inoculation of bacteria into the CSF may occur, with congenital dural defects (dermal sinus or meningomyelocele), neurosurgical procedures (CSF derivation shunts), penetrating wounds, or extension from a suppurative parameningeal focus.

Infants with underlying illnesses such as malignancy, sickle cell disease, agammaglobulinemia, complement deficiency, and acquired immunodeficiency syndrome (AIDS) are predisposed to develop meningitis by both common and uncommon bacterial pathogens.

PATHOPHYSIOLOGY

The intense inflammation within the subarachnoid space as reflected in lumbar CSF and the resulting neurologic damage are not the direct result of the pathogenic bacteria but instead of activation of the host's inflammatory pathways by either the microorganisms or their products (Sáez-Llorens et al., 1990).

Once the meningeal pathogens have entered the central nervous system (CNS), they replicate rapidly and liberate active cell wall or membrane-associated components (i.e., lipoteichoic acid and peptidoglycan fragments of gram-positive organisms and endotoxin of gram-negative bacteria). Effective antimicrobial treatment causes rapid lysis of bacteria, which results in an initial enhanced release of these active bacterial products into CSF. These potent inflammatory substances are capable of stimulating macrophage-equivalent brain cells (e.g., astrocytes, microglia) and/or cerebral capillary endothelium to produce cytokines such as tumor necrosis factor (TNF), interleukin-1 (IL-1), and other inflammatory mediators such as IL-6, IL-8, platelet-activating factor (PAF), nitric oxide, arachidonic acid metabolites (e.g., prostaglandin and prostacycline), and macrophage-derived proteins. The presence of these mediators in CSF of infants and children with bacterial meningitis has been documented by many investigators. The cytokines activate adhesion-promoting receptors on cerebral vascular endothelial cells and leukocytes, resulting in attraction of neutrophils to these sites. Subsequently, leukocytes penetrate the intercellular junctions of the capillary endothelium and release proteolytic products and toxic oxygen radicals. These events result in injury to the vascular endothelium and alteration of blood-brain barrier permeability. Depending on the potency and duration of the inflammatory stimuli, the alterations in permeability result in penetration of low-molecular-weight serum proteins into CSF and in vasogenic edema. Additionally, large numbers of leukocytes enter the subarachnoid space and release toxic substances that contribute to the production of cytotoxic edema. As a result of the high protein and cell content, the increased CSF viscosity contributes to generation of interstitial edema. All these inflammatory events, if not modulated promptly and effectively, eventually cause alteration of CSF dynamics (brain edema, intracranial hypertension), of brain metabolism, and of cerebrovascular autoregulation (decreased cerebral blood flow). Current research focuses on delineating the mechanisms involved in neuronal injury, possibly through the participation of potential mediators such as reactive oxygen and nitrogen substances, and excitatory amino acids. Induction of all these molecular pathways can eventually result in irreversible focal or diffuse brain damage (Pfister et al., 1994).

PATHOLOGY

The gross appearance of the brain in a patient with meningitis is striking. The entire surface and base can be covered by a layer of a thick purulent fibrinous exudate. As a result of generalized vasculitis, thrombosis of vessels and/or sinuses and necrosis of vessel walls can occur, causing compromise of perfusion and cerebral edema.

Histologically, the lesion begins with hyperemia and hemorrhages, followed by a purulent inflammatory reaction in the arachnoid and pia mater. The inflammatory exudate consists of masses of polymorphonuclear leukocytes, fibrin, bacterial clumps, and red blood cells.

As the infection extends to the ventricles, thick pus or adhesions may occlude the various foramina or aqueducts and cause obstructive hydrocephalus. Communicating hydrocephalus results because CSF reabsorption by the arachnoid villi can be impaired because of occlusion of the sagittal or lateral sinuses, high concentrations of CSF protein, or obstruction within the basilar cisterns. The exudate can involve the intracranial portion of the optic nerve, with subsequent neuritis and possible blindness. Involvement of the cochlear aqueduct and/or the internal auditory canal with development of acute suppurative labyrinthitis is considered responsible for the early deafness that commonly occurs in bacterial meningitis.

EPIDEMIOLOGIC FACTORS

The incidence of neonatal meningitis varies greatly among different institutions and geographic areas, with approximate rates of 2 to 10 cases per 10,000 live births (Klein et al., 1986). More than two thirds of all cases of neonatal meningitis in developed countries currently are caused by group B streptococci, viridans streptococci, and gram-negative enteric bacilli. *L. monocytogenes* is encountered occasionally and usually is associated with maternal infection that was acquired from contaminated milk products. In developing countries gram-negative enteric bacilli are the predominant organisms causing bacterial meningitis in newborns; nonetheless, group B streptococci and *L. monocytogenes* have been increasingly isolated in recent years (Moreno et al., 1994). Vertical transmission is the principal mode of acquisition, but nosocomial transmission is also important, especially in low birth weight preterm infants who require long-term intensive care management. Viridans streptococci, enterococci, staphylococci, and nontypeable *H. influenzae* strains can also be implicated. Although virtually all newborn infants are colonized by many of the organisms with which they have contact, sepsis occurs in less than 1% of them. Approximately one fourth of infants with septicemia develop meningitis.

H. influenzae type b meningitis is primarily a disease of infancy. The highest incidence occurs in the first year of life, with most of the cases occurring in children 3 months to 3 years of age. It occurs uncommonly in infants less than 3 months and in children greater than 5 years of age. During the first few months most infants are protected by passively acquired maternal antibodies. Children naturally develop immunity to *H. influenzae* after the third year of life, and concentrations of PRP antibodies reach adult levels by 7 years of age (Dajani et al., 1979). Routine immunization of infants and children with the conjugated vaccines against this organism has resulted in the virtual disappearance of *Haemophilus* meningitis in developed countries (Peltola et al., 1992; Adams et al., 1993). For example, in Dallas County, Texas, the annual incidence of *Haemophilus* disease in children younger than 5 years was reduced from 158 cases per 100,000 person-years in 1983 to 9 cases per 100,000 in 1991 (Murphy et al., 1993).

Meningococcal and pneumococcal meningitis have their highest incidence in the first year of life and rarely occur in infants younger than 3 months of age. Unlike *H. influenzae* infections, these two microorganisms can cause systemic infection at any age in both children and adults.

Although poor living conditions increase the risk of developing meningitis, other factors such as crowding in day-care facilities contribute to the incidence of disease. The increased incidence in certain ethnic groups (American Indians, Eskimos, and blacks) and in families, however, and the observation that siblings of patients with meningitis can have deficient antibody synthesis against *H. influenzae* have suggested that there is also a genetic predisposition to infection.

All types of meningitis occur sporadically; only meningococcal infections occur in epidemic form. Meningococci are transmitted from person to person by nasopharyngeal secretions from a patient or carrier, and transmission usually requires close contact. Major epidemics have occurred in South America, Finland, Mongolia, and sub-Saharan Africa. Outbreaks among military recruits have been observed in training camps and bases during every period of national mobilization.

The risk of acquiring a secondary case of meningococcal or *Haemophilus* disease after household exposure to primary infection is greatly increased compared with that in the normal population. The risk for acquiring *Haemophilus* disease is greatest for unvaccinated infants and children less than 4 years of age, whereas for meningococcal disease the incidence of secondary cases is increased for family members regardless of age. Pneumococcal disease can also occur in families.

CLINICAL MANIFESTATIONS

The clinical findings of acute bacterial meningitis depend principally on the patient's age. The classic manifestations observed in older children and adults are rarely present in infants. In general, the younger the patient, the more subtle and atypical are the symptoms.

Classic Meningitis of Children and Adults

Classic meningitis usually begins with fever, chills, vomiting, photophobia, and severe headache. Occasionally, the first sign of illness is a convulsion that can recur during evolution of the disease. Irritability, delirium, drowsiness, lethargy, and coma can also develop.

The most consistent physical finding is the presence of nuchal rigidity associated with Brudzinski's and Kernig's signs. Brudzinski's sign is elicited by rapid flexion of the neck of the supine patient, followed involuntarily by brisk flexion of the knees in the presence of meningeal irritation. Kernig's sign is present if there is marked resistance to extension of the leg when the patient is in the supine position with the thigh flexed at the hip and the leg flexed at the knee. As the disease progresses, the neck stiffness increases, causing the head to draw backward. Because of the spasm of the back muscles, the patient assumes a position of opisthotonos.

The signs and symptoms just described are common to all types of meningitis. There are other manifestations, however, peculiar to specific infections. Petechial and purpuric eruptions are usually indicative of meningococcemia, although they may be present with *H. influenzae* meningitis. Rashes very rarely occur with pneumococcal infections. The rapid development of multiple hemorrhagic eruptions in association with a shocklike state is almost pathognomonic of meningococcemia (Waterhouse-Friderichsen syndrome). Joint involvement suggests meningococcal or *H. influenzae* infection and can occur early (suppurative arthritis) or late (reactive arthritis) in the illness.

The presence of a chronically draining ear or a history of head trauma with or without skull fracture is most likely associated with pneumococcal meningitis.

Meningitis in Infancy

Infants 3 months to 1 year of age seldom develop the classic picture of meningitis. Fever, vomiting, marked irritability, convulsions, somnolence, and abnormal cry usually characterize the illness. A significant physical finding is a tense, bulging fontanelle, which usually occurs late during the course of illness. Nuchal rigidity may be absent, and Brudzinski's and Kernig's signs are difficult to elicit in this age-group.

Because the highest incidence of meningitis occurs between 6 and 12 months of age, any unexplained, persistent febrile illness in an infant should prompt suspicion of CNS involvement.

Neonatal Meningitis

Meningitis in newborn and premature infants is extremely difficult to recognize. The clinical manifestations are vague and nonspecific. In general, if the diagnosis of sepsis is entertained, the presence of meningitis should be ruled out. Fever is frequently absent. Refusal of feedings, vomiting, excessive irritability or drowsiness, irregular respirations, and jaundice are commonly associated with sepsis and meningitis. At later stages, the fontanelle may be full, tense, or bulging in approximately one third of cases.

DIAGNOSIS

A diagnosis of acute bacterial meningitis cannot be made on the basis of symptoms and signs alone. The classic meningeal findings are frequently minimal or absent or can result from meningismus or from tuberculous or aseptic meningitis. A definitive diagnosis is dependent on CSF examination and culture.

Indications for Lumbar Puncture

A properly performed lumbar puncture is a relatively innocuous procedure. Nevertheless, because of its invasiveness, it should not be done indiscriminately. Whenever the physician suspects meningitis, a lumbar puncture should be performed. Early diagnosis followed by appropriate medical management can have a favorable effect on the outcome; consequently, it is preferable to perform a lumbar puncture that yields normal CSF than to miss an early diagnosis of bacterial meningitis.

In neonates the procedure should be considered when sepsis is suspected, because meningitis accompanies sepsis in 20% to 25% of cases. It may be necessary to postpone the lumbar puncture for hours or several days in some infants with significant cardiopulmonary instability.

In many instances, particularly in infants, fever and convulsions may be the only initial signs of meningitis. It is hazardous to attribute seizures to uncomplicated febrile convulsions. In children older than 2 years of age clinical acumen may enable the skilled physician to identify those children with uncomplicated febrile seizures from those who have meningitis. Nevertheless, it is prudent to perform a lumbar puncture in any infant or child with a febrile convulsion when meningitis cannot be excluded from the diagnosis.

When focal neurologic signs, especially pupillary signs or cardiovascular instability, are present, whether accompanied by papilledema or not, the use of cranial computed tomography (CT) or magnetic resonance imaging (MRI) should be considered before the lumbar puncture to exclude a brain abscess or generalized cerebral edema and to avoid the danger of herniation. If such a procedure will significantly delay treatment, however, antibiotic therapy should be started before the lumbar tap. The subsequent lumbar puncture, when clinically indicated, is conducted under manometric guidance, using a small-gauge needle, with slow removal of the smallest volume of CSF necessary for the diagnostic tests.

Cerebrospinal Fluid Findings

Examination of the CSF of a patient with acute bacterial meningitis characteristically reveals the following: (1) a cloudy appearance, (2) an increased white blood cell count with a polymorphonuclear leukocyte predominance, (3) a low glucose concentration in relation to the serum glucose concentration, (4) an elevated protein concentration, (5) a smear and culture positive for the causative microorganism, and (6) a high manometric pressure. Commonly found CSF findings in patients with bacterial meningitis are shown in Table 17-1.

Cell Count. Normal white blood cell count values depend on the patient's age. During the neonatal period CSF from uninfected infants contains less than 11 leukocytes/mm^3, with an average ± 1 standard deviation of 7.3 ± 14.0 cells/mm^3 (Ahmed et al., 1996). As many as two thirds of those cells can be polymorphonuclear leukocytes. In very low birth weight infants the normal range of values is greater (Rodriguez et al., 1990). By 1 month of age, counts in the range of 0 to 6 cells/mm^3 are noted, and there is rarely more than 1 polymorphonuclear cell/mm^3.

In patients with acute bacterial meningitis the cell count can be extremely variable, but it is usually in the range of 1,000 to 5,000 leukocytes/mm^3. In rare instances, particularly very early in the illness, the cell count may be normal despite a positive CSF culture. In these cases, a lumbar puncture repeated several hours later usually shows characteristic leukocyte values. Although predominance of polymorphonuclear leukocytes is the rule, ap-

Table 17-1 Normal and characteristic abnormal CSF findings in pediatric age-groups with or without bacterial meningitis*

Finding	Neonates† Normal	Neonates† Abnormal	Infants and children Normal	Infants and children Abnormal
Leukocyte count (cells/μl)	<30	>100	<10	>1000
Polymorphonuclear (%)	<60	>80	≤10	>60-80
Protein (mg/dl)	<170	>200	<40	>100
CSF/blood glucose ratio	>0.6	<0.5	>0.5	<0.4
Manometric pressure (mm H$_2$O)	<60	>100	<90	>150

*Patients with aseptic meningitis can have CSF findings that are indeterminant or fit in the abnormal category.
†Normal values may be different in very low birth weight infants (Rodriguez et al., 1990).

proximately 10% of patients with bacterial meningitis show a monocytic pattern, particularly patients with *L. monocytogenes* meningitis.

Glucose. In most patients with bacterial meningitis the CSF glucose concentration is low as a result of increased utilization from metabolic demands. A CSF glucose concentration that is less than half the simultaneously obtained blood glucose concentration usually is considered abnormal. A CSF glucose concentration of less than 20 mg/dl is associated with a higher incidence of hearing impairment. The rapid return of the glucose concentration to near normal is generally a good early index of a favorable response to therapy.

Protein. Protein concentrations usually are elevated in patients with bacterial meningitis. Values less than 40 mg/dl are considered normal in infants and children, and those greater than 100 mg/dl suggest bacterial disease is present. Protein concentrations of more than 100 mg/dl commonly are observed in healthy, uninfected newborn infants, especially premature babies.

Smears. The probability of visualizing bacteria on a gram-stained CSF preparation is dependent on the number of organisms present. In general, a properly prepared smear examined by an experienced person is positive in as many as 80% of cases. The sensitivity is low, however, when *L. monocytogenes* is the cause of meningitis because usually a small number of organisms ($\leq 10^3$ colony-forming units/ml) is present in CSF. Because of the possibility of misidentification, antibiotic therapy should not be tailored for a specific organism on the basis of the stained smear; instead, the results of the culture should be awaited.

CSF Cultures. Culture should be performed routinely on all spinal fluid specimens, even those that are clear on gross inspection and show no increase in the leukocyte count. The yield of positive CSF cultures falls from 70% to 85% to below 50% in patients previously treated with antibiotics, although often there is insignificant change in the CSF inflammatory indices.

CSF Pressure. The mean opening lumbar CSF pressure is generally elevated in patients with bacterial meningitis. Normal values usually do not exceed 50 to 60 mm H$_2$O in newborns and 80 to 90 mm H$_2$O in infants and children (Minns et al., 1989). At the time of diagnosis opening pressures greater than 150 to 200 mm H$_2$O are commonly found in infants and children with bacterial meningitis.

Rapid Diagnostic Tests

Antigen detection by latex particle agglutination has become a routine part of the diagnosis of bacterial meningitis. Identification of the capsular polysaccharide of meningococci, pneumococci, group B streptococci, and *H. influenzae* type b in CSF is possible in many cases. These tests are not meant to replace the CSF culture but are a useful adjunct to the CSF examination and immediate diagnosis. False-negative and rare false-positive tests can occur. A positive antigen test is usually meaningful, but a negative test is unreliable for excluding a diagnosis of bacterial meningitis. The sensitivity of the rapid antigen tests for meningeal pathogens is highest for *H. influenzae* type b.

In patients who have received effective antimicrobial therapy before the first lumbar puncture the CSF findings likely will be modified but still indicative of bacterial meningitis. On the second day of treatment the leukocyte count generally rises.

Thereafter it decreases, and there can be a predominance of lymphocytes by the fifth day or later. Gram-stained smear and culture may be negative in pretreated patients, but antigen detection tests can still be useful. The CSF glucose and protein concentrations generally will remain abnormal for several days despite effective treatment.

DIFFERENTIAL DIAGNOSIS

Acute bacterial meningitis can simulate other inflammatory diseases that involve the meninges either directly or indirectly. Typical cases do not usually pose a diagnostic dilemma. In some instances, however, the spinal fluid findings in patients with bacterial disease do not conform to the typical picture, and confusion can occur in distinguishing viral or mycobacterial meningitis from meningitis caused by the usual bacterial agents.

Aseptic Meningitis

In children with aseptic or proved viral meningitis the spinal fluid commonly shows an increase in lymphocytes and a normal or only slightly decreased glucose concentration, with a slightly elevated protein concentration. Early in the disease the CSF can reveal a large number of polymorphonuclear cells, but a repeat lumbar tap 12 to 24 hours later will demonstrate the typical lymphocyte predominance in CSF. Amplification of genetic material using polymerase chain reaction provides a specific diagnosis within hours, especially for enteroviruses.

Tuberculous Meningitis

Tuberculous meningitis may be clinically indistinguishable from acute bacterial meningitis. The diagnosis is established by (1) an increase in number of CSF leukocytes, usually from 50 to 500 cells/mm^3, with a predominance of lymphocytes, a low glucose, very elevated protein concentrations, and a culture negative for the usual pathogenic organisms but subsequently positive for tubercle bacilli; (2) a positive tuberculin skin test; (3) chest roentgenograms showing evidence of a tuberculous lesion; and (4) a positive history of contact with an active case of tuberculosis.

Brain Abscess

Brain abscess can result from head trauma, chronic otitis media and sinusitis, or septic embolization in children with cyanotic congenital heart disease. The symptoms are usually not as acute as those of meningitis, and focal neurologic signs can be present. Results of the spinal fluid examination are highly variable and can either be normal or show an increase in leukocytes, a normal glucose value, and a slightly elevated protein concentration. The culture of the CSF specimen is usually sterile. Rupture of the abscess into the subarachnoid space or ventricles will result in purulent meningitis with a positive CSF culture. Abscess is frequently associated with *Citrobacter diversus* meningitis of the neonate.

Brain Tumor

The findings with a brain tumor are similar to those with brain abscess except that the course is more insidious, fever is usually absent, and the patient is usually not acutely ill.

Meningismus

Meningismus is characterized by symptoms and signs of meningeal irritation and normal results from spinal fluid examination and culture. It is usually associated with pneumonia, acute otitis media, acute tonsillitis, or other infectious diseases.

Lead Encephalopathy

Lead encephalopathy in infants and children can simulate meningitis. The spinal fluid has a normal glucose concentration, an increased protein concentration, and normal or slightly elevated lymphocyte count. Helpful diagnostic aids include (1) a blood smear showing basophilic stippling, (2) roentgenographic evidence of a line of increased density at the metaphyseal ends of the long bones in growing children, (3) coproporphyrinuria, and (4) an increased blood lead value.

COMPLICATIONS

Complications of acute bacterial meningitis can develop early in the course of illness, either before diagnosis or after several days of the start of treatment.

Systemic Circulatory Manifestations

Systemic circulatory manifestations usually occur during the first hospital day of acute bacterial meningitis. Peripheral circulatory collapse is one of the most dramatic and most serious complications of meningitis. It most frequently is associated with meningococcemia but can accompany other types of infection. Profound shock usually develops early in the course of the illness and, if untreated, progresses rapidly to a fatal outcome. Disseminated intravascular coagulation (DIC) can be an associated finding. Gangrene of the distal extremities can occur in patients with fulminant hemorrhagic meningococcal meningitis. It has been recognized that in some patients antibiotic therapy can initially aggravate these systemic phenomena, probably as a result of release of cell wall or membrane active components such as endotoxin from rapidly lysed microorganisms.

It has been commonly believed that many patients with bacterial meningitis have syndrome of inappropriate antidiuretic hormone (SIADH) secretion requiring fluid restriction in the initial management of patients with neuroinfection. Recent experimental and clinical investigations, however, have suggested that the elevated antidiuretic hormone (ADH) serum concentration is an appropriate host response to unrecognized hypovolemia and that a more liberal use of parenteral fluids can be beneficial (Powell et al., 1990; Tureen et al., 1992; Singhi et al., 1995). In addition, systemic blood pressure must be maintained at levels sufficient to prevent compromise of cerebral perfusion.

Neurologic Complications

Focal neurologic findings such as hemiparesis, quadriparesis, facial palsy, and visual field defects occur early or late in approximately 10% to 15% of patients with meningitis and may correlate with persistent abnormal neurologic examinations on long-term follow-up assessments. Presence of focal signs can be associated with cortical necrosis, occlusive vasculitis, or thrombosis of the cortical veins. Extension of the meningeal inflammatory process can involve the second, third, sixth, seventh, and eighth cranial nerves that course through the subarachnoid space. Inflammation of the cochlear aqueduct and the auditory nerve can lead to reversible or permanent deafness in 5% to 20% of cases. Hydrocephalus of either the communicating or obstructive type is occasionally seen in patients in whom treatment has been either suboptimal or delayed, occurring more often in younger infants. Brain abscesses can rarely complicate the course of meningitis, particularly in newborn infants infected with *C. diversus* or *Proteus* species.

Seizures

Seizure disorders occur before or in the first several days after admission to the hospital in as many as one third of patients with meningitis. Although most of these episodes are generalized, focal seizures are more likely to presage an adverse neurologic outcome. In addition, seizures that are difficult to control or that persist beyond the fourth hospital day and seizures that occur for the first time late in the patient's hospital course have a greater likelihood of being associated with neurologic sequelae.

Subdural Collections of Fluid

Subdural effusions are not generally associated with signs and symptoms, commonly resolve spontaneously, are present in more than one third of patients with meningitis, and usually are not associated with permanent neurologic abnormalities (Snedeker et al., 1990). These collections are less frequently present with meningococcal than with *H. influenzae* or pneumococcal meningitis. Subdural effusions occur principally in infants less than 2 years of age. Indications for performing needle puncture of a subdural effusion include a clinical suspicion that empyema is present (prolonged fever and irritability, stiff neck coupled with CSF leukocytosis), a rapidly enlarging head circumference in a child without hydrocephalus, focal neurologic findings, and/or evidence of increased intracranial pressure.

Arthritis

Joint involvement may be present initially or develop during the course of bacterial meningitis. Early occurrence suggests direct invasion of the joint by the microorganism, usually *H. influenzae* type b, whereas arthritis that develops after the fourth day of therapy is believed to be an immune complex–mediated event that usually involves several joints and is most frequently seen with meningococcal infections.

Other Complications

Buccal or preseptal cellulitis, pneumonia, and pericarditis can also be present in patients with bacterial meningitis, particularly complicating invasive *H. influenzae* infections in infants.

PROGNOSIS

The prognosis in individual patients with bacterial meningitis is correlated with many factors, including (1) age of patient, (2) duration and type of illness before effective antibiotic therapy is instituted, (3) microorganism, (4) number of bacteria or the quantity of active bacterial products in CSF at the time of diagnosis, (5) intensity of the host's inflammatory response, and (6) time needed to sterilize CSF cultures.

As a rule, the younger the patient, the poorer the prognosis. The highest mortality and morbidity rates occur in the neonatal period. Infections caused by group B streptococci, gram-negative enteric bacilli, and pneumococci are associated with poorer outcome from disease. Delay in starting antimicrobial therapy in some patients or in sterilizing CSF cultures has been recognized to increase the rate of adverse outcome. The amount of bacteria or their products correlates with an increased host production of inflammatory mediators such as TNF, IL-1, and prostaglandins. The greater the host's inflammatory response in the subarachnoid space to the microorganism and its products, the greater the likelihood of permanent sequelae.

With prompt and adequate antimicrobial and supportive therapy, the chances for survival today are excellent, especially in infants and children, for whom case fatality rates have been reduced to less than 10%. Long-term sequelae, however, have not been dramatically reduced, despite the advent of extraordinarily active β-lactam antibiotics and highly sophisticated intensive care management. The incidence rate of residual abnormalities in postmeningitic children is approximately 15% (with a range of 10% to 30%). Infants and children who survive bacterial meningitis are more apt to have seizures, hearing deficits, learning and/or behavioral problems, and lower intelligence compared with their siblings who did not have meningitis. Several recent studies have demonstrated that residual neurologic and audiologic abnormalities are reduced in patients who received early dexamethasone therapy (see the following discussion).

TREATMENT

Optimal management of infants and children with bacterial meningitis requires appropriate antimicrobial therapy, fluid and electrolyte adjustments, control of cardiovascular stability and intracranial pressure, and anticonvulsant therapy. The role of corticosteroids has been extensively studied in animal models of meningitis and in patients with bacterial meningitis, and evidence strongly suggests that dexamethasone given before parenteral antimicrobial therapy is beneficial in modulating rapidly the meningeal inflammatory response and in improving long-term outcome in infants and children (Odio et al., 1991; Schaad et al., 1993; Kanra et al., 1995).

Antimicrobial Therapy

Optimal antibiotic therapy entails the selection of appropriate agents that are effective against the likely pathogens and are able to attain adequate bactericidal activity in CSF. The initial empiric regimen chosen for treatment should be broad enough to cover the potential organisms for the age-group involved. Recommended dosages are listed in Table 17-2.

Newborn Infants. In the neonatal period the organisms most often responsible for meningitis are group B *Streptococcus, E. coli* and other gram-negative enteric bacilli, *L. monocytogenes,* and enterococci. The initial empiric regimen used con-

Table 17-2 Daily dosages of recommended antimicrobial agents for treatment of bacterial meningitis in pediatric age-groups*

Drugs	Neonates†		Infants and children
	0-7 Days	**8-28 Days**	
Amikacin‡	15-20 div q12	20-30 div q8	20-30 div q8
Ampicillin	100-150 div q12	150-200 div q8 or 6	200-300 div q6
Cefotaxime§	100 div q12	150-200 div q8 or 6	200-225 div q8
Ceftazidime	60 div q12	90 div q8	150 div q8
Ceftriaxone	—	—	100 once daily
Chloramphenicol‡	25 once daily	50 div q12	75-100 div q6
Gentamicin‡	5 div q12	7.5 div q8	7.5 div q8
Nafcillin/oxacillin	100-150 div q12	150-200 div q8 or 6	200 div q6
Penicillin G	150,000 div q12	200,000 div q8 or 6	250,000 div q6 or 4
Tobramycin‡	5 div q12	6 div q8	6 div q8
Vancomycin‡	30 div q12	45 div q8	60 div q6

*Dosages are expressed in milligrams per kilogram of body weight per day and divided *(div)* for administration every *(q)* 12, 8, 6, or 4 hours. Penicillin is expressed in units per kilogram.

†Daily dosages may be different for very low birth weight infants (Prober et al., 1990).

‡Serum concentrations should be monitored and dosages adjusted accordingly.

§Cefotaxime has been used at dosages up to 360 mg/kg/day for resistant pneumococci.

ventionally has been ampicillin (or penicillin G) and an aminoglycoside. Because of the emergence of aminoglycoside-resistant gram-negative enteric bacilli in some neonatal units, the concern about possible adverse auditory and renal effects, and the relatively low bactericidal activity of aminoglycosides in the CSF, many centers in the United States are now using ampicillin and cefotaxime for initial, empiric treatment of neonatal meningitis. Although cefotaxime is effective for treatment of bacterial meningitis, there is concern that the routine use of a cephalosporin in neonatal intensive care units will lead to rapid emergence of resistant organisms, especially among *Enterobacter cloacae, Proteus* species, and *Serratia* species. By contrast, the use of cefotaxime is advantageous from the standpoint of achieving high CSF bactericidal activity against most coliforms and of avoiding the necessity to monitor serum concentrations of the aminoglycoside to attain safe and therapeutic concentrations. Ceftriaxone, although equivalent in efficacy to cefotaxime, is not recommended for use in the neonatal period because of the potential displacement of bilirubin from albumin-binding sites and its inhibitory effect on growth of the bacterial flora of the intestinal tract. We continue to recommend ampicillin and an aminoglycoside for initial empiric treatment of suspected neonatal meningitis; when the specific pathogen is identified and results of susceptibilities are known, antimicrobial therapy can be modified accordingly. In newborns with meningitis caused by susceptible gram-negative enteric organisms, cefotaxime can be used safely and effectively, either alone or combined with an aminoglycoside. For meningitis caused by group B streptococci or *L. monocytogenes,* ampicillin alone is usually satisfactory after an initial 48 to 72 hours of combined therapy with an aminoglycoside. The possible exception is for disease caused rarely by a tolerant strain (inhibited but not killed by achievable CSF concentrations of ampicillin) of group B *Streptococcus,* in which case combination therapy is continued for the entire course.

The duration of therapy for neonatal meningitis depends on the clinical response and duration of positive CSF cultures after therapy is initiated. Ten to 14 days is usually satisfactory for disease caused by the group B *Streptococcus* and *L. monocytogenes,* and a minimum of 2 weeks of treatment after CSF cultures are sterile is required for gram-negative enteric meningitis. Because of the unpredictable clinical course of illness and the unreliability of the clinical examination in assessing response to therapy in neonates, we believe that the CSF should be examined and cultured at completion of therapy to determine whether additional treatment is required. Additionally, we recommend a cranial CT scan or MRI be performed during treatment to be certain that intracranial complications have not occurred.

One- to Three-Month-Old Infants. Infants 1 to 3 months old are arbitrarily considered as a special category because of the broad array of possible causative agents implicated in meningitis. These agents include the pathogens encountered in neonates and those that usually cause disease in older infants, namely *H. influenzae* type b, *S. pneumoniae,* and *N. meningitidis.* Ampicillin and cefotaxime or ampicillin and ceftriaxone constitute a suitable initial empiric regimen, because in some patients *Listeria* or enterococci (resistant to the cephalosporin) can be the causative agent.

Infants and Children. Therapy with ampicillin and chloramphenicol was effective for many years. Currently, however, cefotaxime and ceftriaxone are widely recommended for treatment of meningitis in infants and children because of their extraordinary in vitro activity against the common meningeal pathogens, their excellent safety record, and their ability to promptly sterilize CSF cultures. Chloramphenicol has been increasingly abandoned because of its unpredictable metabolism in young infants; its pharmacologic interaction when administered concomitantly with phenobarbital, phenytoin, rifampin, or acetaminophen; and the requirement for monitoring its serum concentrations to avoid toxic or subtherapeutic values.

Another reason for using third-generation cephalosporins in the management of meningitis is the fact that currently 20% or more of *S. pneumoniae* strains in the United States are resistant to penicillin. This figure is even higher in some other countries. As many as one half of these strains are moderately resistant (minimum inhibitory concentration [MIC] 0.1 to 1.0 mg/ml), and the rest are considered highly resistant (MIC >1.0 mg/ml). Some of these strains are also resistant to chloramphenicol and to third-generation cephalosporins. Although many of the infections caused by intermedially resistant strains can be successfully treated with either cefotaxime or ceftriaxone (especially in high dosages), we recommend the addition of vancomycin to the initial empiric regimen to ensure eradication of these strains from CSF. Strains of *N. meningitidis* with partial resistance to penicillin have also been encountered in the United States and some other parts of the world. To date, however, no penicillin failures have been reported for these isolates.

We recommend strongly that a repeat lumbar puncture be performed at 24 to 48 hours after admission if a resistant pneumococcus has been isolated from the initial CSF culture and if the patient has not shown dramatic clinical improvement. Modification of antimicrobial regimen should be done according to bacteriologic and clinical findings. Seven days of treatment is satisfactory for most infants and children with uncomplicated meningococcal meningitis, 7 to 10 days for *Haemophilus* disease, and 10 days or longer for pneumococcal meningitis. Performing a lumbar puncture at completion of therapy in a child with uncomplicated meningitis is not recommended, because the information obtained is not useful in predicting which patient will develop bacteriologic relapse (Schaad et al., 1981).

Steroid Therapy

Several prospective, double-blind, placebo-controlled studies evaluating the role of steroids in infants and children with bacterial meningitis have been recently published. In most trials dexamethasone therapy has been associated with improvement in meningeal inflammatory indices, with reduction in CSF cytokine concentrations, and with fewer audiologic and/or neurologic sequelae when compared with placebo recipients. Dexamethasone treatment was not associated with delayed sterilization of CSF cultures nor with a higher incidence of recurrent disease. A few children developed gastrointestinal bleeding while receiving the steroid. Superior outcome versus that in placebo recipients was seen when dexamethasone was given early (i.e., before the first parenteral antibiotic dose) as opposed to late (i.e., after several hours or more of antimicrobial treatment) (Table 17-3). Animal studies have confirmed the critical importance of timing to achieve optimal beneficial effects with dexamethasone therapy. Initial studies used a dexamethasone dosage of 0.15 mg/kg every 6 hours for a total of 4 days. From recent reports it appears that similar beneficial results can be obtained by using a dosage of 0.4 mg/kg every 12 hours for 2 days (Schaad et al., 1993; Syrogiannopoulos et al., 1994).

Although most of the meningitis cases in these prospective studies were caused by *H. influenzae,* data suggest that the salutary effects associated with dexamethasone therapy apply also to pneumococcal meningitis (Kennedy et al., 1991; Kanra et al., 1995). Concern, however, has been raised with the use of steroids in patients with infection caused by resistant pneumococcal strains because of the decreased penetration of antibiotics when dexamethasone is used (Paris et al., 1994). Clinical data, however, suggest that dexamethasone does not interfere with eradication of resistant pneumococci achieved by combined treatment with a third-generation cephalosporin and vancomycin. Based on currently available data, we believe that the ad-

Table 17-3 Long-term sequelae observed in children with meningitis given in 6 randomized, double-blind, placebo-controlled studies of dexamethasone therapy: outcome in relation to timing of the first steroid dose

Author	Number of patients	Antibiotic	Steroid administration in relation to antibiotic	Total sequelae (%) Placebo	Dexamethasone	P-value
Early Dexamethasone Therapy*						
Odio	101	Cefotaxime	15-20 min before	38	14	0.007
Schaad	115	Ceftriaxone	10 min before	16	5	0.066
Kanra	56	Ampicillin Sulbactam	15 min before	27	7	0.062
Late Dexamethasone Therapy†						
Lebel	95	Ceftriaxone	2-3 hours after	20	6	0.065
Wald	143	Ceftriaxone	≤4 hours after	14	9	0.434
King	101	Ceftriaxone	>10 hours after	14	15	1.00

*Sequelae in the early group: steroid: 9%, placebo: 26%; $P = 0.0003$; odds ratio (OR) 0.27 (95% confidence intervals (CI): 0.13-0.57).
†Sequelae in the late group: steroid: 10%, placebo: 16%; $P = 0.14$; OR 0.058 (95% CI: 0.29-1.17).

vantages of dexamethasone therapy, especially when given before the first parenterally administered antibiotic dose, clearly outweigh the possible disadvantages and that its use is strongly recommended for therapy of bacterial meningitis in infants and children. Some physicians do not recommend adjunctive steroid therapy (Kaplan, 1995). Its usefulness in infants younger than 6 weeks has not been established.

SUPPORTIVE THERAPY

Adequate oxygenation, prevention of hypoglycemia and hyponatremia, anticonvulsant therapy, and measures designed to decrease intracranial hypertension and to prevent fluctuation in cerebral blood flow are a crucial part of the management of patients with bacterial meningitis.

Infants and children with alteration of consciousness, pupillary changes, and/or cardiovascular instability should have intracranial pressure monitored. Among measures to reduce abnormal pressures are elevation of the head of the bed to approximately 30 degrees, avoidance of vigorous suctioning and chest physiotherapy, maintenance of normal serum osmolarity, fluid restriction in documented cases of SIADH (dehydration and hypotension should be avoided), and use of mannitol to decrease cerebral edema. A recent report (Kilpi et al., 1995) suggested that glycerol, another hyperosmolar agent given orally, improved significantly the outcome of infants and children as compared with placebo recipients. Further placebo-controlled, blinded studies are required before glycerol can be recommended routinely.

Optimal cerebral perfusion can be maintained by controlling fever to reduce the brain's metabolic demands, by maintaining arterial blood pressures within normal limits, and by hyperventilation to reduce arterial carbon dioxide tension (Pco_2) to a range of 25 to 30 mm Hg (Ross and Scheld, 1989). The use of hyperventilation, however, has been questioned by some authorities who believe that it should not be used in children with bacterial meningitis and evidence of cerebral edema on CT scan, because intracranial pressure would be decreased at the expense of a reduction in cerebral blood flow, possibly approaching ischemic thresholds (Ashwal et al., 1994).

PREVENTION
Vaccination

Immunization is the most effective means of preventing bacterial meningitis in children. Sixty to seventy percent of all *H. influenzae* meningitis cases occur in infants younger than 18 months old. The new conjugated *Haemophilus* vaccines are considerably more immunogenic than the initial polysaccharide vaccine, and studies in Finland and in the United States have demonstrated immunogenicity and protection after initiation of a two- to three-dose vaccine regimen at 2 to 3 months of age (Black et al., 1991; Madore et al., 1990; Makela et al., 1990; Santosham et al., 1991). Vaccination beginning at this age was approved for routine use in the United States in late 1990; depending on the vaccine used, a three- or four-dose regimen is recommended. Routine use of these conjugated vaccines has been associated with disappearance of invasive diseases caused by *H. influenzae* type b organisms in developed areas of the world (Peltola et al., 1992; Adams et al., 1993).

A polyvalent meningococcal vaccine, containing the purified polysaccharide capsules of group A, C, Y, and W-135 organisms, is available but is not recommended for general use in infants and young children. The vaccine is recommended for children older than 2 years of age who are at high risk of infection, such as those with asplenia or with terminal complement deficiencies. Recently, Cuba and Norway have manufactured OMP vaccines against the group B meningococcus. Field trials performed in several parts of the world showed a modest estimated efficacy, with the lowest protection observed in young children (Riedo et al., 1995). It is possible, but unproved, that these vaccines can provide the potential for control of epidemic disease caused by this organism. More immunogenic vaccines directed to multiple meningococcal serotypes are clearly needed to prevent these infections in infants and young children.

The currently manufactured pneumococcal vaccine is composed of purified capsular polysaccharide antigen from 23 pneumococcal serotypes. It is recommended for children older than 2 years of age who are at increased risk of developing pneumococcal disease, including those with asplenia, especially patients with sickle cell hemoglobinopathies, with nephrotic syndrome, and with recurrent meningitis after head trauma. Ongoing research is evaluating promising protein-conjugated polysaccharide pneumococcal vaccines, which have incorporated the 5 to 8 serotypes that most commonly infect young children, aimed at achieving in infants the immunogenicity and efficacy similar to those obtained with *Haemophilus* conjugated vaccines.

Chemoprophylaxis

Intrapartum ampicillin (2 gm initially; 1 to 2 gm every 4 to 6 hours) given to high-risk women with prenatal vaginal or rectal group B streptococcal colonization has been associated with reduced rates of neonatal colonization and of early-onset group B streptococcal sepsis (Gotoff, 1984). Risk factors include preterm labor at less than 37 weeks gestation, premature rupture of membranes beyond 12 to 18 hours, intrapartum fever, multiple births, maternal group B streptococcal urinary tract infection, and previous delivery of a sibling with invasive group B *streptococcus* (GBS) disease. Penicillin-allergic women may be given intravenous clindamycin.

In infants and children, rifampin prophylaxis for *Haemophilus* disease is recommended for all household contacts, irrespective of age, when at least one unvaccinated contact is younger than 4 years of age. The dose is 20 mg/kg daily given for 4 days. The index case should receive rifampin at or near completion of therapy for the *H. influenzae* infection. A recent report, however, suggests that treatment of meningitis with a third-generation cephalosporin effectively eliminates nasopharyngeal carriage of *H. influenzae* organisms, making prophylaxis in the index case unwarranted (Goldwater, 1995). Management of day-care and extended home-care groups must be individualized. The efficacy of rifampin prophylaxis in day-care attendees is unproved, and the difficulties in delivering prophylaxis to many individuals in such centers can be considerable. Accordingly, prophylaxis is recommended only after two cases of disease have occurred among attendees within 2 months in a day-care or home-care setting, provided that many of these children have not been fully vaccinated.

Household and day-care contacts of an index case of meningococcal disease should be given rifampin prophylaxis in a dosage of 10 mg/kg given every 12 hours for four doses or in the same regimen as recommended for *Haemophilus* prophylaxis. Ceftriaxone given in a single intramuscular dose (125 mg for children younger than 12 years; 250 mg for those older than 12 years and adults) has been demonstrated to be more effective than oral rifampin in eliminating meningococcal group A nasopharyngeal carriage, thereby allowing its use when oral rifampin cannot be taken (e.g., during pregnancy) or when compliance with the oral regimen is unlikely (Schwartz et al., 1988). Ciprofloxacin given as a single, oral dose of 500 mg to adults is also effective in eradicating meningococcal carriage.

BIBLIOGRAPHY

Adams WG, Deaver KA, Cochi SL, et al. Decline of childhood *Haemophilus influenzae* type b disease in the Hib vaccine era. JAMA 1993;269:221.

Ahmed A, Hickey SM, Ehrett S, et al. Cerebrospinal fluid values in the term neonate. Pediatr Infect Dis J 1996;15:298.

Appelbaum PC, Scragg JN, Bowen AJ, et al. *Streptococcus pneumoniae* resistant to penicillin and chloramphenicol. Lancet 1977;2:995.

Arditi M, Ables L, Yogev R. Cerebrospinal fluid endotoxin levels in children with *H. influenzae* meningitis before and after administration of intravenous ceftriaxone. J Infect Dis 1989;160:1005.

Ashwal S, Perkin RM, Thompson JR, et al. Bacterial meningitis in children: current concepts of neurologic management. Curr Prob Pediatr 1994;267:84.

Auslander MC, Meskan ME. The pattern and stability of post meningitic hearing loss in children. Laryngoscope 1988;98:940.

Baker CJ. Prevention of neonatal group B streptococcal disease. Pediatr Infect Dis 1983;2:1.

Black SB, Shinefield H, Fireman B, et al. Efficacy in infancy of oligosaccharide conjugate *Haemophilus influenzae* type b (HbOC) vaccine in a United States population of 61,080 children. Pediatr Infect Dis 1991;10:97-104.

Burnes LE, Hodgman JE, Cass AB. Fatal circulatory collapse in premature infants receiving chloramphenicol. N Engl J Med 1959;261:1318.

Converse GM, Gwaltney JM Jr, Strassburg DA, et al. Alteration of cerebrospinal fluid findings by partial treatment of bacterial meningitis. J Pediatr 1973;83:220.

Dajani AS, Asmar BI, Thirumoorthi MC. Systemic *Haemophilus influenzae* disease: an overview. J Pediatr 1979;94:355.

Del Rio M, Chrane D, Shelton S, et al. Ceftriaxone versus ampicillin and chloramphenicol for treatment of bacterial meningitis in children. Lancet 1983;1:1241.

Dodge PR, Swartz MN. Bacterial meningitis. A review of selected aspects. N Engl J Med 1965;272:725.

Feldman HA. Meningococcal disease. JAMA 1966;196:105.

Feldman WE. Concentrations of bacteria in cerebrospinal fluid of patients with bacterial meningitis. J Pediatr 1976;88:549.

Feldman WE. Relation of concentrations of bacteria and bacterial antigen in cerebrospinal fluid to prognosis in patients with bacterial meningitis. N Engl J Med 1977;296:433.

Fishman RA. Brain edema. N Engl J Med 1975;193:706.

Fraser DW, Darby CP, Koehler RE, et al. Risk factors in bacterial meningitis. J Infect Dis 1973;127:271.

Galaid EI, Cherubin CE, Marr JS, et al. Meningococcal disease in New York City, 1973 to 1978 recognition CR groups Y and W-135 as frequent pathogens. JAMA 1980;211:2167.

Gartner JC, Michaels RM. Meningitis from a pneumococcus moderately resistant to penicillin. JAMA 1979;241:1707.

Ginsburg CM, McCracken GH Jr, Rae S, et al. *Haemophilus influenzae* type b disease: incidence in a day care center. JAMA 1977;12:604.

Girgis NL, Farid Z, Makhail IA, et al. Dexamethasone treatment for bacterial meningitis in children and adults. Pediatr Infect Dis J 1989;8:848.

Goldwater PN. Effect of cefotaxime or ceftriaxone treatment on nasopharyngeal *Haemophilus influenzae* type b colonization in children. Antimicrob Agents Chemother 1995;39:2150.

Gotoff SP. Chemoprophylaxis of early onset group B streptococcal disease. Pediatr Infect Dis J 1984;3:401.

Graham DR, Band JD. *Citrobacter diversus* brain abscess and meningitis in neonates. JAMA 1981;245:1923.

Istre GR, Tarpay M, Anderson M, et al. Invasive disease due to *Streptococcus pneumoniae* in an area with a high rate of relative penicillin resistance. J Infect Dis 1987;156:732.

Jacobs MR, Koornhof HJ, Robins-Browne RM, et al. Emergence of multiply resistant pneumococci. N Engl J Med 1978;299:735.

Jacobs RF, His S, Wilson CB, et al. Apparent meningococcemia: clinical features of disease due to *Haemophilus influenzae* and *Neisseria meningitidis*. Pediatrics 1983;72:469.

Kanra GY, Ozen H, Secmeer G, et al. Beneficial effects of dexamethasone in children with pneumococcal meningitis. Pediatr Infect Dis J 1995;14:490.

Kaplan SL. Adjunctive therapy in meningitis. Adv Pediatr Infect Dis 1995;10:167.

Kaplan SL, Feigin RD. Treatment of meningitis in children. Pediatr Clin North Am 1983;30:259.

Kaplan SL, Goddard J, Van Kleeck M, et al. Ataxia and deafness in children due to bacterial meningitis. Pediatrics 1981; 68:8.

Kennedy WA, Hoyt MJ, McCracken GH Jr. The role of corticosteroid therapy in children with pneumococcal meningitis. Amer J Dis Child 1991;145:1374.

Kessler SL, Dajani AS. *Listeria* meningitis in infants and children. Pediatr Infect Dis 1990;9:61.

Kilpi T, Peltola H, Jauhiainen T, et al. Oral glycerol and intravenous dexamethasone in preventing neurologic and audiologic sequelae of childhood bacterial meningitis. Pediatr Infect Dis J 1995;14:270.

King SM, Law B, Langley JM, et al. Dexamethasone therapy for bacterial meningitis: better never than late? Can J Infect Dis 1994;5:219.

Klein JO, Feigin RD, McCracken GH Jr. Report of the task force on diagnosis and management of meningitis. Pediatrics 1986;78:959.

Lebel MH, Freij BJ, Syrogiannopoulos GA, et al. Dexamethasone therapy for bacterial meningitis; results of two double-blind, placebo-controlled trials. N Engl J Med 1988;319: 964.

Lebel MH, Hoyt MJ, McCracken GH Jr. Comparative efficacy of ceftriaxone and cefuroxime for treatment of bacterial meningitis. J Pediatr 1989;114:1049.

Leedom MJ, Inler D, Mathies AW, et al. The problems of sulfadiazine-resistant meningococci. Antimicrob Agents Chemother 1966;6:281.

Linnan MJ, Mascola L, Lou XD, et al. Epidemic listeriosis associated with Mexican-style cheese. N Engl J Med 1988; 319:823.

Madore DV, Johnson CL, Phipps DC, et al. Safety and immunologic response to *Haemophilus influenzae* type b oligosaccharide-CRM 197 conjugate vaccine in 1- to 6-month-old infants. Pediatrics 1990;85:331.

Makela PH, Eskola J, Peltola HO, et al. Clinical experience with *Haemophilus influenzae* type b conjugate vaccines. Pediatrics 1990;85(4S):651.

McCracken GH Jr. Neonatal septicemia and meningitis. Hosp Pract 1976;11:89.

McCracken GH Jr. New developments in the management of children with bacterial meningitis. Pediatr Infect Dis 1984; 3:532.

McCracken GH Jr, Lebel MH. Dexamethasone therapy for bacterial meningitis in infants and children. Am J Dis Child 1989;143:287.

Mertsola J, Ramilo O, Mustafa MM, et al. Release of endotoxin after antibiotic treatment of gram negative bacterial meningitis. Pediatr Infect Dis 1989;8:904.

Minns RA, Engleman KIM, Stirling H. Cerebrospinal fluid pressure in pyogenic meningitis. Arch Dis Child 1989; 64:814.

Moreno MT, Vargas S, Poveda R, Séz-Llorens X. Neonatal sepsis and meningitis in a developing Latin American country. Pediatr Infect Dis J 1994;13:516.

Murphy TV, White KS, Pastor P, et al. Declining incidence of *Haemophilus influenzae* type b disease since introduction of vaccination. J Amer Med Assoc 1993;269:246.

Mustafa MM, Ramilo O, Sáez-Llorens X, et al. Cerebrospinal fluid prostaglandins, interleukin-1β and tumor necrosis factor in bacterial meningitis: clinical and laboratory correlations in placebo and dexamethasone-treated patients. Am J Dis Child 1990;144:883.

Nelson JD. How preventable is bacterial meningitis? N Engl J Med 1982;307:1265.

Nelson JD. Cerebrospinal fluid shunt infections. Pediatr Infect Dis 1984;3:530.

Odio CM, Faingezicht I, Paris M, et al. The beneficial effects of early dexamethasone administration on infants and children with bacterial meningitis. N Engl J Med 1991;324:1525-1531.

Paredes A, Taber LH, Yow MD, et al. Prolonged pneumococcal meningitis due to an organism with increased resistance to penicillin. Pediatrics 1976;58:378.

Paris MM, Hickey SM, Uscher MI, et al. Effect of dexamethasone on therapy of experimental penicillin- and cephalosporin-resistant pneumococcal meningitis. Antimicrob Agents Chemother 1994;38:1320.

Peltola H, Kilpi T, Anttila M. Rapid disappearance of *Haemophilus influenzae* type b meningitis after routine childhood immunization with conjugated vaccines. Lancet 1992;340:592.

Pfister HW, Fontana A, Tauber MG, et al. Mechanisms of brain injury in bacterial meningitis: workshop summary. CID 1994;19:463.

Portnoy JM, Olsen LC. Normal cerebrospinal fluid values in children: another look. Pediatrics 1985;75:484.

Powell KR, Sugarman LI, Eskenazi AE, et al. Normalization of plasma arginine vasopressin concentrations when children with meningitis are given maintenance plus replacement fluid therapy. J Pediatr 1990;117:515.

Prober CG, Stevenson DK, Benitz WE. The use of antibiotics in neonates weighing less than 1200 grams. Pediatr Infect Dis 1990;9:111.

Ramilo O, Sáez-Llorens X, Mertsola J, et al. Tumor necrosis factor α/cachectin and interleukin-1β initiate meningeal inflammation. J Exp Med 1990;172:497.

Rapkin RH. Repeat lumbar punctures in the diagnosis of meningitis. Pediatrics 1974;54:34.

Riedo FX, Plikaytis BD, Broome CV. Epidemiology and prevention of meningococcal disease. Pediatr Infect Dis J 1995;14:643.

Rodriguez AF, Kaplan SL, Mason EO Jr. Cerebrospinal fluid values in the very low birth weight infant. J Pediatr 1990;116:971.

Ross KL, Scheld WM. The management of fulminant meningitis in the intensive care unit. Infect Dis Clin North Am 1989;3:137.

Sáez-Llorens X, Ramilo O, Mustafa MM, et al. Molecular pathophysiology of bacterial meningitis: current concepts and therapeutic implications. J Pediatr 1990;116:671.

Sande MA, Tauber MG, Scheld M, McCracken GH Jr. Pathophysiology of bacterial meningitis: summary of the workshop. Pediatr Infect Dis 1989;8:929.

Santosham M, Wolff M, Reid R, et al. The efficacy in Navajo infants of a conjugate vaccine consisting of *Haemophilus influenzae* type b polysaccharide and *Neisseria meningiditus* outer-membrane protein complex. N Engl J Med 1991; 324:1767-1772.

Schaad UB, Lips U, Gnehm HE, et al. Dexamethasone therapy for bacterial meningitis in children. Lancet 1993;342:457.

Schaad UB, Nelson JD, McCracken GH Jr. Recrudescence and relapse in bacterial meningitis of childhood. Pediatrics 1981;67:188.

Scheld WM, Fletcher DD, Fink FN, et al. Response to therapy in an experimental rabbit model of meningitis due to *Listeria monocytogenes*. J Infect Dis 1979;140:287.

Schwartz B, Al-Ruwais A, As Ashi J, et al. Comparative efficacy of ceftriaxone and rifampicin in eradicating pharyngeal carriage of group A *Neisseria meningitidis*. Lancet 1988;1:1239.

Sell SH. Long term sequelae of bacterial meningitis in children. Pediatr Infect Dis 1983;2:90.

Shapiro ED. Prophylaxis for contacts of patients with meningococcal or *Haemophilus influenzae* type b disease. Pediatr Infect Dis 1982;1:132.

Siegel JD, Shannon KM, DePasse BM. Recurrent infection associated with penicillin-tolerant group B streptococci: a report of two cases. J Pediatr 1981;99:920.

Singhi SC, Singhi PD, Srinivas B, et al. Fluid restriction does not improve the outcome of acute meningitis. Pediatr Infect Dis J 1995;14:495.

Snedecker JD, Kaplan SL, Dodge PR, et al. Subdural effusion and its relationship with neurologic sequelae of bacterial meningitis in infancy: a prospective study. Pediatrics 1990; S6:163.

Syrogiannopoulos GA, Hansen EJ, Erwin AL, et al. *Haemophilus influenzae* type b lipopolysaccharide induces meningeal inflammation. J Infect Dis 1988;157:237.

Syrogiannopoulos GA, Lourida AN, Theodoridou MC, et al. Dexamethasone therapy for bacterial meningitis in children: 2 versus 4 day regimen. J Infect Dis 1994;169:853.

Tauber MC. Brain edema, intracranial pressure, and cerebral blood flow in bacterial meningitis. Pediatr Infect Dis 1989; 8:915.

Tauber MG, Sehibl AM, Hackbarth CJ, et al. Antibiotic therapy, endotoxin concentration in cerebrospinal fluid, and brain edema in experimental *Escherichia coli* meningitis in rabbits. J Infect Dis 1987;156:456.

Tikhomirov E. Meningococcal meningitis: global situation and control measures. World Health Stat Q 1987;40:98.

Toews WH, Bass JW. Skin manifestations of meningococcal infection. Am J Dis Child 1974;127:173.

Tuomanen E. Molecular mechanisms of inflammation in experimental pneumococcal meningitis. Pediatr Infect Dis 1987; 6:1146.

Toumanen E, Liu H, Hengstler B, et al. The induction of meningeal inflammation by components of the pneumococcal cell wall. J Infect Dis 1985;151:859.

Tureen JH, Dworkin RJ, Kennedy SL, et al. Loss of cerebrovascular autoregulation in experimental meningitis in rabbits. J Clin Invest 1990;85:577.

Tureen JM, Tauber MG, Sande MA. Effect of hydration status on cerebral blood flow and cerebrospinal fluid lactic acidosis in rabbits with experimental meningitis. J Clin Invest 1992; 89:947.

Waage A, Halstensen A, Espevik T. Association between tumor necrosis factor in serum and fatal outcome in patients with meningococcal disease. Lancet 1987;1:355.

Wald ER, Kaplan SL, Mason EO, et al. Dexamethasone therapy for children with bacterial meningitis. Pediatrics 1995; 95:21.

Ward JI, Fraser DW, Baroff LJ, et al. *Haemophilus influenzae* meningitis a national study of secondary spread in household contacts. N Engl J Med 1979;301:122.

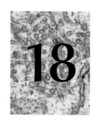

18   MUMPS

Mumps (epidemic parotitis) is an acute contagious disease caused by a paramyxovirus that has a predilection for glandular and nervous tissue. Mumps is characterized most commonly by enlargement of the salivary glands, particularly the parotid glands. One or more of the following manifestations of mumps may be associated with or may occur without parotitis: meningoencephalitis, orchitis, pancreatitis, and other glandular involvement. Inapparent infection occurs in a significant percentage of persons (30% to 40%).

ETIOLOGY

Mumps is caused by a specific virus belonging to the parainfluenza subgroup of the paramyxoviruses. It ranges in size from 90 to 135 nm. It is infective for monkeys and chick embryos and produces cytopathic effects in a variety of tissue cultures of primary monkey kidney, human embryonic kidney, and human diploid fibroblasts. Infectivity is lost as a result of heating at 55° to 60° C for 20 minutes and after exposure to formalin or to ultraviolet light. Infectivity is maintained for years at temperatures of −20° to −70° C. Mumps virus has an antigenic relationship to other members of the myxovirus group, including Newcastle disease virus and parainfluenza viruses.

PATHOLOGY

The mumps-infected parotid gland is rarely available for pathologic examination. The interstitial tissue shows edema and infiltration with lymphocytes. The cells of the ducts degenerate, with accumulation of necrotic debris and polymorphonuclear leukocytes in the lumina. Inclusion bodies are not seen. Mumps orchitis is characterized by edema and a perivascular lymphocytic infiltrate that progresses to involve the interstitial tissue. There are focal hemorrhage and destruction of germinal epithelium, producing plugging of the tubules by epithelial debris, fibrin, and polymorphonuclear leukocytes.

PATHOGENESIS

The current concept of the pathogenesis of mumps stems from experience gained from a variety of epidemiologic, immunologic, clinical, and experimental studies. The virus probably enters through the nose or mouth. Proliferation takes place in either the parotid gland or the superficial epithelium of the respiratory tract. This is followed by viremia, with subsequent localization of virus in glandular or nervous tissue. The parotid gland is most often involved. Mumps virus has been isolated from human saliva, blood, urine, and cerebrospinal fluid (CSF) during the acute phase of the illness. The salivary glands, brain, and spinal cord of experimentally infected monkeys also have yielded virus. The concept of mumps as a generalized infection has been well documented.

CLINICAL MANIFESTATIONS

For a long time the terms *mumps* and *epidemic parotitis* were used interchangeably. Mumps was recognized as primarily an infection of the salivary glands. The isolation of the virus and the development of serologic specific tests, however, have contributed to a better understanding of the pathogenesis and a clarification of the clinical picture of the disease.

Infection with mumps virus usually develops after an incubation period of 16 to 18 days. In approximately 30% to 40% of the patients the resulting infection is inapparent. The remaining 60% to 70% of the patients develop an illness of variable severity, with symptoms that depend on the site or sites of infection. In the majority of instances clinical mumps is characterized only by parotitis, either unilateral or bilateral. Additional relatively common manifestations include submaxillary and sublingual gland infection, orchitis, and meningoencephalitis. Pancreatitis, oophoritis, thyroiditis, and other glandular infections are relatively rare. These various manifestations of mumps may precede, accompany, follow, or occur without parotitis.

Salivary Gland Involvement

The classic illness is ushered in by fever, headache, anorexia, and malaise. Within 24 hours the child complains of an "earache" localized near the lobe of the ear and aggravated by chewing movements of the jaw. The following day the enlarged parotid gland is noticeable and rapidly progresses to its maximum size within 1 to 3 days. The fever usually subsides after a variable period of 1 to 6 days, with the temperature returning to normal before the glandular swelling disappears.

The normal parotid gland is not palpable. It is horseshoe shaped, with the concave portion adjacent to the lobe of the ear (Fig. 18-1). An imaginary line bisecting the long axis of the ear and passing through the ear lobe divides the gland into two relatively equal parts. These anatomic relationships are not altered by the enlarging parotid gland. As the swelling progresses, the lobe of the ear is displaced upward and outward. During the phase of rapid parotid enlargement, the pain and tenderness may be severe. These symptoms subside after the swelling has reached its peak. The enlarged parotid

gland gradually decreases in size over a period of 3 to 7 days. Thus the swelling may be present for possibly 6 to 10 days. Usually one parotid gland enlarges first, and within a few days the other enlarges. Occasionally, both sides swell simultaneously. Approximately 25% of all patients have unilateral parotitis.

The submaxillary swelling, when present, may be seen and palpated beneath the mandible just anterior to the angle of the jaw and directly beneath the anterior portion of the masseter muscle (Fig. 18-2). During the early stages the edema surrounding the submaxillary gland may spread over the mandible onto the cheek and downward toward the neck. When submaxillary mumps occurs without parotitis, it is clinically indistinguishable from cervical adenitis.

Sublingual mumps is usually bilateral and begins as a swelling in the submental region and on the floor of the mouth. Of the three salivary glands, the sublinguals are the least commonly involved.

The clinical picture of mumps just described is the classic one. The disease, however, is extremely variable. Occasionally, the appearance of local glandular swelling and tenderness may be the only manifestation of infection. Fever and constitutional symptoms may be absent.

Frequently, the orifices of the ducts show inflammatory changes. The openings of Stensen's (parotid) and Wharton's (submaxillary) ducts may be reddened and edematous. Patients with exten-

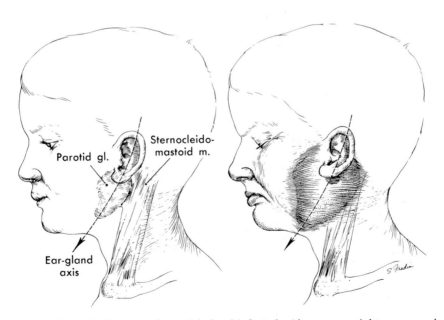

FIG. 18-1 Schematic drawing of parotid gland infected with mumps, *right,* compared with normal gland, *left.* An enlarged cervical lymph node is usually posterior to the imaginary line.

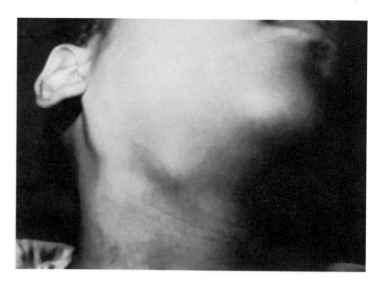

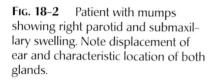

Fig. 18-2   Patient with mumps showing right parotid and submaxillary swelling. Note displacement of ear and characteristic location of both glands.

sive salivary gland involvement may develop edema in the presternal area. It has been postulated that this is caused by an obstruction of the lymphatic vessels by the enlarged salivary glands.

Epididymo-Orchitis

Epididymo-orchitis is the second most common manifestation of mumps infection in the adult male. It usually follows parotitis, but it may precede it or occur as an isolated manifestation of mumps. Epididymitis invariably is associated with the orchitis. Unilateral involvement occurs in 20% to 30% of males who develop the disease after puberty. The incidence of bilateral orchitis is low—approximately 2%. Under epidemic conditions the incidence of orchitis may be higher. In 1959 Philip et al. described an epidemic of 363 cases of mumps in a "virgin" population on St. Lawrence Island in the Bering Sea. The incidence of orchitis in males more than 10 years of age was approximately 35%; bilateral orchitis occurred in approximately 12%. Orchitis develops within the first 2 weeks of infection, most commonly during the first week. In rare instances it may be delayed to the third week. Mumps orchitis may occur in the absence of salivary gland involvement.

Orchitis begins abruptly with fever, chills, headache, nausea, vomiting, and lower abdominal pain. The systemic reaction usually parallels the extent of gonadal involvement. The temperature may vary from normal to over 40° C (104° F). The duration of fever rarely exceeds 1 week. It persists for 3 days or less in approximately 20% of cases, 4 days or less in 50%, and 5 days or less in 80%. The

temperature falls by crisis in approximately half the cases and by lysis in the remainder.

With the appearance of the fever, the testis begins to swell rapidly and becomes very painful and tender. It may increase in size very slightly or to as much as four times that of the normal gland. As the fever subsides, the pain and swelling disappear. The tenderness, however, persists for a longer period. As the testis decreases in size, a change of consistency is noted—loss of turgor. In approximately half of the cases this is subsequently followed by atrophy. However, at least half of the involved glands do return to normal. One of the most important concerns of men with mumps orchitis is the fear that sexual impotence and sterility will follow, but this sequela is rare. Most orchitis is unilateral. Even with bilateral involvement, it would be rare to have complete atrophy of both glands. The extensive experience with mumps orchitis in World Wars I and II failed to demonstrate that impotence and sterility are frequent consequences of this infection.

Meningoencephalitis

Central nervous system (CNS) involvement is another common manifestation of mumps. Symptomatic disease has been estimated to occur in approximately 10% of all cases. In a study by Bang and Bang (1944) 62% of 371 patients with mumps parotitis had cells in the CSF. Of this group 106 (28%) had CNS symptoms. Mumps meningoencephalitis usually follows the parotitis by 3 to 10 days. However, it may precede or even occur in the absence of salivary gland involvement (Fig. 18-3).

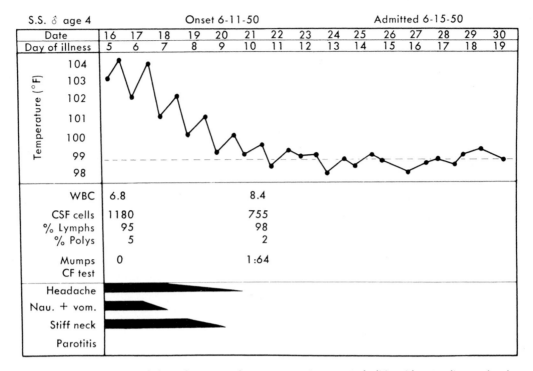

S.S. ♂ age 4   Onset 6-11-50   Admitted 6-15-50

Date	16	17	18	19	20	21	22	23	24	25	26	27	28	29	30
Day of illness	5	6	7	8	9	10	11	12	13	14	15	16	17	18	19

WBC	6.8		8.4
CSF cells	1180		755
% Lymphs	95		98
% Polys	5		2
Mumps CF test	0		1:64

Headache
Nau. + vom.
Stiff neck
Parotitis

FIG. 18-3   Diagram of clinical course of mumps meningoencephalitis without salivary gland involvement. Pleocytosis with predominance of lymphocytes was found. The diagnosis was established by the development of complement-fixing antibody between the fifth and tenth days of illness.

The illness is characterized by fever, headache, nausea, vomiting, nuchal rigidity, change in sensorium, and, only rarely, convulsions. Brudzinski's and Kernig's signs can be elicited. The CSF shows pleocytosis, with a predominance of lymphocytes, normal glucose content, and elevated protein level. Although the glucose content is usually normal, cases with hypoglycorrhachia have been reported (Wilfert, 1969). The temperature usually falls by lysis over a period of 3 to 10 days. As the fever subsides, the symptoms clear, and recovery is usually uneventful. The infection follows the course of benign aseptic meningitis (see Chapter 38) and usually has no sequelae.

Pancreatitis

Pancreatitis is a severe but uncommon manifestation of mumps infection. There is a sudden onset of severe epigastric pain and tenderness associated with fever, chills, extreme weakness, prostration, nausea, and repeated bouts of vomiting. The symptoms gradually subside over a period of 3 to 7 days, and the patient usually recovers completely.

Other Clinical Manifestations

The development of fever, nausea, vomiting, and lower abdominal pain in the female with mumps points to oophoritis. When the right ovary is involved, the signs and symptoms may be indistinguishable from those of acute appendicitis. Many other glands may be involved in the infection. Thyroiditis, mastitis, dacryoadenitis, and bartholinitis are rare manifestations of mumps. In general, except for the symptoms caused by the local swelling, the course is essentially the same as for any other mumps infection.

DIAGNOSIS
Confirmatory Clinical Factors

The following factors should point to mumps as a diagnostic possibility: (1) a history of exposure to mumps 2 to 3 weeks before onset of illness, (2) a compatible clinical picture of parotitis or other glandular involvement, and (3) signs of aseptic meningitis.

In the classic case of so-called epidemic parotitis, confirmatory laboratory procedures are usually unnecessary. In the absence of parotitis or in the presence of recurrent parotitis, however, use of the following specific diagnostic aids may be necessary.

Isolation of Causative Agent

Mumps virus can be recovered from the saliva, mouth washings, or urine during the acute phase of parotitis and from the CSF early in the course of meningoencephalitis. Shedding of virus in the urine may persist for as long as 2 weeks after disease onset. Mumps virus is readily isolated after inoculation of appropriate clinical specimens into a variety of host systems such as rhesus monkey kidney cells and human embryonic lung fibroblasts. Rapid identification of the agent may be accomplished by use of cells grown in shell vials with fluorescein-labeled monoclonal antibodies to identify the virus.

Serologic Tests

A number of serologic tests are used to demonstrate the development of specific mumps antibody: complement fixation (CF), hemagglutination-inhibition (HI), enzyme-linked immunosorbent assay (ELISA), and virus neutralization. The CF and ELISA tests are the most practical and most reliable of these diagnostic procedures.

The formation of mumps CF antibody after infection is shown in Fig. 18-4. The antibody becomes detectable in the blood by the end of the first week, and by the end of the second week a fourfold or greater rise in antibody titer can be demonstrated. When a diagnosis of mumps is suspected, acute and convalescent sera should be tested simultaneously. A fourfold or greater rise in the level of antibody confirms the diagnosis. This test is particularly useful for the diagnosis of mumps meningoencephalitis without parotitis, as is illustrated in Fig. 18-3.

Ancillary Laboratory Findings

The serum amylase level is elevated in both mumps parotitis and pancreatitis. The levels seem to parallel the parotid swelling. The values reach a peak during the first week, gradually returning to normal by the second and third weeks. Serum amylase determinations are abnormal in approximately 70% of cases of mumps parotitis. The finding of normal serum amylase levels may aid in the identification of obscure swellings about the jaw that resemble parotid involvement. The white blood cell count may be normal or slightly elevated. Usually there is a slight predominance of lymphocytes, but at times the reverse is true.

DIFFERENTIAL DIAGNOSIS
Parotitis

Mumps parotitis may be simulated by various conditions affecting the parotid glands or neighboring lymph nodes. Anterior cervical or preauricular

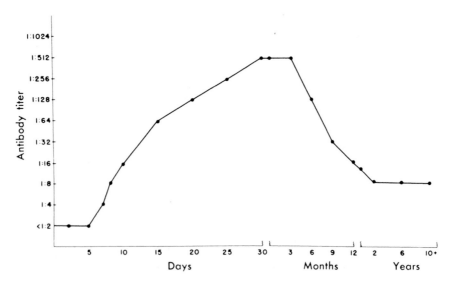

FIG. 18-4 Schematic curve illustrating development of mumps complement-fixing antibody. A significant rise in the level of antibody can be demonstrated in the serum by the end of the second week of illness. The acute and convalescent serum specimens should be tested simultaneously.

adenitis involvement of the lymph nodes, with surrounding edema, may simulate mumps parotitis. The parotid gland can usually be identified by its characteristic location, consistency, and outline. Its anatomic relationship to the ear is illustrated in Fig. 18-1. A line bisecting the long axis and lobe of the ear passes through the center of the gland. It has a brawny consistency with a well-defined posterior border and ill-defined anterior and inferior borders. In contrast, an enlarged lymph node has a well-defined, discrete border, is firm, and does not have the characteristic anatomic relationship to the ear. The appearance of the opening of Stensen's duct does not help very much. An elevated serum amylase level would point to parotid involvement. A mumps antibody test clarifies the diagnosis.

Suppurative Parotitis. In suppurative parotitis the skin over the gland is usually red and hot, and the gland is exquisitely tender. Pus may be expressed from Stensen's duct by massaging the gland. An increase in the number of polymorphonuclear leukocytes is usually present. Although aerobic bacteria such as *Staphylococcus aureus* are the most common cause of acute suppurative parotitis, occasionally anaerobic bacteria *(Bacteroides, Fusobacterium,* and *Peptostreptococcus)* may be responsible (Brook and Finegold, 1978).

Recurrent Parotitis. Recurrent parotitis, a condition of unknown and probably varied causes, is characterized by frequent recurrent swellings of the parotid gland. Infection and hypersensitivity to certain drugs such as iodides and phenothiazines may have a role in the causation of this disease. Roentgenographic studies of the duct system reveal evidence of sialectasia in some cases. The individual attack may be clinically indistinguishable from mumps parotitis. The submaxillary and sublingual glands, which are frequently associated with mumps parotitis, are not involved in recurrent parotitis. The history of previous attacks and a negative or unchanging CF test clarifies the diagnosis.

Calculus. A calculus that obstructs Stensen's duct causes a swelling of the parotid gland that is usually intermittent.

Coxsackie Virus Infection. In 1957 Howlett et al. described a syndrome of parotitis and herpangina caused by Coxsackie virus.

Parainfluenza 3 Virus Infection. In 1970 Zollar and Mufson reported on two children in whom acute parotitis was associated with detection of parainfluenza 3 virus and a significant rise in the level of homologous antibody.

Mixed Tumors, Hemangiomas, and Lymphangiomas of the Parotid. Mixed tumors, hemangiomas, and lymphangiomas of the parotid are responsible for chronic enlargement of the gland and are confused with mumps only during the early stages.

Mikulicz's Syndrome. In Mikulicz's syndrome there is chronic bilateral parotid and lacrimal gland enlargement, usually associated with dryness of the mouth and absence of tears.

Uveoparotid Fever. Uveoparotid fever is a manifestation of sarcoidosis, which may be confused with mumps.

HIV Infection. Bilateral parotid swelling may accompany human immunodeficiency virus (HIV) infection in children, but this condition is chronic, lasting for months to years. Parotitis in HIV-infected children is often associated with pulmonary lymphoid interstitial hyperplasia (LIP).

Meningoencephalitis

Mumps meningoencephalitis without parotitis is clinically indistinguishable from aseptic meningitis caused by Coxsackie virus, ECHO virus, lymphocytic choriomeningitis virus, and a variety of other agents (see Chapter 38). The specific mumps antibody test or virus isolation usually establishes the diagnosis.

COMPLICATIONS
Deafness

Deafness is a very rare but serious complication of mumps. There is usually a sudden onset of vertigo, tinnitus, ataxia, and vomiting followed by permanent deafness. In most cases it is unilateral. The cause has been ascribed to neuritis of the auditory nerve.

Other Neurologic Complications

Other neurologic complications, also very rare, include facial neuritis, myelitis, and postinfectious encephalitis. The latter, like measles encephalitis, may be fatal or complicated by serious sequelae. This type of encephalitis occurs very infrequently.

Myocarditis

Myocarditis as a complication of mumps has occasionally been observed in adults. Electrocardiographic findings indicate that the incidence may be 15%. The development of dyspnea, tachycardia, or bradycardia during the first 2 weeks of illness associated with T-wave changes and prolongation of the PR interval should suggest this diagnosis. The myocarditis is usually followed by an uneventful recovery. More rarely, pericarditis also may occur.

Arthritis

Arthritis also has been described as a rare complication of mumps. It usually appears as migrating polyarthritis involving the larger and smaller joints and clears spontaneously.

Diabetes Mellitus

It has been suggested that some cases of diabetes mellitus may be associated with a previous mumps virus infection. The relationship of mumps virus to diabetes mellitus has been studied epidemiologically and experimentally for many years without clear resolution of the possible role of the virus in the pathogenesis of this disease.

Hepatitis

Hepatitis has been reported as a rare complication of mumps. From the available descriptions, however, it is difficult to determine whether it is truly a complication or possibly a coincident development of viral hepatitis.

Hematologic Complications

Unusual hematologic complications have included thrombocytopenia and hemolytic anemia. They have been severe but self-limited (Graham et al., 1974).

PROGNOSIS

In general, the prognosis of mumps is excellent. Fatalities are very rare. Meningoencephalitis is usually benign and is rarely followed by sequelae. In spite of high incidence of testicular atrophy following orchitis, sterility is extremely rare. In a small percentage of cases permanent deafness may complicate the disease.

IMMUNITY

One attack usually confers lifelong immunity. Mumps may recur, but the rate (4%) cited for second attacks probably reflects errors in diagnosis. Acute cervical adenitis and recurrent parotitis are likely to be erroneously diagnosed as mumps. A survey of 100 patients referred to a communicable disease hospital with a diagnosis of mumps revealed that 5% of the group had cervical adenitis. Permanent immunity is conferred by an attack of any type of mumps infection, including unilateral parotitis, meningoencephalitis without parotitis, or orchitis without parotitis. Indeed, even clinically inapparent infections also confer a lasting immunity. Infants born of mothers who have had mumps have passive immunity that lasts for several months.

A number of tests are available to measure the immune status of a person. These include HI, CF, ELISA, and virus neutralization. Note in Fig. 18-4 that the titer of mumps complement-fixing antibody persists at a low level for many months or years after infection. In a small percentage of cases the antibody level may fall below the detectable range. However, a positive CF test usually indicates past infection.

Several studies have correlated the results of serologic tests with patients who have past histories of a clinical case of mumps. Analysis of the data indicates that 30% to 40% of all susceptible persons exposed to mumps develop the infection in an inapparent form. These conclusions were confirmed experimentally by Henle et al. in 1948 (Fig. 18-5). Of a group of 15 susceptible subjects who were deliberately exposed to mumps, four developed parotitis, two developed submaxillary swelling, and one developed orchitis. The remaining eight subjects developed an inapparent infection as indicated by the isolation of virus and the rise in mumps complement-fixing antibody.

EPIDEMIOLOGIC FACTORS

During the prevaccine era mumps was an endemic disease in most urban populations. In institutions in which crowding favored virus transmission, epidemics occurred frequently. Most cases of mumps occurred in the 5- to 10-year age-group, with approximately 85% of the infections among children less than 15 years of age. It was uncommon in infancy. The age-group affected by mumps was older than those groups affected by measles, varicella, and pertussis. Consequently, there were epidemics

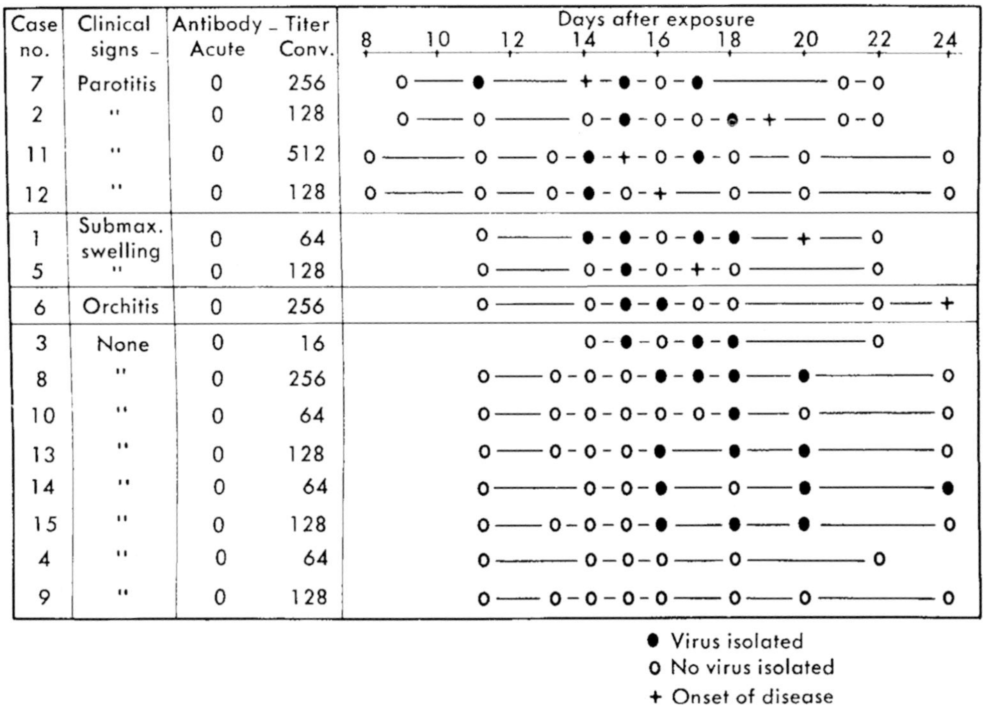

Case no.	Clinical signs	Antibody Titer — Acute	Antibody Titer — Conv.	Days after exposure (8–24)
7	Parotitis	0	256	
2	"	0	128	
11	"	0	512	
12	"	0	128	
1	Submax. swelling	0	64	
5	"	0	128	
6	Orchitis	0	256	
3	None	0	16	
8	"	0	256	
10	"	0	64	
13	"	0	128	
14	"	0	64	
15	"	0	128	
4	"	0	64	
9	"	0	128	

● Virus isolated
○ No virus isolated
+ Onset of disease

FIG. 18-5   Isolation of virus from saliva of patients with apparent and inapparent mumps infection. Virus was detected from 1 to 6 days before onset of salivary gland involvement. Virus was also readily isolated from six to eight patients with inapparent infection. Significant antibody levels developed in all 15 patients who were studied. (From Henle G et al: J Exp Med 1948;88:223.)

among adolescents in boarding schools and among adults in the armed forces. The disease has occurred in persons of all ages, ranging from 1 day to 99 years.

In 1967 when the live attenuated mumps virus vaccine was introduced in the United States, there were 185,691 reported cases of mumps. After routine use of the vaccine was recommended in 1977, there was a progressive decline to an all-time low of 2,982 cases in 1985. The number of reported cases in 1991 was about 4,000, a 97% decrease from 1967.

Mumps is probably acquired through the oropharynx. The source of infection may be saliva or other virus-containing secretions of an infected person. Transmission occurs by direct contact or by droplet infection. The available epidemiologic evidence suggests that the period of infectivity is from several days before the onset of symptoms to the subsidence of the salivary gland swelling. In the average case this represents a period of approximately 7 to 10 days.

The study of experimentally induced mumps infection by Henle et al. (1948) (see Fig. 18-5) has contributed significant data clarifying the period of infectivity. In the patients who developed parotitis 14 to 19 days after exposure, mumps virus was isolated from the saliva as many as 1 to 4 days before onset of parotitis. One patient who developed only submaxillary swelling on the twentieth day yielded mumps virus from the saliva 6 days before. It is of interest that six of the patients with inapparent infection secreted mumps virus in the saliva between the fifteenth and twenty-fourth days after exposure. This is a striking example of how an inapparent case of mumps can be the potential source for the spread of mumps infection. In a later study in 1958 Utz et al. isolated mumps virus in urine as early as the first day of salivary gland involvement and as late as the fourteenth day of illness.

Based on experience with other live attenuated vaccines, it is likely that live attenuated mumps virus vaccine could abort an epidemic in progress. The high incidence of inapparent cases and the infectivity of patients before onset of parotitis both combine to limit the effectiveness of quarantine or isolation. In the past the patient was isolated until the swelling of the salivary gland had subsided. In our opinion, too much time and effort should not be wasted on outmoded rigid isolation and quarantine procedures.

TREATMENT

Mumps is a self-limited infection, the course of which is not altered by use of any of the antimicrobial drugs. Treatment is symptomatic, and supportive measures are used. Acetaminophen will usually control the pain caused by glandular swelling. Warm applications seem to help some patients; others prefer cold. Topical ointments are useless. Parenteral administration of fluids is indicated for the support of patients with persistent vomiting associated with pancreatitis or meningoencephalitis.

PREVENTIVE MEASURES
Passive Protection

Standard immune globulin is ineffective against mumps. The efficacy of mumps-immune globulin is also questionable. During an epidemic of mumps in Alaska, Reed et al. (1967) evaluated the effect of mumps-immune globulin. The attack rate of mumps was 46% among 56 susceptible individuals who received globulin; it was 45% among 185 susceptible persons who did not receive globulin. In addition, under the conditions of this study there was no evidence that the mumps-immune globulin prevented orchitis or meningoencephalitis.

Active Immunization*

Mumps virus vaccine is prepared in chick-embryo cell culture; it was introduced into the United States in December, 1967. The vaccine produces a subclinical, noncommunicable infection with very few side effects. Mumps vaccine is available both in monovalent (mumps only) form and in combinations: mumps-rubella and measles-mumps-rubella (MMR) vaccines.

The vaccine is approximately 95% efficacious in preventing mumps disease, and vaccine-induced antibody is protective and long-lasting, although of considerably lower titer than antibody resulting from natural infection. Estimates of clinical vaccine efficacy ranging from 75% to 95% have been calculated from data collected in outbreak settings using different epidemiologic study designs.

Susceptible children, adolescents, and adults should be vaccinated against mumps, unless vacci-

nation is contraindicated. MMR vaccine is the vaccine of choice for routine administration and should be used in all situations in which recipients are also likely to be susceptible to measles and/or rubella. Persons should be considered susceptible to mumps unless they have documentation of (1) physician-diagnosed mumps, (2) adequate immunization with live mumps virus vaccine on or after their first birthday, or (3) laboratory evidence of immunity. Because live mumps vaccine was not used routinely before 1977 and because the peak age-specific incidence was in 5 to 9 year olds before the vaccine was introduced, most persons born before 1957 are likely to have been infected naturally between 1957 and 1977. Therefore they generally may be considered to be immune, even if they may not have had clinically recognizable mumps disease. However, this cutoff date for susceptibility is arbitrary. Persons who are unsure of their mumps disease history and/or mumps vaccination history should be vaccinated. Testing for susceptibility before vaccination, especially among adolescents and young adults, is not necessary.

Use of immune globulin (IG) has not been demonstrated to be of established value in postexposure prophylaxis and is not recommended. Mumps IG has not been shown to be effective and is no longer available or licensed for use in the United States. Reports of illnesses after mumps vaccination have mainly been episodes of parotitis and low-grade fever. Allergic reactions including rash, pruritus, and purpura have been temporally associated with mumps vaccination but are uncommon and usually mild and of brief duration. The reported occurrence of encephalitis within 30 days of receipt of a mumps-containing vaccine (0.4 per million doses) is not greater than the observed background incidence rate of CNS dysfunction in the normal population. Other manifestations of CNS involvement, such as febrile seizures and deafness, have also been infrequently reported. Complete recovery is usual. Although mumps vaccine virus has been shown to infect the placenta and fetus, there is no evidence that it causes congenital malformations in humans. However, because of the theoretic risk of fetal damage, it is prudent to avoid giving live virus vaccine to pregnant women. Because live mumps vaccine is produced in chick-embryo cell culture, persons with a history of anaphylactic reactions (hives, swelling of the mouth and throat, difficulty breathing, hypotension, or shock) after egg ingestion should be vaccinated only with caution using published protocols.

---

*Abstracted from MMWR 38:388-392, 397-400, June 9, 1989.

Passively acquired antibody can interfere with the response to live, attenuated-virus vaccines. Therefore mumps vaccine should be given at least 2 weeks before the administration of IG or deferred until approximately 3 months after the administration of IG. In theory, replication of the mumps vaccine virus may be potentiated in patients with immune deficiency diseases and by the suppressed immune responses that occur with leukemia, lymphoma, or generalized malignancy or with therapy with corticosteroids, alkylating drugs, antimetabolites, or radiation. In general, patients with such conditions should not be given live mumps virus vaccine. Because vaccinated persons do not transmit mumps vaccine virus, the risk of mumps exposure for those patients may be reduced by vaccinating their close susceptible contacts. An exception to these general recommendations is in children infected with HIV; all asymptomatic HIV-infected children should receive MMR at 15 months of age. Patients with leukemia in remission whose chemotherapy has been terminated for at least 3 months may also receive live mumps virus vaccine.

BIBLIOGRAPHY

Bang HO, Bang J. Involvement of the central nervous system in mumps. Bull Hyg 1944;19:503.

Brook I, Finegold SM: Acute suppurative parotitis caused by anaerobic bacteria: report of two cases. Pediatrics 1978; 62:1019.

Furesz J, Hockin JC. Comment to Champagne S, Thomas E. A case of mumps meningitis: a post-immunization complication? Can Dis Wkly Rep 1987;13:157.

Graham DY, Brown CH, Benrey J, Butel JS. Thrombocytopenia: a complication of mumps. JAMA 1974;227:1162.

Henle G, Henle W, Wendell KK, Rosenberg P. Isolation of mumps virus from human beings with induced apparent or inapparent infections. J Exp Med 1948;88:223.

Howlett JG, Somlo F, Kalz F. A new syndrome of parotitis with herpangina caused by the Coxsackie virus. Can Med Assoc J 1957;77:5.

Lennette E. Laboratory diagnosis of viral infections, ed. 2. New York: Marcel Dekker, 1992.

Nicolai-Scholten S, Ziegelmaier S, Behrens F, et al. The enzyme-linked immunosorbent assay (ELISA) for determination of IgG and IgM antibodies after infection with mumps virus. Med Microbiol Immunol 1980;168:81.

Philip RN, Reinhard KR, Lackmann DB. Observations on a mumps epidemic in a "virgin" population. Am J Hyg 1959;69:91.

Reed D, et al. A mumps epidemic on St. George Island, Alaska. JAMA 1967;199:113.

Sugiura A, Yamada A: Aseptic meningitis as a complication of mumps vaccination. Pediatr Infect Dis J 1991;10:209-213.

Sultz HA, Hart BA, Zielezny M: Is mumps virus an etiologic factor in juvenile diabetes mellitus? J Pediatr 1975;86:654.

Utz JP, Szwed CF, Kasel JA: Clinical and laboratory studies of mumps. II. Detection and duration of excretion of virus in urine. Proc Soc Exp Biol Med 1958;99:259.

Wilfert CM: Mumps meningoencephalitis with low cerebrospinal fluid glucose, prolonged pleocytosis and elevation of protein. N Engl J Med 1969;280:855.

Zollar LM, Mufson MA: Acute parotitis associated with parainfluenza 3 virus infection. Am J Dis Child 1970;119:147.

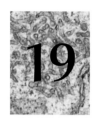

19   OSTEOMYELITIS AND SUPPURATIVE ARTHRITIS

LAURA GUTMAN

Suppurative skeletal infections are relatively uncommon in childhood, but when they occur, they are most likely to afflict young children. More than half of all cases occur in children younger than 5 years of age. This is a time of rapid skeletal growth, so damage to the growth plate or to joints has the potential for lifelong consequences. Skeletal infections are often difficult to recognize or localize early in the course of illness, and many are difficult to manage medically and surgically. Because prompt medical and surgical intervention probably decreases the likelihood of permanent sequelae, physicians who care for children should be aware of the earliest signs and symptoms of suppurative skeletal infections and be aggressive about establishing the diagnosis.

PATHOGENESIS AND EPIDEMIOLOGY

The majority of bone and joint infections are hematogenous in origin. However, infection less commonly can follow penetrating injuries or various medical and surgical maneuvers (e.g., arthroscopy, prosthetic joint surgery, intraarticular steroid injection, and various orthopedic surgeries). Impaired host defenses also can increase the risk of skeletal infection.

Significant blunt trauma is a preceding event in approximately one third of cases of osteomyelitis. Animal models of experimental osteomyelitis involve inflicting trauma to a bone of an animal that is bacteremic. The unique anatomy of the ends of long bones explains the predilection for localization of blood-borne bacteria. In the metaphysis are tiny vascular loops in which blood flow is sluggish. Rupture of some of these vessels as a result of trauma provides a favorable environment for multiplication of bacteria.

In the newborn and young infant there are blood vessels connecting the metaphysis and epiphysis, so it is common for pus from the metaphysis to rupture into the joint space. However, in the latter part of the first year of life the physis (growth plate) forms, there are no transphyseal blood vessels, and purulent infection of the joint occurs only rarely when the synovial attachment allows perforation of the periosteum to occur within the joint space. Bone is not distensible, so pus under pressure, prevented from decompressing into the joint, moves laterally through cortical vascular channels and accumulates under the loosely attached periosteum. After growth ceases, once again blood vessels connect the metaphysis and epiphysis.

Preceding trauma is less common in patients with suppurative arthritis, and the pathogenesis of hematogenous arthritis is poorly understood. The synovium is rich in blood vessels, and insignificant, unremembered trauma may play a role in pathogenesis. Possibly synovial membrane receptors for bacteria play a role in localization. For example, in the era before universal vaccination for *Haemophilus influenzae,* type b accounted for only approximately 10% of cases of osteomyelitis in children in the first 2 years of life (Lebel and Nelson, 1988), but it was the pathogen in 45% of cases of arthritis in that age-group (Fink and Nelson, 1986).

Both conditions are most common in young children (Table 19-1); this is particularly true of arthritis, in which one half of all cases occur in the first 2 years of life and three fourths of all cases by 5 years of age. The figures for osteomyelitis in those two age-groups are approximately one third and one half, respectively.

Skeletal infections consistently occur more commonly in boys than in girls in all reported series. The male-to-female ratio is approximately 2:1 in most series. If trauma is truly an important risk factor, it may be that the life-style of boys predisposes to traumatic events.

Apparently there is no particular predilection for arthritis or osteomyelitis based on race. In most se-

290

Table 19-1   Frequency of disease by age group*

Disease	Number of cases	Age-groups (yr)			
		<2	2-5	6-10	11-15
Osteomyelitis					
Number	399	127	101	108	63
Percent	100	32	25	27	16
Arthritis					
Number	682	362	172	102	46
Percent	100	53	25	15	7

*Based on J Nelson's series of cases.

Table 19-2   Infected bones in 372 patients with monosteal disease and 27 patients with polyosteal disease*

Bone	Monosteal	Polyosteal
Femur	93	12
Tibia	89	18
Humerus	50	8
Fibula	16	10
Phalanx	18	5
Calcaneus	18	0
Radius	13	4
Ischium	14	1
Metatarsus	8	0
Ulna	7	3
Ilium	7	0
Vertebra	7	2
Sacrum	3	0
Skull	3	0
Talus	3	1
Clavicle	2	2
Rib	2	1
Scapula	2	1
Carpal bone	2	0
Cuneiform	2	0
Pubis	3	1
Sternum	3	0
Metacarpus	2	0
One case each: maxilla, mandible, cuboid, bone of pyriform aperture, acetabulum	6	0

*Based on J Nelson's series of cases.

ries the racial distribution of cases reflects that of the local population.

CLINICAL FINDINGS

The earliest signs and symptoms of skeletal infection are often subtle. This is particularly true of the neonate, who characteristically is not ill (Wong et al., 1995). In a report summarizing 83 cases of neonatal osteomyelitis from the literature, 52% had no fever, and only 8% were described as appearing septic or toxic (Nelson, 1983). In infants only pseudoparalysis of an extremity or apparent pain on movement of the affected extremity may be present.

In older infants and children the majority have fever and localized signs. Redness and swelling of skin and soft tissue overlying the site of infection usually are seen earlier in patients with arthritis than in those with osteomyelitis. The exception is with hip involvement in which these signs are usually absent because of the deep location of that joint. In other joints the bulging, infected synovium is relatively near the surface, whereas the metaphyses are located deeper under the soft tissues. Local swelling and redness in a patient with osteomyelitis mean that the infection has spread out of the metaphysis into the subperiosteal space and that there is a secondary soft-tissue inflammatory response.

Nonspecific systemic signs of infection such as nausea, vomiting, diarrhea, and headache are not prominent features of skeletal infections even though many of the patients are bacteremic. If those signs are present, disseminated infection syndrome with multiple foci of disease should be suspected; this is most likely to occur with *Staphylococcus aureus* or group b streptococci.

Long bones are principally involved in osteomyelitis (Table 19-2). The femur and tibia are equally affected and together constitute almost half of all cases (Unkila-Kallio et al., 1993). The bones of the upper extremities account for one fourth of all cases. Flat bones are less commonly affected.

Joints of the lower extremity constitute three quarters of all cases of arthritis. The elbow, wrist, and shoulder joints are involved in approximately 20% of cases, and small joints uncommonly are infected.

A single locus usually is involved in bone or joint infection. Multifocal osteomyelitis and polyarticular arthritis occur in fewer than 10% of cases (Tables 19-3 and 19-4). An exception is gonococcal infection, which is polyarticular in more than half of the cases.

DIAGNOSIS

The differential diagnosis of bone and joint infection includes trauma, cellulitis, pyomyositis, ma-

Table 19-3   Distribution of affected joints in patients with septic arthritis

Joint	Dallas series (646 joints, 591 patients)		Five other series (377 joints, 357 patients)	
	Total joints	Percentage	Total joints	Percentage
Knee	258	40	144	38
Hip	146	23	121	32
Elbow	89	14	21	6
Ankle	85	13	52	14
Wrist	27	4	3	1
Shoulder	28	4	11	3
Hand/foot	8	1	15	4
Other	5	1	10	2

Modified from Fink CW, Nelson JD: Clin Rheum Dis 1986;12:423-435.

Table 19-4   Monarticular and polyarticular involvement in septic arthritis

Joints	Dallas series (591 joints)		Other series (307 joints)	
	Number of patients	Percentage	Number of patients	Percentage
Monarticular	552	93.4	295	96
Two joints	26	4.4	8	2.6
Three joints	10	1.7	3	1
Four joints	3	0.5	1	0.3

Modified from Fink CW, Nelson JD: Clin Rheum Dis 1986;12:423-435.

lignancy, and collagen vascular diseases. It is not unusual for patients with leukemia or neuroblastoma to present with fever and focal signs suggesting bone or joint infection. A biopsy establishes the diagnosis. History and roentgenographic findings help in distinguishing trauma from infection. Pyomyositis is rare outside central Africa and parts of southeast Asia. Sonography and magnetic resonance imaging (MRI) are very helpful in identifying pyomyositis. In most cases the differential diagnosis between cellulitis and similar soft-tissue findings secondary to bone and joint infection becomes obvious during physical examination. When there is doubt, three-phase radionuclide scanning can be helpful. Various collagen vascular diseases may mimic arthritis if the patient has a single joint involved. In most cases multiple joint involvement, disease in other organ systems, failure to respond to antibiotic therapy, and the chronic or remittent nature of the process lead to the correct diagnosis.

Results from routine laboratory tests such as the white blood cell count and differential count, erythrocyte sedimentation rate, and C-reactive protein are nonspecific and not helpful in differentiating skeletal infections from other conditions.

The radiologic assessment of infectious diseases of bones and joints has enjoyed rapid advances over the past decade and continues to be the subject of much research. The application of various radiologic techniques (plain roentgenograms, sonography, radionucleotide imaging, indium-label leukocytes, MRI) have specific uses for specific clinical settings. It is recommended that for the diagnosis of complicated cases of suspected bone/joint infections, advice be sought from an experienced radiologist regarding appropriate use of these modalities (Bloom et al., 1994; Jaramillo et al., 1995).

Plain roentgenograms are useful in selected cases. Distention of the joint space is often visible in the knee and shoulder but seldom is detected in other joints. Distortion of the deep soft tissues around the metaphyses is a very useful radiographic sign when it is present because it is seen only in two other conditions: crush injuries and pyomyositis. Destructive changes in bone are not seen until at least 10 to 14 days after onset of infection (Capitanio and Kirkpatrick, 1970) (Fig. 19-1).

Radionuclide imaging with technetium radiophosphate or gallium bone scintigraphy is useful in selected cases, but there are limitations in sensitiv-

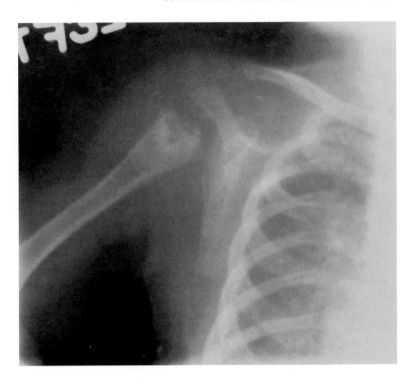

FIG. 19-1 Roentgenogram of a 7-week-old infant with osteomyelitis of the head of the humerus, showing destruction of areas of metaphysis and epiphysis. Pyarthrosis was also present initially.

ity, specificity, and predictive values (Fig. 19-2). In a review of published reports Demopulos et al. (1988) found sensitivities of 84% to 100% and specificities of 70% to 96% in cases of acute osteomyelitis. Imaging is not so successful in cases of acute suppurative arthritis. When three-phase technetium phosphate scans were interpreted "blindly" by radiologists, only 13% of scans of children with proved arthritis were interpreted correctly, and arthritis was incorrectly identified in 32% of children with no evidence of suppurative arthritis (Sundberg et al., 1989). When the radiologists were provided clinical data about each case, the sensitivity rose to 70%, and the specificity was 68%; positive predictive value was 62%, and negative predictive value was 70%. Technetium scans may be uninterpretable in neonates (Asmar, 1992). When a scan is ordered for patients at any age, detailed clinical information should be provided to the radiologist to optimize the interpretation. A negative scan should not rule out bone or joint disease if the clinical findings suggest osteomyelitis or arthritis.

Radionuclide imaging is not necessary in most cases, but it can be useful when there is doubt about the diagnosis or the localization.

Radioactive indium-labeled leukocytes have been used successfully for localizing infection, but the technique is not generally available. Gallium scanning is more sensitive and specific in deter-

mining osteomyelitis than technetium scanning, but it is slower and involves more radiation (Demopulos et al., 1988).

Application of MRI to musculoskeletal disorders has emerged as a major tool for diagnostically challenging situations (Mrazur et al., 1995). Suppurative arthritis, cellulitis, and osteomyelitis can be differentiated (Jacobson, 1989). Further studies are needed.

Ultrasonography has been used to detect fluid in the hip joint (Dorr et al., 1988).

The most recent development in radionuclide scanning for detection of focal infection is the use of indium-labeled intravenous gamma globulin. Successful localization of skeletal infection was achieved in 12 of 13 cases (Rubin et al., 1989).

The ultimate diagnostic tool for skeletal infections is the aspirating needle, and the procedure should be done unless there are unusual circumstances that contraindicate its use. Most joint spaces are easy to enter, but the hip can pose technical problems. Sonographic guidance can facilitate aspiration. If no fluid is obtained, a small amount of air or contrast material is injected and a roentgenogram obtained to confirm the needle tip was in the joint cavity. In cases of osteomyelitis a steel needle is needed to penetrate the cortex into the metaphysis. If pus is encountered in the subperiosteal space, going further is unnecessary. Aspira-

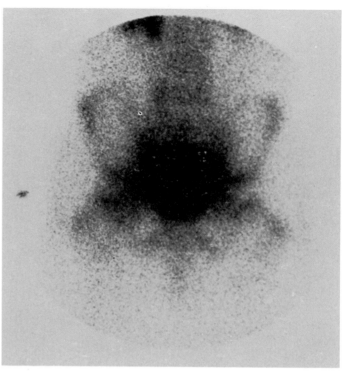

FIG. 19-2   Image intensified technetium pyrophosphate bone scan of the hips and pelvis of a 10-year-old boy with 1 day of point tenderness over the head of the right femur and blood cultures positive for *Staphylococcus aureus.* Roentgenographic areas of radiolucency never appeared.

Right   Left

Table 19-5   Causative agents found in patients with suppurative arthritis

Organism	Dallas data (591 patients)		Other series (343 patients)	
	Number of patients	Percentage found	Number of patients	Percentage found
Staphylococcus aureus	97	17	139	41
Haemophilus influenzae	149	25	41	12
Others	144	25	67	19
Unknown	201	33	96	28

Modified from Fink CW, Nelson JD: Clin Rheum Dis 1986;12:423-435.

tion of joint or bone pus not only serves to confirm the diagnosis of infection but also provides the best specimen for bacteriologic culture.

MICROBIOLOGY

A microbial cause is revealed in approximately two thirds of cases of suppurative arthritis (Table 19-5) and three fourths of cases of osteomyelitis (Table 19-6). Some negative cultures are explained by prior antibiotic therapy and some by the inhibitory effect of pus on microorganisms, but it is possible that some cases that are treated as bacterial arthritis are actually reactive arthritis.

In patients with osteomyelitis *S. aureus* is the most common infecting organism in all age-groups, including the newborn. Group B streptococci and coliform bacilli are also prominent pathogens in the neonate. Group A streptococci are next in frequency but constitute less than 10% of all cases. In the recent past, *H. influenzae* type b has accounted for 7% of cases in children 5 years of age or younger. *Pseudomonas aeruginosa* cases are almost exclusively related to puncture wounds of the foot. After 5 years of age virtually all cases of osteomyelitis are caused by gram-positive cocci except for the *P. aeruginosa* cases.

Table 19-6 Causative agents of osteomyelitis by ages of patients

Organism	Number of cases	Age-groups (yr)		
		<2	2-5	5
Staphylococcus aureus	200	27*	56	64
Streptococci†	44	16	13	6
Haemophilus influenzae type b	16	11	2	0
Pseudomonas aeruginosa	11	2	2	4
Staphylococcus epidermidis	10	6	1	0
Gram-negative enteric bacilli	10	4	4	0.6
S. aureus and group A *Streptococcus*	2	0.8	0	0
Mycobacterium tuberculosis	1	0	1	0
Moraxella kingae	1	0.8	0	0
Brucella abortus	1	0	1	0
Unknown	103	34	20	23
TOTAL	399	127	101	171

*Percent of cases in age group.
†Twenty-nine *S. pyogenes*, eight *S. agalactiae*, six *S. pneumoniae*, one not speciated.

In young patients with suppurative arthritis *H. influenzae* type b outranked *S. aureus* in frequency. The recent control of *H. influenzae* and disease of children through immunization appears greatly to have decreased the incidence of skeletal complications of this infection. After 5 years of age *S. aureus* predominates.

In both conditions occasional cases caused by fungal infection or tuberculosis are encountered, and some viral infections are associated with arthritis.

SPECIAL CONSIDERATIONS
Newborn Infants

The indolent nature of skeletal infections in neonates is noteworthy. Because of the lack of fever and other systemic signs of illness in approximately one half of the neonates, the pain with movement of an extremity is often mistakenly attributed to trauma.

In the series of 83 neonates with osteomyelitis collected from three reports in the literature there was abnormal delivery in 33% and a preceding infection in 46% (Nelson, 1983). Unlike older patients in whom a single bone is involved in more than 90% of cases, polyosteal disease was present in 40% of neonates. Infection of the adjacent joint occurred in 70% of cases. The bacteria involved were *S. aureus* in 53%, streptococci (mostly group B) in 23%, gram-negative enteric bacilli in 13%, and unknown organisms in 11%. Calcaneal osteomyelitis has occurred as a complication of heel puncture (Lilien et al., 1976).

In 23 neonates with suppurative arthritis the pathogens were staphylococci in 9; streptococci in 5; coliform bacilli in 3; *Candida albicans* in 3; and *P. aeruginosa, H. influenzae* type b, and *Neisseria gonorrhoeae* in 1 each. *Candida* infections occur in neonates with central vascular catheters in place who have received prior broad-spectrum antibiotic therapy (Yousefzadeh and Jackson, 1980).

Group B streptococcal infections differ in several respects from other infections (Edwards et al., 1978). The age of onset is later, and the infants have had no preceding infections. Possibly because of trauma during delivery, a single bone is involved, typically the proximal right humerus. Spread to the contiguous joint is less common with group B streptococcal infection than with staphylococcal or coliform infection.

Sickle Cell Anemia

Skeletal infections in patients with sickle cell anemia often are caused by uncommon pathogens, and distinguishing between episodes of aseptic infarction and infection is exceedingly difficult. With infarction there are fever, pain, swelling, redness, leukocytosis, and an increase in acute phase reactants just as with infection, and the progress of roentgenographic changes is the same. However, infarction episodes are far more common than skeletal infections. Gallium and technetium scanning do not discriminate between infection and infarction, probably because infarction also occurs in the presence of infection. If the usual supportive measures for bone infarct episodes do not lead to improvement, osteomyelitis should be suspected and an aspirate of bone taken for culture.

In a series of 14 episodes of osteoarticular infection in 13 sicklemic patients there were eight cases of osteomyelitis and six cases of arthritis (Syrogiannopoulos et al., 1986). The causative bacteria in osteomyelitis were *Salmonella* spp. (four cases) and one case each with *Escherichia coli, Enterobacter aerogenes, H. influenzae* type b, and *S. aureus*. In contrast, the pathogens in arthritis were *Streptococcus pneumoniae* in five cases and *H. influenzae* type b in one case. (Pneumococci are very uncommon causes of arthritis in nonsicklemic patients.)

Hemophilia

Hemarthrosis apparently predisposes to joint infections. It has been calculated that there is a threefold to twelvefold increased risk of suppurative arthritis in hemophiliacs in comparison with the general population (Fajardo et al., 1986). In a review of 139 children with hemophilia four (2.9%) developed joint infection during a 6-year period (Pappo et al., 1989). Just as with sickle cell disease patients, the pneumococcus is the most common pathogen.

Transient Synovitis of the Hip

The syndrome of transient synovitis is the most common cause of hip pain in children. The cause is unknown.

A review of 497 cases during a 30-year period provides useful information, but it is biased toward the more severe cases because all the children were hospitalized (Haueisen et al., 1986). Many children with mild cases are not hospitalized.

The syndrome typically occurs in children 4 to 10 years of age and is twice as common in boys as girls. Approximately half the patients have a preceding upper respiratory infection. Body temperature, leukocyte count, and erythrocyte sedimentation rate are normal or slightly elevated. The most prominent symptoms are thigh pain and a limp or failure to bear weight. Physical examination reveals limitation of internal rotation.

Radiographs of the hip are normal in most children, but a small percentage show a mild increase in joint space size or blurring of deep muscle planes. Of 41 patients who had technetium scans, 22 showed increased uptake of isotope consistent with synovitis. Aspirated joint fluid is serous or serosanguineous.

In mild cases managed as outpatients, symptoms last only a few days. In the 497 hospitalized cases treated with bed rest, with or without Buck's traction, symptoms lasted less than 1 week in 67% and less than 1 month in an additional 21%.

The outcome is excellent in almost all cases. Because an occasional case of Legg-Calvé-Perthes disease mimics toxic synovitis initially, it is recommended that the children be reexamined once or twice during the ensuing 6 months.

Reactive Arthritis

Reactive arthritis is defined as inflammation of one or more joints related to infection at a site distant from the affected joints; no infectious agent can be found within the joint (Fink, 1988). Reiter's syndrome is the best known type of reactive arthritis, but the condition is associated with several types of gastrointestinal infection, group A streptococcal infections, and certain viral infections. Reactive arthritis occurs 3 to 10 days after onset of meningococcal or *Haemophilus* meningitis in 3.5% of patients (Likitnukul et al., 1986).

Results of cell counts and differential counts of synovial fluid are similar in patients with bacterial and reactive arthritis. Some patients with culture-negative arthritis who are treated with antibiotics for presumed bacterial infection probably actually have reactive arthritis.

Large concentrations of tumor necrosis factor alpha and interleukin-1 beta are present in synovial fluid in cases of suppurative arthritis but not in cases of reactive arthritis (Sáez-Llorens et al., 1990). This is a useful discriminating test, but it is available in only a few research laboratories.

Treatment of reactive arthritis is with antiinflammatory drugs.

Acute or Subacute Epiphyseal Osteomyelitis

Acute or subacute epiphyseal osteomyelitis is a little known condition that affects the proximal tibial or distal femoral epiphysis (Green et al., 1981; Rosenbaum and Blumhagen, 1985). The patient presents with signs mimicking arthritis. Roentgenographic changes in the epiphysis are not seen in the acute form; it is likely that some patients are treated with antibiotics for arthritis and the diagnosis of epiphyseal osteomyelitis is never made because follow-up radiographs are not obtained. *S. aureus* sometimes is grown from the synovial fluid, but in most cases the cultures are sterile. The condition responds coincident with administration of antistaphylococcal antibiotics.

Infection Secondary to Trauma

The most common forms of traumatic skeletal infection follow puncture wounds of the feet or compound fractures (Dubey et al., 1988). A great variety of bacteria are involved, and polymicrobial infections are common. Wound cultures fail to predict bone culture results in most patients.

When puncture wounds occur through the soles of sneakers, *P. aeruginosa* osteochondritis often ensues because these organisms can exist in the shoes' foam layer (Fisher et al., 1985). Performing thorough surgical débridement is essential for treating this disease. Even prolonged courses of antipseudomonal therapy fail to eradicate the infection in the absence of surgical débridement (Jacobs et al., 1989). When meticulous surgery is done, a regimen of postoperative antibiotics for only 7 days is effective therapy (Jacobs et al., 1989).

Suppurative Bursitis

Infections of bursae are rare in children. Ten cases were diagnosed in three Denver hospitals during a 25-year period (Paisley, 1982). Eight involved the prepatellar bursa, and there was one each in the olecranon and subacromial bursa. Blunt trauma was a predisposing event in six cases; however, in young infants suppurative bursitis apparently is hematogenous in origin (Meyers et al., 1984). Most cases are manifest by swelling and fluctuance but normal range of motion of the adjacent joint. *S. aureus* and group A streptococci are the usual pathogens.

Chronic Recurrent Multifocal Osteomyelitis

Originally reported as *subacute and chronic symmetrical osteomyelitis* (Giedion et al., 1972), this condition has since been termed *chronic recurrent multifocal osteomyelitis (CRMO)*.

The disease afflicts children and young adults (King et al., 1987; Jurik et al., 1988). It commonly begins between 8 and 12 years of age and affects females twice as often as males. As its name implies, several sites are involved during each episode, and the condition remits and relapses for several years before stopping spontaneously. The metaphyses of long bones are involved, but other bones rarely infected in bacterial osteomyelitis are frequently involved, namely the clavicle and spine. Biopsy stud-

ies of the lesions reveal acute and chronic inflammation, with necrosis and granulation tissue. Sclerosis and hyperostosis are progressive.

Patients with CRMO commonly have chronic inflammatory skin conditions such as palmoplantar pustulosis, psoriasis (Björkstén et al., 1978), and Sweet's syndrome (Majeed et al., 1989). CRMO is considered a noninfectious inflammatory condition that may affect other organ systems such as the lung (Ravelli et al., 1995). However, in one case *Mycoplasma hominis* was cultured from a bone biopsy specimen, and the disease apparently was improved by therapy with clindamycin and later tetracycline (Hummell et al., 1987).

TREATMENT

Optimal treatment of skeletal infections requires collaborative efforts of the pediatrician or family physician, the orthopedic surgeon, and the physiatrist.

Initial Antibiotic Therapy

Initial, empiric antibiotic therapy is based on knowledge of likely bacterial pathogens at various ages, the results of the Gram stain of aspirated material, and special considerations.

In the newborn an antistaphylococcal penicillin such as methicillin or nafcillin and a broad-spectrum cephalosporin such as cefotaxime provide coverage for methicillin-sensitive *S. aureus,* group B streptococcus, and coliform bacilli. An aminoglycoside could be used in place of the cephalosporin, but aminoglycosides have somewhat reduced antibacterial activity in sites with decreased oxygen tension and pH, and these conditions are present in tissue infections. If the neonate is a small premature baby who has been in an intensive care unit for many days or who has a central vascular catheter, the possibility of the presence of nosocomial, multiple antibiotic-resistant gram-negative bacteria, methicillin-resistant staphylococci, or fungi must be considered.

In infants and children up to approximately 4 to 5 years of age the principal pathogens are *S. aureus* and streptococci. Several antibiotics are useful for treating these types of infection. Cephalosporins such as cefuroxime, cefotaxime, or ceftriaxone commonly are used. Most of the experience during the past decade has been with cefuroxime. Beyond 5 years of age, unless there are special circumstances, almost all cases of skeletal infection are caused by gram-positive cocci, so an antistaphylo-coccal antibiotic such as nafcillin can be used.

Some clinical situations dictate special consider-ations about empiric antibiotic selection. In sick-lemic patients with osteomyelitis, coliform bac-teria are common pathogens, so a broad-spectrum cephalosporin such as cefotaxime or ceftriaxone should be used in addition to an antistaphylococcal drug. Arthritis in patients with sickle cell disease is unlikely to be caused by coliform bacteria, so use of the usual antibiotics would be appropriate.

Clindamycin is a useful alternative drug for pa-tients who are expected to have a staphylococcus infection. In addition to good antistaphylococcal activity, clindamycin has broad activity against anaerobes, so it is useful for treatment of infections secondary to penetrating injuries or compound fractures.

In instances of *Pseudomonas* osteomyelitis, which often results from a puncture wound of the foot through tennis shoes, ceftazidime or mezlo-cillin plus an aminoglycoside provide appropriate care. An integral aspect of management is surgical débridement of the lesions (Inaba et al., 1992).

Vancomycin is used in place of a β-lactam when-ever the clinical situation raises the possibility of methicillin-resistant staphylococcal infection.

For immunocompromised patients the potential pathogens are legion. Combination therapy usually is initiated. Use of several combinations of two or three drugs would be rational. Current-ly, vancomycin with ceftazidime or ticarcillin-clavulanate, is used in many places, especially in neutropenic patients.

Subsequent Antibiotic Therapy

When the pathogen has been identified, appropriate adjustments in antibiotics are made if necessary. If a pathogen is not identified and the patient is im-proving, therapy usually is continued with the an-tibiotic selected initially; however, consideration should be given to the possibility of a noninfectious inflammatory condition. Similarly, if a pathogen is not identified and the patient is not improving, con-sideration is given to performing reaspiration or biopsy and to the possibility of a noninfectious condition.

In recent years it has become common practice to change antibiotics from the parenteral route to oral administration when the patient's condition has stabilized after approximately 1 week of par-enteral therapy (Syrogiannopoulos and Nelson, 1988). For the oral antibiotic regimen with β-lactam drugs, a dosage two to three times that used for mild infections is prescribed, and the adequacy of the dosage is assessed by testing serum for bac-tericidal activity or for antibiotic content 45 to 60 minutes after a dose of suspension or 1½ to 2 hours after ingestion of a capsule or tablet, which is the usual time for peak serum concentration. A serum bactericidal titer of 1:8 or greater or a serum con-centration of a β-lactam greater than 20 mg/L is considered desirable. Details of the sequential par-enteral-oral antibiotic regimen have been published (Nelson, 1983).

The oral regimen decreases the risk of nosoco-mial infections related to prolonged intravenous therapy, is more comfortable for the patient, and permits treatment outside the hospital if compli-ance with taking the medicine can be ensured.

Surgical Therapy

No randomized, prospective study has compared two or more surgical procedures in patients with skeletal infections. The measures used derive from training and experience. For example, after arthro-tomy some surgeons leave drains and some do not. Of those who use drains, some use collapsible drains and some use rigid ones. Of those who use rigid drains, some use suction and some do not. None of these things have been evaluated in a con-trolled manner.

Hip joint infection is a surgical emergency be-cause of the vulnerability of the blood supply to the head of the femur. When a penetrating injury has occurred and the presence of a foreign body is likely, surgical intervention is indicated. In other situations the need for surgery is individualized.

For joints other than the hip daily percutaneous needle aspirations of synovial fluid are done. Gen-erally one or two subsequent aspirations suffice. If fluid is still accumulating after 4 to 5 days, arthro-tomy is performed. At the time of surgery the joint is flushed with sterile saline solution. Antibiotics are not instilled because they are irritating to syn-ovial tissue, and adequate amounts of antibiotic are achieved in joint fluid with systemic administration (Nelson, 1971).

If frank pus is obtained from subperiosteal or metaphyseal aspiration, the patient is taken to surgery for drainage through a cortical window. In one series, incision and drainage were done in 36% of cases of arthritis and in 69% of cases of os-teomyelitis (Syrogiannopoulos and Nelson, 1988).

Infected weight-bearing limbs should be pro-tected from the trauma of weight bearing during the initial course of therapy. Good attention to nutrition is essential for satisfactory healing.

Physical Medicine

The major role of physical medicine is a preventive one. If a child is allowed to lie in bed with an extremity in flexion, limitation of extension can develop in a few days. The affected extremity should be kept in extension with sand bags, splints or, if necessary, casts. Casts are indicated when there is a potential for pathologic fracture.

After 2 or 3 days when pain is easing, passive range of motion exercises are started and then continued until the child resumes normal activity.

In neglected cases with flexion contractures, prolonged physical therapy is required.

Duration of Antibiotic Therapy

Prolonged courses of antibiotic therapy have traditionally been recommended, but there has been a trend toward shorter courses.

The Centers for Disease Control guidelines recommend 7 days of therapy for gonococcal tenosynovitis (Centers for Disease Control, 1989). As mentioned previously, 7 postoperative days of treatment is adequate for *Pseudomonas* osteochondritis or arthritis, if surgically débrided. Immunocompromised patients generally require prolonged courses of therapy as do patients with fungal or tuberculous disease.

For the usual case of staphylococcal, streptococcal, or *Haemophilus* infection, treatment is continued for a minimum of 4 weeks provided that the signs of inflammation have disappeared. Duration of antibiotic therapy should be individualized, and if clinical response has been slow, a course of 4 to 6 weeks commonly is used.

PROGNOSIS

Because children are in a dynamic state of growth, sequelae of skeletal infections may not become apparent for months or years, so long-term follow-up is important.

In a series of 40 neonates with osteomyelitis treated during 1970 to 1979 10 had severe sequelae, and six had moderate sequelae (Bergdahl et al., 1985). Major problems relate to retarded growth of an affected bone. Growth disturbance was evident in 20 of 36 nonoperated foci and in 4 of 19 operated foci.

Relapses and chronic infections are uncommon. A group of 50 infants and children with osteomyelitis was followed for an average of 36 months (range, 12 to 56 months) after treatment (Dunkle and Brock, 1982). At diagnosis 32 were classified as acute, 15 as subacute (symptoms for longer than 7 days), and 3 as chronic. Relapses occurred in only two patients, one of whom was originally classified as acute and the other as chronic. In another series (Vaughan et al., 1987) eight of 60 patients did not respond to antibiotics within 48 hours and required surgical drainage. Of the remaining 52 patients, 35 patients were treated with parenteral antibiotics for an average of 21 days, and 17 were treated parenterally for 8 days, followed by 4 weeks of oral antibiotics. Chronic infection ensued in one of the operatively treated patients and in two of the remaining 52.

In 49 patients with suppurative arthritis of weight-bearing joints followed an average of 4.3 years (range, 18 months to 12 years) after treatment 13 patients (27%) had sequelae, and in eight (16%) ambulation was impaired (Howard et al., 1976). Residual damage was more common with hip (40% of cases) and ankle (33%) involvement than with knee joint (10%) disease. Sequelae were equally common after *H. influenzae* and *S. aureus* infection. Evaluation at the time of hospital discharge correctly identified only four of the 13 children with sequelae, and four others who were normal at follow-up had been thought to have permanent damage at discharge. Children with sequelae tended to have been sick longer before diagnosis, and in them drainage of pus was delayed.

Thirty-seven children with hip joint infection treated at the Mayo Clinic from 1943 through 1973 had long-term (mean, 8.3 years) follow-up evaluation (Morrey et al., 1976). Nineteen had satisfactory results, and 18 had unsatisfactory results. "Unsatisfactory" was defined as more than 2.5 cm limb length discrepancy (7 patients), persisting pain (5 patients), limitation of motion (7 patients), or need for secondary surgical procedures (9 patients). Duration of symptoms was the most important prognostic factor. There were no sequelae among the nine patients treated within 4 days of onset of symptoms. Of 11 patients with symptoms for more than 1 week, only two had satisfactory results. Associated metaphyseal osteomyelitis was another bad prognostic sign: only two of 14 had a satisfactory result.

Even with appropriate medical and surgical therapy, there is a potential for permanent disabling sequelae in patients with skeletal infections. Prompt recognition and vigorous medical, surgical, and physical therapy offer the best hope for a satisfactory outcome.

BIBLIOGRAPHY

Adeyokunnu AA, Hendrickse RG. Salmonella osteomyelitis in childhood. Arch Dis Child 1980;55:175-184.

Asmar BI. Osteomyelitis in the neonate. Infect Dis Clin North Am 1992;6:117-132.

Bergdahl S, Ekengren K, Eriksson M. Neonatal hematogenous osteomyelitis: risk factors for long-term sequelae. J Pediatr Orthop 1985;5:564-568.

Björkstén B, Gustavson KH, Eriksson B, et al. Chronic recurrent multifocal osteomyelitis and pustulosis palmo-plantaris. J Pediatr 1978;93:227-231.

Bloom BJ, Miller LC, Tucker LB, et al. Magnetic resonance imaging in staphylococcal osteomyelitis with negative bone scan. Clin Pediatr 1994;33:686-687.

Broderick A, Perlman S, Dietz F. Pseudomonas bursitis: inoculation from a catfish. Pediatr Infect Dis 1985;4:693-694.

Capitanio MA, Kirkpatrick JA. Early roentgen observations in acute osteomyelitis. Am J Roentgenol 1970;108:488-496.

Centers for Disease Control. 1989 sexually transmitted diseases treatment guidelines. MMWR 1989;38(No. S-8):24-25.

Dan M. Septic arthritis in young infants: clinical and microbiologic correlations and therapeutic implications. Rev Infect Dis 1984;6:147-155.

Demopulos GA, Bleck EE, McDougall IR. Role of radionuclide imaging in the diagnosis of acute osteomyelitis. J Pediatr Orthop 1988;8:558-565.

Dorr U, Zieger M, Hauke H. Ultrasonography of the painful hip. Prospective studies in 204 patients. Pediatr Radiol 1988;19:36-40.

Dubey L, Krasinski K, Hernanz-Schulman M. Osteomyelitis secondary to trauma or infected contiguous soft tissue. Pediatr Infect Dis J 1988;7:26-34.

Dunkle LM, Brock N. Long-term follow-up ambulatory management of osteomyelitis. Clin Pediatr 1982;21:650-655.

Edwards MS, Baker CJ, Wagner ML, et al. An etiologic shift in infantile osteomyelitis: the emergence of group B streptococcus. J Pediatr 1978;93:578-583.

Eisenberg JM, Kitz DS. Savings from outpatient antibiotic therapy for osteomyelitis. Economic analysis of a therapeutic strategy. JAMA 1986;255:1584-1588.

Fajardo JE, Mickunas VH, deTriquet JM. Suppurative arthritis and hemophilia. Pediatr Infect Dis 1986;5:593-594.

Fink CW. Reactive arthritis. Pediatr Infect Dis J 1988;7:58-65.

Fink CW, Nelson JD. Septic arthritis and osteomyelitis in children. Clin Rheum Dis 1986;12:423-435.

Fisher MC, Goldsmith JF, Gilligan PH. Sneakers as a source of Pseudomonas aeruginosa in children with osteomyelitis following puncture wounds. J Pediatr 1985;106:607.

Giedion A, Holthusen W, Masel LF, et al. Subacute and chronic "symmetrical" osteomyelitis. Ann Radiol (Paris) 1972;15:329-342.

Goldenberg DL, Reed JI. Bacterial arthritis. N Engl J Med 1985;312:764-771.

Green NE, Beauchamp RD, Griffin PP. Primary subacute epiphyseal osteomyelitis. J Bone Joint Surg (Am) 1981;63:107-114.

Haueisen DC, Weiner DS, Weiner SD. The characterization of "transient synovitis of the hip" in children. J Pediatr Orthop 1986;6:11-17.

Herndon WA, Alexieva BT, Schwindt ML, et al. Nuclear imaging for musculoskeletal infections in children. J Pediatr Orthop 1985;5:343-347.

Howard JB, Highgenboten CL, Nelson JD. Residual effects of septic arthritis in infancy and childhood. JAMA 1976;236:932-935.

Hummell DS, Anderson SJ, Wright PF, et al. Chronic recurrent multifocal osteomyelitis: are mycoplasmas involved? N Engl J Med 1987;317:510-511.

Inaba AS, Zukin DD, Perro M. An update on the evaluation and management of plantar puncture wounds and Pseudomonas osteomyelitis. Pediatr Emerg Care 1992;8:38-44.

Jacobs RF, Adelman L, Sack CM, et al. Management of Pseudomonas osteochondritis complicating puncture wounds of the foot. Pediatrics 1982;69:432-435.

Jacobs RF, McCarthy RE, Elser JM. Pseudomonas osteochondritis complicating puncture wounds of the foot in children: a 10-year evaluation. J Infect Dis 1989;160:657.

Jacobson HG. Musculoskeletal applications of magnetic resonance imaging. JAMA 1989;262:2420-2427.

Jaramillo D, Treves ST, Kasser JR, et al. Osteomyelitis and septic arthritis in children: appropriate use of imaging to guide treatment. Am J Radiol 1995;165:399-403.

Jurik AG, Helmig O, Ternowitz T, et al. Chronic recurrent multifocal osteomyelitis: a follow-up study. J Pediatr Orthop 1988;8:49-58.

King SM, Laxer RM, Manson D, et al. Chronic recurrent multifocal osteomyelitis: a noninfectious inflammatory process. Pediatr Infect Dis 1987;6:907-911.

Lebel MH, Nelson JD. Haemophilus influenzae type b osteomyelitis in infants and children. Pediatr Infect Dis J 1988;7:250-254.

Likitnukul S, McCracken GH Jr, Nelson JD. Arthritis in children with bacterial meningitis. Am J Dis Child 1986;140:424-426.

Lilien LD, Harris VJ, Ramamurthy RS, et al. Neonatal osteomyelitis of the calcaneus: complications of heel puncture. J Pediatr 1976;88:478-480.

Majeed HA, Kalaawi M, Mohanty D, et al. Congenital dyserythropoietic anemia and chronic recurrent multifocal osteomyelitis in three related children and the association with Sweet syndrome in two siblings. J Pediatr 1989;115:730-734.

Meyers S, Lonon W, Shannon K. Suppurative bursitis in early childhood. Pediatr Infect Dis 1984;3:156-158.

Mok PM, Reilly BJ, Ash JM. Osteomyelitis in the neonate. Radiology 1982;145:677-682.

Morrey BF, Bianco AJ, Rhodes KH. Suppurative arthritis of the hip in children. J Bone Joint Surg (Am) 1976;58:388-392.

Morrissy RT, Haynes DW. Acute hematogenous osteomyelitis: a model with trauma as an etiology. J Pediatr Orthop 1989;9:447-456.

Mrazur JM, Ross G, Cummings RJ, et al. Usefulness of magnetic resonance imaging for the diagnosis of acute musculoskeletal infections in children. J Pediatr Orthopaed 1995;15:144-147.

Mustafa MM, Sáez-Llorens X, et al. Acute hematogenous pelvic osteomyelitis in infants and children. Pediatr Infect Dis 1990;9:416-421.

Nelson JD. Acute osteomyelitis in children. Infect Dis Clin North Am 1990;4:513-522.

Nelson JD. Antibiotic concentrations in septic joint effusions. N Engl J Med 1971;284:349-353.

Nelson JD. Bone and joint infections. Pediatr Infect Dis 1983;2:S45-S50.

Nelson JD. A critical review of the role of oral antibiotics in the management of hematogenous osteomyelitis. In Remington JS, Swartz MN (eds). Current clinical topics in infectious diseases. New York: McGraw-Hill, 1983, pp 64-74.

Ogden JA, Lister G. The pathology of neonatal osteomyelitis. Pediatrics 1975;55:474-478.

Paisley JW. Septic bursitis in childhood. J Pediatr Orthop 1982;2:57-61.

Pappo AS, Buchanan GR, Johnson A. Septic arthritis in children with hemophilia. Am J Dis Child 1989;143:1226-1227.

Peltola H, Vahvanen V, Aalto K. Fever, C-reactive protein, and erythrocyte sedimentation rate in monitoring recovery from septic arthritis: a preliminary study. J Pediatr Orthop 1984; 4:170-174.

Rao S, Solomon N, Miller S, et al. Scintigraphic differentiation of bone infarction from osteomyelitis in children with sickle cell disease. J Pediatr 1985;107:685-688.

Ravelli A, Marseglla GL, Viola S, et al. Chronic recurrent multifocal osteomyelitis with unusual features. Acta Paediatr 1995;84:222-225.

Ring D, Johnston CE, Wenger DR. Pyogenic infectious spondylitis in children: the convergence of discitis and vertebral osteomyelitis. J Pediatr Orthopaed 1995;15:652-660.

Rodgriquez W, Ross S, Khan W, et al. Clindamycin in the treatment of osteomyelitis in children. Am J Dis Child 1977; 131:1088-1093.

Rosenbaum DM, Blumhagen JD. Acute epiphyseal osteomyelitis in children. Radiology 1985;156:89-92.

Rubin RH, Fischman AJ, Callahan JR, et al. In-labeled nonspecific immunoglobulin scanning in the detection of focal infection. N Engl J Med 1989;321:935-940.

Rush PJ, Shore A, Inman R, et al. Arthritis associated with *Haemophilus influenzae* meningitis: septic or reactive? J Pediatr 1986;109:412-414.

Sadat-Ali M, Sankaran-Kutty, Kannan Kutty. Recent observations on osteomyelitis in sickle-cell disease. Int Orthop 1985;9:97-99.

Sáez-Llorens X, Mustafa M, Ramilo O, et al. Tumor necrosis factor alpha and interleukin-1 beta in synovial fluid of infants and children with suppurative arthritis, Am J Dis Child 1990; 144:353-356.

Stott NS, Zionts LE, Holtom PD, et al. Acute hematogenous osteomyelitis. An unusual cause of compartment syndrome in a child. Clin Orthopaed Rel Res 1995;317:219-222.

Sundberg SB, Savage JP, Foster BK. Technetium phosphate bone scan in the diagnosis of septic arthritis in childhood. J Pediatr Orthop 1989;9:579-585.

Syrogiannopoulos GA, McCracken GH Jr, Nelson JD. Osteoarticular infections in children with sickle cell disease. Pediatrics 1986;78:1090-1096.

Syrogiannopoulos GA, Nelson JD. Duration of antimicrobial therapy for acute suppurative osteoarticular infections, Lancet 1988;9:37-40.

Unkila-Kallio L, Kalio MJT, Peltola H, et al. Acute haematogenous osteomyelitis in children in Finland. Ann Med 1993; 25:545-549.

Vallejo JG, Ong LT, Starke JR. Tuberculous osteomyelitis of the long bones in children. Pediatr Infect Dis J 1995;14:542-546.

Vaughan PA, Newman NM, Rosman MA. Acute hematogenous osteomyelitis in children. J Pediatr Orthop 1987;7:652-655.

Waldvogel FA, Vasey H. Osteomyelitis: the past decade. N Engl J Med 1980;303:360-370.

Wong M, Isaacs D, Howman-Giles R, et al. Clinical and diagnostic features of osteomyelitis occurring in the first three months of life. Pediatr Infect Dis J 1995;14:1047-1053.

Yousefzadeh DK, Jackson JH. Neonatal and infantile candidal arthritis with or without osteomyelitis: a clinical and radiographical review of 21 cases. Skeletal Radiol 1980;5:77-90.

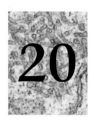

20 OTITIS MEDIA

JEROME O. KLEIN

Acute otitis media and middle ear effusion are among the most common illnesses of childhood. After every episode of acute otitis media, fluid persists in the middle ear for varying periods of time, usually weeks to months. The signs of acute infection resolve with appropriate antibiotic therapy, but the middle ear effusion, now sterile (in episodes of bacterial infection), persists. Conductive hearing loss usually accompanies middle ear effusion, although the extent of the loss varies from child to child. Because of the frequency of acute otitis media and accompanying hearing loss, pediatricians have been concerned that children who suffer from persistent or recurrent middle ear disease might also suffer from delay or impairment of speech, language, or cognitive abilities.

EPIDEMIOLOGY

Otitis media is a disease of infants and young children. The peak age-specific attack rate occurs between 6 and 18 months of age. By 3 years of age, most children have had at least one episode of acute otitis media, and up to one half have had recurrent acute otitis media (three or more episodes). Few children have first episodes of acute otitis media after 3 years of age (Teele et al., 1989). Among the variables associated with acute otitis media are the following host factors: sex (males have more middle ear disease than females); race (there is an extraordinary incidence of infection in some racial groups such as American Indians, Alaskan and Canadian Eskimos, and African and Australian aboriginal children); age at first episode (the earlier in life the first episode occurs, the more likely the child is to have recurrent disease); and sibling or parent history of severe or recurrent acute otitis media (suggesting a genetic basis for the disease). Environmental factors that influence the incidence of acute otitis media include allergy to antigens and pollutants (including atmospheric conditions and

air pollution) (Kim et al., 1996); exposure to smoke (Etzel et al., 1992); breast-feeding (infants who are breast-fed for as little as 3 months have less disease in the first year of life than children who are not breast-fed); season (the incidence of otitis media parallels the seasonal variations of respiratory tract infections); frequent exposure to infectious agents such as occurs in day-care centers (Wald et al., 1988); poverty and associated crowded living conditions and poor sanitation; and access to medical care. Parents with children who have problems with otitis media should be made aware of these risk factors. Although little can be done about most of the host factors, the incidence of otitis media may be reduced by encouraging breast-feeding and discouraging smoking in the household and attendance of the child in large group day care.

ETIOLOGY

The microbiology of otitis media has been documented by appropriate culture of middle ear fluids obtained by needle aspiration (Bluestone and Klein, 1990) (Table 20-1). The findings of bacteriologic studies performed in the United States and Scandinavia are remarkably consistent: *Streptococcus pneumoniae* is the most frequent agent in all age-groups; *Haemophilus influenzae* is the next most frequent pathogen in all age-groups; *Moraxella catarrhalis* is isolated from middle ear fluids with increasing frequency; *Streptococcus pyogenes* has been a significant pathogen in some studies from Scandinavia but not in studies done in the United States; and *Staphylococcus aureus,* gram-negative enteric bacilli, and anaerobic bacteria are infrequent causes of otitis media (see Table 20-1).

Because *S. pneumoniae* is the most important cause of otitis media, investigators have carefully studied the types responsible for infection of the middle ear. The results indicate that relatively few

302

Table 20-1 Bacterial pathogens isolated from middle ear fluids in children with acute otitis media*

Pathogen	Mean (%)	Range (%)
Streptococcus pneumoniae	39	27-52
Haemophilus influenzae	27	16-52
Moraxella catarrhalis	10	2-27
Streptococcus pyogenes	3	0-11
Staphylococcus aureus	2	0-16
None or nonpathogens	28	12-35

*Data from nine reports from United States and Canada, 1980-1987.

Table 20-2 Bacterial pathogens isolated from 169 infants with otitis media during the first 6 weeks of life*

Microorganism	Percent of infants with pathogen
Respiratory bacteria	
Streptococcus pneumoniae	18.3
Haemophilus influenzae	12.4
S. pneumoniae and H. influenzae	3.0
Staphylococcus aureus	7.7
Streptococci, groups A and B	3.0
Moraxella catarrhalis	5.3
Enteric bacteria	
Escherichia coli	5.9
Klebsiella-Enterobacter	5.3
Pseudomonas aeruginosa	1.8
Miscellaneous	5.3
None or nonpathogens	32.0

*Reports from Honolulu, Hawaii (Bland, 1972); Dallas, Texas (Tetzlaff et al., 1977); Denver, CO (Berman et al., 1978); and Huntsville, AL, and Boston, MA (Shurin et al., 1978).

types are responsible for most disease. The eight most common types in order of decreasing frequency are types 19, 3, 6, 23, 14, 1, 18, and 7. All are included in the currently available pneumococcal vaccine. Otitis media caused by *H. influenzae* is associated with nontypeable strains in the vast majority of patients. At one time *H. influenzae* was believed to be of limited importance to otitis media in school-age children and adolescents, but several studies indicate that this organism is a significant cause of otitis media in all age-groups (Grönroos et al., 1964; Howie et al., 1970; Herberts et al., 1971; Schwartz et al., 1977).

Gram-negative enteric bacilli are responsible for approximately 20% of cases of otitis media in young infants (to 6 weeks of age), but these organisms are rarely present in the middle ear effusion of older children. Other than the greater prevalence of otitis media caused by gram-negative bacilli and the presence of other organisms responsible for neonatal sepsis such as group B streptococci and *S. aureus,* the bacteriology of otitis in the infant up to 6 weeks of age is similar to that in older children (Table 20-2) (Bland, 1972; Tetzlaff et al., 1977; Berman et al., 1978; Shurin et al., 1978).

Studies in Cleveland (Shurin et al., 1983) and Pittsburgh (Kovatch et al., 1983) indicate a significant increase in isolation of *M. catarrhalis.* During the period 1980 to 1981, *M. catarrhalis* was isolated from 27% and 19% of children with acute otitis media, respectively. Approximately three fourths of the isolates produced β-lactamase and were therefore resistant to ampicillin. Other bacteria responsible for occasional cases of acute otitis media include group A *Streptococcus, S. aureus,* anaerobic bacteria, and in developing countries,

Mycobacterium tuberculosis, Clostridium tetani, and *Corynebacterium diphtheriae.*

Epidemiologic data suggest that viral infection is associated with acute otitis media (Henderson et al., 1982). Respiratory syncytial virus, influenza virus, rhinoviruses, and enteroviruses with or without concurrent bacterial pathogens (Chonmaitree et al., 1986; Arola et al., 1990) have been isolated from middle ear fluids from some children. In addition, there is evidence of viral infection obtained by enzyme-linked immunosorbent assay (ELISA) techniques that identify viral antigens in middle ear fluids in children with acute otitis media (Klein et al., 1982). Ruuskanen et al. (1991) summarized eight studies published between 1982 and 1990 using immunoassay or isolation; virus was identified in middle ear fluids in 17% of samples.

Only one report of isolation of a mycoplasma *(Mycoplasma pneumoniae)* from middle ear fluid of a child with acute otitis media has been reported (Sobeslavsky et al., 1965).

Chlamydia trachomatis infection results in a mild but prolonged pneumonitis in infants and may be accompanied by otitis media. *C. trachomatis* has been isolated from middle ear fluids of such infants (Tipple et al., 1979).

PATHOGENESIS

The pathogenesis of otitis media must be approached with the understanding that the disease involves a system having contiguous parts, including the nares, nasopharynx, eustachian tube, middle ear, and mastoid antrum and air cells (Fig. 20-1). The middle ear resembles a flattened box, which is approximately 15 mm from top to bottom, 10 mm wide, and only 2 to 6 mm deep. The lateral wall includes the tympanic membrane, and the medial wall includes the oval and round windows. The mastoid air cells lie behind, and the orifice of the eustachian tube is in the superior portion of the front wall.

The eustachian tube connects the middle ear with the posterior nasopharynx, and its lateral one third lies in bone and is open. The medial two thirds are in cartilage, and the walls are in apposition except during swallowing or yawning. In the young infant the eustachian tube is both shorter and proportionately wider than in the older child; the cartilaginous and osseous portions of the tube form a relatively straight line. In an older child the angle of the tube is more acute. These anatomic differences may predispose some infants to early and repeated illness.

The eustachian tube has at least three important physiologic functions with respect to the middle ear: protection of the ear from nasopharyngeal secretions, drainage into the nasopharynx of secretions produced within the middle ear, and ventilation of the middle ear to equalize air pressure within the box with pressure in the external ear canal. When one or more of these functions is compromised, the result may be obstruction of the tube, accumulation of secretions in the middle ear, and, if pyogenic organisms are present, development of suppurative otitis media. Dysfunction of the eustachian tube because of anatomic or physiologic factors apparently is the most important feature of the pathogenesis of infection of the middle ear.

The most likely sequence of events in most episodes of acute otitis media includes an antecedent event (usually caused by an upper respiratory viral infection) that results in congestion of the respiratory mucosa; congestion of the mucosa in the eustachian tube results in obstruction of the narrowest portion of the tube, the isthmus; the obstruction results in negative pressure in the middle ear and then development of middle ear effusion; the secretions of the mucosa of the middle ear, which usually drain through the eustachian tube, now have no egress and accumulate in the middle ear; if pathogenic bacteria that colonize the nasopharynx are present in the middle ear after obstruction of the tube has taken place, the organisms multiply, resulting in an acute suppurative infection.

CLINICAL MANIFESTATIONS

Otalgia (ear pain), otorrhea (ear drainage), hearing impairment affecting one or both ears, and fever suggest infection of the middle ear. However, many children with otitis media do not have these signs. Infants may manifest only general signs of distress, including irritability, bouts of crying, diarrhea, and feeding problems. Less commonly, the patient may exhibit conjunctivitis or complain of vertigo or tinnitus. Swelling about the ear may be a sign of mastoiditis. Acute otitis media is defined by the presence of middle ear effusion accompanied by a sign or symptom of acute illness.

Hyperemia of the tympanic membrane caused by injection of blood vessels is an early sign of otitis media. But redness of the tympanic membrane may be caused by inflammation elsewhere in the system, because the mucous membrane is continuous from the nares and eustachian tube and lines the walls of the middle ear cleft. Thus a "red ear" alone does not establish the diagnosis of otitis media.

Fluid in the middle ear persists for variable periods of time after onset of the acute episode. At the conclusion of a 10- to 14-day course of antimicrobial therapy, approximately two thirds of children still have fluid in the middle ear. The fluid in the middle ear persists in approximately 40% of children at 1 month, 20% at 2 months, and 10% at 3

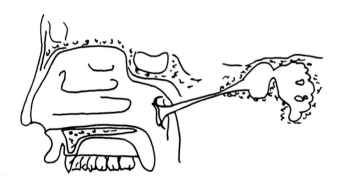

F*IG.* 20-1   Position of the eustachian tube relative to the nasopharynx and the middle ear. The eustachian tube is a double-horned organ with the proximal two thirds lying in cartilage and the distal one third in bone. The segments are connected by the narrow isthmus, the site most vulnerable to obstruction. Thus the system consists of the nares, nasopharynx, eustachian tube, middle ear, and mastoid air cells.

months after onset of acute otitis. Children should be observed until fluid has cleared.

DIAGNOSIS
Clinical

For optimal assessment of the tympanic membrane and its mobility, a pneumatic otoscope should be used. The otoscopic examination should include observation of the following conditions of the tympanic membrane:

- *Position*—normal is slightly convex; bulging indicates increased pressure from positive air pressure or fluid; a retracted drum indicates negative pressure with or without effusion
- *Appearance and color*—the normal color is pearly gray and translucent; congestion of the mucous membrane is indicated by a pink appearance of the membrane; a blue discoloration suggests blood in the middle ear sometimes associated with basal skull fracture; acute suppurative otitis is usually is reflected in a bright red or red-yellow membrane
- *Integrity*—the four quadrants of the membrane should be inspected for perforation, retraction pockets, or cholesteatoma
- *Mobility*—The normal tympanic membrane moves inward with positive pressure and outward with negative pressure (Fig. 20-2). The motion observed is proportional to the pressure applied by gently squeezing and then releasing the rubber bulb attachment on the head of the otoscope. Normal mobility of the tympanic membrane is indicated when positive and then negative pressure is applied and the membrane moves rapidly inward and outward like a sail in a brisk wind. Either presence of fluid in the middle ear or high negative middle ear pressure dampens tympanic membrane mobility.

Tympanometry uses an electroacoustic impedance bridge to record compliance of the tympanic membrane and middle ear pressure. Many instruments are available for use in pediatric practice. After a small probe is inserted into the external canal by means of a snug-fitting cuff, a tone of fixed characteristics is delivered by an oscillator-amplifier through the probe. The compliance of the tympanic membrane is measured by a microphone while the external canal pressure is varied by a pump manometer. The tone is delivered at a given intensity as the air pressure in the canal is varied over a positive and negative range. The recording that results—the tympanogram—reflects the dynamics of the middle ear system, including the tympanic membrane, middle ear, mastoid air cells, and eustachian tube. The technique is reliable, simple, and readily carried out by nonprofessional personnel. However, there are technical problems in applications of presently available instruments to young children, particularly those less than 7 months of age. Tympanometry is of particular value in diagnosis of ambiguous cases of otitis media, in screening for ear disease, and in training of students and young physicians.

The acoustic reflectometry (MDI Instruments, Woburn, MA) is a hand-held instrument that uses principles of reflected energy from the middle ear space to provide information about the presence or absence of middle ear effusion. A microphone located in the probe tip measures the level of transmitted and reflected sound. Acoustic energy is reflected back toward the probe tip from the ear canal and eardrum. The more sound reflected, the greater is the likelihood of the presence of an effusion. In contrast to tympanometry, a seal of the probe is not required, and the reading of reflected sound is almost instantaneous.

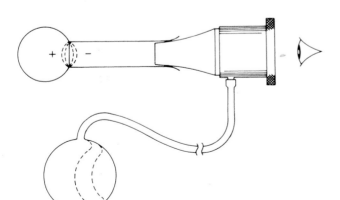

FIG. 20-2   Use of the pneumatic otoscope. The normal tympanic membrane moves inward with positive pressure in the ear canal and outward with negative pressure. The presence of effusion or negative pressure dampens movement of the tympanic membrane.

Radiography

Roentgenographic evaluation of the temporal bone is indicated when complications or sequelae of otitis media are suspect or present. Plain radiographs are of limited value in the diagnosis of mastoiditis or cholesteatoma; computed tomography (CT) and magnetic resonance imaging (MRI) are more precise and should be obtained if a suppurative intratemporal or intracranial complication is suspected.

Microbiology

The results of bacterial cultures of the nasopharynx and oropharynx correlate poorly with those of middle ear fluids. The results are sensitive but not specific for the middle ear pathogen. Thus cultures of the upper respiratory tract are of limited value in specific bacteriologic diagnosis of otitis media. If the child is toxic or has localized infection elsewhere, culture of blood and/or the focus of infection should be performed.

Needle aspiration of a middle ear effusion provides immediate and specific information about the bacteriology of the infection. Although the consistent results of investigations of the bacteriology of acute otitis media provide a guide to the most likely pathogens, *S. pneumoniae* and *H. influenzae,* needle aspiration should be considered in selected children. These children include those who are critically ill at first visit and those who fail to respond adequately to initial therapy and remain toxic and febrile 48 to 72 hours after onset of therapy. Also included are patients with altered host defenses who may be infected with an unusual agent such as those with malignancy or immunosuppressive disease, newborn infants, and those with chronic otitis media. When spontaneous perforation occurs, the exudate in the ear canal is contaminated with flora from the canal. Culture should be obtained, after cleansing the canal with alcohol, by needle aspiration of fluid emerging from the area of perforation or preferably from within the middle ear.

COMPLICATIONS AND SEQUELAE

Suppurative complications of acute infection of the middle ear are now uncommon in areas where children have access to medical care. Contiguous spread of infection, however, may be responsible for mastoiditis, petrositis, labyrinthitis, brain abscess, and meningitis.

Of more concern, at present, is impairment of hearing associated with fluid in the middle ear. Audiograms of children with middle ear effusion usually indicate a mild to moderate conductive hearing loss. The median loss is approximately 25 dB (Fria et al., 1985), which is the equivalent of putting plugs in the ears. The hearing loss is conductive and due to the presence of fluid in the middle ear and is less influenced by the quality of fluid (serous, mucoid, or purulent) than by its volume (partially or completely filling the middle ear space). The conductive hearing impairment is usually reversed with resolution of the middle ear effusion. High negative pressure in the middle ear or atelectasis, both in the absence of middle ear effusion, may also result in conductive hearing loss.

Sensorineural hearing loss is uncommonly associated with otitis media. Permanent sensorineural loss has been described, presumably as a result of the spread of microorganisms or products of inflammation through the round window membrane or because of a suppurative complication of acute otitis media such as labyrinthitis. Permanent hearing loss also may result from irreversible inflammatory changes, including adhesive otitis media and ossicular discontinuity.

The significance of hearing loss associated with acute infection or persistent middle ear effusion is uncertain. Retrospective studies suggest that chronic middle ear disease with effusion occurring during the first few years of life has adverse effects on development of speech and language, hearing, intelligence, and performance in school (Holm and Kunze, 1969; Kaplan et al., 1973; Lewis, 1976; Needleman, 1977; Zinkus et al., 1978, Teele et al., 1990).

Recent longitudinal studies indicate that children who had recurrent episodes of otitis media or persistent middle ear effusion perform less well on tests of speech, language, and cognitive abilities than do their disease-free peers. These data suggest that delay or impairment of development may be an important sequela of otitis media. Boston children observed for ear disease from birth were evaluated at age 7 years by Teele et al. (1990). Estimated time with middle ear effusion during the first 3 years of life was associated significantly with lower scores on tests of cognitive abilities (full-scale, performance, and verbal intelligence quotients), speech and language (articulation and use of morphologic markers), and school performance (lower scores in mathematics and reading).

TREATMENT
Acute Otitis Media

The preferred antimicrobial agent for the patient with otitis media must be active against *S. pneumoniae, H. influenzae,* and *M. catarrhalis.* Group A streptococci and *S. aureus* are infrequent causes of acute otitis media and need not be considered in initial therapeutic decisions. Gram-negative enteric bacilli must be considered when otitis media occurs in the newborn infant, in the patient with a depressed immune response, and in the patient with suppurative complications of chronic otitis media.

In Boston and other centers in the United States, approximately 20% of strains of *S. pneumoniae* are nonsusceptible to penicillin; approximately one third of these strains are resistant (Mason et al., 1992; Welby et al., 1994). Most of the penicillin-resistant strains are also resistant to cephalosporins and include variable patterns of resistance to macrolides, sulfonamides, and tetracyclines. The basis for resistance to penicillins and ephalosporins strains is alteration of the penicillin-binding proteins with less affinity for the drug. The resistance is indicated by increments in the amount of drug required to inhibit the organism, the minimum inhibitory concentration (MIC). Penicillin-susceptible organisms have MICs of ≤ 0.1 µg/ml; intermediate strains are defined as an MIC of 0.1 to 1.0 µg/ml; and resistant strains are 2 or more µg/ml.

Almost all resistance of *H. influenzae* to susceptible penicillins (including penicillins G and V, ampicillin and amoxicillin, and carbenicillin and ticarcillin) is based on production of β-lactamase; the enzyme cleaves the β-lactam ring of susceptible penicillins, rendering the drug inactive against the organism. The vast majority of *M. catarrhalis* strains are β-lactamase producers. The proportion of β-lactamase–producing strains of *H. influenzae* isolated from middle ear fluids varies from 21% in a multicenter study (Doern et al., 1988) to 60% in a report from Northern Virginia and Washington, D.C. (Schwartz and Rodriguez, 1989).

The U.S. Food and Drug Administration has approved 13 products for treatment of acute otitis media (Table 20-3). The manufacturers have provided data indicating clinical efficacy for otitis media but no major clinical advantage for any one drug. Amoxicillin remains the drug of choice because it continues to be effective, safe, and relatively inexpensive. The current incidence of amoxicillin-resistant *H. influenzae* and *M. catarrhalis* due to production of β-lactamase or penicillin-resistant *S. pneumoniae* does not require a change in recommendations for otitis media in most communities (Klein, 1994a).

If an increased number of failures with amoxicillin is noted or laboratory tests indicate a large proportion of β-lactamase–producing strains causing otitis media, other regimens that are β-lactamase stable, such as amoxicillin-clavulanate, a cephalosporin, a sulfonamide, or a macrolide, would be appropriate. If highly resistant *S. pneumoniae* becomes prevalent, physicians will be de-

Table 20-3   Antimicrobial agents for acute otitis media and dosage schedules

Drug (trade name)	No. doses × day	Dosage (kg/day)
cefixime (Suprax)	1/day × 10	6 mg
azithromycin (Zithromax)	1/day × 5	10 mg day 1
		5 mg days 2-5
ceftriaxone* (Rocephin)	1 IM	50 mg
ceftibuten (Cedax)	1/day × 10	9 mg
loracarbef (Lorabid)	2/day × 10	30 mg
cefprozil (Cefzil)	2/day × 10	30 mg
cefpodoxime (Vantin)	2/day × 10	10 mg
cefuroxime axeril (Ceftin)	2/day × 10	30 mg
cefacior (Ceclor)	2-3/day × 10	40 mg
trimethoprim-sulfamethoxazole (Bactrim, Septra)	2/day × 10	8 mg/40 mg
clarithromycin (Biaxin)	2/day × 10	15 mg
amoxicillin (Amoxil)	3/day × 10	40 mg
amoxicillin-clavulanate (Augmentin)	2/day × 10	45 mg
erythromycin-sulfisoxazole (Pediazole)	4/day × 10	40 mg

*Investigational 7/97.

pendent on results of contemporatory antibiotic susceptibility patterns in the community to indicate optimal therapy.

Nasal and oral decongestants, administered either alone or in combination with an antihistamine, are currently among the most popular medications for the treatment of acute otitis media with effusion. The common concept is that these drugs reduce congestion of the respiratory mucosa and relieve the obstruction of the eustachian tube that results from inflammation caused by respiratory infection. The results of clinical trials, however, indicate no significant evidence of efficacy of any of these preparations used alone or in combination for relief of signs of disease or decrease in time spent with fluid in the middle ear after acute infection (Collip, 1961; Fraser et al., 1977; Olson et al., 1978).

Chronic Otitis Media with Effusion

Appropriate management of the child with chronic otitis media remains controversial. The difficulty of arriving at a consensus for management of otitis media with effusion is reflected in an extensive review published by the Agency for Health Care Policy and Research of the U.S. Department of Health and Human Services (Stool et al, 1994b). The major goal of management of persistent middle ear effusion is to achieve and maintain an aerated middle ear that is free of fluid and has a normal mucosa. Current therapies of otitis media with effusion include courses of antimicrobial agents, with or without steroids, myringotomy, adenoidectomy, and use of tympanostomy (ventilating) tubes.

Another 10-day course of a broad-spectrum antimicrobial agent that has activity against β-lactamase–producing organisms should be considered before surgical intervention. Bacterial pathogens are found in approximately one quarter of patients with otitis media with effusion, and a metaanalysis of blinded studies (Stool et al., 1994a) identified resolution of the effusion in 14% of cases after the additional course of antimicrobial agent. Steroid therapy alone or with an antibiotic has been demonstrated to be effective in some children with otitis media with effusion. Berman (1995) recommended a regimen of prednisone, 1 mg/kg/day given orally in 2 doses for 7 days, with an antibiotic for 14 to 21 days.

Before the introduction of antimicrobial agents, myringotomy was the major method of managing suppurative otitis media. Currently, use of myringotomy is limited to the relief of intractable ear pain, hastening resolution of mastoid infection, and drainage of persistent middle ear effusion that is unresponsive to medical therapy. The procedure is of limited value in otitis media with effusion, because the incision heals quickly and before the middle ear mucosa has normalized.

Enlarged adenoids may obstruct the orifice of the eustachian tube in the posterior portion of the nasopharynx and interfere with adequate ventilation and drainage of the middle ear. Recent studies of the use of adenoidectomy in children with prolonged effusions in the middle ear identify a beneficial effect in reducing time spent with effusion in selected children (Gates et al., 1987; Paradise et al., 1990).

Tympanostomy tubes, resembling small collar buttons placed in the tympanic membrane, provide drainage of middle ear fluid and ventilate the middle ear. The effect in children who have impaired hearing because of the presence of fluid is restoration of normal hearing. Placement of the tube treats the effect rather than the cause of the persistent effusion. The criteria for placement of ventilating tubes, management of tubes once they are placed, and long-term benefits, if any, are uncertain. The indications for placement of tympanostomy tubes include persistent middle ear effusions that are unresponsive to adequate medical treatment, persistent tympanic membrane retraction pockets with impending cholesteatoma, and persistent negative pressure with significant hearing loss (Bluestone and Shurin, 1974).

PREVENTION
Advising Parents

Parents of children who have severe and recurrent otitis media or risk factors for middle ear infections should be advised of measures that may reduce the incidence of infection, such as breast-feeding; enrolling children in small rather than large, group day-care centers; and reducing exposure to tobacco smoke.

Chemoprophylaxis

Chemoprophylaxis has been successful in reducing the number of new symptomatic episodes of acute otitis media in children who have a history of recurrent infections. The results of 15 reports of controlled clinical trials of modified courses of antimicrobial agents compared with those in which placebo or historic controls were used were reviewed recently (Klein, 1994b). The majority of studies used a sulfonamide or a broad-spectrum penicillin. All of the reports indicated benefit to the enrollees in reduction of new episodes when they were compared with controls. The interested reader should review selected original studies (Maynard et al., 1972; Perrin et al., 1974, Biedel, 1978; Schwartz et al., 1982; Liston et al., 1983; Schuller, 1983; and Principi et al., 1989). The data are persuasive that children who are prone to recurrent episodes of acute infection of the middle ear are benefited by the following program:

1. Enrollment criteria—children who have had three documented episodes of acute otitis media in 6 months or four episodes in 12 months
2. Drugs and dosage—amoxicillin or sulfisoxazole offers the advantages of demonstrated efficacy, safety, and low cost; the drugs can be administered once a day in one half the therapeutic dosage (sulfisoxazole, 50 mg/kg of body weight; amoxicillin, 20 mg/kg)
3. Duration—approximately 6 months, usually during the winter and spring seasons when respiratory tract infections are most frequent
4. Observation—children should be examined at approximately 1-month intervals when free of acute signs to determine if middle ear effusion is present; management of prolonged middle ear effusion should be considered separately from prevention of recurrences of acute infection

Chemoprophylaxis should be used selectively because a modified dosage schedule of antibiotic used continuously may result in colonization with bacteria resistant to the agent used. Break through episodes should be treated with an alternative antibiotic likely to be effective against resistant strains (see Treatment).

Bacterial Vaccines

Each pneumococcal antigen in the currently available 23-type polysaccharide vaccine produces an independent antibody response. In children 2 years of age and older and adults, antibody develops in about 2 weeks.

Use of pneumococcal vaccine for prevention of recurrences of otitis media in Finnish and American children under 2 years of age resulted in fewer episodes of type-specific infection, but the experience of immunized children with acute otitis media was not significantly different than that of children who received only control materials (Makela et al., 1981; Sloyer et al., 1981; Teele and Klein, 1981). Although some episodes of acute otitis media may have been prevented, the immune response to poly-

saccharide antigens was insufficient to provide significant protection. However, children respond to pneumoccal polysaccharides directly related to age, and the vaccine should be considered in children 2 years of age and older who continue to suffer from otitis media or other respiratory infections. A conjugate pneumococcal polysaccharide vaccine administered as early as 2 months of age is now in clinical trials for safety and efficacy.

Because the vast majority of *H. influenzae* strains responsible for otitis media are nontypeable and current vaccines are prepared from type b capsular polysaccharide, prospects for a vaccine against nontypeable strains lie in the future.

BIBLIOGRAPHY

Arola M, Ruuskanen O, Ziegler T, et al. Clinical role of respiratory virus infection in acute otitis media. Pediatrics 1990; 86:848-855.

Berman S: Otitis media in children. N Engl J Med 1995; 332:1560-1565.

Berman SA, Balkany TJ, Simmons MA. Otitis media in infants less than 12 weeks of age: differing bacteriology among inpatients and outpatients. J Pediatr 1978;93:453-454.

Biedel CW. Modification of recurrent otitis media by short-term sulfonamide therapy. Am J Dis Child 1978;132:681-683.

Bland RD. Otitis media in the first six weeks of life: diagnosis, bacteriology, and management. Pediatrics 1972;49:187.

Bluestone CD, Klein JO. Otitis media, atelectasis, and eustachian tube dysfunction. In Bluestone CD, Stool S (eds). Otitis media in infants and children. Philadelphia: WB Saunders, 1990.

Bluestone CD, Shurin PA. Middle ear disease in children. Pathogenesis, diagnosis, and management. Pediatr Clin North Am 1974;21:379.

Chonmaitree T, Howie VM, Truant AL. Presence of respiratory viruses in middle ear fluids and nasal wash specimens from children with acute otitis media. Pediatrics 1986;77:698.

Collip PJ. Evaluation of nose drops for otitis media in children. Northwest Med 1961;60:999.

Doern GV, Jorgensen JH, Thornsberry C, et al. National collaborative study of the prevalence of antimicrobial resistance among clinical isolates of *Haemophilus influenzae*. Antimicrob Agents Chemother 1988;32:180-185.

Etzel RA, Pattishall EN, Haley NJ, et al. Passive smoking and middle ear effusion among children in day care. Pediatrics 1992;90:228-232.

Fraser JG, Mehta M, Fraser PM. The medical treatment of secretory otitis media: a clinical trial of three commonly used regimens. J Laryngol Otol 1977;91:757.

Fria TJ, Cantekin EI, Eichler JA. Hearing acuity of children with otitis media with effusion. Arch Otolaryngol 1985; 111:10-16.

Gates GA, Avery CA, Prihoda TJ, Cooper JC. Effectiveness of adenoidectomy and tympanostomy tubes in the treatment of chronic otitis media with effusion. N Engl J Med 1987; 317:1444-1451.

Grönroos JA, et al. The etiology of acute middle ear infection. Acta Otolaryngol 1964;58:149.

Henderson FW, Collier AM, Sanyal MA, et al. A longitudinal study of respiratory viruses and bacteria in the etiology of acute otitis media with effusion. N Engl J Med 1982; 306:1377-1383.

Herberts G, Jeppsson PH, Nylen O. Acute otitis media. Pract Otorhinolaryngol 1971;33:191.

Holm VA, Kunze LH. Effect of chronic otitis media on language and speech development. Pediatrics 1969;43:833.

Howie V, Ploussard J, Lester R. Otitis media: a clinical and bacteriologic correlation. Pediatrics 1970;45:29.

Kaplan GJ, et al. Long-term effects of otitis media. A ten-year cohort study of Alaskan Eskimo children. Pediatrics 1973;52:577.

Kim PE, Musher DM, Glezen WP, et al. Association of invasive pneumococcal diseases with season, atmospheric condition, air pollution, and the isolation of respiratory viruses. Clin Infect Dis 1996;22:100-106.

Klein JO. Otitis media. Clin Infect Dis 1994a;19:823-833.

Klein JO. Preventing recurrent otitis: what role for antibiotics? Contemp Pediatr 1994b;11:44-60.

Klein BS, Dollette FR, Yolken RH. The role of respiratory syncytial virus and other viral pathogens in acute otitis media. J Pediatr 1982;101:16-20.

Kovatch AJ, Wald ER, Michaels RH. β-Lactamase–producing Branhamella catarrhalis causing otitis media in children. J Pediatr 1983;102:261-264.

Lewis N. Otitis media and linguistic incompetence. Arch Otolaryngol 1976;102:387.

Liston TE, Foshee WS, Pierson WD. Sulfisoxazole chemoprophylaxis for frequent otitis media. Pediatrics 1983;71:524-530.

Makela PH, Leinonen M, Pukander J, et al. A study of the pneumococcal vaccine in prevention of clinically acute attacks of recurrent otitis media. Rev Infect Dis 1981;3(suppl):124.

Mason EO, Kaplan SL, Lamberth LB, et al. Increased rate of isolation of penicillin-resistant Streptococcus pneumoniae in a children's hospital and in vitro susceptibilities to antibiotics of potential therapeutic use. Antimicrob Agents Chemother 1992;36:1703-1707.

Maynard JE, Fleshman JK, Tschopp CF. Otitis media in Alaskan Eskimo children. JAMA 1972;219:597-599.

Needleman H. Effects of hearing loss from early recurrent otitis media on speech and language development. In Jaffee B (ed). Hearing loss in children. Baltimore: University Park Press, 1977.

Olson AL, Klein SW, Charney E, et al. Prevention and therapy of serous otitis media by oral decongestant: a double-blind study in pediatric practice. Pediatrics 1978;61:679.

Paradise JL, Bluestone CD, Rogers KD, et al. Efficacy of adenoidectomy for recurrent otitis media in children previously treated with tympanostomy-tube placement: results of parallel randomized and non-randomized trials. JAMA 1990; 263:2066-2073.

Perrin JM, et al. Sulfisoxazole as chemoprophylaxis for recurrent otitis media. A double-blind crossover study in pediatric practice. N Engl J Med 1974;291:664.

Principi N, Marchisio P, Massironi E, et al. Prophylaxis of recurrent acute otitis media and middle-ear effusion: comparison of amoxicillin with sulfamethoxazole and trimethoprim. Am J Dis Child 1989;143:1414-1418.

Ruuskanen O, Arola M, Heikkinen T, et al. Viruses in acute otitis media: increasing evidence for clinical significance. Pediatr Infect Dis J 1991;10:425.

Schuller DE. Prophylaxis of otitis media in asthmatic children. Pediatr Infect Dis 1983;2:280-283.

Schwartz R, Rodriguez J, Khan WN, Ross S. Acute purulent otitis media in children older than 5 years: incidence of Haemophilus as a causative organism. JAMA 1977; 238:1032.

Schwartz RH, Puglise J, Rodriguez WJ. Sulfamethoxazole prophylaxis in the otitis media–prone child. Arch Dis Child 1982;57:590-593.

Schwartz RH, Rodriquez WJ. Amoxicillin as the drug of choice for acute otitis media: isn't it time for its reassessment in some areas of the country? Pediatr Infect Dis 1989; 8:806-807.

Shurin PA, Marchant CD, Kim CH, et al. Emergence of beta-lactamase–producing strains of Branhamella catarrhalis as important agents of acute otitis media. Pediatr Infect Dis 1983;2:34-38.

Shurin PA, et al. Bacterial etiology of otitis media during the first six weeks of life. J Pediatr 1978;92:893.

Sloyer JL Jr, Ploussard JH, Howie VM. Efficacy of pneumococcal polysaccharide vaccine in preventing acute otitis media in infants in Huntsville, Alabama. Rev Infect Dis 1981; 3(suppl):119.

Sobeslavsky O, et al. The etiological role of Mycoplasma pneumoniae in otitis media in children. Pediatrics 1965;35:652.

Stool SE, Berg AO, Berman S, et al. Otitis media with effusion in young children. Clinical practice guideline. Number 12. AHCPR Publication No 94-0622. Rockville, Md: Agency for Health Care Policy and Research, Public Health Service, U.S. Department of Health and Human Services, July 1994a, p 52.

Stool SE, Berg AO, Carney CJ, et al. Managing otitis media with effusion in young children. Quick reference guide for clinicians. AHCPR Publication No 94-0623. Rockville, Md: Agency for Health Care Policy and Research, Public Health Service, U.S. Department of Health and Human Services, July 1994b.

Teele DW, Klein JO, Greater Boston Collaborative Study Group. Use of pneumococcal vaccine for prevention of recurrent acute otitis media in infants in Boston. Rev Infect Dis 1981;3(suppl):113.

Teele DW, Klein JO, Chase C, et al. Otitis media in infancy and intellectual ability, school achievement, speech, and language at age 7 years. J Infect Dis 1990;162:685-694.

Teele DW, Klein JO, Rosner B, Greater Boston Otitis Media Study Group. Epidemiology of otitis media during the first seven years of life in children in greater Boston: a prospective, cohort study. J Infect Dis 1989;160:83-94.

Tetzlaff TR, Ashworth C, Nelson ND. Otitis media in children less than 12 weeks of age. Pediatrics 1977; 59:827-832.

Tipple MA, Beem MO, Saxon EM: Clinical characteristics of afebrile pneumonia associated with Chlamydia trachomatis infections in infants less than 6 months of age. Pediatrics 1979;63:192.

Wald ER, Dashefshy B, Byers C, et al. Frequency and severity of infections in day care. J Pediatr 1988;112:540-544.

Welby PL, Keller DS, Cromien JL, et al. Resistance to penicillin and non-beta-lactam antibiotics of Streptococcus pneumoniae at a children's hospital. Pediatr Infect Dis 1994;13:281-287.

Zinkus PW, Gottlieb MI, Schapiro M. Developmental and psychoeducational sequelae of chronic otitis media. Am J Dis Child 1978;132:1100.

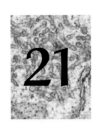

21 PARASITIC: INFECTIONS IN TEMPERATE CLIMATES

HELMINTH INFECTIONS

Children are predisposed to acquiring heavy gastrointestinal worm infections. They therefore suffer greater morbidity from helminth infections compared to less heavily infected adults; whether this predisposition phenomenon has a genetic, immunologic, or behavioral basis is not known. Nevertheless, an increasing body of evidence suggests that children infected with worms suffer from deficits in their physical, intellectual, and cognitive growth. Therefore helminthic diseases (as opposed to asymptomatic helminth infections) have attracted the attention of a new generation of experts interested in the health of children from less-developed countries. In the United States, as well as elsewhere in the industrialized world, the emergence of neurocysticercosis and toxocariasis has also heightened concern about the impact of helminth infections on neuropsychiatric development in children.

Enterobiasis

Infection with the human pinworm, *Enterobius vermicularis,* is one of the most common pediatric problems in the United States. There are no precise recent estimates for the prevalence of enterobiasis; it was reported in 1941 that 19% of the children visiting an outpatient clinic at Children's Hospital of Boston were infected with pinworms (Weller and Sorenson, 1941). Enterobiasis is still very common in elementary schools and day-care centers in the United States (Crawford and Vermund, 1987), although its frequency has probably declined in recent decades (Vermund and MacLeod, 1988). Embryonated eggs of *E. vermicularis* are infectious to humans shortly after being deposited in the perianal area by adult female pinworms. Human enterobiasis results when the eggs are ingested through oral contact with contaminated fingers or fomites (night clothing and bed linen). The eggs may also be swallowed if they become airborne

and associate with household or schoolroom dust particles. Finally, autoinfection resulting from eggs attached to the fingernails (acquired by the child during scratching in an effort to relieve perianal pruritus) comprises a significant number of cases.

The larvae that are liberated from eggs in the gastrointestinal tract migrate to the jejunum and ileum, where they develop into adult male and female pinworms. The adult worms live in the cecum and proximal colon. After mating, the adult female pinworms migrate out and onto the perianal area where they deposit their eggs.

Generally speaking, the larval and adult pinworms do not elicit significant pathology in the large intestine, although Liu et al. (1995) recently reported a case of severe eosinophilic colitis in an 18-year-old homosexual male who acquired a massive inoculum of *E. vermicularis* presumably by direct anal-oral contact. In other rare instances, the adult pinworm may migrate into the appendix or other ectopic sites to cause acute abdominal symptoms that may require surgical intervention (Dalimi and Koshzaban, 1993). However, by far the major clinical feature of pediatric enterobiasis is intense perianal itching (pruritus ani) caused by host inflammation to migrating adult pinworms and their eggs. Bacterial superinfection may exacerbate this process. In girls, migrating pinworms may enter the vagina to cause a vaginitis or even introduce bacteria into the genitourinary tract to cause urinary tract infections (Simon, 1974).

Because pinworm eggs, unlike other intestinal nematode eggs, are not found in the feces, a specific diagnosis of enterobiasis is made on the basis of their recovery from the perianal area. This is usually accomplished by applying adhesive tape first to the perianal skin and then onto a microscope slide. Some investigators believe that the time of highest yield for pinworm egg recovery is early in the morning before a bath or bowel movement.

The goal for treating pediatric enterobiasis is the eradication of adult pinworms. Usually a single dose of either mebendazole (100 mg), albendazole (400 mg), or pyrantel pamoate (11 mg/kg [maximum 1 gm]) is adequate for this purpose (Medical Letter, 1995). However, because newly ingested eggs may be refractory to the anthelminthic, a second dose is required after 2 weeks to eliminate newly developing adult pinworms. The commonly used benzimidazole anthelminthics, mebendazole and albendazole, are embryotoxic and teratogenic in rodents and do not have proven safety in the United States for children less than 2 years of age. However, Biddulph (1990) has reported that widespread use of albendazole and mebendazole in less-developed countries indicates that they are probably safe for infants and children, except for children with blood dyscrasias, leukopenia, and liver disease (Medical Letter, 1995). A frequent problem reported by physicians and nurses is the recurrence of enterobiasis in a child despite two treatment doses of a specific anthelminthic agent. Almost always, this phenomenon occurs as a consequence of reinfection. Therefore it is recommended to treat all members of a household for pinworm infection, and at the time of treatment underwear, bedclothes and towels may be laundered in hot water.

INTESTINAL NEMATODE INFECTIONS (ASCARIASIS, TRICHURIASIS, AND HOOKWORM INFECTION)

Although the giant roundworm *Ascaris lumbricoides,* the whipworm *Trichuris trichiura,* and the two major hookworms *Ancylostoma duodenale* and *Necator americanus* all produce different diseases in children, it is sometimes possible to treat the "unholy trinity" as a single group of pathogens because of the following common features:

1. Each of these nematodes is not directly infectious to humans, but instead requires a period of time in which the egg or larval stages incubate in the soil. For that reason they are sometimes known as soil-transmitted nematodes or geohelminths.
2. The adult stages of each soil-transmitted nematode species live in the intestine, although they tend to occupy distinct niches there. For instance, hookworms usually inhabit proximal portions of the small intestine (duodenum and jejunum), *A. lumbricoides* inhabits all regions of the small intestine, and *T. trichiura* inhabits the colon.

3. Resistance and immunity to the intestinal nematodes are inadequate in childhood so that children tend, on average, to harbor greater numbers of worms than adults (i.e., children appear to be more predisposed to heavy infections).
4. Even among infected children all three nematodes have an aggregated distribution in endemic areas so that many children harbor small numbers of adult worms (light and moderate infections), while a significant minority of children harbor a large number of worms (heavy infections). Moderately and heavily infected children suffer the greatest amount of disease.
5. Moderate and heavy infections with all three nematodes produce similar chronic sequelae, namely physical growth retardation and stunting, as well as intellectual, cognitive, and behavioral deficits.
6. Adult female nematodes produce large numbers of eggs that pass out with the fecal stream. A specific diagnosis of each intestinal nematode infection is made by identifying the characteristic eggs on fecal exam.
7. Mebendazole (Vermox), the most commonly used anthelminthic agent in the United States, is effective against all three nematodes (100 mg b.i.d. for 3 days). Another benzimidazole anthelminthic agent, albendazole (400 mg once, or more for heavy infections), is probably equally effective and has recently became available in the United States. The benzimidazole anthelminthics do not have proven safety in children under 2 years of age, although they have been used extensively for young children in less-developed countries (Biddulph, 1990). Because they are embryotoxic and teratogenic in experimental animals it is advised to weigh the risks versus benefits for these agents. Benzimidazole anthelminthics should be avoided in children with blood dyscrasias or preexisting liver disease. Pyrantel pamoate is a second-line drug available in liquid suspension (11 mg/kg [maximum 1 gm]), which is suitable for *A. lumbricoides* (administered in a single dose) and hookworms (administered in a single dose for 3 successive days), but not for *T. trichiura.* Oxantel (not available in the United States) is suitable for the treatment of trichuriasis; in some countries it is formulated in a liquid preparation with pyrantel pamoate.

There are also important distinct features for each of three major groups of intestinal nematodes. The whipworm *T. trichiura* has the simplest life cycle of the three. Humans become infected with *T. trichiura* by ingesting the embryonated eggs. The larvae hatch in the intestine and penetrate the columnar epithelium. The adult worms reside in the large intestine, where their finely attenuated anterior end creates epithelial tunnels in the mucosa, while their larger posterior end protrudes into the lumen of the large intestine. By this process the adult whipworm disrupts the normal architecture of the colonic epithelium and elicits inflammation. Heavily infected children develop either a *Trichuris* dysentery syndrome (TDS) or *Trichuris* colitis (Bundy and Cooper, 1989). Children with TDS have severe diarrhea with blood and mucus that can result in emaciation and anemia. Mucosal swelling of the rectum can cause an urge to bear down as if stool were present; protracted tenesmus may cause rectal prolapse (Bundy and Cooper, 1989; Despommier et al., 1995). Children with *Trichuris* colitis develop chronic malnutrition, short stature, anemia of chronic disease, and even finger clubbing. Similarities between *Trichuris* colitis and other forms of inflammatory bowel disease such as Crohn's disease and ulcerative colitis have been reported (Bundy and Cooper, 1989). Children with either TDS or *Trichuris* colitis often respond well to specific anthelminthic treatment; afterward they frequently experience impressive catch-up growth.

As in whipworm, humans become infected with *A. lumbricoides* when they ingest embryonated eggs. However, the similarity to the whipworm life cycle ends there, as the emerging larva penetrates the small intestine and enters through the circulatory system before it reaches the lungs. The pulmonary migrations of *A. lumbricoides* larvae elicit a Loeffler's-type of pneumonia consisting of pulmonary infiltrates, wheezing, and eosinophilia. After molting in the lung, the larvae are coughed and swallowed thereby allowing the larvae to enter into the gastrointestinal tract. In the small intestine the larvae become adult worms that grow to lengths of more than 30 cm. *Ascaris* adversely affects the nutritional status of children, resulting in growth retardation (Crompton, 1992). In large numbers, the worms become entangled in a bolus to cause acute intestinal obstruction. Frequently this requires surgical intervention. The adult worms may also migrate into the biliary tree to cause hepatobiliary and pancreatic ascariasis (Despommier et al., 1995). These processes can be precipitated by the administration of certain irritants, possibly including generalized anesthesia.

Unlike the other two members of the "unholy trinity" the infective stages of hookworms are third-stage larvae that either penetrate through the skin *(A. duodenale* and *N. americanus)* or are ingested *(A. duodenale).* Ultimately, the larvae gain entry into the intestine where they molt and grow into adult hookworms. The adult hookworms attach to the mucosal and submucosal layers of the small intestine and lacerate villus capillaries to cause local intestinal hemorrhage—some of the blood is directly ingested by the parasite. Therefore iron deficiency and anemia are the major features of moderate and heavy hookworm infections. Chronic hookworm anemia of childhood results in physical and mental growth retardation (Hotez, 1989; Hotez and Pritchard, 1995). Children often mount a poor immune response to hookworms, so that they remain susceptible to the infection even after receiving anthelminthic chemotherapy (Hotez et al., 1996). An infantile form of infection with *A. duodenale* has been described that causes failure to thrive, melena, and profound anemia. It has been conjectured that infants may sometimes acquire *A. duodenale* larvae by ingesting them in the breast milk from mothers who harbor developmentally arrested larvae.

Toxocariasis

Human toxocariasis resulting in either visceral larva migrans (VLM) or ocular larva migrans (OLM) is a major zoonosis in the United States, Europe, and Japan. Unlike infection with the human ascarid *A. lumbricoides,* accidental infection with a zoonotic ascarid results in significant extraintestinal symptomatology when the larval stages of the parasite migrate through viscera after they fail to complete their development in an aberrant human host. Most commonly humans acquire VLM or OLM by ingesting eggs of the canine ascarid *Toxocara canis,* which are shed in the feces from dogs harboring the adult worms (Hotez, 1995). In many parts of the United States the prevalence of toxocariasis is almost 100% in puppies less than 6 months of age (Hermann et al., 1973). Children between the ages of 1 and 4 years often come into contact with *T. canis* eggs while playing in sandboxes and on playgrounds that were contaminated by a family pet. For that reason, VLM is typically a disease of toddlers and young children (Hotez, 1993). In contrast, OLM caused by *T. canis* often occurs in older children.

Because most of the clinical cases of toxocariasis go undiagnosed, there are no precise estimates for the number of cases in the United States (Schantz, 1989). As Schantz (1989) has pointed out, the prevalence of larva migrans is probably high based on the large number of serum samples that are sent annually to state and local health departments (and forwarded to the Centers for Disease Control and Prevention [CDC]) from patients with a presumptive diagnosis of toxocariasis. The CDC receives an estimated 2,600 to 3,500 specimens every year, of which about 25% to 33% test positive (Schantz, 1989). At least 10,000 individuals in the United States are believed to suffer from toxocariasis (Stehr-Green and Schantz, 1987). The widespread environmental contamination with *T. canis* eggs from some 55 million dogs maintained as pets and another 60 to 80 million unknown dogs in the United States (Elliot et al., 1985; Stehr-Green and Schantz, 1987), together with the intimate play of children with pets, have combined to facilitate relatively high rates of pediatric toxocariasis in the United States, Europe, and Japan (Schantz, 1989, 1991; Petithory et al., 1994; Uga and Kataoka, 1995). In the United States, the seroprevalence of toxocariasis is highest in Puerto Rico and in the Southeast (Schantz, 1989). Among some populations of socioeconomically disadvantaged African-American children the seroprevalence approaches 30% (Herrmann et al., 1973), and among Hispanic children attending a hospital-based primary care clinic in Massachusetts the seroprevalence was reported to be 16% (Bass et al., 1987). Although a proportion of these children live in rural areas, the seroprevalence in inner cities is also high. Of interest is the association between plumbism and *T. canis* infection. Banked sera from inner-city children with elevated serum lead levels have been found to be associated with a high seroprevalence of toxocariasis (Marmor et al., 1987). It has been suggested that the habit of pica (geophagia) is a risk factor for both clinical entities.

The ingestion of *T. canis* eggs can result in either one of two distinct diseases syndromes, VLM and OLM, both of which occur predominantly in children (Hotez, 1993, 1995).

As noted earlier, VLM is primarily a disease of young children. Each ingested *T. canis* egg releases a larva, which invades the intestinal mucosa and migrates through viscera where it both causes mechanical destruction and elicits host inflammation. Eosinophils are a predominant leukocyte involved in the inflammatory responses to the parasite. Classic VLM occurs after the eggs hatch in the gastrointestinal tract and as the larvae migrate through the lungs to cause a pneumonitis, the liver to cause a hepatitis, and the brain to cause a cerebritis. *Toxocara* cerebritis can cause neuropsychiatric disturbances, and there is even some evidence to suggest that *T. canis* is an important etiologic agent of occult epilepsy (Arpino et al., 1990; Nelson et al., 1990). Infected children usually have a leukocytosis, persistent eosinophilia, hyperglobulinemia, and increased serum isohemagglutinins. In addition to identifying the characteristic clinical manifestations, a diagnosis of VLM can be confirmed by enzyme-linked immunosorbent assay (ELISA) that measures specific antibody against *T. canis* larval or egg antigens. ELISA testing on sera from children with a presumptive diagnosis of toxocariasis (with a sensitivity of 85% and a specificity of 92% at a dilution of greater than 1:16) is available from Parasitic Disease Consultants (Tucker, Georgia) or from the CDC. Some newer information suggests that agents of the benzimidazole class, including albendazole, offer promise in the therapy of VLM (Hotez, 1995). For instance, Sturchler et al. (1989) have shown that patients receiving a 5-day treatment course of albendazole (10 mg/kg/day in two divided doses) improved relative to patients who received treatment with an older anthelminthic drug, thiabendazole. Albendazole doses of 400 mg b.i.d. for 3 to 5 days have also been suggested (Medical Letter, 1995). Because mebendazole is poorly absorbed outside of the gastrointestinal tract, high doses may be required to achieve a therapeutic effect in the viscera. In an adult patient, Bekhti (1984) reported success using 1 gm of mebendazole t.i.d. for 21 days. Possible concerns about the use of high-dose benzimidazoles in young children are discussed earlier.

Patients with OLM often have no systemic involvement. Instead, older children (between the ages of 5 and 10 years) are infected with larvae that appear to exclusively invade the retina to cause posterior pole and peripheral pole larval tracks and granulomas. The basis for this phenomenon is not known. However, because there is little systemic (extraocular) involvement the child with OLM does not typically have an eosinophilia. For similar reasons, immunodiagnostic testing on children with OLM is often not helpful. Indeed, only 45% of clinically diagnosed OLM patients have anti-*Toxocara* antibody titers greater than 1:32 (Schantz et al., 1979). Therefore the diagnosis of OLM requires the skill of an ophthalmologist familiar with the characteristic peripheral and posterior pole retinal lesions in a child presenting with a unilateral loss in visual acuity and/or a strabismus (frequently an exotropia). For patients with macular detachment, improvements have been observed after vitrectomy in association with adjunct anthelminthic chemotherapy.

Adult Cestode (Tapeworm) Infections

Despite their large size, adult tapeworms in the intestine of a child do not usually elicit severe symptoms or pathology. All of the major species of human tapeworms are composed of an intestinal attachment organ known as a *scolex* (with suckers, hooks, or grooves) and a chain of egg-containing proglottid segments known as the *strobila*. Tapeworm species identification is made by either recovering the scolex or, in some cases, by examining the proglottid segments and eggs in a fecal sample. Praziquantel is the drug of choice for the treatment of tapeworm infections, having largely replaced niclosamide. For all of the major tapeworm infections except *Hymenolepis nana*, praziquantel is administered in a single dose (5 to 10 mg/kg). The major tapeworm infections of children are discussed in the following sections.

Dipylidiasis. The dog tapeworm *Dipylidium caninum* is acquired by ingesting the cysticercoid larval stage contained within a flea of the genus *Ctenocephalides*. Young children, although often asymptomatic, may experience diarrhea, anorexia, and abdominal pain (Chappell et al., 1990).

Diphyllobothriasis. The fish tapeworm *Diphyllobothrium latum* was at one time endemic among the Scandinavian immigrant populations of Minnesota and Michigan. A related parasite, *D. alascense* occurs among the Inuit. Both tapeworms are acquired by ingesting raw fish; fish become infected when they ingest another crustacean intermediate host containing the larval stage of the parasite. The most dramatic clinical feature of diphyllobothriasis is vitamin B_{12} deficiency, at times even leading to megaloblastic anemia.

Hymenolepiasis. Two major species of the genus *Hymenolepis, Hymenolepsis diminuta* and *H. nana,* are pathogens of humans. Heavy infections with these small tapeworms may cause diarrhea, nausea, anorexia, and abdominal pain (Hamrick et al., 1990). *H. nana,* the dwarf tapeworm, has the interesting feature of being able to complete all

of its life cycle stages from egg to adult tapeworm in humans without requiring an intermediate host. To eradicate the intermediate life cycle stages of *H. nana* that occur in humans, praziquantel may need to be administered in a larger dose (25 mg/kg, once) than necessary for other adult human tapeworm infections.

Taeniasis. Infections with either the beef tapeworm, *Taenia saginata,* or the pork tapeworm, *Taenia solium,* are usually asymptomatic despite their enormous size. However, severe pathology may result when humans serve as the intermediate host of *T. solium* resulting in neurocysticercosis (see the following section). To prevent household transmission of neurocysticercosis, individuals identified by fecal exam as harboring adult *T. solium* in their intestine should be treated with praziquantel.

Neurocysticercosis

In contrast to the benign cestode infections that result when humans serve as the definitive hosts for large tapeworms, far more serious disease occurs in humans who serve as intermediate hosts for the larval stages of tapeworms. Human cysticercosis occurs by ingesting eggs of *T. solium* as a consequence of contact with feces from an individual who harbors the pork tapeworm in the intestine. Once *T. solium* eggs are ingested they liberate oncospheres in the duodenum where they can invade the intestinal mucosa and enter the circulation. From there they disseminate to the muscles and grow into cysticerci *(Cysticercus cellulosae).* Neurocysticercosis occurs when *C. cellulosae* enter the brain and eyes. Cysticercosis is an important emerging infection in the United States, occurring predominantly among families of immigrants from endemic regions of Latin America and Asia. In these countries, family members become infected with the adult tapeworm through ingestion of raw or uncooked pork and then shed *T. solium* eggs in their feces. Children acquire cysticercosis usually through exposure to *T. solium* eggs from immigrant family members or immigrant domestic workers in the household (Schantz et al., 1992). In the United States, neurocysticercosis is currently one of the most common parasitic disease of the central nervous system (CNS) (St. Geme et al., 1993) and a leading cause of epilepsy among Hispanic children living in Los Angeles and other cities along the Mexican border (Richards et al., 1985).

Cysticerci can live for months or years undisturbed in the brain. The pathogenic sequence of events leading to neurocysticercosis is initiated when the cysticercus (a trilaminated "bladder worm" with an invaginated scolex) elicits a vigorous host inflammatory response comprised of lymphocytes, plasma cells, and eosinophils. The observation that inflammation is often greatest around dying cysticerci has significant implications for appropriate specific anthelminthic treatment strategies (see the following section). Host inflammatory responses surrounding dying cysticerci in the brain can trigger seizure foci. In Los Angeles and other U.S. Mexican border cities, children with "simple" neurocysticercosis often present with a solitary inflamed parenchymal mass lesion in association with partial seizures followed by secondary generalization (Mitchell and Crawford, 1988). On contrast-enhanced computed tomography (CT) this type of lesion demonstrates pronounced ring enhancement. Children can also have multiple lesions leading to "complicated" neurocysticercosis. Some investigators believe that complicated disease results from prolonged reexposure in endemic areas. In addition to having multiple cysts these children may also have increased intracranial pressure, meningoencephalitis, arachnoiditis, and hydrocephalus.

Diagnostic imaging with either CT or magnetic resonance imaging (MRI) is usually necessary to diagnose neurocysticercosis. Although either CT or MRI is considered nearly equivalent for this purpose (both modalities require the use of contrast media for complete assessment) there are also some circumstances that might lead the physician to choose one or the other modality (St. Geme et al., 1993). For instance, CT is superior to the MRI for detecting characteristic calcification patterns found in certain types of granulomas, whereas MRI is superior for detecting subarachnoid cysts in the posterior fossa, cysts in the cisterns around the brain stem, intraventricular cysts, and cerebral edema (St. Geme et al., 1993). For confirmation of clinical and radiographic presumptive diagnostic tests, antibodies to cysticercus antigen can be measured either in the serum or CSF using an enzyme-linked immunotransfer blot (EITB) available from the CDC or through a private laboratory (Specialty Laboratories, Inc., Los Angeles, Calif.) (St. Geme et al., 1993). The EITB assay is 100% specific although it has poor sensitivity for children with a solitary lesion. Finally, a fecal examination may reveal the presence of T. solium eggs that could predispose the patient to autoinfection, as well as identify potential family or domestic household carriers.

There is some controversy regarding the optimal treatment for a child with a solitary parenchymal ring-enhancing lesion; such a child may not benefit from specific anthelminthic chemotherapy that targets an already dying larval worm, because these cysts may spontaneously resolve. Anticonvulsants alone may be sufficient for these children, because many remain seizure free after their discontinuation (Mitchell and Crawford, 1988). Others investigators, however, have argued that specific anthelminthic therapy is necessary to eliminate potentially undetected cysts (St. Geme et al., 1993). Certainly, for multiple cysts and other forms of "complicated" neurocysticercosis, anthelminthic chemotherapy is indicated. Both albendazole and praziquantel have been well studied for the treatment of neurocysticercosis and are effective for this purpose. Albendazole (15 mg/kg/day in 2 to 3 doses for 8 to 28 days repeated as necessary [Medical Letter, 1995]) has been shown to be marginally better than praziquantel in terms of cyst resolution and clinical improvement (St. Geme et al., 1993). Patients with three or fewer cysts have been also shown to benefit from a short, 3-day course of albendazole (Alarcon et al., 1989). Because albendazole is not easily available in the United States, therapy with praziquantel (50 mg/kg/day in 3 doses for 15 days [Medical Letter, 1995]) is frequently used first. In addition to anticonvulsant therapy, antiinflammatory adjunct therapy with dexamethasone is beneficial for patients undergoing cysticidal therapy who experience headache, vomiting, or seizures (St. Geme et al., 1993). These children usually require hospitalization. Family members or domestic household contacts found to harbor T. solium tapeworms should be treated with a single dose of praziquantel as described earlier.

PROTIST (PROTOZOAN) INFECTIONS

There is an increasing awareness of parasitic protists (a term that we prefer to protozoa) as major enteropathogens in North America and Europe. Giardia and Cryptosporidium account for the majority of diarrhea cases in some U.S. day-care centers. Other common enteric protozoa that were previously considered commensal may in fact be pathogenic in some children and should be considered as emerging pathogens. Plasmodium falciparum is still the leading killer of children in the world; with increasing international travel, pediatricians should be aware of some basic points in the diagnosis and management of malaria.

Giardiasis

Giardia lamblia is one of the most common enteropathogens of humans and a major cause of pediatric and day-care–associated diarrheas (Pickering et al., 1984). Chronic symptomatic infection with the organism adversely affects the physical growth of children (Farthing, 1995), although it has been suggested that asymptomatic infection may haven an opposite effect (Sagi et al., 1983). After 6 months of age, infants and young children have increased susceptibility to giardiasis; susceptibility is increased even more in children with underlying malnutrition (Sullivan et al., 1991), cystic fibrosis (Roberts et al., 1988), and certain immunodeficiencies such as hypogammaglobulinemia. On the other hand, breast-feeding has a protective effect due not only to passive maternal antibody transfer but also because of direct lytic factors that are present in human milk (Hernell et al., 1986; Reiner et al., 1986).

G. *lamblia* has been generally thought of as a primitive eukaryotic organism belonging to a group of flagellated protozoan parasites. Recent molecular taxonomic data, however, indicate that its classic phylogenetic assignment is in doubt. The organism contains no mitochondria and has prokaryotic-like ribosomal RNA sequences (Sogin et al., 1989). Both features have led some investigators to speculate that the parasite occupies an evolutionary transition between prokaryotes and eukaryotes (Kabnick and Peattie, 1991); Corliss (1994) prefers to use the term *Archeozoa* (instead of the more traditional *Protozoa*) to describe *G. lamblia* and related parasites. Children acquire giardiasis by ingesting the cyst form (7 to 10 microns in length), which is transmitted either from person to person or by fecal contamination of water and food. The inoculum required for infection is small, usually with as few as 10 to 100 cysts (Rendtorff, 1954). The trigger for excystation occurs in response to gastrointestinal fluxes of pH. The excysted trophozoites are binucleated, motile, pear-shaped protists with eight flagellae. The anterior region has a depression in the shape of a ventral disk that facilitates attachment to the intestinal epithelium, a process that is aided by a parasite-derived lectin (Farthing, 1995). The trophozoites respond to bile and other growth factors in the intestinal lumen, dividing by binary fission.

Infection with *G. lamblia* can result in asymptomatic colonization. Other children will experience acute and chronic *Giardia* diarrhea. Despite a large amount of molecular data gathered about this organism, the exact pathogenic mechanisms that result in diarrhea and intestinal malabsorption are still not known. Both parasite and host factors appear to contribute to pathogenicity. Recently, a *Giardia* gene coding for a protein with homology to snake sarafotoxins has been described (Chen et al., 1995). Interestingly, snake poisoning by this class of toxins has been reported to cause cramping, nausea, vomiting, and diarrhea. *Giardia* also causes some direct mucosal damage through the release of proteases and a lectin. The host exacerbates this damage through bacterial overgrowth and a cellular inflammatory response. Children with acute giardiasis present clinically with watery diarrhea. Up to 50% of patients with acute giardiasis develop a chronic, persistent diarrhea with malabsorption (often associated with vitamin A and B_{12} deficiencies), steatorrhea, and weight loss. Secondary lactase deficiency with lactose malabsorption is also common (Farthing, 1995). Chronic giardiasis in children with underlying malnutrition can cause physical growth retardation. Rarely, this can be associated with a protein-losing enteropathy.

Fecal exam by light microscopy of either fresh or polyvinyl alcohol formalin-fixed feces is usually adequate to detect *Giardia* cysts. The sensitivity of diagnosis is increased by identifying the trophozoites in duodenal aspirates. Recently, detection of *Giardia* fecal antigen has been made possible through commercially available ELISA kits that employ either polyclonal or monoclonal antibodies (Addiss et al., 1991).

Three different classes of drugs are available to treat giardiasis (Farthing, 1995). The nitroimidazole derivatives, such as metronidazole (15 mg/kg/day in three doses for 5 days [maximum 750 mg]) and tinidazole (50 mg/kg once [maximum 2 gm]—not marketed in the United States) are highly effective. These two agents require only a brief treatment period and are considered drugs of choice for adolescents. The acridine dye, quinacrine, is also effective for adolescents, but it is less well tolerated and has the disadvantage of causing reversible toxic psychoses and skin disorders. The nitrofuran, furazolidone, is possibly the least effective of the three major drugs for giardiasis, but because it is available in suspension (6 mg/kg/day in four doses for 7 to 10 days) it is widely used in children (Farthing, 1995). Some recent studies suggest that the benzimidazole anthelminthics (e.g., mebendazole and albendazole) may also become effective agents for the treatment of giardiasis. For both nematodes and *Giardia,* these agents target parasite tubulin and microtubules.

Crytosporidiosis and *Cyclospora* Infection

In recent years, *Cryptosporidium parvum* has gained widespread coverage in the lay press as an important water-borne pathogen associated with epidemic diarrhea and as an opportunistic pathogen in human immunodeficiency virus (HIV)-infected patients. New evidence also implicates *C. parvum* as an important cause of diarrhea among young children who attend day-care centers (Alpert et al., 1986; Crawford et al., 1988; Tangermann et al., 1991) and their household contacts (Heijbel et al., 1987). Most studies of patients with diarrhea probably underestimate the true prevalence of cryptosporidiosis because of asymptomatic infections and infections with symptoms too mild to attract medical attention (Kuhls et al., 1994). The seroprevalence of children (ages 5 to 13) and adolescents (14 to 21 years of age) in Oklahoma City was estimated recently to be 38% and 58% respectively (Kuhls et al., 1994). Related coccidia of the genus *Cyclospora* have also been identified as important causes of gastroenteritis among children in less-developed countries, as well as returning travelers (Ortega et al., 1993; Hoge et al., 1995). Emerging infections caused by *Cyclospora* have been identified in the United States and in Europe (Chiodini, 1994).

C. parvum is an intracellular protozoan parasite belonging to the same Apicomplexa phylum that malaria parasites belong to. Hence much of the terminology used to describe the life cycle stages of *C. parvum* is the same as malaria, but the former organism replicates in mammalian intestinal epithelium whereas *Plasmodium* spp. replicates in liver and red blood cells. Human cryptosporidiosis occurs when the host ingests the sporulated oocyst stage. Oocysts may be acquired via human-to-human fecal-oral contact, zoonotic fecal-oral contact (calves, other ruminants, and house pets are major animal reservoirs) (Miron et al., 1991), or through ingestion of contaminated water or unpasteurized milk (Egger et al., 1990). There is also evidence for vertical transmission (Lahdevirta et al., 1987). Excystation of the oocyst in the small intestine (in response to host enzymes and bile salts) causes the release of sporozoites, which attach to the enterocytes of the terminal ileum (Adal et al., 1995). Enterocyte cellular invasion by the sporozoite is fol-

lowed first by intracellular trophozoite formation and then by a process known as *merogony,* in which six to eight merozoites are released. The merozoites invade adjacent enterocytes and develop into a second generation of intracellular parasites. By the second day of the infection, some merozoites can sexually differentiate into microgamonts and macrogamonts. Fertilization of the gamonts results in zygote, and later, new oocyst formation. *Cyclospora* sp. is also a coccidian parasite, closely related to members of the genus *Eimeria* (Relman et al., 1996). Its life cycle has not yet been elucidated but probably resembles *C. parvum.*

The mechanisms by which *C. parvum* causes diarrhea are not well established. A parasite-derived enterotoxin activity has been described but not confirmed (Adal et al., 1995); recently a gene encoding a *Cryptosporidium* hemolysin has been cloned (Steele et al., 1995). Children with cryptosporidiosis typically experience a watery diarrhea accompanied by crampy abdominal pain; nausea and vomiting; and some constitutional symptoms such as anorexia, malaise, and myalgias. Infection often lasts 1 to 2 weeks, but protracted diarrhea with weight loss is also common. An association between immunocompetent children with cryptosporidiosis and subsequent respiratory symptoms has led some investigators to conclude that *C. parvum* is also a pulmonary pathogen (Keren et al., 1987; Egger et al., 1990; Adal et al., 1995). The organism has been recovered in tracheal aspirates of an immunocompetent infant with *Cryptosporidium* diarrhea and laryngotracheitis (Harari et al., 1986). In HIV-infected children with low CD4 cell counts, infection with *C. parvum* often has disastrous consequences. These children can experience a severe and prolonged watery diarrhea with large fluid volume losses and malabsorption. Dehydration and cachexia are often sufficiently severe as to warrant their hospital admission for fluid and nutritional replacement. *C. parvum* infection has been reported to ascend the gastrointestinal tract in children with acquired immunodeficiency syndrome (AIDS) to involve the biliary tree and gallbladder, resulting in cholangitis and cholecystitis.

A laboratory diagnosis of cryptosporidiosis is made in a child by detecting oocysts on fecal examination. Because shedding of oocysts is intermittent, more than one stool sample is often required for diagnosis. It is important for pediatricians to understand that *Cryptosporidium* testing is not always carried out as part of a routine "O & P" examination. Either acid-fast or fluorescent stains are used by many laboratories. At Yale, a modification of the acid-fast stain that uses dimethyl sulfoxide to enhance carbol fuchsin stain penetration (DMSO Modified Acid Fast Stain Kit, Trend Scientific, St. Paul, MN) is used. Both immunofluorescence that uses commercially available monoclonal antibodies and ELISA kits that detect oocyst antigen are being used with increasing frequency. HIV-infected children with cryptosporidiosis of the upper gastrointestinal tract may require endoscopy with aspiration of duodenal fluid or small intestinal brushing to make a diagnosis. *Cyclospora* sp. can be identified by light microscopy of feces and from duodenal or jejunal aspirates as oocysts ranging in size from 8 to 10 microns. The *Cyclospora* oocyts exhibit a characteristic bright blue autofluorescence under ultraviolet light (Chiodini, 1994).

As yet, there is no well-established agent to treat routine pediatric cryptosporidiosis. For the most part, therapy is supportive and includes rehydration and nutritional supplementation. Judicious use of gut motility agents is sometimes warranted. For HIV-infected adults with cryptosporidiosis the non-absorbable aminoglycoside paromomycin to be partially effective. Anectodal information suggests that paromomycin is well tolerated, although it by no means is uniformly successful (Ritchie and Becker, 1994). A frequently used adult dosage of paromomycin for intestinal cryptosporidiosis in adults is 500 mg PO q6h (Ritchie and Becker, 1994). At Yale Children's Hospital we have treated two HIV-infected children with paromomycin doses comparable to those used for luminal amebiasis (30 mg/kg/day divided in three doses). A maintenance dose is often required to prevent relapse. Azithromycin (40 mg/kg PO once daily) has also been used for the treatment of severe *Cryptosporidium* diarrhea in two children with cancer (Vargas et al., 1993) and in four HIV-infected children (Hicks et al., 1996). Some investigators suggest using azithromycin in higher doses to effect a temporary cure. As adjunct therapy, treatment of HIV-infected patients with zidovudine is sometimes associated with resolution of *Cryptosporidium* diarrhea; this effect may be related to transient improvement in immune status (Chandrasekar, 1987; Ritchie and Becker, 1994). Somatostatin and octreotide (long-acting semisynthetic somatostatin analog) are expensive and do not have clearly established efficacy in reducing diarrhea (Cello et al., 1991). Bovine hyperimmune colostrum and bovine transfer factor also have given mixed results in the

treatment of AIDS patients with cryptosporidiosis. Children with *Cyclospora* infections have been successfully treated with a 7-day course of trimethoprim (5 mg/kg) and sulfamethoxazole (25 mg/kg), b.i.d. (Medical Letter, 1995).

Microsporidiosis

The microsporidia are small obligate intracellular parasites of uncertain taxonomy, which infect a variety of both vertebrate and invertebrate hosts. At least four different genera of related organisms have been identified from HIV-infected patients. These include *Encephalitozoon, Nosema, Septata,* and *Enterocytozoon.* Infection occurs when sporoplasm is introduced into a host cell via a unique polar tube. Replication of the organism subsequently occurs in the target cell. Eventually the organisms undergo sporogony and release spores into the environment; transmission may occur through either spore ingestion or inhalation. *Encephalitozoon* infections have been reported from the eye and CNS. *Enterocytozoon* infections are important opportunistic causes of chronic diarrhea and wasting from patients with AIDS (Weber and Bryan, 1994). Typically these patients have CD4 counts below 100 cells/mm^3 and have loose to watery stools, malabsorption, bloating, and anorexia (Asmuth et al., 1994; Dieterich et al., 1994). Coinfection with *Cryptosporidium* and other intestinal pathogens can occur (Weber et al., 1993). Enterocytozoon infections have been reported to respond to therapy with benzimidazoles, including albendazole (Dieterich et al., 1994).

Blastocystis Hominis

As part of a child's workup for diarrhea it is often the case that the pediatrician or nurse practitioner will request a light microscopic examination of the stool as a diagnostic test to look for "ova and parasites." Frequently the parasitology lab will report finding *Blastocystis hominis* in the stool. *B. hominis* is an anaerobic ameobo-flagellate protist that has been assigned to a new proposed subphylum, Blastocysta (Boreham and Stenzel, 1993). Its most characteristic stage is a "vacuolar" form appearing as a thin peripheral band of cytoplasm surrounding a large membrane-enclosed vacuole of unknown function. Its life cycle has yet to be fully elucidated.

High rates of colonization with *B. hominis* have been reported in individuals who (1) live in institutionalized settings, (2) have a recent history of travel, or (3) report recent contact with pets or farm animals. *B. hominis* is also common in preschool and school-age children (Nimri, 1993; O'Gorman et al., 1993; Nimri and Batchoun, 1994). Whether or not *B. hominis* is entirely commensal or if the organism can also invade intestinal mucosa and/or elicit diarrhea is controversial. Inflammation and edema of the colonic mucosa have been reported from patients undergoing sigmoidoscopy and biopsy, although no serologic antibody response to the organism has been demonstrated (Boreham and Stenzel, 1993). The majority of studies investigating the association between *B. hominis* infection and gastroenteritis are based on the identification of clinical laboratory isolates of the organism from patients with abdominal discomfort, cramping diarrhea, and vomiting. Although many of these studies lack adequate case controls, several recent carefully controlled prospective studies have also failed to resolve the controversy. Generally speaking it is recommended that asymptomatic immunocompetent individuals would receive no benefit from antiprotozoan chemotherapy. Some investigators have reported improvements from specific chemotherapy with either metronidazole or tinidazole in *B. hominis*–infected patients having no other identifiable pathogen. Furazolidone and quinacrine also have in vitro activity against *B. hominis,* but there is little if any clinical experience with these drugs for patients with *Blastocystis* (Boreham and Stenzel, 1993).

Imported Malaria and Malaria Chemoprophylaxis

Pediatricians and nurse practitioners are sometimes asked to evaluate febrile children who have recently arrived from a malaria-endemic region. Proper diagnosis, management, and treatment of suspected malaria in these children have a substantial effect on clinical outcome. Malaria caused by *P. falciparum* is the leading killer of children (between the ages of 6 months and 5 years) in the world, causing up to 2 million deaths annually. Therefore, when confronted with a febrile child arriving from a malaria-endemic region, it is essential to determine if the child is infected with *P. falciparum. P. falciparum* has the potential to infect significant percentages of the red blood cells to cause high parasitemias. High parasitemias with this organism can result in severe complications that result in signs and symptoms of shock, including hypoglycemia, severe anemia, adult respiratory distress syndrome, renal failure, and disseminated intravascular coagulation. Cerebral malaria has a high mortality (10% to 40%) and is one of the most

common acute encephalopathies of children (Newton et al., 1991). The sequence of events that leads to cerebral malaria and coma in children with *P. falciparum* is still not known. The sequestration of *P. falciparum*–infected erythrocytes in the cerebral microvasculature (MacPherson et al., 1985), presumably through the adherence of specific parasitized red blood cell–derived ligands to host-endothelial cell receptors (Berendt et al., 1989), is an important precipitating event. These events result in host cytokine release and altered cerebral blood flow. Intracranial pressure, possibly in response to altered cerebral blood flow, is a prominent feature of cerebral malaria; intracranial pressure reduction by osmotic diuresis may be of benefit for these children, although clinical studies are lacking (Newton et al., 1991). The diagnostic benefits of lumbar puncture in a comatose child from the tropics, to rule out the possibility of bacterial meningitis, must be weighed against the risk of herniation (Newton et al., 1991).

The early diagnosis and treatment of children with *P. falciparum* malaria (before the development of severe symptoms) with quinine or quinidine can be life saving. In contrast, *Plasmodium vivax* or *Plasmodium ovale* infects reticulocytes and young red blood cells to cause low parasitemias. Some children with *P. vivax* or *P. ovale* can be managed as outpatients.

Three large children's medical centers located in Toronto (Lynk and Gold, 1989), Chicago (Emanuel et al., 1993), and Washington D.C. (McCaslin et al., 1994) have reviewed their imported malaria cases over 10 years (40 cases), 5 years (20 cases), and 9 years (64 cases), respectively. In the former study 45% of patients received previously incorrect diagnoses and treatments. It was observed in Toronto that *P. falciparum* was the predominant malaria in children from Africa, whereas most of the cases of *P. vivax* were acquired in Asia. In Toronto, most of the *P. falciparum* cases were found within 5 weeks of the patient leaving the endemic area, with a mean of 11 days. Because *P. vivax* (and *P. ovale*) can undergo a period of dormancy in the liver, these infected children present much later after leaving the endemic area, with a mean of 6 months. Children with imported malaria do not reliably show a classic history of periodic fevers. The most common presenting symptoms are daily or irregular fevers, chills, headache, and irritability. The most common presenting signs are splenomegaly, hepatomegaly, pallor, and jaundice. Laboratory findings show anemia and thrombocytopenia. The white blood cell count is not usually elevated. A definitive diagnosis of malaria is usually made on the basis of one or more Giemsa-stained blood smears. A thick smear has increased sensitivity, but it is usually inadequate for species identification. It has been recommended that a well-trained technician should review smears taken every 12 hours until parasites are identified (Lynk and Gold, 1989).

Oral chloroquine phosphate (10 mg base/kg [maximum 600 mg base], then 5 mg base/kg 6 hr later, then 5 mg base/kg at 24 and 48 hrs [Medical Letter, 1995]) is the treatment of choice for children with *P. vivax* or *P. ovale*. Lynk and Gold (1989) report that the standard dose of primaquine (0.3 mg base/kg/day for 14 days [Medical Letter, 1995]) does not always prevent relapse, especially in patients from southeast Asia; doubling of the dose has eliminated this problem. For children unable to tolerate oral chloroquine because of severe illness or vomiting, both parenteral quinidine (see the following) and chloroquine are therapeutic options. Some investigators have reported hypotension and sudden death in children receiving parenteral chloroquine. Guidelines have been suggested to diminish parenteral chloroquine toxicity (Lynk and Gold, 1989).

Two classes of drugs should be administered to children with *P. falciparum* malaria. Generally speaking, imported *P. falciparum* is usually considered chloroquine resistant unless there is certain evidence that the child was infected in a nonresistant endemic area (Lynk and Gold, 1989). Either quinine or quinidine is administered to rapidly diminish the parasitemia. A second, long-acting drug such as pyrimethamine with sulfadoxine (Fansidar), tetracycline, or clindamycin helps prevent recrudescence in the presence of quinine or quinidine. For severely ill children, or those with parasitemias that exceed 5%, parenteral therapy is recommended. Parenteral administration of either quinidine (more commonly available in U.S. hospitals) or quinine is potentially toxic and requires cardiac and blood pressure monitoring. Slow administration of a loading dose of quinidine gluconate (10 mg/kg [maximum 600 mg] in normal saline slowly over 1 to 2 hr) is followed by continuous infusion of 0.02 mg/kg/minute until oral therapy can be started (Medical Letter, 1995). Lynk and Gold (1989) suggest an intravenous loading dose of 14 mg of base/kg of quinidine over 4 hours followed by 7 mg of base/kg given every 8 hours as a 4-hour infusion. Children with parasitemias greater than

5% to 10% or with cerebral malaria have benefited from exchange transfusions (Miller et al., 1989; Phillips et al., 1990), iron chelation therapy (Gordeuk et al., 1992), and glucose replacement (Taylor et al., 1988). Children who are not severely ill and have low parasitemias may be treated with oral quinine sulfate (25 mg/kg/day in three doses for 3 to 7 days).

Parents who bring children to malaria-endemic areas should be cautioned about the need for appropriate chemoprophylaxis and appropriate measures to diminish contact with anopheline mosquitoes (Koumans and Zucker, 1995). Almost all regimens must be initiated before travel, continuing throughout the risk period and then for 4 weeks after return (Table 21-1). Chloroquine alone is a drug of choice for infants and children who travel to areas where no chloroquine-resistant *P. falciparum* malaria transmission occurs. Otherwise, mefloquine is recommended for children greater than 15 kg who travel to chloroquine-resistant *P. falciparum* areas. Children less than 15 kg (and pregnant women) for whom safety of mefloquine has not been established present a special problem in malaria chemoprophylaxis. Chloroquine alone or in combination with proguanil (available overseas) is the commonly used major alternative, although efficacy is questionable. Individuals taking this regimen who are more than 24 hours away from medical care should also consider carrying pyrimethaminesulfadoxine with them as a self-treatment if they become febrile. Under some circumstances young children and pregnant women may require mefloquine when traveling to chloroquine-resistant areas (Koumans and Zucker, 1995). Except for its bitter taste and high association with subsequent vomiting, mefloquine has been administered to very young children less than 15 kg without significant adverse events (Koumans and Zucker, 1995). Doxycycline is as effective as mefloquine for malaria prophylaxis in children greater than 8 years of age. All travelers who need to take malaria chemoprophylaxis should decrease their exposure to anopheline mosquito bites (Table 21-2). These measures include staying in screened rooms between dusk and dawn, using permethrin or deltamethrin-impregnated mosquito nets while sleeping, wearing long-sleeved clothing, and using of repellants containing DEET (young children who use DEET concentrations above 35% may be at risk for drug-associated encephalopathy) (Koumans and Zucker, 1995). A CDC travel hotline (404-332-4555) and fax line (404-332-4565) are available.

Table 21-1   First-line treatment recommendations for common parasitic diseases of childhood[a,b]

Disease	Drug	Dosage
Helminth Infections		
Enterobiasis	Mebendazole	100 mg PO given once
Ascariasis	Mebendazole	100 mg PO b.i.d. × 3 days
Trichuriasis		
Hookworm		
Toxocariasis	Albendazole	10 mg/kg/day in two divided doses × 5 days[c]
Dipylidiasis	Praziquantel	5-10 mg/kg PO given once
Diphyllobothriasis		
Taeniasis		
Hymenolepiasis *(H. diminuta)*		
Hymenolepiasis *(H. nana)*	Praziquantel	25 mg/kg PO given once
Cysticercosis	Praziquantel	50 mg/kg/day in three divided doses × 15 days[d]
Protist (Protozoan) Infections		
Giardiasis	Furazolidone	6 mg/kg/day in four divided doses × 7-10 days[e]
Cryptosporidiosis (HIV infection)	Paromomycin	30 mg/kg/day in three divided doses[f]
	Azithromycin	40 mg/kg/day
Cyclosporiasis	Trimethoprim	5 mg/kg × 7 days[a]
	Sulfamethoxazole	25 mg/kg × 7 days[a]
Microsporidiosis (intestinal)	Albendazole	400 mg b.i.d.[g]
Malaria Treatment		
P. vivax	Chloroquine phosphate	10 mg base/kg (max. 600 mg base)
P. ovale		5 mg base/kg 6 hr later
		5 mg base/kg 24 hr later
		5 mg base/kg 48 hr later
		Total dose = 20-25 mg/kg
		(approx. 300 mg base in a 500 mg tab.)[h]
	Primaquine	0.6 mg base/kg/day × 14 days
P. falciparum	Quinine sulfate	25 mg/kg/day in three doses for 3-7 days
		(max. 650 mg t.i.d.; taken after meals)
	+ Fansidar or tetracycline or clindamycin	
P. falciparum (severe)	Quinidine gluconate[h]	Loading dose:
		10 mg/kg (max 600 mg) in normal saline over 1-2 hr
		Maintenance dose:
		Continuous infusion of 0.02 mg/kg/min until oral therapy can be started

Malaria chemoprophylaxis (see Table 21-2)

[a]Based on agents available in the United States (Medical Letter, 1995).

[b]Discussions about these agents are available in the text.

[c]Albendazole is available from Smith Kline Beecham, Sturchler et al, 1989.

[d]Some studies indicate that albendazole is superior to praziquantel.

[e]Not for use in patients with G6PD deficiency.

[f]Optimal dose and length of therapy not yet established.

[g]Dieetrich et al., 1994.

[h]Children receiving parenteral quinidine gluconate should be intensively monitored (cardiac and blood pressure monitoring). Children with parasitemias greater than 5% to 10% or cerebral malaria can benefit from exchange transfusions, iron chelation therapy, and glucose replacement.

Table 21-2   Chemoprophylaxis for malaria

Drug name	Pediatric dose
Travel to Areas With Chloroquine-sensitive *Plasmodium falciparum*	
Chloroquine phosphate (Aralen; Winthrop New York, NY)	5 mg/kg base (8.3 mg/kg salt) orally once/week up to maximum adult dose of 300 mg base (500 mg salt)
Hydroxychloroquine sulfate (Plaquenil; Winthrop New York, NY)	5 mg/kg base (6.5 mg/kg salt) orally, once/week up to maximum adult dose of 310 mg base (400 mg salt)
Travel to Areas With Chloroquine-resistant *Plasmodium Falciparum*	
Mefloquine (Lariam; Roche, Nutley, NJ)	15-19 kg: ¼ tab once/week; 20-30 kg: ½ tab once/week; 31-45 kg: ¾ tab once/week; >45 kg: 1 tab once/week
Doxycycline (Vibramycin; Pfizer, New York)	>8 yr: 2 mg/kg orally, once/day, up to adult dose of 100 mg/day
Proquanil (Paludrine; ICI Pharmaceuticals, Cheshire, U.K.)	<2 yr: 50 mg once/day; 2-6 yr 100 mg once/day; 7-10 yr: 150 mg once/day; >10 yr: 200 mg once/day*
Prevention of Relapses	
Primaquine	0.3 mg/kg base (0.5 mg/kg salt) orally, once/day for 14 days (maximum 15 mg base, 26.3 salt)
Presumptive Treatment	
Pyrimethamine-sulfadoxine (Fansidar; Roche, Nutley, NJ)	5-10 kg: ½ tab†; 11-20 kg: 1 tab; 21-30 kg: ¼ tab; 31-45 kg: 2 tab; >45 kg: 3 tab single dose

Koumans EAH, Zucker JR: Rep Pediatr Infect Dis 1995;5:1-2.
*In combination with weekly chloroquine.
†Each tablet contains 75 mg pyrimethamine and 1500 mg sulfadoxine.

Malaria prevention in the future may rely on the development of a safe and effective vaccine. The SPf66 malaria vaccine is a chimeric molecule (developed by Manuel Patarroyo and his colleagues at the Instituto de Immunologia in Bogota, Colombia) composed of a polymeric peptide with amino acid sequences derived from *P. falciparum* asexual erythrocytic stage proteins linked by a peptide motif derived from a surface sporozoite protein of the same species (Lopez et al., 1994). Community-based vaccine studies on SPf66 in Latin America have demonstrated its safety, immunogenicity, and protection against clinical attacks of malaria (D'Alessandro et al., 1995). In an African area of intense malaria endemicity, it was determined that SPf66 had a protective efficacy of 31% in at-risk children between the ages of 1 and 5 (Alonso et al., 1994). However, no vaccine efficacy was demonstrated in a similar immunization trial among Gambian infants (D'Alessandro et al., 1995). A vigorous international research effort to identify new malaria vaccine targets is in progress (Hoffman and Franke, 1994; Good, 1994).

BIBLIOGRAPHY

Adal KA, Sterling CR, Guerrant RL. *Cryptosporidium* and related species. In Blaser MJ, Smith PD, Ravdin JI, et al. (eds). Infections of the gastrointestinal tract. New York: Raven Press, 1995.

Addiss DG, Mathews HM, Stewart JM, et al. Evaluation of a commercially available enzyme-linked immunosorbent assay for *Giardia lamblia* antigen in stool. J Clin Microbiol 1991; 29:1137-1142.

Alarcon F, Escalante L, Duenas G, et al. Neurocysticercosis: short course of treatment with albendazole. Arch Neurol 1989;46:1231-1236.

Alonso PL, Smith T, Armstrong Schellenberg JRM, et al. Randomised trial of efficacy of SPf66 vaccine against *Plasmodium falciparum* malaria in children in southern Tanzania. Lancet 1994;344:1175-1181.

Alpert G, Bell LM, Kirkpatrick CE, et al. Outbreak of cryptosporidiosis in a day-care center. Pediatrics 1986;77:152-157.

Arpino C, Castelli Gattinara G, Piergili D, Curatolo P. *Toxocara* infection and epilepsy in children: a case-control study. Epilepsia 1990;31:33-36.

Asmuth DM, DeGirolami PC, Federman M, et al. Clinical features of microsporidiosis in patients with AIDS. Clin Infect Dis 1994;18:819-825.

Bass JL, Mehta KA, Glickman LT, et al. Asymptomatic toxocariasis in children. Clin Pediatrics 1987;26:441-446.

Bekhti A. Mebendazole in toxocariasis. Ann Intern Med 1984; 28:24-28.

Berendt AR, Simmons DL, Tansey J, et al. Intracellular adhesion molecule-1 is an endothelial cell adhesion receptor for *Plasmodium falciparum.* Nature 1989;341:57-59.

Biddulph J. Mebendazole and albendazole for infants. Pediatr Infect Dis J 1990;9:373.

Boreham PFL, Stenzel DJ. *Blastocystis* in humans and animals: morphology, biology, and epizootiology. Adv Parasitol 1993; 32:1-70.

Bundy DAP, Cooper ES. *Trichuris* and trichiuriasis in humans. Adv Parasitol 1989;28:107-173.

Cello JP, Grendell JH, Basuk P, et al. Effect of octreotide on refractory AIDS-associated diarrhea: a prospective, multicenter clinical trial. Ann Intern Med 1991;115:705-710.

Chandrasekar PH. "Cure" of chronic cryptosporidiosis during treatment with azidothymidine in a patient with the acquired immune deficiency syndrome. Am J Med 1987;83:187.

Chappell CL, Enos JP, Penn HM. *Dipylidium caninum,* an underrecognized infection in infants and children. Pediatr Infect Dis J 1990;9:745.

Chen N, Upcroft JA, Upcroft P. A *Giardia duodenalis* gene encoding a protein with multiple repeats of a toxin homologue. Parasitology 1995;423-431.

Chiodini PL. A "new" parasite: human infection with *Cyclospora cayetanensis.* Trans R Soc Trop Med Hyg 1994; 88:369-371.

Corliss JO. An interim utilitarian ("user-friendly") hierarchical classification and characterization of the protists. Acta Protozool 1994;33:1-51.

Crawford FG, Vermund SH. Parasitic infections in day care centers. Pediatr Infect Dis J 1987;6:744.

Crawford FG, Vermund SH, Ma JY, Deckelbaum RJ. Asymptomatic cryptosporidiosis in a New York City day care center. Pediatr Infect Dis J 1988;7:806-807.

Crompton DWT. Ascariasis and childhood malnutrition. Trans R Soc Trop Med Hyg 1992;86:577-579.

D'Alessandro U, Leach A, Drakeley CJ, et al. Efficacy trial of malaria vaccine SPf66 in Gambian infants. Lancet 1995; 346:462-467.

Dalimi A, Khoshzaban F. Comparative study of two methods for the diagnosis of *Enterobius vermicularis* in the appendix. J Helminthol 1993;67:85-86.

Despommier DD, Gwadz RW, Hotez PJ. Parasitic diseases, ed. 3, New York: Springer-Verlag, 1995.

Dieterich DT, Lew EA, Kotler DP, et al. Treatment with albendazole for intestinal disease due to *Enterocytozoon bieneusi* in patients with AIDS. J Infect Dis 1994;169:178-183.

Egger M, Mausezahl D, Odermatt P, et al. Symptoms and transmission of intestinal cryptosporidiosis. Arch Dis Child 1990; 65:445-447.

Elliot DL, Tolle SW, Goldberg L, Miller JB. Pet-associated illness. N Engl J Med 1985;313:985-995.

Emanuel B, Aronson N, Shulman S. Malaria in children in Chicago. Pediatrics 1993;92:83-89.

Farthing MJG. *Giardia lamblia.* In Blaser MJ, Smith PD, Ravdin JI, et al. (eds). Infections of the gastrointestinal tract. New York, Raven Press, 1995.

Fitch CD. Malaria. In Burg FD, Ingelfinger JR, Wald ER, Polin RA (eds). Gellis & Kagan's current pediatric therapy, ed. 15. Philadelphia: WB Saunders, 1995.

Good MF. Antigenic diversity and MHC genetics in sporozoite immunity. Immunol Lett 1994;41:95-98.

Gordeuk V, Thuma P, Brittenham G, et al. Effect of iron chelation therapy on recovery from deep coma in children with cerebral malaria. N Engl J Med 1992;327:1473-1477.

Hamrick HJ, Bowdre JH, Church MT. Rat tapeworm *(Hymenolepis diminuta)* infection in a child. Pediatr Infect Dis J 1990;9:216.

Harari MD, West B, Dwyer B. *Cryptosporidium* as a cause of laryngotracheitis in an infant. Lancet 1986;1:1207.

Heijbel H, Slaine K, Seigel B, et al. Outbreak of diarrhea in a day care center with spread to household members: the role of *Cryptosporidium.* Pediatr Infect Dis J 1987;6:532-535.

Hernell O, Ward H, Blackberg L, et al. Killing of *Giardia lamblia* by human milk lipases: an effect mediated by lipolysis of milk lipis. J Infect Dis 1986;153:715-720.

Hermann N, Glickman LT, Schantz PM, et al. Seroprevalence of zoonotic toxocariasis in the United States: 1971-1973. Am J Epidemiol 1985;122:890-896.

Hicks P, Zwiener RJ, Squires J, Savell V. Azithromycin therapy for *Cryptosporidium parvum* infection in four children infected with human immunodeficiency virus. J Pediatr 1996; 129:297-300.

Hoffman SL, Franke ED. Inducing protective immune responses against the sporozoite and liver stages of *Plasmodium.* Immunol Lett 1994;41:89-94.

Hoge CW, Echeverria P, Ramachandran R, et al. Prevalence of *Cyclospora* species and other enteric pathogens among children less than 5 years of age in Nepal. J Clin Microbiol 1995; 33:3058-3060.

Hotez PJ. Hookworm disease in children. Pediatr Infect Dis J 1989;8:516-520.

Hotez PJ. Visceral and ocular larva migrans. Semin Neurol 1993;13:175-179.

Hotez PJ. *Toxocara canis.* In Burg FD, Wald ER, Ingelfinger JR, Polin RA (eds). Gellis & Kagan's current pediatric therapy, ed. 15. Philadelphia, WB Saunders, 1995.

Hotez PJ, Hawdon JM, Cappello M, et al. Molecular approaches to vaccinating against hookworm disease. Pediatr Res 1996; 40:515-521.

Hotez PJ, Pritchard DI. Hookworm infection. Scient Amer 1995;272:68-75.

Hulbert TV. Congenital malaria in the United States: report of a case and review. Clin Infect Dis 1992;14:922-926.

Kabnick KS, Peattie DA. *Giardia:* a missing link between prokaryotes and eukaryotes. Am Scient 1991;79:34-43.

Keren G, Barzilai A, Barzilay Z, et al. Life-threatening cryptosporidiosis in immunocompetent infants. Eur J Pediatr 1987;146:187-189.

Koumans EHA, Zucker JR. Update on malaria prevention for children and pregnant women. Rep Pediatr Infect Dis 1995;5:1-2.

Kuhls TL, Mosier DA, Crawford DL, Griffis J. Seroprevalence of Cryptosporidial antibodies during infancy, childhood, and adolescence. Clin Infect Dis 1994;18:731-735.

Lahdevirta J, Jokipii AMM, Sammalkorpi K, Jokipii L. Perinatal infection with *Cryptosporidium* and failure to thrive. Lancet 1987;1:48-49.

Liu LX, Chi J, Upton MP, Ash LP. Eosinophilic colitis associated with larvae of the pinworm *Enterobius vermicularis.* Lancet 1995;346:410-412.

Lopez MC, Silva Y, Thomas MC, et al. Characterization of SPf(66)n: a chimeric molecule used as a malaria vaccine. Vaccine 1994;12:585-591.

Lynk A, Gold G. Review of 40 children with imported malaria. Pediatr Infect Dis J 1989;8:745-750.

MacPherson GG, Warrell MJ, White NJ, et al. Human cerebral malaria: a quantitative ultrastructural analysis of parasitized erythrocyte sequestration. Am J Pathol 1985;119:385-401.

Marmor M, Glickman L, Shofer F, et al. *Toxocara canis* infection of children: epidemiologic and neuropsychologic findings. Am J Public Health 1987;77:554-559.

McCaslin RI, Pikis A, Rodriguez WJ. Pediatric *Plasmodium falciparum* malaria: a ten-year experience from Washington, DC. Pediatr Infect Dis J 1994;13:709-715.

Medical Letter on Drugs and Therapeutics. Drug for parasitic infections. Med Letter 1995;37(961).

Miller KD, Greenberg AE, Campbell CC. Treatment of severe malaria in the United States with a continuous infusion of quinidine gluconate and exchange transfusion. N Engl J Med 1989;321:65-70.

Miron D, Kenes J, Dagan R. Calves as a source of an outbreak of cryptosporidiosis among young children in an agricultural closed community. Pediatr Infect Dis J 1991;10:438-441.

Mitchell WG, Crawford TO. Intraparenchymal cerebral cysticercosis in children: diagnosis and treatment. Pediatrics 1988;82:76-82.

Nelson J, Frost JL, Schochet SS. Unsuspected cerebral *Toxocara* infection in a fire victim. Clin Neuropathol 1990;9:106-108.

Newton CRJC, Kirkham FJ, Winstanley PA, et al. Intracranial pressure in African children with cerebral malaria. Lancet 1991; 337:573-576.

Nimri LF. Evidence of an epidemic of *Blastocystis hominis* infections in preschool children in Northern Jordan. J Clin Microbiol 1993;31:2706-2708.

Nimri LF, Batchoun R. Intestinal colonization of symptomatic and asymptomatic schoolchildren with *Blastocystis hominis*. J Clin Microbiol 1994;32:2865-2866.

O'Gorman MA, Orenstein SR, Proujansky R, et al. Prevalence and characteristics of *Blastocystis hominis* infection in children. Clin Pediatr 1993;32:91-96.

Ortega YR, Sterling CR, Gilman RH, et al. *Cyclospora* species—a new protozoan pathogen of humans. N Engl J Med 1993;328:1308-1312.

Petithory J-C, Beddok A, Quedoc M. Zoonoses d'origine ascaridienne: les syndromes de larva migrans viscerale. Bull Acad Natle Med 1994;178:635-647.

Phillips P, Nantel S, Benny WB. Exchange transfusion as an adjunct to the treatment of severe falciparum malaria: case report and review. Rev Infect Dis 1990;12:1100-1108.

Pickering LK, Woodward WE, Dupont HL, et al. Occurrence of *Giardia lamblia* in children in day care centers. J Pediatr 1984; 104:522-526.

Reiner DS, Wang CS, Gillin FS. Human milk kills *Giardia lamblia* by generating toxic lipolytic products. J Infect Dis 1986;154:825-832.

Relman DA, Schmidt TM, Gajadhar A, et al. Molecular phylogenetic analysis of *Cyclospora*, the human intestinal pathogen suggests that it is closely related to *Eimeria* species. J Infect Dis 1996;173:440-445.

Rendtorff RC. The experimental transmission of human intestinal protozoan prasites: II. *Giardia lamblia* cysts given in capsules. Am J Hyg 1954;59:209-220.

Richards FR, Schantz PM, Ruiz-Tiben E, Sorvillo FJ. Cysticercosis in Los Angeles County. JAMA 1985;254:3444-3448.

Ritchie D, Becker ES. Update on the management of intestinal cryptosporidiosis in AIDS. Annal Pharmacother 1994; 28:767-778.

Roberts DM, Craft JC, Mather FJ, et al. Prevalence of giardiasis in patients with cystic fibrosis. J Pediatr 1988;112:555-559.

Sagi EF, Shapiro M, Deckelbaum R. *Giardia lamblia:* prevalence, influence on growth, and symptomatology in healthy nursery children. Isr J Med Sci 1983;19:815-817.

Schantz PM. *Toxocara* larva migrans now. Am J Trop Med Hyg 1989;41:21-34.

Schantz PM. Parasitic zoonoses in perspective. Int J Parasitol 1991;21:161-170.

Schantz PM, Meyer D, Glickman LT. Clinical serologic and epidemiologic characteristics of ocular toxocariasis. Am J Trop Med Hyg 1979;28:24-28.

Schantz PM, Moore AC, Munoz JL, et al. Neurocysticercosis in an Orthodox Jewish community in New York City. N Engl J Med 1992;327:692-695.

Simon RD. Pinworm infestation and urinary tract infection in young girls. Am J Dis Child 1974;128:21-22.

Sogin ML, Gunderson JH, Elwood HJ, et al. Phylogenetic meaning of the kingdom concept: an unusual ribosomal RNA from *Giardia lamblia.* Science 1989;243:75-77.

St. Geme JW III, Maldonado YA, Enzmann D, et al. Consensus: diagnosis and management of neurocysticercosis in children. Pediatr Infect Dis J 1993;12:455-461.

Steele M, Kuhls T, Nida K, et al. Infect Immun 1995;63:3840-3845.

Stehr-Green JK, Schantz PM. The impact of zoonotic diseases transmitted by pets on human health and the economy. Vet Clin N Am Small Animal Pract 1987;17:1-15.

Sturchler D, Schubarth P, Gualzata M, et al. Thiabendazole v. albendazole in treatment of toxocariasis: a clinical trial. Ann Trop Med Parasitol 1989;83:473-478.

Sullivan PB, Marsh MN, Phillips MB, et al. Prevalence and treatment of giardiasis in chronic diarrhoea and malnutrition. Arch Dis Child 1991;66:304-306.

Tangermann RH, Gordon S, Wiesner P, Kreckman L. An outbreak of cryptosporidiosis in a day-care center in Georgia. Am J Epidemiol 1991;133:471-476.

Taylor TE, Molyneux ME, Wirima JJ, et al. Blood glucose levels in Malawian children before and during the administration of intravenous quinine for severe falciparum malaria. N Engl J Med 1988;319:1040-1047.

Uga S, Kataoka N. Measures to control *Toxocara* egg contamination in sandpits of public parks. Am J Trop Med Hyg 1995;52:21-24.

Vargas SL, Shenep JL, Flynn PM. Azithromycin for treatment of severe *Cryptosporidium* diarrhea in two children with cancer. J Pediatr 1993;123:154-156.

Vermund SH, MacLeod S. Is pinworm a vanishing infection? Laboratory surveillance in a New York City medical center from 1971 to 1986. Am J Dis Child 1988;142:566-568.

Weber R, Bryan RT. Microsporidial infection in immunodeficient and immunocompetent patients. Clin Infect Dis 1994; 19:517-21.

Weber R, Sauer B, Luthy R, Nadal D. Intestinal coinfection with *Enterocytozoon bieneusi* and *Cryptosporidium* in a human immunodeficiency virus–infected child with diarrhea. Clin Infect Dis 1993;17:480-483.

Weller TH, Sorenson CW. Enterobiasis: its incidence and symptomatology in a group of 505 children. N Engl J Med 1941; 224:143-146.

Zierdt CH. *Blastocystis hominis*—past and future. Clin Microbiol Rev 1992;4:61-79.

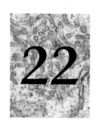

22 PARVOVIRUS INFECTIONS

WILLIAM C. KOCH AND STUART P. ADLER

INTRODUCTION

The Parvoviridae family of viruses are the smallest known DNA-containing viruses. Their genomes contain sufficient DNA to encode only a few proteins. Within the Parvoviridae family is the genus *Parvovirus*. These viruses differ from other Parvoviridae because they replicate their DNA without assistance from a helper virus. Parvoviruses infect many mammalian species, but cross-infection between species does not occur. For example, the canine parvovirus does not infect humans and the human parvovirus does not infect dogs. Similarly, each mammalian parvovirus causes a different illness in its mammalian host, so that parvovirus disease in dogs is very different from that in humans. Parvoviruses were known to cause illness in small mammals long before it was discovered that a parvovirus infected humans. The human parvovirus, called human parvovirus B19, is the only known parvovirus to infect humans, but this single virus causes a wide spectrum of both acute and chronic human diseases.

Cossart et al. (1975) discovered B19 in human sera. They were testing sera for hepatitis B surface antigen and found several sera (one of which was encoded B19) that had small, spherical viral particles with many disrupted fragments and empty shells. They showed that this virus was not hepatitis B virus and that 40% of adults had IgG antibodies to the new viral antigen (Cossart et al., 1975; Paver and Clarke, 1976). The virus subsequently was characterized by genetic and biochemical analysis as being a parvovirus (Summers et al., 1983). Initially B19 was not associated with any specific disease. However, the availability of serologic tests for B19 infection allowed testing of sera from patients, and this eventually led to the discovery of human disease caused by this virus.

CLINICAL MANIFESTATIONS

Since its discovery in 1975, B19 has been associated with a number of diverse clinical syndromes. Recent knowledge of the molecular aspects of B19 infection have shed light on the relationships between these seemingly disparate syndromes. The major syndromes associated with B19 infection are listed in Table 22-1. Asymptomatic infection with B19 also occurs commonly in both children and adults. In studies of large outbreaks, asymptomatic infection is reported in approximately 20% of serologically proven cases (Chorba et al., 1986; Plummer et al., 1985).

Erythema Infectiosum (Fifth Disease)

Erythema infectiosum (EI) is the most common manifestation of infection with parvovirus B19. This is a benign exanthematous illness of childhood that is also known as "fifth disease" because it was the fifth in a numeric classification scheme of common childhood exanthems. This scheme included (1) measles; (2) scarlet fever; (3) rubella; (4) Filatov-Dukes disease (a variant of scarlet fever that is no longer recognized); (5) EI; and (6) roseola. Although the numbering scheme is no longer used, use of the name "fifth disease" for EI has persisted. Anderson first proposed B19 as the cause of EI in 1983, and subsequent studies confirmed this association (Anderson et al., 1983, 1984; Plummer et al., 1985).

EI begins with a mild prodromal phase consisting of low-grade fever, headache, malaise and upper respiratory tract symptoms. This prodrome may be so mild as to go unnoticed. The hallmark of the illness is the characteristic rash. The rash usually occurs in three phases, but these are not always distinguishable (Cherry, 1992). The initial stage consists of an erythematous facial flushing described as a "slapped-cheek" appearance. In the second

Table 22-1 Clinical manifestations of parvovirus B19 infection

Diseases	Patients
Diseases Associated With Acute Infection	
Erythema infectiosum (fifth disease)	Normal children
Polyarthropathy	Normal adolescents and adults
Transient aplastic crisis	Patients with accelerated erythropoiesis
Diseases Associated With Chronic Infection	
Persistent anemia	Immunodeficient/immunocompromised children and adults
Nonimmune hydrops fetalis	Intrauterine infection
Congenital anemia	Intrauterine infection
Chronic arthropathy	Rare patients with B19-induced joint disease
Viral-associated hemophagocytosis	Normal or immunocompromised patients
Vasculitis/purpura	Normal adults and children

Adapted from Brown KE, Young NS. Blood Rev 1995;9:176.

stage the rash spreads quickly or concurrently to the trunk and proximal extremities as a diffuse macular erythema. Central clearing of macular lesions occurs promptly, giving the rash a lacy, reticulated appearance. Palms and soles are usually spared, and the rash tends to be more prominent on the extensor surfaces. Affected children at this point are afebrile and feel well. Adolescents and adult patients often complain of pruritis or arthralgias concurrent with the rash. The rash resolves spontaneously, usually within three weeks, but typically may recur in response to a variety of environmental stimuli such as sunlight, heat, exercise, and stress (Anderson, 1987). Lymphadenopathy is not a consistent feature. Atypical rashes not recognizable as classic EI have also been associated with acute B19 infections; these include morbilliform, vesiculopustular, desquamative, petechial, and purpuric rashes (Anderson, 1987; Török, 1992).

Transient Aplastic Crisis (Erythroid Aplasia)

This was the first clinical syndrome to be definitively linked to B19 infection. An infectious etiology was suspected for the aplastic crisis of sickle cell disease because it usually occurred only once in a given patient, had a well-defined incubation and duration of illness, and occurred in clusters within families and communities (Anderson, 1987). However, attempts to link it to infection with a single agent had repeatedly failed. In 1981 Pattison and colleagues reported six positive tests for B19 (seroconversion or antigenemia) among 600 admissions to a London hospital. All six were

children with sickle cell anemia and aplastic crisis. This association was later confirmed by retrospective studies on the population with sickle cell disease in Jamaica (Serjeant et al., 1981).

In contrast to children with EI, patients with an aplastic crisis are ill at presentation with fever, malaise, and signs and symptoms of profound anemia (pallor, tachypnea, tachycardia, etc.) Rash is rarely present in these patients (Saarinen et al., 1986; Török, 1992). The acute infection causes a transient arrest of erythropoiesis with a profound reticulocytopenia leading to a sudden and often life-threatening fall in serum hemoglobin. Children with sickle hemoglobinopathies may also develop a concurrent vaso-occlusive pain crisis, which further complicates the diagnosis.

Although transient aplastic crises are most common with sickle cell anemia and B19 is the primary cause of the aplastic crisis of sickle cell anemia, any patient with increased red cell turnover and accelerated erythropoiesis can experience an aplastic crisis caused by B19. B19-induced aplastic crises have occurred in many hematologic disorders, including hemoglobinopathies (thalassemia, sickle-C hemoglobin, etc.); red cell membrane defects (hereditary spherocytosis, stomatocytosis); enzyme deficiencies (pyruvate kinase deficiency, glucose-6-phosphate dehydrogenase deficiency, etc.); antibody-mediated red cell destruction (autoimmune hemolytic anemia); and decreased red cell production (iron deficiency, blood loss, etc.) (Török, 1992). B19, however, is not a cause of transient erythroblastopenia of childhood (TEC), another condition of transient red cell hypoplasia that usually occurs in younger, hematologically normal children and follows a more indolent course (Brown and Young, 1995).

Neutropenia and thrombocytopenia also occur during an aplastic crisis, but the incidence varies. In a French study of 24 episodes of aplastic crisis (mostly hereditary spherocytosis), 35% to 40% of patients were either leukopenic or thrombocytopenic, compared to 10% to 15% in a large American study (mainly sickle cell disease) (Lefrere et al., 1986; Saarinen et al., 1986). These transient declines in leukocyte count or platelets follow a similar time course as the reticulocytopenia, although the former are not as severe and recovery is without sequelae. The preservation of leukocytes and platelets in sickle cell anemia compared to other hereditary hemolytic anemias is presumably due to the functional asplenia associated with sickle cell disease (Young, 1988). Varying degrees of neutropenia and thrombocytopenia also occur after natural B19 infection in hematologically normal patients (Anderson et al., 1985). Some cases of idiopathic thrombocytopenic purpura (ITP) and neutropenia in childhood have been associated with acute B19 infection (Saunders et al., 1986; Lefrere et al., 1989). These few reports aside, larger studies have not confirmed B19 as a common cause of either ITP or chronic neutropenia (Brown and Young, 1995).

A typical transient aplastic crisis may be the first manifestation of an underlying hemolytic condition in certain patients who are well compensated and undiagnosed. This is especially well documented in patients with hereditary spherocytosis (Lefrere et al., 1986). The diagnosis of a typical transient aplastic crisis in an otherwise well patient should prompt a thorough hematologic investigation to exclude underlying hemolytic conditions.

Arthropathy

Up to 80% of adolescents and adults have joint symptoms associated with a B19 infection, whereas joint symptoms are uncommon in children (Ager et al., 1966). Arthritis or arthralgia may either be associated with EI or be the only manifestation of infection. Females are more frequently affected than males (Ager et al., 1966; Anderson et al., 1984).

The joint symptoms of B19 infection usually present as the sudden onset of a symmetric peripheral polyarthropathy (Török, 1992). The joints most often affected are the hands, wrists, knees, and ankles, but the larger joints can also be involved (White et al., 1985). The joint symptoms have a wide range of severity, from mild morning stiffness to frank arthritis with erythema, warmth, tenderness, and swelling. Like the rash of EI, the arthropathy has been presumed to be immunologically mediated because the onset of joint symptoms coincides with the development of specific IgM and IgG antibodies. Rheumatoid factor may also be transiently positive, leading to some diagnostic confusion with rheumatoid arthritis in adult patients (Naides and Field, 1988). Fortunately, there is no joint destruction and, in the majority of patients, joint symptoms resolve within 2 to 4 weeks. For some patients, joint discomfort may last for months or, in rare individuals, years. The role of B19 in these more chronic arthropathies is not clear. In patients with symptoms for over 1 year, B19 IgM antibody is usually undetectable and some have evidence of chronic viral infection. Viral DNA has been detected in the bone marrow of four patients with chronic B19 arthropathy (Foto et al., 1993). The viral and host factors involved in disease expression in these patients remain unknown.

Infection in the Immunocompromised or Immunodeficient Host

Patients with impaired humoral immunity are at risk for developing chronic and recurrent infections with parvovirus B19. Persistent anemia, sometimes profound, with reticulocytopenia is the most common manifestation of such infections, which may also be accompanied by neutropenia, thrombocytopenia, or complete marrow suppression. Chronic infections with B19 occur in children with cancer who receive cytotoxic chemotherapy (Koch et al., 1990; Van Horn et al., 1986), children with congenital immunodeficiency states (Kurtzman et al., 1987), children and adults with acquired immunodeficiency syndrome (AIDS) (Frickhofen et al., 1990; Naides and Field, 1988), transplant recipients (Weiland et al., 1989), and even in patients with more subtle and specific defects in IgG class switching who are able to produce measurable antibodies to B19 but are unable to generate adequate neutralizing antibodies (Kurtzman et al., 1989).

B19 has also been linked to viral-associated hemophagocytic syndrome (VAHS) (Koch et al., 1990; Muir et al., 1992). This condition of histiocytic infiltration of bone marrow and associated cytopenias usually occurs in immunocompromised patients. B19 is only one of several viruses that have been implicated as causing VAHS. Thus

VAHS is generally considered a nonspecific response to a variety of viral insults rather than a specific manifestation of a single pathogen.

Intrauterine Infection

Maternal infection with B19 during pregnancy may cause nonimmune fetal hydrops, intrauterine fetal demise, and stillbirth (Anand et al., 1987). The primary pathogenetic mechanism is thought to be a viral-induced red cell aplasia occurring when the fetal erythroid fraction is rapidly expanding. This leads to fetal anemia, hypoxemia, congestive heart failure, fetal hydrops, and fetal death (Török, 1992). Viral DNA is found in infected abortuses, but fetal production of viral-specific IgM is often absent despite documented fetal infection, especially in the first half of pregnancy (Anand et al., 1987; Morey et al., 1991). The fetus seems to be at highest risk during the second trimester (<20 weeks), but fetal losses have occurred in every stage of gestation. Fortunately, the incidence of fetal demise is low and the majority of infants infected in utero deliver normally at term.

The fetal loss rate attributable to B19 has been estimated at between 2% and 9% in prospective studies (Gratacos et al., 1995; Hall and Public Health Laboratory Service, 1990; Rodis et al., 1990). Based on the presence of B19-specific IgM in cord blood or viral DNA in fetal samples, however, the rate of intrauterine infection ranges from 25% to 30% (Gratacos et al., 1995; Hall and Public Health Laboratory Service, 1990; Koch et al., 1993). Even some infants with evidence of intrauterine infection and mild hydrops seen via ultrasound will resolve spontaneously and deliver normally at term (Morey et al., 1991; Török et al., 1992).

Some infants infected in utero develop a chronic or recurrent asymptomatic postnatal infection with B19, the long-term consequences of which are not known (Koch et al., 1993). Recently, several cases of congenital anemia after intrauterine B19 infections have been reported (Brown et al., 1994). Also reported are three children with Diamond-Blackfan anemia (congenital red cell aplasia) who had B19 DNA in their bone marrows (Heegard et al., 1996). There are a few reports of congenital malformations in B19-infected fetuses, but there are no reports to date of liveborn infants with malformations after intrauterine B19 infection (Hartwig et al., 1989). The incidence of birth defects among the children of mothers with a B19 infection during pregnancy has been no higher than for noninfected mothers (Kinney et al., 1988; Török et al., 1992). Thus B19 is unlikely to be a significant cause of birth defects.

Vasculitis and Purpura

There are reports of confirmed acute B19 infections associated with nonthrombocytopenic purpura and vasculitis, including several cases clinically diagnosed as Henoch-Schönlein purpura (HSP), an acute leukocytoclastic vasculitis of unknown etiology in children. Chronic B19 infection has also been associated with a necrotizing vasculitis including cases of polyarteritis nodosa and Wegener's granulomatosis (Finkel et al., 1994). These patients had no underlying hematologic disorder and were generally not anemic at diagnosis. The pathogenesis is unknown but suggests an endothelial cell infection as occurs with other viruses, such as rubella. Parvovirus B19 capsid antigens and DNA were found in a skin biopsy from a patient with EI and this observation lends support to a role for B19 in these vascular disorders (Schwarz et al., 1994). In a controlled study of twenty-seven children with HSP, B19 was not a common cause (Ferguson et al., 1996). Only three of twenty-seven children had B19 IgM, indicating a recent infection. The question of whether B19 is a causative agent in these conditions remains unresolved.

PATHOGENESIS

Because of its small genome, parvovirus B19, like other autonomously replicating parvoviruses, requires a mitotically active host cell for its own replication (Hauswirth, 1984). B19 can only propagate in human erythroid progenitor cells from bone marrow (Ozawa et al., 1987), fetal liver (Yaegashi et al., 1989), peripheral blood (Schwarz et al., 1992), umbilical cord blood (Sosa et al., 1992), and a few leukemic cell lines (Shimomura et al., 1992). The cellular receptor for B19 is globoside, a neutral glycosphingolipid found primarily on erythroid cells, where it is known as the *P blood group antigen* (Brown et al., 1993). This receptor is necessary for B19 infection. Bone marrow from patients who lack the P antigen (p phenotype) cannot be infected in vitro with B19, and individuals without this antigen on their red cells are naturally immune to B19 infection (Brown et al., 1994). The tissue distribution of the cellular receptor explains the predominance of hematologic effects in B19 infection. P antigen is also found on vascular endothelial cells, megakaryocytes, placenta, fetal liver, and fetal myocardial cells, a tissue distribution that may have implications for the pathogenesis of other B19 syndromes (Brown et al., 1993).

The primary target of B19 infection is erythroid progenitor cells in the marrow near the pronormoblast stage (Ozawa et al., 1987). The virus lytically infects these cells, leading to an arrest of erythropoiesis (Young, 1988). Susceptibility to infection appears to increase with increasing differentiation and the pluripotent stem cells are spared (Takahashi et al., 1990). Infected bone marrow cultures are characterized by the presence of giant pronormoblasts, or "lantern cells" (Brown and Young, 1995). These are large, early erythroid cells recognized by their cytoplasmic vacuolization, immature chromatin, and large eosinophilic nuclear inclusion bodies. These cells are also found in bone marrow of clinically infected patients (Kurtzman et al., 1987; Van Horn et al., 1986).

The viral suppression of erythropoiesis by B19 is demonstrated in vitro by its effect on colony assays of erythroid cells. Addition of virus to erythroid colony assays results in near complete inhibition of erythroid colony-forming units (CFU-E) and variable inhibition of erythroid blast-forming units (BFU-E) (Mortimer et al., 1983a). This suppressive effect can be reversed by the addition of convalescent serum containing IgG antibodies to B19. The virus has no effect on colonies of the myeloid cell lines (CFU-GM). B19 has been shown to cause inhibition of megakaryocytopoiesis in vitro without viral replication or cell lysis (Srivastava et al., 1990). Infection of such cells that are nonpermissive for viral replication leads to accumulation of a viral nonstructural protein, NS1, that may itself be toxic to the cell (Ozawa et al., 1988). This mechanism may explain the thrombocytopenia often observed during a B19-induced aplastic crisis.

The neutropenia and leukopenia observed in conjunction with B19 infection is more difficult to explain. Despite the apparent lack of effect of B19 on myeloid colony assays, replicating virus has been isolated from peripheral blood granulocytes in patients with acute B19 infection (Kurtzman et al., 1988). Recently it has been suggested that the development of cell-specific antibodies may play a role in these cytopenias, including neutropenia. Antineutrophil antibodies have been reported in a few cases of childhood neutropenia associated with B19 infection (Murray and Morad, 1994). Destruction of antibody-coated neutrophils in the reticuloendothelial system would then be the pathogenetic mechanism leading to neutropenia in this model. A complete explanation for these nonerythroid cytopenias must await further studies of viral pathogenesis.

For patients with a transient aplastic crisis, this pathophysiologic process makes the clinical presentation understandable. Individuals with conditions of chronic hemolysis and increased red cell turnover are very sensitive to any perturbations in erythropoiesis. Infection with B19 leads to a transient arrest in red cell production and a resultant precipitous fall in serum hemoglobin and hematocrit that usually requires transfusion. The reticulocyte count falls to near zero, reflecting the lysis of infected erythroblasts. Viral-specific IgM appears within 1 to 2 days of the peak of viremia, followed by IgG antibodies to B19, and the infection is controlled. Control of the infection and the relative resistance of the pluripotent stem cells to infection contribute to marrow recovery with a reactive reticulocytosis and rise in serum hemoglobin (Takahashi et al., 1990).

Normal volunteers infected with B19 develop a mild, biphasic illness rather than an aplastic crisis (Anderson et al., 1985). Seven to eleven days after inoculation, such volunteers develop viremia with fever, malaise, and mild upper respiratory tract symptoms. Their reticulocyte counts drop to undetectable levels but, with a normal red cell half-life of 120 days, this results in only a mild, clinically insignificant dip in serum hemoglobin concentration. Their symptoms resolve spontaneously and the reticulocytes return to normal with the appearance of specific antibodies. Some volunteers develop a generalized rash 17 to 18 days after inoculation and arthralgias coincident with the appearance of specific antibodies. Thus some manifestations of B19 infection are a direct result of lytic viral infection (transient aplastic crisis, fetal hydrops), whereas others (EI, arthropathy) are postinfectious phenomena related to the immune response and possibly immune complex development (Anderson, 1990). Skin biopsies from patients with EI have shown only edema and perivascular mononuclear infiltrates (Cherry, 1992). In one skin biopsy, viral capsid proteins and DNA were identified in epidermal cells, suggesting that B19 may have a more direct effect in the production of exanthema (Schwarz et al., 1994).

Like other parvoviruses, B19 crosses the placenta, causing fetal viremia after a primary maternal infection. The fetus is at risk for serious disease because of both its hematologic status and its immature immune status (Anderson, 1990). The fetus has a rapidly expanding red cell mass, a relatively short red cell half-life, and impaired humoral immunity. Intrauterine infection may lead to a profound fetal anemia and consequent high-output cardiac failure. Fetal hydrops ensues and fetal mortality is high. There may also be a direct effect of the virus on the fetal heart, as evidenced by the presence of B19 DNA in myocardial tissue from abortuses and supported by the tissue distribution of the P antigen (Brown et al., 1993; Porter et al., 1988).

IMMUNITY

In the normal host, infection with parvovirus B19 induces a brisk IgM and IgG response. Experimental infection of human volunteers has elucidated the course of the immune response (Anderson et al., 1985). Viremia occurs between 7 and 11 days after inoculation with a peak at 8 to 9 days. IgM antibody to B19 appears 10 to 14 days after infection (generally 1 to 2 days after the peak of viremia) and remains detectable for 6 to 8 weeks but may persist for several months. IgG antibody follows within a few days and persists for life, serving as a marker of prior infection and immunity. The early antibody responses are directed against the major capsid protein, VP2, but, as the immune response matures, reactivity to the minor capsid protein VP1 predominates (Kurtzman et al., 1989b). The immune response to VP1 appears to be crucial for the development of protective immunity: VP1 must be present in recombinant capsids to elicit a neutralizing antibody response in animals (Kajigaya et al., 1991). Some patients with persistent B19 infections have antibody to VP2 but lack antibodies to VP1 (Kurtzman et al., 1989b).

Less is known about the IgA responses to B19 infection. In patients with typical EI, serum IgA appears to parallel IgG response but to a lesser degree, peaking in 1 to 2 weeks and gradually declining over 6 to 12 months (Erdman et al., 1991). No information is available on the secretory IgA response.

Humoral responses appear to control B19 infection. Recovery from infection correlates with the appearance of circulating viral-specific antibody; administration of commercial immunoglobulins appears to cure or ameliorate persistent B19 infections in immunodeficient patients (Frickhofen et al., 1990; Koch et al., 1990; Kurtzman et al., 1989a). Attempts to detect a cellular response to B19 have been generally unsuccessful (Kurtzman et al., 1989b).

DIAGNOSIS

The diagnosis of erythema infectiosum (fifth disease) is usually based on the clinical recognition of the typical exanthem, benign course, and exclusion of other similar conditions. A presumptive diagnosis of a B19-induced transient aplastic crisis in a known sickle cell anemia patient (or a patient of another condition of chronic hemolysis) is based on an acute febrile illness, severe fall in serum hemoglobin, and an absolute reticulocytopenia.

Specific laboratory diagnosis depends on identification of B19 antibodies, viral antigens, or viral DNA. In the immunologically normal patient, determination of anti-B19 IgM is the best marker of recent or acute infection on a single serum sample. IgM antibodies develop rapidly after infection and are generally detectable for 6 to 8 weeks (Anderson et al., 1986). IgG antibodies become detectable a few days after IgM and persist for years and probably life. Seroconversion from IgG-negative to IgG-positive on paired sera also confirms a recent infection. Anti-B19 IgG, however, primarily serves as a marker of past infection or immunity. Patients with EI or acute B19 arthropathy are almost always IgM-positive, so a diagnosis can usually be made from a single serum sample. Patients with B19-induced aplastic crisis may present before antibodies are detectable; however, IgM will be detectable within 1 to 2 days of presentation and IgG will follow within days (Saarinen et al., 1986).

The availability of serologic assays for B19 had previously been limited by the lack of a reliable and renewable source of antigen for diagnostic studies. The development of recombinant cell lines that express B19 capsid proteins promises a more reliable source of antigen suitable for use in commercial test kits. There currently are a few commercial kits available for B19 antibodies, but they use a variety of antigens (recombinant capsid proteins, fusion proteins, synthetic peptides) and their performance in large studies has varied (Cohen and Bates, 1995). Until serologic tests are more standardized and results more consistent, some knowledge of the test method and particular viral antigen used will be necessary for proper interpretation of test results.

In immunocompromised or immunodeficient patients, serologic diagnosis is unreliable because humoral responses are impaired and methods to detect viral particles or viral DNA are necessary to make the diagnosis of a B19 infection. As noted, the virus cannot be isolated on routine cell cultures, so viral culture is not useful. Detection of viral

DNA by DNA hybridization techniques or by polymerase chain reaction is a useful method in these patients (Clewley, 1985, 1989; Koch and Adler, 1990). Both techniques can be applied to a variety of clinical specimens, including serum, amniotic fluid, fresh tissues, bone marrow, and paraffin-embedded tissues (Török, 1992).

Histologic examination is also helpful in diagnosing B19 infection in certain situations. Examination of bone marrow aspirates in anemic patients often reveals giant pronormoblasts against a background of general erythroid hypoplasia. However, the absence of such cells does not exclude B19 infection (Brown et al., 1994; Heegard et al., 1996). Electron microscopy may reveal viral particles in serum of some infected patients and cord blood or tissues of hydropic infants (Caul et al., 1988; Cossart et al., 1975).

DIFFERENTIAL DIAGNOSIS

The differential diagnosis of EI includes rubella, measles, enteroviral infections, scarlet fever, and drug reactions. Rubella is the most clinically similar condition and may be difficult to exclude on physical examination. Measles and scarlet fever should be clinically distinguishable by the significant fever and typical coryzal prodrome of measles and the fever and pharyngitis of scarlet fever. Older children and adolescents presenting with a suggestive rash and joint symptoms should prompt consideration of other rheumatologic disorders such as juvenile chronic arthritis and systemic lupus erythematosus.

Whereas B19 is by far the most common cause of the transient aplastic crisis in sickle cell anemia patients, infection with other pathogens, especially systemic bacterial infections, may cause relative degrees of erythroid hypoplasia and subsequent worsening of the chronic anemia (Cherry, 1992; Serjeant et al., 1981). The degree of suppression of hematopoiesis, however, is much less dramatic; the fall in the reticulocyte count is not as extreme; and other signs of infection are usually present, such as pneumonia, abscess, osteomyelitis, etc.

COMPLICATIONS

In adolescents and adults, erythema infectiosum is often accompanied by arthalgias or arthritis, which may persist after resolution of the rash. Joint symptoms occur in 60% to 80% of adults with EI, whereas the incidence in children (<9 years of age) is less than 10% (Ager et al., 1966; Török, 1992). Before the discovery of B19, neurologic complications of encephalitis and aseptic meningitis were rarely described after EI; subsequently, reports have appeared describing B19-associated meningitis, encephalitis, and also a peripheral neuropathy (Koduri and Naides, 1995; Török, 1992). The majority has resolved without sequelae.

EPIDEMIOLOGY AND TRANSMISSION

B19 is a highly contagious infection. In the United States, 60% or more of white adults are seropositive (have IgG antibodies to B19 in their sera). This indicates a previous infection usually acquired in childhood. Among blacks the rate of seropositivity is lower, about 30%. Transmission of B19 from person to person is probably by droplets from oral or nasal secretions. This is suggested (1) by the rapid transmission among those in close physical contact, such as schoolmates or family members; and (2) by a study of healthy volunteers wherein virus was found in blood and nasopharyngeal secretions for several days beginning a day or two before symptoms appeared. In the volunteer study, no virus was detected in urine or stool.

Because B19 infections are highly contagious and their transmission requires close contact, most outbreaks occur in elementary schools. Seronegative adult school personnel are at high risk for acquiring the infection from students (Adler et al., 1993). Some outbreaks in schools may be epidemic, with many children and staff acquiring the infection and developing symptoms of erythema infectiosum. At other times the infection is often endemic, with transmission occurring slowly and only a few manifesting symptoms.

Other settings where B19 transmission is facilitated include the hospital and the family. B19 can readily be transmitted from infected patients to hospital workers (Bell et al., 1989). Therefore patients with erythrocyte aplasia should be presumed to have a B19 infection until proven otherwise. These patients should receive respiratory and contact isolation while hospitalized. The family is another setting where transmission is rapid, although no intervention is generally necessary to interrupt transmission here.

Outbreaks of B19 also occur in day-care centers, although transmission here is less common than among school-age children. B19 has also been transmitted via infusion of coagulation factors, although this is uncommon (Mortimer et al., 1983b). B19 transmission has not been reported, but is theoretically possible after routine erythrocyte transfusions or organ transplantation.

THERAPY

The only specific therapy currently available is intravenous immunoglobulin. Since most B19 infections are self-limited, therapy mainly has been used in immunocompromised patients with prolonged anemia, for whom red blood cell transfusions may also be necessary. Intrauterine transfusion in the setting of fetal hydrops has been described but is of unknown utility.

PREVENTION

Specific preventive measures are not available. Respiratory and contact isolation of all hospitalized patients with suspected B19 infection is recommended. To reduce the risk of infection to seronegative pregnant school personnel during major school outbreaks, furloughing or transfer of such personnel to jobs without child contact is an option, but of unproven benefit.

BIBLIOGRAPHY

Adler SP, Manganello A-M, Koch WC, et al. Risk of human parvovirus B19 infections among school and hospital employees during endemic periods. J Infect Dis 1993;168:361-368.

Ager EA, Chin TDY, Poland JD. Epidemic erythema infectiosum. N Engl J Med 1966;275:1326-1331.

Anand A, Gray ES, Brown T, et al. Human parvovirus infection in pregnancy and hydrops fetalis. N Engl J Med 1987;316:183-186.

Anderson LJ. Role of parvovirus B19 in human disease. Pediatr Infect Dis J 1987;6:711-718.

Anderson LJ. Human parvoviruses. J Infect Dis 1990;161:603-608.

Anderson LJ, Tsou C, Parker RA, et al. Detection of antibodies and antigens of human parvovirus B19 by enzyme-linked immunosorbent assay. J Clin Microbiol 1986;24:522.

Anderson MJ, Higgins PG, Davis LR, et al. Experimental parvoviral infection in humans. J Infect Dis 1985;152:257-265.

Anderson MJ, Jones SE, Fisher-Hoch SP, et al. Human parvovirus, the cause of erythema infectiosum (fifth disease)? (letter) Lancet 1983;1:1378.

Anderson MJ, Lewis E, Kidd IM, et al. An outbreak of erythema infectiosum associated with human parvovirus infection. Epidemiol Infect 1984;93:83.

Bell LM, Naides SJ, Stoffman P, et al. Human parvovirus B19 infection among hospital staff members after contact with infected patients. N Engl J Med 1989;321:485.

Brown KE, Anderson SM, Young NS. Erythrocyte P antigen: cellular receptor for B19 parvovirus. Science 1993;262:114-117.

Brown KE, Green SW, de Mayolo JA, et al. Congenital anemia after transplacental B19 parvovirus infection. Lancet 1994;343:895-896.

Brown KE, Hibbs JR, Gallinella G, et al. Resistance to parvovirus B19 infection due to lack of virus receptor (erythrocyte P antigen). N Engl J Med 1994;330:1192-1196.

Brown KE, Young NS. Parvovirus B19 infection and hematopoiesis. Blood Rev 1995;9:176-182.

Caul EO, Usher MJ, Burton PA. Intrauterine infection with human parvovirus B19: a light and electron microscopy study. J Med Virol 1988;24:55-66.

Cherry JD. Parvoviruses. In Feigin RD, Cherry JD (eds). Textbook of Pediatric Infectious Diseases. Philadelphia: WB Saunders Co, 1992.

Chorba T, Coccia P, Holman RC, et al. The role of parvovirus B19 in aplastic crisis and erythema infectiosum (fifth disease). J Infect Dis 1986;154:383-393.

Clewley JP. Detection of human parvovirus using a molecularly cloned probe. J Med Virol 1985;15:173.

Clewley JP. Polymerase chain reaction assay of parvovirus B19 DNA in clinical specimens. J Clin Microbiol 1989;27:2647.

Cohen BJ, Bates CM. Evaluation of 4 commercial test kits for parvovirus B19-specific IgM. J Virol Meth 1995;55:11-25.

Cossart YE, Cant B, Field AM, et al. Parvovirus-like particles in human sera. Lancet 1975;1:72.

Erdman DD, Usher MJ, Tsou C, et al. Human parvovirus B19 specific IgG, IgA, and IgM antibodies and serum DNA in serum specimens from persons with erythema infectiosum. J Med Virol 1991;35:110-115.

Ferguson PJ, Saulsbury FT, Dowell SF, et al. Prevalence of human parvovirus B19 infection in children with Henoch-Schönlein purpura. Arthritis Rheum 1996;39:880-881.

Finkel TH, Torok TJ, Ferguson PJ, et al. Chronic parvovirus B19 infection and systemic necrotising vasculitis: opportunistic infection or aetiological agent? Lancet 1994;343:1255-1258.

Foto F, Saag KG, Scharosch LL, et al. Parvovirus B19-specific DNA in bone marrow from arthropathy patients: evidence for B19 virus persistence. J Infect Dis 1993;167:744-748.

Frickhofen N, Abkowitz JL, Safford M, et al. Persistent B19 parvovirus infection in patients infected with human immunodeficiency virus type 1 (HIV-1): a treatable cause of anemia in AIDS. Ann Intern Med 1990;113:926-933.

Gratacos E, Torres P-J, Vidal J, et al. The incidence of human parvovirus B19 infection during pregnancy and its impact on perinatal outcome. J Infect Dis 1995;171:1360-1363.

Hall SM, Public Health Laboratory Service Working Party on Fifth Disease. Prospective study of human parvovirus (B19) infection in pregnancy. Br Med J 1990;300:1166-1170.

Hartwig NG, Vermeij-Keers C, Van Elsacker-Niele AMW, et al. Embryonic malformations in a case of intrauterine parvovirus B19 infection. Teratology 1989;39:295-302.

Hauswirth WW. Autonomous parvovirus DNA structure and replication. In Berns KI (ed). The Parvoviruses. London: Plenum Press, 1984.

Heegard ED, Hasle H, Clausen N, et al. Parvovirus B19 infection and Diamond-Blackfan anaemia. Acta Pediatr 1996;85:299-302.

Kajigaya S, Fujii H, Field A, et al. Self-assembled B19 parvovirus capsids, produced in a baculovirus system, are antigenically and immunologically similar to native virions. Proc Natl Acad Aci. 1991;88:4646-4650.

Kinney JS, Anderson LJ, Farrar J, et al. Risk of adverse outcomes of pregnancy after intrauterine infection with human parvovirus B19 infection. J Infect Dis 1988;157:663-667.

Koch WC, Adler SP. Detection of human parvovirus B19 DNA by using the polymerase chain reaction. J Clin Microbiol 1990;28:65-69.

Koch WC, Adler SP, Harger J. Intrauterine parvovirus B19 infection may cause an asymptomatic or recurrent postnatal infection. Pediatr Infect Dis J 1993;12:747-750.

Koch WC, Massey G, Russell CE, et al. Manifestations and treatment of human parvovirus B19 infection in immunocompromised patients. J Pediatr 1990;116:355-359.

Koduri PR, Naides SJ. Aseptic meningitis caused by parvovirus B19. Clin Infect Dis 1995;21:1053.

Kurtzman G, Frickhofen N, Kimball J, et al. Pure red-cell aplasia of ten years' duration due to persistent parvovirus B19 infection and its cure with immunoglobulin therapy. N Engl J Med 1989a;321:519-523.

Kurtzman GJ, Cohen BJ, Field AM, et al. Immune response to B19 parvovirus and antibody defect in persistent viral infection. J Clin Invest 1989b;84:1114-1123.

Kurtzman GJ, Gascon P, Caras M, et al. B19 parvovirus replicates in circulating cells of acutely infected patients. Blood 1988;71:1448-1454.

Kurtzman GJ, Ozawa K, Cohen B, et al. Chronic bone marrow failure due to persistent B19 parvovirus infection. N Engl J Med 1987;317:287-294.

Lefrere J-J, Courouce A-M, Bertrand Y, et al. Human parvovirus and aplastic crisis in chronic hemolytic anemias: a study of 24 observations. Am J Hematol 1986;23:271-275.

Lefrere J-J, Courouce A-M, Kaplan C. Parvovirus and idiopathic thrombocytopenic purpura (letter). Lancet 1989;i:279.

Morey AL, Nicolini U, Welch CR, et al. Parvovirus B19 infection and transient fetal hydrops (letter). Lancet 1991;337:496.

Mortimer PP, Humphries RK, Moore JG, et al. A human parvovirus-like virus inhibits haematopoietic colony formation in vitro. Nature 1983a;302:426-429.

Mortimer PP, Luban NLC, Kelleher JF, et al. Transmission of serum parvovirus-like virus by clotting-factor concentrates. Lancet 1983b;2:482.

Muir K, Todd WTA, Watson WH, et al. Viral-associated haemophagocytosis with parvovirus B19-related pancytopenia. Lancet 1992;339:1139-1140.

Murray JC, Morad AB. Childhood autoimmune neutropenia and human parvovirus B19 (letter). Am J Hematol 1994;47:336.

Naides SJ, Field EH. Transient rheumatoid factor positivity in acute human parvovirus B19 infection. Arch Intern Med 1988;148:2587-2589.

Naides SJ, Howard EJ, Swack NS, et al. Parvovirus B19 infection in human immunodeficiency virus type 1–infected persons failing or intolerant to zidovudine therapy. J Infect Dis 1993;168:101-105.

Ozawa K, Ayub J, Kajigaya S, et al. The gene encoding the nonstructural protein of B19 (human) parvovirus may be lethal in transfected cells. J Virol 1988;62:2884-2889.

Ozawa K, Kurtzman G, Young N. Productive infection by B19 parvovirus of human erythroid bone marrow cells in vitro. Blood 1987;70:384-391.

Pattison JR, Jones SE, Hodgson J. Parvovirus infections and hypoplastic crisis in sickle-cell anaemia (letter). Lancet 1981;1:664.

Paver WK, Clarke SKR. Comparison of human fecal and serum parvo-like viruses. J Clin Microbiol 1976;4:67.

Plummer FA, Hammond GW, Forward K, et al. An erythema infectiosum–like illness caused by human parvovirus infection. N Engl J Med 1985;313:74-79.

Porter HJ, Quantrill AM, Fleming KA. B19 parvovirus infection of myocardial cells (letter). Lancet 1988;1:535.

Rodis FJ, Quinn DL, Gary GW, et al. Management and outcomes of pregnancies complicated by human B19 parvovirus

infection: a prospective study. Am J Obstet Gynecol 1990; 163:1168-1171.

Saarinen UM, Chorba TL, Tattersall P, et al. Human parvovirus B19-induced epidemic acute red cell aplasia in patients with hereditary hemolytic anemia. Blood 1986;67:1411-1417.

Saunders PWG, Reid MM, Cohen BJ. Human parvovirus induced cytopenias: a report of five cases. Br J Haematol 1986;63:407-410.

Schwartz TF, Roggendorf M, Hottentrager B, et al. Human parvovirus B19 infection in pregnancy (letter). Lancet 1988; 2:566.

Schwarz TF, Serke S, Hottentrager B, et al. Replication of parvovirus B19 in hematopoietic progenitor cells generated in vitro from normal human peripheral blood. J Virol 1992;66:1273-1276.

Schwarz TF, Wiersbitzky S, Pambor M. Case report: detection of parvovirus B19 in skin biopsy of a patient with erythema infectiosum. J Med Virol 1994;43:171-174.

Serjeant GR, Topley JM, Mason K, et al. Outbreak of aplastic crises in sickle cell anaemia associated with parvovirus-like agent. Lancet 1981;2:595-597.

Shimomura S, Komatsu N, Frickhofen N, et al. First continuous propagation of B19 parvovirus in a cell line. Blood 1992;79:18-24.

Sosa CE, Mahoney JB, Luinstra KE, et al. Replication and cytopathology of human parvovirus B19 in human umbilical cord blood erythroid progenitor cells. J Med Virol 1992; 36:125-130.

Srivastava A, Bruno E, Briddell R, et al. Parvovirus B19-induced perturbation of human megakaryocytopoiesis in vitro. Blood 1990;76:1997-2004.

Summers J, Jones SE, Anderson MJ. Characterization of the genome of the agent of erythrocyte aplasia permits its classification as a human parvovirus. J Gen Virol 1983;64: 2527.

Takahashi T, Ozawa K, Takahashi K, et al. Susceptibility of human erythropoietic cells to B19 parvovirus in vitro increases with differentiation. Blood 1990;75:603-610.

Thurn J. Human parvovirus B19: historical and clinical review. Rev Infect Dis 1988;10:1005-1011.

Török TJ. Parvovirus B19 and human disease. Ann Int Med 1992;37:431-455.

Török TJ, Wang Q-Y, Gary GW, et al. Prenatal diagnosis of intrauterine infection with parvovirus B19 by the polymerase chain reaction technique. Clin Infect Dis 1992;14:149-155.

Van Horn DK, Mortimer PP, Young N, et al. Human parvovirus–associated red cell aplasia in the absence of underlying hemolytic anemia. Am J Pediatr Hematol/Oncol 1986; 8:235-239.

Weiland HT, Salimans MMM, Fibbe WE, et al. Prolonged parvovirus B19 infection with severe anaemia in a bone marrow transplant recipient (letter). Br J Haematol 1989;71:300.

White DG, Woolf AD, Mortimer PP, et al. Human parvovirus arthropathy. Lancet 1985;1:419-421.

Yaegashi N, Shiraishi H, Takeshita T, et al. Propagation of human parvovirus B19 in primary culture of erythroid lineage cells derived from fetal liver. J Virol 1989;63:2422-2426.

Young N. Hematologic and hematopoietic consequences of B19 parvovirus infection. Sem Hematol 1988;25:159-172.

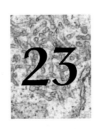

23 PERTUSSIS (WHOOPING COUGH)

EDWARD A. MORTIMER, JR.

Pertussis is a devastating contagious disease of childhood, particularly infancy, that is now well controlled in the United States and other developed countries by immunization. However, at the turn of the century in the United States approximately 5 of every 1,000 infants born alive died of the disease before their fifth birthdays (Mortimer and Jones, 1979). Today, fewer than 10 deaths are reported annually in the United States. Thus the disease remains well controlled in the developed world, although occasional local outbreaks continue to occur. In contrast, in the developing world as recently as the early 1980s, according to the Expanded Programme on Immunization (EPI) in 1992, the rate of childhood pertussis deaths exceeded 7 per 1,000 births. Morbidity and mortality, however, have declined, and it is a remarkable tribute to the efforts of the EPI that by 1992 (in less than 10 years) this rate was reduced by 60% (World Health Organization, 1996).

In the past five years, several other developments related to the control of pertussis have occurred. In the United States there is further confirmation of adults with atypical pertussis as an important reservoir of the disease. The polymerase chain reaction (PCR) has been confirmed as a useful method for identification of the organism in respiratory secretions, although it is not yet available for routine use. However, to date it has not been possible to specify the antigens of *Bordetella pertussis* that induce clinical immunity. Acellular pertussis DTP preparations are now licensed for use in infants, as well as older children, and they are being considered for use as boosters in adults.

The first description of the disease did not appear until the sixteenth century, which is rather curious for an epidemic disorder with such a characteristic clinical picture. An explanatory hypothesis for this curiosity includes the possibility that pertussis was a disease new to humans at that time, perhaps as a consequence of mutation of a somewhat similar organism that affected lower animals. Another hypothesis is that physicians of the past paid less attention to the disease in the presence of many other more devastating diseases. The causative organism, *Bordetella pertussis,* was first recovered by Bordet and Gengou in 1906, and in the mid 1940s effective vaccines became available. Current whole-cell vaccines are essentially the same as those in use 40 years ago, although they are better standardized in terms of immunogenicity and toxicity. Only in recent years has the biologic anatomy of the organism been sufficiently understood to permit development of acellular preparations free of components irrelevant to the production of immunity.

ETIOLOGY

B. pertussis is a gram-negative organism that appears in coccobacillary form on a fresh isolation but in older preparations may be pleomorphic. It is a rather fastidious organism on culture, requiring the addition of 15% to 20% blood or some other substance to neutralize various factors that inhibit its growth. Modified Bordet-Gengou agar medium contains a potato-glycerol base with the addition of blood. A synthetic medium, Stainer-Scholte agar supplemented with cyclodextrin and cephalexin, has a longer shelf life, which facilitates the direct plating of specimens. The organism is hemolytic. Isolates from culture frequently are described as being of phases I through IV. Phase I, or smooth, isolates comprise relatively uniform coccobacillary organisms of high virulence. With repeated transfer the organisms mutate and progressively and irreversibly lose their virulence through phases II, III, and IV. Avirulent phase IV organisms have lost pertussis toxin, adenylate cyclase, and other factors. Failure to limit vaccine production to phase I organisms in the early years of pertussis vaccine development may have contributed to variations in the protective efficacy of different preparations. In nature, *B. pertussis* is pathogenic only for humans, although it is possible to infect some lower animals, including mice and chimpanzees, artificially. Two other organisms of the genus *Bordetella, B. parapertussis* and *B. bronchiseptica,* occasionally produce a pertussislike syndrome in humans.

Antigens

Among the many bacteria that affect humans, *B. pertussis* has been one of the most difficult to study in terms of its biologic anatomy. Indeed, only in the last 20 years or so has it been possible to dissect the organism and relate its various components to disease pathogenesis and immunity in man, although as yet imperfectly. Previously, various physiologic effects and attributes of the organism, recognized in the laboratory and to some extent in humans, could not be assigned to identifiable components. Therefore, from the clinical standpoint the development of an effective subcellular pertussis vaccine, free of potentially toxic components irrelevant to immunity, could not be pursued on any logical scientific basis until recently. A brief review of the constituents of the organism and their probable or possible roles in disease pathogenesis and immunity follows.

Unfortunately, a major problem in determining the efficacy of pertussis vaccines is that, to date, correlation between one or more antibodies with clinical immunity has not been established (Olin, 1995). A component of *B. pertussis* assigned considerable importance in the pathogenesis and immunology of pertussis has been variously designated *pertussis toxin* (PT), *lymphocytosis-promoting factor* (LPF), and *pertussigen,* with the first term used most commonly (Table 23-1). The existence of this component has long been recognized because of its physiologic actions, identified in humans and in laboratory animals; however,

only in the last 20 years has it become evident that these actions are produced by a single molecule. PT is associated with the production of lymphocytosis in humans and experimental animals. It is also the histamine-sensitizing factor (HSF), the effect of which has been long recognized in experimental animals, although this effect is of no apparent consequence in humans. PT also stimulates the release of insulin in humans and animals; in animals, but not in humans, significant hypoglycemia results. PT has a variety of other actions, including (1) mitogenicity for some human and animal cells, and (2) hemagglutination (Wardlaw and Parton, 1988). It is likely that PT plays an important role in the pathogenesis of pertussis. Although sometimes designated as a toxin, it exerts its major effects locally rather than systemically. It appears to facilitate attachment of the organism to respiratory cilia and is an important contributor to respiratory mucosal damage. PT is immunogenic and is a major factor in the induction of immunity in the mouse protection test, which is used as the standard measure of potency for whole-cell pertussis vaccines. Antibodies to PT develop in humans after infection or immunization, and it is highly probable that antibodies to PT are important in clinical immunity to pertussis.

Filamentous hemagglutinin (FHA) is an antigen that apparently plays a single role (that of facilitating attachment of the organism to respiratory cilia) in disease pathogenesis and that also contributes to clinical immunity. It is nontoxic for cells. FHA is vigorously immunogenic, producing measurable antibodies, and there is evidence that these antibodies contribute to clinical protection against pertussis.

Strains of the genus *Bordetella* produce a number of agglutinating capsular antigens. Agglutinogens 1 through 6 are found only in strains of *B. pertussis;* agglutinogen 7 is found in all three members

Table 23-1 Putative roles of constituents of *B. pertussis* in humans

Constituent	Pathogenesis	Immunity
Pertussis toxin	Attachment; cell damage	Important
FHA	Attachment	Probably important
Agglutinogens	Unknown	Possibly important
Pertactin	Unknown	Possibly important
Adenylate cyclase	Cell damage	Unknown
Tracheal toxin	Cell damage	None
Dermonecrotic toxin	Unknown	None
Endotoxin	Probably none	None

of the genus; and factors 14 and 12 occur in *B. parapertussis* and *B. bronchiseptica,* respectively. These agglutinogens apparently are not active in the pathogenesis of pertussis. However, they are immunogenic, and there is seroepidemiologic evidence that they (or some component closely associated with them) play a role in inducing clinical immunity to pertussis. This evidence derives from studies in the United Kingdom suggesting that efficacy of whole-cell pertussis vaccines depends on a match between the agglutinogens present in the vaccine strain and those in strains circulating in the community (Public Health Laboratory Service, 1973). Another component of the organism that has attracted recent attention, particularly in relation to its potential role as a protective antigen, is pertactin, an outer membrane protein, originally called *69K* because of its molecular weight. Pertactin is closely associated with, or may be identical to, agglutinogen 1. It is of interest because serum antibodies to it are found after disease or immunization with the whole-cell vaccine, and these antibodies are protective against respiratory infection with *B. pertussis* in mice (Shahin et al., 1990). Adenylate cyclase is a cellular enzyme that disrupts host cell metabolism and very likely participates in ciliary destruction. It is also immunogenic, but there is no evidence to date that antibodies to this enzyme play a role in clinical immunity.

Another identified component of the organism is tracheal toxin, which very likely plays a role in cell damage. A relatively small molecule, tracheal toxin is not immunogenic. A heat-labile toxin, sometimes known as dermonecrotic toxin, is also produced. It is lethal to animals when given systemically and produces dermonecrosis on local injection. It appears to play no role in clinical immunity, and whether or how it participates in the pathogenesis of the disease is unknown. Like other gram-negative bacteria, *B. pertussis* produces an endotoxin. Compared to the endotoxins of enteric bacilli, the toxicity of this lipopolysaccharide is weak, being one tenth to one hundredth as potent. It is not immunogenic, and there is no evidence that it participates in the pathogenesis of the disease.

EPIDEMIOLOGY

Pertussis is highly contagious, transmitted primarily by intimate respiratory contact. Nearly all nonimmune, exposed household contacts acquire the disease, and approximately 50% of susceptible individuals exposed in school settings develop pertussis. Because there is negligible transplacental immunity, young infants, in whom the disease is most dangerous, are fully susceptible.

In the absence of immunization it is likely that few individuals escape pertussis during life. However, as with many notifiable infections, pertussis is considerably underreported. Indeed, a well-conducted recent study has indicated that as few as one quarter of all cases are actually reported (Sutter and Cochi, 1992). The reasons for lack of notification are multiple and probably include failure to suspect and diagnose the disease (particularly when the manifestations are atypical or mild); the difficulty in laboratory confirmation; and, unfortunately, the failure of some physicians to appreciate the importance of reporting. Curiously, the disease is more often reported in girls than in boys, and mortality rates are higher in girls. An explanation for this phenomenon is not evident; it may be, given that almost every unimmunized child acquires pertussis, that the disease is inexplicably more severe and therefore more recognizable, and thus reported, in females. In the past, pertussis was both endemic and epidemic; major increases in incidence occurred every 3 or 4 years (usually 3). Widespread immunization has not altered this cyclic pattern, although incidence rates, both endemic and peak, are strikingly lower (Cherry, 1984).

Seasonal influences on the incidence of pertussis in the United States are difficult to interpret. There is no unanimity among descriptions of the seasonal epidemiology of pertussis before widespread use of the vaccine. Some reports indicated higher incidence in the summer when young infants probably were in more contact with each other. Others stated that the peak incidence was in late winter and early spring, and some alleged no seasonal variation. However, examination of tabulated deaths from pertussis by month for the 5 years 1936 through 1940, allowing a 4- to 8-week lag between onset and date of death, provides support for the assertion that the incidence of pertussis was highest during the first half of the calendar year, at least in younger children, the group most likely to succumb from the disease. Closer examination of these mortality data shows that this seasonal variation was accounted for by the 2 years (1937 and 1938) when deaths were the highest (70% greater than the other 3 years). Recorded deaths for the 3 years with fewer deaths show no month-to-month variation. This suggests that in colder, temperate zones such as the United States pertussis was endemic year-round before the advent of widespread immunization and that epidemics were more apt to occur in the winter and spring. Remarkably, the seasonal epidemiology of pertussis is presently very different. For the years 1980 through 1989, pertussis was 2 or 3 times more frequent in the late summer or autumn, with a curious disparity between northern and southern states (Farizo, 1992). In southern states the peak occurred in midsummer; in northern states peak months were July to October. In Cincinnati in the years 1989 through 1993, cases of pertussis were far more frequent in the latter half of the year (Christie, 1994). No explanation is available for the past and current seasonality of pertussis or for the apparent shift.

There have also been remarkable changes in the age distribution of pertussis from the prevaccine era to the present, but these changes very likely are explained by widespread immunization beginning in the 1950s. Before World War II approximately half of all reported cases occurred in elementary school–age children, who served as the major reservoir of the disease. Less than 20% of cases occurred in infants under 1 year of age, but 50% to 70% of all deaths occurred in this age group. Fewer than 1% of reported cases occurred in individuals older than 14 years (Dauer, 1943). The present age distribution of pertussis in the United States has changed markedly, very likely as a consequence of several interrelated factors. The first is widespread immunization against the disease. A second factor is the requirement for immunization before school entry in the United States. In some states this requirement includes day-care and preschool classes, but in all states immunization requirements are mandated for entry into elementary school. A factor of indeterminable impact is possible enhanced recognition and reporting of pertussis as a result of augmented interest in the disease and better diagnostic methods. Finally, it is increasingly recognized that pertussis occurs in adolescents and adults, ranging from mild atypical cases to the full-blown syndrome (Mortimer, 1990; Nennig et al.,

1996; Deen et al., 1995; Cherry, 1995; Izurieta et al., 1996). It is uncertain whether this phenomenon (1) has always existed and is now evident because of decreased rates of pertussis in other age groups, (2) is a result of waning of vaccine-induced immunity caused by the declining incidence of pertussis and the consequent lack of reinforcement of immunity caused by casual exposure to the disease, or (3) results from better laboratory methods for diagnosis. It is also important to note that infections may occur in hospital personnel, even as outbreaks (Cherry, 1995). It is logical to assume that these adult infections, whether mild or severe, represent important sources of continuing transmission of *B. pertussis*. Table 23-2 compares the age distributions of pertussis for 1979 through 1981 and 1992 through 1994 in the United States. Because there is firm evidence that partially immune adolescents and adults with pertussis often exhibit mild symptoms, these data probably underestimate the true incidence of infection in older persons. Whatever the reasons, the striking reductions in pertussis morbidity and mortality in the United States have been associated with clear-cut changes in the age distribution of reported cases. These changes have important implications for the control of the disease.

Determining the effects of race on pertussis epidemiology is complicated by a number of factors. In the late 1930s overall pertussis mortality rates for blacks strikingly exceeded those for whites (Dauer, 1943). This was in part a result of the fact that disease incidence rates for blacks compared to whites were considerably higher in infants and very young children, who are at greatest risk of death. Additionally, age-specific mortality rates for blacks were higher in all age groups. These differences in morbidity and mortality are undoubtedly explained in large part by socioeconomic status. Curiously, overall mortality rates from pertussis were always higher in rural areas in the United States; it is likely that this is in part explained by very high mortality

Table 23-2 Age distribution of reported pertussis cases in the United States, 1979–1981 and 1992–1994

Year	Total cases	Percent by age group in years				
		<1	1-4	5-14	15-19	>19
1979-1981	4,601	56	26	12	2	4
1992-1994	14,829	41	20	21	6	12

From Centers for Disease Control from annual summaries published in the *Morbidity and Mortality Weekly Report* for the respective years.

rates in blacks in the rural South. These differences persisted through the first decade or two of the pertussis vaccine era, probably for similar reasons and because of lower rates of immunization in blacks. It is therefore unlikely that any differences in morbidity and mortality by race are related to the genetics of race (Dauer, 1943).

PATHOLOGY

The pathologic findings in patients with pertussis are primarily bronchopulmonary; changes in other organs are of anoxic origin stemming from bronchopulmonary damage. The key changes are bronchial and bronchiolar, with ciliary damage and destruction, edema, and the accumulation of mucoid secretions. Secondary findings are bronchiolar obstruction; atelectasis; areas of bronchopneumonia; and, occasionally, spotty emphysematous changes. Pneumothorax occurs but is uncommon, and secondary bacterial pneumonia such as lobar pneumonia is extremely rare. Mortality from pertussis relates directly to the severity of pulmonary involvement (Lapin, 1943). Other manifestations occur mainly in the brain and are of two varieties. The first comprises edema and other changes characteristic of anoxia. Hemorrhages constitute the other cerebral changes. They may be moderately extensive but usually are small or petechial.

PATHOGENESIS

Knowledge of the actions of the various components of *B. pertussis* permits the development of a hypothesis about the series of pathologic events that occur in the course of whooping cough. Because the likelihood of infection varies directly with the intimacy and duration of contact, it is probable that large numbers of organisms are required to infect the respiratory tract. Attachment of organisms to respiratory cilia is facilitated by PT and FHA. After attachment it is necessary for the organism to evade host defenses; major roles in this process are presumably played by PT and adenylate cyclase. It is logical that tracheal toxin and dermonecrotic toxin participate. Cell damage is a consequence of the actions of PT and adenylate cyclase. It is probable that tracheal and dermonecrotic toxins also contribute (Wardlaw and Parton, 1988). The role of pertactin is uncertain; it may relate to cell adherence. There is no evidence that agglutinogens play a role in pathogenesis. Similarly, there is no evidence that the rather weak endotoxin of *B. pertussis* contributes to disease manifestations (Wardlaw and Parton, 1988). An ob-

vious contribution of PT is the characteristic lymphocytosis of pertussis. There is no evidence that PT induces histamine stimulation of clinical consequence during the illness, nor does the insulin-stimulating activity exert any clinically recognizable effect in humans. *B. pertussis* is noninvasive; accordingly, all the manifestations of pertussis except lymphocytosis may be explained by the unique effects on respiratory endothelium with disruption of function or cell death (Wardlaw and Parton, 1988). As a consequence of ciliary destruction or dysfunction, the normal toilet of the pulmonary tree is compromised. The processes that remove foreign material, cell debris, and secretions are impaired, resulting in the accumulation of viscid mucoid material. Retained secretions obstruct smaller bronchi and bronchioles, with consequent atelectasis and occasional emphysema. Nonspecific bronchopneumonia occurs frequently. The thick ropy secretions that accumulate are very difficult to expel, resulting in episodes of repetitious, paroxysmal coughing, often followed by vomiting. The mechanism of vomiting is probably the accumulation of this viscid material in the pharynx. The characteristic whoop follows a protracted spasm that has nearly emptied the bronchopulmonary tree of air and represents an attempt to inspire through vocal cords that may be partially narrowed because of secretions and consequent spasm. Indeed, it may well be that in some instances inspiration is possible only when some relaxation of vocal cords occurs as a result of severe anoxia. The mechanism of the encephalopathy that sometimes occurs in the course of pertussis, often with permanent brain damage or death, was the subject of considerable debate in the past. A hypothesis often voiced was that one or another toxic product of *B. pertussis* was responsible. No such toxin has been identified; currently, there is general consensus that encephalopathy during the course of pertussis is explained by anoxia engendered by the episodes of paroxysmal coughing and, in some instances, by cerebral hemorrhages of varying extent that result from the combination of increased intracranial pressure during paroxysms and the vascular effects of anoxia. In those children who die of pertussis there are three apparent mechanisms of death that often act in concert. Severe bronchopulmonary disease with bronchopneumonia is of major importance. Often associated with it is the central nervous system damage described earlier. In the past, and perhaps in the developing world today, inanition secondary to repeated emesis following spasms of coughing was undoubtedly a major factor in mortality from whooping cough in infants and children. Additionally, in the past in the United States and presently in the developing world, other underlying disorders such as low birth weight; malnutrition; gastrointestinal infections; and other debilitating conditions, including measles and severe respiratory illnesses, strongly compromise survival of infants and children with whooping cough.

CLINICAL MANIFESTATIONS

The incubation period of pertussis is between 7 and 13 days. In some partially immune individuals it may be a few days longer. The initial symptoms are nonspecific. Throughout the course of the disease, fever is absent or low. There may be mild coryza-like symptoms, plus a mild, dry cough. The cough progresses in frequency and severity, and, approximately 2 weeks after onset, spells of paroxysmal coughing are recognized. The paroxysms progress in severity and frequency; ultimately, dozens of such spells may occur daily. As the paroxysms increase, the characteristic whoop occurs, often followed by vomiting. With severe paroxysms, cyanosis often occurs, the eyes roll back, and the child may appear semiconscious. When a paroxysm terminates, it appears that the respiratory tract has been nearly emptied of air; the characteristic whoop is produced by the initial attempt to inspire through the glottis, which is narrowed by spasm caused by the irritative effects of the secretions and the cough. The vomiting apparently is a consequence of thick mucoid secretions in the pharynx. Frequently, a series of paroxysms may occur in immediate succession. Severe paroxysms are very frightening to the child and to all observers. After an episode the child appears exhausted. In full-blown pertussis, paroxysms with whooping usually persist at least 2 weeks and may continue for 6 weeks. The paroxysms frequently are precipitated by a variety of events, such as feeding, crying, or even hearing another person cough; in the past, when several children with pertussis were in the same hospital room, a paroxysm in one child would precipitate episodes in others. In convalescence the cough gradually disappears over a month or more, although minor exacerbations may occur with exertion or in the course of an intercurrent respiratory infection. The two major and potentially lethal complications of pertussis, bronchopneumonia and encephalopathy, are most apt to occur at the height of the paroxysmal stage. In patients with severe whooping cough it may be difficult to maintain adequate intake of fluid and nourishment because of the vicious cycle of feeding inducing paroxysms and vomiting. In the past, when the incidence of whooping cough was high, particularly in infants, some nurses in contagious disease hospitals were highly valued for their skill and patience in feeding and refeeding infants with severe whooping cough.

DIAGNOSIS

The clinical picture of full-blown pertussis is so characteristic that the disease is readily suspected and recognized by physicians, other health-care personnel, and grandparents who have had prior experience with its manifestations, particularly if a paroxysm is observed. The presence of pertussis in the community or a history of exposure provides strongly supportive evidence; however, the source of infection may be an individual with a mild, atypical illness, particularly a household member with waning immunity. Also strongly supportive of the diagnosis is absolute lymphocytosis, which is usually present at the beginning of the paroxysmal stage and persists for 3 or 4 weeks (Fig. 23-1). However, in infants and in partially immune persons with antibodies to PT, lymphocytosis may not occur.

Proof of the diagnosis of pertussis is achieved by recovery of the organism on culture (Onorato and Wassilak, 1987). The organism is most readily recovered during the catarrhal stage but disappears within 2 or 3 weeks after the onset of paroxysms (see Fig. 23-1). The best source of material for culture is nasopharyngeal mucus obtained by the use of a transnasal swab. Use of cough plates, often the practice in the past, is less frequently successful.

Isolation of *B. pertussis* depends on careful transport and efficient processing of the materials obtained for culture and is particularly enhanced if the clinical microbiologist is experienced with the organism. If the specimen will not be planted for 1 to 2 hours, the swab should be placed in 0.25 to 0.50 ml of casamino acids solution with a pH of 7.2 to prevent drying of the swab. When the specimen will be shipped to another laboratory or when holding time exceeds 2 hours, other organisms may overgrow *B. pertussis*. Therefore swabs should be placed in modified Stuart's medium or Mishulow's charcoal agar. These media are better able to maintain the viability of organisms and to support the growth under the conditions of transport, but there is a decreased recovery rate of *B. pertussis* from

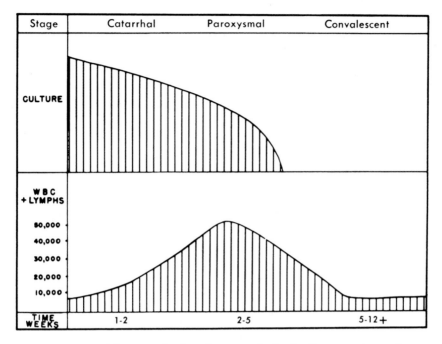

FIG. 23-1   Diagnostic laboratory findings in pertussis. *Bordetella pertussis* may be recovered, usually during catarrhal and early paroxysmal stages (first 4 weeks of illness). The white blood cell count usually is elevated during the paroxysmal stage (second to fifth weeks). Lymphocytes predominate.

transport media as compared to direct inoculation. Modified Bordet-Gengou agar is recommended for primary isolation of the organism. The addition of 0.25 to 0.5 U/ml of penicillin to a second plate is useful in inhibiting the growth of the gram-positive flora of the respiratory tract without affecting growth of *B. pertussis* organisms.

In addition to a specific pattern of biochemical reactions, serologic identification of *B. pertussis* will confirm the isolation. A slide agglutination test can be performed with a standard inoculum of organisms and specific antiserum, which is available commercially (Onorato and Wassilak, 1987). Fluorescent antibody (FA) staining has been used to identify *B. pertussis* from direct smears of nasopharyngeal swabs and for identification of organisms growing on Bordet-Gengou plates. The FA examination of nasopharyngeal swab material is often unreliable even in experienced hands. The FA procedure cannot substitute for cultural isolation of the organism, but it can offer the advantage of more rapid laboratory identification of organisms after isolation. The Analytical Bacteriology Section of the Centers for Disease Control and many of the state bacteriology laboratories are prepared to cul-

ture or examine secretions by FA techniques for *B. pertussis*. In recent years a new approach to the diagnosis of pertussis is the polymerase chain reaction (PCR) (Ewanowich et al., 1993; He et al., 1994; Schlapfer et al., 1995). By PCR the characteristic gene sequences of *B. pertussis* can be identified in respiratory secretions. Requiring relatively few organisms in the specimen, PCR is very sensitive and highly specific. Initially developed as a research tool, it probably will become more widely available.

At present, assessment of antibodies in the serum is usually accomplished by measuring agglutinins, but few laboratories in the United States are prepared to perform tests for *B. pertussis* agglutinin titers. The current microagglutination tests give titers that have not been correlated with protection against disease. Since these agglutinins are not the protective antibodies, they give only an indirect assessment of immunity, although they do reflect prior experience with *B. pertussis* as an infection or as a vaccine. After infection, there may be only a slight rise in agglutinins; this rise tends to occur weeks into the illness. An acute-phase and convalescent-phase pair of sera is needed to define an antibody rise that is indicative of recent contact with antigen.

Other generally available, specific, and reliable serologic measures of infection with *B. pertussis* are needed. Specific tests for antibodies to PT and FHA have been developed, and enzyme-linked immunosorbent assays (ELISAs) for IgG, IgM, and IgA antibodies correlate well with infection and are of considerable use in recognizing culture-negative pertussis, including mild or asymptomatic infections (Granstrom et al., 1988; Steketee et al., 1988). As yet, however, these tests are not available for routine use.

Most instances of the whooping cough syndrome in infants and children represent true pertussis, particularly during outbreaks, although on rare occasions other disorders may mimic whooping cough and result in confusion. Parapertussis, caused by a somewhat similar organism, is usually a milder illness but with many of the same symptoms. Mycoplasmal pneumonia and certain viral infections, notably those caused by adenoviruses and *Chlamydia* spp., may mimic the disease. Confusion occasionally arises in some children with bronchiolitis or protracted bronchopneumonia. Previously unrecognized cystic fibrosis may cause confusion, as may respiratory foreign bodies. In the past, tuberculosis with hilar nodes pressing on the trachea or bronchi occasionally resulted in similar symptoms. Ordinarily, however, there is little confusion, but other conditions should be suspected when confirmatory or supportive evidence such as a positive culture, lymphocytosis, and epidemiologic linkage to a proven case or to an outbreak is lacking.

More important than misclassifying other conditions as pertussis at the present time is the problem of failure to diagnose pertussis in cases that are mild or atypical as a consequence of waning immunity. Such mild illnesses may lack characteristics that distinguish them from a wide variety of other, more common respiratory disorders, and thus pertussis is not suspected. Mild cases in older siblings or parents in a household are often recognized retrospectively when an infant, as yet unimmunized, develops full-blown whooping cough. In individuals with mild disease the diagnosis, even if suspected early, is not easily made. The organism may be more difficult to recover on culture, either because of the lack of copious respiratory secretions or because the number of organisms is small. Additionally, lymphocytosis may be inhibited by residual antibody to PT. Nonetheless, such individuals appear to constitute a major reservoir for pertussis and a source of infection for others.

The need for improved diagnostic criteria for pertussis has been emphasized in recent years by the development of acellular pertussis vaccines. Because there is no established serologic surrogate for immunity to pertussis, controlled field trials designed to assess protection against clinical disease are required (Olin, 1995). Additionally, the mouse protection test, which correlates well with the efficacy of the whole cell vaccine, has not been shown to be valid for the acellular preparation. To ensure the validity and comparability of these trials, standard diagnostic criteria feasible in the field have been developed. For example, for such trials the World Health Organization advocates a combination of at least 21 days of paroxysmal cough plus a positive culture, a significant antibody rise, or household exposure to a culture-proven case. For surveillance in the United States, more liberal (and thus less specific) criteria are employed by the Centers for Disease Control and Prevention.

COMPLICATIONS

There are three major complications of pertussis: respiratory problems, effects on the central nervous system, and malnutrition. Respiratory complications usually comprise varying degrees of atelectasis and nonspecific bronchopneumonia. Localized emphysema may occur, but pneumothorax is rare. True lobar pneumonia is uncommon. In the past, 90% of deaths caused by pertussis resulted from pulmonary complications; this proportion is no doubt reduced considerably at present by modern measures of intensive care, including mechanical ventilation and, perhaps, antimicrobial therapy.

Central nervous system complications occur rarely in the course of pertussis, particularly during the paroxysmal stage, and they may be severe (Litvak et al., 1948). They apparently are secondary to anoxia and cerebral hemorrhages that are usually petechial but may be larger. The clinical findings are those of nonspecific encephalopathy, usually including repeated convulsions and obtunding. Visual disturbances and paralyses may occur. Central nervous system complications are most frequent in young infants. Estimates of the risk of encephalopathy associated with whooping cough are quite imprecise because they are based on hospitalized cases and do not include in the denominator the much larger numbers of children with pertussis who do not require hospitalization. However, from two populations in which it was possible to estimate the total number of cases of pertussis, the apparent risks of severe encephalopathy were 1:11,000 and 1:12,500 (Litvak et al., 1948; Miller et al., 1985). Undoubtedly, the risk is markedly age dependent; it is probably negligible in older children and much higher in young infants. Permanent sequelae—with seizure disorders, developmental retardation, and pareses—frequently ensue. There is also evidence, mostly but not all anecdotal, that milder forms of encephalopathy, insufficiently severe to warrant hospitalization, occur and may be associated with more subtle neurologic disturbances, including developmental disorders. In the past in the United States, malnutrition secondary to repeated vomiting and sometimes progressing to inanition was a major problem, particularly in infants. It remains a serious complication in developing countries, where it is often superimposed on, or concomitant with, other debilitating factors. The combination of large populations of unimmunized children with consequently high rates of pertussis and high case-fatality rates explains the excessive mortality from whooping cough in these countries.

Minor complications of pertussis include otitis media and hemorrhagic phenomena such as epistaxis, petechiae, and subconjunctival bleeding. In infants and children young enough to have lower incisors, ulceration of the frenum may occur because of protrusion of the tongue during coughing spells. Occasionally, a hernia may become manifest because of increased abdominal pressure during coughing spells, and, rarely, prolapse of the rectum occurs.

PROGNOSIS

In the United States the mortality rate has declined remarkably since the turn of the century. At that time approximately 1 of every 200 children born alive died of pertussis before the fifth birthday; in the last decade this risk has been reduced to no more than one in 500,000. This decline cannot be attributed solely to the advent of pertussis vaccines; indeed, by the late 1930s, before pertussis vaccine was available, the mortality rate from pertussis in young children had declined approximately 80% from 1900 (Mortimer and Jones, 1979). This remarkable decline by 1940 must be attributed to a decrease in the case-fatality rate because nearly every child experienced pertussis, a highly contagious disease. Undoubtedly, many factors contributed to this decline in the case-fatality rates. Possible factors include the diminished frequency of diarrheal diseases of infancy as a result

of pasteurization of milk; better nutrition; improved socioeconomic status; and smaller family size, resulting both in decreased exposure of high-risk young infants and in better supportive care of ill infants. With the advent of increasingly widespread immunization against pertussis beginning in the late 1940s, there was a striking acceleration in the decline of mortality from pertussis. A similar decrease was observed in Britain a few years later when pertussis immunization was instituted. Although the vaccine-induced near-elimination of pertussis is clearly the major factor in this accelerated decline, case-fatality rates have undoubtedly also decreased as a result of better supportive care, including respiratory assistance; better nutrition; and, perhaps, the availability of antibiotics (Mortimer and Jones, 1979).

TREATMENT

The treatment of pertussis is largely supportive. In most instances this protracted disease, although fatiguing or exhausting and very unpleasant, can be managed at home. Most patients who require hospitalization are young infants. For children managed at home maintenance of adequate nutrition and hydration is ordinarily easily achieved. Providing high humidity is probably of no value. Cough suppressants, if used at all, should be used in low doses to avoid interference with expulsion of secretions (Bass, 1985).

For those children who must be hospitalized, usually infants, symptomatic management depends on disease manifestations and their severity. The infant or child with severe pertussis must be constantly monitored so that immediate help can be provided for severe paroxysms. A means of suction should be at hand. In patients unable to handle their own secretions, removal of mucoid material is facilitated by placing the child in a head-down position (45 to 60 degrees) to take advantage of gravity. Suction of the oropharynx with a catheter large enough to permit flow of tenacious secretions is required during paroxysms. In a severely ill child, oxygen may be needed. The child's state of hydration must be monitored and maintained at an adequate level. Caloric intake also requires observation, although, during the most severe phase of the disease, optimal intake may not be possible.

Specific therapy is less than satisfactory. Serum immune globulin and hyperimmune antipertussis globulin, no longer available, are of no value, although a recent study of a high-dose experimental preparation suggests the contrary and the need for further study (Granstrom, 1991). *B. pertussis* is susceptible to a number of antibiotics in vitro, but the only agent with useful clinical efficacy is erythromycin. Erythromycin may be expected to eradicate *B. pertussis* from the upper respiratory tract; for this reason all persons with pertussis should receive 14 days of this antibiotic 40 mg/kg daily in 4 divided doses to minimize transmission. Unfortunately, erythromycin has not been shown to exert any effect on the clinical course of full-blown pertussis. Clearly, it will prevent or modify the course of the disease when given promptly to exposed persons or during the incubation period before the onset of symptoms (DeSerres et al., 1995). There is also some evidence that, when given early in the catarrhal stage, it will ameliorate symptoms or shorten the course of the disease. Unfortunately, the potential value of erythromycin is sorely compromised because exposure usually is not recognized and because the symptoms of those with early pertussis in the catarrhal stage are indistinguishable from those with a common respiratory infection. Nonetheless, in a household with a case of recognized pertussis, all family members with or without symptoms should receive a full course of erythromycin promptly in the stated dosage in an effort to prevent further disease and subsequent spread. On the basis of in vitro sensitivity testing it is likely that the newer macrolide antibiotics (clarithromycin and azithromycin) are effective, but no clinical trials are available to date.

IMMUNITY

Immunity to pertussis had once been considered lifelong after a first attack (Mortimer, 1990), but in recent years improved diagnostic methods and enhanced surveillance have shown this belief to be false. The proportion of individuals protected against clinical pertussis by full immunization with the whole-cell vaccine is high but not as high as the proportion protected by the natural disease.

Estimates of vaccine efficacy vary considerably, to a large extent dependent on the stringency of diagnostic criteria and on the type of exposure (household versus community), ranging from about 60% to 95% or more (Onorato et al., 1992; DeSerres et al., 1996). However, as a rule, disease that occurs in immunized persons is distinctly milder. In spite of this apparently low efficacy of whole-cell pertussis vaccine (for example, compared to tetanus toxoid or oral poliovirus vaccines), on a population basis it has reduced mortality and morbidity from pertussis 99% or more over the past 45 years in the United States (Marchant et al.,

1994; Centers for Disease Control, 1994). The logical explanation for this is herd immunity, which decreases transmission of *B. pertussis.*

The likelihood of children acquiring pertussis increases with years elapsed since the last dose. Also, many individuals with waning immunity after immunization may be infected, as measured by serologic studies. They experience conditions ranging from few or no symptoms to the full clinical syndrome. This phenomenon has been observed most often following vaccine-induced immunity but also appears to occur in those who have experienced the natural disease many years previously. This apparent loss of immunity has become particularly evident in recent years because of an increase in the incidence of reported cases of pertussis in adolescents and young adults; the increase is both relative and absolute. This increase has strong implications for future pertussis control because older individuals with the disease, whether full-blown or unrecognized, undoubtedly constitute an important reservoir for disease transmission, particularly to young infants who are as yet unprotected. Therefore one of the reasons for efforts to develop a less reactive, acellular pertussis vaccine is the anticipation that it might be acceptable for use in adults.

PREVENTION

Active immunization is the mainstay of pertussis control worldwide because treatment of pertussis is far from satisfactory, transmission occurs from early or unrecognized infections, and passive immunization is ineffective. (Cherry, 1984; American Academy of Pediatrics, 1994; Mortimer and Jones, 1979). Beginning approximately in 1910, a few years after identification and isolation of the organism, various attempts were made to develop vaccines for primary immunization. For many years these hit-or-miss efforts were largely unsuccessful. Most preparations comprised killed, whole organisms, although around 1940 futile attempts were made to immunize with cell-free filtrates of cultures of the organism. By the early 1940s clinically effective whole-cell preparations were produced, and by 1945 they were licensed and marketed. In the United States, pertussis vaccine was standardized by federal regulation in 1954, and current whole-cell pertussis vaccines are relatively unchanged since that time, except for technical refinements such as better control of the number of organisms required for an immunizing dose.

Early attempts to produce an effective pertussis vaccine were hampered by the lack of a surrogate measure for estimation of clinical efficacy; accordingly, clinical trials were required. This situation was ameliorated to a large extent in the mid-1940s with the development of the mouse protection test, in which mice, immunized with the vaccine in question, are challenged by injecting live pertussis organisms intracerebrally. Quantitation of the immunogenicity of the test vaccine is accomplished by comparing survival rates with those achieved by a standard vaccine of known potency, expressed in "mouse protection units." Each dose contains approximately 4 mouse protection units; a total of 8 or more units in the first 3 primary immunization doses is considered satisfactory. For whole-cell vaccines the mouse protection test correlates with clinical efficacy in man. This test, bizarre as it may seem, has served well over the years in assessing the efficacy of whole-cell pertussis vaccines, thus avoiding the necessity for clinical trials in children.

Today's killed, whole-cell pertussis vaccines are combined with diphtheria and tetanus toxoids and adsorbed onto an aluminum salt, comprising the familiar diphtheria and tetanus toxoids and pertussis vaccine (DTP). Three doses are recommended in infancy, with a reinforcing dose approximately 1 year later and another at entry to elementary school. Because of the alleged reactivity of whole-cell pertussis vaccine in older children and adults, it is not recommended for individuals 7 years and older. Though rarely needed, a monovalent whole-cell pertussis vaccine is available from the Bureau of Laboratories, Michigan Department of Public Health.

Whole-cell pertussis vaccines, widely used in the industrialized world during the past three or four decades, have achieved a remarkable record of success. For the 10 years 1983 through 1992, an average of less than 6 deaths from pertussis was reported annually in the United States. Additionally, during the years 1985 through 1994 an average of about 4,100 cases was reported annually, compared to more than 220,000 four decades ago. Acknowledging that the disease is vastly underreported, even if recognized, this is a remarkable achievement (Sutter and Cochi, 1992).

For many years it has been recognized that DTP is undesirably reactive (Mortimer and Jones, 1979). Most of the reactivity is attributable to the pertussis component (Cody et al., 1981). Local reactions include pain at the site of injection in approximately half of all recipients; redness and swelling are observed in approximately 40%. Systemic reactions include fever of 38° C or more in nearly half of re-

cipients; more than half display irritability. Drowsiness is noted in approximately one third and anorexia in approximately 20%. These systemic symptoms are largely limited to the first 48 hours after injection; fever is most apt to occur between 6 and 12 hours after receipt of the vaccine. Rare but disturbing events that occur after whole-cell DTP injection include so-called hypotensive-hyporesponsive episodes. These episodes usually occur within a few hours of the injection and always within 12 hours. Duration is usually a matter of minutes or 1 or 2 hours but rarely episodes have lasted longer (up to 36 hours). The best estimate of their frequency is 1 per 1,750 doses, but with a wide confidence interval. These episodes are frightening to observe because the child appears cold, clammy, and bluish and responds poorly. Nonetheless, spontaneous recovery occurs, and death has not been observed. The mechanism is unclear; similar episodes have been observed following administration of diphtheria and tetanus toxoids (DT) (Pollock and Morris, 1983).

As would be expected, febrile convulsions occur occasionally after DTP injection but appear to be without sequelae (Baraff et al., 1988; Cody et al., 1981; Shields et al., 1988). The best estimate of their frequency is 1 per 1,750 doses, with a wide confidence interval and variation with age. Occasionally, convulsions after DTP injection occur in the absence of fever; rarely, more complex or protracted seizures may occur with or without fever. It is likely that most, if not all, of these more worrisome convulsive episodes represent the precipitation of overt manifestations of preexisting central nervous system disorders by the systemic effects of DTP. Persistent, inconsolable crying has also been observed after the child is given DTP or, less often, DT. These episodes are without sequelae and probably are caused by pain at the site of injection (Cody et al., 1981). For nearly 60 years, beginning with the original hit-or-miss experimental vaccines, there have been dozens of anecdotal reports suggesting that, on occasion, within 1 or 2 days after injection, pertussis vaccine produces acute, severe encephalopathy, sometimes with permanent brain damage or death (Cherry et al., 1988). Because the disease itself was known to produce encephalopathy and because other vaccines such as those for rabies and smallpox were recognized to cause severe neurologic sequelae, these rare events were accepted as an unfortunate price to pay for the control of a serious disease. As widespread use of the vaccine reduced the threat of the disease markedly, these events became magnified in importance, not only in the United States but also in other industrialized nations, including the United Kingdom, Japan, and Sweden. Widespread publicity about these occurrences caused near boycotts of pertussis vaccine in the United Kingdom and Japan, with reappearance of major outbreaks of the disease (Cherry, 1984; Kanai, 1980; Noble, 1987). In the United States, similar publicity about these alleged injuries exerted only a minor effect on vaccine use, but widespread litigation ensued, resulting in major price increases because of insurance costs. These problems prompted systematic efforts to assess the causative role of pertussis vaccine in severe neurologic disease, both in the United States and in the United Kingdom, with the latter nation being particularly suited to such studies because of the organization of its health-care system.

In the British National Childhood Encephalopathy Study (NCES) over a 3-year period, during which time approximately 2,100,000 doses of DTP were administered, 1,182 children age 3 months to 3 years with acute encephalopathic disorders without obvious causes were studied (Miller et al., 1981, 1985). For each of these children, 2 age-matched controls were selected, and for all case and control children it was determined whether a vaccine had been administered in the prior 28 days and, if so, when. After eliminating from the analysis children with infantile spasms, a disorder shown to bear no causative relationship to DTP in another part of the study (Bellman et al., 1983), it was estimated that the relative risk for acute encephalopathy with permanent brain damage, based on 7 cases, was 4.7%, with a wide confidence interval. Because the approximate number of doses of DTP distributed in the United Kingdom during the period of the study was known, it could be estimated that the risk of acute encephalopathy with permanent brain damage was 1 per 330,000 doses, again with a wide confidence interval (Miller et al., 1981).

The NCES, superbly designed and executed, has been subjected to exhaustive (and exhausting) analysis and reanalysis, not only by the investigators themselves but also by others. A 10-year follow-up of subjects and controls has been performed and continues to show an increased risk of serious neurologic disease after administration of DTP, although the numbers are small (Miller et al., 1993).

Unfortunately, this study has failed to resolve the question of whether pertussis vaccine produces acute encephalopathy with permanent brain damage on rare occasions, and it is unlikely that further analyses will be of help because of the small number of affected subjects who received DTP within 7 days before onset. Further, several of these children showed evidence of other, unrelated disorders. It is also possible that one or more of these children, all apparently normal before administration of DTP, did have some preexisting but unrecognized neurologic impairment, the manifestations of which were brought out by the known systemic effects of DTP. The results are also influenced by whether the analysis is limited to the 3-day interval or the 7-day interval following DTP injection. Differing approaches and assumptions have resulted in analyses of the data with quite disparate results, including some that indicate no risk at all (Bowie, 1990; Miller et al., 1985; Stephenson, 1988).

Four other studies, none of which in itself is of sufficient size to provide a definitive answer, *in toto* provide support for the lack of an association between pertussis vaccine and acute encephalopathy with permanent brain damage (Cherry, 1990). As a result of these various studies, the most conservative statement that can be made is either that pertussis vaccine does not cause acute neurologic disease with permanent sequelae or that, if it does, the rate is too low for measurement and never will be known. It is impossible to prove an absolute negative. Nonetheless, it is very clear that most, if not all, of the various neurologic ills that have been attributed anecdotally to pertussis vaccine represent either coincidence or the precipitation of inevitable events in children with underlying neurologic disorders by the well-known systemic effects of pertussis vaccine, including fever. The estimate of 1 instance of permanent neurologic damage per 330,000 doses of DTP has no validity. Temporal association between DTP administration and the onset of infantile spasms (Bellman, 1983) or the occurrence of sudden infant death syndrome (SIDS) (or an excess of deaths from any other cause) is pure coincidence (Howson and Fineberg, 1992). There is no causative relationship between DTP and other disorders such as hyperactivity; learning problems; infantile autism; behavior problems; transverse myelitis; or other overt, subtle, or slowly progressive neurologic conditions (Butler et al., 1982; Cherry, 1990; Golden, 1990). A detailed review and analysis of the evidence related to reactions to pertussis vaccine has been published (Institute of Medicine, 1991). This special committee report indicates that the evidence is insufficient to conclude that DTP causes chronic neurologic damage, although it may cause acute encephalopathic symptoms. The report also concludes that DTP does not cause SIDS or infantile spasms on the basis of the available data. This report is an authoritative resource for information regarding these and other alleged reactions to DTP, and its conclusions are supported by other authorities (American Academy of Pediatrics, 1996). Unfortunately, the differentiation between association and causation in relation to pertussis vaccine and neurologic injury is not understood by the vast majority of the general public and, indeed, by some physicians. Accordingly, inaccurate portrayals of the risks of pertussis vaccine continue to appear in the media, and litigation over alleged pertussis vaccine injuries continues. The advent of the federally sponsored Vaccine Injury Compensation Program (VICP) originally resulted in an enormous increase in legal claims for alleged injuries. However, this increase involved the compensation program and not civil litigation. The costs were originally far greater than expected because of the imprecision of the congressional act that established the program and because those who adjudicated the claims appeared to assume that temporal association and causation are synonymous and that the expected benign minor symptoms following DTP injection (such as irritability, sleepiness, or decreased appetite) indicate encephalopathy, shock-collapse, or imminent SIDS, as alleged by plaintiff lawyers. In early 1995 the VICP's criteria for compensable injuries were made much more precise and consonant with the facts, and it is anticipated that the costs will diminish strikingly.

ACELLULAR PERTUSSIS VACCINE

The development of acellular pertussis vaccines was made possible by technical advances beginning in the late 1970s. These advances enabled dissection of the organism, isolation of its various components, and determination (as yet incomplete) of their roles in disease pathogenesis and clinical immunity. The obvious, practical purpose of these efforts was to develop a less reactive vaccine, free of components irrelevant to clinical immunity. This endeavor was stimulated by increasing concern about serious sequelae attributed to the whole-cell vaccine, a concern that turned out to be erroneous on the basis of subsequent information. Nonetheless, the whole-cell vaccine is relatively crude compared, for example, to tetanus toxoid, and undoubtedly contains components that may be un-

pleasantly reactive and irrelevant to immunity. Understandable misinterpretation of the effects of this reactivity resulted in, or contributed to, rejection of vaccine acceptance, with consequent recrudescence of epidemic pertussis in Japan, the United Kingdom, and Sweden, as well as major concern and litigation in the United States.

On the basis of antibody responses the first acellular pertussis vaccines (DTaP) for clinical use were licensed and used in Japan in 1981 for children 2 years and older. Infants were excluded because of the assumption that immunization of older children would inhibit transmission to infants; this assumption proved to be false, and in 1988 the age of initiation of DTaP was lowered to 2 months (Kimura and Kuno-Sakai, 1990). Six products, containing two to five antigens, were licensed and appeared to be effective on the basis of household contact studies (Noble et al., 1987). A four-antigen acellular preparation combined with diphtheria and tetanus toxoids that was shown to be clinically protective in Japan (Mortimer et al., 1990) and demonstrated to be less reactive and satisfactorily immunogenic in U.S. children was licensed in the United States in 1991 for the fourth and fifth doses of DTP, and a second two-component DTaP was licensed for the same doses in 1992 (American Academy of Pediatrics, 1994). Because clinical efficacy of DTaP had not been demonstrated in infants, whole-cell DTP was continued for the first 3 doses.

Numerous studies subsequently showed that DTaP is less reactive and both immunogenic and clinically protective when given to young infants (Decker and Edwards, 1995; Edwards and Decker, 1996). Accordingly, in 1996 a DTaP vaccine containing PT, FHA, and pertactin was licensed for children of all ages in the United States (Marwick, 1996). As of July 1997, two other products have been licensed.

In concert with the goals of the worldwide Children's Vaccine Initiative, an effort is being made to simplify vaccine schedules, particularly in relation to the developing world (World Health Organization, 1996). Part of this effort includes combination vaccines to reduce the number of encounters and doses. In the United States, whole-cell DTP combined with conjugated *Haemophilis influenzae* b (Hib) vaccine is licensed; in September 1996 an acellular DTP vaccine combined with Hib vaccine was licensed for the fourth dose of the two vaccines given at 12 to 15 months. In some other countries, whole-cell DTP combined with inactivated po-

Table 23-3 Recommended alternative schedules and preparations for routine immunization against pertussis, United States, July 1997.

Alternative schedules

2 mo	4 mo	6 mo	12-15 mo	5-6 yr
Preparation				
DTP	DTP	DTP	DTP	DTP
(Ac* or Wc†)	(Ac or Wc)	(Ac or Wc)	(Ac or Wc)	(Ac or Wc)
			(or AcDTP Hib‡)	

*Acellular DTP (DTaP). Preferred over whole-cell DTP.
†Whole-cell DTP.

liovirus vaccine is used. A preparation containing whole-cell DTP with hepatitis B vaccine has been developed. Further combinations and, perhaps, other mechanisms of administration may be anticipated.

Table 23-3 illustrates acceptable alternative vaccines for immunization against pertussis in the United States as of October 1996. However, unanswered questions remain (Poland, 1996). It remains uncertain which antigens of *B. pertussis* should be incorporated to the acellular preparations. A surrogate test for clinical immunity is needed. Long-term efficacy of acellular pertussis vaccines is uncertain, which has implications for booster doses, including their use in adults. Also of concern is whether increased reactivity with successive doses occurs, as it has with one acellular preparation (Marwick, 1996). Combinations with other vaccines require studies; these are sorely complicated by the lack of a surrogate test for clinical immunity to pertussis. In spite of these problems and unanswered questions, it is clear that acellular pertussis vaccines represent a major advance.

It is possible that a genetically engineered pertussis vaccine will be developed in the future. This would make the vaccine easier to combine with other vaccines. An oral preparation is within the realm of possibility. Such achievements would facilitate the goal of the Children's Vaccine Initiative to immunize all children with as few doses and as little trauma as possible.

BIBLIOGRAPHY

American Academy of Pediatrics. Pertussis. In Peter G (ed). 1994 Red book: report of the committee on Infectious Diseases, ed 23. Elk Grove Village, Ill: American Academy of Pediatric 1994.

American Academy of Pediatrics, Committee on Infectious Diseases. The relationship between pertussis vaccine and central nervous system sequelae: continuing assessment. Pediatrics 1996;97:279-281.

Baraff LJ, Shields WD, Beckwith L, et al. Infants and children with convulsions and hypotonic-hyporesponsive episodes following diphtheria-tetanus-pertussis immunization: follow-up evaluation. Pediatrics 1988;81:789-794.

Bass JW. Pertussis: current status of prevention and treatment. Pediatr Infect Dis 1985;4:614-619.

Bellman MH, Ross EM, Miller DL. Infantile spasms and pertussis immunization. Lancet 1983;1:1031-1034.

Bowie C. Viewpoint: lessons from the pertussis vaccine court trial. Lancet 1990;335:397-399.

Butler NR, Haslum M, Golding J, Stewart-Brown S. Recent findings from the 1970 child health and education study: preliminary communication. J R Soc Med 1982;75:781-784.

Centers for Disease Control and Prevention. Summary of notifiable diseases, United States, 1994. MMWR 1994;43(53):3-80.

Cherry JD. The epidemiology of pertussis and pertussis vaccine in the United Kingdom and the United States: a comparative study. In Lockhart JD (ed). Current problems in pediatrics. Chicago: Year Book Medical Publishers, 1984.

Cherry JD. "Pertussis vaccine encephalopathy": it is time to recognize it as the myth it is. JAMA 1990;263:1679-1680.

Cherry JD. Nosocomial infections in the nineties. Infect Control Hosp Epidemiol 1995;16:553-555.

Cherry JD, Brunell PA, Golden GS, Karzon DT. Report of the Task Force on Pertussis and Pertussis Immunization—1988. Pediatrics 1988;81(suppl):939-984.

Christie CDC, Marx ML, Marchant CD, Reising SF. The 1993 epidemic of pertussis in Cincinnati: resurgence of disease in a highly immunized population of children. New Engl J Med 1994;331:16-21.

Cody CL, Baraff LJ, Cherry JD, et al. Nature and rates of adverse reactions associated with DTP and DT immunizations in infants and children. Pediatrics 1981;68:650-660.

Dauer CC. Reported whooping cough morbidity and mortality in the United States. Public Health Rep 1943;58:661-676.

Decker MD, Edwards KM (eds). Report of the nationwide multicenter acellular pertussis vaccine trial. Pediatrics 1995; 96(suppl):547-603.

Deen JL, Mink CM, Cherry JD, et al. Household contact study of *Bordetella pertussis* infections. Clin Infect Dis 1995; 21:1211-2119.

DeSerres G, Boulianne N, Duval B. Field effectiveness of erythromycin prophylaxis to prevent pertussis within families. Pediatr Infect Dis J 1995;14:969-975.

DeSerres G, Boulianne N, Duval B, et al. Effectiveness of a whole-cell pertussis vaccine in child-care centers and schools. Pediatr Infect Dis J 1996;15:519-524.

Edwards KM, Decker MD. Acellular pertussis vaccines for infants. New Engl J Med 1996;344:391-392.

Expanded Programme on Immunization. EPI for the 1990s. Geneva: World Health Organization, 1992.

Ewanowich CA, Chui LW-L, Paranchych MG, et al. Major outbreak of pertussis in northern Alberta, Canada: analysis of discrepant direct fluorescent-antibody and culture results by using polymerase chain reaction methodology. J Clin Microbiol 1993;31:1715-1725.

Farizo KM, Cochi SL, Zell ER, et al. Epidemiological features of pertussis in the United States, 1980-1989. Clin Infect Dis 1992;14:708-719.

Golden GS. Pertussis vaccine and injury to the brain. J Pediatr 1990;116:854-861.

Granstrom G, Wretlind B, Salenstedt C-R, Granstrom M. Evaluation of serologic assays for diagnosis of whooping cough. J Clin Microbiol 1988;26:1818-1823.

Granstrom M, Olinder-Neilsen AM, Holmblad P, et al. Specific immunoglobulin for treatment of whooping cough. Lancet 1991;338:1230-1233.

He Q, Mertsola J, Soini H, Vijanen MK. Sensitive and specific polymerase chain reaction assays for detection of *Bordetella pertussis* in nasopharyngeal specimens. J Pediatr 1994;124:421-426.

Howson CP, Fineberg HV. Adverse events following pertussis and rubella vaccines: summary of a report of the Institute of Medicine. JAMA 1992;267:392-396.

Institute of Medicine. Committee report: adverse effects of pertussis and rubella vaccines. Washington D.C.: National Academy Press, 1991.

Izurieta HS, Kenyon TA, Strebel PM, et al. Risk factors for pertussis in young infants during an outbreak in Chicago in 1993. Clin Infect Dis 1996;22:503-507.

Kanai K. Japan's experience in pertussis epidemiology and vaccination in the past thirty years. Jpn J Sci Biol 1980;33:107-143.

Kimura M, Kuno-Sakai H. Developments in pertussis immunization in Japan. Lancet 1990;336:30-32.

Lapin LH. Whooping cough. Springfield, Ill: Charles C Thomas, 1943.

Litvak AM, Gibel H, Rosenthal SE, Rosenblatt P. Cerebral complications in pertussis. J Pediatr 1948;32:357-379.

Marchant CD, Loughlin AM, Lett SM, et al. Pertussis in Massachusetts, 1981-1991: incidence, serologic diagnosis, and vaccine effectiveness. New England J Med 1994;169:1297-1305.

Marwick C. Acellular pertussis vaccine is licensed for infants. JAMA 1996;276:516-517.

Miller D, Madge N, Diamond J, et al. Pertussis immunization and serious acute neurological illness in children. Br Med J 1993;307:1171-1176.

Miller DL, Ross EM, Alderslade R, et al. Pertussis immunisation and serious acute neurological illness in children. Br Med J 1981;282:1595-1599.

Miller D, Wadsworth J, Diamond J, Ross E. Pertussis vaccine and whooping cough as risk factors for acute neurological illness and death in young children. Dev Biol Stand 1985;61:389-394.

Mortimer EA Jr. Perspective: pertussis and its prevention—a family affair. J Infect Dis 1990;161:473-479.

Mortimer EA Jr, Jones PK. An evaluation of pertussis vaccine. Rev Infect Dis 1979;1:927-932.

Mortimer EA Jr, Kimura M, Cherry JD, et al. Protective efficacy of the Takeda acellular pertussis vaccine combined with diphtheria and tetanus toxoids following household exposure of Japanese children. Am J Dis Child 1990;144:899-904.

Nennig ME, Shinefield HR, Edwards KM, et al. Prevalence and incidence of adult pertussis in an urban population. JAMA 1996;275:1672-1674.

Noble GR, Bernier RH, Esber EC, et al. Acellular and whole-cell pertussis vaccine in Japan: report of a visit by U.S. scientists. JAMA 1987;257:1351-1356.

Olin P. Defining surrogate serologic tests with respect to predicting vaccine efficacy: pertussis vaccination. Ann New York Acad Sci 1995;754:273-277.

Onorato IM, Wassilak SGF. Laboratory diagnosis of pertussis: the state of the art. Pediatr Infect Dis J 1987;6:145-151.

Onorato IM, Wassilak SG, Meade G. Efficacy of whole-cell pertussis vaccine in preschool children in the United States. JAMA 1992;267:2745-2749.

Poland GA. Acellular pertussis vaccines: new vaccines for an old disease. Lancet 1996;347:209-210.

Pollock TM, Morris J. A 7-year survey of disorders attributed to vaccination in North West Thames region. Lancet 1983;1:753-757.

Public Health Laboratory Service. Efficacy of whooping-cough vaccines used in the United Kingdom before 1968. Br Med J 1973;1:259-262.

Schlapfer G, Cherry JD, Heininger V, et al. Polymerase chain reaction identification of *Bordetella pertussis* infections in vaccinees and family members in a pertussis vaccine efficacy trial in Germany. Pediatr Infect Dis J 1995;14:209-214.

Shahin RD, Brennan MJ, Li ZM, et al. Characterization of the protective capacity and immunogenicity of the 69-kD outer membrane protein of *Bordetella pertussis*. J Exp Med 1990;171:63-73.

Shields WD, Nielsen C, Buch D, et al. Relationship of pertussis immunization to the onset of neurologic disorders: a retrospective epidemiologic study. J Pediatr 1988;113:801-805.

Steketee RW, Burstyn DG, Wassilak SGF, et al. A comparison of laboratory and clinical methods for diagnosing pertussis in an outbreak in a facility for the developmentally disabled. J Infect Dis 1988;157:441-449.

Stephenson JBP. A neurologist looks at neurological disease temporally related to DTP immunization. Tokai J Exp Clin Med 1988;13:157-164.

Sutter RW, Cochi SL. Pertussis hospitalizations and mortality, 1985-1988: evaluation of the completeness of national reporting. JAMA 1992;267:386-391.

Wardlaw AC, Parton R (eds). Pathogenesis and immunity in pertussis. New York: John Wiley & Sons, 1988.

World Health Organization, Global Programme for Vaccines and Immunization. State of the world's vaccines and immunization. Geneva: World Health Organization, 1996.

24 RABIES (HYDROPHOBIA, RAGE, LYSSA)

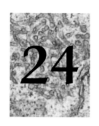

STANLEY A. PLOTKIN

Human rabies is a fatal encephalomyelitis caused by a rhabdovirus that is usually transmitted to man by the bite of a rabid animal. In the United States the disease is rare, the average annual incidence of human rabies having declined from forty cases during the 1940s to zero to two cases per year in the 1980s. Some of the cases are imported; monoclonal serotyping of rabies isolates from four human cases of rabies occurring in the United States in the 1980s revealed viruses similar to those in the country of origin of the patient. The important feature was an incubation period of 11 months to 6 years, with probable acquisition of infection before entry into the United States (Smith et al., 1991). However, in 1995 alone there were four indigenous cases linked to bat exposures, and the difficulty of ascertaining those exposures became evident.

Rabies in domestic animals has decreased in recent years. In 1946 there were more than 8,000 cases of rabies in dogs, compared with 550 cases in all domestic animals in 1988. Rabid domestic animals compose 12% of all rabid animals but are responsible for 64% of exposures requiring treatment. Rabid cats are the most commonly reported rabid domestic species in the United States.

In 1993 there were 8,645 confirmed cases of wildlife rabies in 53 states and territories, of which only 6.4% were in domestic animals (Centers for Disease Control, 1989). These data originate in state and federal laboratories of the United States but reflect the worldwide epizootic in wildlife hosts, extending from the Arctic Circle to the tropics in the Eastern and Western hemispheres. Wild animals currently constitute the most important source of infection for domestic animals in the United States. Skunks and raccoons are the main sources of rabies for domestic animals and the main source of exposure in humans. Transmission from one domestic species to another rarely occurs in the United States (Fig. 24-1).

Pasteur pioneered the development of rabies vaccine in 1895, when, without knowing that the virus was a filterable agent, he managed to transmit it to animals and to chemically attenuate the agent by desiccation. His successful human trials, though based on insufficient animal experimentation, launched the field of vaccine development (Pasteur coined the word "vaccination") and resulted in the worldwide establishment of Pasteur institutes to produce rabies vaccine.

The general treatment of the bite and the question of whether or not to immunize those persons bitten or scratched by animals suspected of being rabid is no longer a difficult decision, now that better tolerated vaccines are available. The decision to immunize must be made immediately after exposure because the likelihood that any prophylactic measure will contribute to the prevention of rabies diminishes rapidly as the interval between exposure and treatment increases.

Although a case of rabies may occasionally develop in persons who receive antirabies treatment, evidence from laboratory and field experience in many parts of the world indicates that postexposure prophylaxis is highly effective when local cleansing, antiserum, and vaccine are appropriately used.

ETIOLOGY

Rabies virus was the first virus transmitted experimentally to a laboratory animal. The rabies virus is classified within the lyssavirus family of rhabdoviruses and shares homology with at least five other viruses (such as Mokola and Duvenhage) that are considerably rarer as causes of disease in man, and about which relatively little is known. Moreover, although there is only one serotype of rabies, the virus varies genetically, and strains coming from different animals and from different geographic areas can be distinguished, facilitating epidemiologic investigation. For example, the fact

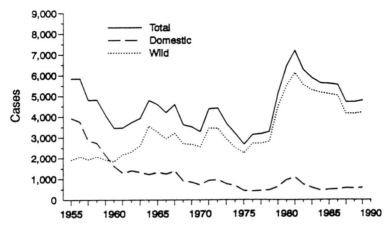

FIG. 24-1   Rabies in wild and domestic animals, by year, in the United States and Puerto Rico, 1955 to 1989. (From MMWR 1990;38:36)

that human rabies cases of occult origin had been acquired from bats was established by molecular epidemiologic studies, as well as the documentation that spread of raccoon rabies to the northeastern United States, had been the result of animal importation for hunting purposes.

Physical and Chemical Properties

Rabies virus is bullet shaped and has a symmetric structure like a beehive. The virus measures 80 to 180 nm in diameter. The negative single-stranded genome is nonsegmented RNA approximately 12,000 nucleotides long. The genome has been cloned and sequenced. The glycoprotein of the spikes on the surface of the virus is encoded by the G gene. This is the attachment protein and is the antigen that elicits neutralizing antibodies. The virulence of the virus is dramatically altered by single amino acid substitutions in the glycoprotein. Monoclonal antibodies against the glycoprotein or the nucleoprotein distinguish strains of virus and have served to clarify the epidemiology of rabies.

Rabies virus survives storage at 4° C for weeks and in the frozen state for much longer periods in the absence of carbon dioxide; therefore in dry-ice cabinets it must be stored in sealed glass ampules. It keeps for years in the dried state at 4° C. Rabies virus is killed by temperatures of 56° C in 1 hour and of 60° C in 5 minutes. It is quickly inactivated by sunlight and ultraviolet light. The virus is resistant to phenol and thimerosal (Merthiolate). It is inactivated by β-propiolactone, ether, formalin, mercury bichloride, and nitric acid.

Host Range

Rabies virus has an extensive host range; all warm-blooded animals are susceptible. Introduction of virus by virtually any route usually gives rise to infection, but intracerebral inoculation with virus from canines almost invariably produces fatal encephalomyelitis. In infected animals, rabies virus is widely distributed. The salivary glands of infected dogs have yielded high titers of virus; lesser quantities have been detected in the lacrimal glands, pancreas, kidney, adrenal glands, and breast tissue. In humans, rabies virus has been recovered from various parts of the central nervous system (CNS), including the olfactory bulbs, horn of Ammon, frontal and occipital cortices, and medulla. It has also been recovered from cervical and abdominal sympathetic ganglia, salivary glands, adrenal glands, myocardium, walls of both small and large intestines, mesenteric lymph nodes, tonsillar and pharyngeal tissues, and lungs.

The term *street virus* is used to designate strains of freshly isolated wild viruses. Such strains are characterized by incubation periods that usually vary from 10 days to several months. However, much longer incubation periods may be observed. Rabies viruses produce either prolonged excitation and viciousness (furious type) or depression and paralysis with early onset (dumb type) or, as occurs in most infected dogs, some manifestations of both types. Street virus rabies is almost always associated with the presence of Negri bodies. The term *fixed virus* refers to laboratory strains transferred in series from brain to brain, usually in the rabbit, characterized by a short and constant incubation period of 4 to 6 days, absence of Negri bodies, and diminished ability to spread centrifugally. The Pasteur strain of fixed virus has been maintained in rabbits since its original isolation in 1882 and is the strain generally used for nerve tissue vaccines.

Rabies virus has also been propagated in chick and duck embryos, in tissue cultures of mouse, in hamster kidneys, in continuous cell lines of African green monkey kidney origin (Vero), and in human diploid cell lines. For immunization of animals, only inactivated virus vaccines prepared from these substrates are used in the United States.

Newer techniques of rabies virus cultivation permitted the development of safer and more immunogenic vaccines for humans, starting in 1957 with one made in duck embryos. Subsequently, cell culture vaccines were developed, and in the 1970s a concentrated, purified rabies virus vaccine was prepared from the supernatants of human diploid cell cultures, thus eliminating the risks of injecting animal proteins, including those originating in the central nervous system.

Immunologic Properties

Both neutralizing and complement-fixing antibodies are formed late in the course of rabies infection, and they may also develop as a result of vaccination. The level of 0.5 IU of neutralizing antibody, which attaches to the viral glycoprotein, is associated with protection against illness. Cell-to-cell spread of virus is prevented by neutralizing antibody in vitro. Postexposure administration of antibody may prevent virus from reaching the CNS.

A measurable cytotoxic T-cell response is generated after vaccination, but the role in pathogenesis or protection is unknown. In vitro the cellular response contributes to clearance of virus from cells, and this can be enhanced by antibody.

PATHOLOGY

The principal changes produced by rabies virus are found throughout the CNS, consisting mainly of neuronal necrosis, which is most pronounced in the thalamus, hypothalamus, substantia nigra, pons, and medulla. The cranial nerve nuclei are severely damaged, and mononuclear cell infiltration is likely to be greater there than elsewhere. The spinal cord shows neuronal changes, especially in the posterior horns. The most distinctive feature of the pathologic changes is the presence of Negri bodies, which are pathognomonic of rabies, although not always present. These specific inclusion bodies are found in the cytoplasm of nerve cells. They consist of acidophilic structures approximately 2 to 10 μm in diameter, are sharply demarcated, and are usually round or oval; they occur most abundantly in the hippocampus (horn of Ammon), basal ganglia, pons, and medulla.

Changes similar to those in the brain may be found in the sympathetic ganglia and dorsal root ganglia of the spinal cord. The salivary glands may show degenerative changes of the acinar cells and neurons; Negri bodies may be found in the latter.

PATHOGENESIS

The attack rate in persons bitten by rabid animals is hard to estimate; it depends on the extent and location of the bites and the dose of virus entering the wound. Lacerations of the head and neck are followed by higher attack rates than are those of the feet and ankles. The amount of virus reaching the nerves is influenced by several additional factors: (1) lack of virus in saliva of 50% of rabid dogs; (2) protection afforded by clothing so that little or no virus enters the wound; and (3) removal or inactivation of virus by soap and water, benzalkonium (Zephiran), and other agents.

Overall, the risk of rabies after human exposures to the bites of rabid animals appears to range from 15% to 40%, with wolf bites to the head exemplifying the high end of the range. Rabies virus in saliva is inoculated into tissue by a bite. Available evidence indicates that rabies virus multiplies initially in the muscle at the inoculation site, reaches neuromuscular junctions, and travels through the axoplasm of peripheral nerves to dorsal root ganglia and the CNS. After multiplication in neurons centrally, the virus travels peripherally along nerve pathways to invade many distal tissues and organs. Host response is limited, perhaps because virus is sequestered from the immune system during the long incubation period, and little inflammatory response or measurable host response can be demonstrated.

CLINICAL MANIFESTATIONS

The incubation period is usually 1 to 2 months, but wide ranges from 10 days to 6 years have been observed. Multiple severe lacerations and the introduction of large doses of virus are associated with short incubation periods.

The illness may begin, as do other kinds of encephalitis, with prodromal symptoms of malaise, fever, headache, anorexia, nausea, sore throat, drowsiness, irritability, and restlessness. The patient may complain of hyperesthesia, paresthesia, or anesthesia in the area of the bite and along the course of the involved peripheral nerves.

Progression of the infection is associated with increased anxiety and hyperexcitability accompanied by mounting fever. Delirium, involuntary twitching movements, and generalized convulsions are often seen. Manic behavior may alternate with periods of lethargy. Violent spasmodic contractions of the muscles of the mouth, pharynx, or larynx when the patient attempts to drink or merely at the sight of water are the striking characteristics that gave rabies its common name—hydrophobia. These painful spasms may be set off by relatively mild stimuli such as noise, light touch, or air currents. The patient may drool profusely from the mouth to avoid swallowing, which is associated with painful spasm.

Within a few days the patient's condition worsens, the pulse rate increases, respirations become more labored or irregular, and the temperature rises steadily. Periods of responsiveness become less frequent, and muscular spasms may give way to paralysis. Peripheral vascular collapse, coma, and death quickly follow. The disease runs its entire course usually in no more than 5 to 6 days and ends fatally.

In 5% to 20% of patients the clinical picture of rabies may be that of an ascending, symmetric, flaccid paralysis without hyperexcitability or spasmodic muscle contractions. This picture resembles that of Guillain-Barré syndrome so that, in the absence of known history of rabies virus exposure, such patients may go through the entire course of illness with no suspicion of the diagnosis of rabies until the characteristic findings are observed at autopsy (Baer, 1975).

The cerebrospinal fluid (CSF) is usually normal: the pressure is normal or slightly increased, the fluid is clear, and in most cases the number of cells is not increased. In patients with pleocytosis the CSF cell count rarely exceeds 100, and the cells are mostly mononuclear leukocytes. There may be a slight increase in the level of protein.

The peripheral white blood cell count shows a slight increase in number of leukocytes that may reach 20,000 to 30,000, with a predominance of polymorphonuclear leukocytes. Abnormal urinary findings may include albumin, casts, reducing substances, and acetone.

■ **CASE 1** An 11-year-old boy was bitten on the forehead by a dog 32 days before onset of the disease; the wound was cauterized, but no antirabies vaccine was given. The patient's illness began with headache, drowsiness, anorexia, and malaise that progressed in 2 days to delirium accompanied by fever and vomiting.

Delirium associated with visual hallucinations and delusions of persecution were the outstanding and persistently recurring features. He was often manic and struck and bit attendants. Except for transient difficulty in swallowing and slurring of speech on the fourth and fifth days, there was a striking absence of localizing neurologic signs. The CSF was normal. The temperature was sustained between 38.9° and 40.3° C (102° and 104.5° F) for 1 week. On the tenth day, irregular respirations were observed, with periods of apnea lasting as long as 45 seconds. He died on the twelfth day from respiratory and circulatory failure. Post mortem touch preparations of the hippocampus showed typical Negri bodies, and rabies virus was isolated from various parts of the brain and other tissues.

DIAGNOSIS

Confirmation of rabies in a biting animal is often the first and crucial step towards the prevention of rabies in humans. All nondomesticated animals and bats should be considered rabid; their heads or, if small, their entire carcasses should be preserved at 0° to 4° C and submitted to state rabies diagnostic laboratories, where rabies virus is sought in brain tissue by fluorescent rabies antibody staining for viral antigen, virus isolation in mice inoculated intracerebrally, and more recently by polymerase chain reaction detection of viral nucleic acid. Negri bodies may be absent, and diagnosis should not depend on their presence.

In a typical human case, rabies is easily recognized. The characteristic history is that of an animal bite followed in several weeks or months by the onset of overwhelming encephalitis; the CNS signs include excitement, anxiety, manic behavior, and delirium associated with spasmodic concentrations of muscles used in swallowing and speech. Clinical laboratory findings are generally of little help. In humans the premortem diagnosis is made best by demonstration of antigen in a skin biopsy. Corneal impressions have been difficult to obtain and unreliable for detection of antigen. During the first week of illness, virus can be isolated occasionally from saliva, CSF, and urine and consistently from the brain. Virus can be demonstrated by immunofluorescence, by identification of Negri bodies, or by inoculation of brain tissue into mice. Primary isolation of virus is accomplished in mice, although cell culture can be used. The presence of IgM antibody in blood and CSF indicates acute infection. Polymerase chain reaction (PCR) may improve sensitivity and specificity of diagnosis.

Tetanus may be confused with rabies. Excitement accompanied by spasms of the laryngeal and pharyngeal muscles is not so common in patients with tetanus and is virtually constant in patients with rabies. Tetanus is characterized by trismus and spasmodic contractions of the muscles of the body.

PROGNOSIS

Rabies was considered 100% lethal until recent years. A small number of cases have now been reported in which survival from rabies infection appears probable, at least in part because of vaccination during the incubation period. However, these cases are rare, and the prognosis in unvaccinated persons is still uniformly fatal.

■ **CASE 2** Probable human rabies with survival. On October 10, 1970, in Lima, Ohio, a 6-year-old boy was bitten on his left thumb by a bat while he was asleep. The bat was captured by the boy's father and was submitted to the Ohio Health Department, where rabies was confirmed on examination of the brain by fluorescent antibody (FA) technique. On October 14 a 14-day course of treatment with duck embryo vaccine (DEV) was begun on the boy.

The boy showed no symptoms until October 30, when he complained of neck pain, and during the next several days he became lethargic and showed malaise and anorexia. His condition worsened, and on November 4 he entered a local hospital with a temperature of 40° C (104° F). During the next 10 days the boy's temperature dropped but he became more lethargic. On November 13 stiffness of the neck developed and the CSF yielded 125 white blood cells. During the next several days the boy's condition deteriorated; he showed total aphasia, weakness of left arm, bilateral Babinski's signs, and coma. A tracheostomy was done because of respiratory difficulty, tachypnea, and increased pharyngeal secretions. The patient was in and out of coma for a week and then gradually began to improve. In December his condition continued to improve, and he was able to walk with assistance and speak in short sentences. As of October 1971 the patient was reported as normal.

Efforts to establish the diagnosis included biopsy of the brain, which was negative for rabies virus by culture, and FA tests. There were no detectable serum antibodies to St. Louis encephalitis, eastern or western equine encephalomyelitis, or leptospirosis. Serum complement–fixing antibody titer to California virus was 1:8 on October 13, and biweekly determinations through December 3 remained the same. Serum–neutralizing antibody titers against rabies were 1:300 on November 13, rose to 1:37,000 on November 27, and remained between 1:39,000 and 1:47,000 during December and January. The question arose whether the 14-day course of treatment with DEV could be responsible for these high antibody titers. It can be stated that rabies antibody titers after a 14-day course of treatment with DEV rarely exceed 1:500 and, therefore, that titers of the magnitude seen in this patient strongly supports the diagnosis of rabies. Indeed, the only aspect of this patient's course not compatible with rabies infection is recovery. The clinical management of this patient included the continuous monitoring of cardiac and pulmonary functions, the prevention of hypoxia by prophylactic tracheostomy, and intensive pulmonary assistance. These measures may have contributed to the arrest of clinical illness and eventual recovery.

EPIDEMIOLOGIC FACTORS

Geographic distribution of rabies includes most of the world. The mammalian host range is so large that areas free of rabies are primarily island nations. The British Isles, Australia, New Zealand, and the Hawaiian Islands are rabies-free through eradication efforts and quarantine to eliminate enzootic cycles. Rabies occurs in any climate and in any season but is most common in Africa and Southwest Asia and is particularly prevalent in India.

The sources of the vast majority of rabies exposures in the high-incidence parts of the world are domesticated dogs and cats. In theory, population control and vaccination of these animals could sharply reduce rabies in humans, but in practice poverty and social customs prevent those measures. In Europe the fox is the main source of human exposure. Recently, vaccination of wild foxes has been practiced in Western Europe with great success using baits containing live viruses—either vaccinia-rabies recombinants or attenuated strains of rabies virus.

In the Americas, canine rabies is still important in Mexico and other parts of Central and South America, and bats (including vampire bats) are important vectors throughout the hemisphere. Although only insectivorous bats are found in the United States, they have recently been implicated in the majority of the rare human cases, presumably because their bites may go undetected in a sleeping individual.

However, the majority of animals confirmed rabid in the United States are skunks, raccoons, and foxes. Rabies in domestic animals has declined to only about 5% of all positives, and the cat is now more likely than the dog to be infected. The recent epidemiology of rabies in the United States has been strongly influenced by the spread of raccoon rabies throughout the Northeast. Introduced into Virginia by the transfer of raccoons from the South for hunting purposes, the epizootic has spread north to New York and to New England, resulting in numerous human exposures. In Canada the fox is the principal species involved by rabies.

Rabies is no respecter of age. The incidence is high in children because of their increased chance of exposure resulting from their friendliness toward animals and their inability to defend themselves against attack. Also, because of their small size, children are more often bitten on the head and face, and thus are more susceptible to infection. Additional factors leading to a higher risk in children include provocative behavior and failure to recognize the signs of rabies in dogs.

Winkler (1968) has pointed out the possibility of airborne respiratory infection acquired in caves inhabited by large numbers of infected bats. Although transmission by inhalation is probably very rare, it must be considered in patients with compatible clinical illnesses who have a history of visits to bat-infested caves. Spelunkers may be listed among those with "high-risk" vocations or avocations for whom preexposure prophylaxis is justified.

Human-to-human transmission of rabies by bite is rare or nonexistent. However, iatrogenic transmission has been reported (Houff et al., 1979), resulting from a corneal transplant to a healthy recipient from a donor who had died of a CNS illness with progressive ascending paralysis similar to Guillain-Barré syndrome. One month after the transplant procedure, the recipient developed an acute fatal meningoencephalitis that was recognized as rabies only at autopsy. Studies of the donor's and the recipient's eyes then demonstrated the presence of rabies virus in both.

PREVENTIVE MEASURES

The prevention of rabies consists either of vaccination preexposure with 3 doses of a cell culture vaccine or postexposure treatment combining local irrigation with administration of antiserum and 5 doses of vaccine.

Attack rates in persons bitten by rabid animals and the effect of specific prophylactic measures are shown in Table 24-1. Sabeti et al. (1964) described the results of treatment of individuals bitten in Iran by wolves proved rabid. The evidence is clear that use of the combination of hyperimmune serum and vaccine was superior to vaccine alone, especially in cases of head bites, which are associated with shorter incubation periods and higher attack rates than are those in which the head and neck are not involved.

In 1964 Veeraraghaven et al. (cited by Johnson, 1965) compared the attack rates in persons bitten by proved rabid animals in India from 1946 to 1962, when a total of 581 persons exposed in this manner were given a complete course of antirabies vaccine; of them, 49 (8.4%) died. In contrast, of 153 persons who were not vaccinated, 77 (50%) died (see Table 24-1).

With use of the new rabies vaccines of the human diploid cell strain (Wiktor et al., 1977), there

Table 24-1 Attack rates in human beings bitten by animals proved to be rabid: effect of specific preventive measures

| Authors | Persons bitten | | Number of rabies deaths | Mortality (%) | Type of prophylaxis |
	Number	On head			
Sabeti et al., 1964*	96	Yes	38	40	Vaccine alone
	71	No	6	8.4	
TOTAL	167		44	26	
	50	Yes	3	6	Serum and
	24	No	0	0	vaccine
TOTAL	74		3	4	
Veeraraghaven et al., 1964*	153	†	77	50	No vaccine
	581	†	49	8.4	Vaccine

*Cited by Johnson HN: Rabies virus. In Horsfall FL Jr, Tamm I (eds). Viral and rickettsial diseases of man, ed 4. Philadelphia: JB Lippincott, 1965.
†No data.

now have been several convincing studies of efficacy in postexposure rabies prophylaxis. Bahmanyar et al. (1976) described the successful protection of eight groups, totaling forty-five persons, who were severely bitten in Iran by six dogs and two wolves that were proved rabid. A total of only 6 doses of vaccine, plus an initial injection of antirabies serum prepared in mules, was administered to each patient. None developed rabies despite deep wounds of the extremities and in some cases the face and head. In Germany all of thirty-one persons bitten by animals that were proved rabid were protected from rabies by a similar vaccine schedule (Kuwert et al., 1976). Extensive United States experience has also shown protection (Anderson et al., 1980; ACIP, 1991).

Vaccines

In recent years, cell culture vaccines have been developed to replace the original nerve tissue vaccines pioneered by Pasteur in 1885, although, unfortunately, even today the majority of human vaccinations in the developing world are done with vaccines produced in the brains of animals.

Cell culture vaccines are highly immunogenic, free of serious reactions, and effective in postexposure prophylaxis, as described previously. They have also been reliable in stimulating high antibody titers when administered in a 3-dose schedule to high-risk individuals before exposure (Plotkin and Wiktor, 1979).

The standard of rabies cell culture vaccines is the one prepared from cultures of human diploid cells, which has been used extensively. However, to reduce the cost of vaccination, other cell culture vaccines have been developed and licensed in some countries, particularly ones prepared in Vero African green monkey kidney cell lines and chick embryo cells. A purified vaccine made from duck embryo cells is also available.

RABIES-IMMUNIZING PRODUCTS

The following information is *abstracted* from the recommendations of the Immunization Practices Advisory Committee (ACIP) (MMWR 1991;40:1-19). Because of space limitations, the following information may be incomplete for certain purposes. Therefore medical personnel intending to use vaccination for rabies prevention are urged to consult the entire original document for complete information.

There are two types of rabies-immunizing products.

1. Rabies vaccines induce an active immune response that includes the production of neutralizing antibodies. This antibody response requires approximately 7 to 10 days to develop and usually persists for more than 2 years.
2. Rabies immune globulins (RIG) provide rapid, passive immune protection that persists for only a short time (half-life of approximately 21 days). In almost all postexposure prophylaxis regimens, both products should be used concurrently.

Two inactivated rabies vaccines are currently licensed for preexposure and postexposure prophylaxis in the United States.

Rabies Vaccine: Human Diploid Cell (HDCV)

The vaccine is inactivated with β-propiolactone and is supplied in forms for the following:

1. Intramuscular (IM) administration (Pasteur-Merieux Sérum et Vaccins, Imovax Rabies, distributed by Connaught Laboratories, Inc., Phone 800. VACCINE). Used at a final diluted volume of 1.0 ml.
2. Intradermal (ID) administration, a single-dose syringe containing lyophilized vaccine (Pasteur-Merieux Sérum et Vaccins, Imovax Rabies I.D., distributed by Connaught Laboratories, Inc.). Used at a final diluted volume of 0.1 ml.

Rabies Vaccine Adsorbed (RVA)

RVA (Michigan Department of Public Health) was licensed in 1988; it was developed by the Biologics Products Program, Michigan Department of Public Health and is currently distributed by Smith Kline Beecham, Philadelphia. The vaccine is prepared from the Kissling strain of Challenge Virus Standard (CVS) rabies virus adapted to fetal rhesus lung diploid cell culture.

Both types of rabies vaccines are considered equally efficacious and safe when used as indicated. The full 1.0-ml dose of either product can be used for both preexposure and postexposure prophylaxis. Only the Imovax Rabies I.D. vaccine (HDCV) has been evaluated by the ID dose and route for preexposure vaccination; the antibody response and side effects after ID administration of RVA have not been studied. Therefore RVA should not be used intradermally.

Rabies Vaccine: Globulins

Rabies immune globulins licensed for use in the United States HRIG (Cutter Biological [a division of Miles, Inc.], Hyperab; and Pasteur-Merieux Sérum et Vaccins, Imogam Rabies, distributed by Connaught Laboratories, Inc.) is an antirabies gamma globulin concentrated by cold ethanol fractionation from plasma of hyperimmunized human donors. Rabies-neutralizing antibody content, standardized to contain 150 IU per ml, is supplied in 2-ml (300 IU) and 10-ml (1,500 IU) vials for pediatric and adult use, respectively.

Both HRIG preparations are considered equally efficacious and safe when used as described in this document.

POSTEXPOSURE PROPHYLAXIS: RATIONALE FOR TREATMENT

Physicians should evaluate each possible exposure to rabies and if necessary consult with local or state public health officials regarding the need for rabies prophylaxis (Table 24-2). In the United States the following factors should be considered before specific antirabies treatment is initiated.

Type of Exposure

Rabies is transmitted only when the virus is introduced into open cuts or wounds in skin or mucous membranes. If there has been no exposure (as described in this section), postexposure treatment is not necessary. The likelihood of rabies infection varies with the nature and extent of exposure. Two categories of exposure (bite and nonbite) should be considered.

Bite. Any penetration of the skin by teeth constitutes a bite exposure. Bites to the face and hands carry the highest risk, but the site of the bite should not influence the decision to begin treatment.

Nonbite. Scratches, abrasions, open wounds, or mucous membranes contaminated with saliva or other potentially infectious material (such as brain tissue) from a rabid animal constitute nonbite exposures.

Although occasional reports of transmission by nonbite exposure suggest that such exposures constitute sufficient reason to initiate postexposure prophylaxis under some circumstances, nonbite exposures rarely cause rabies. The nonbite exposures of highest risk appear to be exposures to large amounts of aerosolized rabies virus, organs (i.e., corneas) transplanted from patients who died of rabies, and scratches by rabid animals.

Other contact by itself—such as petting a rabid animal or contact with the blood, urine, or feces (e.g., guano) of a rabid animal—does not constitute an exposure and is not an indication for prophylaxis.

Table 24-2   Rabies postexposure prophylaxis guide, United States, 1991

Animal type	Evaluation and disposition of animal	Postexposure prophylaxis recommendations
Dogs and cats	Healthy and available for 10 days observation	Should not begin prophylaxis unless animal develops symptoms of rabies*
	Rabid or suspected rabid	Immediate vaccination
	Unknown (escaped)	Consult public health officials
Skunks, raccoons, bats, foxes, and most other carnivores; woodchucks	Regarded as rabid unless geographic area is known to be free of rabies or until animal proven negative by laboratory tests†	Immediate vaccination
Livestock, rodents, and lagomorphs (rabbits and hares)	Consider individually	Consult public health officials. Bites of squirrels, hamsters, guinea pigs, gerbils, chipmunks, rats, mice, other rodents, rabbits, and hares almost never require antirabies treatment

*During the 10-day holding period, begin treatment with HRIG and HDCV or RVA at first sign of rabies in a dog or cat that has bitten someone. The symptomatic animal should be killed immediately and tested.

†The animal should be killed and tested as soon as possible. Holding for observation is not recommended. Discontinue vaccine if immunofluorescence test results of the animal are negative.

Animal Rabies Epidemiology and Evaluation of Involved Species

Wild Animals. All bites by wild carnivores and bats must be considered possible exposures to the disease. Postexposure prophylaxis should be initiated when patients are exposed to wild carnivores unless (1) the exposure occurred in a part of the continental United States known to be free of terrestrial rabies and the results of immunofluorescence antibody testing is available within 48 hours, or (2) the animal has already been tested and shown not to be rabid. If treatment has been initiated and subsequent immunofluorescence testing shows that the exposing animal was not rabid, treatment can be discontinued.

Signs of rabies among carnivorous wild animals cannot be interpreted reliably; therefore any such animal that bites or scratches a person should be killed at once (without unnecessary damage to the head) and the brain submitted for rabies testing. If the results of testing are negative by immunofluorescence, the saliva can be assumed to contain no virus, and the person bitten does not require treatment.

If the biting animal is a particularly rare or valuable specimen and the risk of rabies small, public health authorities may choose to administer postexposure treatment to the bite victim in lieu of killing the animal for rabies testing. Such animals should be quarantined for 30 days.

Rodents (such as squirrels, hamsters, guinea pigs, gerbils, chipmunks, rats, and mice) and lagomorphs (including rabbits and hares) are almost never found to be infected with rabies and have not been known to cause rabies among humans in the United States. However, from 1971 through 1988, woodchucks accounted for 70% of the 179 cases of rabies among rodents reported to CDC. In all cases involving rodents, the state or local health department should be consulted before a decision is made to initiate postexposure antirabies prophylaxis. Exotic pets (including ferrets) and domestic animals crossbred with wild animals are considered wild animals by the National Association of State Public Health Veterinarians (NASPHV) and the Conference of State and Territorial Epidemiologists (CSTE) because they may be highly susceptible to rabies and could transmit the disease. These animals should be killed and tested rather than confined and observed when they bite humans.

Domestic Animals. In areas where canine rabies is not enzootic (including virtually all of the United States and its territories), a healthy domestic dog or cat that bites a person should be confined and observed for 10 days. Any illness in the animal during confinement or before release should be evaluated by a veterinarian and reported immediately to the local health department. If signs suggestive of rabies develop, the animal should be humanely killed and its head removed and shipped, under refrigeration, for examination by a qualified laboratory. Any stray or unwanted dog or cat that bites a person should be killed immediately and the head submitted as described for rabies examination.

In most developing countries of Asia, Africa, and Central and South America, dogs are the major vector of rabies; exposures to dogs in such countries represent a special threat. Travelers to these countries should be aware that >50% of the rabies cases among humans in the United States result from exposure to dogs outside the United States. Although dogs are the main reservoir of rabies in these countries, the epizootiology of the disease among animals differs sufficiently by region or country to warrant the evaluation of all animal bites. Exposures to dogs in canine rabies–enzootic areas outside the United States carry a high risk; some authorities therefore recommend that postexposure rabies treatment be initiated immediately after such exposures. Treatment can be discontinued if the dog or cat remains healthy during the 10-day observation period.

Circumstances of biting incident and vaccination status of exposing animal. An unprovoked attack by a domestic animal is more likely than a provoked attack to indicate that the animal is rabid. Bites inflicted on a person attempting to feed or handle an apparently healthy animal should generally be regarded as provoked. However, in countries where canine rabies is enzootic this rule should be ignored and all bites should be considered as unprovoked.

A fully vaccinated dog or cat is unlikely to become infected with rabies, although rare cases have been reported. In a nationwide study of rabies among dogs and cats in 1988, only one dog and two cats that were vaccinated contracted rabies. All three of these animals had received only single doses of vaccine; no documented vaccine failures occurred among dogs or cats that had received two vaccinations.

POSTEXPOSURE PROPHYLAXIS: LOCAL TREATMENT OF WOUNDS AND VACCINATION

The essential components of rabies postexposure prophylaxis are local wound treatment and the administration, in most instances, of both HRIG and vaccine (Table 24-3). Persons who have been bitten by animals suspected or proven rabid should begin treatment within 24 hours. However, there have been instances when the decision to begin treatment was not made until many months after the exposure because of a delay in recognition that an exposure had occurred, and awareness that incubation periods of >1 year have been reported. In 1977 the World Health Organization (WHO) recommended a regimen of RIG and 6 doses of HDCV over a 90-day period. This recommendation was based on studies in Germany and Iran. When used this way, the vaccine was found to be safe and effective in protecting persons bitten by proven rabid animals and induced an excellent antibody response in all recipients. Studies conducted in the United States by CDC have shown that a regimen of 1 dose of HRIG and 5 doses of HDCV over a 28-day period was safe and induced an excellent antibody response in all recipients.

Immediate and thorough washing of all bite wounds and scratches with soap and water is an important measure for preventing rabies.

Two rabies vaccines are currently available in the United States; either is administered in conjunction with HRIG at the beginning of postexposure therapy. A regimen of 5 doses of 1 ml each of HDCV or RVA should be given intramuscularly. The first dose of the 5-dose course should be given as soon as possible after exposure. Additional doses should be given on days 3, 7, 14, and 28 after the first vaccination. For adults the vaccine should always be administered IM in the deltoid area. For children the anterolateral aspect of the thigh is also acceptable. The gluteal area should never be used for HDCV or RVA injections, since administration in this area results in lower neutralizing antibody titers.

HRIG is administered only once (i.e., at the beginning of antirabies prophylaxis) to provide immediate antibodies until the patient responds to HDCV or RVA by actively producing antibodies. If HRIG was not given when vaccination was begun, it can be given through the seventh day after administration of the first dose of vaccine. Beyond the seventh day, HRIG is not indicated since an antibody response to cell culture vaccine is presumed to have occurred. The recommended dose of HRIG is 20 IU/kg. This formula is applicable for all age groups, including children. If anatomically feasible, at least one half the dose of HRIG should be thoroughly infiltrated in the area around the wound and the rest should be administered intramuscularly in the gluteal area. HRIG should never be administered in the same syringe or into the same anatomic site as vaccine. Because HRIG may partially suppress active production of antibody, no more than the recommended dose should be given.

Table 24-3 Rabies postexposure prophylaxis schedule, United States, 1991

Vaccination status	Treatment	Regimen*
Not previously vaccinated	Local wound cleansing	All postexposure treatment should begin with immediate thorough cleansing of all wounds with soap and water.
	HRIG	20 IU/kg body weight. If anatomically feasible, up to one-half the dose should be infiltrated around the wound(s) and the rest should be administered IM in the gluteal area. HRIG should not be administered in the same syringe or into the same anatomic site as vaccine. Because HRIG may partially suppress active production of antibody, no more than the recommended dose should be given.
	Vaccine	HDCV or RVA, 1.0 ml, IM (deltoid area†), one each on days 0, 3, 7, 14 and 28.
Previously vaccinated‡	Local wound cleansing	All postexposure treatment should begin with immediate thorough cleansing of all wounds with soap and water.
	HRIG	HRIG should not be administered.
	Vaccine	HDCV or RVA, 1.0 ml, IM (deltoid area†), one each on days 0 and 3.

*These regimens are applicable for all age groups, including children.
†The deltoid area is the only acceptable site of vaccination for adults and older children. For younger children the outer aspect of the thigh may be used. Vaccine should never be administered in the gluteal area.
‡Any person with a history of preexposure vaccination with HDCV or RVA; prior postexposure prophylaxis with HDCV or RVA; or previous vaccination with any other type of rabies vaccine and a documented history of antibody response to the prior vaccination.

Table 24-4   Rabies preexposure prophylaxis guide, United States, 1991

Risk category	Nature of risk	Typical populations	Preexposure recommendations
Continuous	Virus present continuously, often in high concentrations. Aerosol, mucous membrane, bite, or nonbite exposure. Specific exposures may go unrecognized.	Rabies research lab worker*; rabies biologics production workers.	Primary course. Serologic testing every 6 months; booster vaccination when antibody level falls below acceptable level.†
Frequent	Exposure usually episodic, with source recognized, but exposure may also be unrecognized. Aerosol, mucous membrane, bite, or nonbite exposure.	Rabies diagnostic lab workers,* spelunkers, veterinarians and staff, and animal-control and wildlife workers in rabies enzootic areas. Travelers visiting foreign areas of enzootic rabies for more than 30 days.	Primary course. Serologic testing or booster vaccination every 2 years.†
Infrequent (greater than population at large)	Exposure nearly always episodic with source recognized Mucous membrane, bite, or nonbite exposure.	Veterinarians and animal-control and wildlife workers in areas of low rabies enzooticity. Veterinary students.	Primary course; no serologic testing or booster vaccination.
Rare (population at large)	Exposures always episodic Mucous membrane, or bite with source unrecognized.	U.S. population at large, including persons in rabies epizootic areas.	No vaccination necessary.

*Judgment of relative risk and extra monitoring of vaccination status of laboratory workers is the responsibility of the laboratory supervisor.

†Minimum acceptable antibody level is complete virus neutralization at a 1:5 serum dilution by RFFIT. Booster dose should be administered if the titer falls below this level.

Table 24-5   Rabies preexposure prophylaxis schedule, United States, 1991

Type of vaccination	Route	Regimen
Primary	IM	HDCV or RVA, 1.0 ml (deltoid area), one each on days 0, 7, and 21 or 28
	ID	HDCV, 0.1 ml, one each on days 0, 7, and 21 or 28
Booster*	IM	HDCV or RVA, 1.0 ml (deltoid area), day 0 only
	ID	HDCV, 0.1 ml, day 0 only

*Administration of routine booster dose of vaccine depends on exposure risk category as noted in Table 24-4.

Preexposure vaccination should be offered to persons among high-risk groups, such as veterinarians, animal handlers, certain laboratory workers, and persons spending time in foreign countries where canine rabies is endemic. Other persons whose activities bring them into frequent contact with rabies virus or potentially rabid dogs, cats,

skunks, raccoons, bats, or other species at risk of having rabies should also be considered for preexposure prophylaxis. Recommended regimens are described in Tables 24-4 and 24-5.

Since the publication of these recommendations, the importance of occult exposure to rabid bats in the United States has become evident. More than half of the viruses isolated from human rabies cases since 1980 have been identified as of bat origin, although in many of these there was no history of bat bite. The mandibles of bats are sufficiently small that bites may be difficult to detect, and the animal may attack sleeping persons. Therefore it is now advised that exposures of sleeping persons, particularly children, to bats be taken more seriously, even if no evidence of bite is found. Thus, in situations in which a bat is found to be present and bite exposure is possible, postexposure prophylaxis should be given unless capture and testing of the bat excludes rabies infection. Obviously this recommendation must be applied with discretion, and it underlines the need for consultation with experts in many instances of putative exposure to rabies.

BIBLIOGRAPHY

Anderson LJ, Nicholson KG, Tauxe RV, et al. Human rabies in the United States, 1960 to 1979: epidemiology, diagnosis, and prevention. Ann Intern Med 1984;100:728-735.

Aoki FY, Rubin ME, Fast MV. Rabies-neutralizing antibody in serum of children compared to adults following postexposure prophylaxis. Biologicals 20:283-287, 1992.

Baer GM (ed). The natural history of rabies. New York: Academic Press, 1975.

Bahmanyar M et al. Successful protection of humans exposed to rabies infection: postexposure treatment with the new human diploid cell rabies vaccine and antirabies serum. JAMA 1976;236:2751.

Bernard KW, Mallonee J, Wright JC, et al. Preexposure immunization with intradermal human diploid cell rabies vaccine: risks and benefits of primary and booster vaccination. JAMA 1987;257:1059-1063.

Bhatt DP et al. Human rabies: diagnosis, complications, and management. Am J Dis Child 1974;127:862.

Centers for Disease Control. Rabies surveillance, United States, 1988. MMWR 1989;38:36.

Eng T, Fishbein DB. Epidemiologic factors, clinical findings, and vaccination status of rabies in cats and dogs in the U.S. in 1988: National Study Group on Rabies. J Am Vet Assoc 1990;197(2):201-209.

Falade E, Andazola-Boyd M, Shingai R, et al. Human rabies: California 1995. MMWR 1996;45(17):353-356.

Hemachuda T. Human rabies: clinical aspects, pathogenesis, and potential therapy. Curr Top Micro Immunol 1994; 187: 121-143.

Houff SA et al. Human-to-human transmission of rabies virus by corneal transplant. N Engl J Med 1979;300:603.

Immunization Practices Advisory Committee (ACIP). MMWR 1991;40:1-19.

Johnson HN. Rabies virus. In Horsfall JL Jr, Tamm I (eds). Viral and rickettsial infections of man, ed 4. Philadelphia: JB Lippincott, 1965.

Kaplan C, Turner GS, Warrell DA. Rabies, the facts. Oxford, UK: Oxford University Press, 1986.

Kuwert EK, Marcus I, Hoher PG. Neutralizing and complement-fixing antibody responses in preexposure and postexposure vaccinees to a rabies vaccine produced in human diploid cells. J Biol Stand 1976;4:249.

Plotkin S, Wiktor TJ. Rabies vaccination. Annu Rev Med 1979;29:583.

Sabeti A, Bahmanyar M, Ghodssi M, Baltazard M. Traitement des mordus par loups enragés en Iran. Ann Inst Pasteur 1964;106:303.

Smith JS. Rabies virus epitopic variation: use in ecologic studies. Adv Virus Res 1989;36:215-253.

Smith JS, Rupprecht CE, Fishbein DB, Clark K. Unexplained rabies in three immigrants in the United States: a virologic investigation. N Engl J Med 1991;324:205-211.

Wiktor TJ, Plotkin SA, Koprowski H. Development and clinical trials of the new human rabies vaccine of tissue culture (human diploid cell) origin. Dev Biol Stand 1977;40:3.

Wilde H, Sirikawin S, Sabchaoren A, et al. Failures of postexposure treatment of rabies in children. Clin Infect Dis 1996;22:228.

Winkler WG. Airborne rabies virus infection. Bull Wildl Dis Assoc 1968;4:37.

Wunner WH, Larson JK, Dietzschold B, Smith CL. The molecular biology of rabies viruses. Rev Infect Dis 1988;10(suppl 4):771-784.

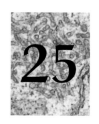

25 RESPIRATORY INFECTIONS AND SINUSITIS

DAVID S. HODES

Acute respiratory tract infections are the most common acute illnesses seen by the American pediatrician. Incidence rates have varied from study to study and from location to location, but rates of about six episodes per year for the first two years of life are reported. The incidence generally declines as children grow older but is boosted by participation in day care and entrance into school.

Whereas the bulk of respiratory infections involve only the upper tract (the anatomy above the epiglottis), are of viral origin, and are self-limited, it is important to remember that lower tract disease is the cause of important morbidity and mortality. Even in the 1990s pneumonia and influenza still account for 1% to 2% of infant mortality in the United States (Guyer et al., 1995). The toll in non-industrialized countries is far greater.

The task of organizing one's thinking about respiratory infections is a formidable one, since it is required to deal with a variety of syndromes (colds, pharyngitis, bronchitis, pneumonia, etc.) and a wealth of causal agents (more than 200 individual agents involved, with probably 90% of them non-bacterial). This chapter attempts to do this by first dealing with individual pathogens and then reviewing clinical syndromes.

VIRUSES

Well over 200 virus serotypes have been implicated as causing respiratory tract disease. Table 25-1 presents a brief summary of these agents and the syndromes they commonly produce.

Orthomyxoviruses and Paramyxoviruses

These respiratory viruses are lipid-enveloped agents containing negative-sense, single-stranded RNA. They mature by budding from host cell membranes and are quite pleomorphic, and they range in size from 100 to 300 nm in diameter. Attachment to the host cell surface is mediated by spikelike viral peptides that project from the surface of the envelope. At least one viral protein is typically applied to the internal surface of the envelope, whereas the nucleocapsid consists of the RNA in conjunction with a nucleoprotein and several other proteins that play roles in the viral transcriptive and replicative processes. The orthomyxoviruses and paramyxoviruses are spread by aerosolized droplets and, on occasion, by the hands (Hall and Douglas, 1981).

Influenza Viruses. Influenza viruses A, B, and C (the only human orthomyxoviruses) were first described in 1933, 1940, and 1949, respectively. The influenza types A and B single-stranded RNA genomes are found in eight segments. The viruses are pleomorphic and usually spherical particles, 80 to 100 nm in diameter (Fig. 25-1). In type A, six each encode a separate virus protein, and the others encode two proteins (Fig. 25-1). Influenza C, clinically the least significant, will likely be reclassified as a separate genus. The surface of the virus (types A and B) is covered by two types of projections 10 to 14 (HA) nm long, one possessing hemagglutinin activity (HA) and the other (NA) neuraminidase activity (NA). The HA spike is responsible for adsorption of the virus to the host cell. In addition, the HA spike is responsible for the characteristic agglutination of erythrocytes by the influenza virus. The NA spike is responsible for the receptor-destroying activity of type A and B viruses. Neuraminidase cleaves neuraminic acid residues on host cell receptors, allowing elution of the virus from the receptors during the viral maturation process and thereby facilitates the cell-to-cell spread of the virus.

Antigenicity and epidemiology. The HA is the major specific envelope antigen, and the differences in this antigen among various strains of virus can be identified by hemagglutination-inhibition

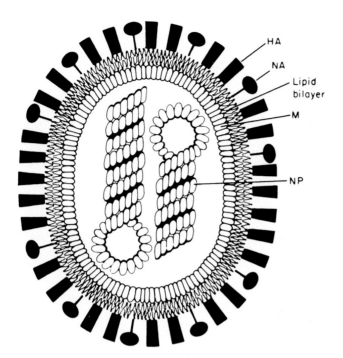

FIG. 25-1 Schematic diagram of the arrangement suggested for the structural components in the influenza virion. The two types of surface projections, hemagglutinin subunits consisting of HA polypeptides and neuraminidase subunits consisting of NA polypeptides, are on the external surface of a lipid bilayer; the mode of their attachment to the bilayer is unknown. On the internal surface of the bilayer is a layer of the membrane polypeptide M, and within it are the ribonucleoprotein composed of NP polypeptides and the viral RNA. The location of the P polypeptides is uncertain. (From Compano RW, Choppin PW: Compr Virol 1975;4:198.)

Table 25-1 Viruses in acute respiratory tract disease

Group of agents	Number of serotypes	Clinical syndromes
Respiratory syncytial virus	2	Bronchiolitis; pneumonia; bronchitis; upper respiratory tract infection
Parainfluenza virus	4	Croup; bronchitis; bronchiolitis; pneumonia
Influenza virus	3	Influenza; croup; upper respiratory tract infection; pneumonia
Coronavirus	3 or more	Common colds in adults
Nonpolio enteroviruses	c.70	Febrile pharyngitis (pediatric age group); colds in military recruits; herpangina; pleurodynia
Rhinovirus	100+	Common colds
Adenovirus	49	Both upper and lower respiratory tract disease in children, infants, and military recruits; bronchiolitis obliterans; pertussis syndrome

(HI) tests. The virus is neutralized by antibody to the HA. In contrast, anti-NA antibody does not neutralize the virus, but it does modify infection, probably by its effect on the release of virus from the cells. Three types of hemagglutinin (H1, H2, H3) and two types of neuraminidase (N1, N2) are recognized. Influenza viruses vary in their antigenic stability. Antigenic changes occur mainly in the HA and NA proteins. Type A virus is least stable and is characterized by frequent minor antigenic changes and occasional major antigenic changes. Type C virus is most stable, and type B is intermediate between A and C, undergoing only minor antigenic changes. The classification of influenza viruses before 1972 was based on the type of ribonucleoprotein antigen, and the subtype was dependent on the hemagglutinin antigen (e.g., A2). However, when it became obvious that neuraminidase undergoes antigenic variation independent of hemagglutinin variation, it was proposed that the influenza virus strain be designated by the antigenic type of its hemagglutinin and neuraminidase—for example, A/Hong Kong/68 (H3N2) (Table 25-2). This designation indicates that the virus was isolated from a person in Hong Kong in 1968 and that it contains HA type 3 and NA type 2 antigens. The term *antigenic drift* describes relatively frequent minor genetic changes

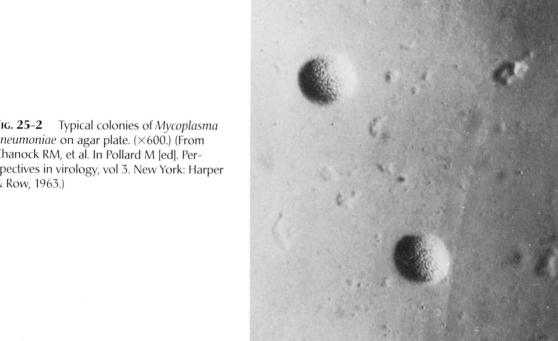

FIG. 25-2 Typical colonies of *Mycoplasma pneumoniae* on agar plate. (×600.) (From Chanock RM, et al. In Pollard M [ed]. Perspectives in virology, vol 3. New York: Harper & Row, 1963.)

in HA or NA that result in the occurrence of annual localized epidemics of influenza type A or B. The various different strains listed in Table 30-2 represent, for the most part, the results of antigenic drift. The term *antigenic shift* refers to the periodic change in the dominant antigenic composition of influenza type A virus. Antigenic shift occurs when there is a major change in the antigenic type of either the HA or NA (e.g., in 1968 the surface antigen shifted from H2N2 to H3N2). It is believed that antigenic shift is effected because two influenza virus particles infecting the same cell can exchange RNA segments (genetic reassortment). By best estimation, the origins of the new segments thus introduced into the human strains are derived from reassortment with strains of influenza from water fowl (Webster et al., 1992). Because a completely novel segment coding for HA or NA is introduced in antigenic shift, the change in antigenicity is far more profound than is seen in the piecemeal mutations of antigenic drift. In each of the four decades between the 1940s and the 1970s major variants emerged with dominant antigens relatively new to most people. When the population at large has no immunity, antigenic shift heralds a pandemic so that localized epidemics of influenza spread worldwide. The last major antigenic shift resulting in pandemic influenza occurred in 1977. Since that time H1N1 and H3N2 strains of influenza type A have cocirculated. As Francis (1961-1962) stated,

Since the breadth of antibody is dependent on experience with strains of varied composition, inexperienced children exhibit the highest incidence of infection by any and all strains and also have the most limited antibody reflection of viral antigens. With the passage of time, antibody to succeeding dominants is acquired, but large gaps exist in the immunity of the community to viral antigens that prevailed when the older segments of the population were young. Such gaps in acquired immunity permit epidemic spread of influenza strains with newly rearranged antigenic composition.

Clinical Manifestations of Disease Caused by Both Influenza A and B. Disease caused by type B probably is generally milder than that caused by type A. The clinical illness is characterized by a sudden rise in temperature, rigors, myalgia, headache, lassitude, and anorexia. Respiratory symptoms include a sore throat, nasal congestion,

Francis T Jr. Problems of acute respiratory disease. Yale J Biol Med 1961-1962; 34:191.

Table 25-2 Designation of influenza type A strains prevalent in the United States[*]

Prototype strain designation	Surface antigens		Years of prevalence
	HA	NA	
A/PR/34	HO	N1	1934-1946
A/FM/47	H1	N1	1947-1956
A/Japan/57	H2	N2	1957-1968
A/Hong Kong/69	H3	N2	1968-1972
A/Philippines/82	H3	N2	1982-1986
A/Chile/83	H1	N1	1983-1984
A/Taiwan/86	H1	N1	1986-1991
A/Sichuan/87	H3	N2	1987-1988
A/Shanghai/87	H3	N2	1989-1990
A/Singapore/88	H1	N1	1988-1991
A/Shanghai/89	H1	N2	1990-1991
A/Texas/91	H1	N1	1991-1996
A/Beijing/89	H3	N2	1991-1993
A/Beijing/92	H3	N2	1994-1995
A/Shendong/93	H3	N2	1995-1996
A/Johannesburg/94	H3	N2	1995-1996
A/Wuhan/95	H3	N2	1996-1997

[*]1971 to 1982 deleted.

conjunctivitis, and a nonproductive cough. The illness generally lasts several days and may be followed by a period of asthenia. Children are more likely to present with croup, bronchiolitis, gastrointestinal complaints, conjunctivitis, and otitis media. Influenza A and B may be complicated by the development of pneumonia. The pneumonia may be caused by the virus itself or by bacterial superinfection. Other complications of influenza include myositis, myocarditis, Reye's syndrome, Guillain-Barré syndrome, and aseptic meningitis. Both myositis and Reye's syndrome have been associated more frequently with influenza B, whereas Guillain-Barré has been associated more frequently with influenza A. Comparatively little is known about influenza virus C.

Pathogenesis. Influenza virus reaches the respiratory tract via droplet infection. After a short incubation period of 1 to 2 days, it is possible to detect virus in the nasopharynx. Viremia is probably a very rare occurrence. The neuraminidase of the virus may decrease the viscosity of the mucus covering of the respiratory tract, thereby exposing the cellular receptors and facilitating the spread of virus-containing fluid to the lower respiratory tract. If specific antibody is present at the portal of entry, the infection may be aborted. This can be achieved

by high levels of serum antibody or the presence of local secretory antibody (IgA). Pathologic changes include evidence of inflammation of the upper respiratory tract with destruction of ciliated epithelial cells. If the infection has progressed to involve the lungs, the findings include interstitial inflammation; necrosis of the bronchiolar and alveolar epithelium; and alveoli filled with red blood cells (RBCs), white blood cells (WBCs), and hyaline membranes. Secondary bacterial infection may be caused by staphylococci, pneumococci, or *Haemophilus influenzae*.

Parainfluenza Viruses. Human parainfluenza viruses (HPIVs) types 1, 2, 3, and 4 were originally so named because they shared with influenza viruses HA and NA activities and a propensity to respiratory disease. Virologically, however, they are clearly distinct and are now grouped in the *Paramyxovirus* (HPIVs 1 and 3) and *Rubulavirus* (HPIVs 2 and 4) genera of the family Paramyxoviridae of the order Mononegavirales. They are pleomorphic with diameters of 150 to 200 nm; the genome is nonsegmented negative-stranded RNA coding for six structural proteins.

Molecular biology. Unlike the influenza viruses, the parainfluenza viruses possess a single surface spike (HN) for both HA and NA. The HN glycoprotein attaches to host cell moieties and initiates infection. A second surface glycoprotein—the F, or fusion, protein—cooperates with the HN to mediate viral envelope fusion to the target cell, penetration, and the fusion of host cells to form syncytia (Moscona and Peluso, 1991.) Proteolytic cleavage of the F glycoprotein by host cell enzymes is required for viral infectivity. The anatomic location of host cell enzymes capable of cleaving the F glycoprotein may help determine the particular tissue tropism of the parainfluenza viruses. Most parainfluenza viruses are readily detected and grown in primary or continuous tissue cultures of monkey and human kidney. Cytopathogenic effects may be scant or lacking in first passage, but the presence of virus can be recognized by adding guinea pig RBCs to the culture and observing adsorption of the red cells to the kidney monolayer (hemadsorption technique).

Clinical syndromes and epidemiology of parainfluenza viruses. Parainfluenza virus types 1, 2, and 3 were recovered from 40% of 2359 infants and children with croup, bronchitis, bronchiolitis, or pneumonia and from 6% of 3,377 children with mild rhinitis, pharyngitis, bronchitis, or a combination of the three (Parrott et al., 1962). Altogether, types 1, 2, and 3 constitute the agents most commonly associated with croup type 3 less prominently. Each of the three types also most frequently manifests as croup. More specifically, parainfluenza virus type 1 has been found chiefly in association with croup and is a major cause of severe croup in young children. Parainfluenza virus type 3 is second only to RSV as the cause of bronchiolitis in young infants. Parainfluenza virus type 4 is isolated infrequently and tends to cause only a mild upper respiratory tract illness. Epidemic outbreaks of croup associated with parainfluenza virus types 1 and 2 generally occur in the autumn of the year. Respiratory infections related to parainfluenza virus type 3 tend to occur endemically throughout the year. Springtime outbreaks of illness secondary to parainfluenza virus type 3 have also been noted.

Serologic studies indicate that primary infection with the parainfluenza virus usually takes place in the first 3 to 5 years of life. Illness associated with primary infection caused by parainfluenza virus types 1 and 2 is most likely to occur in the child older than 2 years of age. The relatively older age at which primary infection occurs with types 1 and 2 suggests a protective role for passively acquired maternal antibody. Illness with primary parainfluenza virus type 3 infection generally occurs in the first year of life. Studies also suggest that infants born with high levels of maternal neutralizing antibody to parainfluenza virus type 3 are at lower risk of having serious illness with type 3 infection.

Most adults have circulating antibodies to parainfluenza virus. The presence of antibody, however, does not preclude reinfection. Severity of illness is related to previous experience with the virus and, accordingly, to age. Thus primary infection is usually expressed as febrile respiratory illness, and approximately one third of the patients have involvement of the lower respiratory tract. Reinfection results in either mild upper respiratory tract disease or no disease. Mild afebrile coldlike illness was observed in adult human volunteers given parainfluenza virus types 1 and 3 experimentally through the nose and throat. Most of the volunteers had specific neutralizing antibody before they were given virus, and there was no difference in serum antibody levels between those in whom illness developed and those who escaped illness. The presence of serum antibody did not prevent illness, but the illness was mild and confined to the upper respiratory tract.

In later studies conducted with human volunteers, Smith et al. (1966) showed that the presence or absence of IgA neutralizing antibody in the nasal secretions was critical in determining whether or not the volunteer would be reinfected after challenge with parainfluenza virus type 1 (Table 25-3). Although an inactivated type 1 parainfluenza virus vaccine stimulated the production of neutralizing antibody in the serum of adult volunteers, the response in their nasal secretions was minimal. The implications of these important studies are (1) that the presence of secretory IgA antibodies in the nasal secretions is a better index of resistance to infection of the upper respiratory tract than the level of serum antibody, and (2) that a live attenuated virus vaccine offers a better chance than inactivated virus vaccine to stimulate the production of neutralizing antibodies in nasal secretions.

Respiratory Syncytial Virus. RSV was first discovered in 1956 by Morris et al., who isolated it from a chimpanzee with coryza. Pioneering work by Chanock and Finberg (1957) established the agent as a cause of pneumonia in children and revealed the characteristic syncytial cytopathology that suggested the agent's name. It was subsequently determined to be the most important single respiratory pathogen in infancy and early childhood and a predominant cause of hospitalization. RSV is estimated to cause 90,000 hospitalizations and 4,500 deaths from lower respiratory tract disease in the United States annually (Institute of Medicine, 1985).

Properties of RSV. RSV is currently classified as a member of the genus *Pneumovirus* within the family Paramyxoviridae. It has the typical pleo-

Table 25-3 Response of volunteers to inoculation with parainfluenza virus type 1

	Presence or absence of virus neutralizing activity in nasal secretions at time of challenge	
	Present	**Absent**
Number of men inoculated	29	51
Virus recovery	2*	33
Upper respiratory tract illness associated with type 1 virus	4*	29
Upper respiratory tract illness not associated with type 1 virus	7	2

Data from Smith CB, et al: N Engl J Med 1966;275:1145.
*$P < 0.01$.

morphic paramyxovirus morphology and a nonsegmented genome of approximately 16 kb. Ten genes have been identified. Prominent are two surface glycoproteins, an attachment glycoprotein (G) and a fusion glycoprotein (F) that seem to mediate viral attachment and cell fusion processes though lacking hemagglutination and neuraminidase properties. Also a matrix protein (M) and a nucleoprotein (N) are found, with the latter being highly conserved. A large polymerase protein (L) is found in the nucleocapsid, along with a phosphoprotein (P). A smaller membrane-associated protein, two nonstructural proteins and another structural protein of uncertain location are also included.

RSV is a delicate virus, being unstable at pH 3 and at temperatures above $37°$ C. It is destroyed by standard ether treatment (which dissolves the lipid membrane) and loses 90% of its infectivity on slow freezing, necessitating rapid freezing and storage at $-70°$ C if preservation is required.

RSV can be shown to replicate in the respiratory tracts of a number of laboratory animals (e.g., hamster, ferret, chinchilla) and clear clinical symptoms are produced in the chimpanzee and cebus and owl monkeys. Histologic lesions resembling those found in human disease can be detected in RSV-infected cotton rats and BALB/c mice, making them useful models for the study of viral pathogenesis. Older individuals of the latter species also develop generic signs of illness such as fur ruffling and decreased activity (Graham et al., 1988). The lamb provides a somewhat more cumbersome model (Lapin et al., 1993).

Tissue culture. RSV can be recovered from clinical specimens by inoculation into a number of tissue culture systems. Human epithelial lines such as HEp-2 and HeLa are the most sensitive, although sensitivity may vary from lot to lot and with the age of the lines. For optimal results it is recommended that inoculation of human fibroblasts and monkey kidney cell lines be carried out as well (Tristram and Welliver, 1995). Typically RSV causes formation of syncytia in the infected cells after 3 to 7 days of incubation. In some cases, cell rounding and degeneration of individual cells also occur.

Antigenic composition. RSV isolates were initially divided into two subgroups, A and B, according to variations in the antigenicity of their G proteins. Nucleotide sequence data now indicate that subgroups A and B of G proteins show only about 50% amino acid identity, whereas other proteins are more conserved. A and B subgroups have been shown to cocirculate within the same community during the same season. Infection with subgroup A induces a broader neutralizing antibody response than does infection with subgroup B, but multiple infection eventually leads to the development of widely reactive neutralizing antibody. Animal models would indicate that antibody to the F protein may result in the evolution of this broad protection (Stott et al., 1987).

Like other negative-sense, nonsegmented RNA genomes, the RSV genome is subject to mutation, and even within a subgroup variability among strains is marked. Thus the G protein genes from different isolates of subgroup A show up to 20% variability in amino acid sequence (Cane et al., 1991). This has made possible a detailed accounting of RSV molecular epidemiology and evolution. Examination of strains over a 40-year period revealed a mutation rate of about 0.25% per year over the entire protein, with clustering occurring on a temporal rather than a geographic basis. Thus some strains arise and die out at different points in time, possibly as the result of immunologic pressure, and identical strains can circulate at the same time at distant spots on the globe (Cane and Pringle, 1995). This variability underscores the concept that RSV epidemics are essentially community based (Anderson, 1991).

Immunologic aspects. Two curious immunologic characteristics of RSV have both raised intriguing questions about its pathophysiology and complicated the development of effective vaccines. The first is the incomplete protection offered by both maternal antibody and by actual infection with the virus. The second is the implication of immunologic mechanisms in the pathogenesis of disease.

The problematic nature of the protection offered by maternal antibody is underscored by the fact that the peak incidence of serious RSV disease is seen in infants aged 2 to 5 months, a time of life when maternal antibody is still circulating within the infant. Nonetheless, some degree of protection is apparently afforded, since infection in the first month is uncommon (Parrott et al., 1973a) and higher levels of maternally derived antibody do seem to correlate with less severe illness (Glezen et al., 1981).

Repeated reinfection with RSV within a year of the previous infection is readily demonstrated in young children (Henderson et al., 1979b; Glezen et al., 1986). Reinfections seem to result in less severe disease, but this resistance may require several repeated infections to develop. Observations in hospital personnel and in the military indicate that both symptomatic and asymptomatic infection of healthy adults is possible (Hall et al., 1978; Johnson et al., 1962b). Family studies produced similar conclusions (Hall et al., 1976).

Studies of the role of cytokines and T-cell responses to RSV have provided new clues to the problem of reinfection. RSV apparently evokes the elaboration from monocytes of inhibitory factors that blunt T-cell proliferation (Preston et al., 1992; Salkind et al., 1991). These factors may impede prompt clearance of reinfecting virus. Induction of IL-10 from RSV-infected alveolar macrophages may also inhibit the immune response (Panuska et al., 1995).

The relationship between subtle RSV genetic mutation (Cane and Pringle, 1995) and the reinfection phenomenon needs further elucidation.

Thinking about RSV immunopathogenesis has been conducted under the pall of the great vaccination incident of the late 1960s. At that time, infants were vaccinated intramuscularly with a formalin-inactivated RSV preparation and were shown to produce both complement-fixing and neutralizing antibodies to the virus. However, when exposed to epidemic wild-type RSV, these infants experienced not protection but, rather, exaggerated disease (Kapikian et al., 1969). An explanation for this phenomenon has been considered of primary importance for future vaccine development, but none has been entirely satisfactory. Damage by antigen-antibody complexes has been suggested, but animal studies have consistently demonstrated vaccine-induced humoral antibody to have a protective effect (Walsh et al., 1987). More attention has recently been paid to the possibility that the vaccination incident was caused by factors unique to the formalinizing process itself. There is evidence that the process may have altered RSV epitopes in such a way as to induce the overproduction of ineffective antibodies rather than neutralizing antibodies (Murphy et al., 1986). A growing body of evidence culled from animal models now indicates that different vaccine formulations may evoke different CD4 helper cell responses and characteristic cytokine elaboration patterns. These unique patterns could possibly result in either protective or pathogenic reactions (Graham, 1995).

Epidemiology. RSV has been isolated globally and in lands of every climate. In temperate areas it appears in seasonal epidemics in the winter and early spring. These outbreaks occur annually with clocklike regularity (Hall and Douglas, 1976). At-

tack rates are high, and it is estimated that 50% of children will be infected during the course of the first RSV epidemic they encounter and virtually all of the rest by the second epidemic. As many of 40% of the infants who first contract RSV in their first 6 months of life will develop disease in the lower respiratory tract, resulting in hospitalization rates of approximately 10 per 1000 infants and emergency room visits of 110 per 1000 (Kim et al., 1973a). This translates into 90,000 hospitalizations and 4500 deaths from lower respiratory tract disease in the United States annually (MMWR, 1995).

RSV is transmitted by direct inoculation of respiratory droplets and thus requires close contact for effective spread. RSV does not appear to be contracted by distant contact with small-particle aerosols. Nonetheless, since RSV is shed profusely by infected infants and may survive for hours on the skin of individuals and on environmental surfaces, it has great potential for nosocomial spread (Hall and Douglas, 1981).

Clinical syndromes associated with RSV. Primary infection with RSV tends to be the most severe, whether this is due to the immunopathologic mechanisms discussed earlier; to immunologic immaturity; or simply to the small, vulnerable airways of the infected infants. The classic syndrome produced is bronchiolitis, which may develop in upwards of 50% of those infected. The syndrome frequently merges into pneumonia. Nonobstructive apnea is a dreaded complication. Also noteworthy are tracheobronchitis and occasional cases of croup. Reinfections of older children and adults are manifested principally as upper respiratory tract infections and tracheobronchitis, although lower respiratory tract disease is noted occasionally, especially in the elderly (Falsey et al., 1992). Otitis media is a common manifestation of RSV infection (Okamoto et al., 1992).

It has long been known that children suffering RSV bronchiolitis early in life are prone to recurrent attacks of reactive airway disease (Rooney and Williams, 1971). Indeed, such children have demonstrated abnormalities of pulmonary function (Pullan and Hey, 1982; Hall et al., 1984). It is indeterminable whether RSV plays a causal role in the production of these abnormalities or whether those congenitally disposed to atopy or abnormal airway anatomy or reactivity are more liable to contract bronchiolitis when first infected with RSV.

Adenoviruses

The adenoviruses were first discovered in 1953 by Rowe et al., who unmasked several agents from adenoids removed from healthy children and grown in tissue culture. Currently, human adenoviruses are included in the genus *Mastadenovirus* along with those of other mammals. Avian adenoviruses form a separate genus. Human adenoviruses are divided into six subgroups on the basis of their hemagglutination reactions and into at least forty-nine different serotypes based on neutralization. Adenoviruses are 80 nm in diameter; possess double-stranded linear DNA; have an icosahedral structure with 252 capsomeres; are resistant to the action of ether and acid but are heat labile, being destroyed at 56° C for 30 minutes; and share a common, but not identical, soluble complement-fixing antigen. The viruses carry many antigenic determinants, including those associated with the hexons (capsomeres surrounded by six neighbors), pentons (capsomeres surrounded by five neighbors), and fibers (elongated structures projecting from the outer surface of the pentons) of the virion. Adenoviruses contain at least eleven structural polypeptides and replicate and produce inclusions within the nuclei of infected cells. The most favorable cultures in vitro have been human lines of epithelial origin (HeLa, KB, HEp-2), primary human embryonic kidney, and fetal diploid lines.

Primary infection with adenoviruses usually occurs in early life, either as an asymptomatic infection or as acute upper respiratory tract disease. Surveillance studies suggest that approximately 5% of acute respiratory tract disease in children less than 5 years of age is due to adenoviruses. (Brandt et al., 1969). Adenovirus is most frequently isolated from children with coryza, otitis media, and pharyngitis (Edwards et al., 1985). Adenovirus-associated pharyngitis is typically exudative and may be difficult to distinguish from streptococcal tonsillitis. Adenovirus types 3, 4, 5, 6, 7, and 14 may be implicated in cases of upper respiratory tract disease with associated pharyngitis and conjunctivitis (pharyngoconjunctival fever). The adenoviruses also can cause diseases of the lower respiratory tract, including croup, bronchiolitis, and pneumonia. Lower respiratory tract illness caused by adenoviruses may be difficult to distinguish from illness caused by other viral respiratory pathogens. Occasionally, fatal pneumonia in very young infants has been described associated with types 3, 4, 7, and 21. In some children, sequelae of adenovirus infection have included bronchiectasis, bronchioloitis obliterans, and unilateral hyperlucent lung (Swyer-James syndrome). Follow-up studies suggest persistent pulmonary damage may occur in a significant number of children with adenoviral pneu-

monia (Simila et al., 1981). The claim that adenovirus, acting alone, can be responsible for a pertussis-like syndrome has been challenged. It is possible that a *B. pertussis* infection merely activates latent adenovirus infection in the respiratory tract (Neumann et al., 1987). Infection caused by adenovirus is generally endemic, with infection occurring throughout the year. Like the other respiratory viruses, the virus is more commonly isolated from October through May. Sporadic outbreaks of respiratory illness caused by adenoviruses have occurred in school-age children living closely together in institutions such as boarding schools and camps.

Although they usually are primarily considered respiratory tract pathogens, adenoviruses may produce viremia, and disease may arise in distant sites. It has also been suggested that the penton protein of the virus may act as an exotoxin, producing systemic effects. Clustered cases of mild keritoconjunctivitis have been caused by many serotypes. Outbreaks of keratoconjunctivitis caused by adenovirus types 8, 11, 19, or 37 have been associated with nosocomial infections caused by ophthalmic instruments and solutions. A more severe form (epidemic kertonconjunctivititis or "shipyard eye") can be more serious, causing corneal opacities (Dawson et al., 1970). Mufson and Belshe (1976) reviewed the association of adenoviruses, especially types 11 and 21, with a syndrome of dysuria, frequency, hematuria, and viruria. The enteric adenoviruses, particularly types 40 and 41, have been significantly associated with community-acquired diarrhea (Kotloff et al., 1989) (see Chapter 9). Adenoviral infection of the central nervous system is rare. Among college students and other adult civilians the incidence of adenoviral infection has been low. Young military recruits, on the other hand, were especially prone in the past to epidemics of acute respiratory disease and atypical pneumonia, often with rubella-like rash caused chiefly by adenovirus type 4 and, to a lesser extent, types 3 and 7. Adenoviruses cause between 5% and 10% of respiratory illnesses in civilians and between 8% and 50% of respiratory illnesses in military recruits.

Picornaviruses

A family of viruses including the rhinoviruses and the enteroviruses (poliovirus, coxsackievirus, and echovirus subgroups) has been designated picornaviruses (*pico* [i.e., very small] RNA). They measure 20 to 30 nm and are characterized by a nucleic acid core of positive, nonsegmented single-stranded RNA; absence of essential lipid as shown by resistance to the action of ether; and cationic stabilization of thermal inactivation (see Chapter 7).

Rhinoviruses. Rhinoviruses can be isolated from the upper respiratory tract and are the principal cause of mild upper respiratory tract illness in adults. Rhinoviruses share many of the properties of enteroviruses, including particle diameter of 20 to 30 nm; RNA core; resistance to ether; and, in general, cytopathic effects in tissue culture. In primary cultures of monkey or human embryonic kidney cells or in human embryonic lung cell lines, rhinoviruses grow best at slightly lower temperatures (33° C) and more acidic pH than enteroviruses. Rhinoviruses differ sharply from the enteroviruses in their sensitivity to acid: all strains of rhinovirus are unstable below pH 6, and enteroviruses are not. From studies published so far, there apparently are at least 102 different serologic types of rhinoviruses.

Rhinovirus colds are one of the most common infections in humans worldwide. They have been the most frequently isolated agents in all epidemiologic studies of upper respiratory tract infections and colds. Their predominance is more pronounced in studies where mild, as well as severe, illnesses are studied (Monto and Cavallaro, 1971). Because isolation of the agents is sometimes difficult, their contribution may be underestimated, but it is likely that they cause a third to a half of all acute respiratory infections. Rhinovirus illness rates are highest for young children and infants and decrease with advancing age. Peaks of infection tend to occur in the spring and fall of the year. Using volunteers, it can be shown that a number of strains will produce colds and that very few virus particles are required for contagion (D'Alessio et al., 1984). Virus can be isolated from nasopharyngeal washings in the first 3 to 5 days of illness. No specific or nonspecific treatment is of proven value.

Enteroviruses. The properties of enteroviruses and their role in causing diverse clinical syndromes, including aseptic meningitis, paralysis, pleurodynia, febrile exanthem, and myocarditis in newborn infants, are described in Chapter 7. There is also a contribution to respiratory illness. Enteroviruses are not usually associated with the common cold syndrome, as are rhinoviruses. Coxsackievirus group A type 21 is an important exception (Johnson et al., 1962a). Nonetheless, enteroviruses often manifest as nonspecific febrile illness complicated by pharyngitis, which may or may not present with an exudate. It is likely that this is the most common presentation of enteroviral infection (Kogon et al., 1969). Group A coxsackieviruses, notably types 1 through 6, 8, 10, and 22 have been etiologically linked with herpangina, an acute illness characterized by fever, vomiting, sore throat, and the appearance of small vesicles or punched-out ulcers in and around the posterior pharynx (Chapter 7). Sporadic reports have implicated many other enteroviruses in this syndrome. Steigman et al. (1962) reported the isolation of group A coxsackievirus type 10 from patients with a summer febrile disease that they called acute lymphonodular pharyngitis. It was characterized by the appearance of discrete, raised, nonulcerative lesions on the anterior pillars, soft palate, and uvula. Another clinical syndrome associated with group A coxsackievirus type 16 was observed in Toronto in 1957 and in California in 1961. The illness was characterized by a vesicular enanthem on the buccal mucosa, tongue, gums, and palate. Another feature, which does not appear with herpan-gina, was a papulovesicular exanthem involving the hands, feet, legs, and buttocks in approximately 25% of the patients. The name *hand-foot-and-mouth disease* is often used to designate this syndrome. It has since been linked to other enteroviruses (mostly coxsackievirus) in addition to group A coxsackievirus type 16. A number of group A and B coxsackieviruses have been associated with other respiratory illnesses. Coxsackieviruses A21 and A24 have been associated with mild upper respiratory tract illness. Pharyngitis caused by coxsackievirus A21 has occurred in outbreaks in military populations. In addition to causing epidemic pleurodynia, which has certain characteristics of a respiratory disease such as cough and chest pain, group B coxsackievirus types 4 and 5 have been implicated in febrile respiratory tract illness accompanied by cough and nasal discharge. These agents have also been associated with influenza-like illness (see Chapter 7).

Echoviruses may also cause human infections characterized by upper respiratory tract and enteric tract diseases and common cold–like illnesses. Echovirus types 1 to 4, 6 to 9, 11, 16, 19, 20, 22, and 25 are known causes of a mild upper respiratory tract illness. Suggestive evidence linking enteroviruses with cases of pneumonia, bronchiolitis, bronchitis, and croup in infants under 2 years of age has been reported. Serious and sometimes fatal cases of enteroviral-associated pneumonia have been described as well, notably in the "Boston exanthem" epidemic of 1959 (Lerner et al., 1960). It

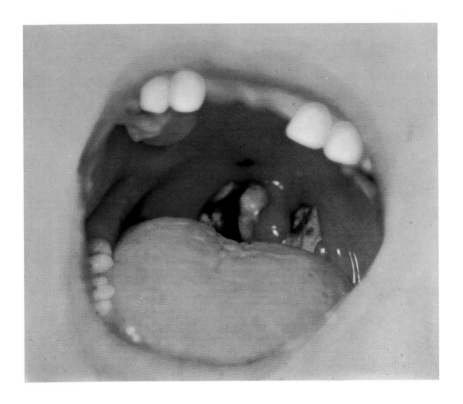

PLATE 1

Tonsillar diphtheria. (Reproduced courtesy of Franklin H. Top, M.D., Professor and Head of the Department of Hygiene and Preventive Medicine, State University of Iowa, College of Medicine, Iowa City, Iowa; and Parke, Davis & Company's *Therapeutic Notes*.)

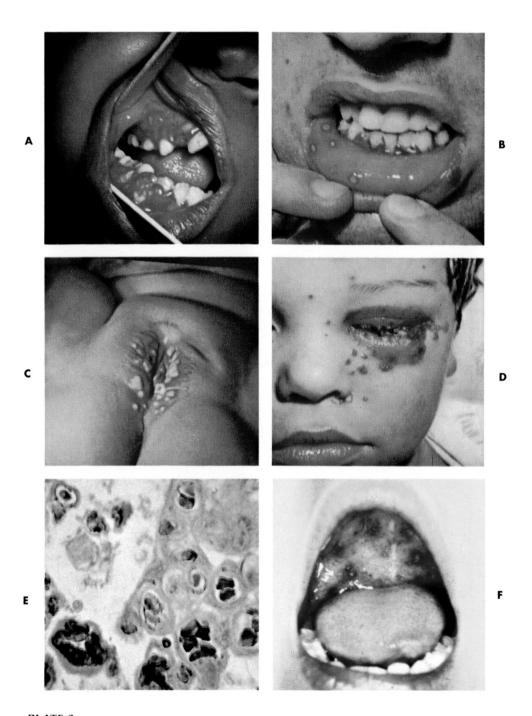

PLATE 2

Herpes simplex infections. **A**, Primary herpetic gingivostomatitis in a child. **B**, Same disease in a young adult. **C**, Primary HSVI vulvovaginitis in an infant. **D**, Primary herpetic kera-toconjunctivitis. **E**, Biopsy of herpetic vesicle. Eosinophilic intranuclear inclusions and giant cells (x800). **F**, Ulcerative lesions on palate and tongue in hand-foot-and-mouth syndrome caused by Coxsackie A-16 virus. (**A** to **E** from Blank H, Rake G. Viral and rickettsial diseases of the skin, eye, and mucous membranes of man. Boston: Little, Brown, 1995. **F** Courtesy James D. Cherry, M.D.)

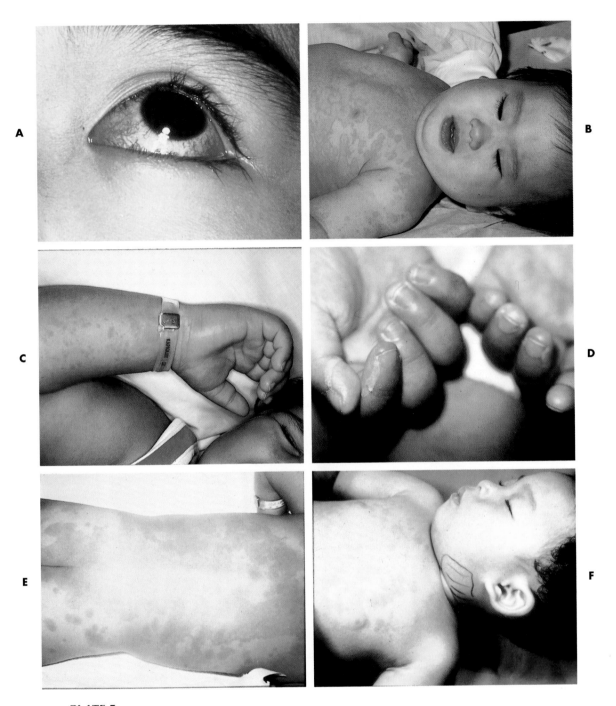

PLATE 3

Some clinical signs of Kawasaki syndrome. **A**, Discrete vascular injection of the bulbar conjunctiva. **B**, Generalized lip erythema with mild edema, cracking, and bleeding fissures. **C**, Diffuse red-purple discoloration of the palm(s). **D**, Desquamation beginning at the fingertips just below the nailbeds. **E**, Diffuse erythematous, nonvesicular and nonbullous, polymorphic rash. **F**, Unilaterally enlarged cervical lymph node.

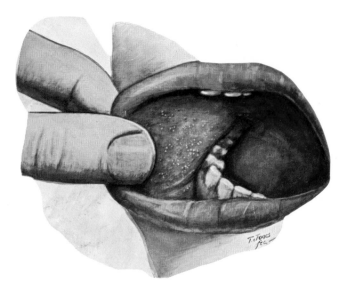

PLATE 4
Koplik's spots. (From Zahorsky J, Zahorsky TS. Synopsis of pediatrics. St. Louis: Mosby, 1953.)

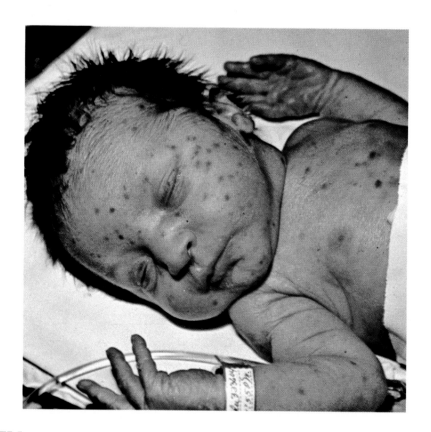

PLATE 5
A 3-day-old infant with generalized macular lesions characteristic of neonatal purpura resulting from congenital rubella. His jaundice is caused by rubella hepatitis. (Courtesy Dr. Kenneth Schiffer, Albert Einstein College of Medicine, New York, NY; from Cooper LZ, et al. Am J Dis Child 1965;110:416.)

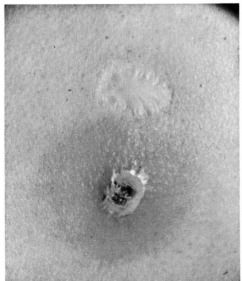

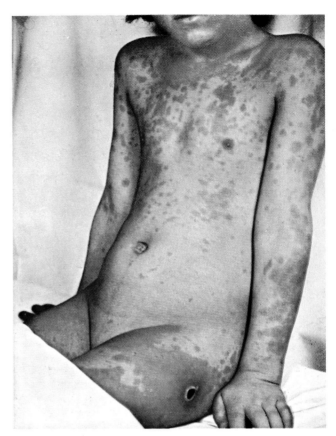

PLATE 6
A, Primary take in a previously vaccinated person. **B**, Toxic eruption complicating vaccinia. (From Top FH, Wehrle PF, eds. Communicable and infectious diseases, ed 8. St Louis: Mosby, 1976.)

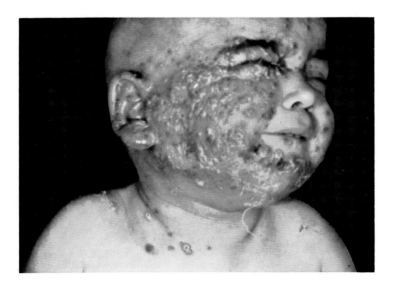

PLATE 7
Eczema vaccinatum. (Courtesy Dr. Otto E. Billo; from Stimson PM, Hodes HLA. Manual of the common contagious diseases. Philadelphia: Lea & Febiger, 1956.)

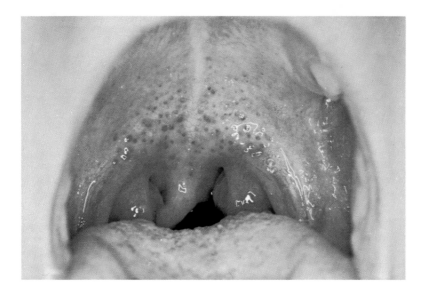

PLATE 8
Marked petechial stippling of the soft palate in scarlet fever. (From Stillerman M, Bernstein SH. Am J Dis Child 1961;101:476.)

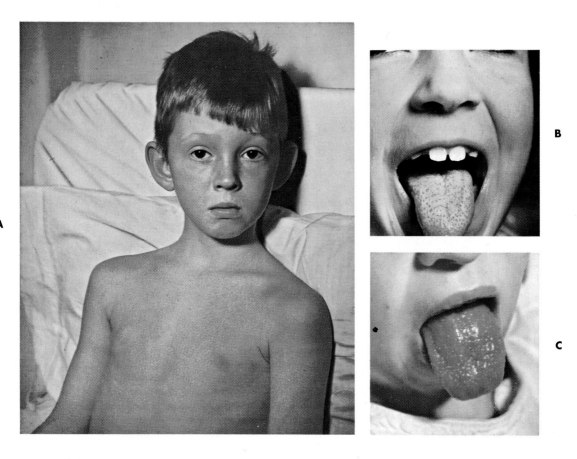

PLATE 9
Scarlet fever. **A**, Punctate, erythematous rash (second day). **B**, White strawberry tongue (first day). **C**, Red strawberry tongue (third day). (Courtesy Dr. Franklin H. Top, Professor and Head of the Department of Hygiene and Preventive Medicine, State University of Iowa, College of Medicine, Iowa City, Iowa; and Parke, Davis & Company's *Therapeutic Notes*.)

may be difficult clinically to distinguish lower respiratory tract disease caused by enteroviruses from other viral lower respiratory tract infections. However, infection caused by enteroviruses typically occurs in the summer and early fall, whereas infection caused by the majority of respiratory pathogens occurs during the winter.

Coronaviruses

The coronaviruses are enveloped, single-stranded, positive-sense RNA viruses. They are medium-sized viruses measuring 100 to 150 nm in diameter. There are two recognized antigenic groups of human respiratory coronaviruses. Other strains, of uncertain pathogencity, have been isolated from human feces. The viruses have been associated with a cold syndrome in adults and children. More serious lower respiratory tract illness has been found on occasion (McIntosh et al., 1974), and outbreaks in military populations have resulted in a high incidence of pneumonia (Wenzel et al., 1974). Coronaviruses tend to cause illness during the winter and spring months. Infection is apparently ubiquitous and incessant, with virtually all adults being seropositive and children showing evidence of infection by 5 years of age. The exact contribution of coronaviruses to respiratory illness is uncertain, since the incidence of diseases seems to vary from year to year and location to location, the means of viral isolation are difficult, and few recent epidemiologic studies are available. An estimate of the contribution at 5% to 10% would seem defensible.

Herpesviruses

Herpes simplex virus types 1 and 2, varicella-zoster virus, cytomegalovirus, and Epstein-Barr virus (EBV) are five of the members of the herpesvirus group for which humans serve as the usual hosts and reservoirs and cause disease of the respiratory tract (Chapters 4, 8, 12, and 37). The herpesvirus group is included in this discussion of respiratory viruses because (1) herpes simplex virus is one of the common causes of acute pharyngitis with vesicles or ulcers; (2) varicella-zoster virus may cause pneumonia, complicating chickenpox, particularly in adults and immunocompromised patients of all ages; (3) involvement of the lungs with pneumonia occurs in cytomegalovirus infection; (4) EBV is a cause of acute tonsillopharyngitis in infectious mononucleosis; and (5) pneumonia is part of a severe systemic illness caused by cytomegalovirus in immunocompromised patients and transplant recipients (Chapter 4).

Hantavirus Pulmonary Syndrome

In May 1993 public health officials in New Mexico were alerted to an outbreak of serious respiratory infection in the Four Corners region of the state. The illness, which mainly affected healthy young adults and some teenagers, was characterized by a prodrome of fever, myalgia, and some gastrointestinal symptoms. This was superseded by respiratory failure and substantial mortality. Postmortem examinations revealed lymphocytic interstitial pulmonary infiltrates and intra-alveolar edema. It is postulated that virus-induced mechanisms result in increased vascular permeability, most notably in the lungs (Duchin et al., 1994).

Using PCR, Nichol and colleagues (1993) were able to implicate an agent now termed *Sin Nombre Virus* (SNV). This virus is a member of the *Hantavirus* genus of the Bunyavirus family. Members of this family are generally spherical, enveloped particles measuring 80 to 120 nm in diameter and containing three strands of negative-sense RNA. At least five genera and 700 species infecting animals and plants are recognized. Other human pathogens belonging to the family include California encephalitis virus, the sandfly fever viruses, and the virus of Korean hemorrhagic fever.

By early 1996, 131 cases of hantavirus pulmonary syndrome (HPS) had been confirmed in the United States (Centers for Disease Control, 1996). Case fatality rates were virtually 50%, which, coupled with an apparently low rate of seroprevalence, would implicate SNV as one of the most pathogenic and virulent of human viruses. The natural host of SNV is the deer mouse, an animal widely spread throughout the United States. Nonetheless, the great bulk of the cases have been clustered in the Southwest. In other areas of the country, HPS has been linked to different but closely related hantavirus species having different rodents as their natural hosts.

RICKETTSIAE

Coxiella burnetii (formerly *Rickettsia burnetii*) is the cause of Q fever, an acute illness characterized by sudden onset of fever, chills, headache, malaise, and weakness that progresses to cough, chest pain, and the clinical picture of atypical pneumonia. The properties of *C. burnetii* and the clinical manifestations of Q fever are described in Chapter 33.

BACTERIA

It is not easy to assess the present-day quantitative role of bacteria in acute respiratory tract disease.

The estimate that the primary cause is nonbacterial in more than 90% of acute respiratory tract infections does not negate the importance of bacteria as both primary and secondary invaders. Patients with lower respiratory tract infections of severity sufficient to require hospitalization are more apt to have bacterial disease than those whose illnesses permit ambulatory care. At the extremes of life, in the newborn and geriatric patient, bacterial pneumonia may be more common, with higher morbidity and mortality. Group A β-hemolytic streptococcus is the most common bacterial cause of acute tonsillopharyngitis with exudate or membrane (Chapter 31).

Although the pathogen is being largely controlled by vaccination (Centers for Disease Control, 1995), acute epiglottitis is the most important respiratory syndrome caused by *H. influenzae* type b (HIB). This disorder generally occurs in the absence of meningitis or other manifestations of infection with *H. influenzae* type b. In addition, epiglottitis occurs at a somewhat later age; the mean age for epiglottitis patients is 40 months, compared to approximately 9 months for patients with meningitis, septic arthritis, and cellulitis caused by the same organism. Pneumonia and empyema caused by HIB have been identified. Identification of the *H. influenzae* type b capsular polysaccharide in serum, exudates, or urine may be of great value in making this diagnosis.

With the multiplicity of different agents, especially viruses, capable of causing any one respiratory syndrome, it is difficult to measure the present-day role of bacteria as the cause of acute respiratory tract disease. To make a precise etiologic diagnosis, the physician must have access to clinical diagnostic laboratories capable of isolating and identifying nonbacterial and bacterial agents. Of available laboratory tests, the quantitative assay for C-reactive protein—although not diagnostic—may be the most closely correlated with bacterial infection. C-reactive protein rises sharply early in the course of pneumonia and other systemic bacterial infections but remains in the normal range during the course of comparable viral infection. The differential diagnosis between viral and nonviral illness is often made on clinical grounds that are imprecise, even though they may include a WBC count and differential, an examination of the polymorphonuclear cells for toxic granulations, an erythrocyte sedimentation rate (ESR), and occasionally the clinical response to a "therapeutic trial" of antibiotic therapy. Definitive diagnosis often depends on the use of invasive procedures to obtain cultures from such normally sterile locations as lung, pleural fluid, or sinus or middle ear cavities.

Potential bacterial pathogens such as pneumococci, *H. influenzae,* and staphylococci frequently are present in the upper respiratory tract as colonizers; such bacteria generally can be identified even in healthy children. Thus isolation of a potential bacterial pathogen in the upper respiratory tract generally does not prove its etiologic involvement in infections such as pneumonia or sinusitis. Respiratory viruses do not cause prolonged carriage but may themselves lead to secondary bacterial infection.

Early in the course of some lower respiratory tract infections a specific bacteriologic diagnosis may be made when appropriate specimens (sputum, pleural fluid, blood) are available for Gram stain and culture or antigenic analysis by techniques such as countercurrent immunoelectrophoresis (CIE). Despite these obstacles to precise definition of etiology, it is clear that bacteria continue to figure prominently in both primary and secondary roles in acute upper and lower respiratory tract illnesses. For example, an inestimable number of cases of streptococcal infections occur annually in the United States; pneumonias complicating epidemic influenza are mostly bacterial and are chiefly responsible for the deaths that follow influenza; and staphylococcal pneumonia with its various complications continues to present a formidable problem, especially in early life.

Hemolytic Streptococci (*Streptococcus Pyrogenes*)

Group A hemolytic streptococci are the main bacterial cause of upper respiratory tract infections, including tonsillopharyngitis with exudate or membrane and febrile nasopharyngitis in infants. *S. pyogenes* is also an occasional cause of otitis media and sinusitis. These organisms are seldom responsible for laryngitis (croup) or pneumonia. The characteristics of hemolytic streptococci and the epidemiologic, immunologic, and pathologic aspects and clinical manifestations of streptococcal infections are discussed in Chapter 31.

Staphylococci

The chief contribution of staphylococci to respiratory tract illness is as the cause of severe pneumonia. Pneumonia caused by *Staphylococcus aureus* is a particularly severe and fulminant bacterial pneumonia that frequently is seen during influenza epidemics or at times when *S. aureus* infections are prevalent in the community. Nosocomial infection was a particular problem in nurseries in the 1950s and 1960s; however, bacterial tracheitis attributed to staphylococcal infection has reemerged as a recognized clinical entity (Nelson, 1984). In addition to the local infection, *S. aureus* involvement of the respiratory tract can produce various toxigenic complications. Toxic shock syndrome, for example, has been reported as a complication of staphylococcal sinusitis in children. The properties of staphylococci and the pathogenesis, pathologic and immunologic aspects, and clinical manifestations of staphylococcal infections are presented in detail in Chapter 30.

Pneumococci

Pneumococci are important agents of pneumonia, sinusitis, otitis media, a syndrome of occult bacteremia, and pyogenic meningitis in children. Control of these infections has been difficult because of their extremely wide distribution, the presence of multiple capsular serotypes without cross-reactivity of the protective antibodies that are produced after infection or colonization, and the relatively poor immunogenicity of the currently available pneumococcal vaccines in infants. Antibiotic resistance is an increasing threat. *Streptococcus pneumoniae* is a gram-positive, lancet-shaped cell surrounded by a polysaccharide capsule. The cell wall is composed of peptidoglycan that is penetrated by teichoic acids. An M protein, specific for each serologic type, is rooted in the cell membrane and extends through the cell wall. A carbohydrate, C substance, is common to all types and is a constituent of teichoic acid. The capsule, acting as a protective shell against phagocytes, provides a significant factor in the virulence of the organism; pneumococci without capsules are avirulent. The presence of type-specific, anticapsular antibody is a critical determinant of immunity to pneumococcal infections. In the immune state, type-specific antibody combines with capsular polysaccharide, thereby promoting phagocytosis. The antibody-polysaccharide reaction is also responsible for the Neufield (quellung) phenomenon under the microscope, wherein it renders the capsule more refractile. Pneumococci are grown on various bacteriologic media, including blood agar and beef infusion broth with 0.5% dextrose and 5% to 10% blood or serum. Pneumococcal cultures are differentiated from other streptococcal species by their bile solubility. Sensitivity to optochin is becoming less reliable (Munoz et al., 1990). On blood agar the colonies are smooth, glistening, 0.5 to 1.5 cm in diameter, and α-hemolytic. Encapsulated pneumococci give a mucoid appearance to their colonies. On the basis of their capsular polysaccharide antigens, at least ninety specific antigenic types of pneumococci have been described. The most frequent types encountered in adults with pneumonia are types 8, 4, 1, 14, 3, 7, 12, 6, 18, 9, 19, and 23, in descending order of frequency, as reported by Austrian et al. (1976) in their collaborative study of more than 3600 patients in the United States. Among children, the serotypes most commonly identified with disease are 19, 23, 14, 3, 6, and 1. Gray et al. (1980) noted similar distributions of pneumococcal types in children with bacteremia, meningitis, and otitis media with one addition, type 18.

Pneumococci are common inhabitants of the normal upper respiratory tract. Factors that may predispose to invasive pneumococcal infection include (1) preceding viral infections; (2) bronchial obstruction and atelectasis; (3) alteration of mucociliary function by allergy, irritants, and other agents; (4) pulmonary congestion with cardiovascular problems; (5) splenectomy, agammaglobulinemia, lymphocytic leukemia, and sickle cell disease; (6) antibody deficiency states; (7) human immunodeficiency virus (HIV) infection; and (8) the absence of acquired immunity, which is present in infants. Among infants and children pneumococci cause pneumonia, otitis media, mastoiditis, and sinusitis as a direct result of colonization in the respiratory tract. More distant foci of pneumococcal illness include meningitis and, infrequently, cellulitis, peritonitis, arthritis, osteomyelitis, endocarditis, and pericarditis. Occult bacteremia is relatively common in febrile children under 2 years, whereas fulminant, overwhelming septicemia may occur in patients with functional or anatomic absence of the spleen.

Most pneumococci remain highly sensitive to penicillin, with minimum inhibitory concentrations (MIC) of 0.05 μg/ml or less. In 1977 resistant strains of *S. pneumoniae* were recovered from South African children with pneumonia, meningitis, or bacteremia. These organisms were resistant to penicillin, ampicillin, methicillin, erythromycin, cephalosporins, tetracycline, aminoglycosides, and chloramphenicol. The only antibiotics to which these virulent organisms were sensitive were rifampin, vancomycin, and bacitracin (Jacobs et al., 1978).

Penicillin resistance involves the emergence of altered penicillin-binding proteins (PBPs). These are cell wall–synthesizing enzymes that are the targets of penicillin action. PBP mutations seem to arise from interspecies recombinatorial events between pneumococcal PBP genes and those of related species. The resultant hybrid PBPs have reduced binding affinity to penicillin and many cephalosporins as well.

International spread of penicillin-resistant (PR) clones of pneumococci has accelerated. By the early 1990s they were predominant, or nearly so, in many parts of Europe and the Middle East. In 1992 some 7% of isolated pneumococcal strains showed some degree of penicillin resistance. By the following year the percentage had doubled and in 1994 some cities were reporting incidences as high as 25% (Hoffman et al., 1995). PR strains, as with the original isolates, have also remained resistant to erythromycin, tetracyclines, and trimethaprim-sulfamethoxazole. Although conventional susceptibility testing finds these strains susceptible to chloramphenicol, their MICs tend to be higher than seen with other strains, and poor results of chloramphenicol treatment of PR pneumococcal meningitis have been reported in South Africa. Although PR strains are generally more sensitive to ceftriaxone and cefotaxime (as opposed to earlier-generation cephalosporins), this generalization appears to be evaporating (Mannheimer et al., 1996). These third-generation cephalosporins can no longer be considered safe monotherapy for life-threatening pneumococcal disease (such as meningitis) caused by PR strains. At this time, vancomycin resistance has not been noted in PR pneumococci, and late-generation quinolones (e.g., clinafloxacin) show promise.

It should be noted that investigators have made a distinction between pneumococci of *intermediate penicillin resistance* (those with MICs between 0.1 and 1 mg/ml) and those of *high resistance* (MICs >2 mg/ml). It is the latter strains that have contributed to deaths from meningitis, and some reports have indicated that penicillin treatment of nonmeningeal illness caused by strains of intermediate resistance is clinically successful. Nonetheless these studies had low statistical power, and trends seem to indicate an increase in highly resistant strains.

Optimal treatment of disease proved or suspected to be caused by a pneumococcus of unknown penicillin sensitivity is uncertain at this time. Rather than present an algorithm, I prefer to suggest that each case be weighed regarding (1) the likelihood that PR strains are involved (local epidemiology); (2) severity of the disease process; and (3) the need to avoid overuse of antibiotics that select for resistant strains. In generally self-limited disease such as otitis media, there is little harm in using penicillin. In most cases of bacteremia or pneumonia, ceftriaxone or cefotaxime would be a reasonable first approximation. In meningitis, vancomycin must be used.

It is further to be emphasized that a number of studies have now linked the casual administration of antibiotics with the emergence of resistance (e.g., Arnold et al., 1996). The need to curb unnecessary antibiotic prescription has seldom been so urgent. Pneumococcus is a ubiquitous pathogen and now only vancomycin, an awkwardly administered and unpleasant agent, stands between us and the preantibiotic era in relation to it in life-threatening cases.

Moraxella (Branhamella) Catarrhalis

This organism, which appears as a plump gram-negative coccus or paired short rods, recently has achieved new recognition as an important respiratory pathogen, being a frequent agent of acute otitis media and sinusitis. In adults, particularly those with chronic lung disease, it seems to be a cause of bronchopulmonary infection. The agent has also been associated with bronchopneumonia in infants with underlying lung damage (Berg and Bartley, 1987). *M. catarrhalis* is a respiratory tract colonizer with no other known reservoir. Carriage of the organism is most common in very young children; is most frequent in the presence of respiratory tract symptoms, although *M. catarrhalis* is not thought to cause such symptoms; and is highly seasonal, with prevalence greatest in the fall and winter. It is remarkable that β-lactamase production by this species was first recognized in the late 1970s and that at about the same time its frequency as an agent of otitis media increased at least threefold. *M. catarrhalis* occurs slightly less frequently than *H. influenzae* in sinus and middle ear aspirates, being found singly or in combination with other agents in 10% to 25% of cases. At present, approximately 85% of *M. catarrhalis* isolates produce β-lactamase and thus are resistant to penicillin and ampicillin. No other resistance factors are found with any frequency. Clinical isolates of *M. catarrhalis* are highly susceptible to erythromycin, to trimethoprim-sulfamethoxazole, and to one orally administered cephalosporin, cefixime. In addition, the β-lactamase produced by this agent may be inhibited by the β-lactamase inhibitors clavulanate and sulbactam; combinations containing these drugs would also be effective in treating infections caused by *M. catarrhalis.* Clinical features of otitis media and sinusitis caused by *M. catarrhalis* have not differed from those associated with other agents. Disseminated infection and pyogenic complications have not been described, even when drugs (such as ampicillin) with limited in vitro activity against the resistant strains are widely used. *M. catarrhalis* is rarely an agent of other infections such as bacteremia, meningitis, endocarditis, and ophthalmia neonatorum.

Haemophilus Influenzae

H. influenzae is a small, gram-negative, pleomorphic bacillus found in encapsulated or nonencapsulated forms. Its biology and pathophysiology are discussed in Chapter 10. Virulent *H. influenzae* possess a type-specific capsular polysaccharide. Six distinct antigenic types, a through f, have been identified by serotypings but more than 90% of serious *H. influenzae* infections in infants and children are caused by type b. Nonencapsulated strains, frequently found in the nasopharynx of normal children and adults, are nontypeable and have been associated with otitis media, sinusitis, and chronic bronchitis. Respiratory tract disease caused by *H. influenzae* type b takes the form of epiglottitis, pneumonia (often with empyema), mastoiditis, sinusitis, and otitis media (Chapters 10 and 20). As with the pneumococci, changes in antibiotic sensitivity have altered the considerations of chemotherapy for *H. influenzae* infections. Since 1974, strains of ampicillin-resistant *H. influenzae* have been recovered from patients throughout the United States and other nations. From 15% to 30% of isolates from children with invasive disease produce β-lactamase (penicillinase) and are therefore resistant to ampicillin therapy. Resistance caused by relatively decreased affinity of the PBPs has also been described (Jorgensen, 1992). Thus cefotaxime, or ceftriaxone, or cefuroxime is currently the initial drug of choice for infants and children with systemic *H. influenzae* infection. These drugs are effective for both the β-lactamase–producing strains and those with altered PBPs. To complicate matters further, a few strains of chloramphenicol-resistant *H. influenzae* have been detected in Europe and the United States, but they are still rare. At present, clinical outcomes reported with chloramphenicol; cefotaxime; ceftriaxone; and, with susceptible strains, ampicillin apparently are identical (Chapter 10).

Bordetella Pertussis

B. pertussis, a common respiratory tract pathogen, is mentioned here because the manifestations in the catarrhal stage of pertussis are those of an upper respiratory tract infection, and often the true cause is unsuspected. Moreover, the severity of pertussis and the mortality in infancy, usually from complicating pneumonia, are not generally appreciated. The characteristics of *B. pertussis* and the clinical manifestations of pertussis are discussed in Chapter 23.

Corynebacterium Diphtheriae

Despite widespread immunization practices, *C. diphtheriae* may occur as the pathogen responsible for membranous tonsillitis and laryngitis. It is mentioned here to emphasize the importance of early recognition of diphtheria because delay in treatment with antitoxin may jeopardize the patient's life. The cause and other aspects of diphtheria are discussed in Chapter 5.

Legionella Pneumophila

As the result of an outbreak of pneumonia in 1976 following a national convention of the American Legion in Philadelphia, a new disease was identified, studied retrospectively and prospectively, associated etiologically with a previously overlooked bacterium, and correlated with a wide spectrum of clinical manifestations. Legionnaires' disease has occurred both in outbreaks and sporadically since initial recognition and examination of sera dating back to 1973. The clinical manifestations range from mild febrile pneumonia to the adult respiratory distress syndrome and may be accompanied by extrapulmonary involvement, including encephalopathy, rhabdomyolysis, and gastrointestinal and renal dysfunction. Cases have been reported throughout the United States and also from England and Spain.

The organism responsible for legionnaires' disease is a gram-negative bacillus, *L. pneumophila.* A natural inhabitant of fresh water, the bacterium becomes concentrated in human-made water delivery systems, where it survives in the presence of optimal temperatures, symbiotic bacteria, and the protozoans that are its natural host (Fields, 1993). Dissemination from these systems is the cause of outbreaks. Despite its ready growth in water systems, *L. pneumophila* is exceedingly fastidious and difficult to grow in vitro. As a result, most diagnostic studies rely on serologic techniques for antibody increases or on direct demonstration of the organism in infected tissues, using special strains. Sputum, pleural fluid, bronchial washings, and lung biopsies or aspirates can all be examined by immunofluorescence and by a modification of the Dieterle spirochete stain (Lattimer et al., 1978). Both in vitro and in vivo the organism may be sensitive to erythromycin, which has been used with some success among patients.

Legionnaire's disease is rare in children. Centers for Disease Control reports usually list fewer than 2% of cases as under 19 years of age. Because the illness occurs with enhanced morbidity and mortality in the aged and in the immunocompromised, more cases may be recognized in pediatric populations with underlying disorders such as cancer, immunodeficiency, and hematologic malignancies (Edelstein, 1993; Kovatch et al., 1984).

Chlamydiae

Chlamydiae are bacteria that are obligate intracellular parasites of eukaryoytic cells. These organisms are discussed in detail in Chapter 28.

Modern nucleic acid sequencing techniques have elucidated a number of species, three of which, *C. psittaci, C. trachomatis,* and *C. pneumoniae,* make a contribuation to human respiratory disease.

C. psittaci, once thought to be confined to parrots, is now appreciated as a pathogen in many species of birds. Spread to humans occurs through handling of avian secretions and excreta and results in a flulike illness complicated by interstitial pneumonia. The recent demonstration that *C. psittaci* can infect cats (Pointon et al., 1991) raises the possibility that these pets may be an unsuspected source of human disease.

The role of *C. trachomatis* in pneumonia during the first months of life has been recognized for some time (Schacter et al., 1975; Beem and Saxon, 1977).

Recently named, *C. pneumoniae* is apparently a major cause of "atypical" or "walking" pneumonia in older schoolchildren, adolescents, and adolescents, and adults (Grayston, 1992). Perhaps 5% to 10% of such cases are caused by this pathogen. The clinical picture is mild and the pneumonia may be associated with upper respiratory involvement manifesting as sore throat or hoarseness. Miller (1991) has reported that the disease may be more severe in children with sickle cell disease.

Chlamydiae are sensitive to a number of antibiotics including erythromycin, tetracyclines, chloramphenicol, and the sulfonamides. Erythromycin given for 2 to 3 weeks is currently the drug of choice for infants and children with chlamydial

pneumonias, although it is possible that shorter treatment with azithromycin may prove an acceptable substitute as it has in chlamydial gential infection (Hammershlag et al., 1993). (See Chapter 28.)

MYCOPLASMA PNEUMONIAE
Biology

The mycoplasmas are ubiquitous, free-living prokaryocytes found in many insects, animals, and plants. They are the smallest free-living forms. Mycoplasmas constitute their own class. They are distinct from viruses in that they contain both DNA and RNA and are capable of growing extracellularly on defined media. They lack a cell wall, but, unlike the L forms of bacteria, they do not revert to walled forms and contain sterols in their cell membranes. Their small genome shows no DNA homology with any known bacteria. Characteristically, they grow down into nutrient agar and produce a "fried egg" appearance with dark centers and a light periphery. An exception, *M. pneumoniae,* grows in "mulberry" colonies. It has been proven to be a highly significant cause of disease in humans. Other class members *(Ureaplasma urealyticum* and *M. hominis)* play a role in human urogenital tract disease and occasionally in systemic or neonatal infections. *M. pneumoniae* is a filamentous, pleomorphic, 10 × 200 nm, moderately motile agent. It has an electron-dense core at one end with a terminal differentiated structure for attachment to host cell membranes—notably those of ciliated and nonciliated epithelial cells. On human ciliated respiratory tract mucosal cells, the bacterium remains extracellular but exerts a toxic effect, possibly via hydrogen peroxide that interferes with ciliary function and mucosal cell metabolism. *M. pneumoniae* is resistant to cell wall–active antibiotics such as penicillin but is sensitive to the tetracyclines and erythromycin, the newer macrolides, and the quinolones.

Much of the knowledge of human respiratory infections caused by mycoplasmas comes from studies begun during World War II of atypical pneumonia among military recruits. Eaton et al. (1944) reported the recovery of an agent from filtered sputum or lung suspensions obtained from patients with mild penicillin-unresponsive forms of pneumonia characterized by prolonged malaise; a patchy consolidation on x-ray; and, frequently, a serologic reaction in which red blood cells are repeatedly agglutinated at 4° C and unagglutinated at 37° C. These pneumonias came to be known as "cold agglutinin-positive primary atypical pneumonias." Material passed to hamsters and cotton rats induced pneumonia that could be prevented by using convalescent patients' serum. In 1957 Liu confirmed Eaton's work by providing unequivocal evidence of infection of humans with the Eaton agent.

In 1962 Chanock et al. grew the agent on artificial medium. The morphologic and staining properties of colonies on agar plates identified the organism as a mycoplasma (Fig. 25-2). With the use of paired serum specimens from patients with *M. pneumoniae* pneumonia, it was observed that acute-phase serum failed to stain the colonies, whereas convalescent-phase serum diluted 1:40 gave rise to intense fluorescence of the colonies (Fig. 25-3).

To complete the etiologic postulates, Chanock et al. (1963) infected human volunteers experimentally. Of twenty-seven volunteers with no detectable antibody, three developed pneumonia; four, febrile respiratory tract illness without pneu-

monia; nine, myringitis with or without bullae and hemorrhage; and four, afebrile respiratory tract illness. All twenty-seven volunteers acquired antibody. Febrile respiratory tract illness without pneumonia developed in other groups of volunteers after administration of *M. pneumoniae* artificially propagated on agar. Of thirty volunteers given these materials, twenty-seven showed development of antibody.

Associated Clinical Syndromes. Community spread of *M. pneumoniae* occurs in protracted outbreaks that may extend through the entire respiratory disease season. Because the organism multiplies slowly, the incubation period is long, averaging 14 days but highly variable. Carriage of viable mycoplasma by individual patients may last up to 3 months. As a result of this extended carriage and the relatively low rate of contagion, the period of spread in households may also last for months. Pediatricians should regard *M. pneumoniae* as the

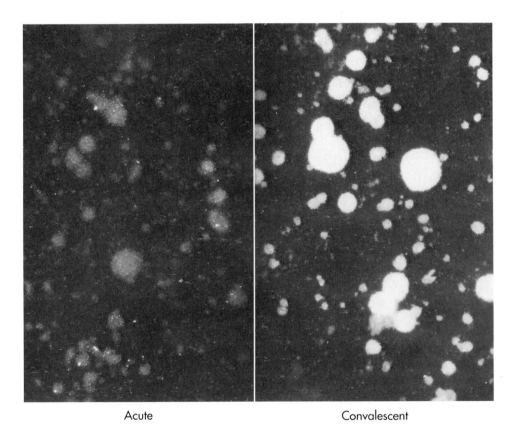

Acute   Convalescent

FIG. 25-3   Agar colonies stained with acute- and convalescent-phase sera from patient with *Mycoplasma pneumoniae* pneumonia. Acute-phase serum fails to stain colonies of *M. pneumoniae*, which indicates absence of antibody; convalescent-phase serum produces intense fluorescence of colonies, indicating presence of antibody. (From Chanock RM, et al. In Pollard M [ed]. Perspectives in virology, vol 3. New York: Harper & Row, 1963.)

most prominent single cause of pneumonia and of prolonged episodes of tracheobronchitis in school-children and adolescents. This is particularly true in otherwise well children who do not have underlying chronic disorders. It should also be considered in wheezing-associated illness (Henderson et al., 1979b). The infection is rarely severe enough to require hospitalization. However, children with sickle cell disease and other conditions may have severe and life-threatening pneumonias in which no other causative agents may be identified. Mycoplasmal infection differs clinically from "typical" pneumococcal pneumonia in having a gradual onset with fever, sore throat, and cough as major complaints. Physical findings of pulmonary infection, rales, and rhonchi may be more severe than would be expected from the general examination. Radiologic findings are generally those of bronchopneumonia involving the lower lobes unilaterally or bilaterally. Hospitalization generally is not required. Children with *M. pneumoniae* infection also may be seen initially with localized tracheobronchitis and with cough and rhonchi in the absence of pulmonary infiltrates. Numerous extrarespiratory signs and symptoms associated with *M. pneumoniae* have been reported. Unfortunately, establishment of a causal connection between *M. pneumoniae* and these findings is difficult. Because this mycoplasma is so common, reports of concurrent, causally unrelated events will be common also. Stevens-Johnson syndrome (erythema multiforme bullosa) is the most frequently observed complication and is the most firmly linked to *M. pneumoniae*. Neurologic syndromes such as meningoencephalitis, transverse myelitis, and Guillain-Barré syndrome have been temporally associated with clinically diagnosed atypical pneumonia. Seeking conclusive evidence of infection—particularly attempting to isolate *M. pneumoniae*—is indicated in the presence of potential neurologic involvement.

Classic diagnostic tests for *M. pneumoniae* infection have included tests for cold agglutinins, for complement-fixing antibody, and for isolation of the organism. None of these provides early confirmation of the diagnosis. Cold agglutinins are antibodies against the altered 1 antigen on the surface of red blood cells of infected patients. They develop 7 to 10 days into the course of infection and are present at a titer of $\geq 1:32$ in approximately 50% of infected children. However, similar titers may be found during infection with respiratory viruses, particularly if cold agglutinins are sought

using less specific bedside methods. Complement-fixing antibody is more specific but, again, requires 1 to 2 weeks to develop. For clinical purposes a fourfold or greater increase in complement-fixing antibody titer between acute- and convalescent-phase serum specimens provides reasonable evidence of infection. Such findings may be useful in guiding treatment of family and community contacts during the course of an outbreak.

M. pneumoniae is not part of the normal respiratory flora. Therefore definitive diagnosis of respiratory infection with this agent may be provided by culture of pharyngeal swabs. Specific antisera are used for identification of compatible organisms grown in culture. Unfortunately, the doubling time of *M. pneumoniae* is over 6 hours (as opposed to 20 minutes for many bacteria), so culture results are seldom available early enough to influence clinical decisions. Culture is thus usually considered only in epidemic situations and in unusually severe cases. Emphasis in the diagnostic laboratory is now shifting to molecular techniques. Antigen capture assays have been applied directly to sputum (Kok et al., 1988) and specific labeled DNA probes employed (Dular et al., 1988).

Erythromycin is effective in shortening the symptomatic course and promoting radiologic resolution of mycoplasmal pneumonia. The oral dose is 50 mg/kg/day divided every 6 hours. Therapy should be given for 7 days. Clinically significant relapses are unusual, even though the organism is not often eradicated by this course of therapy and may be shed for weeks. Other therapeutic options are available. Tetracycline and doxycycline are available for older children and adolescents. The newer macrolides azithromycin and clarithromycin are likely at least as effective as erythromycin and have fewer side effects. They are, however, considerably more expensive. There is also rationale for using the quinolones in older adolescents, but, again, cost is an issue. In addition to causing a major portion of primary atypical pneumonia, *M. pneumoniae* can also give rise to mild upper respiratory tract infection, bronchitis, bronchiolitis, bronchopneumonia, and myringitis bullosa. The incidence of *M. pneumoniae* infection in the children in any given locality may fluctuate widely over a period of years. For example, during 1957 to 1959 in Washington, D.C., *M. pneumoniae* was associated with 10% of all pediatric lower respiratory tract illnesses studied at Children's Hospital, whereas 3 years later only 1% of these conditions were associated with *M. pneumoniae* (Chanock et al., 1963). *M. pneumoniae* plays a major role in respiratory tract disease of school-age children and young adults. Chanock (1965) reported serologic evidence of *M. pneumoniae* infection in 55% of 530 marine recruits with pneumonia and in 28% of 141 recruits with febrile upper respiratory tract infections. Evans and Brobst (1961) found similar evidence of *M. pneumoniae* infection in 25% of 91 university students hospitalized for pneumonia. Although serologic evidence of *M. pneumoniae* infection can be obtained in most persons with cold agglutinin-positive pneumonia, the converse is not true; for example, a sizable proportion of patients with *M. pneumoniae* pneumonia fail to develop cold agglutinins. Thus Chanock observed that, among 239 marines with *M. pneumoniae* pneumonia, cold agglutinins formed in only 46% during convalescence.

Inflammation of the tympanic membrane was observed by Mufson et al. (1961) in four of fifty cases in a military outbreak of *M. pneumoniae* pneumonia. Myringitis with bullae and hemorrhage was observed in nine of twenty-seven volunteers infected experimentally with *M. pneumoniae*. However, *M. pneumoniae* has not been identified as a cause of myringitis or middle ear disease in naturally infected children. *M. pneumoniae* is not known to invade beyond the lining mucosal cells of the respiratory tract.

MISCELLANEOUS AGENTS

Various mycotic infections—including aspergillosis, candidiasis, coccidioidomycosis, and histoplasmosis—are relatively common in certain parts of the world and may be manifested by an influenza-like illness or by atypical pneumonia. *Pneumocystis carinii* may cause an invasive pneumonia with bilateral alveolar disease. *P. carinii* pneumonia is extremely prevalent among patients with immunosuppressive conditions, including HIV infection (Chapter 1). The acquired forms of toxoplasmosis, caused by the protozoan parasite *Toxoplasma gondii*, include a syndrome characterized by fever, maculopapular rash, and pneumonia. These infections have been noted more frequently as opportunistic respiratory pathogens among immunosuppressed hosts. Atypical pneumonia may accompany Q fever caused by *C. burnetii*. Many other organisms play an etiologic role in respiratory tract infection; many of them are listed in Table 25-4. In immunocompromised patients or in normal hosts exposed to special geographic or ecologic settings, fungi must be considered in the differential diagnosis. They include *Blastomyces, Cryptococcus, Histoplasma, Mucor, Coccidioides, Candida,* and *Aspergillus* spp. Other bacteria such as *Yersinia pestis* and *Francisella tularensis* may cause plague and tularemia, respectively, in patients who have been exposed to infected animal hosts *(F. tularensis)* or fleas from infected animals *(Y. pestis)* while camping or hunting. In recent years the gram-negative rods and Enterobacteriaceae have assumed an increasingly important role in pneumonias of children with immune suppression caused by underlying disease or therapeutic protocols and in patients on broad-spectrum antibiotics for other reasons. Aspiration pneumonias may have a predominance of mixed anaerobic bacteria. Infections with *Mycobacterium tuberculosis* are discussed in Chapter 35. More exotic causes must always be considered in the compromised host. Parasites—including *Ascaris, Pneumocystis, Toxoplasma,* and *Strongyloides* spp.—have all been reported to cause pneumonias in such patients. In the immunosuppressed host, lung biopsy may be the only way to establish a definitive diagnosis. Stagno et al. (1981) called attention to the role in pneumonia of infancy of a group of pathogens less often considered. They were cytomegalovirus, *Chlamydia* spp., *Pneumocystis* spp., and *U. urealyticum.*

CLINICAL SYNDROMES

This section describes the clinical signs and symptoms and treatment of acute respiratory tract infections. For clarity, these illnesses have been grouped into nine clinical syndromes and are listed together with their various causative agents in Table 25-4. This arbitrary division, made largely on anatomic grounds, is often inexact; for example, "pure" bronchiolitis without some extension of the process into the peribronchial tissues is probably a rare event. Nevertheless, the clinical picture of bronchiolitis is distinct enough from that of pneumonia that it warrants separate discussion. From a practical point of view, the question of whether or not to treat a patient with antimicrobial agents confronts every physician responsible for the care of persons with respiratory tract infections. The use of antimicrobial agents for viral infections is worthless and may be harmful because the sensitive bacteria will be eliminated, thereby promoting the growth of resistant organisms that may become the secondary bacterial invaders. The danger of fostering the rise of resistant pneumococci has been noted earlier. On the other hand, the same antibiotics may be lifesaving when administered to a patient with severe bac-

Table 25-4   Acute respiratory tract disease—clinical syndromes and causative agents

Clinical syndrome	Causative agents		
	Viruses	Bacteria	Other
Common cold; coldlike illness	Respiratory syncytial Parainfluenza Rhinoviruses Nonpolio enteroviruses Adenoviruses Coronaviruses	*Mycoplasma pneumoniae*	
Febrile nasopharyngitis (in-infants)		Streptococcus, group A Pneumococcus	
Acute tonsillopharyngitis			
With exudate or membrane	Adenoviruses Epstein-Barr	Streptococcus, group A *Corynebacterium diphtheriae*	
With vesicles or ulcers	Herpes simplex Group A Coxsackie		
Acute laryngitis; laryngotracheobronchitis (croup)	Parainfluenza Influenza Adenoviruses Rhinoviruses Respiratory syncytial Measles	*C. diphtheriae*	
Acute epiglottitis		*Haemophilus influenzae* type b	
Bronchiolitis	Respiratory syncytial Parainfluenza Adenoviruses Influenza		
Pneumonia	Respiratory syncytial Parainfluenza Measles Adenoviruses Influenza Cytomegalovirus Varicella-zoster Hantavirus	*M. pneumoniae* *Ureaplasma urealyticum* Staphylococcus Pneumococcus Hemolytic streptococci *H. influenzae* Enterobacteriaceae *Pseudomonas aeruginosa* *Klebsiella pneumoniae* Anaerobes Mycobacteria *Nocardia* *Legionella* *Chlamydia* Others	*Pneumocystis carinii* *Coxiella burnetii* (Q fever) *Toxoplasma gondii* Fungi (*Candida, Aspergillus, Coccidioides, Histoplasma, Blastomyces, Cryptococcus,* etc.)
Influenza-like illness	Influenza Parainfluenza Adenoviruses Lymphocytic choriomeningitis		
Acute sinusitis	Parainfluenza Adenoviruses	Pneumococcus *H. influenzae* *Moraxella catarrhalis* *S. pyogenes* Anaerobes	

terial pneumonia. The difficulties in making a precise etiologic diagnosis complicate matters.

Common Cold, Coldlike Illness, Upper Respiratory Tract Infection

These illnesses are grouped together under the same syndrome because their clinical manifestations overlap widely, and it would be difficult and serve little purpose to make a clinical distinction between them. Moreover, the causes, albeit multiple, are mostly viral.

Clinical Manifestations. The common cold is characterized by varying degrees of nasal congestion and discharge, conjunctivitis, sore throat, cough, and redness of the pharynx and tonsils without exudate. The incubation period is short; the average length is approximately 2 days, with a range of 1 to 6 days. The first symptom in some persons is a scratchy feeling or soreness of the throat. In others the cold starts with a nasal discharge that is typically thin, clear, and profuse; it may be mucoid or serous. Concomitantly, there is a feeling of fullness in the nasopharynx. Swelling of the nasal mucosa soon blocks one or both nostrils. Sneezing attacks are frequent. The eyes water. Some patients have a nonproductive cough. Headache or an uncomfortable feeling of fullness in the head is common. There may be slight fever, but the temperature rarely exceeds 38.3° C (101° F). Chilly sensations, malaise, and muscular aches are not uncommon at the beginning, but they are seldom prominent, nor do they persist in uncomplicated colds.

Examination shows variably inflamed and swollen nasal and pharyngeal mucous membranes. The nasal passages may be occluded. The senses of smell and hearing may be impaired. Enlarged nodules of lymphoid tissue may be seen on the posterior pharyngeal wall. The nasal discharge often becomes mucopurulent in 2 or 3 days, and at this time a postnasal drip may be evident. The cervical lymph nodes may be slightly enlarged or tender. Some persons are likely to develop cold sores caused by herpes simplex virus. Uncomplicated colds seldom last more than a week. The cause of the vast majority of colds and coldlike illnesses is viral. Over 150 different viruses have been implicated, including rhinoviruses (more than 100 types), coronaviruses, RSV, parainfluenza viruses, adenoviruses, and coxsackieviruses A and B. In infants under 6 months of age, group A streptococcus may cause febrile nasopharyngitis, and pertussis in the catarrhal stage may act like an upper respiratory tract infection. The exact contributions of these two bacteria to the total picture is undetermined.

Complications. The common cold may be complicated by an extension of the viral infection or by bacterial infections that include otitis media, sinusitis, tonsillitis, cervical adenitis, laryngitis, bronchitis, bronchiolitis, and pneumonia. Infants and children are particularly likely to develop otitis media; therefore the eardrums should be examined for this complication. Secondary infections may be caused by any pathogenic bacteria in the upper respiratory tract passages. Appropriate antimicrobial therapy has reduced the seriousness of these complications.

Diagnosis. The typical clinical pattern makes the diagnosis easy in most cases. Rhinitis, coryza, sneezing, scratchiness of the throat, and cough—all in the absence of pronounced constitutional symptoms—point to the common cold. There is no practical laboratory test by which the diagnosis can be confirmed. Similar clinical pictures may be presented by various other conditions. Allergic rhinitis may be clinically indistinguishable from the common cold. The presence of eosinophils in the nasal smear and the response to antihistamine drugs may serve to differentiate it. Influenza can be distinguished by the prominence of associated constitutional symptoms and by specific diagnostic tests. Pertussis in the catarrhal stage may be confused with the common cold, as may preeruptive measles. Nasal diphtheria and foreign bodies in the nose rarely may be mistaken for the common cold. Streptococcosis in infants under 6 months of age is characterized by nasopharyngitis associated with a thin mucopurulent discharge and irregular fever. This infection is difficult to distinguish from the common cold except by culture and by its lengthier persistence. A diagnosis of sinusitis should also be considered in the patient with a cold that is more severe or more protracted than is usual.

Treatment. Treatment of colds is entirely symptomatic. Antimicrobial agents do not influence the cold itself and should be reserved for treating bacterial complications such as otitis media, sinusitis, and pneumonia. The occasional case of streptococcal nasopharyngitis should be treated with penicillin. The prophylactic use of antimicrobial agents is unwarranted. Local or systemic use of decongestants such as ephedrine or phenylephrine to shrink the nasal mucosa and prevent middle ear infection is of questionable value. It may be helpful for infants before feeding or at bedtime, but the effect is transitory and a rebound effect may occur. Rest in bed is advisable if the patient has fever or feels ill. It also serves as isolation to reduce the chances of spreading infection to others and acquiring a secondary bacterial infection. Fluids should be given in liberal amounts. The diet is governed best by the patient's appetite. In the patient with a cold, acetaminophen may offer some symptomatic relief. However, acetaminophen may also have an adverse effect on immune function, viral shedding, and the clinical status of patients with colds (Graham et al., 1990).

In volunteers challenged intranasally with rhinovirus type 2, treatment with acetaminophen and other analgesic-antipyretic medications suppressed the neutralizing antibody response. Increased nasal symptoms and a trend toward longer duration of viral shedding were also noted in patients receiving analgesic-antipyretic therapy.

Control Measures. There is no effective method of control of the common cold. Although isolation of the individual patient lowers the risk of spreading the disease, this procedure is not practical on a large scale. It is prudent to keep visitors and other people with colds away from infants and small children.

Acute Otitis Media

Among the most frequent suppurative infections of infancy and childhood are those of the middle ear. They are discussed fully in Chapter 20.

Acute Sinusitis

Historians and sociologists of American pediatrics will someday find an interesting subject in the evolution of the treatment of sinusitis in children during the latter part of the twentieth century. Literally the term means "inflammation of the sinuses, with no regard as to etiology (infectious, allergic, chemically induced, etc.)." The seminal study of Wald et al. (1981)—in which bacteria were grown from the maxillary sinus aspirates of the majority of children "suspected to have acute maxillary sinusitis" who had "abnormal" x-rays—changed this interpretation. The term became synonymous with "invasive bacterial infection of the sinuses," and sinusitis, previously a pediatric nonentity, was transformed into a major cause of outpatient antibiotic prescription. As the threat of resistant pneumo-

cocci begins to loom large, the pendulum is beginning to swing back, and cautious approaches to the ticklish diagnosis are widely advocated editorially (Abbasi and Cunningham, 1996).

None doubt the existence of the entity of invasive bacterial sinusitis in children, and many infectious disease specialists have had the personal experience of seeing this devolve into disastrous intracranial disease. The situation is entirely analogous to otitis media: in the paranasal sinuses and the middle ear a ciliated epithelium lined with mucus sweeps invading bacteria though an opening (ostium or eustachian tube) into the nasopharynx, an area normally colonized with bacteria. If the openings are blocked or the sweeping mechanism fails, bacteria will build up in the normally cleansed environment. The demonstrated pathogens in both otitis media and sinusitis are similar: *S. pneumoniae, H. influenzae,* and *M. catarrhalis.* Bacterial overgrowth leads to potential bacterial tissue invasion, with such complications as mastoiditis and brain abscess representing the extreme cases.

The problem has been a reliable means of diagnosing bacterial tissue invasion without resort to sinus biopsy or other invasive procedures. One by one, many pillars of the noninvasive diagnosis of bacterial sinusitis have fallen. Purulence of nasal discharge has not been proven diagnostic of invasive bacterial disease and may be part and parcel of the cycle of viral rhinitis (Isaacs, 1990). The detection of bacteria in the normal maxillary sinus requires only careful technique (Brook, 1981). Radiographic and CT scan opacities of the sinuses can be demonstrated in uncomplicated colds and in normal children (Gwaltney et al., 1994; Diament et al., 1987).

Wald (1992) has suggested that daytime cough and persistence of rhinitis beyond 10 days suggest bacterial disease, but this figure may be arbitrary and is clouded by the possibility of viral infections repeated one on top of another. Antibiotic intervention in such cases demonstrates only modest success at best (Wald et al., 1986; van Buchen et al., 1997).

Left with these uncertainties, what is currently prudent? One reasonable approach in this era of emerging resistant *S. pneumoniae* is to reserve antibiotic treatment for children showing—in the midst of an upper respiratory infection—high fever, purulent nasal discharge, localized pain around the sinuses, and perhaps some facial swelling. One could expect these symptoms more commonly in older children. The use of expensive x-rays and imaging is, on the basis of current knowledge, to be discouraged. Cases of chronic cough and drainage lasting more than a month may be indication for invasive investigations. An aggressive approach is also likely warranted in the immunosuppressed host.

Acute Tonsillopharyngitis

With Exudate or Membrane. Acute tonsillopharyngitis with exudate or membrane is characterized by fever, sore throat, tonsillar and pharyngeal reddening and edema, and the presence of an exudate or membrane. A varying degree of cervical lymph node enlargement may be present. A frequent cause is group A streptococcus (Chapter 31). Rarely, *C. diphtheriae* is the cause. The special features of disease caused by this pathogen need to be kept in mind to make possible early diagnosis (Chapter 5). Membranous tonsillitis is also a frequent manifestation of infectious mononucleosis (Chapter 8) and is often seen in military recruits, infants, and children up to age 3 years with adenovirus infection. Antimicrobial therapy (discussed in detail in Chapter 31) is indicated for patients with exudative pharyngitis caused by group A hemolytic streptococcus.

Current experience indicates that a 10-day course of penicillin (or erythromycin or, possibly, an oral cephalosporin for patients who are allergic to penicillin) is most effective for routine use. If the diphtheria bacillus is suspected or is proved the responsible agent, therapy with diphtheria antitoxin in addition to penicillin or erythromycin (see Chapter 5) should be instituted. Antibiotics are of no value in the treatment of infectious mononucleosis or adenovirus infection.

With Vesicles or Ulcers. Acute tonsillopharyngitis with vesicles or ulcers is characterized by fever, sore throat, and vesicles or shallow white ulcers 2 to 4 mm in diameter on the anterior fauces, palate, and buccal mucous membrane. It most commonly is caused group A coxsackieviruses. A primary infection with herpes simplex virus is usually characterized by stomatitis and gingivitis rather than tonsillopharyngitis (Chapter 12). Gingivitis is not associated with group A coxsackieviruses (Chapter 7). Antimicrobial agents are of no value in the treatment of these infections.

Infectious Croup

Inflammatory obstruction of the airway produces the characteristic clinical picture in all forms of infectious croup. The severity and extent of the infectious process determine the sites of obstruction in the laryngotracheobronchial tree. Mild laryngitis is characterized by hoarseness and a barking or croupy cough, which is likely to be worse at night. Low-grade fever, loss of appetite, and malaise may be the only constitutional signs. Difficulty in breathing is slight or absent; the condition responds promptly to appropriate treatment and subsides in a few days.

Types

Acute laryngitis (croup). A more severe type of laryngitis begins in the same fashion as mild laryngitis but progresses rapidly to the stage of obstruction. The site of obstruction is usually the subglottic area. Hoarseness is more marked, and breathing becomes rapid and labored, with inspiratory stridor and inspiratory retraction of the suprasternal notch, the supraclavicular spaces, the substernal region, and even the intercostal spaces. The child grows restless, often in spite of high humidity and oxygen levels. For a few moments he may scramble about the crib desperately seeking relief and then lie still briefly, only to be roused again by air hunger. The cycle is repeated until the patient becomes exhausted. Cyanosis is sometimes evident in the nail beds and lips. If the obstruction is unrelieved, the patient's color becomes ashen gray, and he sinks into a relaxed, shocklike state as death approaches. In patients whose infection is limited to the laryngeal area, auscultation of the chest reveals little beyond inspiratory stridor and generally diminished aeration. The pharynx is inflamed, and laryngoscopic examination shows little supraglottic involvement except in *H. influenzae* epiglottis. The main site of obstruction lies below the vocal cords, where the soft subglottic tissues bulge to meet in the midline (Fig. 25-4). The mucosa appears deep red and velvety. A gummy mucopurulent exudate or dry yellow crusts add to the obstruction of the airway.

Acute laryngotracheitis and laryngotracheobronchitis (croup). In a patient with severe acute laryngitis the infection may descend rapidly to the trachea and sometimes the bronchi; this increases the patient's struggle for air, his prostration, and his fever. In laryngotracheobronchitis an expiratory wheeze and various types of bronchitic rales are heard on auscultation of the chest. Aeration of the lungs may be good at one moment and impaired the next. Finding localized areas of suppressed to absent breath sounds, bronchial breathing, and dull-

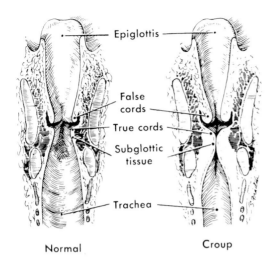

Normal   Croup

Fig. 25-4   Schematic diagram of larynx and trachea in viral croup as compared with normal appearance.

ness to percussion indicates atelectasis resulting from the complete plugging of a bronchus with thick, tenacious exudate. If a main bronchus becomes plugged, air hunger, cyanosis, and restlessness are increased. The heart and mediastinum may be shifted to the affected side. In the presence of obstructive emphysema caused by partial blocking of a bronchus, the heart and mediastinum may be displaced to the opposite side. These various signs and the alarming dyspnea usually disappear after aspiration of the plugged bronchus. The progression of symptoms and signs of acute laryngotracheitis has been described by Forbes (1961) as developing in the following four stages:

Stage 1
  Fever
  Hoarseness of voice
  Croupy cough
  Inspiratory stridor when distributed
Stage 2
  Continuous respiratory stridor
  Lower-rib retraction
  Retraction of soft tissue of the neck
  Activation of accessory muscles of respiration
  Labored respiration
Stage 3
  Signs of anoxia and carbon dioxide retention
  Restlessness
  Anxiety
  Pallor
  Sweating
  Rapid respiration
Stage 4
  Intermittent cyanosis
  Permanent cyanosis
  Cessation of breathing

In patients with mild disease and those whose airway has been improved by treatment, croup rarely progresses beyond stage 1.

Acute epiglottitis. Acute epiglottitis is bacterial in etiology and nearly always is caused by *H. influenzae* type b. The site of the obstruction is supraglottic, in contrast with acute viral laryngotracheitis, in which the obstruction is subglottic (Chapter 10).

Diagnosis. The typical picture of severe epiglottitis or croup is not soon forgotten. Croup begins as an ordinary upper respiratory tract infection. The child then acquires a hoarse voice and a barking cough. This is followed by dyspnea, inspiratory stridor, and retraction of the soft spaces of the thoracic cage. If obstruction is not relieved, the patient shows increasing restlessness, cyanosis, progressive air hunger, and prostration, ending in death. First and foremost, it is important to identify *H. influenzae* epiglottitis because it is a medical emergency that requires immediate therapy. This disease is marked by more rapid development, usually higher temperature, and greater toxicity than seen in most viral croup. The sudden development of obstruction leads to inability to handle secretions, and the child leans forward drooling. Hoarseness is not so prominent as in croup. Diphtheritic laryngitis is now a rare disease. This diagnosis is suggested by the presence of a faucial membrane and evidence of subglottic obstruction. However, even in the absence of a membrane in the pharynx, progression of inspiratory stridor over a 1- to 2-day period in a toxic patient may indicate the presence of diphtheritic laryngitis without evidence of pharyngeal involvement. The diagnosis may be confirmed by culture of the throat and tracheal aspirates.

Differential Diagnosis

Spasmodic croup. Spasmodic croup may simulate infectious croup in many respects. It has traditionally been distinguished from infectious croup by (1) the absence or mildness of signs of inflammation, (2) the typical remissions during the daytime, and (3) the history of previous attacks lasting for 2 or 3 days followed by uneventful recovery. Definitive etiologic investigations are lacking. Allergy is often invoked. Cramblett (1960) described a child with three typical attacks of acute spasmodic croup at 4, 11, and 29 months of age. Each attack was associated with an infection from a virus—parainfluenza virus type 2 in the first attack.

Foreign bodies. An awareness of the capacity of foreign bodies to reproduce the obstructive phenomena is essential. There is often a history of sudden onset of choking and paroxysmal coughing in the absence of signs of infection. Wheezing and the localized absence of breath sounds may be noted. Fluoroscopic and roentgenographic examinations and endoscopy should clarify the diagnosis.

Retropharyngeal abscess. Retropharyngeal abscess might be mistaken for infectious croup or epiglottitis. It occurs in infants and children and is marked by drooling, noisy and difficult mouth breathing, dysphagia, retraction of the head, and enlargement of the cervical lymph nodes. The diagnosis is established by a lateral roentgenogram of the neck and by finger palpation of a fluctuant mass on the posterior pharyngeal wall. Prompt institution of antibiotic therapy and controlled surgical drainage are the cornerstones of treatment.

Angioneurotic edema. Angioneurotic edema, seldom encountered in infants or young children, is characterized by supraglottic swelling in response to a specific food or some other allergen. The diagnosis is confirmed by finding pale red, rounded masses on either side of the superior isthmus of the larynx on direct laryngoscopic examination. Urticaria is an external sign pointing to the likely diagnosis. The rapid response to epinephrine is a good therapeutic test.

Complications. In the course of laryngotracheobronchitis the formation of exudate in the tracheobronchial tree contributes to the development of potentially life-threatening complications. Two factors are believed to promote this condition: (1) breathing air that is not saturated with moisture, and (2) temporary alterations of function of the mucus-secreting glands of the respiratory tract. In any event, crusting of the exudate may lead to further obstruction of the airway and collapse of a segment of the lung. The cough reflex usually is diminished in these patients. Cyanosis develops or increases. Signs of consolidation may be mistaken for pneumonia.

Mediastinal emphysema and pneumothorax are common complications. Extraalveolar thoracic air may be produced through (1) the intrinsic route, in which minute perivascular ruptures occur in the alveoli, leading to pulmonary interstitial emphysema, mediastinal emphysema, pneumothorax, pneumoperitoneum, and subcutaneous emphysema; and (2) the extrinsic route, in which air enters the superior mediastinum behind the pretracheal fascia as a result of tracheostomy. From the superior mediastinum, air can penetrate adjacent areas. Both of these mechanisms may operate to produce mediastinal emphysema and pneumothorax. Tracheostomy is not the only factor nor even necessarily the most important factor, since instances of extraalveolar thoracic air have been observed before or in the absence of tracheostomy.

The presence of pneumothorax may be suspected in a patient with absence of breath sounds and a hyperresonant percussion note on one side of the thorax and displacement of the heart and mediastinum to the opposite side. Roentgenographic examination shows the extent of the pneumothorax and is usually the means of detecting mediastinal emphysema. Subcutaneous emphysema produces a distinctive crackling or crepitus on palpation.

Interstitial bronchopneumonia probably is present in every case of severe croup because the disease process extends to the terminal bronchioles, peribronchial tissues, and alveoli. It is often impossible even by roentgenographic examination to distinguish between patchy areas of atelectasis and interstitial pneumonia. The combination of infection and atelectasis, if persistent, is conducive to bronchiectasis, which may be seen as an end result. Travis et al. (1977) have pointed out the occurrence of pulmonary edema in several patients with laryngotracheitis and epiglottitis.

Prognosis. The prognosis of patients with infectious croup is related to the character and extent of infection and to the amount of obstruction. As the disease progresses downward from simple laryngitis to laryngotracheobronchitis, the mortality rate has been reported to increase (Rabe, 1948). Only one death occurred among 262 patients with viral croup who did not have a tracheostomy. Of 35 patients with fatal cases, six had severe obstruction caused by crusted exudate in the trachea and bronchi (see Chapter 10).

Treatment. The keynote of treatment is to maintain the airway and to combat infection. The patient must be placed promptly in an atmosphere with a high humidity level. In the home this sometimes can be achieved by turning on the hot water taps in a closed bathroom. In the hospital the patient should be placed in a cool (21° to 24° C), humidified atmosphere. Humidified supplemental oxygen (30% to 40%) may be administered by hood, mask, or nasal cannula. Cool mist may relieve stridor by decreasing local inflammation and edema. The patient should have plenty to drink. If fluids cannot be given by mouth, they must be administered parenterally. Rest is of paramount importance. The patient should be spared all needless medical examinations; details of nursing care; and, especially, a succession of diagnostic or therapeutic venipunctures, taking of blood for blood counts, taking of nose and throat cultures, and other tests. Every effort should be made not to disturb a sleeping child. Pulse oximetry offers a noninvasive method of continuously monitoring blood oxygen saturations. Expectorants have been tried and found wanting. Opiates and atropine are contraindicated.

In many cases, especially those in which infection is limited to the upper respiratory tract, a period of breathing supersaturated air, combined with rest, will be followed by no increase in the obstructive symptoms. Hoarseness, dyspnea, and inspiratory retraction or pulling are still present but are no worse. The child is not restless and sleeps from time to time. The color is good, with no cyanosis. Little by little the signs and symptoms disappear, and in a few days the patient progresses to complete recovery. Severe cases with a similar onset are likely not to pursue such a favorable course. The obstructive phenomena are aggravated until it is obvious that the child will suffocate unless an airway is established.

Indications for tracheostomy or intubation. The decision to perform a tracheostomy or intubation for a patient with croup and when to do it call for clinical judgment. If this procedure is indicated, it is best done before the patient becomes exhausted and before it must be done as an emergency, or last-resort, procedure. If despite high humidity and oxygen levels the patient shows increasing duskiness, dyspnea, inspiratory retraction, diminished air entry, and especially restlessness, increasing obstruction to the airway is present and is a clear indication for tracheostomy or intubation. The establishment of an airway is usually followed by immediate and dramatic relief, and the child falls asleep as the tube is being installed.

The teamwork of pediatrician, bronchoscopist, respiratory therapist, and nurse is vitally important for the proper care of the patient. The bronchoscopist should see the patient, if possible, when he is admitted to the hospital, even though there may be no indication for an artificial airway at the moment. Someone with experience should be in attendance at all times. Special nursing care is essential because the tube may become plugged at any time. Frequent aspiration of tracheobronchial secretions is usually necessary. A bronchoscopist should be quickly available to deal with sticky exudates or crusts that cannot be aspirated by a catheter and that give rise to obstruction and pulmonary collapse.

Specific chemotherapy. Since most cases of infectious croup are viral in origin, the indications for administering antimicrobial agents are specific only in patients with *H. influenzae* and *C. diphtheriae* infections.

Corticosteroid therapy. The advocates of corticosteroid therapy postulate that its antiinflammatory effect will reduce edema and improve the airway. The opponents of this therapy point to the equivocal clinical trials and the extensive studies on laboratory animals supported by clinical experience indicating that cortisone enhances susceptibility to infection. Although there is no evidence of harmful effects after the use of these drugs for a period limited to 2 or 3 days, the value of corticosteroids in the treatment of croup remains controversial (Eden et al., 1967; Cherry, 1979; Leipzig et al., 1979). In the absence of a large randomized clinical trial, a metaanalysis of ten previously published reports on the use of steroids supports their use in the treatment of children hospitalized with croup (Kairys et al., 1989). The majority of randomized, blinded trials also report favorable results (Skolnik, 1989). An increased proportion of the steroid-treated children had clinical improvement 12 and 24 hours after initiation of therapy. A reduced incidence of endotracheal intubation was also noted among steroid-treated children. A prudent approach would be to limit the use of steroids in croup to those children who both are hospitalized and have severe disease.

Other therapy. Nebulized racemic epinephrine appears helpful, in the experience of some clinicians (Taussig et al., 1977; Westley et al., 1978). Treatments given at 2- to 4-hour intervals may produce acute beneficial results, but patients must continue under close observation because there may be a "rebound phenomenon," with relapse within several hours of the initial improvement. The dose is 0.5 ml of 2.25% racemic epinephrine in 2.5 ml of normal saline solution dispensed as a nebulized treatment.

Acute Bronchiolitis

Clinical Picture. Bronchiolitis usually begins as an ordinary upper respiratory tract infection with nasal discharge, cough, slight fever, fretfulness, and loss of appetite. In a day or so the infant gets rapidly worse and presents an alarming picture of rapid labored breathing, with retraction of the intercostal spaces, use of accessory respiratory muscles, cyanosis, and prostration. Increasing obstruction leads to progressive hypoxemia, which, if unrelieved, may be followed by exhaustion and death. Respirations are rapid, shallow, difficult, and often wheezy, with a rate of 60 to 80 or more per minute. Inspiratory retraction is seen in the suprasternal notch and the intercostal and subcostal spaces. The cough is frequent, distressing, and often paroxysmal. Cyanosis appears or is intensified during coughing or crying and probably is continuous if the obstruction is severe. The patient is prostrate and takes little interest in his surroundings.

Physical findings, often changeable, are those of overinflated lungs; that is, the percussion note is hyperresonant, the diaphragm is depressed, and expiration is prolonged. Early, the breath sounds are diminished, and often no rales are heard. Later, fine, dry, or sibilant rales are audible. Roentgenographic examination of the chest shows that the lung fields are abnormally transparent, with increased bronchovascular markings. The diaphragm is depressed, and the intercostal spaces are widened. Atelectatic areas are usually small and difficult to recognize in the roentgenogram. Occasionally, one or more segments are collapsed. Arterial blood gas determinations can be very helpful in assessing the patient's respiratory exchange, the need for further support, and the response to treatment. The anticipated findings are an initial hypoxemia, which may be followed by respiratory acidosis and hypercapnia as deterioration occurs.

The nonbacterial cause of bronchiolitis, long suspected on clinical grounds, became more clearly defined as a result of the studies of Parrott et al. (1962). RSV is the most important single agent causing bronchiolitis, followed by parainfluenza virus types 3 and 1, adenoviruses, rhinoviruses, and influenza virus. Measles virus occasionally may cause bronchiolitis. In school-age children similar illnesses, wheezing-associated respiratory infections, are more often caused by *Mycoplasma pneumoniae* (Henderson et al., 1979b). RSV bronchiolitis and bronchopneumonia may be found as nosocomial infections among infants and children in nurseries and pediatric wards and may also occur among day-care center residents (Wenzel et al., 1977).

Determination of a specific viral diagnosis is crucial for the institution of infection control procedures and for the consideration of specific antiviral therapy. The agent responsible for an episode of bronchiolitis frequently can be determined by virus isolation or vital antigen detection. Virus isolation takes several days.

Detection of viral antigen can be accomplished in several hours and thereby offers a means by which a rapid viral diagnosis can be ascertained. Techniques widely used for the detection of RSV antigen in respiratory epithelial cells include the indirect immunofluorescent method and the enzyme-linked immunosorbent assay (ELISA). Tests for influenza, parainfluenza, and adenoviruses, as well as the longer-established test for RSV, are now commercially available.

The treatment of acute bronchiolitis should aim at (1) relieving bronchiolar obstruction, (2) correcting hypoxemia and acidosis, (3) controlling potential cardiac complications, (4) providing supportive measures, and (5) combating any secondary bacterial infection.

The patient should breathe air high in oxygen content and well saturated with water vapor, to render exudates less sticky. Oxygen tends to dry bronchial secretions and is used only in conjunction with water vapor. There is some support for the use of inhaled albuterol (Shuh et al., 1990), but no evidence supports the use of steroids either alone or as a supplement to B-agonists (Klassen et al., 1997). Cardiovascular support and drugs may be required in the presence of manifestations of developing heart failure such as enlargement of the liver, gallop rhythm, change in quality of heart sounds, tachycardia, and pulmonary edema. If the patient has very severe bronchiolitis that progresses in spite of these measures, it may be necessary to provide assisted ventilation and all the support available in an intensive care unit.

Because of the viral cause of bronchiolitis, antimicrobial therapy is of no benefit. The routine prophylactic or therapeutic use of antimicrobial agents is contraindicated.

Ribavirin, given by inhalation over periods of 12 to 20 hours for 2 to 5 days, is a widely employed treatment in children hospitalized with severe RSV infections. Special procedures must be taken for patients requiring mechanical ventilation since the formulation can lead to mechanical failures otherwise. Recent nonrandomized studies and studies of children whose disease has progressed to the point of mechanical ventilation have questioned the value of ribavirin and dampened enthusiasm for its use (Wheeler et al., 1993; Moler et al., 1996). Nonetheless a carefully controlled randomized study has pointed to a definite, if only modest, benefit (Hall et al., 1983).

Ribavirin has its advocates and opponents. Although the subject of much controversy, ribavirin is expensive and inconvenient to use. The risk it poses to hospital personnel who inhale it has remained more of a supposition than an established fact.

Ribavirin should be considered in selected groups of infants hospitalized with lower respiratory tract disease caused by RSV. Infants with cardiopulmonary diseases, immunodeficiency diseases, neurologic or metabolic diseases, or prematurity or severely ill infants (oxygen saturation less than 90%) are possible candidates for ribavirin therapy. (Committee on Infectious Diseases, American Academy of Pediatrics, 1996).

Pneumonia

The term *pneumonia* is used to describe a variety of reactions of the lung to various infectious and noninfectious agents. This discussion is limited to infectious pneumonia—bacterial and nonbacterial—that affects chiefly infants and children. The clinical manifestations vary greatly, depending on the causative agent, the age of the patient, systemic reaction to the infection, the presence of any underlying compromise of host defense, and the degree of bronchial and bronchiolar obstruction.

Bacterial Pneumonia. Most children with bacterial pneumonia are treated and recover without use of diagnostic procedures that would differentiate viral from bacterial pneumonia and document the specific bacterial cause. Nevertheless, viral pneumonia occurs far more frequently than bacterial pneumonia. Among bacterial causes, the pneumococcus and the mycoplasma remain the most frequent agents of pneumonia. *H. influenzae* type b, now on the decline; *S. pyogenes* (group A); and *S. aureus* are also important causes of pneumonia in otherwise normal children. Staphylococcal pneumonia may present as a nosocomial problem, particularly in neonates, or as a complication of other respiratory infections such as influenza.

The lack of availability of sputum or other materials for culture from the lower respiratory tract makes the causative diagnosis of bacterial pneumonia very difficult to establish with certainty in infants and young children. In most patients the diagnosis is based on clinical assessment and judgment.

Occasionally, however, the following findings may be helpful: positive blood culture, empyema fluid available for sampling, positive bacterial antigen assay (latex agglutination test), or characteristic chest roentgenogram findings such as pneumatoceles in patients with staphylococcal pneumonia. Leukocytosis with shift to the left, toxicity, grunt-

ing respirations, or splinting caused by pleural irritation may be clues to a bacterial cause. More invasive diagnostic procedures may be required in children who fail to respond to appropriate therapy and in those who are immunocompromised. These procedures include bronchoscopy with the flexible fiberoptic bronchoscope, bronchoalveolar lavage, lung aspiration, and open lung biopsy.

Pneumococcal Pneumonia.

Clinical picture. The onset of pneumococcal pneumonia is typically sudden in a child who has been well or who has had an upper respiratory tract infection. In infants, vomiting or a convulsion may be the first manifestation. An older child may complain of a headache, abdominal pain, or chest pain. Examination reveals a temperature of 38.9° to 40° C (102° to 104° F), rapid pulse, rapid shallow respirations, hot dry skin, and little else. In infants the possibility of central nervous system involvement must be considered, even in the absence of obvious neurologic or meningeal signs. This also should be considered in those infants with high fever, convulsions, restlessness, stupor, stiff neck, bulging anterior fontanelle, or Brudzinski's sign; examination of the CSF often is required to differentiate meningismus from meningitis. The course of pneumococcal pneumonia in a 9-year-old child is shown in Fig. 25-5.

By about the second day of illness, cough, expiratory grunt, dilation of the nostrils, suppression of breath sounds, and inconstant rales over the involved portion of the lungs point to the true nature of the disease. A pleural friction rub may be heard. Later, dullness and bronchial breathing indicate the area of consolidation, which may be confirmed by roentgenography. Resolution begins approximately 24 hours after appropriate antimicrobial treatment is started. Complications such as empyema, pericarditis, meningitis, arthritis, and peritonitis are seldom seen today. Otitis media is common but should be easily controlled. The causative diagnosis may be confirmed by culturing pneumococci from sputum, blood, or empyema fluid. Pleural effusions, when present in sufficient quantity, provide an important diagnostic opportunity. Active accumulations of cell (exudates), such as seen in malignancy or infection can be differentiated from passive serum ultrafiltrates (transudates) (Table 25-5). Gram stain should never be overlooked, since it gives an instant indication of the diagnosis. Antigen detection in pleural fluids has been positive for pneumococcal antigens, even when blood

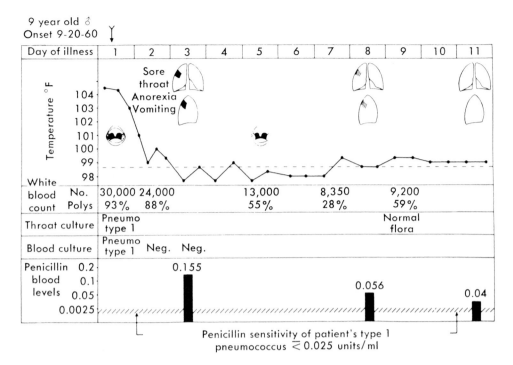

FIG. 25-5 Treatment of type 1 pneumococcal tonsillitis and pneumonia with a single injection of a penicillin preparation containing 600,000 units of aqueous procaine penicillin and 600,000 units of benzathine penicillin G. Note the dramatic subsidence of fever, the clearing of the exudative tonsillitis and pulmonary consolidation, and the rapid elimination of the type 1 pneumococci from the throat and blood. The penicillin blood level at 11 days (0.04 unit per milliliter) still exceeded the sensitivity of the patient's type 1 pneumococcus (<0.025 unit of penicillin per milliliter). (From Krugman S: Pediatr Clin North Am 1961;8:1199.)

Table 25-5 Clinical manifestations of infection with *Mycoplasma pneumoniae*

Respiratory tract	Other
Coryza	Erythema multiforme, other rashes
Pharyngitis	
Tracheobronchitis	Meningoencephalitis, cerebellar ataxia
Bullous myringitis	
Pneumonia	Guillain-Barré syndrome
Pleural effusion	Myocarditis, pericarditis
	Autoimmune hemolytic anemia, thrombocytopenia
	Migratory polyarthritis, hepatitis

cultures have been negative (Siegel et al., 1978). In evaluating children with pneumococcal pneumonia, it is important to remember that as many as 25% may have a predisposing underlying condition (Burman et al., 1985). These conditions include sickle cell disease, HIV infection, splenectomy, congenital heart disease, leukemia, immunoglobulin deficiency, asthma, galactosemia, and other metabolic disorders, especially in those children with hepatic damage. The peak incidence of pneumococcal disease is in the first 2 years of life, so some of these disorders may not yet have been detected.

Treatment. The quandary of antibiotic treatment of pneumococcal or presumed pneumococcal disease in the era of penicillin resistance has been touched on earlier. Although penicillin remains the treatment of choice if the strain is sensitive, pneumococcal pneumonia is a potentially life-threatening disease, and physicians may prefer to use vancomycin when the child is toxic. Adjustments can be made if the organism is isolated and antibiotic sensitivities become known. In penicillin-allergic patients, erythromycin, choramphenicol, and sulfonamides, as well as vancomycin, are alternatives when sensitivities are favorable. The response to therapy usually is observed within 1 to 2 days. The treatment should be continued for at least 5 days or more if the clinical findings warrant it. Only one drug is necessary.

Atypical Pneumonia.

Syndromes and agents. clinical manifestations of nonbacterial pneumonia (atypical pneumonia or viral pneumonia) are diverse. The onset is usually gradual but may be sudden. Systemic signs, especially fever, may be striking or inconspicuous. A mild respiratory tract illness usually precedes the more acute episode. Cough, fever, chilliness, headache, malaise, anorexia, listlessness, and irritability are common manifestations. Anorexia may be prominent. Cough appears early, is often severe and relentless, and interferes with sleep. Sputum, if obtainable, is mucoid or mucopurulent and may be blood streaked. Physical signs are variable; the child appears listless but only mildly or moderately ill. This may provide contrast with the child with bacterial pneumonia, where the picture is often one of prostration and anxiety. The temperature may be normal or elevated; respirations are usually normal. Chest findings are minimal, often limited to medium sticky rales and slight impairment of percussion note and breath sounds. The pneumonia frequently is discovered only on roentgenographic examination. The latter reveals a picture that also is not distinctive and varies from enlarged hilar shadows to patchy consolidation. Shifting areas of consolidation may be seen. The clinical course is irregular but usually benign, with complete recovery normally occurring in 1 to 3 weeks. Laboratory findings include a normal or slightly increased WBC count. Standard bacteriologic cultures are noncontributory.

Immunocompromised. Patients may develop pneumonias from unusual causes such as *Pneumocystis* spp., cytomegalovirus (Chapter 4), toxoplasmosis (Chapter 34), or tuberculosis (Chapter 35). Fungal pneumonias may also be associated with impaired host defenses or with exposure in endemic geographic areas. Blastomycosis has been reported in the valleys of the St. Lawrence, Ohio, and Mississippi rivers and in the southeastern United States. Histoplasmosis is endemic in certain parts of the United States, particularly the Ohio River valley. Coccidioidomycosis is endemic in the southwestern United States and in Argentina.

The wide spectrum of agents that may cause pneumonia in immunocompromised patients presents a serious diagnostic challenge. This diagnostic problem is of growing concern given the increasing incidence of the acquired immunodeficiency syndrome among children. Viral (cytomegalovirus, herpes simplex, parainfluenza); protozoal *Pneumocystis* spp.); fungal (*Candida,* *Aspergillus, Cryptococcus,* and *Zygomycetes* spp.); and unusual bacterial (*Nocardia* spp., gram-negative bacilli, *Staphylococcus* spp.) agents may be the causative culprits. Every case must be considered on its own individual features, but a precise diagnosis of pneumonia is often essential to successful intervention. Therefore performing invasive techniques, ranging from fiberoptic bronchoscopy to open lung biopsy, may be necessary if antigen detection and cultures of blood, sputum, or other sources are not helpful. Empiric therapy with amphotericin B—or fluconazole acyclovir, trimethoprim-sulfamethoxazole, or other drugs—may be initiated on the basis of clinical clues before test results are received.

Treatment. Most atypical pneumonias are viral in origin and are not influenced by antimicrobial therapy. Some atypical pneumonias are caused by fastidious bacteria, including *Chlamydia* and *Mycoplasma* spp. Patients with pneumonia caused by *C. trachomatis* or *C. psittaci* should receive erythromycin or tetracycline.

Erythromycin or the newer macrolides are recommended for *M. pneumoniae* pneumonia. General therapeutic measures include bed rest and maintenance of fluid intake. Oxygen is indicated for patients who are cyanotic and dyspneic, and a moist atmosphere is helpful for those with obstructive bronchitis or bronchiolitis.

Because of the lack of correlation between the results of bacterial and fungal upper respiratory tract cultures and the infecting microbes of the lower respiratory tract, the etiology of pneumonia and other lower respiratory infections of infancy and childhood is often uncertain. The severity of illness (especially in infants) is often masked, and the clinician is pressed to intervene with less than satisfying documentation of cause. For this reason, antibiotics are often prescribed with a halfhearted zeal—"in case there is secondary bacterial invasion" superimposed on a likely viral infection. The small infant has a number of liabilities that predispose him to respiratory failure with an infection that in an older child might be relatively benign (Pagtakhan and Chernick, 1982). These liabilities include the following: obligatory nasal breathing, immature musculature of the chest wall, tiny diameters and collapsibility of airways, limited collateral ventilatory pathways, increased tendency for parenchymal collapse, fragility of metabolic and energy balances, and easy fatigability.

The survival of infants with bronchopulmonary dysplasia has augmented the population of infants for whom a "minor respiratory infection" may become life threatening and who may require a temporary period of mechanical ventilatory support. Similarly at high risk are infants with congenital heart disease (MacDonald et al., 1982) or with severe asthma.

Unusual pneumonias such as those of fungal or protozoal origin require the use of drugs with special problems of toxicity. Amphotericin B, which is effective for many of the fungi, should be used only with careful attention to its potential for nephrotoxicity, febrile reactions, anemia, hypokalemia, cardiac arrhythmias, and other adverse effects. *P. carinii* pneumonia generally responds well to treatment with trimethoprim-sulfamethoxazole, although success is not guaranteed. Patients with HIV infection have higher rates of adverse reactions to therapy, with Stevens-Johnson syndrome being a dreaded complication. Pentamidine isothionate, itself a cause of renal damage and hypoglycemia, is the best-tested alternative.

Aspiration Pneumonia. Pneumonias in children with central nervous system or neuromuscular disease or in those incapable of handling respiratory secretions represent a special case. Such children often present to the emergency rooms of general or children's hospitals referred from chronic care facilities because of fever, toxicity, or respiratory distress. Aspiration of food or secretions is almost always the source of the problem. The breath may be fetid. Therapy should be directed against the gingival and oropharyngeal aerobic and anaerobic flora in community-acquired cases. Many physicians choose a broad spectrum agent such as ampicillin-sulbactam, but high doses of penicillin G (300,000 units/kg/day) are an alternative. In patients who have been on prolonged antibiotic therapy, the addition of coverage for such agents as gram-negative aerobic bacilli and staphylococci may be warranted. Therapy may be prolonged, particularly if abscess formation occurs, but surgical drainage is seldom mandatory.

Influenza-Like Illness

The syndrome termed *influenza-like illness* is characterized by sudden onset, chills or chilliness, fever, headache, marked prostration, muscular pains in the back and extremities, respiratory symptoms, and lack of any clear-cut abnormal physical findings outside the upper respiratory tract. This syndrome may be caused by several viruses in addition to the influenza viruses A and B:

parainfluenza virus types 1, 2, and 3; adenoviruses; and a number of enteroviruses, especially coxsackieviruses. The incubation period is short, usually 24 to 72 hours. Nausea and vomiting may occur. Pain or a burning sensation in the eyes may be present. Constitutional symptoms are more prominent, as a rule, than are respiratory symptoms. There is commonly a hacking cough accompanied by substernal soreness, which suggests tracheobronchitis. Dryness or scratchiness of the throat may occur together with hoarseness. Rhinitis, sneezing, and nasal discharge usually appear later. The physical findings are characteristically scanty and ill defined. In those patients who have fever, the temperature may go as high as 39.4° to 40° C (103° to 104° F). The temperature is more likely higher in children than in adults. The pulse rate is usually in proportion to the degree of fever. The face may appear flushed, and the conjunctivae may be injected. The throat may look normal, or it may be reddened and show glistening hypertrophied lymphoid nodules on the posterior pharyngeal wall. The lungs are usually clear. Signs of consolidation are not present in uncomplicated influenza-like illness.

The clinical laboratory findings are usually normal. The WBC count occasionally shows moderate leukopenia. The sedimentation rate is increased. Blood cultures are sterile. Results of roentgenographic examination of the chest are usually normal.

Like most other viral diseases, influenza-like illness is a self-limited infection. The course of the disease is usually one of rapid and progressive improvement. After severe infections, some patients tend to show persistent prostration and sweating, and they are easily tired for several days after the temperature comes down to normal. Prompt and complete recovery is the rule in ordinary epidemics, and complications rarely are seen outside a pandemic. When complications do occur, they most frequently arise in the respiratory tract, manifesting as either otitis media or pneumonia. The pneumonia may be either viral or a result of secondary bacterial superinfection. Other complications of influenza include myositis, myocarditis, Reye's syndrome, and Guillain-Barré syndrome.

Amantadine is an oral antiviral drug that inhibits the uncoating of influenza A virus. The clinical usefulness of amantadine is limited to influenza type A and does not extend to treatment of illness caused by influenza type B. When administered early in the course of influenza type A disease, amantadine shortens the illness and alleviates symptoms in patients; however, there is no evidence to suggest that therapy with amantadine is effective in preventing complications of influenza type A infection. Treatment with amantadine should be considered for patients with severe disease or for those with an underlying condition that puts them at high risk of having a severe or complicated course. The dose of amantadine for children 9 years or younger or for children who weigh less than 45kg is 4 to 8 mg/kg/day given orally in 1 or 2 doses (not to exceed 150 to 200 mg/day). For older children and for children who weigh more than 45 kg, it is 200 mg/day in 2 divided doses. Treatment should be started as soon as possible after the onset of symptoms and should be continued for 2 to 7 days, depending on the clinical response.

Otherwise, treatment of influenza-like illness is largely symptomatic. Bed rest is recommended. Complications rarely are encountered and are best dealt with as they arise. The routine prophylactic use of antibacterial agents is discouraged. Antipyretics are usually effective in alleviating symptoms. Salicylates are customarily avoided because of the association of Reye's syndrome with their use and the syndrome's clear link with influenza epidemics. Fluids should be given freely. The diet is best governed by the patient's appetite.

CONTROL OF RESPIRATORY DISEASE

The development of the measles, polio, rubella, and mumps vaccines in the 1950s and 1960s produced a heady feeling in the pediatric community. Renewed optimism is swelling as the new hepatitis B, hepatitis A, and varicella vaccines have further raised expectations. The vaccine approach is looked at as a solution for everything from AIDS to cancer. The record of vaccination in respiratory disease, however, is sobering: influenza virus vaccines are not completely effective; the history of RSV vaccination (see foregoing discussion) has been punctuated with tragedy, and, despite brilliant initiatives, it is still a story of frustration; the record of pneumococcal vaccines is spotty. There are several traditional reasons for expecting that the road to effective vaccines against respiratory agents will be a difficult one. There are also developments in modern molecular biology that may illuminate past problems and indicate future ones. There are also applications of modern techniques and evocations of old-fashioned strategies.

Traditional reasons for the disappointing performance of respiratory infection prophylaxis are several. First, microbes are considered most vulnerable when their pathophysiology requires blood stream invasion. Of course not all systemically invading agents are exquisitely sensitive to immunologic clearance (HIV and malaria come to mind), but pathogens that remain, like respiratory pathogens, at the body-environment interface flourish in a milieu that is only partially controlled by programmed responses. Second, vaccination is most successful when only a limited number of pathogenic serotypes (genotypes) are capable of producing disease. This is not the case with many respiratory pathogens. Finally, as Chanock has emphasized on numerous occasions, when natural infection does not provide effective permanent immunity, providing immunity by vaccination is difficult.

Influenza

Current influenza vaccines are not live agents. Although live attenuated vaccines have great theoretic advantage in the case of respiratory viruses (they could replicate in the upper respiratory tract mucosa and stimulate local, as well as systemic, immunity), no such stable vaccine strain capable of being produced in timely response to an influenza epidemic has yet been devised.

Nevertheless, the current inactive vaccines are produced as promptly as possible each influenza season. As noted earlier, antibodies to the influenza HA and NA proteins seem to be crucial in interrupting the viral replication cycle. These antigens, as noted, are subject to antigenic shift and antigenic drift. Such mutations render strains less susceptible to immune mechanisms mounted against their ancestral strains, which means that vaccines with contemporary HA and NA proteins need to be prepared for each successive influenza season.

Vaccine production begins with selection of the most recent epidemiologic strains. Strains of influenza A H3N2 and H1N1 are selected along with a strain of influenza B. Virus is grown in embryonated eggs for vaccine preparation. If the currently circulating wild-type strains grow poorly, gene reassortment techniques can be used to improve the yield (Robertson et al., 1992). Coinfection of cells with wild-type virions and those of a strain well-adapted to growth in eggs will result in reassortant progeny that exhibit the current HA and NA antigens from the wild-type strain and the growth capacity of the coinfecting strain. Two types of inactivated vaccine may then be produced. Whole-virus vaccines are prepared by purifying intact virus particles from allantoic fluid by such means as industrial-scale column chromatography and rate-zonal centrifugation. These processes rid the final vaccine preparation of extraneous antigens and reduce untoward reactions. The virus is then inactivated with formalin or β-propiolactone. A vaccine dose contains roughly 10^{10} virions. As opposed to whole-virus vaccine preparations, the split-virus vaccines are prepared by solubilizing the intact virus particles with detergents before chemical inactivation. These vaccines are less reactogenic than the whole-virus vaccines.

In infants and children, influenza virus vaccines may be somewhat less immunogenic and doses producing a response may be more reactogenic than in adults. Only the split-virus vaccine should be used for children under 12 years of age. Either the split-virus or whole-virus vaccine may be used for children 12 years of age and older.

Even in the best of circumstances, the protection provided by the administration of inactivated influenza virus vaccines is incomplete. Efficacy rates range from 60% to 80%, and attenuation of illness is a prime benefit. For this reason, and for the theoretic reasons noted earlier, development of practical live-attenuated influenza vaccines remains an important goal. Temperature-sensitive mutant vaccines—which have the added safety advantage of being unable to cause lower respiratory tract disease because of their inability to replicate at core body temperature—have been developed, as have cold-adapted mutants. Because *de novo* annual development of such vaccines using the contemporary influenza strains is impractical, molecular biologic approaches are now being investigated. Reassortment technologies are envisioned to package the genes for the HA and NA proteins from currently circulating strains into virions whose other genes are donated by pre-prepared attenuated strains (Murphy, 1993). It is thus hoped that the HA

and NA antigens can be introduced into the host by a virus strain already weakened by its other mutations. Even more sophisticated techniques involve generation of the cDNA of the H gene, introduction of a specific mutation into the DNA, generation of the corresponding RNA, and transfection of this RNA into cells. Coinfecting such cells with a helper influenza strain will generate reassortment mutants with the desired HA mutation (Enami et al., 1990).

Annual immunization with the current vaccine strains is recommended for targeted high-risk children and for close contacts of high-risk patients. High-risk children are those with chronic cardiopulmonary diseases, sickle cell disease and other hemoglobinopathies, diabetes, chronic renal or metabolic diseases, or HIV infection; children receiving long-term aspirin therapy who may be at risk of Reye's syndrome; or children receiving immunosuppressive therapy. Close contacts of high-risk patients may include hospital personnel, household contacts, and children who are members of the patients' households.

The vaccine is administered intramuscularly and should be given in the autumn before the start of influenza season. Previously unimmunized children should receive 2 doses of vaccine timed 1 month apart to achieve a satisfactory response. The dosage of vaccine given varies according to the age of the child (Table 25-6). There is no available information about the safety, reactivity, or immunogenicity of influenza vaccine in children under 6 months of age. Immunization is not routinely recommended for children less than 6 months of age. Side effects include fever and myalgias. These begin 6 to 12 hours after vaccination and last for a day or two. Immediate-type hypersensitivity reactions have been noted in people with severe aller-

Table 25-6   Influenza vaccine dosage, by patient age

Age group	Product[*]	Dosage	No. doses	Route[†]
6-35 mo	Split virus only	0.25 ml	1 or 2[‡]	IM
3-8 yr	Split virus only	0.50 ml	1 or 2[‡]	IM
9-12 yr	Split virus only	0.50 ml	1	IM
≥12 yr	Whole or split virus	0.50 ml	1	IM

[*]Modified from Centers for Disease Control. Recommendations of the advisory committee on immuzation practices. MMR 1996; 45:44. Because of the lower potential for causing febrile reactions, only split-virus vaccines should be used for children. They may be labeled as "split," "subvirion," or "purified-surface-antigen" vaccine. Immunogenicity and side effects of split- and whole-virus vaccines are similar for adults when vaccines are used at the recommended dosage.

[†]The recommended site of vaccination is the deltoid muscle for adults and older children. The preferred site for infants and young children is the anterolateral aspect of the thigh.

[‡]Two doses are recommended for children <9 years of age who are receiving influenza vaccine for the first time.

gies. For these reasons it is recommended not to administer influenza vaccines to people with febrile illnesses or to those with known allergies to eggs. The 1976 vaccination program for swine influenza was associated with an increased incidence of Guillain-Barré syndrome. This association has not been noted subsequently. Amantadine, an antiviral agent that apparently blocks the release of the active influenza A transcriptive complex, has been used successfully in the prophylaxis of type A influenza strains in epidemic settings. It also has some therapeutic effect. Monto et al. (1979) reported a favorable result among University of Michigan students during the 1978 outbreak of H1N1 influenza. The drug was given orally, once daily, for at least 6 weeks. Their results showed a 70% efficacy in prevention of illness and infection in contrast to a placebo-control group. The available data on amantadine's effects and toxicity in the pediatric age group are more limited. A daily dose of 100 mg/day in children weighing more than 20 kg is an effective prophylactic dose. For children less than 20 kg the prophylactic regimen is the same as that described previously for treatment. Indications for amantadine prophylaxis include the following: individuals at high risk who were vaccinated after influenza A activity had begun in the community; nonimmunized persons caring for high-risk individuals; immunodeficient individuals likely to respond poorly to a vaccine; and persons for whom vaccine is contraindicated (persons with anaphylactic hypersensitivity to egg protein).

Respiratory Syncytial Virus

The inactivated vaccine incident prompted attempts to develop live attenuated vaccines that would better mimic natural infection. As in the case of influenza vaccines, temperature-sensitive and cold-adapted mutants have theoretical advantages. The problem of genetic stability of vaccine strains when administered to infants, however, is a real one (Kim et al., 1973b; Wright et al., 1982; Chanock et al., 1992).

Hopes are raised, however, by the delineation of the RSV genome. This has led to the detailed analysis of hyperattenuated mutants and will perhaps lead to more stable vaccines (Connors et al., 1995). It is possible that the cDNA-controlled mutation strategy may be applicable to RSV as well as influenza. Other avenues include the use of purified RSV F and G proteins as immunizing agents (Tristram et al., 1993) and the Jennerian strategy attempting to use the bovine variant of RSV as a vac-

cine. None of these approaches will be satisfactory, however, if the recently elucidated genetic variability of RSV means that protective immunity is highly strain-specific.

One old modality of protection that is currently being reexamined is the use of immune globulin. Preparations of immune globulin with enhanced activity against RSV are now available. They have apparently provided significant protection to infants at high risk for disease when infused intravenously at intervals throughout the RSV season (Groothuis, et al. 1995), and there are grounds for believing this approach has therapeutic as well as prophylactic potential (Hemming et al., 1995). It should be noted, however, that the use of hyperimmune globulin has so far been limited to infants with heart and lung problems. Repeated infusions were performed and fluid overload was an occasional problem. This approach is clearly not applicable to the general population, is expensive, and requires careful monitoring by physicians.

Pneumococcus

The importance of type-specific antibody to the capsular polysaccharide of the pneumococcus has been recognized. This antibody is thought to interact with the complement system to facilitate phagocytosis of the invading bacteria. Modern vaccines have been combinations of the capsular polysaccharide antigens of a number of different pneumococcal strains. They have shown partial effectiveness in adults. However, the antibody response to polysaccharide antigens of children under the age of 2 years is poor. These antigens elicit a relatively T cell-independent response in which B cell production or antibody occurs with a low requirement for T cell mediation. T cell-independent antigens are poor inducers of immunologic memory and induce antibodies of low avidity that do not demonstrate isotypic shift. The T cell-independent response is poorly developed in children under 2 years of age. Pneumococcal polysaccharide vaccine is therefore not recommended for children.

Currently available pneumococcal vaccines contain purified capsular polysaccharide antigens of 23 sterotypes of pneumococci, which comprise about 90% of the serotypes causing invasive disease in children. The pneumococcal vaccines are of proven use in children with sickle cell disease and asplenia (Amman et al., 1977) and may well be of use in normal populations of older children where the disease is endemic (Riley et al., 1986). Vaccination is targeted at children at high risk for invasive pneumococcal disease (American Academy of Pediatrics, 1994). These include children over 2 years of age with sickle cell disease, functional or anatomic asplenia, nephrotic syndrome, renal failure, immunosuppression for organ transplantation or cancer, or HIV infection. Patients undergoing elective splenectomy should receive vaccination at least 2 weeks before undergoing the procedure. Revaccination should be considered for children 10 years old or younger and 6 years or more after initial vaccination for older children.

Because of the emergence of penicillin-resistant strains of pneumococcus, the search for an effective pneumococcal vaccine generally applicable to the pediatric age group is a high priority. The problem of poor infant response to polysaccharide antigens is being tackled by coupling of bacterial polysaccharides to protein carriers to enhance immunogenicity (Käyhty and Eskola, 1996), which converts the polysaccharide antigen to a T cell-dependent antigen in which B cell production of antibody is mediated by T helper cells. T cell-dependent responses are far better developed in infants than are T cell-independent ones. A number of such conjugate vaccines are currently in development and are reaching phase-III trials. In these vaccines 7 or 8 polysaccharide antigens from the clinically most important strains are linked to a protein carrier.

Chemoprophylaxis constitutes a second avenue of approach to the protection of children at high risk of pneumococcal infection. The administration of daily penicillin V or G to children with functional or anatomic asplenia is of demonstrated value (Gaston et al., 1986). Prophylaxis is begun by age 4 months and administered as 125 mg twice a day. This dose is to be doubled after age 5, but there are indications, at least in sickle cell disease, that penicillin may not be needed beyond this age when vaccine has been given (Falletta et al., 1995).

BIBLIOGRAPHY

Abbasi S, Cunningham AS. Are we overtreating sinusitis? Contemp Pediatr 1996;13:49-62.

Adair JC, Ring WH. Management of epiglottitis in children. Anesth Analg 1975;54:622.

Adams JM, Imagawa DT, Zide K. Epidemic bronchiolitis and pneumonitis related to respiratory syncytial virus. JAMA 1961;176:1037.

Almeida JD, Tyrrell DAJ. The morphology of three previously uncharacterized human respiratory viruses that grow in organ culture. J Gen Virol 1967;1:175.

Amman AJ, et al. Polyvalent pneumococcal-polysaccharide immunization of patients with sickle-cell anemia and patients with splenectomy. N Engl J Med 1977;297:897.

Anas N, Boettrich C, Hall CB, et al. The association of apnea and respiratory syncytial virus infection. J Pediatr 1982; 101:65.

Anderson KC, Maurer MJ, Dajani AS. Pneumococci relatively resistant to penicillin: a prevalence survey in children. J Pediatr 1980;97:939.

Anderson LJ, et al. Antigenic characterization of respiratory syncytial virus strains with monoclonal antibodies. J Infect Dis 1985;151:626-633.

Anderson LJ, et al. Multicenter study of strains of respiratory syncytial virus. J Infect Dis 1991;163:687-692.

Andrewes CH. The taxonomic position of common cold viruses and some others. Yale J Biol Med 1961-1962;34:200.

Andrewes CH, Bang FB, Chanock RM, Zhdanov VM. Parainfluenza virus 1, 2, 3: suggested names for recently isolated myxoviruses. Virology 1959;8:129.

Arnold KE, Leggiadro RJ, Breiman RF, et al. Risk factors for carriage of drug-resistant *Streptococcus pneumoniae* among children in Memphis, Tennessee. J Pediatr 1996;128:757-764.

Arth C, Von Schmidt BV, Grossman M, Schachter J. Chlamydial pneumonitis. J Pediatr 1978;93:447.

Austrian R. Pneumococcal infection and pneumococcal vaccine. N Engl J Med 1977;297:938.

Austrian R, et al. Prevention of pneumococcal pneumonia by vaccination. Trans Assoc Am Phys 1976;89:184.

Beale J, McLeod DL, Stackiw W, Roads AJ. Isolation of cytopathic agents from respiratory tract in acute laryngotracheobronchitis. Br Med J 1958;1:302.

Beare AS, Craig JW. Virulence for man of a human influenza A virus antigenically similar to "classical" swine viruses. Lancet 1960;2:4.

Beaty HN, et al. Legionnaires' disease in Vermont, May to October 1977. JAMA 1978;240:127.

Beem M, et al. Association of the chimpanzee coryza agent with acute respiratory disease in children. N Engl J Med 1960; 263:523.

Benfield GFA. Recent trends in empyema thoracis. Br J Dis Chest 1981;75:358.

Berg FA, Bartley DL. Pneumonia associated with *Branhamella catarrhalis* in infants. Pediatr Infect Dis J 1987;6:569-573.

Beschamps GJ, Lynn HB, Wenzl JE. Empyema in children: review of Mayo Clinic experience. Mayo Clin Proc 1970; 45:43.

Bloom HH, Forsyth BR, Johnson KM, Chanock RM. Relationship of rhinovirus infection to mild upper respiratory disease. I. Results of a survey in young adults and children. JAMA 1963;186:38.

Bloom HH, Johnson KM, Jacobsen R, Chanock RM: Recovery of parainfluenza viruses from adults with upper respiratory illnesses. Am J Hyg 1961;74:50.

Bock BV, et al. Legionnaires' disease in renal-transplant recipients. Lancet 1978;1:410.

Bradburne AS, Tyrrell DA. Coronaviruses of man. In Melnick JL (ed). Progress in medical virology, vol 12. New York: S Karger, 1970.

Brandt CD, et al. Infections in 18,000 infants and children in controlled study of respiratory tract disease. I. Adenovirus pathogenicity in relation to serologic type and illness syndromes. Am J Epidemiol 1969;90:484.

Brook I. Anaerobic and aerobic normal flora of maxillary sinuses. Laryngoscope 1981;91:372-376.

Bryson YJ. The use of amantadine in children for prophylaxis and treatment of influenza A infections. Pediatr Infect Dis 1982;1:44-46.

Burman LA, Norrby R, Trollfors B. Invasive pneumococcal infections; incidence, predisposing factors, and prognosis. Rev Infect Dis 1985;7:133.

Burrows B, Knudson RG, Lebowitz MD. The relationship of childhood respiratory illness to adult obstructive airway disease. Am Rev Respir Dis 1977;115:751.

Cane PA, Matthews DA, Pringle CR. Identification of variable domains of the attachment (G) protein of subgroup A respiratory syncytial viruses. J Fen Virol 1991;72:2091-2096.

Cane PA, Pringle CR. Evolution of subgroup A respiratory syncytial virus: evidence of progressive accumulation of amino acid changes in the attachment protein. J Virol 1995;69:2918-2925.

Carson JL, Collier AM, Clyde WA Jr. Ciliary membrane alterations occurring in experimental *Mycoplasma pneumoniae* infection. Science 1979;206:349.

Carson JL, Collier AM, Hu SS. Acquired ciliary defects in nasal epithelium of children with acute viral upper respiratory infections. N Engl J Med 1985;312:463.

Cattaneo SM, Kolman JW. Surgical therapy of empyema in children. Arch Surg 1973;106:564.

Centers for Disease Control. Hantavirus pulmonary syndrome —United States, 1995 and 1996. MMWR 1996;45:291-295.

Centers for Disease Control. Progress toward elimination of *Haemophilus influenzae* type b disease among infants and children—United States, 1993-1994. MMWR 1995;44:545-550.

Centers for Disease Control. Multiple-antibiotic resistance of pneumococci—South Africa. MMWR 1977;26:285.

Chandler FW, Hicklin MD, Blackmon JA. Demonstration of the agent of Legionnaires' disease in tissue. N Engl J Med 1977;297:1218.

Chanock RM. Mycoplasma infections of man. N Engl J Med 1965;273:1199.

Chanock RM, Bell JA, Parrott RH. Natural history of parainfluenza infection. In Pollard M (ed). Perspectives in virology, vol 2. Minneapolis: Burgess Publishing, 1961.

Chanock RM, Finberg L. Recovery from infants with respiratory illness of a virus related to chimpanzee coryza agent (CCA). II. Epidemiologic aspects of infection in infants and young children. Am J Hyg 1957;66:291.

Chanock RM, Hayflick L, Barile MD. Growth on artificial medium of an agent associated with atypical pneumonia and its identification as a PPLO. Proc Natl Acad Sci USA 1962;48:41.

Chanock RM, Parrott RH, Connors M et al. Serious respiratory tract disease caused by respiratory syncytial virus: Prospects for improved therapy and effective immunization. Pediatrics 1992;90:137-143.

Chanock RM, et al. Respiratory syncytial virus. I. Virus recovery and other observations during 1960 outbreak of bronchiolitis, pneumonia, and minor respiratory diseases in children. JAMA 1961;176:647.

Chanock RM, et al. Biology and ecology of two major lower respiratory tract pathogens—RS virus and Eaton PPLO. In Pollard M (ed). Perspectives in virology, vol 3. New York: Harper & Row, 1963, p 257.

Chany C, et al. Severe and fatal pneumonia in infants and young children associated with adenovirus. Am J Hyg 1958;67:3967.

Chaudhary S, Bilisnky SA, Hennessy JL, et al. Penicillin V and rifampin for the treatment of group A streptococcal pharyngitis. J Pediatr 1985;106:481.

Cherry JD. The treatment of croup: continued controversy due to failure of recognition of historic, ecologic, etiologic and clinical perspectives. J Pediatr 1979;94:352.

Committee on Infectious Diseases, American Academy of Pediatrics. Reassessment of the indications for ribavirin therapy in respiratory syncytial virus infections. Pediatr 1996;97:137-140.

Connors M, Crowe JE Jr, Firestone CY, et al. A cold-passaged, attenuated strain of human respiratory syncytial virus contains mutations in the F and L genes. Virology 1995;208:478-484.

Cowan MH, et al. Pneumococcal polysaccharide immunization in infants and children. Pediatrics 1978;62:721.

Cradock-Watson JE, McQuillin J, Gardner PS. Rapid diagnosis of respiratory syncytial virus infection in children by the immunofluorescent technique. J Clin Pathol 1971;24:347.

Cramblett HG. Croup: present day concept. Pediatrics 1960;25:1071.

D'Alessio DJ, Meschievitz CK, Peterson JA, et al. Short duration exposure and transmission of rhinovirus colds. J Infect Dis 1984;150:1189-1194.

Dawson CR, Hanna L, Wood TR, et al. Adenovirus type 8 keratoconjunctivitis in the United States. Am J Ophtholmol 1970;69:473-480.

Denny FW, Clyde WA. Acute lower respiratory tract infections in nonhospitalized children. J Pediatr 1986;108:635-646.

Denny FW, Clyde WA Jr, Glezon WP. *Mycoplasma pneumoniae* disease: clinical spectrum pathophysiology, epidemiology, and control. J Infect Dis 1971;123:74.

Diament MJ, Senac MO Jr, Gilsanz V, et al. Prevalence of incidental paranasal sinuses opacification in pediatric patients: a CT study. J Comp Assist Tomog 1987;11:426-431.

Dolin R, et al. A controlled trial of amantadine and rimantadine in the prophylaxis of influenza A infection. N Engl J Med 1982;307:580-583.

Duchin JS, Koster FT, Peters CJ, et al. Hantavirus pulmonary syndrome: a clinical description of 17 patients with a newly recognized disease. N Engl J Med 1994;330:449-455.

Dular R, Kajioka R, Kasatiya S. Comparison of Gen-Probe commercial kit and culture technique for diagnosis of *Mycoplasma pneumoniae* infection. J Clin Microbiol 1988;26:1068-1069.

Eaton MD, Meiklejohn G, van Herrick WJ. Studies on etiology of primary atypical pneumonia: filtrable agent transmissible to cotton rats, hamsters, and chick embryos. J Exp Med 1944;79:649.

Edelstein PH. Legionnaires' disease. Clin Infect Dis 1993;16:741-747.

Eden AN, Kaufman A, Yu R. Corticosteroids and croup: controlled double blind study. JAMA 1967;200:133.

Edwards KM, Thompson J, Paolini BS, Wright PF. Adenovirus infections in young children. Pediatrics 1985;76:420-424.

Eliasson R, Mossberg B, Camner R, Afzelius BA. The immotile cilia syndrome. N Engl J Med 1977;297:1.

Enami M, Luytjes W, Krystal M, et al. Introduction of site-specific mutations into the genomes of influenza virus. Proc Nat Acad Schi USA 1990;87:3802-3805.

Escobar JA, et al. Etiology of respiratory tract infections in children in Cali, Colombia. Pediatrics 1976;57:123.

Evans AS, Brobst M. Bronchiolitis, pneumonitis, and pneumonia in University of Wisconsin students. N Engl J Med 1961;265:401.

Faden HS. Treatment of *Haemophilus influenza* type b epiglottitis. Pediatrics 1979;63:402.

Falletta JM, Woods GM, Verter JI, et al. Discontinuing penicillin prophylaxis in children with sickle cell anemia. J Pediatr 1995;127:685-690.

Falsey AR, Treanor JJ, Betts RF, et al. Viral respiratory infections in the institutionalized elderly: clinical and epidemiologic findings. J Am Geriatr Soc 1992;40:115-119.

Fernald GW, Collier AM, Clyde WA Jr. Respiratory infections due to *Mycoplasma pneumoniae* in infants and children. Pediatrics 1975;55:327.

Fields BS. *Legionella* and protozoa: interaction of a pathogen and its natural host. In Barbaree JM, Breiman RF, Dufour AP (eds). *Legionella* —current status and emerging perspectives. Washington, D.C.: American Society for Microbiology, 1993.

Finland M. Pneumonia and pneumococcal infections, with special reference to pneumococcal pneumonia. Am Rev Respir Dis 1979;120:481.

Fogel JM, Berg IJ, Gerber MA, Sherter CB. Racemic epinephrine in the treatment of croup: nebulization alone versus nebulization with intermittent positive pressure breathing. J Pediatr 1982;101:1028-1031.

Forbes JA. Croup and its management. Br Med J 1961;1:1389.

Fox JP, Cooney MK, Hall CE. The Seattle virus watch. V. Epidemiologic observations of rhinovirus infections in families with young children. Am J Epidemiol 1975;101:122.

Fox JP, et al. The virus watch program: a continuing surveillance of viral infections in metropolitan New York families. VI. Observations of adenovirus infections: virus excretion patterns, antibody response, efficiency of surveillance, patterns of infection, and relation to illness. Am J Epidemiol 1969;89:25.

Francis T Jr. Factors conditioning resistance to epidemic influenza. Harvey Lect 1942;37:39.

Francis T Jr. Problems of acute respiratory disease. Yale J Biol Med 1961-1962;34:191.

Fraser DW. Legionnaires' disease: description of an epidemic of pneumonia. N Engl J Med 1977;296:1150.

Freij BJ, Kusmiesz H, Nelson JD, et al. Parapneumonic effusions and empyema in hospitalized children: a retrospective review of 227 cases. Pediatr Infect Dis 1984;3:578.

Friis B, Andersen P, Brenoe E, et al. Antibiotic treatment of pneumonia and bronchiolitis: a perspective randomized study. Arch Dis Child 1984;59:1038.

Frommell G, Bruhn FW, Schwartzman JD. Isolation of *Chlamydia trachomatis* from infant lung tissue. N Engl J Med 1977;296:1150.

Gardner PS. How etiologic, pathologic, and clinical diagnoses can be made in a correlated fashion. Pediatr Res 1977;11:254.

Gardner PS, McQuillin J, Court SDM. Speculation on pathogenesis in death from respiratory syncytial virus infection. Br Med J 1970;1:327.

Gardner PS, et al. Death associated with respiratory tract infections in children. Br Med J 1967;4:316.

Gaston MH, Verter JI, Woods G, et al. and the Prophylactic Penicillin Study Group. Prophylaxis with oral penicillin in children with sickle cell anemia: a randomized trial. N Engl J Med 1986;314:1593-1599.

Ginsberg CM, Howard JB, Nelson JD. Report of 65 cases of *Haemophilus influenzae* b pneumonia. Pediatrics 1979; 64:283.

Glezen WP. Pathogenesis of bronchiolitis: epidemiologic considerations. Pediatr Res 1977;11:234.

Glezen WP, Denny FW. Epidemiology of acute lower respiratory disease in children. N Engl J Med 1973;228:498.

Glezen WP, Frank AL, Taber LH, Kasel JA. Parainfluenza virus type 3: seasonality and risk of infection and reinfection in young children. J Infect Dis 1984;150:851-857.

Glezen WP, Paredes A, Allison JE, et al. Risk of respiratory syncytial virus infection for infants from low-income families in relationship to age, sex, ethnic group, and maternal antibody level. J Pediatr 1981;98:708-715.

Glezen WP, Taber LH, Frank AL, Kasel JA. Risk of primary infection and reinfection with respiratory syncytial virus. Am J Dis Child 1986;140:543-546.

Glezen WP, Wilfert CM. Your role in the war against flu. Contemp Pediatr 1988;86-98.

Glezen WP, et al. Epidemiologic patterns of acute lower respiratory disease in children in a pediatric group practice. J Pediatr 1971;78:397.

Glicklich M, Cohen RD, Jona JZ. Steroids and bag and mask ventilation in the treatment of acute epiglottitis. J Pediatr Surg 1979;14:247.

Goldman AS, Schochet SS Jr, Howell JT: The discovery of defects in respiratory cilia in the immotile cilia syndrome. J Pediatr 1980;96:244.

Graham BS. Pathogenesis of respiratory syncytial virus vaccine-augmented pathology. Am J Respir Crit Care Med 1995;152;S63-S66.

Graham BS, Perkins MD, Wright PT, et al. Primary respiratory syncytial virus infection in mice. J Med Virol 1988;26:153-162.

Graham NM et al. Adverse effects of aspirin, acetaminophen, and ibuprofen on immune function, viral shedding, and clinical status in rhinovirus-infected volunteers. J Infect Dis 1990;162:1277-1282.

Graman PS, Hall CB. Nosocomial viral respiratory infections. Sem Resp Infect 1989;4:253-260.

Gray BM, Converse GM III, Dillon HC Jr. Serotypes of *Streptococcus pneumoniae* causing disease. J Infect Dis 1980; 140:979.

Grayston JT. Infections caused by *Chlamydia pneumoniae* strain TWAR. Clin Infect Dis 1992;15:1757-1763.

Groothuis JR, Gutierrez KM, Lauer BA. Respiratory syncytial virus infection in children with bronchopulmonary dysplasia. Pediatrics 1988;82:199-203.

Groothuis JR, Simoes EAF, Hemming VG, et al. Respiratory syncytial virus (RSV) infection in preterm infants and the protective effects of REV immune globulin. Pediatrics 1995; 95:463-467.

Guyer B et al. Annual summary of vital statistics—1994. Pediatrics 1995;96:1029-1039.

Gwaltney JM Jr, Phillips CD, Miller RD, et al. Computed tomographic study of the common cold. N Engl J Med 1994; 330:25-30.

Hackstadt T, Rocky DD, Heinzen RA, et al. *Chlamydia trachomatis* interrupts an exocytic pathway to acquire endogenously synthesized sphingomyelin in transit from the Golgi apparatus to the plasma membrane. EMBOJ 1996;15: 964-967.

Hall CB, Douglas RG Jr. Respiratory syncytial virus and influenza: practical community surveillance. Am J Dis Child 1976;130:615-620.

Hall CB, Douglas RG Jr. Modes of transmission of respiratory syncytial virus. J Pediatr 1981;99:100-103.

Hall CB, Geiman JM, Biggar R, et al. Respiratory syncytial virus infections within families. N Engl J Med 1976;294: 414-419.

Hall CB, Hall WJ, Gala CL, et al. A long-term prospective study in children following respiratory syncytial virus infection. J Pediatr 1984;105:358-364.

Hall CB, McBride JT, Walsh EE, et al. Aerosolized ribavirin treatment of infants with respiratory syncytial virus infection: a randomized double-blind study. N Engl J Med 1983; 308:1443-1447.

Hall CB, et al. Neonatal respiratory syncytial virus infection. N Engl J Med 1979;300:393.

Hall CB, et al. Respiratory syncytial viral infection in children with compromised immune function. N Engl J Med 1986; 315:77-80.

Hall CB, et al. Risk of secondary bacterial infection in infants hospitalized with respiratory syncytial viral infection. J Pediatr 1988;113:266-271.

Hall WJ, Hall CB, Speers DM. Respiratory syncytial virus infections in adults: clinical virologic and serial pulmonary function studies. Ann Inter Med 1978;88:203-205.

Hammershlag MR, Golden NH, Oh MK. Single dose of azithromycin for the treatment of genital chlamydial infections in adolescents. J Pediatr 1993;122:961-965.

Hammerschlag MR, et al. Prospective study of maternal and infantile infection with *Chlamydia trachomatis*. Pediatrics 1979;64:142.

Harlap S, Davies AM. Infant admissions to hospital and maternal smoking. Lancet 1974;1:529.

Harrison HR, English NG, Lee CK, Alexander ER. *Chlamydia trachomatis* infant pneumonitis: comparison with matched controls and other infant pneumonitis. N Engl J Med 1978;298:702.

Hemming VG, Prince GA, Groothuis JR, et al. Hyperimmune globulins in prevention and treatment of respiratory syncytial virus infections. Clin Microbiol Rev 1995;8:22-33.

Henderson FW. Pulmonary infections with respiratory syncytial virus and the parainfluenza viruses. Sem Resp Infect 1987;2:112-121.

Henderson FW, Collier AM, Clyde WA Jr, Denny FW. Respiratory syncytial virus infections, reinfections, and immunity: a prospective longitudinal study in young children. N Engl J Med 1979a;300:530-534.

Henderson FW, et al. The etiologic and epidemiologic spectrum of bronchiolitis in pediatric practice. J Pediatr 1979b;95:183.

Hierholzer JC, Hirsch MS. Croup and pneumonia in human infants associated with a new strain of respiratory syncytial virus. J Infect Dis 1979;140:926.

Hilleman MR, et al. Appraisal of occurrence of adenovirus caused respiratory illness in military populations. Am J Hyg 1957;66:29.

Hilleman MR, et al. Polyvalent pneumococcal polysaccharide vaccines. J Infect 1979;1(suppl 2):73.

Hirst GK. Studies of antigenic differences among strains of influenza A by means of red cell agglutination. J Exp Med 1943;78:407.

Hoffman E. Empyema in childhood. Thorax 1961;16:128.

Hoffman J, Cetron MS, Farley MM, et al. The prevalence of drug-resistant *Streptococcus pneumoniae* in Atlanta. N Engl J Med 1995;333:481-486.

Institute of Medicine. Appendix N: prospects for immunizing against respiratory syncytial virus. In New vaccine development: establishing priorities. Volume 1: diseases of importance in the United States. Washington, D.C.: National Academy Press, 1985.

Isaacs D. Cold comfort for the catarrhal child. Arch Dis Child 1990;65:1295-1296.

Jackson GG. Sensitivity of influenza A virus to amantadine. J Infect Dis 1977;136:301.

Jacobs JW, et al. Respiratory syncytial and other viruses associated with respiratory disease in infants. Lancet 1971;1:871.

Jacobs MR, et al. Emergence of multiply resistant pneumococci. N Engl J Med 1978;299:735.

Johnson KM, Bloom HH, Forsyth B, et al. Relative role of identifiable agents in respiratory disease. II. The role of enteroviruses in respiratory disease. Am Rev Resp Dis 1962; 88:2240-2245.

Johnson KM, Bloom HH, Mufson MA, Chanock RM. Natural reinfection of adults by respiratory syncytial virus. N Engl J Med 1962b;267:68-72.

Johnson KM, et al. Acute respiratory disease associated with coxsackie A21 virus infection. I. Incidence in military personnel: observations in a recruit population. JAMA 1962c; 179:112.

Jorgensen JH. Update on mechanisms and prevalence of antimicrobial resistance in *Haemophilus influenzae*. Clin Infect Dis 1992;14:1119-1123.

Kairys SW, Olmstead EM, O'Connor GT. Steroid treatment of laryngotracheitis: a metaanalysis of the evidence from randomized trials. Pediatrics 1989;83:683-693.

Kapikian AZ, et al. An epidemiologic study of altered clinical reactivity to respiratory syncytial (RS) virus infection in children previously vaccinated with an inactivated RS virus vaccine. Am J Epidemiol 1969;89:405-421.

Kaye HS, Marsh HB, Dowdle WR. Seroepidemiologic survey of coronavirus (strain OC 43) related infections in a children's population. Am J Epidemiol 1971;94:43.

Käyhty H, Eskola J. New vaccines for the prevention of pneumococcal infections. Emerg Infect Dis 1996;2:289-298.

Kevy SV. Current concepts: croup. N Engl J Med 1964;270:464.

Kim HW, Arrobio JO, Brandt CD, et al. Epidemiology of respiratory syncytial virus infection in Washington D.C. I. Importance of the virus in different respiratory tract disease syndromes and temporal distribution of infection. Am J Epidemiol 1973a;98:216-225.

Kim HW, Arrobio JO, Brandt CD, et al. Safety and antigenicity of temperature sensitive (ts) mustuant respiratory syncytial virus (RSV) in infants and children. Pediatrics 1973b;52: 56-63.

Kim HW, et al. Respiratory syncytial virus neutralizing activity in nasal secretions following natural infection. Proc Soc Exp Biol Med 1969;131:658.

Klassen TP, Sutcliffe T, Watters LK, et al. Dexamethasone in salbutamol-treated inpatients with acute bronchiolitis: a randomized, controlled trial. J Pediatr 1997;130:191-196.

Klein BS, Dollete FR, Yolken RH. The role of respiratory syncytial virus and other viral pathogens in acute otitis media. J Pediatr 1982;101:16-20.

Kogon A, Spigland I, Frothingham TE, et al. The virus watch program: a continuing surveillance of viral infections in metropolitan New York families. VII. Observations on viral excretion, seroimmunity, intrafamilial spread and illness association in Coxsackie and echovirus infections. Am J Epidemiol 1969;89:51-61.

Kok TW, Varkanis G, Marmion BP, et al. Laboratory diagnosis of *Mycoplasma pneumoniae* infection. I. Direct detection of antigen in respiratory exudates by enzyme immunoassay. Epidemiol Infect 1988;101:669-684.

Komaroff AL, Aronson MD, Pass TM, et al. Serologic evidence of chlamydial and mycoplasmal and pharyngitis in adults. Science 1983;222:927-929.

Koren G, Frand M, Barzilay Z, et al. Corticosteroid treatment of laryngotracheitis v spasmodic croup in children. Am J Dis Child 1983;137:941.

Kosloske AM, Cushing AH, Shuck JM. Early decortication for anaerobic empyema in children. J Pediatr Surg 1980; 15:422.

Kotloff KL, et al. Enteric adenovirus infection and childhood diarrhea: an epidemiologic study in three clinical settings. Pediatrics 1989;84:219-225.

Kovatch AL, Jardin DS, Dowling JN, et al. Legionellosis in children with leukemia in relapse. Pediatrics 1984;73:811.

Lamprecht CL, Krause HE, Mufson MA. Role of maternal antibody in pneumonia and bronchiolitis due to respiratory syncytial virus. J Infect Dis 1976;134:211-217.

Lang WR, et al. Bronchopneumonia with severe sequelae in children with evidence of adenoviruses in the etiology of acute hemorrhagic cystitis. J Urol 1969;1:73.

Lapin CD, Hiatt PW, Langston C, et al. A lamb model for human respiratory syncytial virus infection. Pediatr Pulmonol 1993;15:151-156.

Lattimer CL, McCrone C, Galgon J. Diagnosis of Legionnaires' disease from transtracheal aspirate by direct fluorescent antibody staining and isolation of the bacterium. N Engl J Med 1978;299:1172.

Leipzig B, et al. A prospective randomized study to determine the efficacy of steroids in treatment of croup. J Pediatr 1979; 94:194.

Lerner AM, Klein JO, Finland M. Infections due to coxsackievirus group A type 9 in Boston, 1959, with special reference to exanthems and pneumonia. N Engl J Med 1960;263: 1265-1272.

Li KI, Kiernan S, Wald ER, et al. Isolated uvulitis due to *Haemophilus influenzae* type b. Pediatrics 1984;74:1054.

Light RW, Girard WM, Jenkinson SG, et al. Parapneumonic effusions. Am J Med 1980;69:507.

Lin J-SL. Human mycoplasmal infections: serologic observations. Rev Infect Dis 1985;7:216.

Lindsay MI Jr, et al. Hong Kong influenza: clinical, microbiologic, and pathologic features in 127 cases. JAMA 1970;214:1825.

Lionakis B, Gray SW, Skandalakis JE, et al. Empyema in children; a 25-year study. J Pediatr 1958;53:719.

Liu C. Studies on primary atypical pneumonia. J Exp Med 1957;106:455.

Loda FA, Glezen WP, Clyde WA Jr. Respiratory disease in group day care. Pediatrics 1972;49:428.

Loda FA, et al. Studies on the role of viruses, bacteria, and *M. pneumoniae* as causes of lower respiratory tract infections in children. J Pediatr 1968;72:161.

MacDonald NE, Hall CB, Suffin SC, et al. Respiratory syncytial virus infection in infants with congenital heart disease. N Engl J Med 1982;307:397.

Mannheimer SB, Riley LW, Roberts RB. Association of penicillin-resistant pneumococci with residence in a chronic care facility. J Inf Dis 1996;174:513-519.

Marmion BP, Goodburn GM. Effect of an organic gold salt on Eaton's primary atypical pneumonia agent and other observations. Nature 1961;189:247.

Martin AJ, Gardner PS, McQuillin J. Epidemiology of respiratory viral infection among pediatric inpatients over a 6-year period in northeast England. Lancet 1978;2:1035.

McClung HW, Knight V, Gilbert BE, et al. Ribavirin aerosol treatment of influenza B virus infection. JAMA 1983; 249:2671.

McConnochie KM, Roghmann KJ. Bronchiolitis as a possible cause of wheezing in childhood: new evidence. Pediatrics 1984;74:1.

McIntosh K, Chao RT, Brause HE, et al. Coronavirus infection in acute lower respiratory tract disease in children. J Infect Dis 1974;130:502-507.

McIntosh K, et al. The immunologic response to infection with respiratory syncytial virus in infants. J Infect Dis 1978; 138:24.

McLaughlin FJ, Goldman DA, Rosenbaum DM, et al. Empyema in children: clinical course and long-term follow-up. Pediatrics 1984;73:587.

Melnick JL, et al. Picornaviruses: classification of nine new types. Science 1963;141:153.

Miller ST, Hammerschlag MR, Chirgwin K, et al. Role of *Chlamydia pneumoniae* in acute chest syndrome of sickle cell disease. J Pediatr 1991;118:30-33.

Mills JL, et al. The usefulness of lateral neck roentgenograms in laryngotracheobronchitis. Am J Dis Child 1979;133:1140.

Mintz L, et al. Nosocomial respiratory syncytial virus infections in an intensive care nursery: rapid diagnosis by direct immunofluorescence. Pediatrics 1979;64:149.

MMWR. Update: respiratory syncytial virus activity—United States, 1995-96. 1995;44:900-902.

Moler FW, Steinhart CM, Ohmt ST, et al. Effectiveness of ribavirin in otherwise well infants with respiratory syncytial virus–associated respiratory failure. J Pediatr 1996;128:422-428.

Molteni RA. Epiglottitis: incidence of extraepiglottic infection: report of 72 cases and review of the literature. Pediatrics 1976;58:526.

Monto AS, Cavallaro JJ. The Tecumseh study of respiratory illness. II. Patterns of occurrence of infection with respiratory pathogens, 1965-1969. Am J Epidemiol 1971;94:280-289.

Monto AS, et al. Prevention of Russian influenza by amantadine. JAMA 1979;241:1003.

Morris JA, Blount RE, Savage RE. Recovery of cytopathogenic agent from chimpanzees with coryza. Proc Soc Exp Biol Med 1956;92:544-549.

Moscona A, Peluso RW. Fusion properties of cells persistently infected with human parainfluenza virus type 3: participation of hemagglutinin-neuraminidasein membrane fusion. J Virol 1991;65:2773-2777.

Mufson MA. Pneumococcal infections. JAMA 1981;246:1942.

Mufson MA, Belshe RB. A review of adenoviruses in the etiology of acute hemorrhagic cystitis. J Urol 1976;115:191.

Mufson MA, et al. Eaton agent pneumonia: clinical features. JAMA 1961;178:369.

Munoz R, Fenoll A, Vicioso D, et al. Optochis resistant variants of *Streptococcus pneumoniae*. Diag Microbiol Infect Dis 1990;13:63-66.

Murphy BR. Use of live attenuated cold-adapted influenza A reassortant virus vaccines in infants, children, young adults, and elderly adults. Infect Dis Clin Pract 1993;2:174-181.

Murphy BR, Prince GA, Walsh EE, et al. Dissociation between serum neutralizing antibody responses of infants and children who received inactivated respiratory syncytial virus vaccine. J Clin Microbiol 1986;24:197-202.

Murphy BR, et al. Current approaches to the development of vaccines effective against parainfluenza and respiratory syncytial viruses. Virus Res 1988;11:1-15.

Murphy D, Lockhart CH, Todd JK. Pneumococcal empyema. Am J Dis Child 1980;134:659.

Murphy TF, Henderson FW, Clyde WA, et al. Pneumonia: an 11-year study in a pediatric practice. Am J Epidemiol 1981;113:12.

Neligan GA, et al. Respiratory syncytial virus infection of the newborn. Br Med J 1970;3:146.

Nelson WE. Bacterial croup: a historical perspective. J Pediatr 1984;105:52.

Neumann R, Gensersch B, Eggers HJ. Detection of adenovirus nucleic acid sequences in human tonsils in the absence of infectious virus. Virus Res 1987;7:93-97.

Nichol ST, Spiropoulos CF, Morzunov S, et al. Genetic identification of a hantavirus associated with an outbreak of acute respiratory illness. Science 1993;262:914-917.

Okamoto Y, Kudo K, Shirotori K, et al. Detection of genomic sequences of respiratory syncytial virus in otitis media with effusion in children. Ann Otol Rhinol Laryngol 1992; 157(suppl):7-10.

Ort S, Ryan JL, Barden G, et al. Pneumococcal pneumonia in hospitalized patients. JAMA 1983;249:214.

Outwater KM, Crone RK. Management of respiratory failure in infants with acute viral bronchiolitis. Am J Dis Child 1984; 138:1071.

Pagtakhan RD, Chernick V. Respiratory failure in the pediatric patient. Pediatr Rev 1982;3:247.

Panuska JR, Merolla R, Rebert NA, et al. Respiratory syncytial virus induces interleukin-10 by human alveolar macrophages: suppression of early cytokine production and implications for incomplete immunity. J Clin Invest 1995;96:2445-2453.

Parrott RH, et al. Respiratory diseases of viral etiology. Am J Publ Health 1962;52:907-917.

Parrott RH, Kim HW, Arrobio JO, et al. Epidemiology of respiratory syncytial virus infection in Washington, D.C. II Infection and disease with respect to age, immunologic status, race, and sex. Am J Epidemiol 1973a;98:289-300.

Parrott RH, et al. Epidemiology of respiratory syncitial virus infection in Washington, D.C. Am J Epidemiol 1973b;52:907.

Pedreira FA, Guandolo VL, Feroli EJ, et al. Involuntary smoking and incidence of respiratory illness during the first year of life. Pediatrics 1985;75:594.

Pointon AM, Nicholls JM, Neville S, et al. Chlamydia infection among breeding cattle in south Australia. Austral Vet Pract 1991;21:58-63.

Postma DS, Jones RO, Pillsbury HC. Severe hospitalized croup: treatment trends and prognosis. Laryngoscope 1984;94:1170-1175.

Preston FM, Beier PL, Pope JH. Infectious respiratory syncytial virus (RSV) effectively inhibits the proliferative T-cell response to inactivated RSV in vitro. J Infect Dis 1992; 165:819-825.

Pullan CR, Hey EN. Wheezing, asthma, and pulmonary dysfunction 10 years after infection with respiratory syncytial virus in infancy. Brit Med J 1982;248:1665-1669.

Rabe EF. Infectious croup. I. Etiology. II. "Virus" croup. III. *Haemophilus influenza* type b croup. Pediatrics 1948;2:255, 415, 559.

Radowski MA, Kransler JK, Beem MO, et al. *Chlamydia* pneumonia in infants: radiography in 125 cases. Am J Roent 1981;137:703-706.

Report of the Committee on Infectious Diseases, ed 23. Elk Grove, Ill.: American Academy of Pediatrics, 1994.

Richardson LS, et al. Enzyme-linked immunosorbent assay for measurement of serological response to respiratory syncytial virus infection. Infect Immun 1978;20:660-664.

Riley ID, Alpers MP, Gratten H, et al. Pneumococcal vaccine prevents death from acute lower-respiratory-tract infections in Papua New Guinean children. Lancet 1986;2:877-881.

Robertson JS, Nicholson C, Newman R, et al. High-growth reassortant influenza vaccine viruses: new approaches to their control. Biologicals 1992;20:213-220.

Rooney JC, Williams HE. The relationship between proven viral bronchiolitis and subsequent wheezing. J Pediatr 1971; 79:744-747.

Rowe WP, et al. Isolation of a cytopathogenic agent from human adenoids undergoing spontaneous degeneration in tissue culture. Proc Soc Exp Biol Med 1953;84:570.

Salkind AR, McCarthy DO, Nichols JE, et al. Interleukin-1 and interleukin-1 inhibitor activity induced by respiratory syncytial virus: Abrogation of virus-specific and alternate human lymphocyte proliferative responses. J Infect Dis 1991; 193:71-77.

Sanford JP. Legionnaires' disease: the first thousand days. N Engl J Med 1979;300:654.

Santosham M, Yolken RH, Zuiroz E, et al. Detection of rotavirus in respiratory secretions of children with pneumonia. J Pediatr 1983;103:583.

Sanyal SK, Mariencheck WC, Hughes WT, et al. Course of pulmonary dysfunction in children surviving *Pneumocystis carinii* pneumonitis: a prospective study. Am Rev Respir Dis 1981;124:161.

Schachter J. Chlamydial infections. N Engl J Med 1978; 298:428, 490, 540.

Schachter J, Sugg N, Sung M. Psittacosis: the reservoir persists. J Infect Dis 1978;137:44.

Schachter J, et al. Pneumonitis following inclusion blennorrhea. J Pediatr 1975;87:779.

Schachter J, et al. Prospective study of chlamydial infections in neonates. Lancet 1979;2:377.

Shands KN, Ho JL, Meyer RD, et al. Potable water as a source of Legionnaires' disease. JAMA 1985;253:1412.

Shapiro ED, Berg AT, Austrian R, et al. The protective efficacy of polyvalent pneumococcal polysaccharide vaccine. N Engl J Med 1991;325:1453-1460.

Shope RE. The influenza of swine and man. Harvey Lect 1935-1936;31:183.

Shuh S, Canny G, Reisman JJ, et al. Nebulized albuterol in acute bronchiolitis. J Pediatr 1990;117:633-637.

Siegel JD, Gartner JC, Michaels RH. Pneumococcal empyema in childhood. Am J Dis Child 1978;132:1094.

Siegel ST, Wolff LJ, Baehner RL, et al. Treatment of *Pneumocystis carinii* pneumonitis. Am J Dis Child 1984;138:1051.

Simila S, Linna O, Lenning P, et al. Chronic lung damage caused by adenovirus type 7: a 10-year follow-up study. Chest 1981;80:127-131.

Skolnik NS. Treatment of croup: a critical review. Am J Dis Child 1989;143:1045-1049.

Smit P, et al. Protective efficacy of pneumococcal polysaccharide vaccines. JAMA 1977;238:2613.

Smith CB, Purcell RH, Bellanti JA, Chanock RM. Protective effect of antibody to parainfluenza type 1 virus. N Engl J Med 1966;275:1145.

Smith W, Andrewes CH, Laidlaw PO. A virus obtained from influenza patients. Lancet 1933;2:66.

Stagno S, Brasfield DM, Brown MB, et al. Infant pneumonitis associated with cytomegalovirus, chlamydia, *Pneumocystis,* and *Ureaplasma:* a prospective study. Pediatrics 1981; 68:322.

Stagno S, Pifer LL, Hughest WT, et al. *Pneumocystis carinii* pneumonitis in young immunocompetent infants. Pediatrics 1980;66:56-62.

Steen-Johnsen J, Orstavik I, Attramadal A. Severe illnesses due to adenovirus type 7 in children. Acta Paediatri Scand 1969;58:157.

Steigman AJ, Lipton MM, Brapennicke H. Acute lymphonodular pharyngitis: a newly described condition due to coxsackie A virus. Am J Dis Child 1962;102:713.

Stephens RS. Molecular mimicry and *Chlamydia trachomatis* infection of eukaryotic cells. Trends Microbiol 1994;2:99-101.

Stiles QR, Lindesmith GG, Tucker BL, et al. Pleural empyema in children. Ann Thorac Surg 1970;10:37.

Stott EJ, Ball LA, Anderson K, et al. Immune and histopathological responses in animals vaccinated with recombinant vaccinia viruses that express individual genes of human respiratory syncytial virus. J Virol 1987;61:3855-3861.

Stuart-Harris C. Swine influenza virus in man. Lancet 1976;2:31.

Sussman SJ, Magoffin RL, Lennette EH, Schieble J. Cold agglutinins, Eaton agent, and respiratory infections of children. Pediatrics 1966;38:571.

Taussig LM, Castro O, Beaudry PH, et al. Treatment of laryngotracheobronchitis (croup): use of intermittent positive-pressure breathing and racemic epinephrine. Am J Dis Child 1975;129:790-793.

Taussig LM, et al. Treatment of laryngotracheobronchitis (croup). Am J Dis Child 1977;238:2613.

Taylor-Robinson D, Tyrrell DA. Serotypes of viruses (rhinoviruses) isolated from common colds. Lancet 1962;1:452.

Terranova W, Cohen MI, Fraser DW. 1974 outbreak of Legionnaires' disease diagnosed in 1977, clinical and epidemiological features. Lancet 1978;2:122.

Travis KW, Todrez ID, Shannon DC. Pulmonary edema associated with croup and epiglottitis. Pediatrics 1977;59:695.

Tristram DA, Welliver RC, Mohar CK, et al. Immunogenicity and safety of respiratory syncytial virus subunit vaccine in seropositive children 18-30 months old. J Infect Dis 1993;167:191-195.

Tristram DA, Welliver RC. Respiratory syncytial virus. In Murray PR et al. (eds.). Manual of clinical microbiology, ed 6. Washington, D.C.: ASM Press, 1995.

Turner JAP, Corkey CWB, Lee JYC, et al. Clinical expressions of immotile cilia syndrome. Pediatrics 1981;67:805.

Turner RB, Hayden FG, Hendley JO. Counterimmunoelectrophoresis of urine for diagnosis of bacterial pneumonia in pediatric outpatients. Pediatrics 1983;71:780.

Unger A, Tapia L, Mimnich LL, et al. Atypical neonatal respiratory syncytial virus infection. J Pediatr 1982;100:762.

Valenti WM, Clarke TA, Hall CB, et al. Concurrent outbreaks of rhinovirus and respiratory syncytial virus in an intensive care nursery: epidemiology and associated risk factors. J Pediatr 1982;100:722.

Van Buchen FL, Knottnervs JA, Schrijnemaators VJJ. Primary care-based randomised placebo-controlled trial of antibiotic treatment in acute maxillary sinusitis. Lancet 1997;341:683-687.

Van der Veen J, Oei KG, Abarbanal MFW. Patterns of infections with adenovirus types 4, 7, and 21 in military recruits during a 9-year survey. J Hyg (Camb) 1969;67:255-268.

Wald ER. Sinusitis in children. N Engl J Med 1992;326:319-323.

Wald ER, Chiponis D, Ledesma-Medina J. Comparative effectiveness of amoxacillin and amoxacillin-clavulanate potassium in acute paranasal sinus infection in children: a double-blind, placebo-controlled trial. Pediatrics 1986;77:795-800.

Wald ER, Milmoe GJ, Bowen A, et al. Acute maxillary sinusitis in children. N Engl J Med 1981;304:749-754.

Walsh EE, Hall CB, Briselli M, et al. Immunization with glycoprotein subunits of respiratory syncytial virus to protect cotton rats against viral infection. J Infect Dis 1987;155:1198-1203.

Wang EL, Prober CG, Manson B, et al. Association of respiratory viral infections with pulmonary deterioration in patients with cystic fibrosis. N Engl J Med 1984;311:1653.

Weber ML, et al. Acute epiglottitis in children: treatment with nasotracheal intubation. Pediatrics 1976;57:152.

Webster RG, Bean WJ Jr, Gorman OT, et al. Evolution and ecology of influenza A viruses. Microbiol Rev 1992;56:152-179.

Welliver RC. Detection, pathogenesis, and therapy of respiratory syncytial virus infections. Clin Micro Rev 1988;1:27-39.

Welliver RC, Kaul A, Ogra PL. Cell-mediated immune response to respiratory syncytial virus infection: relationship to the development of reactive airway disease. J Pediatr 1979;94:370.

Welliver RC, Sun M, Rinaldo D, Ogra PL. Predictive value of respiratory syncytial virus specific IgE responses for recurrent wheezing following bronchiolitis. J Pediatr 1986;109:776-780.

Welliver R, Wong DT, Choi TS, Ogra PL. Natural history of parainfluenza virus infection in childhood. J Pediatr 1982;101:180-187.

Welliver RC, et al. Role of parainfluenza virus specific IgE in pathogenesis of croup and wheezing subsequent to infection. J Pediatr 1982;101:889-896.

Wenzel RP, Hendley JO, Davies JA, et al. Coronavirus infections in military recruits. Am Rev Resp Dis 1974;109:621-624.

Wenzel RP, et al. Hospital-acquired viral respiratory illness on a pediatric ward. Pediatrics 1977;60:367.

Westley CR, Cotton EK, Brooks JG. Nebulized racemic epinephrine by IPPB for the treatment of croup. Am J Dis Child 1978;132:484.

Wheeler JG, Wofford J, Turner RB. Historical cohort evaluation of ribavirin efficacy in respiratory syncytial virus infection. Ped Inf Dis J 1993;12:209-213.

Winterbauer RH, Dreis DF. Thoracic empyema: handling a dangerous infection wisely. J Respir Dis 1983;116.

Wolfe WG, Spock A, Bradford WD. Pleural fluid in infants and children. Am Rev Respir Dis 1968;98:1027.

Wright PF, Belshe RB, Kim HW, et al. Administration of a highly attenuated live respiratory syncytial virus vaccine to adults and children. Infect Immun 1982;37:397-400.

Yunis EJ, et al. Adenovirus and ileocecal intussusception. Lab Invest 1975;33:347.

Zollar LM, Krause HE, Mufson MA. Microbiologic studies on young infants and lower respiratory tract disease. Am J Dis Child 1973;126:56.

Zuravleff JJ, Yu VC, Shonnard JW, et al. Diagnosis of Legionnaires' disease. JAMA 1983;250:1981.

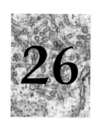

26 RUBELLA (GERMAN MEASLES)

Rubella is an acute infectious disease characterized by minimal or absent prodromal symptoms; a 3-day rash; and generalized lymph node enlargement, particularly of the postauricular, suboccipital, and cervical lymph nodes. Before 1941 rubella was important chiefly because it was responsible for epidemics in schools and military installations and because it was frequently confused with measles and scarlet fever. Since 1941 a great deal of interest has been focused on this disease because of the association of rubella during pregnancy with an increased incidence of congenital malformations. Since the widespread use of live attenuated rubella vaccine in the United States beginning in the late 1960s, rubella has become an unusual disease occurring mainly in irregular mini-epidemics, especially among the unvaccinated.

ETIOLOGY

Rubella is caused by a specific virus that is present in the blood and nasopharyngeal secretions of patients with the disease. Based on his transmission studies with rhesus monkeys, Hess postulated in 1914 that rubella was caused by a virus. This observation was not confirmed until 1938, when Hiro and Tasaka produced the disease in children by inoculating them with filtered nasal washings obtained from patients during the acute phase of rubella. In 1942 Habel et al. also successfully transmitted rubella to the rhesus monkey, using nasal washings and blood. Reports by Anderson in 1949 and by Krugman et al. in 1953 confirmed Hiro and Tasaka's findings. Krugman et al. (1953) and Krugman and Ward (1954) also demonstrated that virus was present in the blood 2 days before and on the first day of rash and proved conclusively that rubella can occur without a rash. The cultivation of rubella virus in tissue culture was reported independently and simultaneously by two groups. In 1962 Weller and Neva observed a cytopathic effect

in human amnion cells. At the same time, Parkman et al. (1962) isolated the virus in cultures of African green monkey kidney tissue. Cells infected with rubella virus remained normal in appearance in spite of challenge with echovirus type 11, which characteristically causes a cytopathic effect.

Rubella virus is a moderately large single-stranded RNA virus. On the basis of its biochemical, biophysical, and ultrastructural properties, rubella virus is classified in the family Togavirus, which embraces the genus *Alphavirus* (which includes many arboviruses), and the genus *Rubivirus,* of which rubella virus is the only agent. The clinical and laboratory behavior of rubella virus, however, is more like that of the paramyxoviruses. It does not require a vector for transmission, and there is no RNA sequence homology between rubella virus and other togaviruses. Its nucleocapsid is 30 nm in diameter, and it is surrounded by a lipid envelope, 60 to 70 nm in diameter, that contains glycoproteins. The nucleocapsid protein consists of four polypeptides. The envelope glycoprotein consists of E1 and E2 glycopeptides. Hemagglutination inhibition and neutralizing antibodies react with the E1 peptides (Dorsett et al., 1985).

Rubella virus is highly sensitive to heat, to extremes of pH, and to a variety of chemical agents. It is rapidly inactivated at 56° C and at 37° C. However, at 4° C the virus titer is relatively stable for 24 hours. For long-term preservation of the virus, a temperature of −60° C is much better than the usual deep-freeze temperature of −20° C. It is inactivated by a pH below 6.8 or above 8.1, ultraviolet irradiation, ether, chloroform, formalin, β-propiolactone, and other chemicals. It is resistant to thimerosal (Merthiolate) (1:10,000 solution) and antibiotics.

Rubella virus has been cultivated in a variety of tissue cultures. In general, the virus produces interference with growth of certain other viruses (which

402

is used as a marker for growth of rubella virus) without a cytopathic effect in the following primary tissue culture cells: African green monkey kidney, bovine embryo kidney, guinea pig kidney, rabbit kidney, human amnion, and human embryonic kidney. Interference without a cytopathic effect has also been observed in rhesus monkey and human diploid cell lines. Cytopathic effect has been observed in a variety of continuous cell lines, including rabbit kidney (RK13), rabbit cornea, and hamster (BHK-21). Rubella virus strains belong to one serologic type. Hemagglutination and complement-fixing antigens have been prepared in several tissue culture systems. The inhibition of these antigens by specific rubella antisera has formed the basis for practical serologic tests.

POSTNATALLY ACQUIRED RUBELLA
Clinical Manifestations

The first symptoms of rubella occur after an incubation period of approximately 16 to 18 days, with a range of 14 to 21 days. The typical clinical course is illustrated in Fig. 26-1. In the child the first sign of illness is the appearance of the rash. In adolescents and adults, however, the eruption is preceded by a 1- to 5-day prodromal period characterized by low-grade fever, headache, malaise, anorexia, mild conjunctivitis, coryza, sore throat, cough, and lymphadenopathy. These symptoms rapidly subside after the first day of rash. The enanthem of

rubella, described by Forschheimer in 1898, may be observed in many patients during the prodromal period or on the first day of rash. It consists of reddish spots, pinpoint or larger in size, located on the soft palate. In patients with scarlet fever the soft palate may be covered with punctate lesions, and in patients with measles it may have a red, blotchy appearance; these lesions are indistinguishable from the enanthem of rubella. Obviously, the so-called Forschheimer spots are not pathognomonic for rubella and do not have the same diagnostic significance as Koplik's spots in measles.

Lymph Node Involvement. Observations on patients with experimentally induced rubella or during epidemics indicate that lymph node enlargement may begin as early as 7 days before onset of rash (Fig. 26-2). There is generalized lymphadenopathy, but the suboccipital, postauricular, and cervical nodes are most commonly involved. The swelling and tenderness are most apparent and severe on the first day of rash. Subsequently, the tenderness subsides within 1 or 2 days, but the palpable enlargement of the nodes may persist for several weeks or more. As indicated in Table 26-1, the extent of the lymphadenopathy may be extremely variable; occasionally it may even be absent. At times, splenomegaly also may be noted during the acute stage of the disease. Nevertheless, involvement of the suboccipital, postauricular, and cervical lymph nodes is not pathognomonic for rubella. Lymphadenopathy is associated with diseases such as measles, chickenpox, adenovirus infections, and infectious mononucleosis.

Exanthem. The rash, particularly in children, may be the first obvious indication of illness. It appears first on the face and then spreads downward rapidly to the neck, arms, trunk, and extremities. The eruption appears, spreads, and disappears more quickly than does the rash of measles (Fig. 26-3). By the end of the first day the entire body may be covered with the discrete pink-red maculopapules. On the second day, the rash begins to disappear from the face, and the lesions on the trunk may coalesce to form a uniform red blush that may resemble the rash of mild scarlet fever. The lesions on the extremities, however, remain discrete and generally do not coalesce. In the typical case the rash has disappeared by the end of the third day. If the eruption has been intensive, there may be some fine, branny desquamation; usually there is none.

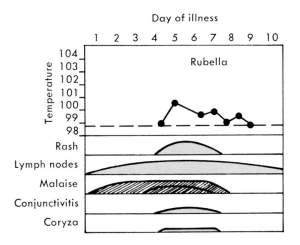

FIG. 26-1 Schematic diagram illustrating typical course of rubella in children and adults. Lymph nodes begin to enlarge 3 to 4 days before rash. Prodromal symptoms (malaise) are minimal in children *(shaded area)*. In adults there may be a 3- to 4-day prodrome *(hatched area)*. Conjunctivitis and coryza, if present, are usually minimal and accompany the rash.

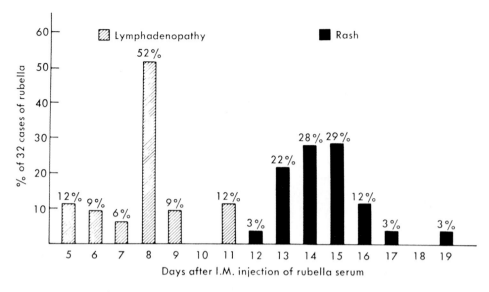

Fig. 26-2   Time of onset of lymphadenopathy and rash in 32 cases of experimentally transmitted rubella. Note appearance of lymphadenopathy 5 to 7 days before onset of rash. (From Green RH et al.: Am J Dis Child 1965;110:348.)

Table 26-1   Clinical aspects of experimental rubella in children

Patient	Maximum temperature (F°)	Rash	Lymph node enlargement	Leukopenia
C.R.	100.4	+	++	0
J.G.	101.6	0	+	0
P.K.	100.8	0	++	++
N.K.	99.6	++	+	++
E.T.	101.6	+++	+++	0
K.L.	100.4	++	+	+
J.S.	99.0	++	+	0
S.E.	99.4	++	0	0
G.O.	99.8	++	++	0
C.N.	99.4	+++	+++	—
P.A.	99.6	+++	++	—
T.B.	99.2	+	+	—
M.I.	99.4	++	+++	—

From Krugman S, Ward R: J Pediatr 1954;44:489.
+, Mild; ++, moderate; +++, marked; *0*, none; —, not done.

The characteristic pink-red lesions of rubella differ from the purple-red lesions of measles and the yellow-red lesions of scarlet fever. In rubella the lesions are generally discrete and may or may not coalesce; if they do, a diffuse erythematous blush results. In contrast, the lesions of measles, particularly around the head and neck, tend to coalesce and form irregular blotches with crescentic margins. The similarities and differences between the eruptions of rubella and those of scarlet fever have been referred to previously. The circumoral area also differs in these two diseases; in rubella the rash involves this area, and in scarlet fever there is circumoral pallor.

The duration and extent of the rash may be variable. The eruption, which as a rule lasts for 3 days, may persist for 5 days or may be so evanescent that it disappears in less than a day. In an unknown num-

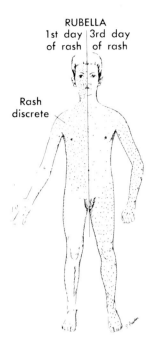

RUBELLA
1st day | 3rd day
of rash | of rash

Rash
discrete

FIG. 26-3 Schematic drawing illustrating development and distribution of rubella rash.

ber of instances, rubella may even occur without a rash. The existence of rubella without rash has been established. In thirteen cases of experimentally induced rubella that we studied in 1954 (see Table 26-1), the rash was extensive in three, moderate in six, mild in two, and absent in two. In 1965 Green et al. studied twenty-four children who were intimately exposed to rubella. A rise in rubella virus–neutralizing antibody titer was observed in twenty-two of the children. Rubella without rash occurred in eight of the twenty-two infected children. These two studies suggest that the incidence of subclinical rubella infections is approximately 25%.

Fever. In children the temperature may be either normal or slightly elevated. Fever, if present, rarely persists beyond the first day of rash and is usually low grade. A typical temperature course is illustrated in Fig. 26-1. During epidemics, patients with rubella occasionally have temperatures as high as 40° C (104° F). In adolescents and adults there may be low-grade fever during both the prodromal period and the first day of rash. The maximum temperature in a group of thirteen children with experimentally induced rubella is listed in Table 26-1; in eight the temperature was normal, and in five it ranged between 38° and 38.7° C (100.4° and 101.6° F).

Hematologic Manifestations. Generally, the white blood cell count is low. As indicated in Table 26-1, however, the white blood cell count may be normal. An increased number of plasma cells and Türk's cells also have been described in rubella. Occasionally there may be an increased percentage of abnormal lymphocytes or a decrease in platelets.

Diagnosis

Confirmatory Clinical Factors. A diagnosis of rubella is suggested by the appearance of a maculopapular eruption beginning on the face, progressing rapidly downward to the trunk and extremities, and subsiding within 3 days. Prodromal symptoms are minimal or absent, fever is low grade or absent, and lymphadenopathy precedes the appearance of the rash. A history of exposure, if available, is helpful.

Detection of Causative Agent. As indicated in Fig. 26-4, rubella virus may be recovered from the pharynx as early as 7 days before the onset of rash and as late as 14 days after onset of rash. The availability of virus isolation procedures has provided an important laboratory tool for the precise diagnosis of rubella. As indicated in Fig. 26-4, virus may be recovered from the pharynx with regularity within 5 days after the onset of rash; in contrast, viremia that is present before the onset of rash is rarely observed after the onset of rash.

Serologic Tests. The pattern of appearance and persistence of rubella virus–neutralizing, complement-fixing (CF), and hemagglutination-inhibition (HI) antibody is shown in Fig. 26-4. Antibody is usually detectable by the third day of rash, and peak levels are reached approximately 1 month later. CF antibody may be short lived, declining to nondetectable levels within a year or more after infection. Neutralizing and HI antibodies usually persist for life. The HI antibody test has the advantages of high sensitivity and early availability of results. The most commonly used test today is an enzyme-linked immunosorbent assay (ELISA), which can be used to measure IgG and IgM antibodies to rubella. For serologic diagnosis the acute-phase serum should be obtained as early as possible after onset of rash, and convalescent-phase serum should be collected 2 to 4 weeks later. Acute rubella may be diagnosed by a fourfold or greater rise in titer of IgG antibodies in paired acute-phase and convalescent-phase serum specimens or by the presence of rubella-specific IgM antibodies in one

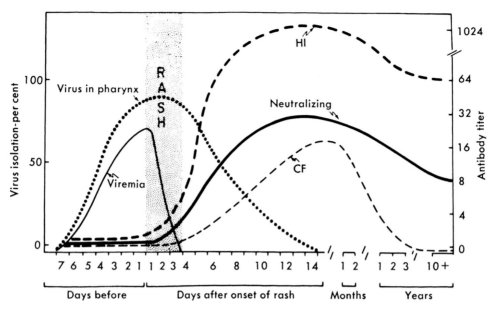

Fig. 26-4   Natural history of postnatal rubella. Pattern of virus excretion and antibody response. (Modified from Cooper LZ, Krugman S: Arch Ophthalmol 1967;77:434.)

serum specimen. False-negative and false-positive IgM reactions may occur, however. In addition, true positive IgM reactions may be demonstrated in primary infections and reinfections.

Differential Diagnosis. Other diseases that may mimic rubella include toxoplasmosis, scarlet fever, modified measles, roseola (caused by human herpesvirus–6 infection), fifth disease (erythema infectiosum, caused by parvovirus infection), and enteroviral infections. Additional information is discussed in Chapter 40.

Complications

Rubella in childhood is rarely followed by complications. Secondary bacterial infections, which are so common in measles, are not encountered in rubella. The following complications have been observed, especially during epidemics.

Arthritis. Joint involvement in adolescents and adults with rubella is much more common than is generally appreciated. It usually develops just as the rash is fading on the second to third day of illness. Either one or more of the larger and smaller joints may be involved. The arthritis may be manifested by a return of fever and either transient joint pain without swelling or massive effusion into one or more joint spaces. These manifestations usually clear spontaneously within 5 to 10 days but may on

occasion take several weeks to resolve. However, chronic arthritis that lasts for longer periods following rubella is exceedingly rare.

Rubella arthritis with involvement of the knees, ankles, or elbows may simulate the polyarthritis of rheumatic fever. When there is fusiform swelling of the fingers, it may resemble rheumatoid arthritis. In a study of ten female patients with rubella arthritis of the small- and medium-sized joints that lasted 1 week, positive latex fixation tests for rheumatoid factor were demonstrated in nine of the ten patients with arthritis as compared with only two of seven patients who had rubella without arthritis (Johnson and Hall, 1958). In another study of fourteen women observed for a 2- to 5-year follow-up period after experiencing rubella arthritis, however, none showed any clinical manifestations suggesting rheumatoid disease (Kantor and Tanner, 1962). During an epidemic of rubella in a London suburb, Fry et al. (1962) observed arthritis in 15% of seventy-four adults with rubella; they detected arthritis in 33% of forty females and in 6% of thirty-four males. During an epidemic of rubella in Bermuda in 1971, joint manifestations were observed in 25% of children under the age of 11 years and in 52% of patients 11 years of age or older (Judelsohn and Wyll, 1973). Rubella virus has been isolated from joint fluid taken from patients with acute rubella arthritis and from peripheral blood of those with chronic rubella arthritis.

Encephalitis. Complications of rubella in the central nervous system (CNS) are extremely rare. Encephalitis is less commonly encountered after rubella than after measles or varicella. The incidence usually cited is 1 in 6,000 cases of rubella. The clinical manifestations are similar to those observed in other types of postinfectious encephalitis. Complete recovery is generally the rule, but fatalities have been reported. Observations by Kenny et al. in 1965 indicated that demyelinization apparently is not a feature of rubella encephalopathy. Neurologic abnormalities are minor and occur infrequently, and intellectual function is generally unaffected if the patient survives. However, electroencephalographic abnormalities are relatively common and persistent.

Purpura. Thrombocytopenic and nonthrombocytopenic purpura may, in rare instances, complicate rubella. In addition to a reduction in platelet count, there is usually prolonged bleeding time and increased capillary fragility. In some reported cases the clinical manifestations have included one or more of the following disorders: cutaneous hemorrhages; epistaxis; bleeding gums; hematuria; bleeding from the intestinal tract; and, rarely, cerebral hemorrhage. Most patients become symptom-free within 2 weeks, and the platelet count returns to normal values. Thrombocytopenia may last from weeks to months; it may be associated with long-term sequelae if there is bleeding into organs such as the eye and the brain.

Prognosis

The prognosis is almost uniformly excellent. Rubella is one of the most benign of all infectious diseases in children. However, the rare complications of encephalitis and thrombocytopenic purpura may alter the prognosis. Many reported deaths attributed to rubella infection reflect errors in diagnosis. Immunosuppressed patients have not been reported to be at increased risk from rubella, as they are for measles.

Immunity

Active Immunity. One attack of rubella is generally followed by permanent immunity. Although some so-called second attacks represent errors in diagnosis, it is now recognized that clinical reinfection can occur, although rarely, with this virus. Viremia is believed to be rare in reinfections. Active immunity is induced by infection after natural exposure or immunization. As indicated in Fig. 26-4, rubella-neutralizing antibody may persist for many years after infection.

Passive Immunity. Neutralizing antibodies for rubella are present in gamma globulin and in convalescent-phase serum. Rubella, like measles and mumps, is rarely observed in the early months of life because of transplacentally acquired immunity.

Epidemiologic Factors

Rubella is worldwide in distribution. It is endemic in most large cities where vaccination is not routine. In such areas, localized epidemics occur at irregular intervals compared to the fairly consistent periodicity of measles. During the prevaccine era, major epidemics occurred at 6- to 9-year intervals. Rubella outbreaks usually occur during the spring months in the temperate zones. The extensive and routine use of live attenuated rubella vaccine since licensure in 1969 has had a major impact on the epidemiology of the disease. The last epidemic in the United States occurred in 1964. During the subsequent 28 years there was a progressive decrease in the number of reported cases of rubella. Major epidemics of the disease have been eliminated in the United States.

The age distribution of rubella during the prevaccine era was striking. It was rare in infancy and uncommon in preschool-age children. There was an unusually high incidence of the disease in older children, adolescents, and young adults. Rubella was a constant problem in boarding schools, colleges, and military installations. A significant number of workdays were lost as a result of outbreaks among military personnel.

Rubella is probably spread via the respiratory route. Studies of human volunteers have confirmed this impression. The disease has been transmitted with nasopharyngeal secretions obtained from patients with rubella on the first day of the rash. The period of infectivity probably extends from the latter part of the incubation period to the end of the third day of the rash.

Isolation and Quarantine

Isolation and quarantine precautions generally are not warranted. However, outbreaks of rubella have been a problem among hospital and medical personnel in several states, including New York (McLaughlin and Gold, 1979), California, and Colorado (Edell et al., 1979). During the New York experience a male physician with rubella exposed 170 persons, including susceptible pregnant patients. These episodes created a difficult problem for institutions and staff—a problem that is prevented today by the following measure: (1) routine screening of both male and female medical personnel caring for patients who may be pregnant, and (2) immunization of those with no detectable rubella antibody.

Treatment

Symptomatic Treatment. In many instances, rubella is asymptomatic and requires no treatment at all. Even if the child has a low-grade fever, bed rest may be unnecessary. Headache, malaise, and pain in the lymph nodes can be easily controlled with acetaminophen. No specific antiviral therapy is available.

Treatment of Complications. Arthritis is usually well controlled by aspirin. Bed rest is advised if there is fever or involvement of the weight-bearing joints. A patient with encephalitis should be treated in the same way as a patient with measles encephalitis (p. 259). Corticosteroid therapy and platelet transfusions may be indicated in severe cases of thrombocytopenic purpura.

CONGENITAL RUBELLA

Congenital rubella was identified as a clinical entity more than a century after the disease was first recognized. In 1941 Gregg reported the occurrence of congenital cataracts among seventy-eight infants born after maternal rubella infection acquired during the 1940 epidemic in Australia. More than half of these infants had congenital heart disease. Since 1941 Gregg's report of the rubella syndrome has been amply confirmed. The occurrence of rubella during the first trimester of pregnancy has been associated with a significantly increased incidence of congenital malformations, stillbirths, and abortions. The epidemic of rubella in the United States in 1964 was followed by the birth of many thousands of infants with the congenital rubella syndrome. Today there are typically less than ten cases of congenital rubella reported annually in the United States.

Pathogenesis

Studies by many investigators have provided evidence to support the following concept of the natural history of congenital rubella. As indicated in Fig. 26-4, viremia is present for several days before onset of rash. Maternal viremia may be followed by a placental infection and subsequent fetal viremia, leading to a disseminated infection involving many fetal organs. Timing is the crucial element in the pathogenesis of congenital rubella. A fetal infection probably will be chronic and persistent if it is acquired during the early weeks and months of pregnancy. However, after the fourth month of gestation, the fetus apparently is no longer susceptible to the chronic infection that is characteristic of intrauterine rubella during the first 8 to 12 weeks.

The pathogenesis of rubella embryopathy is not entirely clear. Studies in human embryonic tissue culture cells have indicated that rubella infection was associated with inhibition of mitosis and an increased number of chromosomal breaks (Plotkin et al., 1965). Autopsies of infants with congenital rubella revealed hypoplastic organs with a subnormal number of cells (Naeye and Blanc, 1965). Consequently, it is likely that rubella embryopathy may be caused by (1) inhibition of cellular multiplication; (2) chronic, persistent infection during the crucial period of organogenesis; or (3) a combination of both factors.

Clinical Manifestations

The classic rubella syndrome described by Gregg and others in the 1940s was characterized by intrauterine growth retardation, cataracts, microcephaly, deafness, congenital heart disease, and mental retardation. Extensive studies of this syndrome during the 1964 rubella epidemic in the United States shed new light on this problem. The availability of specific virus isolation and serologic techniques provided information that revealed a broader spectrum of this disease. Intrauterine rubella infection may be followed by spontaneous abortion of the infected fetus, a stillbirth, live birth of an infant with single or multiple malformations, or birth of a normal infant. The various manifestations of congenital rubella are listed in Box 26-1. It is clear that the consequences of rubella infection during pregnancy are varied and unpredictable. Virtually every organ may be involved—singly, multiply, transiently, or progressively and permanently.

Neonatal Manifestations. A variety of clinical manifestations may be present during the first weeks of life. Low birth weight in relation to period of gestation is common. Thrombocytopenic purpura characterized by a petechial and purpuric eruption may occur in association with other transient conditions, such as hepatosplenomegaly, hepatitis, hemolytic anemia, bone lesions (metaphyseal rarefac-

---

BOX 26-1

MANIFESTATIONS OF CONGENITAL RUBELLA

Growth retardation (low birth weight)
Eye defects
    Cataracts
    Glaucoma
    Retinopathy
    Microphthalmia
Deafness
Cardiac defects
    Patent ductus arteriosus
    Ventricular septal defect
    Pulmonary stenosis
    Myocardial necrosis
Central nervous system defects
    Psychomotor retardation
    Microcephaly
    Encephalitis
    Spastic quadriparesis
    Cerebrospinal fluid pleocytosis
    Mental retardation
    Progressive panencephalitis
Hepatomegaly
Hepatitis
Thrombocytopenic purpura
Splenomegaly
Bone lesions
Interstitial pneumonitis
Diabetes mellitus
Psychiatric disorders
Thyroid disorders
Precocious puberty

---

fants have tolerated the cardiac lesions with little difficulty; others have developed congestive heart failure in the first months of life.

Eye Defects. Cataracts, unilateral or bilateral, are common consequences of congenital rubella. They appear as pearly white nuclear lesions, frequently associated with microphthalmia. The cataracts may be too small at birth to be visible on casual examination. A careful ophthalmoscopic examination with a +8 lens held 15 to 20 cm from the eye may reveal an early cataract. Rubella glaucoma is a less common eye lesion, and it may be clinically indistinguishable from hereditary infantile glaucoma. It may be present at birth, or it may appear after the neonatal period. The cornea is enlarged and hazy, the anterior chamber is deep, and ocular tension is increased. Glaucoma that requires prompt surgical therapy must be differentiated from transient corneal clouding. Retinopathy is the most common eye manifestation of congenital rubella. It is characterized by discrete, patchy, black pigmentation that is variable in size and location. Retinopathy does not affect visual acuity if the lesions do not involve the macular area. The presence of this lesion is a valuable aid in the clinical diagnosis of congenital rubella.

Hearing Loss. Deafness may be the only manifestation of congenital rubella. It may be unilateral but is usually bilateral. It is probably caused by maldevelopment and possibly by degenerative changes in the cochlea and organ of Corti. Hearing loss may be severe or so mild that it is overlooked unless detected by an audiometric examination. Severe bilateral hearing loss is responsible for speech defects.

Central Nervous System Involvement. Psychomotor retardation is a common manifestation of congenital rubella. In severe cases the brain is the site of a chronic, persistent infection, as indicated by the presence of pleocytosis, increased concentration of protein, and rubella virus in the CSF for as long as 1 year after birth. Microcephaly is a well-known manifestation (Desmond et al., 1967). The most common consequence of CNS involvement is mental retardation (mild or profound). Behavioral disturbances and manifestations of minimal cerebral dysfunction also are common. Less common are severe spastic diplegia and autism.

Progressive rubella panencephalitis was described in four patients with congenital rubella

tion), and bulging anterior fontanelle with or without pleocytosis in the cerebrospinal fluid (CSF). These transient manifestations may occur in association with the classic cardiac, eye, hearing, and CNS defects. An infant with neonatal thrombocytopenic purpura characterized by the typical "blueberry muffin" skin lesions is shown in Plate 5.

Cardiac Defects. Patent ductus arteriosus, with or without pulmonary artery stenosis, and atrial and ventricular septal defects are the most common cardiac lesions. Clinical evidence of congenital heart disease may be present at birth or delayed for several days. Other cardiac manifestations include myocardial involvement, as indicated by electrocardiographic findings, and necropsy evidence of extensive necrosis of the myocardium. Many in-

(Townsend et al., 1975; Weil et al., 1975). Severe, progressive, neurologic deterioration was noted during the second decade of life. In two patients there was progression of spasticity, ataxia, intellectual deterioration, seizures, and subsequent fatality. Other findings included (1) high levels of rubella antibody in serum and CSF, (2) increased levels of CSF protein and gamma globulin, (3) histopathologic changes in the brain, and (4) isolation of rubella virus from a brain biopsy of one of the patients. In some ways this syndrome resembled subacute sclerosing panencephalitis, a rare complication of measles.

Diagnosis

The presence of congenital rubella should be suspected under the following circumstances: (1) a history of possible rubella or exposure to rubella during the first trimester of pregnancy, and (2) the presence of one or more of the various manifestations of congenital rubella listed in Box 26-1. However, final confirmation of the diagnosis is dependent on virus isolation or immunologic procedures.

Demonstration of the Virus. Rubella virus has been cultured from pharyngeal secretions, urine, CSF, and virtually every tissue and organ in the body. Infants with congenital rubella may re-

main chronically infected for many weeks or months. As indicated in Fig. 26-5, the incidence of virus shedding decreases with advancing age. Most infants with congenital rubella are no longer shedding virus and have a normal pattern of serum immunoglobulins by 1 year of age. However, infants with severe dysgammaglobulinemia may shed virus for a more prolonged period. Isolation of virus from the blood is very rare. Viremia has been observed chiefly in infants with immunologic disorders. Biopsied tissues or blood and cerebrospinal fluid have also been used to demonstrate rubella antigens with monoclonal antibodies and for detection of rubella RNA by in situ hybridization and polymerase chain reaction (PCR).

Immunologic Response. The immunologic response to an intrauterine infection is shown in Fig. 26-6. It differs significantly from the response to rubella acquired postnatally. The chief difference lies in the pattern of virus excretion and antibody response. In rubella acquired after birth, virus excretion is transient, rarely persisting for more than 2 or 3 weeks (see Fig. 26-4); in contrast, virus shedding may persist for many months after birth in congenital rubella. As indicated in Fig. 26-6, the serum of an infant with congenital rubella contains actively acquired IgM-specific antibody and pas-

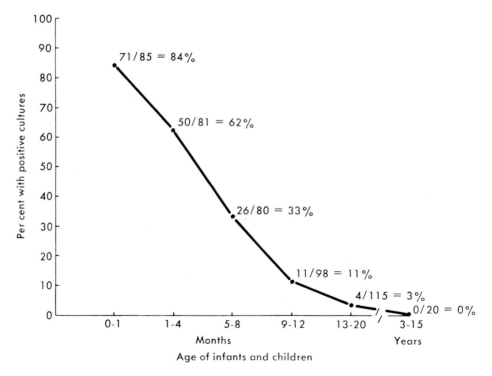

Fig. 26-5 Incidence of rubella virus excretion by age in infants with congenital rubella. (From Cooper LZ, Krugman S: Arch Ophthalmol 1967;77:434.)

RUBELLA (GERMAN MEASLES)

sively acquired maternal IgG antibody. Several months later, transplacentally acquired IgG is no longer detectable, and high levels of IgM may be present. By the end of 1 year, actively acquired IgG apparently is the dominant rubella antibody. Consequently, the presence and persistence of rubella antibody in the serum of an infant 5 to 6 months of age or older and the identification of the antibody in early infancy as IgM are indicative of congenital rubella infection.

The pattern of persistence of HI antibody following congenital rubella is different from that following naturally acquired infection. Detectable levels of antibody persist for many years in most children after a natural rubella infection. However, approximately 20% of children with congenital rubella by age 5 years may no longer have detectable rubella HI antibody (Cooper et al., 1971).

Differential Diagnosis

Cytomegalovirus infection, congenital toxoplasmosis, and congenital syphilis also may be characterized by the following manifestations of congenital rubella: thrombocytopenic purpura, jaundice, hepatosplenomegaly, and bone lesions. Herpes simplex virus infection shows the same manifestations, with the exception of bone lesions and a vesicular skin rash. The diagnosis may be clarified by the presence of other findings more compatible with congenital rubella, such as congenital cataract, glaucoma, patent ductus arteriosus, or maternal history of rubella. The precise diagnosis should be confirmed by specific laboratory tests.

Prognosis

Neonatal thrombocytopenic purpura carries a poor prognosis. The mortality rate exceeded 35% after the first-year follow-up of a large group of infants (Cooper and Krugman, 1967). The usual causes of death were sepsis, congestive heart failure, and general debility. In the absence of purpura the mortality rate was approximately 10%. Deaths usually occurred during the first 6 months of life. The prognosis is excellent for children with minor defects.

There has been a long-term follow-up of approximately 500 children born with the congenital rubella syndrome in New York City during the epidemic from 1964 to 1965. In their twenties, these patients could be divided into three groups: approximately one third were relatively normal; one third were mildly to moderately incapacitated; and the remainder were profoundly handicapped, requiring institutional care. Patients with congenital rubella syndrome have had difficulty in developing social skills, especially after leaving special educational units as young adults. Suicide attempts have not been uncommon. Approximately 15% of patients with congenital rubella syndrome have developed insulin-dependent diabetes, presumably as a result of an autoimmune mechanism. Long-term follow-up studies from Australia have yielded similar findings (McIntosh et al., 1992).

Epidemiologic Factors

The incidence of congenital rubella is dependent on the immune status of women of childbearing

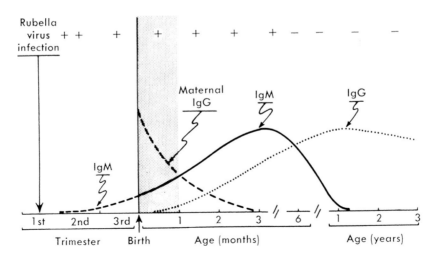

Fig. 26-6 Natural history of congenital rubella. Pattern of virus excretion and antibody response.

age and the occurrence of significant epidemics. In the United States approximately 15% of young women have no detectable rubella antibody. During the 1964 epidemic, 3.6% of pregnant women had rubella; in contrast, the infection rate was 0.1% to 0.2% during interepidemic years (Sever, 1967). Congenital rubella is a contagious disease. The infected newborn infant may disseminate the virus to close contacts for many months. This reservoir may provide a source for maintaining the virus in nature from year to year. The risk associated with maternal rubella infection has been variously estimated. An evaluation of several prospective studies indicates that the risk of congenital malformations after maternal rubella is as follows: (1) 30% to 50% during the first 4 weeks of gestation, (2) 25% during the fifth to eighth weeks of gestation, and (3) 8% during the ninth to twelfth weeks of gestation. The overall risk of malformations from rubella during the first trimester is approximately 20%. There is a slight risk of deafness when rubella occurs during the thirteenth to sixteenth weeks.

Isolation and Quarantine

Isolation of Infants with Congenital Rubella. The primary aim of isolation procedures is to prevent rubella infection in susceptible pregnant women. Infants with congenital rubella may shed virus for many weeks or months after birth. Intimate contact is generally required for the transmission of rubella. Accordingly, potentially susceptible pregnant women should avoid close exposure to these infants.

Isolation in the Hospital. Infants suspected of having congenital rubella should be admitted to a separate room designated as the isolation unit. Personnel assigned to this area should be selected on the basis of their childbearing potential and immune status. Isolation should be continued until the infant is ready to go home.

Isolation in the Home. No special precautions are necessary for the parents and young sibling contacts. Potentially susceptible female visitors to the home should avoid physical contact with the infant during the contagious period. If laboratory facilities are available for identification of rubella virus, infants should be considered contagious until negative cultures have been obtained. As indicated in Fig. 26-5, evidence of virus shedding may disappear by 1 month of age in some infants; on the other hand, it may persist for a year or

more in a small number of infants. If laboratory facilities are not available, the data shown in Fig. 26-5 may be used as a guide for the estimation of period of contagion. In general, there is some correlation between the severity of the infection and the duration of virus shedding. Infants with severe involvement usually shed virus much longer than infants with minimal involvement.

PREVENTIVE MEASURES

Live attenuated rubella vaccine was licensed in the United States in 1969; the vaccine currently available is RA 27/3, which is propagated in human diploid cells and is more immunogenic (particularly with regard to stimulation of secretory immunity) than previously licensed vaccines. The current vaccine strategy is to immunize all infants at 12 to 15 months of age with measles-mumps-rubella (MMR) vaccine and to administer a second dose of MMR during childhood. Two doses of monovalent rubella vaccine may also be administered to anyone who is thought to be susceptible to the infection and is not pregnant. It is especially important that hospital workers of either sex be immune to rubella to avoid possible nosocomial transmission. It is likely that, years following immunization, antibody titers may be undetectable but that protection against infection is the rule. At present there is little if any evidence of significant waning immunity to rubella years after immunization. Although rubella vaccine has not been associated with the congenital syndrome, vaccination is contraindicated in pregnant women and pregnancy should be avoided for at least 3 months following rubella vaccination. Rubella-susceptible children whose mothers are also rubella-susceptible should be immunized, since individuals who are vaccinated do not shed rubella virus or transmit the virus to susceptibles. Although it is not recommended that rubella vaccine be given to immunosuppressed persons, no adverse effects of rubella vaccine have been reported in such individuals who have been vaccinated. Rubella vaccine has been safely given to children with HIV infection. Occasionally, rubella vaccine may be associated with arthralgia or arthritis, especially in young women. Rubella vaccination can result in a chronic arthritis on very rare occasion; episodes of arthritis in vaccinees are usually self-limited, lasting only about 1 week.

Although vaccine-induced titers are generally lower than those following natural rubella, vaccine-induced immunity usually protects against both clinical illness and viremia after natural exposure. Occasional reports have indicated that viremic reinfection following exposure may occur in vaccinated individuals with low levels of detectable antibody, but there are also rare reports of clinical reinfection and fetal infection following natural immunity.

Persons can be considered immune to rubella only if they have documentation of (1) laboratory evidence of rubella immunity or (2) adequate immunization with at least 1 dose of rubella vaccine on or after the first birthday. Clinical diagnosis of rubella is not reliable and should not be considered in assessing immunity to rubella.

BIBLIOGRAPHY

ACIP. Recommendations of the Immunization Practices Advisory Committee (ACIP). MMWR 1990;39:3-18.

Anderson SG. Experimental rubella in human volunteers. J Immunol 1949;62:29.

Bosma TJ, Corbett KM, Eckstein MB, et al. Use of PCR for prenatal and postnatal diagnosis of congenital rubella. J Clin Micro 1995;33:2881.

Boué A, Nicolas A, Montagnon B. Reinfection with rubella in pregnant women. Lancet 1971;1:1251.

Burke JP, Hinman AR, Krugman S (eds). International symposium on prevention of congenital rubella infection. Rev Infect Dis 1985;7(suppl 1):1.

Buser F, Nicolas A. Vaccination with RA 27/3 rubella vaccine. Am J Dis Child 1971;122:53.

Chantler JK, et al. Persistent rubella virus infection associated with chronic arthritis in children. N Engl J Med 1985; 313:1117.

Cooper LZ, Florman AL, Ziring PR, Krugman S. Loss of rubella hemagglutination inhibition antibody in congenital rubella. Am J Dis Child 1971;122:397.

Cooper LZ, Krugman S. Clinical manifestations of postnatal and congenital rubella. Arch Ophthalmol 1967;77:434.

Cooper LZ, et al. Neonatal thrombocytopenic purpura and other manifestations of rubella contracted in utero. Am J Dis Child 1965;110:416.

Cooper LZ, et al. Transient arthritis after rubella vaccination. Am J Dis Child 1969;118:218.

Cusi MG, et al. Serological evidence of reinfection among vaccinees during rubella outbreak. Lancet 1991;336:1071.

Davis WJ, et al. A study of rubella immunity and resistance to reinfection. JAMA 1971;215:600.

Desmond MM, et al. Congenital rubella encephalitis. J Pediatr 1967;71:311.

Dorsett PH, Miller DC, Green KY, et al. Structure and function of rubella virus proteins. Rev Infect Dis 1985;7:S150.

Edell TA, et al. Rubella in hospital personnel and patients, Colorado. MMWR 1979;28:325.

Enders JF. Rubella vaccination. N Engl J Med 1970;283:161.

Fleet WF Jr, et al. Exposure of susceptible teachers to rubella vaccines. Am J Dis Child 1972;123:28.

Fleet WF Jr, et al. Fetal consequences of maternal rubella immunization. JAMA 1974;227:621.

Forchheimer F. Enanthem of German measles. Philadelphia Med 1898;2:15.

Fry J, Dillane JB, Fry L. Rubella, 1962. Br Med J 1962;2:833.

Grayston JT, Watten RH. Epidemic rubella in Taiwan, 1957-1958. III. Gamma globulin in the prevention of rubella. N Engl J Med 1959;261:1145.

Green RH, et al. Studies on the natural history and prevention of rubella. Am J Dis Child 1965;110:348.

Gregg NM. Congenital cataract following German measles in the mother. Trans Ophthalmol Soc Aust 1941;3:35.

Gregg NM, et al. Occurrence of congenital defects in children following maternal rubella during pregnancy. Med J Aust 1945;2:122.

Habel K, et al. Transmission of rubella to Macacus mulatta monkeys. Public Health Rep 1942;57:1126.

Halstead S, Diwan AR. Failure to transmit rubella virus vaccine: a close contact study in adults. JAMA 1971;215:634.

Hermann KL, et al. Rubella immunization: persistence of antibody four years after a large-scale field trial. JAMA 1976; 235:2201.

Hess AF. German measles (rubella): an experimental study. Arch Intern Med 1914;13:913.

Hill AB, Doll R, Galloway T McL, Hughes JPW. Virus diseases in pregnancy and congenital defects. Br J Prev Soc Med 1958;12:1.

Hiro Y, Tasaka S. Die Röteln sind eine Virus-krankheit. Monatsschr Kinderheilkd 1938;76:328.

Horstmann DM, et al. Rubella: reinfection of vaccinated and naturally immune persons exposed in an epidemic. N Engl J Med 1970;283:771.

Houser HG, Schalet N. Prevention of rubella with gamma globulin. Clin Res 1958;6:281.

Ingalls TH. Progress in pediatrics: German measles and German measles in pregnancy. Am J Dis Child 1957;93:555.

Jackson ADM, Fisch L. Deafness following maternal rubella: results of a prospective investigation. Lancet 1958;2:1241.

Johnson RE, Hall AP. Rubella arthritis: report of cases studied by latex tests. N Engl J Med 1958;258:743.

Judelsohn RG, Wyll SA. Rubella in Bermuda: termination of an epidemic by mass vaccination. JAMA 1973;223:401.

Kantor TG, Tanner M. Rubella arthritis and rheumatoid arthritis. Arthritis Rheum 1962;5:378.

Kenny FM, Michaels RH, Davis KS. Rubella encephalopathy: later psychometric, neurologic, and encephalographic evaluation of seven survivors. Am J Dis Child 1965;110:374.

Kilroy AW, et al. Two syndromes following rubella immunization: clinical observations and epidemiological studies. JAMA 1970;214:2287.

Klock LE, et al. A clinical and serological study of women exposed to rubella vaccinees. Am J Dis Child 1972;123:465.

Korones SB, et al. Congenital rubella syndrome: study of 22 infants. Am J Dis Child 1965;110:434.

Krugman S (ed). Proceedings of the international conference on rubella immunization. Am J Dis Child 1969;118:1.

Krugman S. Present status of measles and rubella immunization in the United States: a medical progress report. J Pediatr 1971;78:1; J Pediatr 1977;90:1.

Krugman S, Ward R. The rubella problem. J Pediatr 1954; 44:489.

Krugman S, Ward R, Jacobs KG, Lazar M. Studies on rubella immunization. I. Demonstration of rubella without rash. JAMA 1953;151:285.

Landrigan PJ, Stoffels MA, Anderson E, Witte JJ. Epidemic rubella in adolescent boys. JAMA 1974;227:1283.

Lee SH, et al. Resurgence of congenital rubella syndrome in the 1990s. JAMA 267:2616, 1992.

Levin MJ, et al. Diagnosis of congenital rubella in utero. N Engl J Med 1974;290:1187.

Lock FR, Gatling HB, Mauzy CH, Wells HB. Incidence of anomalous development following maternal rubella. Am J Obstet Gynecol 1961;81:451.

Lündström R. Rubella during pregnancy: a follow-up study of children born after an epidemic of rubella in Sweden, 1951, with additional investigations on prophylaxis and treatment of maternal rubella. Acta Paediatr 1962;51(suppl 133):1-110.

MacFarlane DW, Boyd RD, Dodrill CB, Tufts E. Intrauterine rubella, head size, and intellect. Pediatrics 1975;55:797.

McIntosh ED, et al. A fifty-year follow up of congenital rubella. Lancet 340:414, 1992.

McLaughlin MD, Gold LH. The New York rubella incident: a case for changing hospital policy regarding rubella testing and immunization. Am J Public Health 1979;69:287.

Mellinger AK, et al. High incidence of congenital rubella syndrome after a rubella outbreak. Ped Infect Dis J 1995;14:573.

Menser MA, Forrest JM, Bransby RD. Rubella infection and diabetes. Lancet 1978;1:57.

Meyer HM Jr, Parkman PD, Panos TC. Attenuated rubella virus. II. Production of an experimental live-virus vaccine and clinical trial. N Engl J Med 1966;275:575.

Modlin JF. Surveillance of the congenital rubella syndrome, 1969-73. J Infect Dis 1974;130:316.

Modlin JF, et al. A review of five years experience with rubella vaccine in the United States. Pediatrics 1975;55:20.

Naeye RL, Blanc W. Pathogenesis of congenital rubella. JAMA 1965;194:1277.

Neff JM, Carver DH. Rubella immunization: reconsideration of our present policy. Am J Epidemiol 1970;92:162.

O'Shea S, et al. Rubella reinfection; role of neutralizing antibodies and cell-mediated immunity. Clin Diagn Virol 1994; 2:349.

Parkman PD, Buescher EL, Artenstein MS. Recovery of rubella virus from army recruits. Proc Soc Exp Biol Med 1962; 111:225.

Parkman PD, Meyer HM Jr, Kirschstein RL, Hopps HE. Attenuated rubella virus. I. Development and laboratory characterization. N Engl J Med 1966;275:569.

Pitt DB. Congenital malformations and maternal rubella. Med J Aust 1957;1:233.

Plotkin SA, Boué A, Boué JG. The in vitro growth of rubella virus in human embryonic cells. Am J Epidemiol 1965;81:71.

Redd S, et al. The measles-mumps-rubella vaccination program in Finland. N Engl J Med 332:1102, 1995.

Robinson J, et al. Congenital rubella after anticipated maternal immunity: two cases and a review of the literature. Ped Infect Dis J 1994;13:812.

Schiff GM, Donath R, Rotte T. Experimental rubella studies. I. Clinical and laboratory features of infection caused by the Brown strain rubella virus. II. Artificial challenge studies of adult rubella vaccinees. Am J Dis Child 1969;118:269.

Schiff GM, et al. Rubella vaccines in a public school system. Am J Dis Child 1974;128:180.

Scott HD, Byrne EB. Exposure of susceptible pregnant women to rubella vaccinees: serologic findings during the Rhode Island immunization campaign. JAMA 1971;215:609.

Shaffner W, et al. Polyneuropathy following rubella immunization. Am J Dis Child 1974;127:684.

Sennett RA, Copeman WSC. Notes on rubella, with special reference to certain rheumatic sequelae. Br Med J 1940; 1:924.

Sever JL. Epidemiology of rubella. Washington DC: Pan American Health Organization, World Health Organization, May 1967, Scientific Publication No 147, p 366.

Smith CA, et al. Rubella virus and arthritis. Rheum Dis Clin North Amer 1987;13:810.

Stewart GL, et al. Rubella virus hemagglutination-inhibition test. N Engl J Med 1967;276:554.

Tingle AJ, Allen M, Petty RE. Rubella-associated arthritis. I. Comparative study of joint manifestations associated with natural rubella and RA 27/3 rubella immunization. Ann Rheum Dis 1986;45:110-114.

Townsend JJ, et al. Progressive rubella panencephalitis: late onset after congenital rubella. N Engl J Med 1975;292:990.

Vesikari T, Buimovici-Klein E. Lymphocyte responses to rubella antigen and phytohemagglutinin after administration of the RA 27/3 strain of live attenuated rubella vaccine. Infect Immunol 1975;11:748.

Warkany J, Kalter H. Congenital malformations. N Engl J Med 1961;265:1046.

Weil ML, et al. Chronic progressive panencephalitis due to rubella virus stimulating SSPE. N Engl J Med 1975;292:994.

Weller TH, Neva FA. Propagation in tissue culture of cytopathic agents from patients with rubella-like illness. Proc Soc Exp Biol Med 1962;111:215.

Wesselhoeft C. Rubella (German measles). N Engl J Med 1947;236:943, 978.

Wilkins J, Leedon JM, Portnoy B, Salvatore MA. Reinfection with rubella virus despite live vaccine–induced immunity. Am J Dis Child 1969;118:275.

Ziring PR, Florman AF, Cooper LZ. The diagnosis of rubella. Pediatr Clin North Am 1971;18:87.

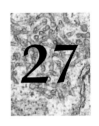

27 SEPSIS IN THE NEWBORN

MORVEN S. EDWARDS AND CAROL J. BAKER

Classically defined, neonatal sepsis or septicemia is a clinical syndrome in the infant less than 29 days of age manifested by systemic signs of infection and isolation of a pathogen from the bloodstream (Baker, 1986). Both clinical and laboratory definitions have been proposed (Gaynes et al., 1996). Primary bloodstream infection may occur in some asymptomatic newborns (Wiswell et al., 1995) and clinical sepsis without bacteremia in others, especially if the mother has received antimicrobial agents before delivery. The improved survival of very low birth weight infants has rendered the postnatal age limit of 29 days impractical. It is recognized that "neonatal" sepsis occurs at least until the postconceptual age of 1 month postterm and occasionally longer in the extremely low birth weight infant. For the purpose of this review, the neonatal period will include both the first 4 weeks of life for the term infant and 4 weeks after hospital discharge for those infants born prematurely. The clinical presentation and management of sepsis will include both types of infants.

Reported incidence rates for proven neonatal sepsis range from 1 to 8 cases per 1,000 live births (Stoll et al., 1996b). The incidence and the fatality rates each are inversely related to birth weight and to gestational age. Fatality rates have fallen dramatically in the past quarter of a century in association with improved early recognition and technologic and therapeutic advances in care of newborn infants, especially those born before 37 weeks of gestation.

Two patterns based on age at onset of signs of sepsis have been recognized historically. The designations early-onset and late-onset neonatal sepsis, originally applied to neonatal group B streptococcal infections, were applied to neonatal listeriosis and subsequently to other pathogens. These remain useful designations, because there are distinctives in risk factors, source of acquisi-

tion of infecting organisms, and clinical presentation that vary with the postnatal age at onset (Table 27-1). Recently, the term *late, late-onset* has come into increasingly common use to designate a third category of neonatal sepsis. These infants are usually survivors of extremely low birth weight who are more than 30 days of age but remain hospitalized for several weeks after birth in the intermediate or intensive care unit setting. The major risk factor for these infants is the ongoing violation of anatomic and mucosal barriers to infection by the intravascular access catheters that are required for their care in the setting of immature host defense mechanisms. Despite the frequency with which late, late-onset infection occurs, the associated fatality rate is low, estimated at less than 5%.

ETIOLOGY

Ongoing surveillance for the past three quarters of a century have documented shifts in the etiologic agents causing neonatal sepsis. Group A *Streptococcus* was the predominant pathogen in the 1930s and 1940s; this was replaced in the 1950s by *Escherichia coli*. The late 1950s and early 1960s witnessed outbreaks of *Staphylococcus aureus* sepsis (Freedman et al., 1981). *E. coli* experienced a resurgence in the late 1960s and group B *Streptococcus,* a newly recognized human pathogen, appeared. In the 1970s several centers noted that the overall incidence of neonatal sepsis had increased, as group B *Streptococcus* joined rather than supplanted *E. coli.*

For the past 30 years group B *Streptococcus* has remained the single most frequent pathogen causing early-onset neonatal sepsis (Table 27-2). The overall prevalence of *E. coli* sepsis has declined, but it remains the second most common causative agent and the most frequent gram-negative organism. Recognition that shifts do occur has prompted ongoing surveillance of bloodstream isolates in the

415

Table 27-1   Patterns of neonatal sepsis

Characteristic	Early-onset	Late-onset	Late, late-onset
Onset	Less than 7 days of age (usually first 48 hr)	7 to 30 days	30 days to discharge
Gestation	25% <37 weeks	Often full term	Usually <32 weeks
Risk factors	Maternal intrapartum complications common	Often none	Prematurity
Source of organism	Maternal genital tract	Maternal genital tract, nosocomial or community	Nosocomial, community
Usual clinical presentation	Nonspecific signs or respiratory distress	Focal or nonspecific signs	Focal or nonspecific signs
Case-fatality ratio	10%-20%	5%-10%	<5%

Table 27-2   Etiologic agents in early-onset neonatal sepsis

Organism	Percent of patients by year studied		
	1966 to 1978*	1979 to 1988†	1991 to 1993‡
Gram-Positive Organisms			
Group B *Streptococcus*	46	55	31
Enterococcus	3	4	0
Streptococcus viridans	1	2	9
Other streptococci	3	3	7
Staphylococcus aureus	2	1	3
Coagulase-negative staphylococci	0	1	7
Gram-Negative Organisms			
Escherichia coli	23	14	16
Klebsiella or *Klebsiella-Enterobacter*	5	1	5
Haemophilus pneumoniae	6	8	11
Other gram-negatives	4	4	10
Other, Mixed, or Nonspecified	7	7	1
TOTAL **(Number of Infants)**	100 (137)	100 (93)	100 (147)

*Data from Freedman et al. Am J Dis Child 1981;135:140. Refers to infants born at Yale-New Haven Hospital who were less than 48 hours of age at time of culture.

†Data from Gladstone et al. Pediatr Infect Dis J 1990;9:820. Refers to infants born at Yale-New Haven Hospital who were 4 days of age or less at time of culture.

‡Data from Stoll et al. J Pediatr 1996a;129:72. Refers to very low birth weight infants (≤1500 gm) from whom cultures were obtained within 72 hours of life.

newborn (Gladstone et al., 1990). Among gram-positives, *group B* streptococci dominated in the early 1980s and now account for less than 35% of early-onset cases. Other streptococci, including an occasional group A, C, or G streptococci and *Streptococcus pneumoniae,* are less frequent causal agents.

Among gram-negatives, a recently published multicenter report of very low birth weight neonates (401 to 1500 gm) admitted to the 12 National Institute of Child Health and Human Devel-

opment (NICHD) Neonatal Research Network centers during a 32-month period from 1991 to 1993 noted *E. coli* to be the predominant early-onset pathogen (Stoll et al., 1996b). Nontypeable *Haemophilus influenzae* was recognized as an early-onset pathogen in the 1970s, and it accounts for approximately 6% to 8% of cases.

In the 1990s, a shift in serotype prevalence among group B streptococci occurred. A newly recognized serotype, type V, has been observed and causes approximately 15% to 20% of cases of in-

Table 27-3 Etiologic agents in late-onset neonatal sepsis

Organism	Percent of patients by year studied		
	1966 to 1978*	1979 to 1988†	1991 to 1993‡
Gram-Positive Organisms			
Coagulase-negative staphylococci	0	21	55
Staphylococcus aureus	9	7	9
Enterococcus/group D *Streptococcus*	3	9	5
Group B *Streptococcus*	10	6	2
Other	0	5	2
Gram-Negative Organisms			
Enterobacter or *Klebsiella-Enterobacter*	23	16	8
Escherichia coli	37	21	4
Pseudomonas	4	6	2
Other	2	2	4
***Candida* Species**	0	6	7
Other, Mixed, or Nonspecified	12	1	2
TOTAL **(Number of Infants)**	100 (197)	100 (110)	100 (2355)

*Data from Freedman et al. Am J Dis Child 1981;135:140. Refers to infants born at or transported to Yale-New Haven Hospital who were more than 48 hours and less than 30 days at time of culture.

†Data from Gladstone et al. Pediatr Infect Dis J 1990;9:820. Refers to infants who were 5 or more days of age when cultures were obtained.

‡Data from Stoll et al. J Pediatr 1996a;129:63. Refers to very low birth weight infants (≤1500 gm) who were more than 72 hours of age when cultures were obtained.

fection overall in both adults and newborn infants (Blumberg et al., 1996) and a decline in type II group B streptococcal strains has been observed. It remains to be seen whether the emergence of type V will herald a change in the overall incidence of group B streptococcal infections.

Listeria monocytogenes is conspicuously absent from listings of agents causing early-onset neonatal sepsis. Although it is a "classic" pathogen, it remains an uncommon one. In our inborn delivery service of approximately 8,000 infants yearly, one or two cases of listeriosis are documented. Some of these are linked epidemiologically to contaminated dairy products. Although it is eclipsed in frequency by the more common pathogens, it is important to include listeriosis as an etiologic consideration because its clinical and epidemiologic features are distinctive.

In contrast to the relatively modest shifts in early-onset etiologic agents, the pathogens causing late-onset sepsis in the newborn infant have changed dramatically in the past 30 years (Table 27-3). Coagulase-negative staphylococci have become the major cause of late-onset sepsis (Battisti et al., 1981; Placzek and Whitelaw, 1983; Gaynes et al., 1996). In the series reported by Gladstone et al. (1990), coagulase-negative staphylococci ac-

counted for 19% of all late-onset and 43% of late, late-onset infection. Coagulase-negative staphylococci comprised a majority of all isolates in the NICHD Neonatal Research Network centers from 1991 to 1993 (Stoll et al., 1996b). It is likely that this shift has been caused by a change in the population at risk and not because of a change in the intrinsic virulence of these commensals.

S. aureus continues to be an important cause of late-onset neonatal sepsis, especially when focal signs are clinically evident. Although its prevalence has not changed, the likelihood that infecting isolates are methicillin resistant has increased. This concern is nursery specific, and it requires ongoing surveillance of susceptibility patterns of isolates from nursery patients. Enterococci, also commensals like coagulase-negative staphylococci, may be the emerging late-onset pathogens of the 1990s. These intrinsically low virulence organisms are increasingly encountered in infants with late-onset sepsis (Dobson and Baker, 1990; McNeeley et al., 1996). Their plasmid-mediated and intrinsic capacities to acquire resistance to commonly employed antimicrobials, including vancomycin, pose a substantial threat to the newborn (Murray, 1990). Already debilitated hosts, such as those with necrotizing enterocolitis or needing central vascular access, are at high risk for enterococcal infection. Group B streptococci causing late-onset sepsis may have been acquired vertically at time of delivery or may be nosocomially-acquired through hand-to-hand contact in the nursery (Noya et al., 1987).

Taken as a group, gram-negative organisms are less likely to cause late-onset sepsis than in the past. Those commonly encountered, including *Enterobacter, Klebsiella, Pseudomonas,* or *Serratia* species, may exhibit multiple antibiotic resistance patterns. Nosocomial acquisition is the rule, and each of these organisms has been documented as a cause of nursery outbreaks (Cook et al., 1980; Campbell et al., 1992).

Fungal infections, including those caused by *Candida* and *Aspergillus,* are encountered with increasing frequency in the nursery as late-onset pathogens. Although *Candida albicans* is most common, other species such as *Candida tropicalis* and *Candida parapsilosis* also have been reported (Butler and Baker, 1988). *Aspergillus* species may cause a sepsislike presentation or a focal infection, such as a distinctive invasive dermatitis (Rowen et al., 1992). Because the presenting features often are indistinguishable from bacterial disease, they should be considered as potential pathogens and appropriate diagnostic procedures should be initiated promptly.

PATHOLOGY

Newborn infants with serious, overwhelming early-onset sepsis often have such a rapidly fatal course that there has been insufficient time elapsed for evidence of an inflammatory response histologically. The cause of death in these patients usually is irreversible shock. Accompanying findings may include periventricular leukomalacia and intraventricular hemorrhage, scattered areas of hepatic necrosis, and renal or adrenal hemorrhage or necrosis (Klein and Marcy, 1995). The histopathologic findings in the lungs of newborns with fatal early-onset sepsis have been defined for infection caused by group B streptococci. The organisms may colonize hyaline membranes without accompanying pneumonitis. Alternatively there may be histologic evidence of extensive acute pneumonia or of mild diffuse or focal pneumonia with or without evidence of surfactant deficiency.

With late-onset infection, focal inflammation in affected organ systems often is evident. The most important of these is meningitis in which exudate may be found around the base of the brain and involving the ependymal and subependymal tissues.

Often widespread vasculitis, hemorrhage, and venous thrombosis are found. Gram-negative enteric pathogens may cause central nervous system devastation, with hemorrhagic meningoencephalitis often followed by widespread necrosis and liquefaction of the brain.

PATHOGENESIS

The pathogenesis of neonatal sepsis is modulated by factors that are *extrinsic* or external to the infant and by those that are *intrinsic* or internal. For early-onset infection, maternal obstetric events are key extrinsic factors that affect infection risk, whereas for late-onset infection, the iatrogenic factors required to sustain life dominate.

Extrinsic Factors

Heading the list of extrinsic factors that predispose to early-onset infection is preterm delivery. The risk of early-onset sepsis is increased 10 to 15 times if gestation is less than 37 weeks. This relates in part to the role of transplacentally-acquired maternal IgG, because active IgG transport does not occur until 32 to 34 weeks of gestation. Risk to the infant also is inversely related to duration of rupture of membranes. Rupture of more than 18 hours predisposes to acquisition of infection by the ascending route. An infant born to a woman with intraamniotic infection has a 1% to 5% chance of becoming infected. This risk increases to 5% to 15% if prematurity or prolonged rupture of membranes coexist. Preterm premature rupture of membranes before onset of labor at any gestation also increases infant risk for sepsis. Intrapartum maternal fever, before delivery or within 24 hours after delivery, often heralds maternal infection including chorioamnionitis, bacteremia, endometritis, or urinary tract infection, with organisms that also may cause early-onset sepsis.

Maternal urinary tract infection during pregnancy, usually manifested as asymptomatic bacteriuria, enhances neonatal risk for early-onset group B streptococcal infection. Urinary tract infection, usually coexisting with heavy maternal colonization, is associated with a significantly increased risk for group B streptococcal sepsis in the neonate (Ancona et al., 1980). Sepsis risk also is enhanced when infants are born to women less than 20 years of age or to those who have received no prenatal care (Schuchat et al., 1994). A cohort study in greater metropolitan Atlanta and a multistate case-control study both documented a higher incidence of early-onset group B streptococcal disease among African Americans (Schuchat et al., 1990, 1994). However, a multivariate analysis indicated that race was not an independent risk factor, and variables such as maternal age and perinatal complications were more closely associated with neonatal disease (Schuchat et al., 1990).

Intrauterine monitoring devices or abrasions resulting from obstetric forceps may provide a portal of entry for colonizing organisms to invade. The actual risk probably is quite small. Because internal monitors are nearly always used in the setting of other potential maternal risk factors, such as prolonged labor or membrane rupture, separating the risk attributable to this variable is difficult.

A consideration of extrinsic factors for late-onset sepsis differs when the neonate is admitted to the hospital from the community. These infants usually were born at term, without known maternal risk factors for infection, and were discharged home to be readmitted with signs of sepsis at age 2 to 4 weeks. In contrast, the long-term nursery resident usually has required numerous invasive procedures including endotracheal intubation, umbilical vessel catheterization, central or percutaneous vascular device, scalp vessel catheterization, transcutaneous oxygen monitoring, feeding tube placement, and frequent blood sampling. Each of these may promote bloodstream invasion by organisms colonizing skin or mucous membrane surfaces. In addition, the frequent use of antimicrobial agents, often in multiple courses, may enhance the risk for overgrowth of commensals (including *Candida*) and colonization with microorganisms resistant to these agents (e.g., ampicillin, cephalosporins, gentamicin).

Intrinsic Factors

Humoral immunity in the newborn consists almost entirely of maternal IgG, providing an array of antibodies qualitatively similar to and quantitatively slightly higher than maternal. This is proportionately decreased in the preterm infant. Although passive transport of maternal IgG occurs as early as 8 weeks of gestation, active transport does not begin until about 32 weeks of gestation. Very low birth weight (<1500 gm) infants have relatively low IgG concentrations that decline to less than 100 mg/dl by age 3 to 4 months. IgA and IgM are not transported transplacentally, but the fetus has the capacity to synthesize these immunoglobulins in response to intrauterine infection.

Complement proteins are important in humoral immune defense, particularly against bacterial pathogens. These proteins are not transplacentally transferred but are synthesized in the fetal liver as early as the first trimester. At term, classical complement pathway component concentrations in serum are similar to or slightly lower than those in older infants or adults. Levels of alternative pathway components, including B and properdin, range from 30% to 60% of adult normal values in term infants and are proportionately lower in preterm infants. Because the classical pathway usually is initiated by antigen-antibody complexes, deficient function may be caused by the lack of an appropriate initiating factor. However, deficient function has been observed even for pathogens that can initiate antibody-independent function of the classic pathway (i.e., type Ia group B streptococci) (Edwards et al., 1983). Although the integrity of the complement pathways may be intact in the neonate, varying degrees of functional impairment have been described. For example, aberrant function of the thioester bond has been proposed as an explanation for low quantities of functional C3 in term and preterm newborns (Zach and Hostetter, 1989).

The monocyte-macrophage system consists of circulating monocytes and tissue macrophages of the reticuloendothelial system. The function of macrophages in the reticuloendothelial system of the neonate has not been extensively studied. However, damaged erythrocytes are not removed efficiently from the circulation. Because the terminal saccharides of some neonatal pathogens (*E. coli* and group B streptococci) and senescent red blood cells are quite similar, a deficiency in reticuloendothelial system–mediated bacterial clearance is presumed. The number of circulating monocytes is normal, but their chemotaxis is impaired. The production of proinflammatory cytokines, such as leukotriene B_4 and interleukin-8, in response to a bacterial stimulus also is impaired when the function of monocytes from newborn infants is compared with that from adults (Rowen et al., 1995). In contrast, comparable amounts of tumor necrosis factor alpha and interferon gamma are synthesized by monocytes from neonates and adults.

The number of circulating neutrophils is elevated in both premature and term infants at birth, peaking at 12 hours and returning to baseline by 72 hours of age. Increased numbers of immature neutrophils are found in neonatal sepsis. These reflect release from the neutrophil storage pool, which is more rapidly depleted in the newborn than in the older infant and in the premature than the term infant (Christensen et al., 1982). A number of functional defects have been described for neonatal neutrophils, including adherence, aggregation, movement, phagocytosis, and intracellular killing (Hill, 1987). The current consensus is that "stressing" of neutrophils by insults such as sepsis or hypoxemia decreases phagocytic activity for gram-negative and bactericidal activity for both gram-positive and gram-negative organisms. A myriad of developmental defects in signal transduction, cytoskeletal rigidity, oxidative metabolism, and cell surface receptor upregulation, to name several, contribute to the observed abnormalities in functional capacity of the neonatal neutrophil.

CLINICAL MANIFESTATIONS

The clinical manifestations of neonatal sepsis are characteristically subtle and generalized (Table 27-4). Even minimal deviation from baseline state should be viewed as a sign of possible infection. Even when focal infection exists, this often is not evident early in the course, and repeated physical examinations with special attention to the skin, soft tissues, joints, and abdomen are necessary.

Alterations in Temperature

In contrast to older children, fever is not reliably present in neonates with septicemia. Among the 455 infants comprising the four case series summarized in Table 27-4, fever was a presenting feature in only one half. The generally accepted definition of fever is a rectal temperature exceeding 38.0° C (100.4° F). Bonadio (1987) found that none of the

Table 27-4 Clinical signs of neonatal sepsis in 455 newborn infants

Clinical sign	Percentage of infants with sign
Hyperthermia	51
Hypothermia	15
Lethargy	25
Irritability	16
Respiratory distress	33
Apnea	22
Cyanosis	24
Jaundice	35
Hepatomegaly	33
Anorexia	28
Vomiting	25
Abdominal distention	17
Diarrhea	

From Klein JO, Marcy SM. Bacterial sepsis and meningitis. In Remington JS, Klein JO (eds). Infectious diseases of the fetus and newborn infant, ed. 4. Philadelphia: WB Saunders, 1995.

54 infants less than 4 weeks of age with a history of fever, but afebrile at evaluation in the emergency department, had sepsis. In contrast, 15% of infants with documented fever at presentation had serious bacterial infection. As with older children, the magnitude of fever is predictive of serious bacterial infection (Bonadio et al., 1990). A substantial subset of newborns, particularly premature infants, is more likely to develop hypothermia as a manifestation of sepsis. Often hypothermia persists despite all attempts to correct potential external contributing factors. Taken together, two thirds of neonates with sepsis can be expected to manifest alterations in the core body temperature.

Nonspecific Signs of Sepsis

Often it is a mother or nursing personnel who first observe that an infant is "off his feeds," "sleeping more than usual," "fussy," or "just not right." The very nonspecificity of these signs is a hallmark of neonatal sepsis. Tachycardia or bradycardia, hypotension, or poor peripheral perfusion are later and more ominous, sometimes irreversible, signs suggesting neonatal sepsis. Although these on occasion may suggest focal infection involving the myocardium or pericardium, more often they indicate generalized sepsis without cardiac disease.

Respiratory Signs

Signs of respiratory distress, including tachypnea, grunting, retractions, cyanosis, and nasal flaring, are suggestive of sepsis, either in the presence or absence of coexisting pulmonary immaturity. In early-onset sepsis, these findings may be reflected in a 5-minute APGAR score of 6 or less (Baker, 1978). Apnea in an otherwise asymptomatic term infant is a sensitive, although late, sign of early-onset sepsis caused by group B streptococci.

Hepatic Signs

Jaundice, usually manifested as unconjugated hyperbilirubinemia, is a frequent finding, being observed in one third of neonates with proven gram-positive or gram-negative sepsis. Hepatomegaly, often striking, is observed with the same frequency. One must remember that a liver edge palpable up to 2 cm below the right costal margin is normal for term newborns.

Gastrointestinal Signs

Gastrointestinal signs are common in neonates with sepsis. Decreased feeding, weak suck, vomiting, or gastric residuals after tube feeding often are observed (see Table 27-4). Abdominal distention is possibly related to intestinal ileus. Early in the course, it may be difficult to distinguish between infants who have sepsis without an intestinal focus and those with an intraabdominal process, such as necrotizing enterocolitis. Diarrhea is relatively uncommon, but guaiac-positive stools may be observed either with necrotizing enterocolitis or with sepsis.

Central Nervous System Signs

Meningitis is less frequent in neonates with sepsis than was reported a decade ago; this most likely is a result of earlier empiric therapy (Shattuck and Chonmaitree, 1992). In describing the changing spectrum of group B streptococcal infection, Yagupsky et al. (1991) documented meningitis in only 15% of infants. Most infants with early-onset meningitis have nonspecific findings, including episodes of tachycardia or bradycardia, acidosis, irritability, or lethargy. Specific central nervous system signs, such as seizures, hypertonia or hypotonia, or bulging of the anterior fontanelle, are found in a minority. These are observed proportionately more often in late-onset meningitis. Overall, seizures occur in 40% of infants with meningitis, bulging or full fontanelle in 28%, and nuchal rigidity in 15% (Klein, 1994).

Cutaneous and Mucous Membrane Signs

The skin and mucous membranes should be examined carefully for the clues that accompany infection in a minority of infants. These are distinctive enough that their presence often establishes a provisional diagnosis. Careful examination may reveal a pustular lesion, suggesting staphylococcal infection, or a focus of infection such as an abscess, omphalitis, or arthritis, focal sites from which a specimen for culture may be obtained. The nodular or necrotic-centered lesions typical of ecthyma gangrenosum suggest gram-negative sepsis caused by *Pseudomonas aeruginosa* or *Serratia marcescens.* However, similar lesions also have been observed in disseminated fungal infection. On occasion, these nodular lesions may have the appearance of a "cold abscess." A distinctive cutaneous presentation consisting of erythematous plaquelike or scaly lesions is characteristic of invasive fungal dermatitis caused by *C. albicans* or *Aspergillus* in premature infants (Rowen et al., 1992). Listeriosis may be accompanied by small, noninflammatory pustular or papular, well-circumscribed cutaneous lesions. The finding of vesicular lesions on the skin

or mucous membranes is virtually pathognomonic of herpes simplex, although similar lesions may be observed with neonatal varicella or coxsackie-virus infections. Petechial and purpuric lesions are more often manifestations of generalized sepsis with thrombocytopenia or disseminated intravascular coagulopathy than of embolic phenomena, especially in premature infants with fragile blood vessels and thin integument.

DIAGNOSIS
Microbiologic Techniques

The gold standard establishing the diagnosis of neonatal sepsis is the isolation of a microorganism from one or more blood cultures. The minimum volume that will yield the diagnosis depends on the intensity of bacteremia (inoculum size). In newborn infants this is at least 1.0 ml (Neal et al., 1986). Documentation of sepsis will be "missed" in 10% to 15% of infected infants when only one blood culture specimen is processed, leading some investigators to advocate deferring therapy while a second blood specimen is obtained (Wiswell and Hachey, 1991). This approach is neither practical nor feasible. In those infants with a clinical course consistent with sepsis and a single sterile blood culture, sepsis is presumed and therapy is continued.

Improvements in laboratory devices to monitor incubating blood cultures from newborn infants allow detection of positives by 48 hours of incubation (Rowley and Wald, 1986). If the laboratory only reports cultures on a daily basis, however, this may occur on the third day of therapy. In one study, only 4 of 111 positive blood cultures obtained before antibiotic therapy required more than 48 hours of incubation to become positive (Pichichero and Todd, 1979). In another, virtually all organisms (28 of 29) categorized as definite pathogens were identified by day 2 of processing (Kurlat et al., 1989).

Because the most frequent signs in neonates with proven meningitis are nonfocal, a lumbar puncture is recommended in the evaluation of possible sepsis. If the infant's condition is unstable, the procedure can be deferred and the infant should be treated as if there were coexistent meningitis until the clinical condition permits its exclusion. In one review, 6 of 39 infants (38%) with culture-proved meningitis caused by group B streptococci, *S. aureus,* or gram-negative rods had negative blood cultures (Visser and Hall, 1980).

It has been noted that meningitis is infrequently documented in asymptomatic infants evaluated at birth because maternal risk factors are reported (Fielkow et al., 1991) or in preterm infants with symptoms of respiratory distress (Weiss et al., 1991). Some experts propose omission of the lumbar puncture in evaluating such infants. However, Wiswell et al. (1995) observed that up to one third of cases of meningitis in neonates less than 7 days of age would have had the diagnosis missed or delayed if examination of the cerebrospinal fluid had been omitted. The decision is one that requires consideration of the limited risk of the procedure against the benefit of documenting the diagnosis of meningitis. Based on currently available data, we believe that a lumbar puncture should always be performed to exclude meningitis, ideally when the infant undergoes initial evaluation for sepsis or after appropriate specific and supportive therapy is initiated for the presumptive diagnosis of meningitis.

Culture of urine is not recommended in evaluation of early-onset sepsis, because positive cultures reflect bacteremia rather than true infection or anatomic abnormalities of the urinary tract. In contrast, urine obtained by catheterization or suprapubic bladder aspiration should always be a part of the evaluation of infants for late-onset infection because this may be the primary source of sepsis (Visser and Hall, 1979). Cultures from body surfaces, such as the ear canal, nasopharynx, umbilicus, or rectum, have no role in the evaluation of possible neonatal sepsis. They are poorly predictive of blood culture results and add unnecessary expense (Evans et al., 1988).

Laboratory Aids

Because clinical signs of sepsis are subtle and culture results require up to 48 hours, a number of sepsis screening tests, employed singly or together, have been proposed to aid in the diagnosis of neonatal sepsis. Although these may provide useful information, none has proved sufficiently sensitive to reliably predict infection. Clinical judgment ultimately dictates which infants require evaluation and empiric treatment for neonatal sepsis. However, the screening tests summarized in Table 27-5 may provide information to assist in the decision to evaluate or to observe an individual neonate.

The complete blood count (CBC) is the most thoroughly evaluated and easily performed sepsis screening test. White blood cell (WBC) count reference values are defined and provide range of normal values within the first hours and days of age (Klein and Marcy, 1995). When considered independently of age, a WBC more than $20,000/mm^3$ or less than $5,000/mm^3$ identifies infants at risk for sepsis. A low total neutrophil (PMN) count of less than $4,000/mm^3$ suggests depletion of bone marrow reserves and may be an early indicator of overwhelming sepsis. The sensitivity of the ratio of the absolute number of immature to total PMNs (I:T ratio) is modest, but its negative predictive value is high. Nonetheless, initiation of empiric antimicro-

Table 27-5 Sepsis screening tests: uses and limitations

Test	Findings supporting possible infection	Comment(s)
Total white blood cell (WBC) count	$<5,000/mm^3$ or $>20,000/mm^3$	Less than half of those with finding have proved infection
Total neutrophil (PMN) count	$<4,000/mm^3$	Particularly useful in first hours of life
Total immature PMN count	$>1,100/mm^3$ (cord blood); $>1,500/mm^3$ (12 hr); $>600/mm^3$ (>60 hr)	Relatively insensitive; finding unusual in uninfected infants
Immature to total PMN ratio (I:T ratio)	>0.2	Sensitivity 30%-90%; good negative predictive value
Platelet count	$<100,000/mm^3$	Insensitive, nonspecific, and late finding
C-reactive protein (CRP)	>1.0 mg/dl	Sensitivity 50%-90%
Erythrocyte sedimentation rate (ESR)	>5 mm/hr (first 24 hr); age in days plus 3 mm/hr (through age 14 days); 10-20 mm/hr (>2 wk of age)	Individual laboratories must establish normal values; normal value varies inversely with hematocrit
Fibronectin	<120-145 μg/ml	Sensitivity 30%-70%
Haptoglobin	>10 mg/dl (cord blood); >50 mg/dl (after delivery)	Unreliable due to poor sensitivity

From Edwards MS, Baker CJ. Bacterial infections in the neonate. In Long SS, Pickering LK, Prober CG (eds). Principles and practice of pediatric infectious diseases. New York: Churchill Livingstone, 1997.

bial therapy in a healthy, term neonate for one of the above abnormalities is infrequent. Thus these WBC indices should be used in the context of obstetric risk factors, infant gestational age, and clinical status.

Hepatocytes stimulated by interleukin-1 rapidly synthesize large amounts of proteins collectively known as *acute phase reactants* (Klein, 1994). Some have been studied extensively in the evaluation of neonatal sepsis and are included in Table 27-5. None is a sufficiently sensitive indicator of neonatal sepsis to advocate its routine use.

The proinflammatory cytokines, including interleukin-1 β, interleukin-6, interleukin-8, tumor necrosis factor-α, and leukotriene B_4, are elicited early in the course of bacterial infection being produced by peripheral blood monocytes, macrophages, and neutrophils. Several investigators have documented elevations of one or more of these cytokines or their receptors in neonatal sepsis (Williams et al., 1993; Spear et al., 1995; Vallejo et al., 1996). Whether these responses occur early and reliably enough in the course of neonatal sepsis to warrant their use as diagnostic tests awaits additional study.

TREATMENT

Treatment for suspected neonatal sepsis should be initiated promptly once diagnostic studies have been obtained. Initial therapy is dictated by the infant's age and physical location at onset of signs (community or nursery) and by focus of infection (Table 27-6). Antimicrobial agents are chosen by most likely pathogens and their expected susceptibility patterns. The dosages suggested and their intervals of administration take into account the expected renal immaturity of neonates, especially very low birth weight infants.

Nonbacterial agents that may cause a sepsis syndrome also should be considered. If disseminated herpes simplex infection is a consideration in the infant 5 to 14 days of age, acyclovir (10 to 15 mg/kg/8 hr) should be initiated immediately while viral culture results are pending. Cultures usually yield the virus within 48 to 72 hours, and if the diagnosis is excluded, acyclovir therapy can be discontinued. If disseminated candidiasis is a diagnostic consideration in the neonate with late-onset infection, amphotericin B therapy usually can be deferred until blood cultures confirm this diagnosis. Exceptions to this include neonates with inva-

Table 27-6 Empiric antimicrobial therapy for suspected neonatal sepsis

Clinical presentation	Antibiotic(s) (dose/kg) IV	Interval (hours)	Expected duration
Sepsis, early-onset	Ampicillin (50 mg) plus	q8	7-10 days
	gentamicin (2.5 mg)*	q12	
Sepsis, late-onset (term infant, community-acquired)	Ampicillin (50 mg) plus	q6-8	7-10 days
	gentamicin (2.5 mg)*	q8-12	
Sepsis, late-onset (inpatient)	Vancomycin (10-15 mg) plus	q8	10-14 days
	gentamicin (2.5 mg)* or amikacin (15 mg)†	q8	
Meningitis, early-onset	Ampicillin (100 mg) plus	q8	14-21 days
	gentamicin (2.5 mg)* plus	q8	
	cefotaxime (50 mg)	q12	
Meningitis, late-onset	Ampicillin (75 mg) plus	q6	14-21 days
	gentamicin (2.5 mg)* or amikacin (15 mg)† plus	q8	
	cefotaxime (50 mg)‡	q6-8	
Bone or joint infection	Nafcillin (50 mg) or vancomycin plus	q6-8	3-6 weeks
	gentamicin (2.5 mg)*	q8	
Suspected gastrointestinal infection	Include clindamycin (10 mg) or	q6-8	10-14 days
	piperacillin (50 mg) with an aminoglycoside	q6-8	

From Edwards MS, Baker CJ. Bacterial infections in the neonate. In Long SS, Pickering LK, Prober CG (eds). Principles and practice of pediatric infectious diseases. New York: Churchill Livingstone, 1997.

*For birth weight <1,500 gm, interval may be longer. For birth weight <1,500 gm, unit dosage usually is 2.5 mg/kg and interval is determined by serum levels. If given more than 72 hours, monitor serum levels to achieve a peak of 5-10 μg/ml and a trough of <2.0 μg/ml.

†For birth weight <1,500 gm, interval may be longer. Monitor serum levels to achieve a peak of 25-40 μg/ml and a trough of 5-15 μg/ml. Monitor serum levels to achieve a peak of 20-35 μg/ml and a trough of <10 μg/ml.

‡Interval is q12h (first week of life), q8h (7-28 days of age), q6h (>28 days of age).

sive fungal dermatitis and necrotizing enterocolitis with fungal hyphae present by stains. When used, the initial dose of amphotericin B is 0.5 mg/kg given over a 1- to 2-hour interval, and subsequent daily doses are 1 mg/kg (higher doses are necessary if aspergillosis is proved).

The initial empiric treatment of early-onset sepsis should include ampicillin and gentamicin. This same regimen is appropriate for infants admitted from the community with presumed late-onset sepsis without an evident focus. Gentamicin serum levels need not be obtained unless therapy is continued for more than 72 hours, renal function is abnormal or unstable, or the infant has a birth weight of <1500 gm. Serum level determination should be deferred until the fifth dose to allow for steady state distribution equilibrium. This combination therapy provides empiric coverage for the expected pathogens causing early-onset and community-acquired late-onset infection, including group B streptococci, *E. coli,* enterococci, and *L. monocytogenes.*

The empiric treatment of late-onset sepsis in neonates who remain hospitalized depends in part on the nosocomial pathogens in a specific nursery. Since coagulase-negative staphylococci are the most frequent gram-positive organisms isolated from these infants, vancomycin should be initiated pending results of cultures. This choice also is appropriate empiric therapy for those nurseries in which methicillin-resistant *S. aureus* is endemic, as well as for group B streptococci, enterococci, and alpha hemolytic streptococci. The choice of aminoglycoside depends on the gram-negative pathogens common in the nursery and their susceptibility to gentamicin or amikacin. If blood culture surveillance for the nursery indicates uniform susceptibility to gentamicin, this considerably less expensive agent should be employed. If amikacin is initiated empirically and a gentamicin-susceptible gram-negative is isolated, gentamicin should be substituted for continuation of therapy.

Routine use of third-generation cephalosporins for empiric therapy of neonatal sepsis is not recommended. Their use as empiric therapy for neonatal sepsis has been associated with outbreaks of infection caused by multiply antibiotic-resistant enteric pathogens (McCracken, 1985). When employed selectively, some third-generation cephalosporins have an important role in treatment of neonatal infection. When lumbar puncture suggests meningitis, cefotaxime should be added to the regimen to provide an extended spectrum for gram-negative enterics and to provide good cerebrospinal fluid concentrations during the interval when aminoglycosides may not have attained therapeutic levels. Because ceftriaxone may cause biliary sludging and contribute to hyperbilirubinemia, use of this agent is not appropriate in the newborn.

Several caveats apply to choice of empiric therapy when a presumed or potential focus of infection accompanies sepsis. First, ampicillin in doses appropriate for meningitis should be employed until lumbar puncture results exclude meningeal infection. Second, ampicillin should be added to a vancomycin-aminoglycoside regimen if listeriosis or group B streptococcal meningitis is suspected, because spread to the meninges may occur when when vancomycin is the sole gram-positive agent employed. Third, an antistaphylococcal agent, either nafcillin or vancomycin, should be provided as part of the regimen whenever a bone or joint focus of infection is suspected. Finally, if necrotizing enterocolitis or another abdominal focus of infection is suspected, the empiric regimen should include an antimicrobial agent with reliable activity against anaerobes.

Once a pathogen has been identified and its antibiotic susceptibility determined, therapy can be modified and simplified (Table 27-7). Penicillin G remains the drug of choice for proved group B streptococcal infection. The suggested dose is 200,000 units/kg/day for nonmeningeal and 400,000 to 500,000 units/kg/day for meningeal infections. Because the median minimal inhibitory concentration of group B streptococci to penicillin is 0.05 µg/ml, some tenfold higher than that of group A streptococci, these doses are chosen to optimize adequate penetration into all tissues. Because enterococci are only moderately susceptible to ampicillin and because synergy with gentamicin has been demonstrated for many strains, the combination should be continued to complete the course of therapy. Ampicillin alone is sufficient to complete therapy for *L. monocytogenes* infections. An antistaphylococcal penicillin should always be used rather than vancomycin for staphylococcal strains susceptible to oxacillin, both for ease of administration and to minimize development of vancomycin-resistant enterococci.

Monotherapy may be used to complete treatment for many enteric gram-negative infections. For example, ampicillin may be employed for susceptible *E. coli* strains. Often an aminoglycoside is appropriate for the treatment of *Klebsiella* infections. Because strains of *Enterobacter cloacae* or *Serra-*

Table 27-7   Antimicrobial therapy of proved newborn sepsis

Organism	Antibiotics of choice
Group B streptococci	Penicillin
Enterococci	Ampicillin plus gentamicin
Listeria monocytogenes	Ampicillin ± gentamicin
Staphylococci, coagulase-positive	Vancomycin
Staphylococcus epidermidis	Vancomycin
Escherichia coli, Klebsiella, Citrobacter	Ampicillin or aminoglycoside or cefotaxime
Enterobacter, Serratia	Aminoglycoside alone or in combination with a β-lactam antibiotic
Pseudomonas aeruginosa	Aminoglycoside plus ticarcillin or ceftazidime
Anaerobic enteric organisms	Clindamycin or piperacillin

tia marcescens rapidly may develop resistance to β-lactam antibiotics, treatment regimens should consist of an aminoglycoside alone or in combination with a β-lactam, such as cefotaxime or piperacillin. However, the β-lactam should not be employed as monotherapy. Similarly, combination therapy consisting of an aminoglycoside and an antipseudomonal penicillin or cephalosporin (i.e., ceftazidime) is indicated for the treatment of infections caused by *P. aeruginosa.*

Therapy should be continued for a total of 10 days for clinically suspected and proved neonatal sepsis. A minimum of 14 days' therapy is appropriate if meningitis is documented, and 21 days usually is required if the etiology is a gram-negative organism. A blood culture should be performed to document sterility after 24 to 48 hours of antibiotic therapy. Persistent bacteremia suggests an ongoing focus of infection or inadequate therapy.

The duration of amphotericin B treatment for invasive fungal infection is a total dose of 25 to 30 mg/kg. Newborn infants usually tolerate amphotericin B without complications, but renal function should be monitored. The serum potassium should be monitored daily during the first several days of amphotericin B therapy, because renal tubular wasting of potassium may occur. When potassium levels are stable, monitoring can be liberalized to twice weekly. If the diagnosis of disseminated fungal infection can be excluded by renal ultrasound, ophthalmologic examination, and echocardiogram to exclude a large vessel thrombus at the tip of a catheter site, and if all blood cultures are sterile after catheter removal, a shorter course of amphotericin B therapy (approximately 10 mg/kg) is sufficient for catheter-related fungemia. Other antifungal agents have not been studied sufficiently to provide guidance regarding optimal dose and interval, safety, and efficacy; thus their use should be considered experimental.

Supportive Therapy

Supportive therapy is important in the management of neonatal sepsis. Fluids and electrolytes should be carefully monitored, and hypovolemia and electrolyte abnormalities should be corrected. Shock, hypoxia, and metabolic acidosis should be identified and managed appropriately. Anticipatory ventilatory support should be employed so that adequate oxygenation of tissues is ensured. Hypoglycemia should be treated promptly. Monitoring for hyperbilirubinemia should be carried out so that phototherapy can be initiated early enough to obviate the need for exchange transfusion. Adequate caloric intake, sometimes as parenteral nutrition, is required to provide positive nitrogen balance so that tissue healing can be optimized.

Neonatal sepsis may be complicated by the development of disseminated intravascular coagulopathy (DIC). Monitoring of prothrombin and partial thromboplastin times, platelet count, hemoglobin, and fibrin-split products is important so that fresh frozen plasma, platelet transfusion, red blood cell, or whole blood transfusion can be judiciously employed.

Neutropenia caused by neutrophil storage pool depletion is associated with a poor prognosis in neonatal sepsis (Christensen et al., 1982). Clinical trials employing neutrophil transfusion met with variable results (Baley, 1988; Cairo, 1989). However, this adjunctive therapy is rarely employed today given concerns regarding possible transmission of infectious agents and logistics in providing 24-hour-a-day processing. Recent technologic advances suggest that stimulation of neonatal hematopoiesis through the administration of granulocyte colony stimulating factors (G-CSF) and granulocyte-monocyte colony stimulating factors (GM-CSF) may promote improvement of neonatal neutrophil number and function. Meanwhile these growth factors should be considered experimental.

The adjunctive treatment of neonatal sepsis with intravenous immunoglobulin (IVIG) containing specific antibodies is a promising therapeutic adjunct. Development of "pathogen-specific" products would permit administration of small volumes but at potentially effective doses. Such products are under development.

PREVENTION

Potential approaches for the prevention of neonatal sepsis include prenatal interventions that would promote delivery of term rather than premature infants, intrapartum or postpartum chemoprophylaxis, and immunoprophylaxis to confer IgG-mediated passive immunity for infants during the interval of maximum risk from maternal or nosocomial pathogens.

Although provision of prenatal care as a measure to reduce prematurity is conceptually simple, its implementation is socially complex. A decline in the rate of preterm deliveries would reliably reduce the incidence of early-onset neonatal sepsis and would substantially drop the rates for late-onset nosocomial sepsis. Regarding the latter, infection control measures to minimize risk from disruption of skin and mucous membrane defense barriers and transmission of nosocomial agents should be encouraged.

Intrapartum maternal chemoprophylaxis has been the focus of preventive measures for group B streptococcal infection (American Academy of Pediatrics, 1992). This approach is based on the randomized, controlled trial reported by Boyer and Gotoff (1986) in which intrapartum ampicillin given to high-risk women who were carriers of group B streptococci significantly reduced both early-onset disease and vertical transmission of group B streptococci. These and other data provided the basis for formulating guidelines for use of maternal chemoprophylaxis to prevent early-onset group B streptococcal disease (ACOG, 1993; CDC, 1996). These recently have been modified and expanded (ACOG, 1996; CDC, 1996). Selection of women for intrapartum chemoprophylaxis is based either on culture screening (vaginal and rectal sites) at 35 to 37 weeks gestation or on the presence of one or more risk factors (without culture screening) enhancing risk for early-onset group B streptococcal disease in the neonate. These factors include labor onset or membrane rupture before 37 weeks gestation, intrapartum fever, or rupture of membranes more than 18 hours before

delivery. Women with either previous delivery of an infant with group B streptococcal disease or group B streptococcal bacteriuria during pregnancy would always receive prophylaxis. The proportion of disease theoretically prevented would increase using the culture-based approach, because group B streptococcal carriers without risk factors (accounting for about 30% of cases) would be offered chemoprophylaxis. The regimen consists of intravenous penicillin G (5 million units initially then 2.5 million units every 4 hours) until delivery. Penicillin-allergic women would receive either intravenous clindamycin or erythromycin. Prophylaxis should be initiated as soon as possible, because efficacy is improved when the duration before delivery is more than 4 hours (i.e., more than two doses).

Management of asymptomatic infants born to women receiving chemoprophylaxis depends on the duration of prophylaxis before delivery and gestational age, but every infant should be observed in the hospital for a minimum of 48 hours. A detailed algorithm of infant management is summarized in the revised guidelines from the American Academy of Pediatrics (Cairo, 1989). However, asymptomatic infants of 35 weeks of gestation or more whose mothers have received two or more doses of penicillin G require neither diagnostic evaluation nor empiric treatment.

Information is limited concerning chemoprophylaxis for prevention of early-onset gram-negative sepsis. One trial conducted in Central America evaluated the effect of a single 1-gm dose of intrapartum ceftriaxone compared with no treatment (Sáez-Llorens et al., 1995). Infants born to women given ceftriaxone were colonized with gram-negative bacilli (as well as group B streptococci) at a lower rate than untreated women, and there was a trend toward a lower incidence of culture-proved early-onset sepsis. Additional data are required before this approach can be recommended.

The frequent occurrence of catheter-related late-onset infection caused by coagulase-negative staphylococci has prompted the evaluation of low-dose vancomycin added to parenteral alimentation solution to prevent nosocomial gram-positive infection (Kacica et al., 1994; Spafford et al., 1994). Although a dramatic and significant reduction in the rate of catheter-related sepsis was observed, this form of chemoprophylaxis is not recommended. Concerns for development of vancomycin-resistance outweigh any potential advantage of this approach.

The use of immunoprophylaxis to prevent neonatal sepsis is attractive. This approach is preferable to chemoprophylaxis, because it obviates concerns regarding complications of antimicrobial use and development of resistance. A number of promising studies preceded the assessment in two prospective large clinical trials designed to determine the role of IVIG prophylaxis in reducing nosocomial infections in very low birth weight infants. One study found that prophylactic use of IVIG failed to reduce the incidence of hospital-acquired infections in infants weighing <1300 gm at birth (Fanaroff et al., 1994), whereas the other showed that treatment with IVIG effected a significant reduction in the risk of nosocomial infection (Baker et al., 1992). Differences in the characteristics of the cohort, as well as the antibody, profiles of the immune globulin preparations employed may account for the conflicting conclusions of these two trials. Currently, IVIG is not recommended in the routine prophylaxis of very low birth weight infants, although some nurseries employ it selectively.

Even if 100% efficacious, any postpartum immunoprophylactic approach to prevention of neonatal sepsis will have little if any impact on early-onset disease. The use of maternal immunization to impart passive protection for the neonate is a realistic goal. Clinical trials of protein-polysaccharide vaccines for group B streptococci have been initiated (Kasper et al., 1996). The model of maternal immunization for prevention of neonatal sepsis has seen success in the prevention of neonatal tetanus, and it holds promise for application not only to group B streptococcal disease but also for other bacterial pathogens causing sepsis in the newborn infant.

BIBLIOGRAPHY

American Academy of Pediatrics Committee on Infectious Diseases and Committee on Fetus and Newborn. Guidelines for prevention of group B streptococcal (GBS) infection by chemoprophylaxis. Pediatrics 1992;90:775-778.

American College of Obstetricians and Gynecologists. Group B streptococcal infections in pregnancy: ACOG's recommendations. ACOG Newsletter 1993;37:1.

American College of Obstetricians and Gynecology. Prevention of early-onset group B streptococcal disease in newborns. ACOG committee opinion. Am Int J Gynaecol Obstet 1996;173:1-12.

Ancona RJ, Ferrieri P, Williams PP. Maternal factors that enhance the acquisition of group B streptococci by newborn infants. J Med Microbiol 1980;3:273-280.

Baker CJ. Early onset group B streptococcal disease. J Pediatr 1978;93:124-125.

Baker CJ. Neonatal sepsis: an overview. Clinical use of intravenous immunoglobulins. London: Academic Press, 1986.

Baker CJ, Melish ME, Hall RT, et al. Intravenous immune globulin for the prevention of nosocomial infection in low-birth-weight neonates. N Engl J Med 1992;327:213-219.

Baley JE. Neonatal sepsis: the potential for immunotherapy. Clin Perinatol 1988;15:755-771.

Battisti O, Mitchison R, Davies PA. Changing blood culture isolates in a referral neonatal intensive care unit. Arch Dis Child 1981;56:775-778.

Blumberg HM, Stephens DS, Modansky M, et al. Invasive group B streptococcal disease: the emergence of serotype V. J Infect Dis 1996;173:365-373.

Bonadio WA. Incidence of serious infections in afebrile neonates with a history of fever. Pediatr Infect Dis J 1987;6:911-914.

Bonadio WA, Romine K, Gyuro J. Relationship of fever magnitude to rate of serious bacterial infections in neonates. J Pediatr 1990;116:733-735.

Boyer KM, Gotoff SP. Prevention of early-onset neonatal group B streptococcal disease with selective intrapartum chemoprophylaxis. N Engl J Med 1986;314:1665-1669.

Butler KM, Baker CJ. Candida: an increasingly important pathogen in the nursery. Pediatr Clin North Am 1988;35:543-563.

Cairo MS. Neutrophil transfusions in the treatment of neonatal sepsis. Am J Pediatr Hematol Oncol 1989;11:227-232.

Campbell JR, Diacovo T, Baker CJ. *Serratia marcescens* meningitis in neonates. Pediatr Infect Dis J 1992;11:881-886.

Centers for Disease Control and Prevention. Prevention of perinatal group B streptococcal disease: a public health perspective. MMWR 1996;45:1-24.

Christensen RD, Rothstein G, Anstall HB, et al. Granulocyte transfusions in neonates with bacterial infection, neutropenia, and depletion of mature marrow neutrophils. Pediatrics 1982;70:1-6.

Cook LN, Davis RS, Stover BH. Outbreak of amikacin-resistant Enterobacteriaceae in an intensive care nursery. Pediatrics 1980;65:264-268.

Dobson SRM, Baker CJ. Enterococcal sepsis in neonates: features by age at onset and occurrence of focal infection. Pediatrics 1990;85:165-171.

Edwards MS, Baker CJ. Bacterial infections in the neonate. In Long SS, Pickering LK, Prober CG (eds). Principles and practice of pediatric infectious diseases. New York: Churchill Livingstone, 1997.

Edwards MS, Buffone GJ, Fuselier PA, et al. Deficient classical complement pathway activity in newborn sera. Pediatr Res 1983;17:685-688.

Evans ME, Schaffner W, Federspiel CF, et al. Sensitivity, specificity, and predictive value of body surface cultures in a neonatal intensive care unit. JAMA 1988;259:248-252.

Fanaroff AA, Korones SB, Wright LL, et al. A controlled trial of intravenous immune globulin to reduce nosocomial infections in very-low-birth-weight infants. N Engl J Med 1994;330:1107-1113.

Fielkow S, Reuter S, Gotoff SP. Cerebrospinal fluid examination in symptom-free infants with risk factors for infection. J Pediatr 1991;119:971-973.

Freedman RM, Ingram DL, Gross I, et al. A half century of neonatal sepsis at Yale, 1928 to 1978. Am J Dis Child 1981;135:140-144.

Gaynes RP, Edwards JR, Jarvis WR, et al. Nosocomial infections among neonates in high-risk nurseries in the United States. Pediatrics 1996;98:357-361.

Gladstone IM, Ehrenkranz RA, Edberg SC, et al. A ten-year review of neonatal sepsis and comparison with the previous fifty-year experience. Pediatr Infect Dis J 1990;9:819-825.

Hill HR. Biochemical, structural, and functional abnormalities of polymorphonuclear leukocytes in the neonate. Pediatr Res 1987;22:375-382.

Kacica MA, Horgan MJ, Ochoa L, et al. Prevention of gram-positive sepsis in neonates weighing less than 1500 grams. J Pediatr 1994;125:253-258.

Kasper DL, Paoletti LC, Wessels MR, et al. Immune response to type III group B streptococcal polysaccharide-tetanus toxoid conjugate vaccine. J Clin Invest 1996;98:2308-2314.

Klein JO. Neonatal sepsis. Semin Pediatr Infect Dis 1994;5:3-8.

Klein JO, Marcy SM. Bacterial sepsis and meningitis. In Remington JS, Klein JO (eds). Infectious diseases of the fetus and newborn infant, ed 4. Philadelphia: WB Saunders, 1995.

Kurlat I, Stoll BJ, McGowan JE Jr. Time to positivity for detection of bacteremia in neonates. J Clin Microbiol 1989;27:1068-1071.

McCracken GH Jr. Use of third-generation cephalosporins for treatment of neonatal infections. Am J Dis Child 1985;139:1079-1080.

McNeeley DF, Saint-Louis F, Noel GJ. Neonatal enterococcal bacteremia: an increasingly frequent event with potentially untreatable pathogens. Pediatr Infect Dis J 1996;15:800-805.

Murray BE. The life and times of the Enterococcus. Clin Microbiol Rev 1990;3:46-65.

Neal PR, Kleiman MB, Reynolds JK, et al. Volume of blood submitted for culture from neonates. J Clin Microbiol 1986;24:353-356.

Noya FJD, Rench MA, Metzger TG, et al. Unusual occurrence of an epidemic of type Ib/c group B streptococcal sepsis in a neonatal intensive care unit. J Infect Dis 1987;155:1135-1144.

Pichichero ME, Todd JK. Detection of neonatal bacteremia. J Pediatr 1979;94:958-960.

Placzek MM, Whitelaw A. Early and late neonatal septicaemia. Arch Dis Child 1983;58:728-731.

Rowen JL, Correa AG, Sokol DM, et al. Invasive aspergillosis in neonates: report of five cases and literature review. Pediatr Infect Dis J 1992;11:576-582.

Rowen JL, Smith CW, Edwards MS. Group B streptococci elicit leukotriene B_4 and interleukin-8 from human monocytes: neonates exhibit a diminished response. J Infect Dis 1995;172:420-426.

Rowley AH, Wald ER. Incubation period necessary to detect bacteremia in neonates. Pediatr Infect Dis 1986;5:590-591.

Sáez-Llorens X, Ah-Chu MS, Castaño E, et al. Intrapartum prophylaxis with ceftriaxone decreases rates of bacterial colonization and early-onset infection in newborns. Clin Infect Dis 1995;21:876-880.

Schuchat A, Deaver-Robinson K, Plikaytis BD, et al. Multistate case-control study of maternal risk factors for neonatal group B streptococcal disease. Pediatr Infect Dis J 1994;13:623-629.

Schuchat A, Oxtoby M, Cochi S, et al. Population-based risk factors for neonatal group B streptococcal disease: results of a cohort study in metropolitan Atlanta. J Infect Dis 1990;162:672-677.

Shattuck KE, Chonmaitree T. The changing spectrum of neonatal meningitis over a fifteen-year period. Clin Pediatr 1992;31:130-136.

Spafford PS, Sinkin RA, Cox C, et al. Prevention of central venous catheter-related coagulase-negative staphylococcal sepsis in neonates. J Pediatr 1994;125:259-263.

Spear ML, Stefano JL, Fawcett P, et al. Soluble interleukin-2 receptor as a predictor of neonatal sepsis. J Pediatr 1995;126:982-985.

Stoll BJ, Gordon T, Korones SB, et al. Early-onset sepsis in very low birth weight neonates: a report from the National Institute of Child Health and Human Development Neonatal Research Network. J Pediatr 1996a;129:72-80.

Stoll BJ, Gordon T, Korones SB, et al. Late-onset sepsis in very low birth weight neonates: a report from the National Institute of Child Health and Human Development Neonatal Research Network. J Pediatr 1996b;129:63-71.

Vallejo JG, Baker CJ, Edwards MS. Interleukin-6 production by human neonatal monocytes stimulated by type III group B streptococci. J Infect Dis 1996;174:332-337.

Visser VE, Hall RT. Lumbar puncture in the evaluation of suspected neonatal sepsis. J Pediatr 1980;96:1063-1066.

Visser VE, Hall RT. Urine culture in the evaluation of suspected neonatal sepsis. J Pediatr 1979;94:635-638.

Weiss MG, Ionides SP, Anderson CL. Meningitis in premature infants with respiratory distress: role of admission lumbar puncture. J Pediatr 1991;119:973-975.

Williams PA, Bohnsack JF, Augustine NH, et al. Production of tumor necrosis factor by human cells in vitro and in vivo, induced by group B streptococci. J Pediatr 1993;123:292-300.

Wiswell TE, Baumgart S, Gannon CM, et al. No lumbar puncture in the evaluation for early-onset neonatal sepsis: will meningitis be missed? Pediatrics 1995;95:803-806.

Wiswell TE, Hachey WE. Multiple site blood cultures in the initial evaluation for neonatal sepsis during the first week of life. Pediatr Infect Dis J 1991;10:365-369.

Yagupsky P, Menegus MA, Powell KR. The changing spectrum of group B streptococcal disease in infants: an eleven-year experience in a tertiary care hospital. Pediatr Infect Dis J 1991;10:801-808.

Zach TL, Hostetter MK. Biochemical abnormalities of the third component of complement in neonates. Pediatr Res 1989;26:116-120.

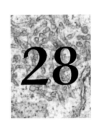

28 SEXUALLY TRANSMITTED DISEASES

MARGARET R. HAMMERSCHLAG, SARAH A. RAWSTRON, AND KENNETH BROMBERG

Sexually transmitted diseases (STDs) comprise a wide range of infections and conditions that are transmitted mainly by sexual activity. The "classic" STDs, gonorrhea and syphilis, currently are being overshadowed by a new set of STDs that are not only more common, but more difficult to diagnose and treat. These "new" STDs include infections caused by *Chlamydia trachomatis,* human papillomavirus, and human immunodeficiency virus (HIV). Physicians are confronted by particularly complex social and clinical problems caused by STDs in neonates and infants, in abused older children, and in adolescents. Rapid application of new technology to the diagnosis of STDs has led to a growing array of diagnostic laboratory tests that require critical evaluation. This chapter presents a comprehensive overview of STDs in neonates, infants, older children, and adolescents.

SEXUALLY TRANSMITTED DISEASES AND SEXUAL ABUSE OF CHILDREN

Sexual assault is a violent crime that affects men, women, and children of all ages. STDs can be transmitted during sexual assault. In children the isolation of a sexually transmitted organism may be the first indication that abuse has occurred. However, most sexually abused children are not initially seen with genital complaints. Unfortunately, the presence of an STD is frequently viewed as a short-cut to prove abuse. Although the presence of a sexually transmissible agent in a child beyond the neonatal period is suggestive of sexual abuse, exceptions do occur. For example, rectal and genital infection with *C. trachomatis* in young children may be due to persistent perinatally acquired infection, which may persist for up to 3 years. The use of STDs as indicators of sexual abuse is further complicated by inappropriate use of certain diagnostic tests such as tests for *C. trachomatis* antigen or misidentification of other bacteria as *Neisseria*

gonorrhoeae. A much higher standard of accuracy must be used for children than for adults since identification of an STD in a child will have legal and social, as well as medical implications.

Epidemiology of Sexual Abuse in Children

The incidence and prevalence of sexual abuse of children are difficult to estimate, in major part because much sexual abuse in childhood escapes detection. Several relatively extensive studies of sexual abuse of children in the United States have examined sex, race, and age-dependent variables. Patterns of childhood sexual abuse appear to depend on the sex and age of the victim (Glaser et al., 1989). Approximately 80% to 90% of abused children are female, with mean ages of 7 to 8 years. Most, 75% to 85%, were abused by a male assailant—adult or minor—known to the child. This individual is most likely a family member, especially the father or father substitute (stepfather, mother's boyfriend), uncles, and other male relatives (Rimsza and Niggemann, 1982). Victims of unknown assailants usually are older than the children abused by a known person, and the abuse usually involves only a single episode. In contrast, abuse by family members or acquaintances usually involves multiple episodes over periods of time ranging from 1 week to years. Most victims describe a single type of sexual activity, but more than 20% have experienced multiple types of forced sexual acts. Vaginal penetration occurs in approximately 50% and anal penetration in one third of female victims. More than 50% of male victims have experienced anal penetration. Other types of sexual activity include orogenital contact (in 20% to 50% of victims) and fondling. Children who are abused by a known assailant usually experience less trauma than victims of assault by a stranger.

Risk of Infection

An accurate determination of the risk of sexually transmitted conditions in victims of sexual abuse has been hindered by a variety of factors. First, the prevalence of sexually transmitted infections may vary regionally and among different populations within the same region. Second, few studies have attempted to differentiate between infections existing before the abuse. The presence of preexisting infection in adults is usually related to prior sexual activity (Jenny et al., 1990). In children, preexisting infection may be related to prolonged colonization after perinatal acquisition, inadvertent nonsexual spread, prior peer sexual activity, or prior sexual abuse (Glaser et al., 1989). Finally, incubation periods for STDs range from a few days for *N. gonorrhoeae* to several months for human papillomavirus. The incubation periods and timing of an examination after an episode of abuse are critically important in detecting infections. Multiple episodes of abuse increase the risk of infection, probably by increasing the number of contacts with an infected individual. In most cases the site of infection is consistent with the child's history of assault (Rimsza and Niggemann, 1982). Rates of infection also vary with the type of assault initially described. Vaginal or rectal penetration is more likely to lead to detectable infection than is fondling (Tilelli et al., 1980; White et al., 1983). However, the majority of children who are abused have no physical complaints related to either trauma or infection.

GONORRHEA

Until 1995, when infection with *Chlamydia trachomatis* became a reportable disease to the Centers for Disease Control (CDC), gonorrhea was the most frequently reported infectious disease in the United States. Since 1995, gonorrhea has become the second most frequently reported infectious disease after chlamydial infection. The World Health Organization estimates that there are approximately 100 million gonorrheal infections each year throughout the world. The reported number of cases of gonorrhea in the United States in 1994 was 418,068. This number has been decreasing yearly since a peak of 1 million cases in 1978 (Centers for Disease Control, 1994). Many cases escape detection and contribute to the silent reservoir of infection in males and females. In 1994, gonococcal infections were most common in the 15- to 19-year age group (Centers for Disease Control, 1994), making this a significant pediatric infection, and

not solely an adult infection. Gonorrhea is an inflammatory disease of the mucous membranes of the genitourinary tract that occurs only in humans. It is caused by *N. gonorrhoeae,* which first was described by Neisser in 1879. The most common portal of entry is the genitourinary tract, and the organism may then cause various inflammatory diseases of adjacent tissues such as cervicitis, salpingitis, and vulvovaginitis in children. The newborn may acquire the organism during delivery when direct contact with contaminated vaginal secretions leads to conjunctivitis. Bacteremia may occur, leading most commonly to the arthritis-dermatitis syndrome and, rarely, endocarditis and meningitis. Other manifestations of infection in children include gonococcal proctitis and pharyngitis. However, many gonococcal infections (15% to 44%) in children are asymptomatic (Ingram et al., 1992; De Jong, 1986).

Bacteriology

N. gonorrhoeae is a nonmotile non–spore forming, gram-negative coccus that characteristically grows in pairs (diplococci), with flattened adjacent sides in the configuration of "coffee beans." All *Neisseria* species, including *N. meningitidis,* rapidly oxidize dimethyl- or tetramethyl-paraphenylene diamine, the basis of the diagnostic oxidase test. The cell envelope of *N. gonorrhoeae* is similar to that of other gram-negative bacteria. Specific surface components of the envelope have been related to adherence, tissue and cellular penetration, cytotoxicity, and evasion of host defenses, both systemically and at the mucosal level.

Pili. Pili are filamentous projections that traverse the outer membrane of the organism and are composed of repeating protein subunits (pilin). When *N. gonorrhoeae* is grown on translucent agar, various colonial morphologies can be seen. Fresh clinical isolates initially form colony types P+ and P++ (formerly called T1 and T2). These organisms have numerous pili extending from the cell surface. After 20 to 24 hours, P− (formerly T3 and T4) colonies—in which the cells are nonpiliated—predominate. These nonpiliated organisms are not virulent. The shift between P+ or P++ and P− colony types is termed *phase variation* and is mediated by chromosomal rearrangement (Segal et al., 1985). The protein that constitutes pili (pilin) has regions of considerable antigenic variability between strains of *N. gonorrhoeae.* Single strains of *N. gonorrhoeae* also can produce pili of different antigenic composition (antigenic variation), which has made the possibility of a pilus-based vaccine against *N. gonorrhoeae* less feasible. Piliated gonococci are better able to attach to human mucosal surfaces than nonpiliated organisms. Pili also contribute to killing by neutrophils (Britigan et al., 1985).

Outer Membrane. The gonococcus has a cell envelope like other gram-negative bacteria; it consists of three layers: an inner cytoplasmic membrane, a middle peptidoglycan cell wall, and an outer membrane. The outer membrane contains lipooligosaccharide (LOS), phospholipid, and a variety of proteins. One of them is protein I, which functions as a porin and is believed to play an important role in pathogenesis. Preliminary data suggest that it may facilitate endocytosis of the organism or otherwise trigger invasion. Protein I is also the basis of the most commonly used gonococcal serotyping system because there is consistent antigenic variation between different strains (Knapp et al., 1984). Certain *N. gonorrhoeae* protein I serovars are associated with resistance of the organism to the bactericidal effect of normal nonimmune serum and an increased propensity to cause bacteremia. Gonococcal LOS is an endotoxin that differs from the polysaccharide of most gram-negative bacteria in that it lacks O-antigenic side chains. Some components of LOS are also related to resistance of *N. gonorrhoeae* to serum bactericidal activity. LOS also demonstrates interstrain antigenic variations, which are the basis of another serotyping system (Apicella, 1976).

Strain Typing

Characterization of gonococcal strains recently has been based on two primary methods—auxotyping and serology. Auxotyping is based on the differing requirements for specific nutrient or cofactors, which are genetically stable characteristics. It is done by examining the ability of strains of the organism to grow on chemically defined media that lack these factors (Catlin, 1973). More than thirty auxotypes have been identified. Common types include prototrophic (Proto) strain, also known as *zero* or *wild-type* strain; proline-requirement (Pro) strain; and strains that require arginine, hypoxanthine, and uracil (AHU strain). The most widely based serotyping system is based on protein I, as described previously. There are two major subgroups—IA and IB—which can be classified further into serovars based on coagglutination with a panel of monoclonal antibodies (Knapp et al., 1984). Combining typing strains with auxotyping and serology has been helpful in studying the epidemiology of gonococcal infection both geographically and temporally (Ahmed et al., 1992). It has been especially helpful in analyzing patterns of antibiotic resistance (Hook et al., 1987).

Genetics

Many strains of *N. gonorrhoeae* possess a 24.5 mD conjugative plasmid and can therefore conjugally transfer other non–self transferable plasmids. Many strains also carry a plasmid that specifies production of a TEM-1 type β-lactamase; the two most common plasmids of this type have molecular weights of 3.2 and 4.4 mD. Gonococci that carry the 24.5 conjugative plasmid with the tetM transposon inserted have high-level resistance to tetracycline, with minimum inhibitory concentration (MIC) greater than 16 mg/L, and this can be readily transferred to other gonococci. This tetM determinant functions by encoding for a protein that protects ribosomes from the effect of tetracycline. All gonococci also contain a small cryptic plasmid (2.6 mD) whose function is unknown.

Antibiotic resistance in *N. gonorrhoeae* may also be mediated by chromosomal mutations, which are not transferable by plasmids. Chromosomal resistance to β-lactam antibiotics and the tetracyclines appears to result from a series of minor mutations that reduce the permeability of the outer membrane or alter penicillin-binding protein 2, reducing its affinity for penicillin (Johnson et al., 1988).

Diagnosis

The Gram stain is considered to be positive if typical gram-negative diplococci are seen in association with polymorphonuclear leucocytes. A positive Gram stain from a male urethral specimen is highly sensitive and specific for gonococcal infection. However, in females, the adult cervix and the vagina of prepubertal children may be colonized with other *Neisseria* species, rendering the Gram stain less reliable. Similarly, gram-stained smears of rectum and pharynx are not useful to determine infection at these sites.

In younger children, because of medical and legal implications, the importance of an accurate microbiologic diagnosis cannot be overemphasized. Gram stain of the vaginal discharge in a child with suspected gonorrhea is not accurate and has a poor predictive value for the diagnosis of gonorrhea. Diagnostic specimens of the pharynx, rectum, and vagina or urethra should be taken and immediately plated onto selective media appropriate for isolation of *N. gonorrhoeae* (e.g., Thayer-Martin media) and then placed in an atmosphere enriched with carbon dioxide, which is done most easily using an extinction candle jar. Isolation of gonococci from sites containing many saprophytic organisms (vagina, cervix, pharynx, and rectum) is enhanced if selective media containing antibiotics (e.g., Thayer-Martin media) are used; these media inhibit most of the normal flora and permit only the growth of gonococci and meningococci. Specimens from other usually sterile sites (blood, synovial fluid, or cerebrospinal fluid) should only be inoculated onto nonselective (antibiotic-free) media such as enriched chocolate agar. *N. gonorrhoeae* are gram-negative, oxidase-positive diplococci, and their presence should be confirmed with additional tests, including rapid carbohydrate tests, enzyme-substrate tests, and rapid serologic tests. Failure to perform appropriate confirmatory tests may lead to misidentification of other organisms as *N. gonorrhoeae.* Whittington et al. (1988) found that 14 of 40 presumptive gonococcal isolates sent to the Centers for Disease Control (CDC) for confirmation had been misidentified as *N. gonorrhoeae.* Misidentified organisms included other *Neisseria* species, *Moraxella catarrhalis,* and *Kingella dentrificans.* The CDC (1993) recommends that confirmation of an organism as *N. gonorrhoeae* should include at least two procedures that use different principles (e.g., biochemical and enzyme-substrate or serologic). In addition, it is recommended that isolates be preserved to allow additional or repeated analyses.

Pathology and Pathogenesis

Stratified squamous epithelium can resist invasion by the gonococcus, whereas columnar epithelium is susceptible to it. This difference accounts for the absence of lesions in the adult vagina and on the external genitalia of both sexes. The susceptibility of columnar epithelium leads to infection of the urethra, prostate gland, seminal vesicles, and epididymis in males. In females, infection occurs primarily in the urethra, Skene's and Bartholin's glands, cervix, and fallopian tubes. Gonorrhea can occur in males or females without signs or symptoms (Amstey and Steadman, 1976). The primary infection can also occur in the rectal or pharyngeal mucosa of either sex. The alkaline pH of secreted mucus and the lack of estrogen permit vaginal in-

fections with overt vulvovaginitis to occur in the prepubertal girl (Hook and Holmes, 1985). Gonococci attach to the mucosal epithelium and then penetrate between and through the epithelial cells to reach the subepithelial connective tissue by the third or fourth day of infection. An inflammatory exudate quickly forms beneath the epithelium. In the acute phase of infection, numerous leukocytes (many with phagocytosed gonococci) are present in the lumen of the urethra, causing a characteristic profuse yellow-white discharge in males. In the absence of specific treatment the inflammatory exudate in the subepithelial connective tissue is replaced by macrophages and lymphocytes. Direct extension of the infection occurs through the lymphatic vessels and less often through the blood vessels. Acute urethritis is the most common manifestation in males, and the infection can then spread to the posterior urethra, Cowper's glands, seminal vesicles, prostate, and epididymis, which leads to perineal, perianal, ischiorectal, or periprostatic abscesses. Rarely, in young boys (Fleisher, 1980) and in adults, penile edema may be seen. In teenage and adult males, acute prostatitis can result in prostatic abscess or chronic prostatitis. Acute epididymitis is the most frequent complication of gonococcal infection.

In females, primary infection most frequently affects the columnar epithelium of the postpubertal cervix, and the histopathologic appearance resembles that of the male urethra. Spread of infection to the fallopian tubes may be acute or subacute, without signs and symptoms, and sometimes it is extremely difficult to diagnose. Acute stages can result in peritonitis. As a rule, the infection is confined to the pelvis. The end result of untreated or inadequately treated salpingitis is complete or partial obstruction of the tubes, which often leads to tubal pregnancy or sterility. Pelvic inflammatory disease (PID) is an especially common complication of gonorrhea in female adolescents, and when it occurs in this age range, it is especially likely to result in infertility (see Pelvic Inflammatory Disease and Salpingitis, next section) (Hook and Holmes, 1985).

Clinical Manifestations

In Pregnancy. The effects of gonococcal disease on the infant may begin before delivery, since there is evidence that gonococcal disease in pregnant women may have an adverse effect on both the mother and the infant. Edwards et al. (1978) observed nineteen women with intrapartum gonorrhea. They had a significantly greater occurrence of premature rupture of membranes, prolonged rupture of membranes, chorioamnionitis, and premature delivery. Other studies have shown an alarming incidence of perinatal deaths and abortions. In addition to the effect on the fetus, postpartum complications in the mother are common. Therefore the diagnosis of gonococcal disease should be sought and controlled during pregnancy. To obtain control, the following issues should be considered:

1. Recurrent infection after an initial episode during pregnancy is very common. Therefore specimens for culture should be obtained in later pregnancy from the woman who is infected in early pregnancy.
2. Many mothers conceive their first child while they are teenagers, an age range in which gonococcal disease has a particularly high prevalence and in which the young women may look to their pediatrician for medical care.
3. Gonococcal disease is especially dangerous to women because PID is a relatively frequent complication (see Pelvic Inflammatory Disease and Salpingitis).

In Infancy. Gonococcal ophthalmia is the most common form of gonorrhea in infants and results from perinatal contamination of infants by their infected mothers during parturition. Transmission rates of 42% have been observed (Laga et al., 1986). An initially nonspecific conjunctivitis with serosanguinous discharge is rapidly replaced by a thick, purulent exudate. Corneal ulceration and iridocyclitis appear unilaterally or bilaterally. Unless therapy is initiated promptly, perforation of the cornea may occur, leading to blindness. Ophthalmia neonatorum, formerly a leading cause of blindness, has been controlled by prophylaxis with silver nitrate or with antimicrobial agents such as erythromycin and tetracycline. Crede's original study in 1881 reported that 2% silver nitrate prophylaxis reduced the incidence of gonococcal ophthalmia from 10% to 0.5%. Neonatal ocular prophylaxis is not 100% effective; failures do occur (Laga et al., 1988; Rothenberg, 1979; Bernstein et al., 1983). The infant possibly is more likely to acquire the infection despite prophylaxis if there has been premature rupture of membranes (Handsfield et al., 1973). A more recent study of neonatal ocular prophylaxis in the United States suggests that prenatal screening and treatment of pregnant women has had a significant impact on the prevention of gonococcal ophthalmia (Hammerschlag et al., 1989). Bacitracin and sulfonamides are ineffective for prophylaxis (Rothenberg, 1979).

Other manifestations seen in newborns are other local infections such as scalp abscesses (associated with scalp electrodes) or systemic infections caused by gonococcemia and subsequent seeding of the organism to other areas—for example, sepsis, arthritis, meningitis and pneumonia. Gonococcal infections may also be asymptomatic, with cultures positive from oropharynx, vagina, and rectum.

In Young Children. Gonococcal vulvovaginitis is the most common gonococcal disease in children. It must be distinguished bacteriologically from vulvovaginitis caused by other agents by isolating *N. gonorrhoeae* from a vaginal swab; an endocervical culture is not necessary. In preadolescent females the vaginal exudate may be minimal and may be confused with a benign discharge (Michalowski, 1961). Symptoms referable to the urinary tract (dysuria) may predominate. Infection with *N. gonorrhoeae* is the most common sexually transmitted disease found in sexually abused children (Schwarcz and Whittington, 1990); a positive culture for *N. gonorrhoeae* from any site in a child without prior peer sexual activity is strongly suggestive of sexual abuse (Branch and Paxton, 1965). *N. gonorrhoeae* rarely may be spread by sexual play among children, but the index case has usually been a victim of abuse (Potterat et al., 1986). *N. gonorrhoeae* has been found in approximately 5% of children suspected of having been sexually abused (see Table 25-1). It may cause purulent vulvovaginitis in girls or urethritis in boys. Gonococcal ophthalmia may also occur as a result of autoinoculation from a genital site. However, as many as 20% to 25% of children with genital cultures containing *N. gonorrhoeae* may be asymptomatic, and an even higher number of rectal and pharyngeal infections are asymptomatic (Groothius et al., 1983; De Jong, 1986; McClure et al., 1986). Ascending pelvic infection may occur in prepubertal females (Burry, 1971), and it may occur in the absence of significant vaginal discharge. The main signs of early disease are dysuria and vaginal discharge. When gonococcal infection spreads from the cervix into the fallopian tubes, it is characterized by lower abdominal pain. The onset of acute salpingitis, or PID, may be abrupt and must be distinguished from acute appendicitis, cystitis, pyelonephritis, cholecystitis, and ectopic pregnancy (see Pelvic Inflammatory Disease and Salpingitis).

In Adolescents. Gonococcal infections are now most common in the 15- to 19-year age group (Centers for Disease Control, 1996a). Among adolescent girls, the most frequent presenting symptoms are those of cervicitis (vaginal discharge and intermenstrual bleeding) and urethritis (dysuria). However, many girls have only mild symptoms, and many infections are asymptomatic (32% in one study of adolescent girls [Biro et al., 1995]). Coinfection with *Chlamydia trachomatis* is common (about one third of gonococcal infections are coinfected with *C. trachomatis* [Biro et al., 1995]). Abdominal pain is usually a manifestation of PID, and is not associated with uncomplicated gonococcal infection.

In teenage males the onset of gonococcal urethritis is marked by sudden burning on urination occurring 2 days to 2 weeks after sexual exposure, similar to the presentation in adult males. This is followed by a mucopurulent discharge from the urethra. Involvement of the prostate gland is manifested by retention of urine, pain, and fever. Epididymitis may also occur, characterized by severe pain, tenderness, and swelling. Asymptomatic infection can also occur and is seen in approximately 2% of asymptomatic adolescent boys screened for gonorrhea (Hein et al., 1977; Smith et al., 1986).

Extragenital Manifestations

Disseminated Gonococcal Infection. Disseminated gonococcal infection (DGI) results from gonococcal bacteremia and occurs in 0.5% to 3% of patients with gonorrhea (Holmes et al., 1971). The strains of *N. gonorrhoeae* associated with DGI are usually very susceptible to penicillin, are resistant to the bactericidal action of nonimmune serum, have the AHU−auxotype, and belong to several specific protein 1A serovars (Knapp and Holmes, 1975). Individuals with deficient terminal components of complement (C5, C6, C7, or C8) are more susceptible to disseminated gonococcal infection and meninogoccal bacteremia (Petersen et al., 1979). Approximately 5% of patients with disseminated gonococcal infection have this deficiency. Other host risk factors apparently associated with an increased risk of dissemination include female sex, menstruation, pharyngeal gonorrhea, and pregnancy (Holmes et al., 1971). DGI can result from a primary infection at any site including cervix, urethra, anal canal, pharynx, and conjunctiva. The most common clinical manifestation of disseminated gonococcal infection is the arthritis-dermatitis syndrome. Joint symptoms are seen at initial presentation of DGI in more than 90% of patients (Handsfield, 1975). The arthralgias may be migratory and may involve more than one joint. The most commonly involved joints are the knees, ankles, wrists, elbows, and the small joints of the hands and feet. The symptoms range from mild to severe and include arthralgias with no inflammation to arthritis with synovial effusion and even joint destruction. Tenosynovitis is frequent (O'Brien et al., 1983). A characteristic rash consisting of discrete papules and pustules, often with a hemorrhagic or necrotic component, are also present in 50% to 75% of patients. Usually five to forty lesions are present, occurring primarily on the extremities, and ranging from 1 to 20 mm (Barr and Danielsson, 1971). The polyarthropathy and dermatitis frequently resolve spontaneously if not treated. However, arthritis may persist and progress, usually in one or two joints, most commonly the knee, ankle, elbow, or wrist. At this stage the clinical picture is that of septic arthritis. Disseminated gonococcal infection is the leading cause of infective arthritis in young adults. Studies of septic arthritis in children have found that *N. gonorrhoeae* is the third most frequent organism in children over 3 years of age and the most frequent in children over 11 years of age (Nelson, 1972). Some patients can develop gonococcal septic arthritis without prior polyarthritis or dermatitis. Most clinical manifestations of disseminated gonococcal infection are secondary to the bacteremia, although immune complexes and other immunologic mechanisms may be contributory to some cases. Patients usually have fever and some systemic toxicity, although it is frequently mild and often absent. It has been hypothesized that DGI consists of an early bacteremic stage that leads to a septic joint stage if left untreated (Handsfield, 1975; O'Brien et al., 1983), although not all patients fit this picture. Some bacteriologic findings are consistent with this hypothesis; for example, blood cultures are often positive in the early phase, and joint fluid may be culture positive in the later stage. Positive blood and synovial fluid cultures are almost always mutually exclusive (O'Brien et al., 1983). The organism may also be detected by immunochemical methods in biopsy specimens from about 60% of the skin lesions (Tronca et al., 1974), but cultures and Gram stains are positive in only 10% of cases. Overall, approximately 50% of patients with disseminated gonococcal infection will have positive cultures of the blood or synovial fluid, but *N. gonorrhoeae* can be recovered from a mucosal site (e.g., pharynx, rectum) in at least 80% of patients, an important consideration when evaluating a child with suspected septic arthritis. The differential diagnosis of disseminated gonococcal infection includes meningococcemia; other infectious arthritis; and an entire range of inflammatory arthritides, including Reiter's syndrome. Infrequent but serious complications of disseminated gonococcal infection include infective endocarditis, meningitis, osteomyelitis, and pneumonia.

Perihepatitis. Gonococcal perihepatitis (Fitz-Hugh-Curtis syndrome) results from extension of infection from salpingitis to the capsule and outer surface of the liver. It should be considered in females with right upper quadrant pain, palpable liver, abnormal liver function tests, and adnexal and uterine cervical tenderness. A positive endocervical culture for *N. gonorrhoeae* supports the diagnosis.

Conjunctivitis. Conjunctivitis beyond the newborn period follows direct spread of the gonococcus, usually via fingers contaminated with genital secretions. It rarely results from gonococcemia. Conjunctivitis is often severe with profuse purulent discharge, chemosis, eyelid edema, and ulcerative keratitis, and presentations may mimic orbital cellulitis (Lewis et al., 1990).

Oropharyngitis. Gonococcal oropharyngitis is common among homosexuals (Weisner et al., 1973) and among children who are victims of sexual abuse. Infection follows orogenital contact. Pharyngitis is usually asymptomatic and is detected on routine screening (Groothius et al., 1983). Pharyngeal cultures are positive in 15% (Nelson et al., 1976) to 54% (Groothius et al., 1983) of children with genital gonococcal infections. Rarely, pharyngeal infections are symptomatic (Abbott, 1973).

Anorectal Gonorrhea. Rectal infections are common in girls, probably because of the proximity of the vagina and the possibility of contamination of the anus with vaginal discharge. Rectal cultures may be positive in up to 50% of girls with positive vaginal cultures (Nelson et al., 1976). Most rectal infections are asymptomatic and are detected by routine screening, but occasionally there are symptoms (Speck, 1971). The symptoms are a purulent rectal discharge with rectal pain, blood, or mucus in the stool and perianal itching or burning.

Treatment

During the 20 years before 1976, all *N. gonorrhoeae* were sensitive to penicillin, but a gradual increase had been noted in the mean MIC. In March 1976 reports appeared of the first clinical isolations of penicillinase-producing *N. gonorrhoeae* (PPNG) arising in the Far East. PPNG strains have accounted for more than 30% of isolates of *N. gonorrhoeae* in the United States (Schwarcz et al., 1990). Since children acquire their infections from adults, parallel increases in PPNG infections in children were also found (Rawstron et al., 1989). There has also been a similar increase in tetracycline-resistant *N. gonorrhoeae* (TRNG). The CDC (1987) defines any area that has a rate of PPNG higher than 3% over a 3-month period as a hyperendemic area for PPNG and recommends that all infections be treated with penicillinase-resistant antibiotics. These resistant strains cause the same disease spectrum as penicillin-sensitive organisms. In 1983 an outbreak of chromosomally mediated penicillin-resistant gonococci was reported from North Carolina; subsequently, it has occurred in other areas of the country (Hook et al., 1987). These organisms, which do not produce penicillinase, are rare in children. Quinolone-resistant *N. gonorrhoeae* have emerged in Southeast Asia (Kam et al., 1996); in the United States, strains of *N. gonorrhoeae* with decreased susceptibility to fluoroquinolones have been detected (Centers for Disease Control, 1994), although this is not yet a widespread problem. Although strains of *N. gonorrhoeae* with decreased susceptibility to ceftriaxone do occur (Schwebke et al., 1995), no documented clinical treatment failures have been observed related to decreased gonococcal susceptibility to ceftriaxone in the United States (Gorwitz et al., 1993).

Prevention of Neonatal Infection. Endocervical cultures for gonococci should be obtained from all pregnant women as an integral part of prenatal care at the first prenatal visit. A second culture late in pregnancy should be obtained from women who are at high risk of gonococcal infection.

Prevention of Gonococcal Ophthalmia. Routine preventive prophylaxis of gonococcal ophthalmia includes (1) 1% silver nitrate (with no irrigation with saline solution, which might reduce efficacy); or (2) ophthalmic ointments containing tetracycline (1%) or erythromycin (0.5%) (Centers for Disease Control, 1993; American Academy of

Pediatrics, 1994). Use of bacitracin ointment (not effective) and penicillin drops (sensitizing) is not recommended.

Management of Infants Born to Mothers with Untreated Gonococcal Infection. The infant born to a mother with untreated gonorrhea should have orogastric and rectal cultures taken routinely and blood cultures taken if the infant is symptomatic. A term infant should receive a single injection of ceftriaxone (50 mg/kg intravenously [IV] or intramuscularly [IM], not to exceed 125 mg). Although ceftriaxone is not usually given to newborn infants, it is indicated in this specific setting.

Neonatal Disease

Gonococcal Ophthalmia. Infants with gonococcal ophthalmia should be hospitalized. They should receive a single dose of ceftriaxone (25 to 50 mg/kg/day, maximum dose 125 mg IV or IM) (Laga et al., 1986; Centers for Disease Control, 1993). Cefotaxime (25 mg/kg IV or IM every 12 hours for 7 days) is an alternative treatment. Infants with gonococcal ophthalmia should receive eye irrigations with buffered saline solution until the discharge is cleared. Additional topical therapy is not indicated. Simultaneous infection with *C. trachomatis* has been reported and should be considered in infants who do not respond satisfactorily. Both mother and infant should be tested for chlamydial infection.

Complicated Infection. Infants with arthritis, abscess, and septicemia should be treated by hospitalization and administration of ceftriaxone at 25 to 50 mg/kg IV or IM once daily for 7 days. Meningitis should be similarly treated with ceftriaxone, with treatment extending for 10 to 14 days.

Childhood Disease Beyond Infancy

Children with uncomplicated gonococcal vulvovaginitis, cervicitis, urethritis, pharyngitis or proctitis should be treated with ceftriaxone (125 mg IM once) (Centers for Disease Control, 1993) whether lighter or heavier than 45 kg. Using lidocaine as a diluent for the ceftriaxone injection reduces the pain of the injection (Schichor et al., 1994). Children who cannot tolerate ceftriaxone may be treated with spectinomycin (40 mg/kg, maximum 2 g) IM in a single dose (Rettig et al., 1980). Spectinomycin is not as effective in treating pharyngeal gonorrhea (Judson et al., 1985). The source of the infection must be identified, which may be facili-

tated by hospitalization (Ingram et al., 1982). Children with disseminated gonococcal infection (bacteremia or arthritis) should be treated with ceftriaxone (50 mg/kg, maximum 1 g, once daily for 7 days). Meningitis requires the same therapy, except the maximum dose is 2 g and duration of therapy is 10 to 14 days. All children with rectogenital gonorrhea should also be evaluated for coinfection with chlamydia. The newer expanded-spectrum oral cephalosporins such as cefixime are effective as a single dose (oral) in adults but have not yet been evaluated in children.

Gonococcal Infections in Adolescents

Single-dose efficacy is a major consideration in treatment of gonococcal infections, especially in adolescents. Another important factor is coinfection with *C. trachomatis,* which can be documented in up to 45% of adolescents with gonorrhea in some populations. For teenagers more than 12 years of age, treatment should follow the recommended regimens for adults with one exception: quinolones are not approved for use in children up to 18 years of age. The first-line regimens for treatment of uncomplicated gonococcal infection adults recommended by the CDC (1993) include: single-dose ceftriaxone (125 mg IM); cefixime (400 mg orally, single dose); ciprofloxacin (500 mg orally, single dose); ofloxacin (400 mg orally, single dose). Each regimen should also include a regimen effective against possible coinfection with *C. trachomatis* (Stamm et al., 1984) such as doxycycline (100 mg orally, 2 times a day for 7 days). Ciprofloxacin or ofloxacin may be used only if the adolescent is more than 16 years old. Alternative injectable regimens for individuals who cannot tolerate ceftriaxone are spectinomycin (2 g IM in a single dose); cefotaxime (500 mg IM once); ceftizoxime (500 mg IM once); cefotetan (1 g IM once); and cefoxitin (2 g IM once). All these regimens should be followed by a 7-day course of doxycycline. Tetracyclines cannot be used as a single drug for gonorrhea and chlamydia because of the increasing prevalence of TRNG strains.

PELVIC INFLAMMATORY DISEASE AND SALPINGITIS

Vaginal infection of females who are adolescent or younger may progress to involve the fallopian tubes or may disseminate to the pelvis. Pelvic inflammatory disease (PID) comprises a spectrum of inflammatory disorders of the upper genital tract in women and may include endometritis, salpingitis, tuboovarian abscess, and pelvic peritonitis. *N. gonorrhoeae* and *C. trachomatis* are implicated in most cases; however, microorganisms that can be part of the vaginal flora, such as anaerobes, *Gardnerella vaginalis, Haemophilus influenzae,* enteric gram-negative rods, and *Streptococcus agalactaie* are also involved (Eschenbach et al., 1975; Mardh, 1980). Some experts also believe that genital mycoplasmas such as *Mycoplasma hominis* and *Ureaplasma urealyticum* also play a role in the etiology of PID.

PID in adolescents is particularly likely to result in infertility and is the single most common cause of infertility in young women (Shafer et al., 1982; Westrom, 1980; Gates, 1984). A confirmed diagnosis of salpingitis and a more accurate bacteriologic diagnosis are made by laparoscopy. Since laparoscopy is not always available, the diagnosis of PID is often based on imprecise clinical findings and culture of specimens from the lower genital tract. Cultures of women with acute PID have recovered *N. gonorrhoeae* from the endocervix from approximately 35% to 80% of cases and from a smaller proportion of samples of fallopian tube aspirates (Eschenbach et al., 1975).

Risk factors for PID and acute salpingitis include young age at acquisition of gonococcal disease, a history of previous PID, multiple sexual partners, and use of an intrauterine device (IUD) for contraception. Approximately 15% of teenagers who develop gonorrhea progress to PID (Westrom, 1980). Diagnosing PID may be difficult, and the differential diagnosis includes numerous other conditions of the lower abdomen, including appendicitis, ectopic pregnancy, cholecystitis, mesenteric adenitis, pyelonephritis, and septic abortion. Misdiagnosis of PID is common, and it is one of the more common causes of medically nonindicated laparotomy. As mentioned previously, laparoscopy assists in establishing a diagnosis. The clinical diagnosis of PID is imprecise. Data indicate that a clinical diagnosis of symptomatic PID has a positive predictive value for salpingitis of 65% to 90% when compared with laparoscopy as the standard. Recommendations by Shafer et al. (1982) suggest that a clinical diagnosis of PID be supported by presence of lower abdominal pain and tenderness, cervical motion tenderness, and adnexal tenderness. Fever, leukocytosis, elevated sedimentation rate, and adnexal mass observed through abdominal ultrasound support the diagnosis. Culdocentesis, if performed, may reveal evidence of purulent reaction in the peritoneal cavity. The outcome for fertility probably is improved with prompt and vigorous therapy.

The Centers for Disease Control (1993) recommends that empiric treatment of PID should be instituted on the basis of the presence of all of the following three minimum clinical criteria for pelvic inflammation and in the absence of a cause other than PID:

Lower abdominal tenderness

Adnexal tenderness

Cervical motion tenderness

When severe clinical signs are present a more elaborate diagnostic evaluation is warranted. These additional criteria may be used to increase the specificity of the diagnosis:

Routine criteria

Oral temperature > 38.3° C

Abnormal cervical or vaginal discharge

Elevated erythrocyte sedimenation rate

Elevated C-reactive protein

Laboratory documentation of infection with *N. gonorrhoeae* or *C. trachomatis*

Elaborate criteria

Histopathologic evidence of endometritis on endometrial biopsy

Tubo-ovarian abscess on sonography or other radiologic tests

Laparoscopic abnormalities consistent with PID

Treatment and Prevention of Salpingitis and Pelvic Inflammatory Disease. Detailed recommendations are contained in the "Sexually Transmitted Diseases Treatment Guidelines," published by the CDC as a supplement to the *Morbidity and Mortality Weekly Report.* The last edition was published in 1993, and the following recommendations are based on this edition. Treatment regimens must provide empiric, broad-spectrum coverage of likely pathogens. Antimicrobial coverage should include *N. gonorrhoeae, C. trachomatis,* gram-negative facultative bacteria, anaerobes, and streptococci. In female adolescents treatment of gonorrhea with drug regimens that are effective against gonococci but not chlamydiae has led to a high incidence of residual salpingitis and, in males, of urethritis, both associated with continued disease caused by chlamydia (Stamm et al., 1984). No single therapeutic regimen has been established for women with PID. Selection of a regimen depends on availability of a drug, cost, patient acceptance, and regional differences in antimicrobial susceptibility of the likely pathogens.

Many experts recommend that all patients with PID be hospitalized so that therapy with parenteral antibiotics can be given under supervision. Indications for hospitalization for therapy of PID include the following:

1. Noncompliance.
2. All adolescents (compliance with therapy among adolescents is unpredictable).
3. Diagnostic uncertainty (appendicitis or ectopic pregnancy cannot be excluded).
4. Pelvic abscess is suspected.
5. Patient has HIV infection.
6. Severe illness or nausea and vomiting preclude outpatient treatment.
7. Patient is unable to follow or tolerate an outpatient regimen.
8. Failure to respond clinically to an outpatient regimen.
9. Clinical follow-up within 72 hours of starting therapy cannot be arranged.

The first-line inpatient regimen recommended by CDC is cefoxitin, 2 g IV every 6 h; or cefotetan, 2 g IV every 12 hours, plus doxycycline, 100 mg orally or intravenously every 12 hours for at least 48 hours after the patient demonstrates substantial clinical improvement, after which doxycycline, 100 mg orally, bid, should be continued for a total of 14 days. The alternate regimen is clindamycin, 900 mg IV q8h plus gentamicin, loading dose IV or IM (2 mg/kg) followed by a maintenance dose (1.5 mg/kg) every 8 h. This regimen should also be continued for 48 hours after the patient demonstrates substantial clinical improvement, after which doxycycline, 100 mg orally, bid, or clindamycin, 450 mg, po qid, for a total of 14 days. For children less than 8 years of age, erythromycin is substituted for the doxycycline. These regimens are effective in adolescent and adult women (Wasserheit et al., 1986; Wolner-Hanssen et al., 1986; Walters and Gibbs, 1990).

Follow-up. Because of the risk of persistent *C. trachomatis* infection, patients should be retested 7 to 10 days after completing treatment. Some experts also recommend screening for *C. trachomatis* and *N. gonorrhoeae* 4 to 6 weeks after completion of treatment. Evaluation and treatment of the sex partners of women with PID is very important because of the risk of reinfection. There is a high likelihood of urethral gonococcal or chlamydial infection in the partner. The CDC (1993) recommends that sex partners should be treated empirically with regimens effective against *C. trachomatis* and gonorrhea regardless of the apparent etiology of PID in their partner.

SYPHILIS

Primary and secondary syphilis continue to decline after having reached epidemic proportions in the United States. The incidence of 20.1 cases per 100,000 persons in 1990 was the highest since 1949. In 1995 that rate declined to 6.3 cases per 100,000 persons (Centers for Disease Control, 1996a). These changes are typical of the fluctuations seen with syphilis.

The number of babies with congenital syphilis is known to parallel closely the rates of primary and secondary syphilis among women of childbearing age. Indeed, the number of babies with congenital syphilis reported to the CDC had risen steadily from a low of 104 in 1978 to 4410 in 1991, a 1-year lag from the peak of primary and secondary syphilis. In 1995 the number had declined to 1548 (Centers for Disease Control, 1996b). In the past the number of reported cases of congenital syphilis was considered an underestimate of true disease (Rathbun, 1983). However, in 1988 the reporting definitions for congenital syphilis recommended by the CDC were changed (see surveillance definition in Centers for Disease Control, 1990). Therefore the number of babies with congenital syphilis increased after 1988, partly because of the change in definition (Cohen et al., 1990) and partly because of a true increase in numbers. Statistics after 1988, using the new definition, are at a baseline rate several times that of the pre-1988 figures but have fallen since 1991, consistent with the relationship between early maternal syphilis and congenital syphilis. The epidemiology of syphilis had also changed in 1990. The rates of early syphilis increased most for heterosexual minorities, predominantly blacks. One reason for this increase of syphilis was the increases of crack and cocaine use among the urban poor, with an associated exchange of sex for drugs (Centers for Disease Control, 1988). Unfortunately, because much of this sexual activity is anonymous, contact tracing and treatment of sexual partners—the usual methods of containing syphilis—have become increasingly difficult, undoubtedly impeding elimination of this disease. Recently emphasis has been placed on a persistent focus of syphilis in the south (St. Louis, 1996).

Children of any age can have syphilis, which may be congenital or acquired. Physicians taking care of children should be aware of the signs and symptoms of acquired and congenital syphilis.

Bacteriology

Treponema pallidum is the causative agent of syphilis. It is a thin, delicate organism, varying in length from 5 to 15 μm, with a width of 0.15 μm, which means it is not visible by light microscopy.

T. pallidum has tight spirals every 1.1 μm along its length, appearing like a helical coil (Hovind-Hougen, 1983). When seen through dark-field microscopy, it exhibits a spiral movement, with flexion around its midportion. The organism divides slowly, only every 30 hours, and cannot be cultured on artificial media. Tissue culture does not sustain the growth of *T. pallidum* for long periods (Jenkin and Sander, 1983), and inoculation into rabbits is the only reliable means for cultivating this organism. Humans are the only natural host, although several mammals (including rabbits and monkeys) can be infected.

Pathogenesis

The central problem in understanding the pathogenesis of syphilis is that, although there is a vigorous host response to infection, treated disease has a minimal effect on resistance to reinfection, and the infection may persist for life. The treponemes initially invade the body through microscopic abrasions produced by sexual intercourse or other physical activity. Approximately one third of people who have sex with infected partners will become infected. The treponemes attach to the cells by one end, although no specialized receptor site has been seen on electron microscopy (Hovind-Hougen, 1983). Once inside the epithelial layer, the organisms replicate locally. The host responds first with an influx of polymorphonuclear neutrophil leukocytes (PMNs). The *T. pallidum* undergoes rapid phagocytosis (Musher et al., 1983), probably because host IgG is present on the surface of the organism (Alderete and Baseman, 1979). Lymphocytes soon replace the PMNs (Baker-Zander and Sell, 1980). By the time the patient comes to clinical attention, a variety of antibodies usually are detected. However, the occurrence of secondary syphilis at the same time that the antibody titers are their highest indicates that the host response to infection is not effective, since the localized disease comes under control at the same time that the manifestations of generalized infection appear. However, at this time the host is immune to intradermal challenge with *T. pallidum* (Musher, 1984). The host eventually suppresses the infection, and there are no clinically apparent lesions, although the organism is not necessarily eradicated from the body; *T. pallidum* can be isolated from patients years after infection.

Acquired Syphilis

Acquired syphilis in childhood appears to follow a course similar to that in adults. Although most recognized syphilitic disease of children is congenital, syphilis can be acquired at any age. Acquired syphilis in preadolescent children represents the result of sexual abuse or assault until proven otherwise, although sexually active adolescents may acquire the disease through consenting sexual activity.

Primary Syphilis. Primary syphilis is characterized by a painless chancre that appears at the site of contact 10 to 90 days after exposure (average, 21 days). A chancre looks like a rounded, firm ulcer with a rubbery base and well-defined margins. The lesion is usually single and most commonly is found on the glans penis of the male and on the cervix or external genitalia of the female. It can also be found on the scrotum, anus, rectum, lips, tongue, tonsil, nipple, and fingers. Primary lesions in women often go unnoticed, since they may not be visible. Chancres persist for 3 to 6 weeks, then heal spontaneously. They usually are accompanied by regional lymphadenopathy. The lymph nodes are painless, not fluctuant, not tender, rubbery in consistency, and often bilaterally enlarged with genital lesions.

The diagnosis of primary syphilis can be made definitively by a positive dark-field examination or a positive direct fluorescent antibody test for *T. pallidum* (DFA-TP). In addition, serologic tests for syphilis should be performed. However, nontreponemal serologic tests are positive in less than 80% of patients presenting with primary syphilis. The treponemal tests (e.g., FTA-ABS) become positive earlier, with approximately 90% of patients initially seen with primary syphilis having positive tests (Duncan et al., 1974). Therefore, if primary syphilis is suspected, the laboratory should be instructed to perform the treponemal test even if the nontreponemal or reagin test (RPR or VDRL) is nonreactive. However, patients with a previously reactive treponemal test may be reactive for life, so the results may not be specific for a particular episode of genital ulcer disease (Romanowski et al., 1991).

Secondary Syphilis. The secondary manifestations usually appear 3 to 6 weeks after the appearance of the chancre and 6 weeks to several months after the initial contact. The primary lesion may still be evident or may have healed when the secondary lesions appear. Signs and symptoms commonly include local or generalized rash, generalized adenopathy, malaise, fever, headache, and pharyngitis. Less common manifestations are condylomata lata, mucous patches of the mouth, and alopecia. This is a systemic infection, and it is not unusual to find pleocytosis or increased protein in the cerebrospinal fluid (CSF) of patients with secondary syphilis. Lukehart et al. (1988) isolated *T. pallidum* from ten (30%) of thirty-three patients with secondary syphilis, with four of these patients having normal CSF values. Therefore patients with central nervous system (CNS) involvement with *T. pallidum* can have normal CSF values. Nevertheless, it is neither routine nor recommended to perform lumbar punctures on patients with secondary syphilis, since CNS involvement is so common it is considered a part of the disease.

The skin rash is usually macular or maculopapular and rarely pustular. The rose-pink rash spreads to involve the whole body, including palms and soles, and darkens to a dull red color; it is usually not pruritic. *T. pallidum* can be demonstrated in any mucous or cutaneous lesion but is found most easily in moist lesions. The diagnosis is usually confirmed by serology during this stage, and serologic tests are virtually always positive with high titers (>1:16). Secondary syphilitic manifestations usually resolve in 3 to 12 weeks.

Other conditions that may resemble primary and secondary syphilis include carcinoma, scabies, lichen planus, psoriasis, drug reactions, Behçet's syndrome, Reiter's syndrome, pityriasis rosea, and tinea versicolor. Since the rash is so similar, when a diagnosis of pityriasis rosea is made, a test should be performed to exclude syphilis.

Latent Syphilis. After the secondary lesions resolve, the stage of latent syphilis begins. The latent stage is arbitrarily divided into early latency (syphilis of less than 1 year's duration) and late latency (syphilis of more than 1 year's duration). During early latency approximately 25% of patients with untreated syphilis will have relapses of secondary syphilis. Late latency is the stage during which tertiary manifestations can occur. By definition, latent syphilis is clinically inapparent, and the diagnosis is usually made by a positive serologic finding in the absence of any primary or secondary symptoms. All untreated cases of syphilis are latent at some time during the course of the disease; indeed, the disease may be latent for the duration of the infection or the life of the patient. Approximately one third of infected untreated individuals develop late syphilitic manifestations, with characteristic central nervous system (CNS), cardiovascular, or gummatous lesions. Approximately two thirds of untreated infected individuals do not have any problems later, although more than half remain serologically positive. However, these patients do have a life expectancy that is shorter than normal. Patients who have latent syphilis for more than 4 years are rarely contagious to their sexual partners, but pregnant women can transmit the disease to the fetus even after having latent syphilis for many years. The likelihood of transmission is directly related to the duration of infection, with secondary syphilis being the most infectious.

Late Syphilis. Late syphilis is an uncommon entity in the postantibiotic era among adults and is extremely uncommon in children. Late syphilis is asymptomatic in the majority of people but may present as neurosyphilis, cardiovascular syphilis, or gummas. Gummas probably represent a hypersensitivity phenomenon. The other lesions of late syphilis are those of a vascular disease, with obliterative endarteritis of terminal arterioles and small arteries, which results in inflammatory and necrotic changes. Patients can have more than one late manifestation of syphilis.

Neurosyphilis. The essential pathologic process of all types of neurosyphilis is obliterative endarteritis, usually of terminal vessels, with associated parenchymatous degeneration. Neurosyphilis may be divided into the following groups, depending on the type and degree of CNS pathologic condition: asymptomatic; meningeal; meningovascular; and parenchymatous, consisting of paresis or tabes dorsalis. Optic atrophy is a serious complication of neurosyphilis and is detected by examination of the peripheral visual fields. Pupillary changes may be seen in late neurosyphilis; the classic change is the Argyll Robertson pupil, which is small and irregular and fails to react to light but responds normally to accommodation effort.

Asymptomatic. The patient with asymptomatic neurosyphilis is usually seen because of a positive serologic finding without signs or symptoms of CNS involvement. However, the CSF shows an increase in number of cells and total amount of protein and a reactive CSF VDRL for syphilis.

Meningeal. Acute syphilitic meningitis usually appears within a year of infection as acute hydrocephalus, cranial nerve palsies, or focal cerebral involvement. The CSF shows pleocytosis, increased protein, and a positive CSF VDRL.

Meningovascular. In patients with meningovascular neurosyphilis, definite signs and symptoms of

CNS damage are present, indicating cerebrovascular occlusion; infarction; and encephalomalacia with focal neurologic signs, depending on the size and location of the lesion. The CSF is always abnormal, with pleocytosis, increase in amount of protein, and a reactive CSF VDRL.

Parenchymatous. This form of neurosyphilis appears as paresis or tabes dorsalis. The manifestations of paresis can be myriad and are always indicative of widespread damage to the parenchyma. Personality changes range from minor ones to obvious psychosis. Focal neurologic signs are uncommon. Results of the CSF studies are invariably abnormal, the number of cells and the concentration of protein are increased, and the CSF VDRL is positive.

Cardiovascular Syphilis. The damage in patients with cardiovascular syphilis is caused by medial necrosis of the aorta, with aortic dilation often extending into the valve commissures. The essential signs are those of aortic insufficiency or saccular aneurysm of the thoracic aorta.

Syphilitic Gummas. Gummas are nonspecific granulomatous-like lesions. They most commonly are found in skin or bone and less commonly in mucosae, viscera, and muscle. They are usually benign, although they may cause serious problems if located in vital areas.

Congenital Syphilis

Congenital syphilis is a disease caused by maternal syphilis. Infection results from transplacental infection of the developing fetus from a mother with spirochetemia. An untreated syphilitic pregnant woman can transmit infection to the fetus at any clinical stage of her disease, although transmission is more likely with early infection. Fiumara et al. (1952) found that 50% of mothers with untreated primary or secondary syphilis had babies with congenital syphilis. The transmission to the fetus declined to 40% in early latent syphilis and 10% in late latent syphilis. Stillbirth is a frequent outcome of untreated syphilitic pregnancies. Wendel (1988) found that one half of babies with congenital syphilis were stillborn. Rawstron (1997) found that most stillbirths associated with reactive maternal syphilis serologic conditions during an outbreak had detectable *T. pallidum,* thus proving infection. However, evidence of fetal damage such as abortion is rare before the eighteenth week of gestation. Pathologic examination of tissues obtained from

therapeutic abortions before 12 weeks of gestation have shown that treponemal organisms are present in fetuses from mothers who have untreated syphilis (Harter and Benirschke, 1976). No inflammatory response has been seen unless gestation is 15 weeks or more. Fetal immunoimmaturity and the inability to recognize *T. pallidum* antigens are probably responsible for the lack of damage caused by syphilis in fetuses less than 18 weeks' gestation.

Babies have congenital syphilis usually because of lack of prenatal care in the mother (Mascola et al., 1984a). This is a preventable disease if the mother receives appropriate therapy early in pregnancy. However, treatment does not guarantee that the baby will not be infected, particularly if therapy is given late in pregnancy (Mascola et al., 1984b; Rawstron, and Bromberg, 1991a). A woman who has been adequately treated with penicillin and followed with quantitative serologic testing and has no evidence of reinfection does not need retreatment with each subsequent pregnancy. However, if any doubt exists about the adequacy of previous treatment or the presence of active infection, a course of treatment should be given to prevent congenital syphilis. Women who have been treated for syphilis in the past may become reinfected, and their babies can develop congenital syphilis.

The signs and symptoms of congenital syphilis are divided arbitrarily into early manifestations, which appear in the first 2 years of life, and late manifestations, which emerge any time thereafter. The outcome of untreated fetal infection is variable. Intrauterine death (stillbirth) occurs in an estimated 25% to 50% of infections. Historically, perinatal death has occurred in another 25% to 30% of untreated infected babies, although perinatal death is less common now, since many deaths in the past were due to prematurity (Wendel, 1988). Those infants who survive have a broad spectrum of manifestations.

Early Congenital Syphilis. The abnormal physical and laboratory findings in patients with early congenital syphilis are varied. The onset may be before birth to approximately 3 months of age, with most cases occurring within the first 5 weeks of age. Some babies are so severely infected that they are stillborn, and some die in the early neonatal period despite the use of antibiotics. However, not all babies become symptomatic. A baby with congenital syphilis may appear normal at birth only to appear later (delayed onset) with multiorgan system involvement (Taber and Huber, 1975). Some neonates have only hepatosplenomegaly, with or without jaundice, and some are totally asymptomatic but have evidence of bone involvement on roentgenograms or abnormal lumbar puncture results. Since most congenital syphilis is now discovered during the newborn hospital stay because of suspicion raised by a reactive serologic finding in the mother or baby, the current presentation of congenital syphilis is different than that described formerly in the literature (Fiumara, 1975). More babies who are asymptomatic but have abnormal tests indicative of infection are found. In the past these infants probably would have presented later with symptoms. Recent publications have downplayed the value of bone roentgenograms and CSF examinations in the diagnosis of congenital syphilis (Beeram, 1996; Risser, 1996), but it is likely that the incidence of congenital syphilis in these populations was low. During epidemics of syphilis, women of childbearing age can remain seropositive for long periods of time if not treated early in their infection. In addition, information about this treatment may not be easily available, giving the false impression that these women have untreated syphilis. Since these studies did not employ either *T. pallidum* detection or specific IgM determination, their conclusions should be suspect. It is reasonable to accept the utility of roentgenograms (Ingraham, 1935) and CSF VDRL determinations based on their sensitivity and specificity from both the preantibiotic era and other epidemics. Only studies that create an independent standard for congenital syphilis diagnosis can be used to refute the historically determined utility of these recommended tests.

Skeletal system. The roentgenographic changes in the bones are of diagnostic value because of their frequency and early appearance. They are present in approximately 50% to 95% of babies with congenital syphilis (Hira et al., 1985). The changes often are present at birth but may not appear until the first few weeks of life. Some have suggested that roentgenograms would be of most value at 1 month of age but this suggestion is not usually practical. The bony changes include osteochondritis and periostitis; metaphyseal changes are most common. The findings are symmetric and self-limited and heal in approximately 6 months, with or without therapy. The skeletal lesions are usually asymptomatic but are occasionally painful, so much so that the child will refuse to move the affected limb (pseudoparalysis of Parrot). The femur and tibia are most often involved, and a radiologic study of the knee is recommended when screening for syphilis. On x-ray films the earliest changes are revealed in the metaphysis and are seen as transverse, saw-tooth, radiodense bands of provisional calcification, with an underlying zone of osteoporosis, which is seen as radiolucent bands. Irregular areas of increased density and rarefaction produce the moth-eaten appearance of the x-ray film. The classic Wimberger's sign consists of a focal defect in the medial proximal tibial epiphysis and is caused by destructive osteitis. Periostitis appears later than osteochondritis and is seen on x-ray films as multiple layers of periosteal new bone formation. Radiologic findings in patients with congenital syphilis are shown in Figs. 28-1, 28-2, and 28-3.

Rhinitis. Rhinitis was a common manifestation historically but is uncommon now. It is not usually

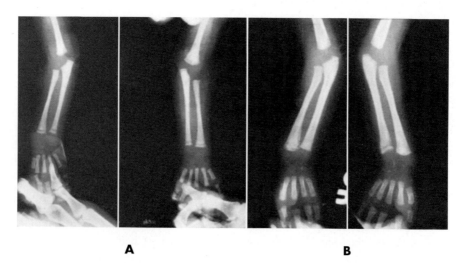

A   **B**

FIG. 28-1   Congenital syphilis. **A,** Typical wide horizontal metaphyseal radiolucent bands. **B,** Destructive syphilitic metaphysitis of the radius and ulna in a 6-week-old infant. Note subperiosteal reaction.

present at birth but appears after the first week of life. It initially is seen as severe and intractable rhinorrhea, which is often bloody and may be associated with a hoarse cry caused by laryngitis.

Rash. Historically, the syphilitic rash typically appeared 1 or 2 weeks after the rhinitis, but it is more common now to see the rash without preceding rhinitis. The typical eruption is maculopapular and consists of small, dark-red spots, but bullous eruptions can also occur. The rash commonly is present on the back, perineum, extremities, palms, and soles. The rash lasts 1 to 3 months without treatment, and the lesions may be covered by a fine, silvery scale and be followed by desquamation. The rash usually fades to leave coppery residual pigmentation.

Constitutional symptoms. The most common finding with early congenital syphilis is hepatosplenomegaly. Jaundice may be associated with it because of hepatic dysfunction, which is manifest by an increase in conjugated bilirubin (Srinivasan et al., 1983). Generalized lymphadenopathy may occur, although it is more common in historical cases. Infants may have fevers and occasionally nephrosis or nephritis. Choroiditis and iritis are uncommon.

The laboratory findings include a Coombs-negative hemolytic anemia with leukopenia or leukocytosis and thrombocytopenia. Congenital syphilis is one of the causes of a leukemoid reaction. Lumbar puncture may reveal a positive CSF VDRL, with increased protein and pleocytosis, although most babies clinically have no findings of CNS involvement. Sanchez et al. (1992) described five infants with congenital syphilis, four of whom had *T. pallidum* recovered from the CSF by rabbit infectivity tests. Three of the babies had a positive CSF VDRL, but one asymptomatic baby had normal CSF findings, although *T. pallidum* had been recovered from the CSF. We have detected *T. pallidum* in the unremarkable CSF of infants with congenital syphilis by immunofluorescent antigen detection.

The congenital syphilis of neonates and infants may resemble other intrauterine infections, including toxoplasmosis, rubella, cytomegalovirus, and herpes simplex virus. Other conditions that may resemble congenital syphilis in newborns include bacterial sepsis, blood group incompatibility, battered child syndrome, "periostitis" of prematurity, neonatal hepatitis, and osteomyelitis.

The placenta is a useful organ to examine when looking for congenital syphilis. The presence of

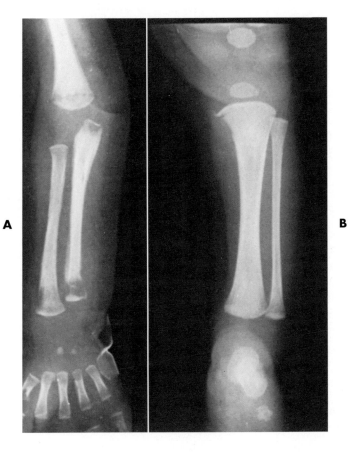

A

B

FIG. 28-2   Congenital syphilis. **A,** Panosteitis in an infant 9 weeks old. Metaphysitis is present and subperiosteal bone is appearing. **B,** Radiolucent area of the medial aspect of the proximal tibial metaphyses. This is called Wimberger's sign.

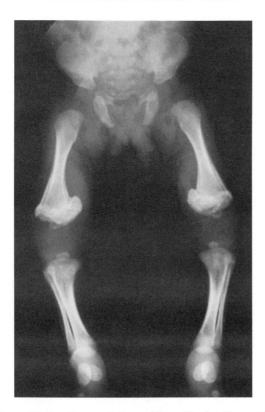

FIG. 28-3 Congenital syphilis. Diaphysitis with abundant callus formation secondary to pathologic fractures through the metaphyseal lesions. The lesions healed, and there were no sequelae.

necrotizing funisitis suggests congenital syphilis (Fojaco et al., 1989). The placenta may also be large and bulky and have the characteristic findings of focal villitis, endovascular and perivascular proliferation of vessels, and relative immaturity of villi (Russell and Altshuler, 1974). *T. pallidum* seen in tissue specimens is the only accepted method for making a confirmed diagnosis of congenital syphilis.

Late Congenital Syphilis. Late manifestations of congenital syphilis are the result of scarring from the early systemic disease and include involvement of the teeth, bones, eyes, and eighth nerve (Fiumara and Lessell, 1983); gummas in the viscera, skin, or mucous membranes; and neurosyphilis (Digre et al., 1991; Wolf and Kalangu, 1993). Late syphilis is very rare in the antibiotic era.

Teeth. Characteristic changes are found in the permanent upper-central incisors, which present a notched appearance of the biting edges; these are called *Hutchinson's teeth.* First molars with malde-

velopment of the cusps are known as *mulberry* or *Moon's molars* (Figs. 28-4 and 28-5).

Interstitial keratitis. Interstitial keratitis is the most common late lesion. It may appear at any age between 4 and 30 years or later, but characteristically it appears when the patient is close to puberty. It first is seen as unilateral photophobia, pain, and blurred vision. A ground-glass appearance may develop in the cornea, accompanied by vascularization of the adjacent sclera. These changes become bilateral and lead to blindness. Penicillin treatment is ineffective, but steroid treatment can help prevent loss of vision.

Eighth nerve deafness. Hearing loss is usually sudden and appears around 8 to 10 years of age. Hutchinson's triad consists of interstitial keratitis accompanied by neural deafness and typical Hutchinson's teeth (Karmody and Schuknecht, 1966).

Neurosyphilis. The same manifestations of neurosyphilis seen in patients with acquired syphilis can occur in those with congenital syphilis, although symptomatic neurosyphilis is very rare. Paresis is seen more frequently and tabes dorsalis less frequently in the congenital form than in the acquired form of the disease.

Bone changes. Bone changes include sclerosing lesions, saber shins, frontal bossing, and the gummatous or destructive lesion of saddle nose. Perforation of the hard palate is almost pathognomonic of congenital syphilis.

Clutton's joint. Clutton's joint is painless arthritis of the knees and, rarely, other joints. It usually is first seen around puberty.

Cutaneous lesions. Rhagades represent scarring from persistent rhinitis during infancy and are rarely seen today.

Laboratory Procedures in the Diagnosis of Syphilis

There are two main ways of diagnosing syphilis. The first is to detect treponemes using dark-field or immunofluorescent methods. The second is to detect antibodies formed in response to a treponemal infection, using nontreponemal and treponemal antibody tests.

Dark-Field Examination. The diagnosis of syphilis can be made by a positive dark-field examination of appropriate specimens. This test requires a compound microscope equipped with a dark-field condenser with which the specimen is illuminated by reflected light against a dark background. A positive diagnosis can be made by an experienced worker on the basis of characteristic morphologic

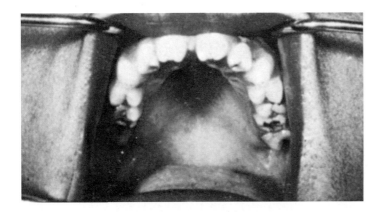

FIG. 28-4   Hutchinson's teeth. Note the notched edges and screwdriver shape of the central incisors.

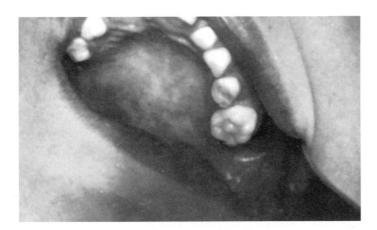

FIG. 28-5   Mulberry or Moon's molar.

aspects and motility. Dark-field examination is most productive during primary, secondary, and early congenital syphilis when lesions are present. Gloves should be worn when examining suspected syphilitic lesions and when performing dark-field examinations. Lesions should be cleaned thoroughly with physiologic saline solution with no additives. The lesion should then be squeezed and scraped firmly to collect serum rather than blood. Aspirated material from involved regional lymph nodes also can be examined for *T. pallidum*. The specimen must be viewed within 5 to 10 minutes to detect motile treponemes. If the result of the initial dark-field examination is negative, it should be repeated on at least 2 successive days to confirm a negative result.

Immunofluorescent Antigen Detection.
Alternative methods to detect *T. pallidum* in lesions are direct and indirect fluorescent antibody tests for *T. pallidum*. These tests use either monoclonal or polyclonal antibodies against *T. pallidum* that are directly fluorescein tagged or use a second fluorescein-tagged antibody to detect the primary antibody-antigen complex (Yobs et al., 1964). The ad-

vantage of immunofluorescent methods over dark-field microscopy is that slides are more permanent and can be mailed to reference laboratories for review by experts if the volume of patients seen is too small to warrant having a dark-field microscope (Bromberg et al., 1993).

Reaginic Tests.
The serologic diagnosis of syphilis uses two general types of tests: reaginic and treponemal. The reaginic tests use cardiolipin and lecithin as antigen. The antibody measured has been termed *reagin*, which has no relationship to the reaginic IgE in allergic patients. Antibody appears in the blood 1 to 3 weeks after the chancre appears or approximately 4 to 6 weeks after the infection. The reaginic tests commonly used today are the VDRL test and the rapid plasma reagin (RPR) test. The RPR test uses a modified VDRL antigen. The RPR test is inexpensive and quantitated and can be well controlled. The height of the titer tends to correlate with disease activity, rising with new infection and falling after treatment. A change of one doubling dilution is within laboratory error and therefore not significant. Changes of

two dilutions (fourfold changes) are considered significant when assessing disease activity. However, these tests are not specific for syphilis and may also be reactive in patients with collagen-vascular disease, liver disease, and other conditions.

Positive serologic results are found in approximately 80% of patients with primary syphilis, 100% of patients with secondary syphilis, and 95% of those with early latent syphilis, but only 70% of patients with late latent or late (tertiary) syphilis (Sparling, 1971). Thus false-negative serologic findings using reaginic tests is a problem in very early and again in later stages of untreated syphilis. With adequate treatment the reaginic tests should become nonreactive 6 to 12 months after primary syphilis and 12 to 24 months after secondary syphilis (Fiumara, 1980). Romanowski et al., (1991) found that it took much longer for titers to become nonreactive. Patients with later stages of syphilis who are treated take longer for their titers to fall and may never revert to nonreactive on nontreponemal tests; thus they may remain with low titers for life or "serofast."

Treponemal Tests. The fluorescent treponemal antibody absorption (FTA-ABS) test is an indirect antibody test that uses *T. pallidum* as the antigen. The FTA-ABS test is quite sensitive and specific (Deacon et al., 1966). It is technically more difficult than the nontreponemal tests and is used for confirmation of positive nontreponemal tests. The results of this test are reported as reactive, minimally reactive, or nonreactive, and they are not quantitated. The treponemal tests become reactive earlier in primary syphilis than do nontreponemal tests and, once positive, can remain so for life, even after appropriate therapy.

The microhemagglutination assay for antibodies to *T. pallidum* (MHA-TP) is a qualitative hemagglutination test that uses sheep erythrocytes as carriers for the *T. pallidum* antigen. False-positive tests are very uncommon with both FTA-ABS and MHA-TP when they are used to confirm a reactive nontreponemal test. When treponemal tests are used as screening tests, they have lower specificity. Patients with lupus may have false-positive FTA-ABS, MHA-TP, and nontreponemal tests.

T. pallidum IgM tests are useful in diagnosing congenital syphilis because, unlike IgG, IgM does not cross the placenta. Therefore detection of specific IgM in a baby is a strong indication of infection. There are various kinds of *T. pallidum* IgM tests, but none is widely available. The original *T.*

pallidum IgM, an immunofluorescent test described by Scotti and Logan (1968), had too many false-positive (10%) and false-negative (up to 35%) results for widespread clinical use (Kaufman et al., 1974). A newer IgM-FTA test is performed by the CDC, although its usefulness has not been evaluated fully. It is more widely used in Europe. Western blot tests have been used for research purposes and apparently are sensitive and specific for evaluating babies with congenital syphilis, although only small numbers of babies have been evaluated using this technique (Sanchez et al., 1989, 1992, 1993; Grimprel et al., 1991). None of these IgM tests can detect all babies with syphilis, since some babies are so recently infected that they have no IgM present at delivery. Thus a combination of antigen or DNA detection along with IgM might present the best strategy for diagnosis identifying them (Bromberg et al., 1993).

Diagnosis of Congenital Syphilis. The diagnosis of congenital syphilis in the newborn period can be difficult. Both the nontreponemal and treponemal tests measure IgG antibody and therefore do not distinguish disease in the infant from maternally derived antibody. The minority of babies with congenital syphilis are symptomatic at birth. Although some infants will develop symptoms later if left untreated, some may never become symptomatic. Unfortunately, there is no "gold standard" test for congenital syphilis. A combination of physical findings, radiologic results, laboratory tests, and ancillary tests is used to screen for and diagnose congenital syphilis. In the past clinicians waited for the development of symptoms, but in present-day practice this is unwise because of the high probability of losing the patient to follow-up. In the diagnosis of congenital syphilis, therefore, it is best to err on the side of overdiagnosis and overtreatment (see Box 28-1). The 1993 CDC guidelines recommend that infants should be evaluated for congenital syphilis if they are born to mothers with positive nontreponemal and treponemal tests and the mothers fit any of the following criteria:

1. Have untreated syphilis.
2. Were treated for syphilis during pregnancy with a nonpenicillin regimen (e.g., erythromycin).
3. Were treated for syphilis less than 1 month before delivery.
4. Did not have the expected decrease in nontreponemal titers after treatment of syphilis (fourfold decline).

BOX 28-1
CONGENITAL SYPHILIS

Clinical Description

A condition caused by infection in utero with *Treponema pallidum.* A wide spectrum of severity exists, and only severe cases are clinically apparent at birth.

An infant (<2 years) may have signs such as hepatosplenomegaly, characteristic skin rash, condyloma lata, snuffles, jaundice (nonviral hepatitis), pseudoparalysis, anemia, or edema (nephrotic syndrome and/or malnutrition). An older child may have stigmata such as interstitial keratitis, nerve deafness, anterior bowing of shins, frontal bossing, mulberry molars, Hutchinson's teeth, saddle nose, rhagades, or Clutton's joints.

Laboratory Criteria for Diagnosis

Demonstration of *T. pallidum* by darkfield microscopy, fluorescent antibody, or other specific stains in specimens from lesions, placenta, umbilical cord, or autopsy material.

Case Classification

Presumptive: the infection of an infant whose mother had untreated or inadequately treated* syphilis at delivery regardless of signs in the infant; or the infection of an infant or child who has a reactive treponemal test for syphilis and any one of the following:

Any evidence of congenital syphilis on physical examination.

Any evidence of congenital syphilis on long bone roentgenogram.

A reactive cerebrospinal fluid (CSF) VDRL.

An elevated CSF cell count or protein (without other cause).

A reactive test for fluorescent treponemal antibody absorbed-19S-IgM antibody.

Confirmed: a case (among infants) that is laboratory confirmed.

Comment

Congenital and acquired syphilis may be difficult to distinguish when a child is seropositive after infancy. Signs of congenital syphilis may not be obvious, and stigmata may not yet have developed.

Abnormal values for CSF VDRL, cell count, and protein, as well as IgM antibodies, may be found in either congenital or acquired syphilis. Findings on long bone roentgenograms may help, since roentgenographic changes in the metaphysis and epiphysis are considered classic for congenitally acquired disease. The decision may ultimately be based on maternal history and clinical judgment. The possibility of sexual abuse should be considered.

For reporting purposes, congenital syphilis includes cases of congenitally acquired syphilis among infants and children, as well as syphilitic stillbirths.

Syphilitic Stillbirth
Clinical case definition

A fetal death that occurs after a 20-week gestation or in which the fetus weighs >500 g, and the mother had untreated or inadequately treated* syphilis at delivery.
Comment

For reporting purposes, syphilitic stillbirths should be reported as cases of congenital syphilis.

From Centers for Disease Control, October 19, 1990.
*Inadequate treatment consists of any nonpenicillin therapy or penicillin given <30 days before delivery.

---

5. Did not have a well-documented history of treatment for syphilis.
6. Were treated appropriately during pregnancy but had insufficient serologic follow-up during pregnancy to assess disease activity.

It is also recommended that an infant not be released from the hospital until the serologic status of its mother is known because one third of babies born to mothers with positive serologic findings have nonreactive cord blood serologic findings (Miller et al., 1960; Rawstron, 1991b). Therefore maternal serologic testing is preferred over cord

blood testing in screening for congenital syphilis at delivery.

Infants whose mothers fit the criteria in the foregoing list should be evaluated with a physical examination, looking for evidence of congenital syphilis. The infants should have a nontreponemal antibody titer evaluation and a lumbar puncture, with analysis for CSF VDRL, cells, and protein. They should also have long-bone radiologic studies performed. Roentgenograms of the knee are preferred for screening. Treponemal IgM tests should be performed if available. Although not specifically recommended by the CDC, a complete blood count and a serum alanine aminotransferase (ALT) level to screen for hepatitis are useful when trying to determine if infection is present in an asymptomatic baby.

Treatment

T. pallidum is exquisitely sensitive to penicillin with an MIC of 0.005 to 0.01 μg/ml as defined by rabbit experimentation (Eagle et al., 1950). Effective therapy of syphilis has been aimed at maintaining an MIC of 0.03 units/ml (0.018 μg/ml) for 7 to 10 days (Idsoe et al., 1972) because of the slow dividing time of *T. pallidum* (every 30 hours). Thus therapy is designed to achieve and maintain several times the necessary inhibitory levels. Penicillin remains the drug of choice because there is no evidence of resistance of *T. pallidum* to penicillin, and it has minimal toxicity and established efficacy in treating syphilis.

Congenital Syphilis. Who should be treated? The decision to treat rests on the results of the evaluation described previously. Infants with abnormalities on evaluation or those born to mothers with inadequately treated syphilis should be treated. Even when the diagnosis is "normal," babies should be treated if their mothers had untreated syphilis at delivery or have evidence of relapse or reinfection after treatment, as shown by a rising nontreponemal titer or a titer that has not fallen within an appropriate time. If the infants do not undergo a full evaluation, it is recommended they be treated as if they had congenital syphilis.

How they should be treated? Treatment of congenital syphilis is the same regardless of whether or not there are CSF abnormalities, since patients can have neurosyphilis and normal CSF values. Treatment should be with aqueous crystalline penicillin G (50,000 units/kg/dose) administered every 12 hours during the first week of life and then every 8 hours (100,000 to 150,000 units/kg/day). This dose is increased compared with previous recommendations. An alternative, which perhaps is preferable because of its ease of administration, is procaine penicillin (50,000 units/kg/day), given as 1 intramuscular dose daily (McCracken and Kaplan, 1974). The length of therapy for both regimens is 10 to 14 days. If more than 1 day of therapy is missed, the entire therapy should be restarted. Therapy for neonatal sepsis that includes penicillin or ampicillin in appropriate doses for meningitis should be counted as part of the therapy for congenital syphilis.

There is a small group of infants who are at low risk of infection but who should receive therapy if their follow-up cannot be ensured. Babies who fit the criteria for evaluation but do not fit the criteria for congenital syphilis should be treated if they cannot be followed. For these babies one dose of benzathine penicillin G (50,000 units/kg) is recommended by the CDC. Some experts, however, do not like to use benzathine penicillin G in babies with congenital syphilis because CSF levels are subtherapeutic (Speer et al., 1977) and treatment failures, although not common, have been documented (Beck-Sague and Alexander, 1987). If follow-up of these patients is a problem, they should be treated with procaine penicillin for 10 days. Some programs have treated these infants with procaine penicillin at home administered by visiting nurses. These programs have the secondary benefit of providing needed parenting education.

Treatment Beyond the Newborn Period. After the newborn period, all children with syphilis should have a lumbar puncture performed. Any child who is thought to have congenital syphilis or who has neurologic involvement should be treated with aqueous crystalline penicillin G (50,000 units/kg/dose) every 4 to 6 hours for 10 to 14 days. Older children with acquired syphilis and normal neurologic results may be treated with benzathine penicillin G (50,000 units/kg IM) up to the adult dose of 2.4 million units. If the child has latent syphilis of unknown duration, 3 doses of benzathine penicillin (50,000 units/kg/dose [maximum 2.4 million units per dose]) at weekly intervals should be given. Penicillin is the only recommended treatment for children with syphilis; therefore, if there is a history of penicillin allergy, children and all pregnant women should be skin tested and desensitized if necessary (Zenker and Rolfs, 1990; Wendel et al., 1985).

Adolescents with Syphilis. Treatment of adolescents with syphilis should be similar to that of adults at the same stage of disease. Primary, secondary, and early latent syphilis of less than 1 year's duration should be treated with benzathine penicillin G (50,000 units/kg), with a maximum of 2.4 million units IM in 1 dose. Alternative regimen for penicillin-allergic patients is doxycycline (100 mg orally twice a day for 2 weeks).

Adolescents with late latent syphilis of more than 1 year's duration should be treated with benzathine penicillin G (150,000 units/kg total, with a maximum of 7.2 million units total) administered as 3 doses of 50,000 units/kg IM (maximum 2.4 million units) given 1 week apart for 3 consecutive weeks. Alternative therapy for penicillin-allergic patients is doxycycline in the same doses used for patients with early syphilis but given for 4 weeks instead of 2 weeks.

Neurosyphilis. Recommended treatment for neurosyphilis in adults is aqueous penicillin G, 2 to 4 million units every 4 hours IV (12 to 24 million units per day) for 10 to 14 days. Alternative therapy is procaine penicillin (2 to 4 million units IM daily) with probenicid (500 mg orally 4 times a day) for 10 to 14 days. Many experts also recommend benzathine penicillin G (2.4 million units IM weekly for 3 doses) after finishing either of the foregoing treatment regimens.

Jarisch-Herxheimer Reaction. Jarisch-Herxheimer reaction is an acute febrile reaction that may occur after any therapy for syphilis. The reaction consists of a fever, which is usually accompanied by headache and myalgia, that commonly lasts less than 24 hours. Pregnant women may have associated contractions and should be warned about this possibility. There is no treatment recommended except for antipyretics if necessary.

Follow-up. Infants with congenital syphilis should be followed with serologic tests at 3, 6, and 12 months of age. If the baby did not receive therapy, follow-up should also include serologic testing at 1 and 2 months to ensure that titers are falling. Nontreponemal titers usually disappear by 6 months of age in the absence of infection. If titers are stable or increasing, the child should be reevaluated and retreated. Treponemal titers are usually negative by 1 year of age in the absence of infection. If the treponemal titers are still positive at 12 months, this is strong evidence that the child was truly infected with syphilis. If the child received adequate therapy in the newborn period and the nontreponemal titer is nonreactive, the child does not need retreatment. Infants who were never treated for congenital syphilis should be evaluated—including performance of a lumbar puncture—and treated. Lumbar punctures should be repeated every 6 months for 3 years or until the CSF examination is normal in infants with a positive CSF VDRL in the newborn period.

Syphilis and HIV Disease

There have been reports of adult patients with neurosyphilis and HIV disease and of one case of a patient with secondary syphilis who had a nonreactive VDRL test result on several occasions before the re-

sult became positive. Musher et al. (1990) found that HIV coinfection with syphilis has caused the following: failure to respond to treatment within the expected time; relapse after treatment; and the frequent appearance of early neurosyphilis, especially after conventional doses of benzathine penicillin. There have been no documented treatment failures among either pregnant women who are HIV positive with syphilis or their offspring. At this time the CDC recommends no change in therapy for patients with early syphilis in HIV-infected patients, although some experts have recommended CSF examination and treatment appropriate for neurosyphilis for all patients with HIV and syphilis (Musher et al., 1990). Recommended penicillin regimens do not always attain treponemicidal CSF levels (Dunlop et al., 1979; Frenz et al., 1984), although most patients do well with these regimens. These patients should be followed very closely for signs of treatment failure. Any patient with syphilis should have HIV testing, since both of these diseases may be present in the same patient. In regard to the management of infants born to HIV positive and RPR positive mothers, although there are no data, it is our recommendation to treat these infants as if they had central nervous system involvement.

Syphilis and Sexual Abuse

Syphilis is not commonly found among sexually abused children (Table 28-1). However, it has been reported in a few instances. White et al. (1983) detected 6 cases among 108 of 409 prepubertal children on whom serologic tests were performed. Five children were asymptomatic and had additional sexually transmitted disease, and only 1 was symptomatic with chancres. De Jong (1986) found only 1 out of 532 abused children had a positive serologic test for syphilis. Children are seen with the same signs and symptoms as adults with syphilis. Ginsberg (1983) described 3 patients with acquired syphilis, 1 of whom was initially seen with a primary chancre and 2 with rashes of secondary syphilis. Similar findings have been described by Ackerman et al. (1972), who observed 3 abused children first seen with rashes of condylomata lata of secondary syphilis. It is recommended that a serologic test for syphilis be performed on every child suspected of being sexually abused and that the test also be repeated after 12 weeks.

CHLAMYDIA TRACHOMATIS

The genus *Chlamydia* comprises a group of obligate intracellular parasites with a unique developmental cycle with morphologically distinct infec-

Table 28-1 Prevalence of syphilitic, gonorrheal, and chlamydial infections in sexually abused children

Study (year)	Number tested	Number (%) positive		
		Syphilis	Gonorrhea	Chlamydia
Rimsza and Niggemann (1982)	285	0	21 (7)	NS
White et al. (1983)	409	6 (1)	46 (11)	NS
De Jong (1986)	532	1 (0.2)	25 (5)	NS
Hammerschlag et al. (1984)	51	0	5 (10)	2 (4)
Ingram et al. (1984)	50	NS	10 (20)	3 (6)
Ingram et al. (1992)	1538	1 (0.1)	41 (3)	18 (1)

Ns, Not stated.

tious and reproductive forms. All members of the genus have a gram-negative envelope without peptidoglycan, share a genus-specific lipopolysaccharide antigen, and use host adenosine triphosphate (ATP) for the synthesis of chlamydial protein. The genus now contains four species, *Chlamydia trachomatis; C. psittaci; C. pneumoniae; and C. pecorum,* which was recently speciated off from *C. psittaci.* Infection with *C. pecorum* has been described in cattle and sheep. There are fifteen known serotypes of *C. trachomatis* (Table 28-2).

The chlamydial developmental cycle involves an infectious, metabolically inactive extracellular form (elementary body [EB]) and a noninfectious, metabolically active intracellular form (reticulate body) (Fig. 28-6). EBs, 200 to 400 nm in diameter, attach to the host cell by a process of electrostatic binding and are taken into the cell by endocytosis that is not dependent on the microtubule system. Within the host cell the EB remains within a membrane-lined phagosome. Fusion of the phagosome with the host cell lysosome does not occur. The EBs then differentiate into reticulate bodies that undergo binary fission. After approximately 36 hours, the reticulate bodies differentiate into EBs. At approximately 48 hours, release may occur by cytolysis or by a process of exocytosis or extrusion of the whole inclusion, leaving the host cell intact. Infection can proceed without causing significant cellular damage. Thus there is a biologic basis for the prolonged subclinical infection, which is a hallmark of human chlamydial disease. Because the organisms are obligate intracellular parasites, they are actively infecting cells rather than simple colonizers, which have no interaction with the host cells.

C. trachomatis is the most prevalent sexually transmitted infection in the United States today. The CDC estimates that the number of new *C. trachomatis* infections exceeds 4 million annually. The prevalence of chlamydial infection is more weakly associated with socioeconomic status, ur-

Table 28-2 Serovars of *Chlamydia trachomatis*

Serovar	Disease
A, B, Ba, C	Hyperendemic blinding trachoma
D, E, F, G, H, I, J, K	Neonatal inclusion conjunctivitis
	Infantile pneumonitis
	Nongonococcal urethritis
	Mucopurulent cervicitis and salpingitis
	Proctitis
	Epididymitis
L1, L2, L3	Lymphogranuloma venereum

ban or rural residence, and race or ethnicity than gonorrhea and syphilis. Prevalences of *C. trachomatis* infection are consistently greater than 5% among sexually active, adolescent, young adult women attending outpatient clinics, regardless of the region of the country, location of the clinic (urban or rural), or the race or ethnicity of the population (Table 28-3). Prevalences commonly exceed 10%. Decreasing age at first intercourse and increasing age at marriage have contributed much to the higher prevalence of *C. trachomatis* infection. Infection with *C. trachomatis* is usually asymptomatic and of long duration. If a pregnant woman has active infection during delivery, the infant can acquire the infection and is at risk to develop either conjunctivitis or pneumonia (Alexander and Harrison, 1983). Rarely, children acquire chlamydial infection as a result of sexual abuse.

Infections in Adolescents and Adult Males

C. trachomatis is the single most frequently identifiable cause of nongonococcal urethritis in men, accounting for 30% to 40% of all episodes, or 1.5 million episodes annually. The usual incubation pe-

Table 28-3   Studies on prevalence of STDs in adolescents

Study (date)	Location	Infection	Sex	Number infected (%)
Chacko and Lovchik (1984)	Baltimore	*C. trachomatis*	M	35
			F	23
Golden et al. (1984)	Brooklyn	*C. trachomatis*	F	10.2
		Gonorrhea	F	9.7
		Syphilis	F	3
Saltz et al. (1981)	Cincinnati	*C. trachomatis*	F	22
		Gonorrhea	F	3
Fraser et al. (1982)	Oklahoma City	*C. trachomatis*	F	8
		Gonorrhea	F	12
Fisher et al. (1987)	Suburban New York City	*C. trachomatis*	F	14.5
Chambers et al. (1987)	San Francisco	*C. trachomatis*	M	30
		Gonorrhea	M	4
Blythe et al. (1988)	Indianapolis	*C. trachomatis*	F	25
		Gonorrhea	F	5.5
Moscicki et al. (1990)	San Francisco	*C. trachomatis*	F	8
		HPV	F	18
Fisher et al. (1991)	Suburban New York City	HPV	F	32
Hammerschlag et al. (1993)	Brooklyn	*C. trachomatis*	F	21.8
	Birmingham, AL	*C. trachomatis*	F	18.5
			M	9.4

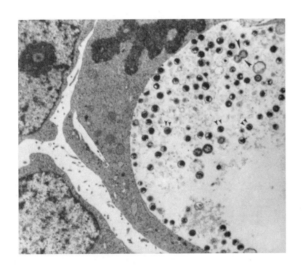

FIG. 28-6   Electron micrograph of *Chlamydia trachomatis* inclusions at 48 hours, demonstrating reticulate body undergoing binary fission (arrows) and elementary bodies (double arrows).

riod is 5 to 10 days. Nongonococcal urethritis generally causes less dysuria and less profuse, less purulent urethral exudate than gonorrhea. However, in the individual patient it may be difficult to differentiate between chlamydial and gonococcal infection (Chacko and Lovchik, 1984). Most men develop symptoms after *C. trachomatis* infection, but a large proportion may have prolonged, clinically

inapparent infection. The presence of four or more polymorphonuclear leukocytes (PMNs) per high-power field (hpf) on a Gram stain of an intraurethral smear or more than 15 PMNs per hpf in the sediment of a first-voided urine specimen is evidence of urethritis even in the absence of frank discharge (Chambers et al., 1987).

C. trachomatis can also cause proctitis among homosexual men. If the infection is due to a lymphogranuloma venereum strain, the individual may develop proctocolitis that is difficult to differentiate from Crohn's disease both clinically and histopathologically. *C. trachomatis* can also cause epididymitis in young men. It has been estimated that one diagnosed case of epididymitis caused by *C. trachomatis* occurs for every eighteen diagnosed episodes of uncomplicated chlamydia-related urethritis in men aged 15 to 34 years. Overall, *C. trachomatis* causes 50% of epididymitis among men 15 to 34 years of age (Hammerschlag, 1989).

Infections in Adolescent and Adult Females

Nonpregnant Women. Most cervical infections with *C. trachomatis* in women are asymptomatic and of long duration (Eagar et al., 1985). Sexually active adolescent women have one of the highest reported rates of chlamydial infection, often exceeding 10% to 15%. A recent study from Canada found that after implementation of a chlamydia control program in 1987, the annual incidence of chlamydial infection was highest among females from 15 to 24 years of age (3,418 cases per 100,000 residents) (Orr et al., 1994). Recurrent infection occurred in 13.4% of patients and was also more common in women and patients from 15 to 24 years of age. In the United States, Blythe et al. (1992) found that 38.4% of adolescent women had recurrent infection within 9 months of their initial chlamydial infection. Although *C. trachomatis* has been associated with mucopurulent cervicitis, the majority of women have no specific physical clinical findings.

Among the many possible complications of chlamydial infection, the most important in female patients is acute salpingitis. Several studies and histopathologic reports from Scandinavia indicate a very strong causal association between *C. trachomatis* and salpingitis (Mardh, 1980). Later clinical and animal studies from the United States using aggressive culture methods, including cultures from the fallopian tubes, have confirmed the European experience (Patton, 1985; Bowie and Jones, 1981; Wasserheit et al., 1986). The organism is probably responsible for at least 20% of salpingitis cases in the United States. Studies from Sweden and the United States indicate that approximately one in four patients admitted to the hospital with acute salpingitis has upper genital tract infection with *C. trachomatis,* confirmed by isolation of the organism from the fallopian tubes. The presence of *C. trachomatis* in the cervix of a woman with PID does not necessarily imply that the organism will be present in the tubes, but it is very suggestive. Investigators from Sweden found that nineteen of fifty-three women with salpingitis had cervical chlamydial infection and that of those who had cervical infection and laparoscopy, six of seven grew *C. trachomatis* from the fallopian tubes (Mardh, 1980). Why ascending infection develops in some women with cervical infection is not known. Salpingitis is 10 times more likely to occur in a sexually active 15-year-old girl than in a sexually active 25-year-old woman (Westrom, 1980). In addition to being more prevalent than gonococcal infections, chlamydial salpingitis apparently has a more severe clinical outcome. Compared with patients with gonococcal salpingitis or nonchlamydial, nongonococcal salpingitis, patients with chlamydial salpingitis have a less acute presentation, are less often febrile, have a longer history of symptoms, have a higher erythrocyte sedimentation rate, and have more tubal inflammation (Cromer and Heald, 1987). In addition,

chlamydial salpingitis is more likely to lead to infertility. Infertility rates of 13% after one episode of salpingitis, 36% after two episodes, and 75% after three or more episodes have been reported (Westrom, 1980). Case-control studies have documented a consistent association between high titers of antibody to *C. trachomatis* and tubal obstruction (Westrom, 1980; Brunham et al., 1986). Studies in animals have shown that *C. trachomatis* infects and subsequently destroys the tubal mucosa (Patton, 1985). A similar microscopic and pathologic appearance of the tubes has been found in several patients from whom *C. trachomatis* was isolated. This pattern of repeated infections leading to fibrosis and eventual scarring is also seen in another human chlamydial infection—trachoma. A recent study has demonstrated that screening women 18 to 34 years of age for cervical chlamydial infection and treating them will prevent subsequent pelvic inflammatory disease (Scholes et al., 1996). This study showed a nearly 60% reduction in disease in the women who were screened and treated compared to a group of women that was not offered routine screening.

Another serious complication of chlamydial salpingitis is an increased risk of ectopic pregnancy, which is related directly to the oviduct damage. Many women who have had an ectopic pregnancy give no history of PID, but over 20% have histopathologic and serologic evidence of chlamydial infection (Brunham et al., 1986).

Pregnant Women. In the United States the prevalence of *C. trachomatis* infection in pregnant women ranges from a low of 2% to more than 30%, depending on the population studied (Hammerschlag, 1989). Chlamydial infection during pregnancy has been inconstantly linked to prematurity. The overall relationship, when found, has been weak, and the mechanism is not understood (Harrison et al., 1983). Late (72+ hours) endometritis occurs consistently in 10% to 30% of women with chlamydial infections after induced abortion. *C. trachomatis* apparently is an important cause of postabortion complications.

Infections in Infants

Pregnant women who have cervical infection with *C. trachomatis* can transmit the infection to their infants, who may subsequently develop neonatal conjunctivitis or pneumonia. Epidemiologic evidence strongly suggests that the infant acquires chlamydial infection from the mother during vaginal delivery (Alexander and Harrison, 1983). Infection after cesarean section is rare and usually occurs after early rupture of the amniotic membrane. No evidence supports the idea of postnatal acquisition from the mother or other family members. Approximately 50% to 75% of infants born to infected women will become infected at one or more anatomic sites, including the conjunctiva, nasopharynx, rectum, and vagina.

Conjunctivitis. Inclusion conjunctivitis, or inclusion blennorrhea, is probably the major clinical manifestation of perinatally acquired chlamydial infection. The risk of developing chlamydial conjunctivitis after vaginal delivery in an infant born to a mother with active cervical chlamydial infection ranges from 20% to 50% (Alexander and Harrison, 1983). *C. trachomatis* is also the most common identifiably infectious cause of neonatal conjunctivitis in the United States, accounting for 17% to more than 40% of cases.

The incubation period is usually 5 to 14 days but may be shorter if the membranes rupture prematurely. The clinical presentation is variable, ranging from minimal conjunctival injection with scant mucopurulent discharge to a more severe presentation with chemosis, pseudomembrane formation, and marked palpebral swelling. The conjunctivae are frequently very friable and may bleed when stroked with a swab. Although conjunctivitis may initially be unilateral, it frequently becomes bilateral. If not treated,the infection may persist for weeks. Chlamydial conjunctivitis in infants is not a follicular conjunctivitis as seen in classic endemic trachoma. Approximately 50% of infants with chlamydial conjunctivitis are also infected in the nasopharynx.

Pneumonia. The nasopharynx is the most frequent site of perinatally acquired chlamydial infection. Approximately 70% of infected infants have positive cultures at that site. Most of these nasopharyngeal infections are asymptomatic and may persist for 3 years or more. *C. trachomatis* pneumonia develops in approximately 30% of infants with nasopharyngeal infection. In those who develop pneumonia the presentation and clinical findings are very characteristic. The children usually are initially seen at 4 to 12 weeks of age. A few cases have been seen initially as early as 2 weeks of age, but no infant cases have been seen beyond 4 months. The infants frequently have a history of cough and congestion, with an absence of fever. On physical examination the infant is tachypneic, and rales are heard on auscultation of the chest; wheezing is distinctly uncommon. There are no specific radiographic findings except hyperinflation (Fig. 28-7) (Beem and Saxon, 1977; Harrison et al., 1978). A review of chest roentgenograms of 125 infants with *C. trachomatis* pneumonia found bilateral hyperinflation and diffuse infiltrates (with a variety of radiographic patterns, including interstitial, reticular, and nodular ones); atelectasis; and bronchopneumonia. Lobar consolidation and pleural effusions were not seen (Radkowski et al., 1981). Significant laboratory findings include peripheral eosinophilia (>300 cells/cm^3) and elevated serum immunoglobulin levels.

C. trachomatis is rarely isolated from the lungs of infants with chlamydia pneumonia, leading some to believe that an immune mechanism is involved in pathogenesis (Alexander and Harrison,

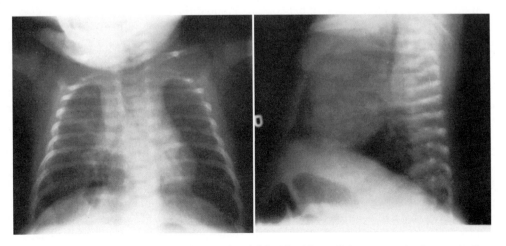

FIG. 28-7   Roentgenographic findings of a child with chlamydial pneumonia demonstrating hyperinflation and atelectasis.

454 KRUGMAN'S INFECTIOUS DISEASES OF CHILDREN

1983). Histopathologic studies have not revealed any characteristic features. Biopsy material has shown pleural congestion and near-total alveolar and partial bronchiolar mononuclear consolidation with occasional eosinophils, granular pneumocytes, and focal aggregations of neutrophils. Marked necrotic changes are evident in the bronchioles. Follow-up studies have suggested that infantile chlamydial pneumonia may be associated with pulmonary function test abnormalities and respiratory symptoms 7 to 8 years after recovery from the acute illness (Weiss et al., 1986).

Infections in Older Children

C. trachomatis has not been associated with any specific clinical syndrome in older infants and children. It has been suggested that the isolation of *C. trachomatis* from a rectal or genital site in children without prior sexual activity may be a marker of sexual abuse. Although evidence for other modes of spread such as through fomites is lacking for this organism, perinatal maternal-infant transmission resulting in vaginal or rectal infection has been documented, with prolonged infection lasting for periods up to 2 years. Pharyngeal infection for up to 3 years has also been observed. Schachter et al. (1986a) have detected subclinical rectal and vaginal infection in 14% of infants born to chlamydia-positive women; some infants were still culture-positive at 18 months of age.

Reporting of vaginal infection with *C. trachomatis* in prepubertal children was uncommon before 1980. The possibility of sexual contact frequently was not discussed. In 1981 Rettig and Nelson reported concurrent or subsequent chlamydial infection in nine of thirty-three (27%) prepubertal children with gonorrhea. This rate compares with those of 11% to 62%, depending on the study, of concurrent infection in men and women. *C. trachomatis* was not found in any of thirty-one children presenting with urethritis or vaginitis that was not gonococcal. No information was given about possible sexual activity.

Recent studies have identified rectogenital chlamydial infection in 1.2% to 13% of sexually abused children when the children were routinely cultured for the organism (see Table 28-1). Most of those with chlamydial infection were asymptomatic. In two studies that had control groups, similar percentages of control patients were infected (Hammerschlag et al., 1984; Ingram et al., 1984). The control group in one study comprised children who were referred also for evaluation of possible sexual abuse but were found to have no history of sexual contact and siblings of abused children. The mean age of this group was 4½ years as compared to 7½ years for the group with a history of sexual contact, thus suggesting a bias related to the inability to elicit a history of sexual contact from young children. In the second study the control group was selected from a well-child clinic. Three girls in this group had positive chlamydial cultures; two who had positive vaginal cultures were sisters who had been sexually abused 3 years previously and had not received interim treatment with antibiotics. The implication of this observation was that these children were infected for at least 3 years and were totally asymptomatic. The remaining control child had *C. trachomatis* isolated from her throat and rectum; no history of sexual contact could be elicited. Ingram et al. (1992) reviewed the results of *C. trachomatis* cultures among 1538 children, 1 to 12 years of age, being evaluated for possible sexual abuse who were seen between May 1981 and November 1991. The overall rate of chlamydial infection during this period was 1.2%. Most were asymptomatic and almost all had a definite history of sexual contact. One 31-month-old girl had no history of sexual contact; *C. trachomatis* was isolated from her rectal and vaginal specimens. Her mother was known to have chlamydial infection when she was pregnant, and her daughter had culture-positive chlamydial conjunctivitis at 8 weeks of age. This probably represents persistent perinatally acquired infection.

The possibility of prolonged vaginal or rectal carriage in the sexually abused group was minimized in the study of Hammerschlag et al. (1984) because the chlamydial cultures obtained at the initial examination were negative and the infection was detected only at follow-up examination 2 to 4 weeks later. However, the two abused girls who developed chlamydial infection were victims of a single assault by a stranger. In the setting of repeated abuse by a family member over long periods of time, development of infection would be difficult to demonstrate.

Lymphogranuloma Venereum

Lymphogranuloma venereum (LGV) is a systemic, sexually transmitted disease caused by the LGV biovars of *C. trachomatis* (L1, L2, L3). Approximately twenty cases of LGV have been reported in children. Fewer than 1000 cases are reported in adults in the United States each year. Unlike the trachoma biovar, LGV strains have a predilection for lymph node involvement. The clinical course of LGV can be divided into three stages: (1) the primary lesion, a painless papule on the genitals, which usually is very transient; (2) lymphadenitis or lymphadenopathy; and (3) the tertiary stage. Most patients present during the second stage with enlarging, painful buboes, usually in the groin. The nodes may break down and drain. Males are more likely to have this presentation. In females the lymphatic drainage of the vulva is to the retroperitoneal nodes. Fever, myalgia, and headache are also common. The tertiary stage includes the genitoanorectal syndrome, with rectovaginal fistulas, rectal strictures, and urethral destruction. Diagnosis can be made by culture of *C. trachomatis* from a bubo aspirate or serologically. Most patients with LGV have complement fixation (CF) titers greater than 1:16. The recommended therapy is 2 to 3 weeks of either tetracycline or sulfisoxazole.

Diagnosis

The definitive diagnosis of genital chlamydial infection in adolescents and adults is isolation of the organism in tissue culture—from the urethra in men and the endocervix in women. Care should be taken to obtain cells, not discharge. The most commonly used tissue culture system is McCoy cells treated with cycloheximide. After a 48- to 72-hour incubation period the cultures are confirmed by staining the inclusions, preferably with a fluorescein-conjugated monoclonal antibody, although iodine can also be used. Characteristic intracytoplasmic inclusions should be visible. Although many centers now perform *C. trachomatis* cultures, there is no standardization of methods or designated reference laboratories. Alternately, a nonculture method can be used. The types of test currently available are a direct fluorescent antibody (DFA) test, in which chlamydial EBs are identified directly on a specimen smear stained with a conjugated antichlamydial monoclonal antibody, enzyme immunoassays (EIA) test, DNA probe, and polymerase chain reaction (PCR). The DFA, EIA, and DNA probes are best for screening in high-prevalence populations (prevalence of infection >7%) (Centers for Disease Control, 1993). Sensitivities compared to culture range from 60% to 80% for these assays. Several DNA amplification assays are now available (PCR-Amplicor, Roche Molecular Diagnostics; ligase chain reaction [LCR], Abbott Diagnostics) or will be in the near future (transcription mediated amplification

[TMA], GenProbe). Preliminary data with the commercially available PCR suggest very high sensitivities and specificities (Leoffelholz et al., 1992); however, it is more expensive. PCR appears to be sufficiently sensitive to detect *C. trachomatis* in urine from men and women (Quinn et al., 1996). As other DNA amplification assays for *C. trachomatis* are approved, costs will probably decrease.

Serologic testing is not helpful for the diagnosis of chlamydial infections in adults. Since most infections in adolescents and adults are asymptomatic, it would be difficult to demonstrate either seroconversion or rises in titers. Serosurveys of populations of sexually active adults have found prevalences of antichlamydial antibody in more than 20% of individuals. The most widely available serologic test is the complement fixation (CF) test. This genus-specific test is most useful for the diagnosis of LGV. Unfortunately, it is not sensitive enough for use in oculogenital infections caused by the trachoma biovar in adults or children. The microimmunofluoresence (MIF) test is species-specific and sensitive but is available only at a limited number of research laboratories.

Chlamydial Conjunctivitis and Pneumonia in Infants.
Culture of chlamydia from the conjunctivae or nasopharynx is diagnostic. The nasopharyngeal specimens can be obtained with a posterior swab or by aspirate. The use of Dacron-tipped swabs with either wire or plastic shafts is preferred. The diagnosis of conjunctivitis can be made by examination of Giemsa-stained conjunctival scrapings, but this method has only had a 30% sensitivity compared to that of culture in several studies. The DFA and EIA tests can also be used for conjunctival and nasopharyngeal specimens. These tests perform very well with conjunctival specimens, with sensitivities and specificities exceeding 90% (Hammerschlag, 1994). Performance with nasopharyngeal specimens has not been as good; sensitivity compared to culture can be as low as 30%. Preliminary evaluation of PCR suggests that this assay is as sensitive as culture for diagnosis of *C. trachomatis* conjunctivitis (Hammerschlag et al., 1997). Diagnosis of chlamydial pneumonia also can be made serologically; an IgM titer greater than 1:32 with the MIF test is very suggestive (Harrison et al., 1978).

Chlamydial Infections in Older Children.
Because of the medical and legal implications, culture is the only approved method for the diagnosis

of rectal and genital chlamydial infections in pre-pubertal children (Centers for Disease Control, 1993). Culture means isolation of the organism in tissue culture with confirmation by visual identification of the characteristic inclusions, preferably with fluorescent antibody (FA) staining. Nonculture methods cannot be used in this setting. Very little data are available about the use of these tests in rectal and genital specimens from prepubertal children, and what is available suggests that they are neither sensitive nor specific (Hammerschlag et al., 1988; Hauger et al., 1988; Porder et al., 1989).

Treatment

Because of its long growth cycle, treatment of chlamydial infections requires multiple-dose regimens. None of the currently recommended single-dose regimens for gonorrhea are effective against *C. trachomatis*.

Uncomplicated Genital Infection in Adolescent and Adult Males and Nonpregnant Women. The treatment of choice is doxycycline (100 mg orally, twice a day for 7 days) or azithromycin (1 g as a single oral dose) (Centers for Disease Control, 1993). Azithromycin has a 30-hour half-life in serum. A single 1-g oral dose of azithromycin is equivalent to 7 days of doxycycline for the treatment of uncomplicated genital chlamydial infection in men and nonpregnant women (Martin et al., 1992; Hammerschlag et al., 1993).

C. trachomatis in Pregnancy. The CDC currently recommends four different erythromycin regimens—none of which have been extensively evaluated—for treating *C. trachomatis* in pregnant women. Poor tolerance may reduce the compliance to 50% or less in some populations (Schachter, 1986b). The primary regimen is erythromycin base, 500 mg 4 times a day orally for 7 days. If not tolerated, the dosage can be reduced to 250 mg 4 times a day orally for 14 days. If erythromycin is not tolerated, amoxicillin (500 mg 3 times a day orally for 7 days) is as effective and is associated with significantly fewer side effects (Turrentine and Newton, 1995).

Chlamydial Conjunctivitis and Pneumonia in Infants. Oral erythromycin suspension (ethylsuccinate or stearate; 50 mg/kg/day for 10 to 14 days) is the therapy of choice for chlamydial conjunctivitis and pneumonia in infants. It provides better and faster resolution of the conjunctivitis and treats any concurrent nasopharyngeal infection, which will prevent the potential development of pneumonia. Additional topical therapy is not needed (Heggie et al., 1985). Erythromycin administered at the same dose for 2 to 3 weeks is the treatment of choice for pneumonia and results in clinical improvement and elimination of the organism from the respiratory tract. Although clarithromycin and azithromycin pediatric suspensions are now available, there are no data on the use of these agents for treatment of *C. trachomatis* infection in infants.

Although an initial study suggested that neonatal ocular prophylaxis with erythromycin ointment would prevent the development of chlamydial ophthalmia, subsequent studies have not confirmed this (Bell et al., 1987; Hammerschlag et al., 1989). It appears that neither ocular prophylaxis with silver nitrate nor erythromycin and tetracycline ointments or drops are effective for the prevention of neonatal chlamydial conjunctivitis or pneumonia. The identification and treatment of pregnant women before delivery is the optimal method of prevention of chlamydial infection in infants (Centers for Disease Control, 1993a).

Older Children. Chlamydial infections in older children can be treated with oral erythromycin (50 mg/kg/day, 4 times a day orally to a maximum of 2 g/day for 7 to 14 days). Children older than 8 years of age may be treated with doxycycline (2 to 4 mg/kg/day divided into 2 doses orally for 7 days). Azithromycin may be used in adolescents 15 years of age and older.

BACTERIAL VAGINOSIS

Bacterial vaginosis (nonspecific vaginitis) is a polymicrobial infection characterized by the overgrowth of *Gardnerella vaginalis* and several anaerobic bacteria and by depletion of *Lactobacillus* species. The diagnosis of bacterial vaginosis is made by examination of the vaginal secretions for clue cells (vaginal epithelial cells heavily covered with bacteria) (Fig. 28-8), the development of a fishy odor after the addition of 10% potassium hydroxide to vaginal secretions ("whiff test"), and a vaginal pH greater than 4.5 (Amsel et al., 1983; Thomason et al., 1990).

Although bacterial vaginosis is very common in adult women, it has been diagnosed infrequently in children (Table 28-4). One possible reason is that prior studies of pediatric populations have concen-

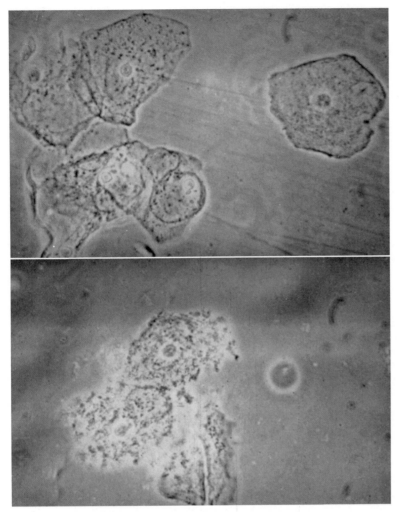

FIG. 28-8   **A**, Photomicrograph of a wet mount, demonstrating normal vaginal epithelial cells; **B**, photomicrograph of wet mount containing clue cells, which are epithelial cells studded with bacteria.

Table 28-4   Prevalence of trichomoniasis and bacterial vaginosis in sexually abused children

Study (year)	Number tested	Cause	Number (%) positive
White et al. (1983)	409	Trichomoniasis	4 (1)
De Jong (1983)	25*	Trichomoniasis	0
		Bacterial vaginosis	3 (12)
Hammerschlag et al. (1985)	31	Trichomoniasis	2 (6)
		Bacterial vaginosis	6 (19)
Ingram et al. (1992)	141*	Trichomoniasis	3 (2)
	99*	Bacterial vaginosis	7 (7)

*Only patients with signs suggestive of vaginitis were evaluated.

trated on the isolation of *G. vaginalis* and have not routinely examined vaginal secretions for clue cells or odor. The CDC has stated that cultures for *G. vaginalis* are not useful and are not recommended for the diagnosis of this syndrome. Studies in children have suggested that *G. vaginalis* may be part

of the normal vaginal flora (Hammerschlag et al., 1985). Bartley et al. (1987) examined a group of sexually abused children and a group of control children. Although *G. vaginalis* was isolated from the vaginal cultures of 14.6% of the abused girls, it was also found in 4.2% of the controls. Presence of

G. vaginalis was not associated with vaginal discharge in these children. Another study reported finding G. vaginalis in vaginal specimens from 37% of non–sexually active postmenarcheal girls (median age, 15.9 years; range, 13 to 21 years) (Shafer et al., 1985). Ingram et al. (1992) isolated G. vaginalis from 5.3% of a group of children with confirmed sexual contact and/or gonorrhea or chlamydial infection; 4.9% of a group of children evaluated for possible abuse, but not confirmed; and 6.4% of a group of normal children seen as controls. Although some practitioners have suggested that the presence of G. vaginalis is an indicator of sexual abuse, the preceding data suggest otherwise.

Data from adults suggest that acquisition of bacterial vaginosis is related to sexual activity. In a major study, Amsel et al. (1983) diagnosed bacterial vaginitis in 69 of 397 females consecutively coming to a student health center gynecology clinic. They failed to demonstrate the disease among 18 patients who had no history of previous sexual intercourse. Four of these sexually inexperienced patients had positive vaginal cultures for G. vaginalis, which suggests that other organisms or factors are involved in the sexual transmission of bacterial vaginitis. Other investigators have found that male partners of women with bacterial vaginosis have a high prevalence of urethral colonization with G. vaginalis.

Minimal data exist on the prevalence of bacterial vaginosis in sexually abused female children. Hammerschlag et al. (1985) obtained paired vaginal wash specimens from thirty-one girls within 1 week and 2 or more weeks after sexual assault. None had bacterial vaginosis as defined by the presence of both clue cells and a positive whiff test at the initial examination. Vaginal pH was not used as a diagnostic criterion because the normal pH range in prepubertal girls is not well defined. At follow-up examination, four (13%) of the thirty-one girls had bacterial vaginosis. Two girls were asymptomatic. Treatment with metronidazole was followed by clinical improvement. None of the twenty-three controls (nonabused children) had bacterial vaginosis.

Bacterial vaginosis apparently is also a common cause of vaginal discharge in children without sexual contact. Samuels et al. (1985) examined vaginal washes from twenty-nine girls 3 months to 1 year of age with symptomatic vulvovaginitis. Bacterial vaginosis was diagnosed in nine (31%) of these children. All had a discharge, which was uni-

formly thin and ranged from grey-white to yellow in color, and only three (33%) of these girls had a history of sexual abuse; N. gonorrhoeae also was isolated from a pharyngeal culture from one child. Treatment with metronidazole resulted in reversion of the vaginal secretions to normal on follow-up examination. The relatively common occurrence of bacterial vaginosis in children may be due in part to the frequent colonization of the prepubertal vagina with anaerobes, especially Bacteroides species.

Treatment

Oral metronidazole (15 mg/kg/day, 3 times a day for 7 days) apparently is effective for the treatment of bacterial vaginosis in children. Ampicillin or amoxicillin has been recommended as an alternative regimen when the use of metronidazole is contraindicated, but these are less effective. The combination of amoxicillin and clavulanate (Augmentin) may be effective since it offers better coverage for anaerobic bacteria, especially Bacteroides species.

TRICHOMONIASIS

Trichomonas vaginalis is a flagellated protozoan that inhabits the urogenital systems of both males and females and is considered a pathogen (Fig. 28-9). The trophozoites (the only stage) are found in the urine of both sexes, in vaginal secretions, and in prostatic secretions. Approximately 5 million women in the United States have trichomoniasis, and roughly 1 million men may harbor the parasite. The infection in males is generally asymptomatic, but 25% to 50% of infected women exhibit symptoms, which include dysuria; vaginal itching and burning; and, in severe infections, a foamy, yellowish-green discharge with a foul odor.

Although nonsexual transmission of T. vaginalis has been reported between infected mothers and their infants at delivery, the exact risk of the infant's acquiring the infection is unknown (Al-Salihi et al., 1974). The presence of this organism in vaginal specimens from prepubertal girls strongly suggests sexual abuse; but, as with other sexually transmitted diseases, perinatally acquired infection can be an important confounding variable. The duration of perinatally acquired trichomoniasis has been assumed to be very short—2 to 3 months after birth. Recently we saw two female infants with well-documented neonatal trichomonal infection that persisted for 6 and 9 months before the infants were finally treated. In most reports of infection with T. vaginalis in prepubertal children published

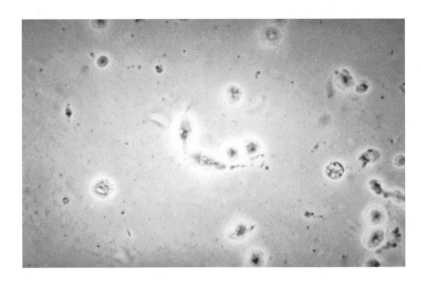

Fig. 28-9 Photomicrograph of wet mount, demonstrating *Trichomonas vaginalis* trophozoites.

before 1978, the possibility of sexual activity or abuse is not discussed (Neinstein et al., 1984). In one study of unselected girls who went to a well-child clinic, *T. vaginalis* was identified in two girls; both were postmenarcheal and one was sexually active. They both were symptomatic (Hammerschlag et al., 1978).

In most reported studies, wet mount examinations have been performed infrequently in asymptomatic sexually abused children and often are not performed in abused girls who have not had a vaginal discharge. Patients with trichomoniasis may be asymptomatic and have negative results from wet mount preparations (Wolner-Hanssen et al., 1989). In one study in which both wet mount examinations and cultures were used, trichomoniasis was found in two of thirty-one abused children at follow-up, but not at an initial examination (see Table 28-4). *T. vaginalis* was not identified in the children who served as controls. Trichomonads are not infrequently seen in urine collected for other purposes. If the specimen is obtained with a urinary collection bag—as is done frequently in young children, especially girls—the trichomonads may have originated in the vagina or may represent fecal contamination.

T. hominis, a commensal species that can inhabit the colon, is considered nonpathogenic. The only way the two *Trichomonas* species can be differentiated is by the presence of an undulating membrane that extends most of the length of the organism in *T. hominis* but only half the length of the organism in *T. vaginalis.* Old urine specimens may also be contaminated with *Bodo* species or other free-living flagellates, especially if the urinary collection

vessel is open to the air and is not sterile. The presence of a trichomonad in a vaginal specimen has greater significance.

Diagnosis

Although some workers believe wet mount examinations are as efficient as culture for the diagnosis of *T. vaginalis* infection, current evidence suggests that cultivation methods are superior (Fouts and Kraus, 1980). Several culture media are available commercially. A conjugated monoclonal antibody stain has been developed that apparently is both sensitive and specific, but available clinical data are limited. It has not yet been evaluated as an assay for the diagnosis of trichomoniasis in children (Kruger et al., 1988).

Treatment

Trichomoniasis in adult women can be successfully treated with a single oral dose (2 g) of metronidazole or with 250 mg taken orally 3 times daily for 7 days, but there are no published studies of its use in children. The few cases of trichomoniasis in prepubertal girls reported in the literature were treated with 7-day courses of oral metronidazole (15 to 35 mg/kg/day) (Jones et al., 1985).

HUMAN PAPILLOMAVIRUS INFECTION

Human papillomavirus (HPV), a double-stranded DNA virus, is the organism responsible for common warts and venereal warts, or condylomata acuminata. Genital papillomas in adults are transmitted by sexual intercourse. The majority are caused by human papillomavirus type 6 (HPV-6) or type 11 (HPV-11); smaller numbers are caused by types 16 (HPV-16) and 18 (HPV-18). Common skin warts and genital warts do not share HPV types.

HPV is becoming recognized as one of the most frequently occurring STDs. In the San Francisco Bay area, Moscicki et al. (1990) reported that 18% of sexually active females tested positive for HPV DNA. HPV represented the most common STD in that age group, followed by *C. trachomatis,* with a prevalence rate of 8%. A similar study of adolescents in suburban New York City reported an HPV prevalence rate of 33% (Fisher et al; 1991). More than 80% of male partners of females with HPV are infected with HPV; most of these infections are subclinical. The cause of genital papillomas in children is less well studied, but sexual abuse by an infected adult or, less likely, contact with warts at other body sites has been suggested. Human papillomaviruses can also be transmitted to infants at birth, causing laryngeal papilloma (Boyd, 1990). The condylomata may affect the vulva, perineum, vaginal introitus, and periurethral areas. Girls apparently are affected twice as frequently as boys, although this may reflect a difference in patterns of reporting rather than a true epidemiologic observation (Davis and Emans, 1989; Boyd, 1990).

Clinical Manifestations

The lesions of condylomata acuminata are usually flesh-colored to purple papillomatous growths. These warts are often multiple and commonly coalesce into larger masses. In females, condylomata acuminata lesions usually occur at the posterior part of the introitus, the adjacent labia minora, and the rest of the vestibule. Less commonly, they can be found on the clitoris, perineum, vagina, cervix, anus, and rectum. In males, venereal warts are usually localized to the penis, including the shaft, prepuce, frenulum, corona, and glans. The meatus, anus, and scrotum may also be involved. Anal warts are seen most commonly in patients who have engaged in anal intercourse. In contrast, many females with anal warts report no history of anal sex, suggesting autoinoculation as a mode of transmission. The anatomic distribution may be different in prepubertal children, especially males. Male children are less likely to have involvement of the penile shaft, prepuce, or glans—3% vs. 18% to 52%—and are more likely to have perianal disease—77% vs. 8% (Boyd, 1990). Female disease patterns show fewer age-related differences. Recently a new clinical and histologic type of HPV infection has been described as subclinical HPV in-

fection. The lesions with this type cannot be seen with the naked eye and require colposcopy, acetowhitening, or cytologic studies for diagnosis. They can occur anywhere in the anogenital tract. In women they occur predominantly on the cervix; in males they can occur anywhere on the penis and on the perianal area, scrotum, and urethra. Recently, increasing attention has been focused on the association between HPV infection and the various genital carcinomas, particularly cervical carcinoma in women. HPV structural antigens and DNA have been found in the lesions of cervical intraepithelial neoplasia, which precedes the development of frank cervical carcinoma. HPV antigens and DNA have also been found in invasive carcinoma specimens and in specimens of anal, vulvar, vaginal, and penile carcinomas. Studies of adolescents in San Francisco have found infection with oncogenic-related HPV types is very common (Moscicki et al., 1990).

The risk of developing genital warts in sexually abused children has not been adequately assessed because no studies have included data on long-term follow-up. However, one half of the cases of genital warts in children reported since 1976 were related to sexual abuse (Seidel et al., 1979; De Jong et al., 1982; Neinstein et al., 1984). Rock et al. (1986) examined the genital tract papillomas by molecular hybridization in five children for the presence of HPV DNA. Papillomavirus DNA was detected in each sample and contained either HPV-6, HPV-11, or HPV-16. These types are the same as those responsible for genital warts in adults. Sexual abuse was thought likely to have occurred in three of these children. Although there was no history of maternal condylomata at the time of birth in the remaining two children, many congenital infections in women are subclinical, and flat warts of the vulva and vagina may go unnoticed by the affected individual and the physician (Bender, 1986). DNA typing in four subsequent studies reported that 5% to 20% of anogenital warts in children have skin HPV types (HPV-2, HPV-3), suggesting possible nonsexual acquisition (Cohen et al., 1990; Gibson et al., 1990; Obaleck et al., 1990; Padel et al., 1990). Gutman et al. (1992), examining vaginal washes, found HPV DNA in five of fifteen sexually abused girls 2 to 11 years of age, compared to none of seventeen controls (3 months to 5½ years of age). The HPV types were 6, 11, and 15. The results of the wash did not correlate with the presence or absence of external anogenital warts. This was also a very small, selected population. The children in the control group were significantly younger than the cases. Additional studies should be done evaluating the predictive value of the method for the diagnosis of HPV infection in the setting of suspected sexual abuse.

The major confounding variable in linking the presence of genital warts with sexual abuse is ruling out perinatal acquisition. Maternal HPV infection may be more common than previously thought. One study found evidence of HPV, as defined by DNA probes, in 4% of male infants undergoing routine circumcision. The prolonged incubation period, or period of latency, before clinical condylomata are evident further complicates this issue. It is impossible to define the longest latency period between viral infection at delivery and the presence of clinical disease. The average latency period apparently is approximately 3 months, but it may range up to 2 years. A child who is first found to have perianal condylomata at 20 months of age may have had visible disease that could have been detected on close inspection (with colposcopy) 6 months earlier. Most cases of childhood condylomata occurring beyond the plausible incubation period (2 years) after acquisition at delivery probably are due to child abuse. Other means of transmission are unlikely. It is theoretically possible to transfer anogenital condylomata inadvertently from caretakers during activities such as shared bathing, but this has never been proven conclusively. The prolonged incubation period would also make it difficult to determine when abuse occurred.

Diagnosis

Until the recent recognition that HPV infection can be inapparent, the diagnosis of condylomata acuminata was usually based on the history and appearance of the lesions. Anogenital warts must be differentiated from other papillomatous lesions, including benign and malignant neoplasms, anatomic variants, and other infectious conditions. Of the latter, the most important lesions to differentiate are condylomata lata of secondary syphilis. Because these may coexist condylomata acuminata, obtaining serologic tests for syphilis and dark-field microscopy of suspicious or ulcerating lesions is strongly recommended. Genital lesions of molluscum contagiosum also can be confused with genital warts.

In adolescent and adult women the Papanicolaou (Pap) test commonly is used to diagnose HPV infection. The koilocyte ("balloon cell") can be seen on a Pap smear and is pathognomic for HPV. However, there is a subjective component to reading smears, and the sampling error presents a problem. A negative Pap smear result does not rule out HPV infection. Performing a biopsy should be considered for any puzzling lesion.

Electron microscopy can be used to identify HPV particles in biopsy specimens and may be especially useful in identifying lesions from children. More recently, antigen detection and molecular hybridization techniques have shown promise in detecting HPV in scrapings and biopsies of lesions (Bauer et al., 1991). However, the same problems encountered with Pap smears occur with these newer methods. Their diagnostic use may be compromised because of sampling error, insufficient material, or interference by large numbers of red or white blood cells that obscure visualization of the cervical epithelial cells. None of these methods have been evaluated in prepubertal children.

Treatment

None of the currently available therapies is completely satisfactory for the treatment of genital warts in adults, and less information is available about treatment for children. Children have been treated with local application of podophyllin, cryosurgery, electrosurgery, ablation with carbon dioxide laser, and 75% trichloroacetic acid. Treatment of genital warts in children can be complicated and should be carried out in consultation with an expert.

OTHER INFECTIONS

Several other STDs deserve mention. Chancroid is caused by *H. ducreyi,* a small, nonmotile, gram-negative, non–spore forming rod. Clinically, chancroid usually is seen initially as a small, inflammatory papule on the preputial orifice or frenulum in men and on the labia, fourchette, or perianal region in women. The lesion becomes pustular and ulcerative within 2 to 3 days. An associated painful, tender inguinal adenopathy occurs in over 50% of cases. Unlike that of lymphogranuloma venereum, the characteristic ulcer of chancroid is concurrent with lymphadenopathy. Recently, reported cases of chancroid have increased dramatically in the United States, especially in urban areas such as Los Angeles, New York, and Miami (Schmid, 1990). Although no reports of chancroid in children have been found in the literature, chancroid may appear with the increasing incidence in reports about the adult population.

Infection with hepatitis B virus (HBV) is also a sexually transmitted disease and may be a complication of sexual abuse (Szmuness et al., 1975) (see Chapter 11). It has been recommended that male victims of homosexual rape be screened for HBV infection. Although homosexual behavior is a well-recognized risk factor for acquiring HBV infection, a similar increased risk exists among heterosexuals with multiple sex partners. Screening for HBV probably should also be included in the medical evaluation of the child victim of sexual assault.

Consideration should also be given to screening for HIV infection in victims of sexual assault, including children (Gellert et al., 1990). Although no available studies document the risks of transmission in this situation, individual reports have noted acquisition of HIV infection through sexual assault (Leiderman and Grimm, 1986; Gutman et al., 1991). Since HIV, like HBV, can be transmitted through homosexual or heterosexual activity, screening for infection may be indicated in both instances.

Investigators in Newark, New Jersey, have reported some children with probable perinatally acquired HIV first seen with the infection at 8 to 9 years of age. Although the apparent usual incubation period is 18 months, it is possible that it may extend for years in some individuals. The group in

Newark now screens all sexually abused children for HIV—not for forensic purposes, but because they believe that sexual abuse is an epidemiologic risk factor for HIV infection in their population. The risk factors for HIV infection are similar to those for sexual abuse: drug abuse in parent, alcoholism, and poverty. Gellert et al. (1993) reviewed the results of HIV testing of 5622 children suspected of being sexually abused; 28 (0.5%) were infected with HIV and lacked any alternative transmission route to that of sexual abuse. Sexual abuse must be considered as a potential, although infrequent, mode of transmission of HIV infection in children. (Herpes simplex virus [HSV] infections are discussed in Chapter 12.)

Laboratory studies that are indicated as part of the evaluation of sexually assaulted children at initial and follow-up examinations are presented in Box 28-2.

BOX 28-2

LABORATORY STUDIES INDICATED AS PART OF EVALUATION OF SEXUALLY ASSAULTED CHILDREN AT INITIAL AND FOLLOW-UP EXAMINATIONS

Gram stain of any genital or anal discharge

Cultures for *N. gonorrhoeae* (rectogenital and throat) and *C. trachomatis* (rectogenital)

Serologic tests for syphilis

Wet mount preparation for trichomonads and clue cells (girls)

Whiff test (girls)

Vaginal culture for *T. vaginalis,* if available (girls)

Serum sample (save frozen)

Cultures of lesions for herpes simplex virus

Hepatitis B surface antigen*

Human immunodeficiency virus antibody*

HSV culture

Studies should be repeated 7 days later, except for syphilis and hepatitis B serologic tests, which should be obtained 12 weeks later.

---

*Obtain if there is supportive epidemiologic evidence.

BIBLIOGRAPHY

Sexually transmitted diseases and sexual abuse of children (general)

Centers for Disease Control. 1993 sexually transmitted diseases treatment guidelines. MMWR 1993;42(RR-14).

De Jong AR. Sexually transmitted diseases in sexually abused children. Sex Transm Dis 1986;13:123-126.

Glaser JB, Hammerschlag MR, McCormack WM. Epidemiology of sexually transmitted diseases in rape victims. Rev Infect Dis 1989;11:246-254.

Hammerschlag MR. Sexually transmitted diseases in sexually abused children. Adv Pediatr Infect Dis 1988;3:1-18.

Hammerschlag MR, Alpert S, Rosner I, et al. Microbiology of the vagina in children: normal and potentially pathogenic organisms. Pediatrics 1978;62:57-62.

Ingram DL, Everett D, Lyna PR, et al. Epidemiology of adult sexually transmitted disease agents in children being evaluated for sexual abuse. Pediatr Infect Dis J 1992;11:945-950.

Jenny C, Hooton TM, Bowers A, et al. Sexually transmitted diseases in victims of rape. N Engl J Med 1990;322:713-716.

Neinstein LS, Goldenring J, Carpenter S. Nonsexual transmission of sexually transmitted diseases: an infrequent occurrence. Pediatrics 1984;74:67-75.

Rimsza ME, Niggemann EH. Medical evaluation of sexually abused children: a review of 311 cases. Pediatrics 1982;69:8-14.

Schwarcz SK, Whittington WL. Sexual assault and sexually transmitted diseases: detection and management. Rev Infect Dis 1990;12:5682-5690.

Tilelli JA, Turek D, Jaffe AC. Sexual abuse of children: clinical findings and implications for management. N Engl J Med 1980;302:319-323.

White ST, Coda FA, Ingram DA, et al. Sexually transmitted diseases in sexually abused children. Pediatrics 1983;72:16-21.

Gonorrhea

Abbott SL. Gonococcal tonsillitis-pharyngitis in a 5-year-old girl. Pediatrics 1973;52:287-289.

Ahmed HJ, Ilardi I, Antognoli A, et al. An epidemic of *Neisseria gonorrhoeae* in a Somali orphanage. Int J STD & AIDS 1992;3:52-53.

American Academy of Pediatrics. Gonococcal infections. In Peter G (ed). 1994 Red Book: Report of the Committee on Infectious Diseases, ed 23. Elk Grove Village, Ill: American Academy of Pediatrics, 1994.

Amstey MS, Steadman KT. Asymptomatic gonorrhea and pregnancy. J Am Vener Dis Assoc 1976;3:14.

Apicella MA. Serogrouping the *Neisseria gonorrhoeae:* identification of four immunologically distinct acidic polysaccharides. J Infect Dis 1976;134:377.

Barr J, Danielsson D. Septic gonococcal dermatitis. Br Med J 1971;1:482-485.

Bernstein GA, Davis JP, Katcher ML. Prophylaxis of neonatal conjunctivitis: an analytic review. Clin Pediatr 1983;21:545-550.

Biro FM, Rosenthal SL, Kiniyalocts M. Gonococcal and chlamydial genitourinary infections in symptomatic and asymptomatic adolescent women. Clin Peds 1995;34:419-423.

Branch G, Paxton R. A study of gonococcal infection among infants and children. Public Health Rep 1965;80:347-352.

Britigan BE, Cohen MS, Sparling PF. Gonococcal infections: a model of molecular pathogenesis. N Engl J Med 1985;312:1683-1694.

Burry VF. Gonococcal vulvovaginitis and possible peritonitis in prepubertal girls. Am J Dis Child 1971;21:536-537.

Catlin BW. Nutritional profiles of *Neisseria gonorrhoeae, Neisseria meningitidis,* and *Neisseria lactamica* in chemically defined media and the use of growth requirements for gonococcal typing. J Infect Dis 1973;128:178-194.

Centers for Disease Control. Antibiotic-resistant strains of *Neisseria gonorrhoeae.* MMWR 1987;36(suppl 5):1S-18S.

Centers for Disease Control. 1993 Sexually transmitted diseases treatment guidelines. MMWR 1993;42(RR-14):56-67.

Centers for Disease Control. Summary of notifiable diseases, United States, 1994;43(53).

Centers for Disease Control. Decreased susceptibility of *Neisseria gonorrhoeae* to fluoroquinolones—Ohio and Hawaii, 1992-1994. MMWR 1994;43:325-327.

DeJong AR. Sexually transmitted diseases in sexually abused children. Sex Transm Dis 1986;13:123-126.

Edwards LE, et al. Gonorrhea in pregnancy. Am J Obstet Gynecol 1978;132:637.

Fleisher G, Hodge D, Cromie W. Penile edema in childhood gonorrhea. Ann Emerg Med 1980;9:314-315.

Gorwitz RJ, Nakashima AK, Knapp JS. Sentinel surveillance for antimicrobial resistance in *Neisseria gonorrhoeae*— United States, 1988-1991. MMWR 1993;42(SS-3):29-39.

Groothius J, Bischoff MC, Javrequi LE. Pharyngeal gonorrhea in young children. Pediatr Infect Dis 1983;2:99-101.

Hammerschlag MR, Doraiswamy B, Alexander ER, et al. Are rectogenital chlamydial infections a marker of sexual abuse in children? Pediatr Infect Dis 1984;3:100-104.

Hammerschlag MR, Cummings C, Roblin PM, et al. Efficacy of neonatal ocular prophylaxis for the prevention of chlamydial and gonococcal conjunctivitis. N Eng J Med 1989;320:769-772.

Handsfield HH. Disseminated gonococcal infection. Clin Obstet Gynecol 1975;18:131-142.

Handsfield HH, Hodson EA, Holmes KK. Neonatal gonococcal infection. JAMA 1973;225:697.

Hein K, Marks A, Cohen MI. Asymptomatic gonorrhea: prevalence in a population of urban adolescents. J Pediatr 1977;90:634-635.

Holmes KK, Counts GW, Beaty HN. Disseminated gonococcal infection. Ann Intern Med 1971;74:979.

Hook EW III, Holmes KK. Gonococcal infections. Ann Intern Med 1985;102:229-243.

Hook EW III, Judson FN, Handsfield HH. Auxotype/serovar diversity and antimicrobial resistance of *Neisseria gonorrhoeae* in two mid-sized American cities. Sex Transm Dis 1987;14:141-146.

Ingram DL, Everett D, Lyna PR, et al. Epidemiology of adult sexually transmitted disease agents in children being evaluated for sexual abuse. Pediatr Inf Dis J 1992;11:945-950.

Ingram DL, Runyan DK, Collins AD, et al. Vaginal *Chlamydia trachomatis* infection in children with sexual contact. Pediatr Infect Dis 1984;3:97-99.

Ingram DL, White ST, Durfee MR, et al. Sexual contact in children with gonorrhea. Am J Dis Child 1982;136:994-996.

Johnson SR, Morse SA. Antibiotic resistance in *Neisseria gonorrhoeae:* genetics and mechanisms of resistance. Sex Transm Dis 1988;15:217-224.

Judson FN, Ehret JM, Handsfield HH. Comparative study of ceftriaxone and spectinomycin for treatment of pharyngeal and anorectal gonorrhea. JAMA 1985;253:1417-1419.

Kam KM, Wong PW, Cheung MM, et al. Quinolone-resistant *Neisseria gonorrhoeae* in Hong Kong. Sex Transm Dis 1996;23:103-108.

Knapp JS, Holmes KK. Disseminated gonococcal infections caused by *Neisseria gonorrhoeae* with unique nutritional requirements. J Infect Dis 1975;132:204.

Knapp JS, Tam MR, Nowinski RC, et al. Serological classification of *Neisseria gonorrhoeae* with use of monoclonal antibodies to gonococcal outer membrane protein I. J Infect Dis 1984;150:44-48.

Laga M, Naamara W, Brunham RC, et al. Single-dose therapy of gonococcal ophthalmia neonatorum. N Engl J Med 1986;315:1382-1385.

Laga M, Nzanze H, Brunham RC, et al. Epidemiology of ophthalmia neonatorum in Kenya. Lancet 1986;2:1145-1149.

Laga M, Plummer FA, Piot P, et al. Prophylaxis of gonococcal and chlamydial ophthalmia neonatorum. N Engl J Med 1988;318:653-657.

Lewis LS, Glauser TA, Joffe MD. Gonococcal conjunctivitis in prepubertal children. Am J Dis Child 1990;144:546-548.

McClure EM, Stack MR, Tanner T, et al. Pharyngeal culturing and reporting of pediatric gonorrhea in Connecticut. Pediatrics 1986;78:509-510.

Michalowski B. Difficulties of diagnosis and treatment of gonorrhea in young girls. Br J Vener Dis 1961;37:142-144.

Nelson JD. The bacterial etiology and antibiotic management of septic arthritis in infants and children. Pediatrics 1972;50:437-440.

Nelson JD, Mohs E, Dajani AS, Plotkin SA. Gonorrhea in preschool and school-aged children: a report of the prepubertal gonorrhea cooperative study group. JAMA 1976; 236:1359.

O'Brien JP, Goldenberg DL, Rice P. Disseminated gonococcal infection: a prospective analysis of 49 patients and a review of the pathophysiology and immune mechanisms. Medicine 1983;62:395-406.

Petersen BH, Lee TJ, Synderman R, et al. *Neisseria meningitidis* and *Neisseria gonorrhoeae* bacteremia associated with C6, C7, or C8 deficiency. Ann Intern Med 1979;90:917-920.

Potterat JJ, Markewich GS, King RD, et al. Child-to-child transmission of gonorrhea: report of asymptomatic genital infection in a boy. Pediatrics 1986;78:711-712.

Rawstron SA, Hammerschlag MR, Gullans C, et al. Ceftriaxone treatment of penicillinase-producing *Neisseria gonorrhoeae* infections in children. Pediatr Infect Dis 1989;8:445-448.

Rettig PJ, Nelson JD, Kusmiess H. Spectinomycin therapy for gonorrhea in prepubertal children. Am J Dis Child 1980; 134:559-563.

Rothenberg R. Ophthalmia neonatorum due to *Neisseria gonorrhoeae:* prevention and treatment. Sex Transm Dis 1979; 6:187-191.

Schichor A, Bernstein B, Weinerman H, et al. Lidocaine as a diluent for cetriaxone in the treatment of gonorrhea. Arch Pediatr Adolesc Med 1994;148:72-75.

Schwarcz SK, Whittington WL. Sexual assault and sexually transmitted diseases: detection and management in adults and children. Rev Infect Dis 1990;12:S682-S690.

Schwebke JR, Whittington W, Rice RJ, et al. Trends in susceptibility of *Neisseria gonorrhoeae* to ceftriaxone from 1985 through 1991. Antimicrob Agents Chemother 1995;39:917-920.

Schwarz SK, Zenilman JM, Schnell D, et al. National surveillance of antimicrobial resistance in *Neisseria gonorrhoeae*. JAMA 1990;264:1413-1417.

Segal E, Billyard E, So M, et al. Role of chromosomal rearrangement in *Neisseria gonorrhoeae* pilus phase variation. Cell 1985;40:293-300.

Smith JA, Linder CW, Jay S. Isolation of *Neisseria gonorrhea* from the urethra of asymptomatic adolescent males. Clin Peds 1986;25:566-568.

Speck WT, Lawsky AR. Symptomatic anorectal gonorrhea in an adolescent female. Am J Dis Child 1971;122:438-439.

Stamm WE, Guinan ME, Johnson C, et al. Effect of treatment regimens for *Neisseria gonorrhoeae* on simultaneous infection with *Chlamydia trachomatis*. N Engl J Med 1984; 310:545-549.

Tronca E, Handsfield HH, Weisner PJ, Holmes KK. Demonstration of *Neisseria gonorrhoeae* with fluorescent antibody in patients with disseminated gonococcal infection. JID 1974; 129:583-586.

Weisner PJ, Tronca E, Bonin P, et al. Clinical spectrum of pharyngeal gonococcal infection. N Engl J Med 1973;288:181-185.

Whittington WL, Rice RJ, Biddle JW, Knapp JS. Incorrect identification of *Neisseria gonorrhoeae* from infants and children. Pediatr Infect Dis 1988;7:3-10.

Pelvic inflammatory disease and salpingitis

Bowie WR, Jones H. Acute pelvic inflammatory disease in outpatients: association with *Chlamydia trachomatis* and *Neisseria gonorrhoeae*. Ann Intern Med 1981;95:685-688.

Cromer BA, Heald FP. Pelvic inflammatory disease associated with *Neisseria gonorrhoeae* and *Chlamydia trachomatis:* clinical correlates. Sex Transm Dis 1987;14:125-129.

Eschenbach DA, Buchanan TM, Pollock HM, et al. Polymicrobial etiology of acute pelvic inflammatory disease. N Engl J Med 1975;293:166-171.

Gates W. Sexually transmitted organisms and infertility: the proof of the pudding. Sex Transm Dis 1984;11:113-116.

Mardh PA. An overview of infectious agents of salpingitis, their biology, and recent methods of detection. Am J Obstet Gynecol 1980;138:933-951.

Patton DL. Immunopathology and histopathology of experimental chlamydial salpingitis. Rev Infect Dis 1985;7: 746-753.

Scholes D, Stergachis A, Heidrich FE. Prevention of pelvic inflammatory disease by screening for cervical chlamydial infection. N Engl J Med 1996;334:1362-1366.

Shafer M-A, Irwin CE, Sweet RL. Acute salpingitis in the adolescent female. J Pediatr 1982;100:339-350.

Walters MD, Gibbs RS. A randomized comparison of gentamicin-clindamycin and cefoxitin-doxycycline in the treatment of acute pelvic inflammatory disease. Obstet Gynecol 1990;75:867-872.

Wasserheit JN, Bell TA, Kiviat NB, et al. Microbial causes of proven pelvic inflammatory disease and efficacy of clindamycin and tobramycin. Ann Intern Med 1986;104:187-193.

Westrom L. Incidence, prevalence, and trends of acute pelvic inflammatory disease and its consequences in industrialized countries. Am J Obstet Gynecol 1980;138:880-892.

Wolner-Hanssen P, Eschenbach D, Paavonen J, et al. Treatment of pelvic inflammatory disease: use of doxycycline with an appropriate B-lactam while we wait for better data. JAMA 1986;256:3262-3263.

Syphilis

Ackerman AB, Goldfaden G, Cosmides JC. Acquired syphilis in early childhood. Arch Dermatol 1972;106:92-93.

Alderete JF, Baseman JB. Surface-associated host proteins on virulent *Treponema pallidum*. Infect Immunol 1979; 26:1048.

Baker-Zander S, Sell S. A histopathologic and immunologic study of the course of syphilis in the experimentally infected rabbit: demonstration of long-lasting cellular immunity. Am J Pathol 1980;101:387.

Beck-Sague C, Alexander ER. Failures of benzathine penicillin G therapy in early congenital syphilis. Pediatr Infect Dis 1987;6:1061-1064.

Beeram MR, Chopde N, Dawood Y, et al. Lumbar puncture in the evaluation of possible asymptomatic congenital syphilis in neonates. J Pediatr 1996;128:125-129.

Bromberg K, Rawstron S, Tannis G. Diagnosis of congenital syphilis by combining *Treponema pallidum*–specific IgM detection with immunofluorescent antigen detection for *T. pallidum*. J Infect Dis 1993;168:238-242.

Centers for Disease Control. Sexually transmitted diseases treatment guidelines. MMWR 1993;42:1-102.

Centers for Disease Control. Continuing increase in infectious syphilis, United States. MMWR 1988;37:35-37.

Centers for Disease Control. Case definitions for public health surveillance. MMWR 1990;39(RR-13):36.

Centers for Disease Control. Summary of notifiable diseases, United States 1995. MMWR 1996a;44:53.

Centers for Disease Control, Division of STD Prevention. Sexually transmitted disease surveillance 1995. U.S. Department of Health and Human Services, Public Health Service. Atlanta: Centers for Disease Control and Prevention, 1996b.

Cohen DA, Boyd D, Pabhudas I, Mascola L. The effects of case definition, maternal screening, and reporting criteria on rates of congenital syphilis. Am J Public Health 1990;80: 316-317.

Deacon WE, Lucas JB, Price EV. Fluorescent treponemal antibody-absorption (FTA-ABS) test for syphilis. JAMA 1966; 198:624.

Digre KA, White GL, Cremer SA, Massanari RM. Late-onset congenital syphilis: a retrospective look at University of Iowa hospital admissions. J Clin Neuroophthalmol 1991;11:1-6.

Duncan WC, Knox JM, Wende RD. The FTA-ABS test in dark field–positive primary syphilis. JAMA 1974;228:859-860.

Dunlop EMC, Al-Egaily MB, Houang ET. Penicillin levels in blood and CSF achieved by treatment of syphilis. JAMA 1979;241:2538.

Eagle H, Fleischman R, Muselman AD. The effective concentration of penicillin in vitro and in vivo for streptococci, pneumococci, and *Treponema pallidum*. J Bacteriol 1950; 59:625-643.

Fiumara NJ. Syphilis in newborn children. Clin Obstet Gynecol 1975;18:183-189.

Fiumara NJ. Treatment of primary and secondary syphilis. Serological response. JAMA 1980;243:2500-2502.

Fiumara NJ, Fleming WL, Downing JG, Good FL. The incidence of prenatal syphilis at the Boston City Hospital. N Engl J Med 1952;247:48-52.

Fiumara NJ, Lessell S. The stigmata of late congenital syphilis: an analysis of 100 patients. Sex Transm Dis 1983;10: 126-129.

Fojaco RM, Hensley GT, Moskowitz L. Congenital syphilis and necrotizing funisitis. JAMA 1989;261:1788-1790.

Frenz G, Hideon PB, Esperson F, et al. Penicillin concentrations in blood and spinal fluid after a single intramuscular injection of penicillin G benzathine. Eur J Clin Microbiol 1984;3:147.

Ginsberg CM. Acquired syphilis in prepubertal children. Pediatr Infect Dis 1983;2:232-234.

Grimprel E, Sanchez PJ, Wendel GD, et al. Use of polymerase chain reaction and rabbit infectivity testing to detect *Treponema pallidum* in amniotic fluid, fetal and neonatal sera, and cerebrospinal fluid. J Clin Microbiol 1991;29:1711-1718.

Harter CA, Benirschke K. Fetal syphilis in the first trimester. Am J Obstet Gynecol 1976;124:705.

Hira SK, Bhat GJ, Patel JB, et al. Early congenital syphilis: clinico-radiologic features in 202 patients. Sex Transm Dis 1985;12:177-183.

Hovind-Hougen K. Morphology. In Shell RF, Musher DM (eds). Pathogenesis and immunology of treponemal infection. New York: Marcel Dekker, 1983.

Idsoe O, Guthie T, Willcox RR. Penicillin in the treatment of syphilis. Bull World Health Organ 1972;47(suppl):1-68.

Ingraham NR. The diagnosis of infantile congenital syphilis during the period of doubt. Am J Syph Neurol 1935;19: 547-580.

Jenkin HW, Sander PL. In vitro cultivation of *Treponema pallidum*. In Shell RF, Musher DM (eds). Pathogenesis and immunology of treponemal infection. New York: Marcel Dekker, 1983.

Karmody CS, Schuknecht HP. Deafness in congenital syphilis. Arch Otolaryng 1966;83:44-53.

Kaufman RE, Olansky DC, Wiesner PJ. The FTA-ABS (IgM) test for neonatal congenital syphilis: a critical review. J Am Venereol Dis Assoc 1974;1:79-84.

Lukehart SA, Hook EW III, Baker-Zander SA, et al. Invasion of the central nervous system by *Treponema pallidum:* implications for diagnosis and treatment. Ann Intern Med 1988; 109:855-862.

Mascola L, Pelosi R, Blount JH, et al. Congenital syphilis: why is it still occurring? JAMA 1984a;252:1719-1722.

Mascola L, Pelosi R, Alexander CE. Inadequate treatment of syphilis in pregnancy. Am J Obstet Gynecol 1984b;150: 945-947.

McCracken GH Jr, Kaplan JM. Penicillin treatment for congenital syphilis. JAMA 1974;228:855.

Miller JL, Meyer PG, Parrott NA, Hill JH. A study of the biologic falsely positive reactions for syphilis in children. J Pediatr 1960;57:548-552.

Musher DM. Biology of *Treponema pallidum*. In Holmes KK, Mardh PA, Sparling PF, Wiesner PJ (eds). Sexually transmitted diseases. New York: McGraw-Hill, 1984.

Musher DM, et al. The interaction between *Treponema pallidum* and human polymorphonuclear leucocytes. J Infect Dis 1983; 147:77.

Musher DM, Hamill RJ, Baughn RE. Effect of human immunodeficiency virus (HIV) infection on the course of syphilis and on the response to treatment. Ann Intern Med 1990; 113:872-881.

Rathbun KC. Congenital syphilis. Sex Transm Dis 1983;10: 93-99.

Rawstron SA, Bromberg K. Failure of recommended maternal therapy to prevent congenital syphilis. Sex Transm Dis 1991a;18:102-106.

Rawstron SA, Bromberg K. Comparison of maternal and newborn serologic tests for syphilis. Am J Dis Child 1991b; 145:1383-1388.

Rawstron SA, Jenkins S, Blanchard S, et al. Maternal and congenital syphilis in Brooklyn, NY. Epidemiology, transmission, and diagnosis. Am J Dis Child 1993;147:727-731.

Risser WL, Hwang LY. Problems in the current case definition of congenital syphilis. J Pediatr 1996;129:499-505.

Romanowski B, Sutherland R, Fick GH, et al. Serologic response to treatment of infectious syphilis. Ann Intern Med 1991;114:1005-1009.

Russell P, Altshuler G. Placental abnormalities of congenital syphilis. Am J Dis Child 1974;128:160-163.

Sanchez PJ, McCracken GH Jr, Wendel GD, et al. Molecular analysis of the fetal IgM response to *Treponema pallidum* antigens: implications for improved serodiagnosis of congenital syphilis. J Infect Dis 1989;159:508-517.

Sanchez PJ, Wendel GD, Norgard MV. IgM antibody to *Treponema pallidum* in cerebrospinal fluid of infants with congenital syphilis. Am J Dis Child 1992;146:1171-1175.

Sanchez PJ, Wendel GD Jr, Grimprel E, et al. Evaluation of molecular methodologies and rabbit infectivity testing for the diagnosis of congenital syphilis and neonatal central nervous system invasion by *Treponema pallidum*. J Infect Dis 1993;167:148-157.

Scotti AT, Logan LL. A specific IgM antibody test in neonatal congenital syphilis. J Pediatr 1968;73:242-243.

Shah AM, Boby KFJ, Karande SC, et al. Late onset congenital syphilis. Indian Pediatr 1995;32:795-798.

Sparling PF. Diagnosis and treatment of syphilis. N Engl J Med 1971;284:642.

Speer ME, Taber LH, Clark DB, Rudolph AJ. Cerebrospinal fluid levels of benzathine penicillin G in the neonate. J Pediatr 1977;9:996.

Srinivasan G, Ramamurthy RS, Bharathi A, et al. Congenital syphilis: a diagnostic and therapeutic dilemma. Pediatr Infect Dis 1983;2:436-441.

St. Louis ME, Farley TA, Aral SO. Untangling the persistence of syphilis in the South. Sex Transm Dis 1996;23:11-14.

Taber LH, Huber TW. Congenital syphilis. Prog Clin Biol Res 1975;3:183.

Wendel GD. Gestational and congenital syphilis. Clin Perinatol 1988;15:287-303.

Wendel GD Jr, Sanchez PJ, Peters MT, et al. Identification of *Treponema pallidum* in amniotic fluid and fetal blood from pregnancies complicated by congenital syphilis. Obstet Gynecol 1991;78(5 pt 2):890-895.

Wendel GD, Stark BJ, Jamison RB, et al. Penicillin allergy and desensitization in serious infections during pregnancy. N Engl J Med 1985;312:1229-1232.

Wolf B, Kalangu K. Congenital neurosyphilis revisited. Eur J Pediatr 1993;152:493-495.

Yobs AR, Brown L, Hunter EF. Fluorescent antibody technique in early syphilis. Arch Pathol 1964;77:220-225.

Zenker PN, Rolfs RT. Treatment of syphilis, 1989. Rev Infect Dis 1990;12(suppl 6):S590.

Zenker PN, Rolfs RT. Congenital syphilis: trends and recommendations for evaluation and management. Pediatr Infect Dis J 1991;10:516-522.

Chlamydia trachomatis infections

Alexander ER, Harrison HR. Role of *Chlamydia trachomatis* in perinatal infection. Rev Infect Dis 1983;5:713-719.

Beem MO, Saxon EM. Respiratory tract colonization and a distinctive pneumonia syndrome in infants infected with *Chlamydia trachomatis.* N Engl J Med 1977;296:306-310.

Bell TA, Sandstrom KI, Gravett MG, et al. Comparison of ophthalmic silver nitrate solution and erythromycin ointment for prevention of natally acquired *Chlamydia trachomatis.* Sex Transm Dis 1987;14:195-200.

Blythe MJ, Katz BP, Batteiger BE, et al. Recurrent genitourinary chlamydia infection in sexually active adolescents. J Pediatr 1992;121:487-493.

Blythe MJ, Katz BP, Caine VA. Historical and clinical factors associated with *Chlamydia trachomatis* genitourinary tract infection in female adolescents. J Pediatr 1988;112:1000-1004.

Brunham RC, Binns B, McDowell J, Paraskevas M. *Chlamydia trachomatis* infection in women with ectopic pregnancy. Obstet Gynecol 1986;67:722-726.

Centers for Disease Control. Recommendations for the prevention and management of *Chlamydia trachomatis* infections, 1993. MMWR 1993;42(RR-12).

Chacko MR, Lovchik JC. *Chlamydia trachomatis* infection in sexually active adolescents: prevalence and risk factors. Pediatrics 1984;73:836-840.

Chambers CV, Shafer MA, Adger H, et al. Microflora of the urethra in adolescent boys: relationship to sexual activity and nongonococcal urethritis. J Pediatr 1987;110:314-321.

Chernesky MA, Mahony JB, Castriciano S, et al. Detection of *Chlamydia trachomatis* antigens by enzyme immunoassay and immunofluorescence in genital specimens from symptomatic and asymptomatic men and women. J Infect Dis 1986;154:141-148.

Eagar RM, Beach RK, Davidson AJ. Epidemiologic and clinical factors of *Chlamydia trachomatis* in black, hispanic and white female adolescents. West J Med 1985;143:3-41.

Fisher M, Swenson PD, Risucci D, Kaplan MH. *Chlamydia trachomatis* in suburban adolescents. J Pediatr 1987;111:617-620.

Fraser JJ, Rettig PJ, Kaplan DW. Prevalence of cervical *Chlamydia trachomatis* and *Neisseria gonorrhoeae* in female adolescents. Pediatrics 1982;71:333-336.

Golden N, Hammerschlag M, Neuhoff S, Gleyzer A. Prevalence of *Chlamydia trachomatis* cervical infection in female adolescents. Am J Dis Child 1984;138:562-564.

Hammerschlag MR. Chlamydial infections. J Pediatr 1989;114:727-734.

Hammerschlag MR. *Chlamydia trachomatis* in children. Pediatr Ann 1994;32:349-353.

Hammerschlag MR, Cummings C, Roblin P, et al. Efficacy of neonatal ocular prophylaxis for the prevention of chlamydial and gonococcal conjunctivitis. N Engl J Med 1989;320:769-772.

Hammerschlag MR, Doraiswamy B, Alexander ER, et al. Are rectogenital chlamydial infections a marker of sexual abuse in children? Pediatr Infect Dis 1984;3:100-104.

Hammerschlag MR, Golden NH, Oh MK, et al. Single dose of azithromycin for the treatment of genital chlamydia infections in adolescents. J Pediatr 1993;122:961-965.

Hammerschlag MR, Rettig PJ, Shields ME. False-positive results with the use of chlamydial antigen detection tests in the evaluation of suspected sexual abuse in children. Pediatr Infect Dis 1988;7:11-14.

Hammerschlag MR, Roblin PM, Cummings C, et al. Comparison of enzyme immunoassay and culture for diagnosis of chlamydial conjunctivitis and respiratory infections in infants. J Clin Microbiol 1987;25:2306-2308.

Hammerschlag MR, Roblin PM, Gelling M, et al. Use of polymerase chain reaction for the detection of *Chlamydia trachomatis* in ocular and nasopharyngeal specimens from infants with conjunctivitis. Pediatr Infect Dis J, 1997, (in press).

Harrison HR, Alexander ER, Weinstein L, et al. Cervical *Chlamydia trachomatis* and mycoplasmal infections in pregnancy: epidemiology and outcomes. JAMA 1983;250:1721-1727.

Harrison HR, English MG, Lee CK, Alexander ER. *Chlamydia trachomatis* infant pneumonia. N Engl J Med 1978;298:702-708.

Hauger SB, Brown J, Agre F, et al. Failure of MicroTrak to detect *C. trachomatis* from genital tract sites of prepubertal children at risk for sexual abuse. Pediatr Infect Dis 1988;7:660-661.

Heggie AD, Jaffe AC, Stuart LA, et al. Topical sulfacetamide vs oral erythromycin for neonatal chlamydial conjunctivitis. Am J Dis Child 1985;139:564-566.

Heggie AD, Lumicao GG, Stuart LA, et al. *Chlamydia trachomatis* infection in mothers and infants. Am J Dis Child 1981;135:507-511.

Ingram DL, Runyan DK, Collins AD, et al. Vaginal *Chlamydia trachomatis* infection in children with sexual contact. Pediatr Infect Dis 1984;3:97-99.

Loefflelholz MJ, Lewinski CA, Silver SR, et al. Detection of *Chlamydia trachomatia* in endocervical specimens by polymerase chain reaction. J Clin Microbiol 1992;30:2847-2851.

Martin DH, Mroczkowski TF, Dalu ZA, et al. A controlled trial of a single dose of azithromycin for the treatment of chlamydial urethritis and cervicitis. N Engl J Med 1992;327:921-925.

Orr P, Sherman E, Blanchard J, et al. Epidemiology of infection due to *Chlamydia trachomatis* in Manitoba, Canada. Clin Infect Dis 1994;19:876-883.

Porder K, Sanchez N, Roblin PM, et al. Lack of specificity of Chlamydiazyme for detection of vaginal chlamydial infection in prepubertal girls. Pediatr Infect Dis 1989;8:358-360.

Quinn TC, Welsh L, Lentz A, et al. Diagnosis by Amplicor PCR of *Chlamydia trachomatis* infection in urine samples from women and men attending sexually transmitted disease clinics. J Clin Microbiol 1996;34:1401-1406.

Radkowski MA, Kranzler JK, Beem MO, Tippk MA. Chlamydia pneumonia in infants: radiography in 125 cases. Am J Roentgenol 1981;137:703-706.

Rettig PJ, Nelson JD. Genital tract infection with *Chlamydia trachomatis* in prepubertal children. J Pediatr 1981;99:206-210.

Roblin PM, Hammerschlag MR, Cummings C, et al. Comparison of two rapid microscopic methods and culture for detection of *Chlamydia trachomatis* in ocular and nasopharyngeal specimens from infants. J Clin Microbiol 1989;27:968-970.

Saltz GR, Linnemann CC, Brookman RR, et al. *Chlamydia trachomatis* cervical infections in female adolescents. J Pediatr 1981;98:981-985.

Schachter J, Grossman M, Sweet RL, et al. Prospective study of perinatal transmission of *Chlamydia trachomatis*. JAMA 1986a;255:3374-3377.

Schachter J, Sweet RL, Grossman M, et al. Experience with the routine use of erythromycin in pregnancy. N Engl J Med 1986b;314:276-279.

Shafer MA, Vaughan E, Lipkin ES, et al. Evaluation fluorescein-conjugated monoclonal antibody test to detect *Chlamydia trachomatis* endocervical infections in adolescent girls. J Pediatr 1986;108:779-783.

Turrentine MA, Newton ER. Amoxicillin or erythromycin for the treatment of antenatal chlamydial infection: a metaanalysis. Obstet Gynecol 1995;86:1021-1025.

Weiss SG, Newcomb RW, Beem MO. Pulmonary assessment of children after chlamydial pneumonia of infancy. J Pediatr 1986;108:661-664.

Bacterial vaginosis

Amsel R, Tolter PA, Spiegel CA, et al. Nonspecific vaginitis: diagnostic criteria and microbial and epidemiologic associations. Am J Med 1983;74:14-22.

Bartley DL, Morgan L, Rimsza MA. *Gardnerella vaginalis* in prepubertal girls. Am J Dis Child 1987;141:1014-1017.

Hammerschlag MR, Cummings M, Doraiswamy B, et al. Nonspecific vaginitis following sexual abuse in children. Pediatrics 1985;75:1028-1031.

Ingram DL, White ST, Lyna PR, et al. *Gardnerella vaginalis* infection and sexual contact in female children. Child Abuse Neglect 1992;16:847-853.

Samuels P, Hammerschlag MR, Cummings M, et al. Nonspecific vaginitis is an important cause of vaginitis in children. Presented at the 25th Interscience Conference on Antimicrobial Agents and Chemotherapy, 1985, Minneapolis (abstract 391).

Shafer M-A, Sweet RL, Ohm-Smith MJ, et al. Microbiology of the lower genital tract in postmenarcheal adolescent girls, differences by sexual activity, contraception, and presence of nonspecific vaginitis. J Pediatr 1985;107:974-981.

Spiegel CA, Amsel R, Holmes KK. Diagnosis of bacterial vaginosis by direct Gram stain of vaginal fluid. J Clin Microbiol 1983;18:170-177.

Thomason JL, Velbart SM, Anderson RJ, et al. Statistical evaluation of diagnostic criteria for bacterial vaginosis. Am J Obstet Gynecol 1990;162:155-160.

Trichomoniasis

Al-Salihi FL, Curram JP, Wang JS. Neonatal trichomonas vaginalis: report of three cases and review of the literature. Pediatrics 1974;53:196-200.

Fouts AC, Kraus SJ. Trichomonas vaginalis: reevaluation of its clinical presentation and laboratory diagnosis. J Infect Dis 1980;141:137-143.

Jones JG, Yamauchi T, Lambert B. *Trichomonas vaginalis* infestation in sexually abused girls. Am J Dis Child 1985;139:846-847.

Kruger JN, Tam MR, Stevens CE, et al. Diagnosis of trichomoniasis: comparison of conventional wet-mount examination with cytologic studies, cultures, and monoclonal antibody staining of direct specimens. JAMA 1988;259:1223-1227.

Wolner-Hanssen P, Krieger JN, Stevens CE, et al. Clinical manifestations of vaginal trichomoniasis. JAMA 1989;261:571-576.

Human papillomavirus infection

Bauer HM, Greer CE, Chambers JC, et al. Genital human papillomavirus infection in female university students as determined by a PCR-based method. JAMA 1991;265:472-477.

Bender ME. New concepts of condyloma acuminata in children. Arch Dermatol 1986;122:1121-1124.

Boyd AS. Condylomata acuminata in the pediatric population. Am J Dis Child 1990;144:817-824.

Cohen BA, Honig P, Androphy E. Anogenital warts in children. Arch Dermatol 1990;126:1575-1580.

Davis AJ, Emans SJ. Human papillomavirus infection in the pediatric and adolescent patient. J Pediatr 1989;115:1-9.

DeJong AR, Weiss JC, Brent RL. Condyloma acuminata in children. Am J Dis Child 1982;136:704-706.

Fisher M, Rosenfeld WD, Burk RD. Cervicovaginal human papillomavirus infection in suburban adolescents and young adults. J Pediatr 1991;119:821-825.

Gibson PE, Gardner SD, Best SJ. Human papillomavirus types in anogenital warts of children. J Med Virol 1990;30:142-145.

Gutman LT, St Claire KK, Hermann-Giddens ME, et al. Evaluation of sexually abused and nonabused young girls for intravaginal human papillomavirus infection. Am J Dis Child 1992;146:694-699.

Moscicki A-B, Palefsky J, Gonzales J, et al. Human papillomavirus infection in sexually active adolescent females: prevalence and risk factors. Pediatr Res 1990;28:507-513.

Obaleck S, Jablonska S, Favre M, et al. Condylomata acuminata in children: frequent association with human papillomaviruses responsible for cutaneous warts. J Am Acad Dermatol 1990;23:205-213.

Padel AF, Venning VA, Evans MF, et al. Human papillomaviruses in anogenital warts in children; typing by DNA hybridization. Brit Med J 1990;300:1491-1494.

Rock B, Noghashfar Z, Barnett N, et al. Genital tract papillomavirus infection in children. Arch Dermatol 1986;122:1129-1132.

Seidel J, Zonana J, Tolten E. Condylomata acuminata as a sign of sexual abuse in children. J Pediatr 1979;95:553-554.

Other infections

Gellert GA, Durfee MJ, Berkowitz CD. Developing guidelines for HIV antibody testing among victims of pediatric sexual abuse. Child Abuse Neglect 1990;14:9-17.

Gellert GA, Durfee MJ, Berkowitz CD, et al. Situational and sociodemographic characteristics of children infected with human immunodeficiency virus from pediatric sexual abuse. Pediatrics 1993;91:39-44.

Gutman LT, St Claire KK, Weedy C, et al. Human immunodeficiency virus transmission by child sexual abuse. Am J Dis Child 1991;145:137-141.

Leiderman BA, Grimm KT. A child with HIV infection. JAMA 1986;256:3094.

Schmid GP. Treatment of chancroid, 1989. Rev Infect Dis 1990;12:80:S580-S589.

Szmuness W, Much MI, Prince AM, et al. On the role of sexual behavior in the spread of hepatitis B infection. Ann Intern Med 1975;83:489-495.

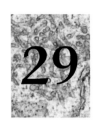

29 SMALLPOX AND VACCINIA

Two decades have passed since the eradication of smallpox, and we have once again deliberated the justification for devoting a chapter in this tenth edition to variola and vaccinia. A full discussion of smallpox (variola) and vaccinia was included in Chapter 28 of the seventh (1981) edition of this book. Therefore we have chosen to restrict this chapter to brief general sections, comments on contemporary issues, remarks on related viruses and illnesses, and a list of significant references for those readers who choose to explore further this fascinating example of human conquest of a disease.

For more than 3,000 years smallpox was a widespread illness with serious morbidity and mortality. Nations in Africa and the Asian subcontinent reported hundreds of thousands of cases annually as recently as 1967. In that year the World Health Organization (WHO) began its 10-year program of smallpox eradication. On October 26, 1977, Ali Maow Maalin, a cook in the district hospital at Merka, Somalia, had the onset of his smallpox rash. He is recorded in history as the last known patient with endemic smallpox. In the years after Maalin's recovery the only known smallpox victims acquired their infection as the result of a laboratory contamination in Birmingham, England.

Several hundred episodes of suspected endemic smallpox have been reported to WHO since the case of Ali Maow Maalin, but none has been verified. Instead, they proved to be chickenpox, herpes simplex, monkeypox, drug eruptions, or other skin disorders. Of special note is monkeypox, which has been reported with regularity from West and Central Africa. Originally recovered from monkeys who became ill in captivity, the virus has been responsible for human illness closely resembling smallpox, usually in children with no history of previous smallpox vaccination. Secondary spread among humans is quite unusual, but several cases

have been documented. Sporadic cases of human monkeypox are reported and may result from direct transmission in handling the carcasses of monkeys who have died from the infection or from eating infected squirrels. A recent cluster of cases has been investigated in Zaire (Ivker, 1997) by teams from the Centers for Disease Control and Prevention (CDC) and WHO.

The WHO Assembly on May 8, 1980, certified the final global eradication of smallpox (WHO, 1980). This is an achievement unique in the history of mankind's interaction with the microorganisms of the environment (Fenner et al., 1988). Smallpox virus exists today only in the deep freezers of two selected laboratories.

The two laboratories that maintain stocks of variola virus are at the CDC in Atlanta, Georgia, and the Research Institute for Viral Preparations in Moscow, Russia. They participate in the smallpox eradication surveillance and research program of WHO. Current plans call for destruction of the remaining stocks of smallpox virus in June 1999 (Donohoe 1996; Fox, 1996), an event postponed repeatedly since its original 1993 date. This has been a matter of continued controversy. Proponents of virus destruction express concern about inadvertent or deliberate escape of variola from these two repositories and resultant biologic hazards or warfare (Mahy et al., 1993). Opponents of the destruction of these virus stocks point to far more efficient agents of biologic warfare (e.g., anthrax, botulinus toxin) and highlight the unique aspects of virus-host interactions and molecular pathogenesis that remain to be fully elucidated with such a host-specific agent (Joklik et al., 1993). The complete genome of smallpox virus has been cloned into plasmids and sequenced (Massung et al., 1994; Shchelkunov, 1995), enabling research to continue using the cloned genes.

SMALLPOX (VARIOLA MAJOR; VARIOLA MINOR OR ALASTRIM; VARIOLOID)

Smallpox was an acute, highly contagious, preventable disease caused by the variola virus, family Poxviridae, genus *Orthopoxvirus*. Other members of the family include vaccinia, monkeypox, cowpox, camelpox, and ectromelia (mousepox). Smallpox was characterized by a 3- to 4-day prodromal period of chills, high fever, headache, backache, vomiting, and prostration. The temperature began to subside as the eruptive stage commenced on the third or fourth day. The eruption progressed from macular to papular to vesicular to pustular and finally to crusting during an 8- to 14-day period. The temperature rose again, and the constitutional symptoms intensified during the pustular stage. The rash had a characteristic peripheral or centrifugal distribution, with lesions at the same stage in any one regional area.

Variola major, variola minor or alastrim, and varioloid were the three chief forms of the disease. *Variola major* was classic smallpox. It had a high mortality rate that varied with the type of lesions as follows: ordinary-discrete, less than 10%; ordinary-semiconfluent, 25% to 50%; ordinary-confluent, 50% to 75%; flat, greater than 90%; hemorrhagic, nearly 100% (Koplan and Foster, 1979). In general, infants, pregnant women, and elderly patients had higher fatality rates. *Variola minor,* or alastrim, was a mild type of smallpox occurring in nonvaccinated persons. It was caused by a less virulent strain of the virus that bred true. The mortality rate was usually less than 1% except in rare instances when the rash became confluent or hemorrhagic. *Varioloid* was a mild form of smallpox occurring in previously vaccinated persons who had partial immunity. This mild disease was caused by a virulent strain of the virus capable of causing variola major in a nonimmunized contact (Mazumder et al., 1975; Koplan and Foster, 1979).

Variola and monkeypox are the two members of the poxvirus group that caused generalized disease in man. A third human pathogen, molluscum contagiosum virus, ordinarily produces a benign self-limited rash disease with multiple, umbilicated papules on the trunk and face. However, in severely immunocompromised patients, such as those with acquired immunodeficiency syndrome (AIDS), molluscum contagiosum may be far more extensive and prolonged (Hughes and Parham, 1991). Other poxviruses that can infect man (cowpox, orf, buffalopox, bovine papular stomatitis, pseudocowpox, sealpox, tanapox, yabapox) may cause only a localized nodular and/or pustular skin lesion most often as a result of direct contact with the lesions of an infected animal.

Etiology

The poxviruses are a family of large, ellipsoid, complex DNA viruses. They include more than 20 mammalian viruses plus groups of bird (avipox) and insect (entomopox) viruses. A number of the group can initiate human infection, but only variola (smallpox) has been of worldwide significance. Humans are the only host for variola virus so that eradication of human infection left no sylvan or other occult reservoir from which virus could be reintroduced.

The poxviruses are unique in a number of their features: they are the largest of all viruses with a double-stranded DNA genome from 130 to 375 kbp in length coding for 150 to 300 proteins, replicating in the cell's cytoplasm, and encoding dozens of enzymes, several of which are enclosed in the intact virion. The viruses are assembled intracytoplasmically and when mature are released from the infected cell. Both enveloped and nonenveloped particles are infectious, the former released by exocytosis while the latter exit with cell disruption (Fenner, 1997).

Smallpox and vaccinia viruses are morphologically indistinguishable and closely related immunologically. The elementary bodies can be identified in smears of vesicular fluid stained by the Paschen, Giemsa, or Gutstein method. As viewed with an electron microscope, they are brick shaped or ovoid and approximately 200×400 nm in size. Aggregates of these bodies in infected host cells form the so-called Guarnieri's bodies, which are intracytoplasmic inclusions measuring approximately 10 μm in diameter. The viral genome is contained within a central core that in turn is enclosed by an external coat of lipid and protein surrounding two lateral bodies as well. Research continues on the classification and genetic relatedness of the many poxviruses and their interrelationships. All poxviruses apparently share a common inner core nucleoprotein antigen.

Ropp et al. (1995) have reported the rapid identification and differentiation of smallpox and other members of the orthopox genus by Polymerase chain reaction (PCR) using primers based on genome sequences encoding the hemagglutinin (HA) protein.

Infection with smallpox and vaccinia viruses stimulates the production of at least four types of antibody: antihemagglutinin, complement-fixing antibodies, neutralizing antibodies, and antibodies that inhibit agar gel precipitation. Levels of antihemagglutinin and complement-fixing antibodies rise significantly by the end of the second week of illness or vaccination; they persist for several months. Neutralizing antibodies develop later but persist for years.

Pathogenesis, pathology, clinical manifestations, diagnosis, differential diagnosis, complications, prognosis, immunity, epidemiologic factors, treatment, preventive measures, isolation, quarantine, and control are discussed in Chapter 28 of the seventh edition and in references listed at the end of this chapter (Behbehani, 1983; Fenner et al., 1988).

VACCINIA

Two centuries ago on May 14, 1796, Edward Jenner performed his historic experiment inoculating 8-year-old James Phipps with "matter" taken from the lesion of a milkmaid, Sarah Nemes, infected by a cow. When challenged on July 1, 1796, with virulent smallpox virus, James proved fully resistant.

Although the pedigree of later vaccinia strains became confused by their mixture with variola and an equine virus, standard vaccines since the last of the nineteenth century have been labeled *vaccinia* (Baxby, 1977).

Vaccinia is an acute infectious disease induced by deliberate smallpox vaccination or by the accidental contact of abraded skin with infective material. It is characterized by the development of a localized lesion that progresses in sequence from papule to vesicle to pustule to crust. Fever and regional lymphadenitis may develop during the vesicular or pustular stage. The infection stimulates the production of antibodies that are protective against smallpox.

Clinical Manifestations

The clinical manifestations of vaccinia are dependent for the most part on the immune status of the individual. Two types of reactions may result from a successful vaccination: a "major" response (pustular lesion or an area of definite induration or congestion surrounding a central lesion, scab, or ulcer 6 to 8 days after vaccination) or an "equivocal" response.

Major Response. Three days after vaccination, the inoculated site becomes reddened and pruritic. It becomes papular on the fourth day and vesicular by the fifth or sixth day. A red areola surrounds the vesicle, which becomes umbilicated and then pustular by the eighth to the eleventh day. By this time the red areola has enlarged markedly. The pustule begins to dry, the redness subsides, and the lesion becomes crusted between the second and third week. By the end of the third week, the scab falls off, leaving a permanent scar that at first is pink in color but eventually becomes white.

At the end of the first week, between the vesicular and pustular phases, there may be a variable amount of fever, malaise, and regional lymphadenitis. These symptoms usually subside within 1 to 2 days and are more likely to occur in older children and adults than in infants.

Accelerated, Modified, or Vaccinoid Reaction. Revaccination of a partially immune person is followed by an attenuated form of vaccinia with the following characteristics: (1) usually there is no fever or constitutional symptoms; (2) a papule appears by the third day, becomes vesicular by the fifth to seventh day, and dries shortly thereafter; (3) the vesicle and its red areola are relatively small; and (4) the scar, if present, is usually insignificant and disappears within 1 or 2 years.

Accelerated reactions may also result from scratching and autoinoculation with the vesicular fluid of a primary vaccinia pox. The accelerated lesions mature simultaneously with the initial primary lesion and heal without scarring as a rule.

• • •

The absence of a reaction does *not* mean that the person is immune. In most instances either the vaccine is not potent or the technique is at fault. Occasionally, a papule may result from needle trauma. To evaluate a vaccination, it would be ideal to inspect the lesion daily. When this is not practical, the optimal times of inspection are the third, seventh, and fourteenth days.

Vaccination Procedures

Methods. The most commonly used method of vaccination is the multiple pressure method.

Precautions. Because vaccination is generally an elective procedure, it should be postponed in instances of intercurrent infection. Primary vaccination of individuals with eczema or other types of exfoliative dermatitis may be complicated by eczema vaccinatum, a severe and potentially fatal disease. Vaccination should be deferred until the skin lesions clear.

It is recommended that vaccination, in those few instances when indicated, be given as *one* inoculation over the *deltoid* area, with the *multiple pressure* or *multiple puncture technique* and a fully potent vaccine.

Immunity

Immunity develops between the eighth and eleventh days after vaccination. Antihemagglutinin, complement-fixing, and virus-neutralizing antibodies are demonstrable between the tenth and thirteenth days. Duration of immunity is extremely variable; it may range between 2 and 10 years. Revaccination at 3-year intervals is generally adequate to maintain optimal immunity (El-Ad et al., 1990).

Complications

Until May 1983 when it was withdrawn by Wyeth Laboratories (the sole U.S. producer) from general availability, smallpox vaccine occasionally was administered to patients with recurrent herpes simplex or papillomas in the mistaken expectation that doing so would interfere with development of new lesions or would accelerate the resolution of older ones. Because some of these patients suffered from underlying immunodeficiency disorders, they acquired life-threatening progressive vaccinia caused by unarrested local replication of vaccinia virus.

Currently, smallpox vaccine is available only from the CDC in Atlanta, Georgia, and is recommended only for laboratory workers who may be engaged in surveillance or research involving nonvariola orthopoxviruses (CDC, 1991). It seems appropriate and prudent to retain the following paragraphs on the possible complications of vaccination.

Secondary Bacterial Infection. The local lesion may become secondarily infected with staphylococci or streptococci, causing cellulitis.

Accidental Infection. Autoinoculation by means of scratching an active lesion may produce secondary pocks over various parts of the body. The severity of this complication is governed by the site of inoculation. For example, a lesion of the eye with corneal involvement can result in ulceration, scarring, and blindness.

Toxic Eruptions. An erythema multiforme type of eruption occasionally occurs between the seventh and tenth days at the height of the vaccinia re-

action. The rash may be generalized or localized to a particular area. It usually clears within 3 to 5 days. It is considered a sensitivity reaction (Plate 6). This rash was most often seen in infants vaccinated before their first birthday.

Generalized Vaccinia. This potentially serious complication arose between the seventh and fourteenth days after vaccination. A generalized eruption develops, with crops of lesions simulating a primary vaccination. Healing without scars takes place rapidly, being completed at the same time as the healing of the primary vaccinia lesion.

The possibility of serious consequences from the administration of recombinant vaccinia viruses or conventional vaccinia to human immunodeficiency virus (HIV)–infected individuals has been exemplified in case reports (Redfield et al., 1987; Guillaume et al., 1991).

Eczema Vaccinatum. This potentially fatal complication of vaccinia develops in patients with eczema or other forms of exfoliative dermatitis who have been either vaccinated or exposed to an active case of vaccinia. The disease is characterized by high fever, severe toxicity, and an extensive vesicular and pustular eruption chiefly confined to the area of dermatitis (Plate 7 and Fig. 29-1). Healthy areas of skin also may become involved. The mortality may be significant.

Progressive Vaccinia (Vaccinia Necrosum; Prolonged Vaccinia; Vaccinia Gangrenosa). Progressive vaccinia, a highly fatal complication, is fortunately rare. The initial vaccinal lesion fails to heal and progresses to involve more and more areas of adjacent skin. The necrosis of the tissues contin-

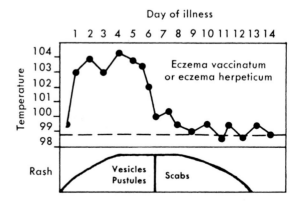

FIG. 29-1 Schematic diagram of the clinical course of eczema herpeticum or eczema vaccinatum.

ues to extend, often over a period of months. Metastatic lesions may develop in other parts of the skin, bones, and viscera. This complication has been observed in patients with immunologic disorders. The common denominator has been depression of T-lymphocyte function, either congenital or acquired. Progressive vaccinia is also likely to occur in patients with immunologic deficits caused by malignant disease of the lymphatic system (leukemia or lymphomas) and/or their therapy. Treatment has been attempted with vaccinia-immune globulin (VIG), N-methylisatin-β-thiosemicarbazone (methisazone, marboran), interferon, transfer factor, acyclovir, and rifampin. Cases have been too infrequent to evaluate therapy in a controlled study.

Postvaccinal Encephalitis. Postvaccinal encephalitis is a serious but rare complication. The incidence of postvaccinal encephalitis in Sweden from 1947 to 1954 was 1.9 per 100,000. Surveillance of complications of smallpox vaccination in the United States in 1968 revealed 2.9 cases of encephalitis per 1 million primary vaccinations; the highest incidence, 6.5 per 1 million, was observed in infants less than 12 months old (Lane et al., 1969; Goldstein et al., 1975).

The clinical picture is the same as in other postinfectious encephalitides. The usual manifestations include fever, headache, vomiting, meningeal signs, paralysis, drowsiness, coma, and convulsions. The spinal fluid may contain an increase in number of mononuclear cells and amount of protein. Pathologically, the brain shows the same type of perivascular infiltration and demyelination as occur in encephalitis complicating measles and chickenpox. The mortality rate may be as high as 30% to 40%.

Treatment

Primary vaccinia requires no treatment. Dressings are unnecessary except to prevent the possible transmission of virus to susceptible contacts. Fever and pain in the arm may be treated with appropriate doses of antiinflammatory drugs. Superimposed pyogenic infections may require hot compresses and appropriate antimicrobial therapy. Patients with eczema vaccinatum need intensive supportive therapy; they should receive VIG, 0.6 ml per kilogram of body weight intramuscularly. The same dose would be indicated for patients with vaccinia necrosum. In general, the treatment of encephalitis is the same as that of any infectious or postinfectious encephalitis (see Chapter 38).

Preventive Measures

Most complications of vaccinia are preventable. Vaccination is contraindicated under the following circumstances: evidence of eczema or other chronic forms of exfoliative dermatitis in the vaccinated person or a close contact; or altered immune status from disease or immunosuppressive therapy.

In 1971 the United States Public Health Service accepted the recommendation of its Advisory Committee on Immunization Practices that *routine* smallpox vaccinations in the United States be discontinued. In 1976 the former recommendations of routine smallpox vaccination for hospital employees was also rescinded. Since that time the sole civilian group for whom vaccine has been indicated is laboratory workers directly involved with orthopoxviruses.

It is worth noting a renaissance of interest in widespread vaccinia administration. Smith et al. (1983) reported the successful incorporation into the vaccinia virus genome of coding sequences for the hepatitis B surface antigen. Gene portions from many other human viral pathogens have similarly been exploited to provide a vaccinia vector that could serve to induce immunity to a number of viral infections (Moss, 1991). The most active research with recombinant vaccinia viruses has focused on preparations expressing HIV envelope glycoproteins (Cooney et al., 1991), which have already been used in human clinical trials. This promises to be an active area of investigation in the coming years.

BIBLIOGRAPHY
Smallpox

Bauer DJ, St Vincent L, Kempe CH, Downie AW. Prophylactic treatment of smallpox contacts with N-methylisatin-β-thiosemicarbazone (compound 33T57). Lancet 1963;2:494.

Bauer DJ, et al. Prophylaxis of smallpox with methisazone. Am J Epidemiol 1970;90:130.

Behbehani AB. The smallpox story: life and death of an old disease. Microbiol Rev 1983;47:455-509.

Breman JG, Arita I. The confirmation and maintenance of smallpox eradication. N Engl J Med 1980;303:1263-1273.

Cho CT, Wenner HA. Monkeypox virus. Bacteriol Rev 1973;37:1.

Donohoe MT. A call for the destruction of smallpox virus stores. Am J Public Health 1996;86:268.

Fenner F. Poxviruses. In Richman DD, Whitley RJ, Hayden FG (eds). Clinical virology. New York: Churchill Livingstone, 1997.

Fenner F, Henderson DA, Arita I, et al (eds). Smallpox and its eradication. Geneva, Switzerland: World Health Organization, 1988, pp 581-583.

Fox JL. WHO resolves to send smallpox stocks to a 1999 grave. Nature Med 1996;2:729.

Henderson DA. The eradication of smallpox. Sci Am 1976;235:25.

Hughes WT, Parham DM. Molluscum contagiosum in children with cancer or acquired immunodeficiency syndrome. Pediatr Infect Dis J 1991;10:152-156.

Ivker R. Human monkeypox hits beleaguered Zaire. Lancet 1997;349:709.

Joklik WK, Moss B, Fields BN, et al. Why the smallpox virus stocks should not be destroyed. Science 1993;262:1225-1226.

Koplan JP, Foster SO. Smallpox: clinical types, causes of death, and treatment. J Infect Dis 1979;140:440.

Mahy BW, Almond JW, Berns KI, et al. The remaining stocks of smallpox virus should be destroyed. Science 1993;262:1223-1224.

Massung RF, Lin LI, Qi J, et al. Analysis of the complete genome of smallpox variola major virus strain Bangladesh 1975. Virology 1994;201:215-240.

Mazumder DNG, De S, Mitra AC, Mukherjee MK. Clinical observations on smallpox: a study of 1233 patients admitted to the Infectious Diseases Hospital, Calcutta, during 1973. Bull WHO 1975;52:301.

Murphy FA, Faquet CM, Bishop DHL, et al. Virus taxonomy. Classification and nomenclature of viruses. Poxviridae. Arch Virol 1995;10:S79-S91.

Ricketts TF, Byles JB. The diagnosis of smallpox, vols I and II. Reprinted from the 1908 London edition. U.S. Department of Health, Education, and Welfare, Bureau of Disease, Prevention and Environmental control, Division of Foreign Quarantine, 1966.

Ropp SL, Jin Q, Knight JC, et al. PCR strategy for identification and differentiation of smallpox and other orthopoxvirus. J Clin Microbiol 1995;33:2069-2076.

Shchelkunov SN. Functional organization of variola major and vaccinia virus genomes. Virus Genes 1995;10:53-71.

Walls HH, Ziegler DW, Nakano JM. Characterization of antibodies to orthopoxviruses in human sera by radioimmunoassay. Bull WHO 1981;59:253-262.

World Health Organization. Declaration of global eradication of smallpox. Weekly Epidemiol Rec 1980;55:145-152.

Vaccinia

Baxby D. The origins of vaccinia virus. J Infect Dis 1977;136:453.

Centers for Disease Control. Contact spread of vaccinia from a recently vaccinated Marine—Louisiana. MMWR 1984;33:37-38.

Centers for Disease Control. Contact spread of vaccinia from a National Guard vaccinee—Wisconsin. MMWR 1985;34:182-183.

Centers for Disease Control and Prevention. Vaccinia (smallpox) vaccine recommendations of the Immunization Practices Advisory Committee (ACIP). MMWR 1991;40(RR-14):1-10.

Cooney EL, Collier AC, Greenberg PD, et al. Safety of and immunological response to a recombinant vaccinia virus vaccine expressing HIV envelope glycoprotein. Lancet 1991;337:567-572.

El-Ad B, Roth Y, Winder A, et al. The persistence of neutralizing antibodies after revaccination against smallpox. J Infect Dis 1990;161:446-448.

Goldstein JA, Neff JM, Lane JM, Koplan JP. Smallpox vaccination reactions, prophylaxis, and therapy of complications. Pediatrics 1975;55:342.

Guillaume JC, Saiag P, Wechsler J, et al. Vaccinia from recombinant virus expressing HIV genes (letter). Lancet 1991;377:1034-1035.

Jenner E. An inquiry into the causes and effects of the variolae vacciniae, a disease discovered in some of the western counties of England, particularly Gloucestershire, and known by the name of cowpox. Reprinted by Cassell and Co, Ltd, 1896. Available in Pamphlet vol 4232, Army Medical Library, Washington, DC.

Kempe CH. Studies on smallpox and complications of smallpox vaccination. Pediatrics 1960;26:176.

Lane JM, Ruben FL, Neff JM, Millar JD. Complications of smallpox vaccination, 1968. N Engl J Med 1969;281:1201.

Moss B. Vaccinia virus: a tool for research and development. Science 1991;252:1662-1667.

Neff JM, et al. Complications of smallpox vaccination. National survey in the United States, 1963. N Engl J Med 1967;276:125.

Redfield RR, Wright DC, James WD, et al. Disseminated vaccinia in a military recruit with human immunodeficiency virus (HIV) disease. N Engl J Med 1987;316:673-676.

Smith GL, Mackett M, Moss B. Infectious vaccinia virus recombinants that express hepatitis B virus surface antigens. Nature 1983;302:490-495.

Tyzzer EE. The etiology and pathology of vaccinia. J Med Res 1904;11:180.

Zagury D, Leonard R. Fouchard M, et al. Immunization against AIDS in humans. Nature 1987;326:249-250.

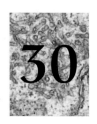

30 STAPHYLOCOCCAL INFECTIONS

ALICE S. PRINCE

Staphylococcus aureus is a major cause of infection in infants, children, and adults. It is particularly common in the pediatric population as a cause of skin and soft tissue infection, ranging from impetigo, furuncles, and wound infections to septic arthritis and osteomyelitis. Staphylococci are also frequently associated with such life-threatening infections as septicemia, endocarditis, and toxic shock syndrome. Coagulase-negative staphylococci are an increasingly common clinical problem and are currently the most frequent cause of bacteremia in hospitalized patients, particularly in the neonate or child with an indwelling intravascular device.

ETIOLOGY
Microbiology

Staphylococci are catalase-producing gram-positive organisms that often grow in clusters, as suggested by the term *staphylococci,* which is derived from the Greek, meaning "bunch of grapes." These are hardy organisms that can persist on nonphysiologic surfaces for long periods of time and grow well on artificial media under both aerobic and anaerobic conditions. Colonies often produce a yellow pigment. *S. aureus* ferments a variety of sugars, including mannitol, under anaerobic conditions and tolerates high concentrations of NaCl. The ability to produce coagulase differentiates *S. aureus* from the less virulent coagulase-negative staphylococci such as *S. saprophyticus, S. hemolyticus,* and *S. epidermidis.*

The cell wall of *S. aureus* is composed primarily of peptidoglycan, which is composed of repeating subunits of N-acetyl muramic acid and N-acetyl glucosamine, and teichoic acid, a polymer of repeating units of glycerol-phosphate and protein A. The cell wall components of *S. aureus* are important in pathogenesis because they can elicit specific responses by the host immune system. Peptidogly-

can can activate, complement, and stimulate antibody production, as well as elicit IL-1 production by monocytes. Many strains also express a capsular polysaccharide that may contribute to virulence; organisms that express certain capsular polysaccharides (types 5 and 8) are more frequently associated with bacteremia and sepsis (Soell et al., 1995).

PATHOGENESIS

Staphylococci are ubiquitous organisms that may be considered as part of the commensal flora in some settings or may act as virulent pathogens. The expression of specific bacterial virulence factors and the nature of the host immune response contribute to the nature of the pathogen-host interaction. Staphylococci express several classes of adhesins. They bind to the RGD (arginine-glycine-aspartate) sequence of fibronectin. This receptor allows colonization of mucous membranes. Staphylococci also can bind to several components of the extracellular matrix, including collagen, laminin, vitronectin, and fibrinogen (Hienz et al., 1996). Upon exposure to *S. aureus,* endothelial cells and mononuclear leukocytes are stimulated to initiate a cascade of cytokine production in a manner analogous to that following lipopolysaccharide stimulation by gram-negative organisms, with the elaboration of interleukin-1β and interleukin-6 (IL-1β and IL-6) (Yao et al., 1995, Soell et al., 1995). Because of their expression of exoproducts, organisms cause local tissue damage and disseminate via the blood stream once infection is established.

Staphylococci are capable of causing disease by three major mechanisms: direct destruction of tissue via the activity of numerous secreted exoenzymes, production of intoxication syndromes in which staphylococcal exotoxins enter the circulation and act at sites in the host distant from the source of the infection, and induction of multisystem disease by widespread T-cell activation and cytokine release resulting from the expression of staphylococcal superantigens.

The hallmark of staphylococcal infection is suppuration. Much of the pathology associated with staphylococcal infection is due to expression of secreted exoproducts, including lipase; phospholipase; the hemolysins α, β, γ, and Δ; and hyaluronidase, enzymes that enable the organism to break down host tissues, including the extracellular matrix components. Coagulase, an enzyme that triggers the final steps in the coagulation cascade to produce fibrin, is produced by *S. aureus,* enabling the organism to wall itself off from the blood supply of the host. These bacteria produce numerous factors that impede phagocytosis. Protein A, a major component of staphylococcal cell walls, binds the Fc portion of immunoglobulin chains, thereby blocking the ligand for internalization of organisms by phagocytic cells and effectively thwarting efficient phagocytosis. Staphylococci also produce catalase, which converts H_2O_2 to water and oxygen, destroying one of the important antibacterial products generated by neutrophils. In patients with chronic granulomatous disease of childhood, who are unable to generate superoxide, catalase production allows *S. aureus* to persist in the absence of effective phagocytic killing. Other defects in phagocytic function—such as Job's syndrome, Chediak-Higashi syndrome, and Wiskott-Aldrich syndrome—similarly predispose to staphylococcal infections.

Staphylococcal toxins that cause exfoliation have been well characterized. The exfoliatins (ETA and ETB) are responsible for dermatologic lesions characterized by erythema and desquamation caused by the splitting of the desmosomes that link epidermal cells. Exfoliatin (ETB) is usually produced by organisms of phage group II and is plasmid encoded. ETB is associated with staphylococcal scalded skin syndrome, a disease of infants and young children. ETA is a chromosomal enzyme and found in several different phage groups.

Staphylococci also produce several toxins that act as superantigens. These are antigens that bind to MHC class II molecules and interact with specific Vβ chains of the T-cell receptor (Kappler et al., 1989). These antigens do not require processing and are able to interact superficially with components of the Vβ chain alone, not in the context of the usual antigen binding groove of the T-cell receptor. Thus these antigens can activate entire classes of T cells bearing specific Vβ domains. This T-cell activation results in the amplification of

these clones; the activation of monocytes; and the release of numerous cytokines, including IL-2; IL-4; IL-6; interferon-γ (IFN-γ); tumor necrosis factor-α (TNF-α); and IL-1β, with consequent effects on multiple organ systems. The staphylococcal toxins TSST-1 and TSST-2 associated with toxic shock syndrome (described later in the chapter) and the staphylococcal enterotoxin B, a cause of staphylococcal food poisoning, are superantigens. The expression of these toxins is highly regulated. TSST-1, for example, is expressed under conditions of low Mg^{++}, thus staphylococci in a milieu in which the divalent cations are depleted, as might occur in proximity to a hyperabsorbent synthetic tampon, upregulate the expression of these genes.

EPIDEMIOLOGY

The usual source of staphylococcal infection is colonization of the nares. Clinical studies in surgical patients have demonstrated that preoperative nasal colonization with this organism is associated with a significantly higher rate of surgical wound infection (Kluytmans et al., 1995). The organisms can be aerosolized from the anterior nares, or more commonly it is spread by interpersonal contact. Small breaks in the skin can become infected, or the organism can disseminate in a nosocomial setting from hospital personnel to patients. Careful handwashing is of utmost importance in preventing spread of infection.

Numerous molecular techniques have been developed to track the epidemiology of hospital outbreaks of staphylococcal infection. These have been of great importance in nursery epidemics of staphylococcal disease, such as scalded skin syndrome, pustulosis, or bullous impetigo. Historically, phage typing was used to trace the source of these organisms. However, since staphylococci often contain numerous transferable genetic elements, such as plasmids, transposons, and phages, more recent studies have utilized restriction endonuclease polymorphisms, pulsed field gel electrophoresis, or ribotype analysis to follow and characterize the organisms from patients who are epidemiologically linked.

CLINICAL SYNDROMES CAUSED BY S. *AUREUS*
Skin and Soft Tissue Infections

One of the most common presentations of *S. aureus* infection is localized infection of the skin. These include small, localized infections such as impetigo, paronychia, and furuncles. Organisms gain access to the skin structures following nasal colonization or from small breaks in the skin. Local replication of organisms producing the exoproducts and toxins described earlier causes a localized infection of the contiguous connective tissue. The peptidoglycan of *S. aureus* heralds a brisk immunologic response with the local accumulation of macrophages and polymorphonuclear leukocytes. Thrombosis of the small surrounding blood vessels occurs with the deposition of fibrin, a consequence of staphylococcal coagulase. As this process continues, a central area of necrotic tissue with dead and dying phagocytes and bacteria is surrounded by a fibrinous capsule, that is, the formation of a small abscess. Thus a small localized infection such as impetigo may progress to cellulitis and development of an abscess.

Impetigo. Impetigo, particularly bullous impetigo, is most often caused by *S. aureus*. The infection usually begins with a small area of erythema that progresses into bullae filled with cloudy fluid. These rupture and heal with crust formation. Impetigo is most common in the summer months in temperate climates and is a common complication of insect bites and varicella. Topical treatment with mupirocin is usually adequate; however, children with extensive impetiginized varicella are at significant risk for superinfection with *S. aureus* or group A streptococci, which require systemic therapy.

Folliculitis. It is another common superficial staphylococcal infection involving the hair follicle. Clinically, folliculitis presents as a tender pustule surrounding a hair follicle and can usually be managed with local treatment.

Staphylococcal Furuncles and Carbuncles. They represent more extensive local staphylococcal infections of the skin, which traditionally involve areas of the skin with hair follicles, such as the neck, axillae, and buttocks. These localized infections extend into the subcutaneous tissues and are actually small abscesses containing abundant amounts of purulent material. They respond promptly to drainage.

Hydradenitis Suppurativa. An infection of the sweat glands of the skin, hydradenitis suppurativa usually is caused by *S. aureus*. This is most often seen in moist areas such as the axillae or in the folds in the perineal and genital region. These lesions may spontaneously rupture and heal with scarring.

Mastitis. *S. aureus* is a well-recognized cause of mastitis, which presents both in nursing mothers (animals and human), as well as newborn infants. The ability of most strains of *S. aureus* to produce lipase is thought to contribute to the pathogenesis of this infection. The patients present with erythema, swelling, and tender induration of the breast and some may progress to have systemic symptoms of fever and malaise. These infections occasionally evolve to frank abscess formation and require prompt systemic antistaphylococcal therapy.

Staphylococcal Lymphadenitis. A common infection in children, it presents as a tender, erythematous mass in the cervical chain of lymph nodes with accompanying fever (Hieber and Davis, 1976). Cervical adenitis was traditionally considered a complication of streptococcal pharyngitis; however, staphylococci are now frequently the cause of these infections, although the possibility of mycobacterial infection should also be considered. Surgical drainage of staphylococcal lymphadenitis is preferable if lesions are fluctuant. More often the involved area is indurated and not amenable to drainage. In these cases, treatment with antistaphylococcal antibiotics is usually successful, although complete resolution of all swelling may take weeks.

Skin Diseases Caused by Staphylococcal Toxins

Staphylococcal scalded skin syndrome was originally described as an exfoliative dermatitis of infants by Ritter von Rittershain. The disease is caused by staphylococci of phage group II, which produce an exfoliative toxin (Melish and Glasgow, 1970; Albert et al., 1970). The specific phage group 71 is most often associated with this disease. Infants present with generalized erythema, which progresses to bullae formation, followed by generalized desquamation (Gooch and Britt, 1978) (see Figs. 30-1 and 30-2). The skin becomes extremely friable and even gentle stroking leads to desquamation (Nikolsky's sign). Histopathologically, the skin separates intradermally at the stratum granulosum layer. Clinically, staphylococcal scalded skin syndrome is similar to a disease in adults characterized by Lyell and termed *toxic epidermal necrolysis* (TEN), and analogous pathology can be seen in some drug hypersensitivity reactions as well. However, TEN can be differentiated from SSS by intraepithelial splitting at the dermoepidermal junction. In SSS disease, cultures of the skin are usually

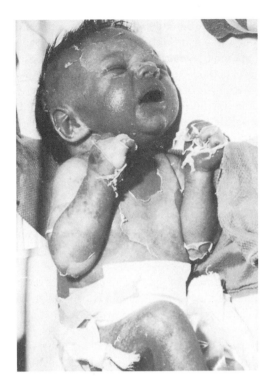

FIG. 30-1 Newborn infant with scalded skin syndrome in exfoliative stage. (From Melish ME, Glasgow LA. Reprinted by permission of New England Journal of Medicine 1970;282:1114.)

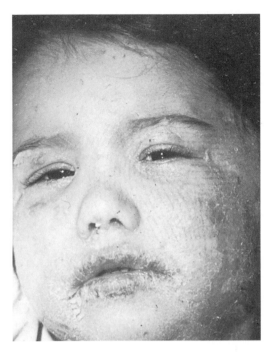

FIG. 30-2 Two-year-old girl in the resolving phase of the scalded skin syndrome undergoing secondary desquamation. Large, thick flakes of dried skin are concentrated particularly about the mouth. (From Melish ME and Glasgow LA. Reprinted by permission of the New England Journal of Medicine 1970;282:1114.)

negative for staphylococci, although a distant site of infection, such as the umbilical stump or the nasopharynx, may yield the organism. The infants have systemic signs of infection with fever and irritability and occasionally may be septic. Treatment involves the administration of antistaphylococcal antibiotics and supportive care with attention to the fluid deficits caused by loss of the epidermal barrier.

Diseases Caused by Staphylococcal Superantigens

Staphylococcal toxic shock syndrome was first characterized by Todd, who observed seven children with a severe multisystem illness characterized by high fever, scarlatiniform rash, vomiting, diarrhea, renal and hepatic dysfunction, disseminated intravascular coagulation (DIC), and shock (Wiesenthal and Todd, 1984; Davis et al., 1980). This syndrome is similar to the previously described staphylococcal scarlet fever syndrome. A large increase in cases was noted in young, previously healthy women who use hyperabsorbent tampons (Parsonnet, 1989). These women present during their menses while using tampons, with fever, vomiting, diarrhea, myalgias, and a characteristic "sunburn" type of rash. This rash progresses to a generalized desquamation, usually involving the palms and soles. *S. aureus* is isolated from the tampon or vagina, or from another site in the cases of non–menstrual associated TSS, as originally described by Todd. These staphylococci produce a toxin (Schlievert et al., 1981), TSST-1 or TSST-2, which acts as a superantigen, activating whole classes of T cells bearing specific Vβ chains, without specificity for the α chain or the antigen binding groove of the T-cell receptor. TSST-1 can also induce the expression of IL-1β and TNF-α by mononuclear cells. Thus the manifestations of the disease are those of excessive T-cell activation and cytokine release. The diagnosis can be made clinically in a patient with fever, rash, hypotension, and signs of multisystem involvement. Treatment of TSS should focus on reversing shock and hypotension, removing the focus of the staphylococcal infection, and treatment with antistaphylococcal antibiotics to prevent further expression of the toxin.

Staphylococcal Enterotoxins

Staphylococcal enterotoxin type B is another superantigen that is associated with outbreaks of gastrointestinal disease. This is typically described in outbreaks in which a common food source is contaminated by an individual carrying the staphylococci. The toxin-producing organisms proliferate in food that is uncooked or only partially cooked (custards, potato salad) and not properly refrigerated. Patients present with an acute onset of vomiting and watery diarrhea 2 to 6 hours after ingestion. Symptoms are generally self-limited, and supportive therapy is usually sufficient. Antimicrobial agents are not necessary. The staphylococcal enterotoxins can also be associated with a TSS-like syndrome.

Illnesses Caused by S. Aureus

Septicemia. Caused by *S. aureus*, it can occur both in normal (Hieber et al., 1977; Hodes and Barzilai, 1990; Sheagren, 1984) and immunocompromised hosts (Ladisch and Pizzo, 1978). As ubiquitous organisms, staphylococci gain access to the blood after colonization of indwelling plastic catheters or other foreign bodies, through breaks in the skin, or from frank infection of wounds. Once the organisms reach the vascular endothelium, they are able to induce the expression of cytokines, including IL-6 and IL-1β (Yao et al., 1995). Thus, in a manner analogous to that of the gram-negative organisms, in which LPS or endotoxin triggers the expression of inflammatory mediators, in vitro data suggest that staphylococcal cell wall peptidoglycan fragments can similarly initiate an immune response by the endothelium. High-grade bacteremia follows, with the usual signs of fever and tachycardia in an acutely ill patient. Although uncomplicated staphylococcal bacteremia may occur in previously well patients, including adolescents (Shulman and Ayoub, 1976), the organisms can seed other sites, causing local complications.

Endocarditis. Endocarditis is a major complication of staphylococcal septicemia (Bayer, 1982). In a recent review of endocarditis in the pediatric age group, *S. aureus* was the most common pathogen isolated, accounting for 39% of sixty-two cases, and was associated with central nervous system complications and the need for surgical intervention more often than other pathogens (Saiman et al., 1993). Although *S. aureus* endocarditis was originally described as a disease of intravenous drug users, it is also a well-known complication of congenital heart disease. This entity can present in

a previously well child with asymptomatic cardiac pathology such as mitral valve prolapse, or with an asymptomatic ventricular septal defect. These lesions (1) produce turbulent blood flow that causes a reactive focus on the cardiac endothelium, provide a nidus for fibrin and platelet deposition; and (2) expose fibronectin receptors (Hamill, 1987). During transient bacteremia, staphylococci can lodge in these fibrinous lesions, bind to fibronectin, and proliferate. Patients present acutely ill, often with septic shock and petechiae, and are found to have positive blood cultures for *S. aureus*. Embolic phenomena are common with this disease and may include pulmonary emboli; renal emboli; and central nervous system involvement with significant sequelae, including stroke (Saiman et al., 1993) (Fig. 30-3). Treatment of these patients includes detailed hemodynamic assessment and two-dimensional echocardiography, which may help to document the nature and size of vegetations. Since *S. aureus* endocarditis can be a fulminant disease that results in destruction of the infected valve, valvular re-

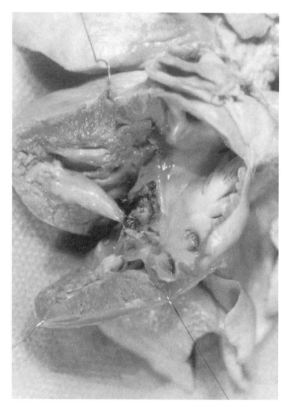

FIG. 30-3 Vegetation on the systemic (tricuspid) valve of a 15-month-old patient with hypoplastic left-heart syndrome. The cause of death was a cerebral vascular accident caused by septic emboli and a mycotic aneurysm.

placement can be an important therapeutic option. For hemodynamically stable patients not actively embolizing from their infection, treatment with antimicrobial agents can be curative.

Another group of patients at risk for staphylococcal endocarditis are those with indwelling vascular access devices (Decker and Edwards, 1988; Saiman, Prince 1993). This is a common problem in oncology patients receiving chemotherapy and neonates who are dependent on such catheters for parenteral nutrition. Infections can occur at the skin site of the intravascular device and then seed the catheter, or they may occur on the catheter itself. Some of these infections can be managed without removal of the catheter. Patients who are acutely ill and at risk of embolizing from this source should be treated with prompt removal of the catheter and a course of antistaphylococcal drugs. Infections caused by the coagulase-negative staphylococci, as discussed later, are not usually as fulminant as those caused by *S. aureus*.

Pulmonary Infections. Pulmonary infections caused by *S. aureus* can arise as complications of septicemia or may result from aspiration of these organisms, often in a nosocomial setting. In young infants, staphylococcal pneumonia usually presents with high fever, respiratory distress, and pulmonary infiltrates. The radiographic findings progress to dense consolidation, followed by pneumatocele formation, consisting of multiple thin-walled abscesses with air fluid levels (Chartrand and McCracken, 1982). Areas of consolidation may extend to the pleura, causing empyema (Fig. 30-4, *A-B*). The management of empyema is a topic of some controversy (Pont and Rountree, 1963). Several methods are available to evacuate purulent material from the pleural space, to reexpand the lung, and to control the infection. Chest tube drainage, under ultrasound or computed tomography guidance, is often effective if performed early in the course of the disease, before multiple loculated areas develop. The instillation of urokinase to act as a thrombolytic agent has recently been advocated, since nonantigenic, nonpyrogenic preparations of urokinase are available. It is also possible to perform video-assisted thoracoscopy to lyse adhesions and facilitate drainage of purulent material (Bryant and Salmon, 1996). This is likely to be a safe and effective procedure preferable to a formal decortication, and there is increasing experience with children. This is a less invasive procedure that still enables the surgeon, under direct visualization, to lyse adhesions and irrigate the pleural space.

Thoracoscopy may be performed early in the course of empyema, before extensive adhesions develop. These therapeutic alternatives provide much more flexibility in the management of empyema than the relatively rigid guidelines offered for decortication in traditional teachings. Resolution of fever and pleural reaction may take weeks. An open thoracotomy and decortication is still an alternative therapy that may be needed less often as physicians accrue experience in treating children with alternative, less invasive techniques.

Bone and Joint Infections. A common complication of staphylococcal bacteremia in children, 90% of the cases occur in patients under 15 years of age (Faden and Grossi, 1991, Waldvogel et al., 1982). Staphylococcal osteomyelitis occurs most often in the metaphyseal portions of the long bones, particularly the tibia, femur, and humerus. It is proposed that organisms lodge in the long capillary loops that perfuse the metaphysis, where there is relatively sluggish blood flow and few phagocytic cells. Organisms slowly replicate and symptoms are often delayed until there is a significant degree of bone destruction. Children present with fever and bony tenderness; infants present with irritability, limpness, or refusal to walk. Laboratory data is not usually diagnostic. The white blood cell count may not be elevated, although the erythrocyte sedimentation rate is usually high. The diagnosis of acute hematogenous osteomyelitis can be made by radionuclide scan using ^{99}Tc phosphonate, which demonstrates areas of bone turnover, or by magnetic resonance imaging (MRI) (see Fig. 30-5, *A-C*). Plain radiographs of the involved area do not show the classic changes of periosteal new bone formation until the infection has been present for 10 to 14 days (Ledesma-Medina and Newman, 1989). Rupture of a focus of osteomyelitis into a contiguous joint space can result in a septic arthritis, as in the hip or shoulder. Patients have local signs of soft tissue swelling and limited range of movement. Diagnosis is made by aspiration of the joint. Because of the virulence of *S. aureus,* septic arthritis of the hip usually requires open drainage to prevent destruction of the joint (Bray and Schmid, 1986). Repeated needle aspirations of the knee may provide adequate drainage.

Septic Arthritis. It may also present as an acutely swollen joint with signs of erythema, warmth, tenderness, and swelling without any bony involvement. The joint space is seeded by the hematogenous route. This diagnosis is confirmed

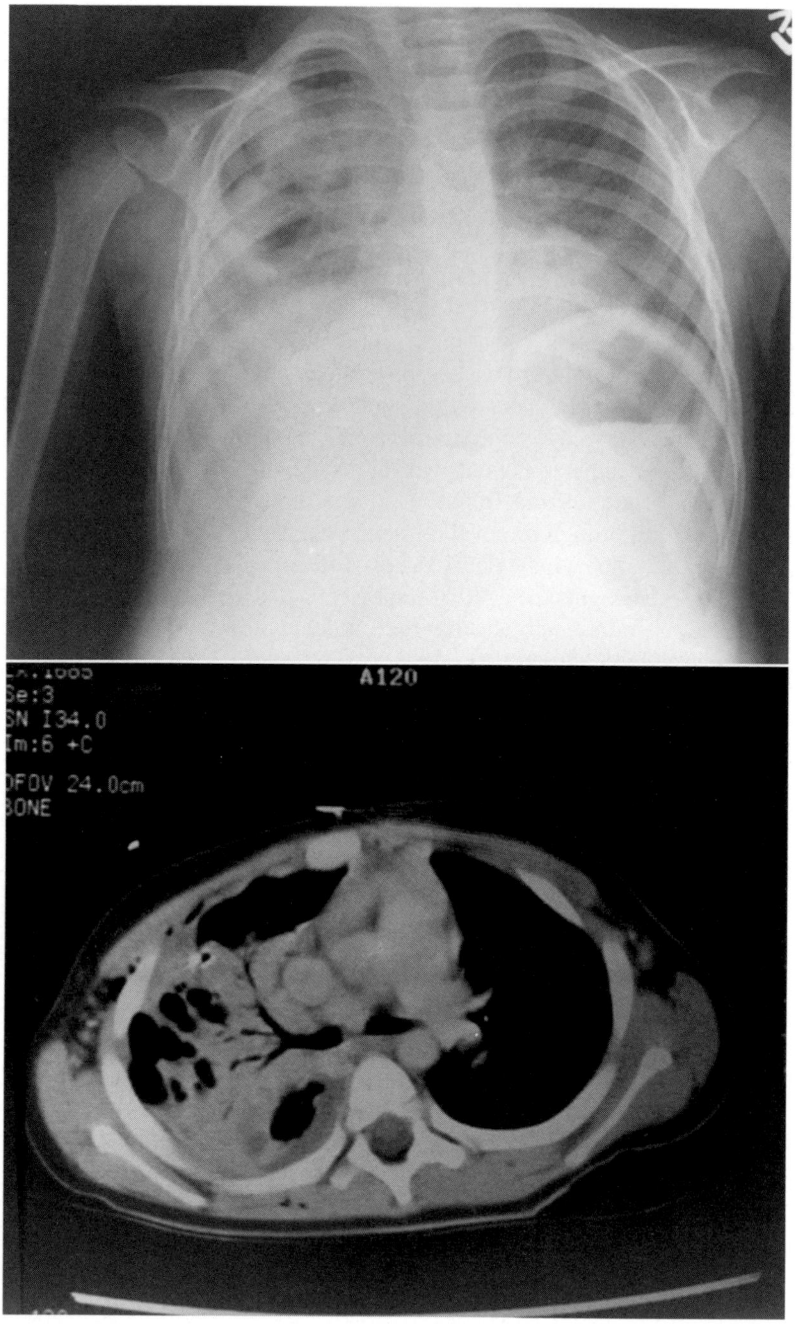

FIG. 30-4   **A**, Chest radiograph demonstrating staphylococcal empyema with areas of consolidation scattered throughout the right lung. **B**, Mediastinal windows on an axial CT scan at the level of the take-off of the right middle lobe bronchus shows areas of consolidation and abscess (pneumatocoele) formation. The top of the empyema can be seen adjacent to the spine.

by the aspiration of purulent joint fluid with polymorphonuclear leukocytes, a high protein content, and the recovery of staphylococci. However, in cases of hematogenous septic arthritis, the plain radiographs and ^{99}Tc scans of the surrounding bones are negative. Prompt drainage and antibiotic treatment usually results in excellent cure rates. Several studies have demonstrated excellent cure rates for staphylococcal bone and joint infections using oral antimicrobial agents if the organisms are suscepti-

ble to the usual antistaphylococcal agents and if patients are compliant with therapy (Tetzlaff et al., 1978).

Pyomyositis. Another soft-tissue infection, it is often caused by *S. aureus*. Although this entity is most often described in tropical regions, it is also seen in normal and immunocompromised patients in temperate climates (Christin, 1992). This is a primary infection of the skeletal muscle, most often

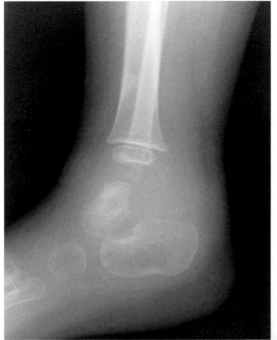

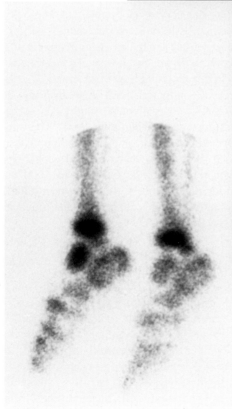

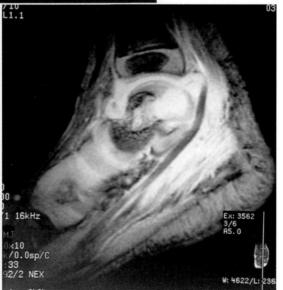

FIG. 30-5 Radiologic imaging of staphylococcal osteomyelitis of the right talus. **A,** A plain radiograph of the ankle demonstrates bony destruction and an irregular border of the talus; **B,** ^{99}Tc bone scan shows an area of increased uptake of the radionuclide in the right talus; **C,** the appearance of the bone by magnetic resonance imaging demonstrates bone destruction surrounded by a dense inflammatory response and fluid collection.

involving the larger muscles of the extremities; it is thought to arise in areas of traumatized skeletal muscle. Patients present with muscle tenderness, cramping, pain, and fever. The diagnosis can be suggested by ultrasonography, although computed tomography and especially magnetic resonance imaging will differentiate hematomas, tumors, and abscesses. Treatment consists of appropriate antibiotics and usually is expedited by drainage.

Methicillin-Resistant S. Aureus. Since first described in 1961 (Jevons, 1961), methicillin-resistant *S. aureus* (MRSA) has become an increasingly common cause of nosocomial infection and thus a problem of increasing importance. These organisms are frequently associated with infections at the sites of indwelling catheters or in patients who are hospitalized for prolonged periods of time (Romero-Vivas et al., 1995). Patients with nasal carriage of MRSA are at increased risk of developing an infection caused by these organisms (Kluytmans et al., 1995). In addition, MRSA may be isolated from the sputum of cystic fibrosis patients who have been treated with multiple courses of antistaphylococcal antibiotics.

MRSA expresses *mecA,* a gene that encodes a mutant penicillin-binding protein, PBP2b, not found in methicillin-susceptible strains of staphylococci (Hartmann and Tomacz, 1984). This altered penicillin binding protein has diminished affinity for penicillin. Thus the usual concentrations of the antistaphylococcal penicillins do not significantly impair the activity of PBP2b, and the organism is not killed. The gene mecA is part of a transposon and can be found in methicillin-resistant coagulase-negative staphylococci as well (Spratt, 1994). As discussed in the following section, therapy of infections caused by MRSA requires treatment with antibiotics that do not interact with these mutant target sites.

THERAPY OF INFECTIONS CAUSED BY *S. AUREUS*

There are numerous antimicrobial agents with activity against the staphylococci. Because staphylococcus is a major pathogen, there has been a long standing interest in the development of effective antistaphylococcal therapy. These agents include parenteral drugs, oral compounds, topical agents, fixed combinations, and antimicrobial glycopeptides with activity against MRSA and coagulase-negative staphylococci. Since virtually all strains of *S. aureus* produce β-lactamase with penicilli-

nase activity, the antistaphylococcal agents must be stable to these enzymes. The antistaphylococcal penicillins for parenteral use (methicillin, oxacillin, and nafcillin) all contain bulky side groups to protect the integrity of the β-lactam ring. Each has slightly different pharmacologic properties and side effects, but they have essentially equivalent activity against most clinical isolates. The addition of a β-lactamase inhibitor such as clavulanate, sulbactam, or tazobactam to the penicillins amoxicillin, ticarcillin, ampicillin, or piperacillin, respectively, results in broad-spectrum penicillins that are also highly active against β-lactamase–producing staphylococci. Oral agents such as augmentin (clavulanic acid + amoxicillin), cloxacillin, and dicloxacillin are available for therapy of infections that can be treated with oral drugs.

Most first- and some second-generation cephalosporins (including cephalothin, cefazolin, cefamandole, and cefuroxime) also have excellent antistaphylococcal activity by virtue of the poor activity of most staphylococcal β-lactamases against the cephalosporin nucleus. Any of these parenteral β-lactam agents should be effective against serious staphylococcal infections caused by susceptible organisms. Imipenem, a carbapenem, is also highly active against most strains of *S. aureus*. There are numerous oral cephalosporin derivatives that have excellent antistaphylococcal activity (Rodriguez and Wiedermann 1994). These include cephalexin, cefaclor, and cefuroxime. The newer second- and third-generation oral cephalosporins, in general, have less antistaphylococcal activity than the older drugs. Cefuroxime acetil does have good antistaphylococcal activity and is available in a liquid form.

Other classes of antimicrobial agents also possess excellent antistaphylococcal activity. The macrolides (including erythromycin, clarithromycin, azithromycin, and clindamycin) can all be used for the oral therapy of staphylococcal infection. Similarly the fluoroquinolones, particularly ciprofloxacin, have excellent antistaphylococcal activity and have been used in selected settings where a β-lactam antibiotic cannot be used. Several of these agents can be used parenterally, as well as by the oral route. The addition of rifampin, an antibiotic that interferes with RNA polymerase activity, also may be considered for the therapy of difficult staphylococcal infections, since it is lipid soluble and penetrates widely throughout the intracellular compartments and the central nervous system (Gombert et al., 1981). However, resistance to rifampin develops rapidly and it should never be used as a single agent. The aminoglycosides, such as gentamicin, also have excellent antistaphylococcal activity but in general are only used for an additive or synergistic effect in infections that are difficult to treat, or they are occasionally used topically.

For severe life-threatening infections, particularly in areas in which MRSA is found, vancomycin is the drug of choice for presumptive treatment of staphylococcal infection until an organism is isolated and its susceptibility established. (Kline and Mason, 1988; Storch and Rajagpolan, 1986). Although the β-lactam agents are considered to be the drugs of choice for serious staphylococcal infection, the increased numbers of strains with altered penicillin-binding proteins and the hyperexpression of penicillinases have resulted in the widespread use of vancomycin for staphylococcal infections. Newer glycopeptide antibiotics with activity against MRSA are currently being developed. For the treatment of endocarditis or other infections with persistent bacteremia, combination therapy may be useful, such as adding rifampin (which can accumulate within phagocytic cells) to vancomycin or a β-lactam agent. Aminoglycosides can be used similarly although there is increased nephrotoxicity when both vancomycin and aminoglycosides are used together.

INFECTIONS CAUSED BY COAGULASE-NEGATIVE STAPHYLOCOCCI
Microbiology

Coagulase-negative staphylococci such as those belonging to the *S. epidermidis* group are considered to be part of the commensal flora. However, they can become significant nosocomial pathogens in the patient with an indwelling intravascular device or in immunocompromised patients in intensive care units, and they are especially important as a cause of infection in neonates (Kloos and Bannerman, 1994). As such, they have received remarkably little attention as pathogens and little is known about their virulence factors or how the host responds to these organisms. The coagulase-negative staphylococci are differentiated from *S. aureus* on the basis of their lack of coagulase, lack of β-hemolysis of blood agar plates, and inability to ferment mannitol. They often contain extrachromosomal DNA and can exchange plasmids and transposons with *S. aureus*; the mecA gene, which confers methicillin resistance in *S. aureus*, is also found at a high frequency in coagulase-negative staphylococci. Since these staphylococci are being

isolated from normally sterile sites with increasing frequence, clinical laboratories now are able to speciate many of the strains previously grouped only as "coagulase-negative staphylococci." *Staphylococcus epidermidis, S. saprophyticus,* and *S. haemolyticus* have been recognized as causes of human disease, along with other members of this group.

Nosocomial Infections

These ubiquitous organisms are the most frequent cause of nosocomial bacteria and are responsible for significant morbidity and increased cost of hospitalization (Kloos and Bannerman, 1994; Patrick, 1990; Rupp and Archers, 1994). The vast majority of these infections are attributed to infections of intravascular devices, most commonly intravenous catheters in neonates (Noel and Edelson, 1984). Because of the indolence of these infections, they can go undetected for relatively long periods of time. Organisms associated with catheter infections may produce an exopolysaccharide, which facilitates adherence to the plastic catheters, although its role in virulence has not been well established (Diaz-Mitoma et al., 1987; Goldmann and Pier, 1993). It is possible that the exopolysaccharide is produced during the "colonization" phase of the infection while the organisms form microcolonies. However, it has not been established whether the organisms bind to human proteins or extracellular matrix components that coat these plastic catheters. Virtually all indwelling catheters do become colonized by these organisms, but symptomatic infections are infrequent. It is postulated that bacteremia occurs when large numbers of organisms are present and are intermittently shed into the bloodstream (Hodes and Barzilai, 1990). This bacteremia may be accompanied by clinical signs of fever or hypothermia, cardiovascular instability, or glucose intolerance. These findings are particularly common in premature neonates with bacteremia and sepsis caused by coagulase-negative staphylococci. Older patients with bacteremia caused by these organisms may have transient fever but generally have few clinical signs indicative of a systemic infection. Treatment of these infections without removal of the indwelling catheter is often successful using vancomycin because these organisms invariably have altered penicillin-binding proteins with low affinity for the β-lactam antibiotics (Archer, 1988).

The coagulase-negative staphylococci are a common source of bacteremia in neonates—particularly low birth weight, premature infants (Gray, 1995). Epidemiologic studies suggest that, like *S. aureus*, specific endemic strains of coagulase-negative staphylococci can cause clusters of nosocomial infections in neonatal intensive care units (Low, 1992; Lyytikainen et al., 1995). In addition to the clinical symptoms caused by bacteremia, infections caused by the coagulase-negative staphylococci are a significant cause of neonatal morbidity, prolonging the length and cost of hospitalization of the small infants.

Endocarditis

While increasing numbers of pediatric patients with congenital heart disease undergo operative repair, there has been a corresponding increase in the prevalence of endocarditis caused by coagulase-negative staphylococci (Saiman et al., 1993). These organisms do not generally infect native valves but cause an indolent, subacute picture in patients with prosthetic valves and conduits. Unlike the fulminant infections associated with *S. aureus*, these bacteremias may be difficult to document because of the intermittent administration of antibiotics in these high-risk patients. In addition, single positive blood cultures for coagulase-negative staphylococci are often considered contaminants if endocarditis is not considered to be part of the differential diagnosis. Thus, if this diagnosis is to be entertained, it is important to draw several blood cultures and use echocardiography (including two-dimensional techniques) and esophageal leads to try to make a diagnosis. These patients can also present with worsening congestive heart failure and embolic phenomena, although this is less common than in the adult population. Children with central venous catheters, particularly neonates, can also develop cardiovascular infections caused by coagulase-negative staphylococci in the presence of native valves. This can be a complication of a patent ductus arteriosus, or it can be secondary to jet flow lesions and endothelial damage accompanying unrepaired ventricular septal defects.

Central Nervous System Infections

Coagulase-negative staphylococci are the most common cause of CSF shunt infection, accounting for more than 50% of incidences. It is likely that most of these infections are caused by organisms that colonize the shunt at the time of surgery, although infection tracking up from the sutures at an infected wound site can also occur. CSF shunts in young infants are most commonly infected, and most infections occur within the first few months following placement (Pople et al., 1992). Nosocomial strains of *S. epidermidis* are most commonly isolated from the CSF and can cause a relatively indolent infection characterized by fever and shunt malfunction but only rarely with signs of meningismus or peritonitis. Examination of the CSF usually reveals pleocytosis, and cultures are positive for the staphylococci. Particularly in infants, increased protein and low glucose levels may be present but are milder than expected in infection caused by other bacterial species. Treatment invariably requires removal of the infected hardware and high doses (vancomycin at 60 to 70 mg/kg of body weight) to achieve levels in the CSF in the absence of a brisk inflammatory response. Some clinicians advocate the use of rifampin plus vancomycin, since rifampin perfuses freely into the CSF.

Urinary Tract Infection

S. saprophyticus has been recognized to be a common cause of urinary tract infection (UTI) in adolescent girls (Jordan et al., 1980); *S. saprophyticus* UTIs lead to the same signs and symptoms as the more widely recognized infections caused by *E. coli*. Patients present with dysuria and are found to have pyuria and hematuria. *S. saprophyticus* can be differentiated from other staphylococcal species by resistance to novobiocin, production of urease, and specific pattern of carbohydrate utilization. It is rarely a cause of UTI outside of this group of young, healthy, sexually active women. However, when *S. saprophyticus* is recovered from the urine in this setting it should not be considered commensal flora, but instead treated as a pathogen. These organisms are usually susceptible to several antimicrobial agents, including trimethoprim-sulfamethoxasole.

PREVENTIVE MEASURES

Because staphylococci are ubiquitous organisms, it is difficult to prevent the infections associated with them. Careful handwashing is of paramount importance in preventing person-to-person spread of the organism from contaminated secretions. It is important to consider the susceptibility of different hosts to these bacteria. The risk of nosocomial staphylococcal infection is much greater and is of greater consequence in a neonatal nursery than among older children. Patients in intensive care units with multiple venous access devices or large surgical incisions are also at greater risk for hospital-acquired staphylococcal infection. Control of nosocomial outbreaks of staphylococcal disease requires the coordinated efforts of all medical personnel involved and the input of the hospital epidemiologist.

BIBLIOGRAPHY

Albert S, Baldwin R, Czekajewski S, et al. Bullous impetigo due to group II *Staphylococcus aureus*. Amer J Dis Child 1970; 120:10-13.

Archer GL. Molecular epidemiology of multiresistant *Staphylococcus epidermidis*. J Antimicrob Chemother 1988; 21(suppl):133-138.

Bayer AS. Staphylococcal bacteremia and endocarditis: state of the art. Arch Int Med 1982;142:1169-1177.

Bray SB, Schmid FR. A comparison of medical drainage (needle aspiration) and surgical drainage (arthrotomy or arthroscopy) in the initial treatment of infected joints. Clin Rheum Dis 1986;12:501-522.

Bryant RE, Salmon CJ. Pleural empyema. Clin Inf Dis 1996;22:747-764.

Chartrand SA, McCracken GH. Staphylococcal pneumonia in infants and children. Ped Inf Dis 1982;1:19-23.

Christin L, Sarosi GA. Pyomyositis in North America: case reports and review. Clin Inf Dis 1992;15:668-77.

Davis JP, Chesney PJ, Wand PJ, LaVenture M. Toxic-shock syndrome: epidemiologic features, recurrence, risk factors, and prevention. N Engl J Med 1980;303:1429-1435.

Decker MD, Edwards KM. Central venous catheter infections. Pediatr Clin NA 1988;35:579-612.

Diaz-Mitoma F, Harding GKM, Hoban DJ, et al. Clinical significance of slime production in ventriculoperitoneal shunt infections caused by coagulase-negative staphylococci. J Inf Dis 1987;156:555-560.

Faden H, Grossi M. Acute osteomyelitis in children: reassessment of etiologic agents and their clinical characteristics. Am J Dis Child 1991;145:65-69.

Goldmann DA, Pier GB. Pathogenesis of infections related to intravascular catheterization. Clin Microbiol Rev 1993; 6:176-192.

Gombert ME, Landesman SH, Corrado ML, et al. Vancomycin and rifampin therapy for *Staphylococcus aureus* meningitis associated with CSF shunts. J Neurosurg 1981;55:633-635.

Gooch JJ, Britt EM. *Staphylococcus aureus* colonization and infection in newborn nursery patients. Am J Dis Child 1978;132:893-896.

Gray JE. Coagulase-negative staphylococi bacteremia among very low birth weight infants: relation to admission illness severity, resource use, and outcome. Pediatrics 1995;95:225-230.

Hamill RJ. Role of fibronectin in infective endocarditis. Rev Inf Dis 1987;9:S360-S371.

Hartmann BM, Tomacz A. Low-affinity penicillin binding protein associated with β-lactam resistance in *Staphylococcus aureus*. J Bacteriol 1984;158:513-518.

Hieber JP, Davis AT. Staphylococcal cervical adenitis in young infants. Pediatrics 1976;57:424-428.

Hieber JP, Nelson JA, McCracken GH. Acute disseminated staphylococcal disease in childhood. Am J Dis Child 1977; 131:181-185.

Hienz SA, Schennings T, Heimdahl A, Flock J. Collagen binding of *Staphylococcus aureus* is a virulence factor in experimental endocarditis. J Infect Dis 1996;174:83-88.

Hodes DS, Barzilai A. Invasive and toxin-mediated *Staphylococcus aureus* diseases in children. Adv Ped Inf Dis 1990; 5:35-68.

Jevons, MP "Celbenin"-resistant staphylococci. Br Med J 1961; 14(1):124-125.

Jordan PA, Irvani A, Richard GA, et al. Urinary tract infection caused by *Staphylococcus saprophyticus*. J Infect Dis 1980; 142:510-515.

Kappler J, Kotzin B, Herron J, et al. V beta-specific stimulation of human T cells by staphylococcal toxins. Science 1989;244:811-813.

Kline MW, Mason EO Jr. Methicillin-resistant *Staphylococcus aureus*: a pediatric perspective. Pediatr Clin NA 1988;35:613-624.

Kloos WE, Bannerman TL. Update on clinical significance of coagulase-negative staphylococci. Clin Microbiol Rev 1994;7:117-140.

Kluytmans JA, Mouton JW, Ijzerman EP, et al. Nasal carriage of *Staphylococcus aureus* as a major risk factor for wound infections after cardiac surgery. J Infect Dis 1995;171:216-219.

Ladisch S, Pizzo PA. *S. aureus* sepsis in children with cancer. Pediatrics 1978;61:231-234.

Ledesma-Medina J, Newman B. Use of imaging techniques in the diagnosis of infectious diseases of children. Adv Pediatr Inf Dis 1989;4:1-50.

Low DD. An endemic strain of *Staphylococcus haemolyticus* colonizing and causing bacteremia in neonatal intensive care unit patients. Pediatrics 1992;89:696-700.

Lyytikainen O, Saxen H, Ryhanen R, et al. Persistence of a multiresistant clone of *Staphylococcus epidermidis* in a neonatal intensive care unit for a four-year period. Clin Inf Dis 1995;20:24-29.

Melish ME, Glasgow LA. The staphylococcal scalded skin syndrome: development of an experimental model. N Engl J Med 1970;282:1114.

Noel GJ, Edelson PJ. *Staphylococcus epidermidis* bacteremia in neonates: further observations and the occurrence of focal infection. Pediatrics 1984;74:832-837.

Parsonnet J. Mediators in the pathogenesis of toxic shock syndrome: overview. Rev Infect Dis 1989;11(suppl 1):S263-S269.

Patrick CC. Coagulase-negative staphylococci: pathogens with increasing clinical significance. J Pediatr 1990;116:497-507.

Pont ME, Rountree WC. The medical and surgical treatment of staphylococcal pneumonia. Diseases of the Chest 1963; 43:176-185.

Pople IK, Bayston R, Haywood R. Infection of cerebrospinal fluid shunts in infants: a study of etiological factors. J Neurosurg 1992;77:29-36.

Rodriguez WJ, Wiedermann BL. The role of newer oral cephalosporins, fluoroquinolones, and macrolides in the treatment of pediatric infections. Adv Ped Inf Dis 1994;9:125-140.

Romero-Vivas J, Rubio M, Fernandez C, Picazo JJ. Mortality associated with nosocomial bacteremia due to methicillin-resistant *Staphylococcus aureus*. Clin Inf Dis 1995;21:1417-1423.

Rupp ME, Archer GL. Coagulase-negative staphylococci: pathogens associated with medical progress. Clin Inf Dis 1994;19:231-245.

Saiman L, Prince A, Gersony W. Pediatric infective endocarditis in the modern era. J Pediatr 1993;122:847-853.

Schlievert PM, Shands KN, Dan BB, et al. Identification and characterization of an exotoxin from *S. aureus* associated with toxic-shock syndrome. J Infect Dis 1981;143:509.

Sheagren JN. *S. aureus* the persistent pathogen. New Engl J Med 1984;310:1368-1374,1437-1440.

Shulman ST, Ayoub EM. Severe staphylococcal sepsis in adolescents. Pediatrics 1976;58:59-66.

Soell M, Diab M, Haan-Archipoff G, et al. Capsular polysacharide types 5 and 8 of *Staphylococcus aureus* bind specifically to human epithelial (KB) cells, endothelial cells, and monocytes and induce release of cytokines. Infect Immun 1995;63:1380-1386.

Spratt B. Resistance to antibiotics mediated by target alterations. Science 1994;264:388-393.

Storch GA, Rajagpolan L. Methicillin-resistant *Staphylococcus aureus* bacteremia in children. Pediatr Inf Dis 1986; 5:59-67.

Tetzlaff TR, McCracken GH, Nelson JD. Oral antibiotic therapy for skeletal infections of children. J Pediatr 1978; 92:485.

Waldvogel FA, Medoff G, Swartz MN. Osteomyelitis: a review of clinical features, therapeutic considerations, and unusual aspects. I. Hematogenous osteomyelitis. N Engl J Med 1970;282:198.

Waldvagel FA, Vasey H: Osteomyelitis: the past decade, N Engl J Med 1980;303:360-370.

Wiesenthal AM, Todd JK. Toxic shock syndrome in children aged 10 years or less. Pediatrics 1984;74:112-117.

Yao, L, Bengualid V, Lowy FD, et al. Internalization of *Staphylococcus aureus* by endothelial cells induces cytokine gene expression. Infect Immun 1995;63:1835-1839.

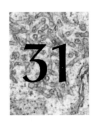

31 STREPTOCOCCAL INFECTIONS

Edward L. Kaplan

Group A β-hemolytic streptococcal infections are among the most common bacterial infections in children. Although usually causing no more threatening problems than uncomplicated tonsillitis or pharyngitis, they may result in serious and life-threatening suppurative and nonsuppurative complications. Scarlet fever, erysipelas, toxic shock syndrome, acute poststreptococcal glomerulonephritis, and acute rheumatic fever compose only a partial list of the complications caused by the group A β-hemolytic streptococcus. Streptococcal infections have become particularly important because, during the latter part of the 1980s and continuing into the 1990s, complications of group A streptococcal infections appear to have become more common than in the previous decades; serious sequelae are more frequently reported (Kaplan, 1993).

MICROBIOLOGY

Although other β-hemolytic streptococci such as those of Lancefield groups B, C, and G can cause serious infections in humans, the group A hemolytic streptococcus is the most frequent to cause human infections. These microorganisms are characterized by their tendency to grow in chains. The capsules are composed largely of hyaluronic acid.

The serologic grouping of hemolytic streptococci is based on the presence of group-specific polysaccharide antigens. Lancefield (1933) initially identified twelve serologic groups, A through L; others have also been initially identified. Serologic grouping of hemolytic streptococci is achieved by the precipitin technique of Lancefield (Lancefield, 1933) and also by commercially available typing reagents. A fluorescent antibody (FA) technique is not as widely used as it was in the past.

A major component of the bacterial cell wall is the group-specific carbohydrate, which in the case of group A organisms has antigenic components that cross-react with glycoprotein from human car-

diac valves (Goldstein et al., 1968) and has been hypothesized to be important in the pathogenesis of rheumatic fever.

Group A streptococci may be presumptively differentiated from other groups by a nonserologic procedure described in 1953 by Maxted, who used a special bacitracin disk in a simple antibiotic plate method (Maxted, 1953). Group A strains are more frequently (>95%) sensitive to bacitracin than other groups of β-hemolytic streptococci. Growth of most group A strains is inhibited by a special 0.04 unit bacitracin disk. In an analysis of 12,560 strains, there was very good agreement between the bacitracin test and the precipitin test in 95.8% of cases (Moody, 1972).

The most important surface protein is the M protein; it determines the type specificity of group A streptococci. More than eighty distinct types have been identified, but many more remain to be characterized. In addition, M proteins play an important role in virulence. They inhibit the phagocytosis of streptococci by host leukocytes. This antiphagocytic effect can be neutralized by type-specific antibody for the infecting serotype. Cross-protection between different types does not occur. Two additional protein antigens, T and R, have no known role in the virulence of the organism or in eliciting protective type-specific immunity.

The inner layer of the cell wall is composed of mucopeptide, or peptidoglycan. Experimental injection of this material into rabbits has induced carditis (Rotta and Bednat, 1969), but whether it is involved in the pathogenesis of acute rheumatic fever remains unknown because no experimental animal model exactly mimics acute rheumatic fever in humans.

Group A hemolytic streptococci secrete a number of extracellular toxins and enzymes, such as streptokinase; nucleases (A, B, C, D); hemolysins (streptolysins S and O); hyaluronidase; and several pyrogenic exotoxins. Streptolysins cause the hemolysis observed on blood agar plates. Streptolysin O is oxygen-labile, so the surface hemolysis on the plate is due to streptolysin S. Infection with group A streptococci is followed by the production of specific antibodies for the extracellular antigens (e.g., antistreptokinase, antideoxyribonuclease B, antistreptolysin O, hyaluronidase).

The erythrogenic toxins are responsible for the rash of scarlet fever. The identification of at least three immunologically distinct rash-producing toxins explains the reported occurrences of several distinct episodes of scarlet fever in the same person (Zabriskie, 1964; Watson and Kim, 1970). Production of erythrogenic toxin is mediated by lysogeny (Zabriskie, 1964). A role for these toxins has also been proposed in the pathogenesis of the streptococcal toxic shock syndrome; this is especially true for SPEA (streptococcal pyrogenic exotoxin A). Although the mechanism has not been precisely defined, an activation with the cytokine system has been proposed as a part of the pathogenesis of this severe complication of group A streptococci.

EPIDEMIOLOGY

Group A streptococci are spread primarily by the respiratory route. Individuals with acute group A streptococcal upper respiratory tract infection, especially those who harbor large numbers of organisms in their anterior nares, are especially likely to transmit this organism to close contacts (family or schoolmates). In contrast, many individuals who are "carriers" and tend to harbor small numbers of organisms with the upper respiratory tract infection are less likely to spread the organism to contacts. Contaminated foods (especially milk, ice cream, other dairy products, and eggs or egg products) have been responsible for a number of well-documented food-borne epidemics of pharyngitis.

Although the pediatric age group is most frequently infected, people of all ages are susceptible to group A streptococcal infections. The incidence varies with age according to the clinical type of infection. In general, however, these infections are least frequent in infancy, begin to rise gradually at about age 4 to 5 years, and reach a peak between the ages of 5 and 15 years. Although the incidence of group A streptococcal upper respiratory tract infection is lower among preschool-age children, outbreaks of group A streptococcal upper respiratory tract infections have been documented in day-care facilities (Smith et al., 1989).

Although the incidence of group A streptococcal upper respiratory tract infection was once thought

higher in temperate climates, it is now recognized that these infections and their sequelae occur widely in the tropics. However, a number of prevalence studies have indicated that groups C and G β-hemolytic streptococci are also commonly found in the upper respiratory tract in tropical climates. These organisms do not cause rheumatic fever. Whether their presence is indicative of true infection or only colonization is not completely understood.

Streptococcal infections of the skin (impetigo, pyoderma) are more common in preschool-age children but may occur in any age group. The geographic distribution of skin infections seems to favor warmer or tropical climates, and infections occur mainly in summer or early fall in temperate climates. However, streptococcal impetigo occurs even in winter months in temperate zones. In temperate zones such as North America and Europe, group A streptococcal pharyngitis occurs most often during late winter and early spring.

IMMUNITY

Group A hemolytic streptococci are composed of numerous somatic antigens that also produce a number of extracellular antigens. Some of these antigens—type-specific M protein and the erythrogenic toxins—stimulate the production of antibodies that provide a person with immunity. Type-specific immunity (against specific M-serotypes of group A streptococcus) is long lasting (several decades).

It has been postulated that the development of immunity and hypersensitivity may play a role in the increase of streptococcal disease with advancing age. Atypical group A streptococcal infections in infants may result from the initial response to the microorganism.

Antibacterial immunity is largely due to the specific M protein of group A hemolytic streptococci. A person who is infected with one of the approximately fifty recognized specific serotypes of group A streptococci develops antibodies against strains of the homologous type only. Thus infection with type 4 streptococcus is followed by development of antibodies against type 4, but not against heterologous types.

The current concept of type-specific antibacterial immunity is supported by data obtained from many immunologic and epidemiologic studies. During a lifetime the average individual experiences multiple group A streptococcal infections, some apparent and others inapparent. Each infection is likely caused by a different serotype of group A streptococcus. It has been demonstrated that the sera of infants and young children usually contains only a limited number of these type-specific antibodies. As a person's age increases, a larger number of these type-specific antibodies develops as a result of repeated infections. However, second attacks of streptococcal infection with the same type are not unknown. The capacity of early antibiotic therapy to decrease the immune response to various streptococcal antigens may explain some of these second attacks. This reduced response has prompted controversy about whether early antibiotic treatment can be detrimental to the patient. However, recent evidence suggests that this is not true (Gerber et al., 1990).

In summary, the immune status of a person may affect the type of infection acquired after exposure to a particular pathogenic strain of streptococcus. The hypothetical example in Fig. 31-1, which assumes exposure to type 4 group A streptococci, illustrates this graphically. It may be noted that (1) type 4 antibacterial immunity prevents clinical disease regardless of the antitoxic status; (2) when type 4 antibacterial immunity is absent but antitoxic immunity is present, streptococcal pharyngitis or tonsillitis may develop, but scarlet fever likely will not occur; and (3) when neither type 4 antibacterial nor antitoxic immunity is present, scarlet fever may develop.

CLINICAL MANIFESTATIONS

The clinical manifestations of group A streptococcal infection are governed by many factors, the most important being the portal of entry, the pa-

tient's age, and the immune status of the host. An effect of type-specific immunity has been discussed. Powers and Boisvert (1944) emphasized the importance of the age factor in relation to the clinical infection. They clearly described the manifestations of streptococcal infections, or "streptococcosis," for three pediatric age groups: under 6 months, 6 months to 3 years, and 3 to 12 years.

Streptococcosis in Infants Less Than 6 Months of Age

Streptococcosis in infants under 6 months of age is characterized by nasopharyngitis associated with a thin mucopurulent nasal discharge and usually low-grade temperature. Frequently there are impetigious excoriations around the nares. The acute symptoms last for approximately 1 week, but persistent nasal discharge and irritability may continue for as long as 6 weeks. The disease may be clinically indistinguishable from the common cold. It can be confirmed only by means of a culture of the nasal discharge, which will reveal large numbers of group A streptococci.

Streptococcosis in Children 6 Months to 3 Years of Age

In streptococcosis in children 6 months to 3 years of age, there is an insidious onset of low-grade fever, mild constitutional symptoms, and mild nasopharyngitis. The nasal discharge can be clear. The anterior cervical lymph nodes are usually enlarged and tender. It should be remembered, however, that the "classic" streptococcal upper respiratory tract infection can occur in young children.

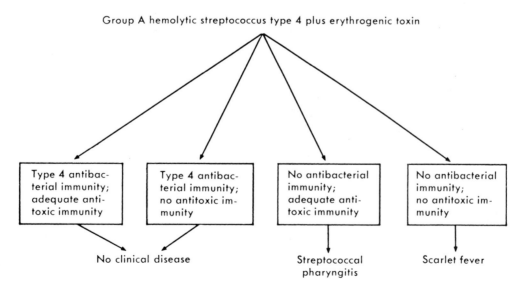

FIG. 31-1 Effect of immune status on streptococcal infections.

Sinusitis and otitis media may accompany pharyngitis or tonsillitis. The low-grade fever and symptoms may persist for as long as 4 to 8 weeks. This type of streptococcal infection is clinically similar to various nonspecific respiratory tract infections. Diagnosis can best be established by throat culture, as well as culture of the anterior nares.

Group A Streptococcal Upper Respiratory Tract Infection in Children 3 to 12 Years of Age

In children 3 to 12 years of age, group A streptococcal upper respiratory tract infection usually is manifested as acute onset of tonsillitis or pharyngitis, with or without scarlet fever. Streptococcal tonsillitis is essentially scarlet fever without a rash. The clinical picture, complications, prognosis, and treatment are identical to those of scarlet fever; consequently, they are considered in the discussion of scarlet fever (see the following section).

Scarlet Fever

The average incubation period for scarlet fever is 2 to 4 days, with a range of 1 to 7 days. The disease is ushered in abruptly by fever; vomiting; sore throat; and constitutional symptoms such as headache, chills, and malaise. Within 12 to 48 hours after onset, the typical rash appears. It is not unusual for abdominal pain to be an early and prominent symptom. In fact, the association of this manifestation with vomiting may suggest the possibility of a surgical abdomen. The combination of vomiting and abdominal pain in streptococcal tonsillitis without rash is also frequently seen. The significant findings are fever, enanthem, and exanthem.

Fever. In the typical case (Fig. 31-2) the temperature rises abruptly to 39.4° C (103° F) and reaches its peak by about the second day. It then gradually falls to normal within 5 or 6 days. Severe cases have a higher and more protracted temperature course. Occasionally, in mild scarlet fever, the temperature may be low (under 38.3° C; 101° F) or normal. The pulse rate may be increased out of proportion to the fever. The fever often drops precipitously to normal or near normal within 24 hours after antibiotic therapy is begun.

Enanthem. The enanthem includes lesions on the tonsils, pharynx, tongue, and palate. The tonsils are enlarged, edematous, reddened, and covered with patches of exudate. The pharynx also is edematous and beefy red in appearance. In mild cases the tonsils and pharynx show moderate erythema and little or no exudate. Severe cases may be characterized by membranous ulcerative tonsillitis, sometimes similar to that seen in patients with diphtheria (Plate 8). The tongue changes in appearance as the disease progresses. During the first 1 or 2 days the dorsum has a white "fur coat," and the tip and edges are reddened. As the papillae become reddened and edematous, they project through the coat, producing the so-called white strawberry tongue. By the fourth or fifth day the white coat has peeled off. The red, glistening tongue, studded with prominent papillae, presents the appearance of a red strawberry (Plate 9). The palate is usually covered with erythematous punctiform lesions and occasionally with scattered petechiae. The uvula and the free margin of the soft palate are reddened and edematous (Plate 8).

Exanthem. The rash usually appears within 12 hours after onset of the illness; occasionally it may be delayed for 2 days. The rash is an erythematous punctiform eruption that blanches on pressure. The punctate lesions, pinhead in size, give the skin a rough, sandpaper-like texture. The rash of scarlet fever resembles a "sunburn with goose pimples" (Plate 9).

FIG. 31-2 Schematic diagram of a typical case of untreated uncomplicated scarlet fever. The rash usually appears within 24 hours of onset of fever and sore throat.

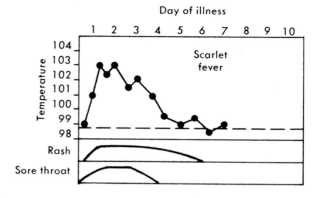

The exanthem (Fig. 31-3) has the following distinctive features:

1. It becomes generalized very rapidly, usually within 24 hours.
2. The punctiform lesions are usually not present on the face. The forehead and cheeks are red, smooth, and flushed, and the area around the mouth is pale (circumoral pallor).
3. It is more intense in skin folds such as the axillae and the groin and at sites of pressure such as the buttocks.
4. It has areas of hyperpigmentation, occasionally with tiny petechiae in the creases of the folds of the joints, particularly in the antecubital fossae. These lesions form transverse lines (Pastia's sign) that persist for a day or so after the rash has faded.
5. If the eruption is severe, minute vesicular lesions (miliary sudamina) may be scattered over the abdomen, hands, and feet.
6. It desquamates several days later.

The rash, fever, sore throat, and other clinical manifestations clear up by the end of the first week. The period of desquamation follows shortly thereafter.

Desquamation. Desquamation is one of the most characteristic features of scarlet fever. The extent and duration of the desquamation are directly proportional to the intensity of the rash. It becomes apparent initially on the face, at the end of the first week, as fine branny flakes. Then it spreads to the trunk and finally to the extremities, becoming generalized by the third week (Fig. 31-4). The desquamating skin of the trunk comes off in larger, thicker flakes. Frequently, circular areas of epidermis of variable size peel off, giving the skin a punched-out or pinhole appearance. The hands and feet usually are the last to desquamate, becoming involved between the second and third weeks after onset. The tips of the fingers characteristically show splitting of the skin at the free margins of the nails. In severe cases an epidermal cast of the fingers, hands, or feet may be shed. In mild cases of scarlet fever the process of desquamation may be complete in 3 weeks; in severe cases it may persist for as long as 8 weeks. Sometimes a retrospective diagnosis may be made on the basis of peeling skin and a history of a sore throat associated with a rash several weeks before. Occasionally the eruption may be missed entirely. Not infrequently, the rash of scarlet fever is confused with the rash of Kawasaki disease.

Surgical Scarlet Fever

The portal of entry in patients with classic scarlet fever is the nasopharynx. Occasionally, however, hemolytic streptococci may infect the site of a wound, a burn, or other type of skin lesion. Under these circumstances, so-called surgical scarlet fever may develop. The clinical manifestations are identical to those described earlier except that the pharyngeal and tonsillar involvement are absent. However, there may be local inflammatory signs at the wound or operative site.

Streptococcal Sepsis

Although most group A streptococcal infections occur as surface infections of the respiratory tract or skin, they can cause serious invasive disease in otherwise normal infants and children. These are usually fulminant bacteremic or septicemic infections with pneumonia, empyema, osteomyelitis, endometritis, meningitis, or soft-tissue abscesses (Burech et al., 1976).

Since the late 1980s an increasing number of cases of fulminant group A streptococcal bacteremia associated with a toxic shock syndrome have been reported. Such streptococcal infections have a high mortality rate (reported as high as 30%). One important risk factor for invasive infection in children is varicella. This has continued into the 1990s (Stevens 1992, 1995).

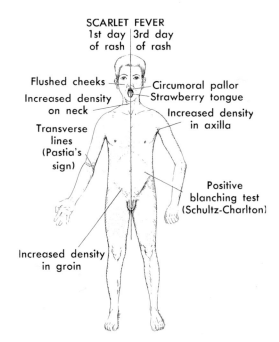

SCARLET FEVER
1st day | 3rd day
of rash | of rash

Flushed cheeks
Increased density on neck
Transverse lines (Pastia's sign)

Circumoral pallor
Strawberry tongue
Increased density in axilla

Positive blanching test (Schultz-Charlton)

Increased density in groin

FIG. 31-3 Schematic drawing illustrating development and distribution of scarlet fever rash.

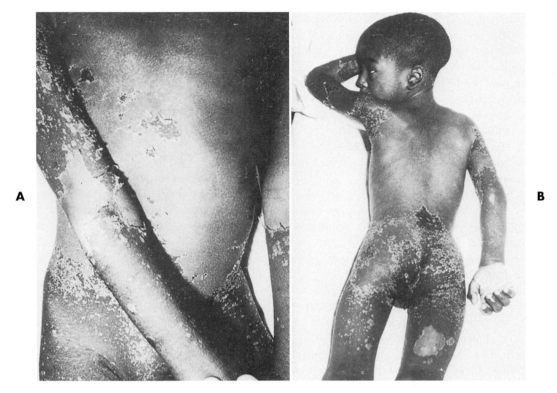

FIG. 31-4   Desquamation in a patient 16 days after onset of severe scarlet fever. **A,** Typical circular punched-out areas in groin and upper thighs; **B,** sequence of spread from face to trunk and finally to extremities.

The streptococcal toxic shock syndrome (with or without necrotizing fasciitis) results in multiorgan failure. The diagnostic criteria are listed in Box 31-1.

Streptococcal Infections of the Skin

Impetigo or Pyoderma. The characteristic superficial purulent crusting lesions of streptococcal pyoderma are relatively easy to recognize. The vesicular stage of streptococcal impetigo may be transient, and the vesicles are small (1 to 2 mm in diameter). The typical lesion is a thick, adherent, amber-colored crust on an erythematous base; there can be an associated local lymphadenopathy (Wannamaker, 1970). On the other hand, bullous impetigo is usually caused by staphylococci. These vesicular lesions are larger (1 to 2 cm in diameter); they rupture, and thin crusts are formed. There usually is no accompanying lymphadenopathy.

Group A streptococcal impetigo is usually associated with different serotypes of streptococci than are commonly found in upper respiratory tract infections (Wannamaker, 1970). These strains often are of the high serotype numbers (49 and above) and frequently initially can be isolated from the skin and skin lesions before they colonize the upper respiratory tract.

Erysipelas. Erysipelas, formerly very common, is relatively rare today. It is characterized by a red, indurated thickening of the skin. It begins as a small lesion that spreads marginally for approximately 4 to 6 days. The margins have a raised, firm, tender, palpable border. On the face the rash may assume a butterfly distribution. The skin lesion is usually associated with fever and constitutional symptoms that subside when the rash stops progressing.

Histologically, there is evidence of an inflammatory reaction involving the superficial lymph vessels. The lymph channels are filled with fibrin, leukocytes, and streptococci. The progressively diffuse lymphatic involvement accounts for the peculiar spread and evolution of the lesion.

Eczema Streptococcum. Children and infants with weeping eczematoid lesions are prone to develop secondary infections, particularly with hemolytic streptococci. The resulting lesion shows

---

BOX 31-1

**THE STREPTOCOCCAL TOXIC
SHOCK SYNDROME***

I. Isolation of *Streptococcus pyogenes*
   A. From a normally sterile site
   B. From a nonsterile site
II. Clinical Signs
   A. Hypotension *and*
   B. Multiorgan involvement (At least 2 of
      the following)
      1. Renal impairment
      2. Coagulopathy
      3. Liver involvement
      4. Adult respiratory distress syndrome
         (ARDS)
      5. Generalized erythematous macular
         rash that may desquamate.
      6. Soft tissue necrosis including necro-
         tizing fasciitis, myositis, or gan-
         grene.

(Modified from JAMA 1993;269:390-391 and from
Kaplan EL. The Report on Pediatric Infectious Diseases 1996; 6:17-18.)
Note: Definite case includes criteria I-A and II (A
and B). Probable case includes I-B and II (A and B)
in the absence of another identified etiology.

---

extensive erythema, serosanguineous exudate,
crusting, weeping, and regional adenopathy.

DIAGNOSIS OF GROUP A
STREPTOCOCCAL INFECTIONS

The diagnosis of group A streptococcal upper respiratory tract infections, including scarlet fever,
can be suspected and confirmed by (1) characteristic clinical features, (2) isolation of the causative
agent, (3) serologic tests, and (4) other less specific
laboratory tests (Wannamaker, 1972).

Clinical Features of Streptococcal
Upper Respiratory Tract Infection
and Scarlet Fever

The triad of fever, vomiting, and sudden onset of
severe sore throat associated with an exudative tonsillitis or pharyngitis and an erythematous punctiform eruption strongly suggests scarlet fever. The
same symptoms and signs without a rash point to
streptococcal tonsillitis or pharyngitis.

    Stillerman and Bernstein (1961) observed that
groups of symptoms and signs are better indicators

of streptococcal pharyngitis than single symptoms
and signs. The following four syndromes were associated with positive cultures in more than 70% of
the cases:

1. Moderate redness of the oropharynx, exudate over
the tonsils, and cervical adenitis (75%)
2. Marked redness of the oropharynx with or without
tonsillar exudate, and cervical adenitis (74%)
3. Moderate or marked redness of the oropharynx, no
tonsillar exudate, and petechiae on the palate, with
or without cervical adenitis (95%)
4. Moderate or marked redness of the oropharynx,
tonsillar exudate, and petechiae on the palate, with
or without cervical adenitis (100%)

    Wannamaker (1972) described differences in the
typical clinical picture of group A streptococcal upper respiratory tract infections in different age
groups. The classical presenting complaints of
older children and adults with group A streptococcal upper respiratory tract infection are much less
commonly encountered in infants and toddlers. The
latter group often presents with a more subacute illness, often with low-grade fever and malaise. This
may make the clinical diagnosis more difficult, especially in day-care centers with many young children present; it is easy to confuse this syndrome
with upper respiratory tract infections of viral
origin.

LABORATORY DIAGNOSIS
Isolation of the Causative Agent

The throat culture remains the most reliable confirmatory laboratory test. One of the most valuable
reasons for performing a throat culture is to rule out
the presence of group A streptococcal infection and
thus eliminate unnecessary antibiotic therapy.

    Group A β-hemolytic streptococci may be iso-
lated from the throat, the anterior nares, the nasopharynx, or an infected wound. It is rare to isolate
this organism from the blood in patients with only
upper respiratory tract infection. A positive throat
culture may indicate an acute streptococcal infection, but it may also indicate the presence of the
group A streptococcal upper respiratory tract "carrier" state (Kaplan, 1980). A quantitative throat
swab culture often, but *not always,* reveals a correlation between the isolation of large numbers of
streptococci and the presence of true streptococcal
pharyngitis (Breese et al., 1972). Studies by Bell
and Smith (1976) revealed a heavy growth of *Streptococcus pyogenes* in 71% of throat swabs taken
from 1054 children with pharyngitis, as compared

with 1.7% of 462 normal children who were carriers. There is considerable overlap, so quantitation of the throat culture is not a totally reliable method for differentiating the two conditions. Diagnosis of streptococcal impetigo is made by isolation of the organism from a skin lesion.

Rapid Antigen Detection Tests

Several rapid antigen detection tests for confirming the presence of group A streptococci on throat swabs are commercially available. In general, the specificity of these tests has been reported to be better than their sensitivity (Kaplan, 1988). These tests can, however, be helpful in the rapid diagnosis of group A streptococcal upper respiratory tract infections and also in establishing a streptococcal cause in patients with pyoderma (Kaplan et al., 1989). Because of published reports describing reduced sensitivity of some streptococcal rapid antigen detection tests, most clinicians who find a negative rapid antigen detection test in a patient who has symptoms compatible with this infection then obtain a conventional throat culture for confirmation. The throat culture remains the "gold standard" for the laboratory diagnosis of group A streptococcal upper respiratory tract infections, although the technology of many rapid antigen detection tests has improved. It should also be remembered that rapid antigen detection tests do not identify non–group A hemolytic streptococci such as serologic groups C and G, organisms that have been associated with pharyngitis.

Streptococcal Antibody Tests

The measurement of antibodies to group A streptococcal antigens is useful as an aid in diagnosis of previous infections and sequelae. However, antibody tests are *not* helpful in the acute diagnosis of these infections, since the time required to develop antibodies is such that the tests are of no immediate value.

Antistreptolysin O (ASO) titers are elevated in the serum of most patients recovering from a recent group A streptococcal upper respiratory tract infection. The anti–streptolysin O test is not as helpful in individuals who have group A streptococcal pyoderma before acute poststreptococcal glomerulonephritis. This is due to the cholesterol present in skin; the antigenicity of streptolysin O is reduced by the presence of free cholesterol (Kaplan and Wannamaker, 1976). On the other hand, the antideoxyribonuclease B (anti-DNase B) test is appropriate for documenting a previous group A streptococcal infection either of the upper respiratory tract or of the skin. This test is also commercially available. The peak antistreptolysin O titer is reached between 3 and 6 weeks after infection; the peak anti-DNase B test is reached later—between 6 and 8 weeks after the onset of infection. Another commercially available streptococcal antibody test is the anti-hyaluronidase (AH) test. It is not as widely used. The kinetics of the immune response to this extracellular antigen are similar to those for antibody to streptolysin O. An agglutination test that is said to measure several different antibodies at the same time (the Streptozyme test) has been available for almost 20 years, but technical problems have been reported with this test. Batch-to-batch variation in the reagents and difficulty in reading the agglutination have led to published reports expressing concern about its usefulness.

Antibody titers to group A streptococcal extracellular antigens (ASO, anti-DNase B, etc.) vary with age, season of the year, and site of infection. Antibody levels also are dependent on the interval since the preceeding group A streptococcal infection. For example, the peak for the antistreptolysin O titer usually is reached 3 to 6 weeks after an infection, whereas the peak for the antideoxyribonuclease B titer occurs somewhat later, approximately 6 to 8 weeks after infection. The results of the laboratory test are influenced by when the serum is obtained. Early eradication of hemolytic streptococci by antimicrobial therapy may suppress the development of antibodies. For most school-age children, antistreptolysin O titers of 250 and greater can be considered abnormal. Anti-DNase B titers of 250 to 300 or greater can be considered abnormal. It is best to determine a rise in titer between acute-phase and convalescent-phase sera to document a previous group A streptococcal infection; single titers can sometimes be misleading.

Less-Specific Laboratory Tests

In patients with acute streptococcal infection, leukocytosis with a predominance of polymorphonuclear leukocytes is usually present. It is not uncommon to see an increase in number of eosinophils to between 5% and 10% of the total white blood cell count in patients with scarlet fever. The erythrocyte sedimentation rate is often elevated.

DIFFERENTIAL DIAGNOSIS OF GROUP A STREPTOCOCCAL INFECTIONS

The differential diagnosis of scarlet fever is discussed in detail in Chapter 36. A number of other infectious agents are associated with pharyngitis

(Bisno, 1996). Some of the conditions that may be confused with this disease are rubella, rubeola, exanthem subitum, erythema infectiosum, Lyme disease, infectious mononucleosis, staphylococcal scalded skin syndrome, Kawasaki syndrome, and toxic shock syndrome. Sunburn in a child with nonspecific pharyngitis may be confused with scarlet fever; the absence of eruption in the bathing suit area clarifies the diagnosis. Heat rash (miliaria) also may simulate a scarlatiniform eruption.

The differential diagnosis of exudative and membranous tonsillitis is covered in the chapters on diphtheria (Chapter 5) and Epstein-Barr virus infections (infectious mononucleosis; Chapter 8).

Wannamaker in 1970 and Peter and Smith in 1977 described the comparative features of streptococcal infections of the throat and skin. The serotypes of group A streptococci causing disease in these two organ systems are different. For example, serotypes that classically cause pharyngitis are relatively rarely isolated from the skin lesions (Anthony et al., 1969). The features of these infections are listed in Table 31-1.

COMPLICATIONS OF GROUP A STREPTOCOCCAL INFECTION

Complications following group A streptococcal infections may occur early or late in the course of the disease.

Early Complications

Early complications are generally the result of an extension of the streptococcal infection; they usually occur during the first week of illness. Thus extension of the infection to the regional lymph nodes results in cervical adenitis. Progression of the infection into the middle ear results in acute otitis media. Sinusitis also may be caused by hemolytic streptococci.

Bronchopneumonia is a rare early complication of group A streptococcal infection involving the upper respiratory tract. Early bacterial complications rarely occur in adequately treated patients. Other uncommon complications include mastoiditis, septicemia, and osteomyelitis. A toxic shock syndrome (not related to the staphylococcal toxic shock syndrome discussed in Chapter 27) is an uncommon but often very severe infection with high morbidity and mortality (Stevens et al., 1989; Stevens, 1992).

Late Complications

The late or nonsuppurative sequelae of group A streptococcal infections are acute rheumatic fever and acute poststreptococcal glomerulonephritis.

The pathogenetic mechanisms responsible for the development of these nonsuppurative sequelae remain incompletely explained. Generally speaking, they are believed to result from an abnormal host immune response to one or more as yet undefined group A streptococcal somatic or extracellular antigens. Although numerous hypotheses implicating various specific antigens have been described, confirmatory evidence is lacking. These nonsuppurative sequelae usually develop after a latent period of 1 to 3 weeks and may follow both evident or inapparent infections.

Rheumatic Fever. Although the disease was very common in North America and Europe before, during, and immediately after World War II, the incidence of acute rheumatic fever in these industrialized countries declined remarkably during the late 1960s and 1970s. Rheumatic fever incidence figures of less than 1 case per 100,000 people per year were common in the United States by the late 1970s. In contrast, in developing countries of the world, rheumatic fever and rheumatic heart disease remain very significant public health problems (World Health Organization Study Group, 1988). Very high prevalence rates of rheumatic heart disease have been described in schoolchildren in a number of developing countries around the world, making this nonsuppurative sequel of group A streptococcal infections a major cardiovascular problem in the world today.

In the mid-1980s an unexpected "resurgence" of acute rheumatic fever occurred in the United States, affecting not only schoolchildren, but also military recruits (Markowitz and Kaplan, 1989, Kaplan 1993). The exact reasons for this resurgence are not completely understood, but the increase likely was associated with the introduction and spread of specific group A streptococci (M types 1, 3, 5, 6, and 18 were most often recovered from these patients). Many were a mucoid phenotype.

It has been suggested that certain serotypes are "rheumatogenic," but no rheumatogenic antigen or toxin has yet been definitely linked to the onset of rheumatic fever. Indeed, it may be that only certain strains of a given serotype have the capacity to cause rheumatic fever.

There has always been evidence to suggest that, in addition to the need for a group A streptococcal upper respiratory tract infection, there appears to be a genetic predisposition to developing rheumatic fever. Many factors have been studied, but the mechanism is not yet fully explained. Most likely it is related to abnormal immunologic processing of

Table 31-1   General features of streptococcal infections at different sites

	Streptococcal pharyngitis and tonsillitis	Streptococcal impetigo and pyoderma
Clinical features		
Erythema	Usually present and generalized	Often minimal and localized to immediate area around lesion
Vesicular stage	Absent	Typical of early lesion but transient
Pustular stage	Patchy exudate; pustules sometimes confluent	Pustules usually discrete; flora often mixed
Crusted stage	Absent	Frequent and characteristic
Local pain	Common; may be intense	Usually absent
Systemic reaction	Fever, headache, and malaise common	Unusual
Regional adenitis	Common	Less common, but adenopathy frequently seen
Deep-seated cellulitis	May occur	Perhaps less common
Bacteremia	Rare	May be relatively more frequent
Scarlatiniform rash	Sometimes present	Rare
Course	Typically acute except in infants	Often chronic; lesions may become ecthymatous
Laboratory findings		
Leukocytosis	Usually present	Often absent
Bacterial agent	Group A streptococci	Group A streptococci; often also large numbers of staphylococci
Serologic types of group A streptococci	Many different types	Few types predominate
Antistreptolysin O response	Common	Uncommon
Epidemiologic factors		
Seasonal occurrence	Winter and spring	Late summer and early fall
Common-source epidemics	May occur	Not described
Geographical distribution	More common in temperate or cold climates	Common in hot or tropical climates
Age	Young school-age children	Children of preschool age
Sex	Equal incidence	Equal incidence
Transmission	Direct spread from human reservoirs, particularly nasal carriers	Unknown; insects may be mechanical vectors
Carrier state	Common in pharynx of many populations	Unusual on skin except in certain situations
Preceding trauma	Not present	May predispose to natural or experimental infection
Preceding viral infection	Uncommon	Uncommon
Complications		
Acute nephritis	Occurs; partially preventable (50%)	Occurs; preventability unknown
Acute rheumatic fever	Occurs; preventable	Does not occur
Treatment		
Local	Not important	Removal of crusts and scrubbing with hexachlorophene soap
Systemic	Single intramuscular injection of benzathine penicillin G or oral administration of penicillin for 10 days	May not be necessary; extensive lesions may require intramuscular injection of benzathine penicillin G

From Wannamaker LW. N Engl J Med 1970;282:23.

one or more group A streptococcal antigens. Recent evidence suggests that some individuals who are susceptible can be identified by abnormal markers on their peripheral non–T lymphocytes. However, these findings require confirmation by large prospective studies.

Rheumatic fever is a serious complication of group A streptococcal infections; its incidence is approximately 3% after exudative group A streptococcal pharyngitis. Rheumatic fever does not follow streptococcal impetigo. With optimal antibiotic therapy for the preceding streptococcal upper respiratory tract infection, the attack rate is reduced to almost zero. Recurrent attacks of rheumatic fever, on the other hand, are a relatively frequent complication of group A streptococcal infection, but essentially can be prevented by continuous administration of prophylactic penicillin or sulfadiazine (secondary prophylaxis). Rheumatic fever is rare in children under 3 years of age; the initial attack occurs most often in children 5 to 15 years of age.

The diagnosis of rheumatic fever requires fulfilling the Jones criteria. More specific findings such as pancarditis and migratory polyarthritis are given more weight than are nonspecific (called "minor") findings such as fever and arthralgia. Box 31-2 shows the updated Jones criteria from the most recent revision in 1992 (American Heart Association, Special Writing Group, 1992). Two major criteria—or one major and two minor criteria—plus evidence of a preceding streptococcal infection are needed to suggest rheumatic fever. It is important to recognize that in patients who fulfill the Jones criteria but do not have evidence of a preceeding group A streptococcal infection, the diagnosis of rheumatic fever should be made with extreme caution.

Acute Poststreptococcal Glomerulonephritis. The incidence of acute nephritis is variable. Certain serotypes of group A hemolytic streptococci—for example, types 12, 49, 55, and 57—are "nephritogenic," and infections with these microorganisms may be followed by an attack of nephritis. Nephritis, unlike rheumatic fever, can follow infection of either the throat or of the skin. Nephritis is usually manifested by fever, bloody urine, peripheral edema, and, occasionally, hypertension and azotemia. In contrast to the clinical course of rheumatic fever, only one attack usually occurs; recurrences occur but are unusual. The rarity of recurrences may be a result of the relatively limited number of nephritogenic serotypes of streptococci. Although residua of acute poststreptococcal nephri-

---

BOX 31-2

THE JONES CRITERIA FOR RHEUMATIC FEVER, UPDATED 1992

Major Criteria

Carditis
Migratory polyarthritis
Syndenham's chorea
Subcutaneous nodules
Erythema marginatum

Minor Criteria

Fever
Arthralgia
Prolonged PR interval
Elevated acute-phase reactants
Evidence of a recent group A streptococcal infection

Modified from American Heart Association, Special Writing Group 1992; 268:2069-2072.

---

tis have been suspected in adult patients, it is generally believed that the long-term prognosis for children with acute streptococcal nephritis is excellent. Residual renal disease is very uncommon.

PROGNOSIS FOR PATIENTS WITH GROUP A STREPTOCOCCAL INFECTION

The prognosis for patients with adequately treated uncomplicated group A streptococcal upper respiratory tract infections is excellent. Serious septic complications usually can be prevented. Appropriate antibiotic therapy will also reduce the incidence of rheumatic fever, thereby improving the prognosis. Deaths caused by scarlet fever and other streptococcal infections, very common some decades ago, are now extremely rare. However, severe group A streptococcal suppurative infections have a relatively high mortality rate. Mortality rates of 30% to greater than 50% have been reported in patients with group A streptococcal necrotizing fasciitis.

TREATMENT OF GROUP A STREPTOCOCCAL UPPER RESPIRATORY TRACT INFECTION
Antimicrobial Therapy

Penicillin remains the preferred drug for treatment of group A streptococcal upper respiratory tract infections. Strains of group A hemolytic streptococci are uniformly susceptible to penicillin (Coonan and

Kaplan, 1994). Penicillin therapy is usually followed by a subsidence of fever and constitutional symptoms. Some researchers (Breese et al., 1972; Hall and Breese, 1984) have indicated that administering antibiotics reduces the symptoms of streptococcal sore throat more rapidly than no treatment. Indeed, several other recent studies have confirmed that prompt therapy is associated with more prompt resolution of the symptoms, allowing children to return to school and parents to work at an earlier time (Nelson, 1984).

Optimal antibiotic treatment eradicates the group A streptococci from the site of infection, usually prevents septic complications, and drastically reduces the risk of rheumatic fever. However, it is uncertain whether the development of nephritis is affected by early antibiotic therapy. Therapy also rapidly alleviates symptoms (Gerber et al., 1990).

Optimal antibiotic management of group A streptococcal respiratory tract infections can be achieved using a variety of regimens. Because of the absence of documented resistance to penicillin by group A streptococci, it continues to be recommended as the therapy of choice by the American Heart Association, the American Academy of Pediatrics, and the World Health Organization.

The objective in treating streptococcal upper respiratory tract infection is to eradicate the organism. This usually can be accomplished by either 10 days of oral therapy (250 to 500 μg of penicillin V taken 2 to 4 times a day) or by a single injection of intramuscular benzathine penicillin G, a repository form of the antibiotic. Oral therapy may not always be as effective because of a lack of patient compliance. The use of intramuscular benzathine penicillin G (600,000 units for children weighing <60 pounds and 1,200,000 units for children weighing >60 pounds) virtually eliminates the problem of compliance. Mixtures of benzathine penicillin G with procaine penicillin G are available. However, the total penicillin dosage should be based on the amount of benzathine penicillin G in the mixture, because the other forms are rapidly excreted.

Although penicillin remains the treatment of choice, treatment failures (failure to eradicate the organism from the upper respiratory tract) have been documented (Kaplan, 1985; Markowitz et al., 1993). Since group A streptococci are uniformly sensitive to penicillin and the MICs for these organisms have not changed (Coonan and Kaplan, 1994), the reasons for failure to eradicate the organism have not been completely defined. In addition to lack of compliance, other possible explanations include the streptococcal "carrier" state, production of β-lactamase by normal flora of the upper respiratory tract, and even tolerance to penicillin. Additional careful documentation is needed to resolve this very practical problem.

An alternative antibiotic for use in penicillin-allergic patients is erythromycin. It can be given at a dosage of 40 mg/kg/day in 3 or 4 divided doses. The maximum dosage is 1 gram per 24 hours. Unlike with penicillin, erythromycin resistance does occur. It was widespread in Japan during the 1960s and 1970s, but resistance in that part of the world has decreased recently. However, reports in the early 1990s from Finland demonstrate that this is still a possibility; clinicians and clinical microbiologists must be aware of the possibility. Current information from the United States and most parts of the world suggest that erythromycin (and other macrolide antibiotic resistance) is present in less than 5% of recovered and tested group A streptococcal isolates.

Recently a number of other antimicrobial agents have been studied for their efficacy to eradicate group A streptococci from the upper respiratory tract. Efficacy has been shown for a number of cephalosporins. However, attempts to demonstrate superiority of the cephalosporins have often shown equivalency rather than significant superiority. When cephalosporins are used for this indication, most health professionals generally choose a first-generation cephalosporin. It is generally accurate to state that most, if not all, of the newer antibiotics available for the treatment of group A streptococcal upper respiratory tract infections are more expensive than penicillin.

Several newer oral antibiotics (both cephalosporins and macrolides) have been given for less than 10 days. Reports have suggested that they may be equivalent to oral penicillin, but confirmatory studies to clearly document this are required.

There are several special situations that may require additional considerations in treating group A streptococcal upper respiratory tract infections. There are some instances in which a patient either cannot be bacteriologically "cured" or continues to contract new clinically distinct documented (by culture) group A infections. In these instances, studies have shown that antibiotics such as clindamycin (10 days); a combination of oral amoxicillin and clavulanic acid for 10 days; oral dicloxacillin given for 10 days; or intramuscular benzathine penicillin G (accompanied by 4 days of oral rifampin) may be successful.

For severe systemic group A infections, including the streptococcal toxic shock syndrome and necrotizing fasciitis, there are theoretical reasons to use clindamycin (usually intravenously), either alone or in combination with parenteral (usually intravenous) penicillin. There is little or no place for the use of oral antibiotics when the diagnosis of severe group A systemic infection has been established. When there is accompanying fasciitis or myositis, frequent and extensive surgical debridement is indicated.

Group A streptococcal impetigo or pyoderma, especially if it involves more than a few lesions, is best treated with systemic antibiotics. Penicillin V, semisynthetic penicillins, oral first-generation cephalosporins, and macrolides have been used successfully. In preliminary studies it has also been shown that intramuscular benzathine penicillin G not only eradicates existing lesions, but also provides some degree of protection against the development of new lesions for approximately 4 weeks.

Topical agents such as bacitracin ointment or mupericin have been used successfully in patients with pyoderma. Generally the place for topical therapy is limited to those with relatively few lesions on a small surface area of the body.

Supportive Therapy for Group A Streptococcal Infections

Although bed rest may sometimes be necessary during the febrile period of group A streptococcal pharyngitis, it is virtually impossible to keep most children in bed when they feel well. Acetaminophen is indicated for relieving sore throat and malaise. An adequate fluid intake should be encouraged during the febrile period. A regular diet should be offered when tolerated. The use of nonsteriodal antiinflammatory agents has been questioned in patients suspected of have systemic group A streptococcal infections.

ANTIBIOTICS FOR PREVENTION OR CURTAILMENT OF EPIDEMICS

Penicillin remains the drug of choice for secondary prevention of recurrent attacks of rheumatic fever. The widespread prophylactic use of antibiotics, specifically penicillin, to prevent streptococcal infections in epidemic conditions has been recommended. Clear-cut indications for prophylaxis for entire populations in the midst of epidemics have not been established.

In situations where there is a documented community-wide outbreak of severe streptococcal infections with sequelae, the use of widespread prophylaxis often has been successful in terminating the outbreak. Ideally the results of a throat culture should resolve the question of whether or not to treat an individual patient, but this often is not practical in a large population in an epidemic. Examples of populations in which widespread prophylaxis has been administered include schools, military populations, or other populations living in close quarters (residential facilities).

With the resurgence of severe group A streptococcal infections, questions also have been raised regarding the efficacy of prophylactic antibiotics in special situations where there has been unusually close contact with a patient with a severe infection such as streptococcal toxic shock or necrotizing fasciitis. Definitive studies are not yet available, but many physicians recommend prophylactic penicillin or a similar antibiotic (first-generation cephalosporin) for family members who are found to be culture-positive. Medical personnel who have come in close contact with a patient with this infection or with secretions should be cultured and, if positive, treated. There are those who would, in these instances, empirically treat close family or other contacts with antibiotics without obtaining a culture.

To provide long-term secondary rheumatic fever prophylaxis for prevention of recurrent attacks of rheumatic fever, regular injections of intramuscular benzathine penicillin G have proven most effective. Injections of 1,200,000 every 4 weeks are adequate in most instances. Recent data have suggested, however, that in high-risk patients or in those countries where the risk of recurrence is quite high, injections given every 3 weeks may be indicated (Lue, 1994). Although sulfadiazine can be used for secondary rheumatic fever prophylaxis, it cannot be used for treatment of group A streptococcal infections. In patients who can take neither sulfadiazine nor penicillin, erythromycin has been used successfully for secondary prevention.

The duration of secondary rheumatic fever prophylaxis varies. Usually this can be given until the patient is 18 to 21 years of age or for 5 years after the last attack, whichever is longer. However, variables such as whether or not the patient has valvular involvement and whether the patient is considered to be at "high risk" will also influence the decision.

BIBLIOGRAPHY

American Heart Association, Special Writing Group. Guidelines for the diagnosis of rheumatic fever: Jones criteria, 1992 update. JAMA 1992; 268:2069-2073.

American Heart Association. Committee on Rheumatic Fever, Endocarditis, and Kawasaki Disease. Prevention of rheumatic fever. 1995.

Anthony BF, Kaplan EL, Wannamaker LW, et al. Attack rates of acute nephritis after type 49 streptococcal infection of the skin and of the respiratory tract. J Clin Invest 1969;48:1697-1704.

Bell SM, Smith DD. Quantitative throat swab culture in the diagnosis of streptococcal pharyngitis in children. Lancet 1976; 2:61.

Bisno AL. Acute pharyngitis: etiology and diagnosis. Pediatrics 1996;97:949-954.

Breese BB, et al. Beta-hemolytic streptococcal infection: the clinical and epidemiologic importance of the number of organisms found in culture. Am J Dis Child 1972;124:352.

Burech DL, Koranyi KI, Haynes RE. Serious group A streptococcal diseases in children. J Pediatr 1976;88:972.

Coonan KM, Kaplan EL. In vitro susceptibility of recent North American group A streptococcal isolates to eleven oral antibiotics. Pediatr Infect Dis J 1994;13:630-635.

Gerber MA, Randolph MF, DeMeo KK, Kaplan EL. Lack of impact of early antibiotic therapy for streptococcal pharyngitis on recurrence rates. J Pediatr 1990;117:853-858.

Goldstein I, Rebeyotte P, Parlebas J, et al. Isolation from heart valves of glycopeptides which share immunological properties with *Streptococcus haemolyticus* group A polysaccharides. Nature 1968;219:866-868.

Hall CB, Breese BB. Does penicillin make Johnny's strep throat better? Pediatr Infect Dis J 1984;3:7-9.

Kaplan EL. The group A streptococcal upper respiratory tract carrier state: an enigma. J Pediatr 1980;97:337-345.

Kaplan EL. Benzathine penicillin for treatment of group A streptococcal pharyngitis: a reappraisal in 1985. Pediatr Infect Dis 1985;4:592-596.

Kaplan EL. The rapid identification of group A β-hemolytic streptococci of the upper respiratory tract. Pediatr Clin North Am 1988;35:535-342.

Kaplan EL. Global assessment of rheumatic fever and rheumatic heart disease at the close of the century, the influences and dynamics of population and pathogens: a failure to realize prevention? (The T. Duckett Jones Memorial Lecture). Circulation 1993;88:1964-1972.

Kaplan EL, Reid HFM, Johnson DR, Kunde CA. Rapid antigen detection in the diagnosis of group A pyoderma: influence of a "learning curve effect" on sensitivity and specificity. Pediatr Infect Dis J 1989;8:591-593.

Kaplan EL, Wannamaker LW. Suppression of the antistreptolysin O response by cholesterol and by lipid extracts of the rabbit skin. J Exp Med 1976;144:754-767.

Lancefield RC. A serological differentiation of human and other groups of hemolytic streptococci. J Exp Med 1933;57:571.

Lue HC, Wu MH, Wang JK, et al. Long-term outcome of patients with rheumatic fever receiving benzathine penicillin G prophylaxis every 3 weeks vs every 4 weeks. J Pediatr 1994;125:812-816.

Markowitz M, Gerber MA, Kaplan EL. Treatment of streptococcal pharyngotonsillitis: reports of penicillin's demise are premature. J Pediatr 1993;123:679-685.

Markowitz M, Kaplan EL. Reappearance of rheumatic fever. Adv Pediatr 1989;36:39-66.

Maxted WR. The use of bacitracin for identifying group A haemolytic streptococci. J Clin Pathol 1953;6:224.

Moody MD. Old and new techniques for rapid identification of group A streptococci. In Wannamaker LW, Matsen JM (eds). Streptococci and streptococcal diseases: recognition, understanding, management. New York: Academic Press, 1972.

Nelson JD. The effect of penicillin therapy on the symptoms and signs of streptococcal pharyngitis. Pediatr Infect Dis 1984;3:10-13.

Peter G, Smith AL. Group A streptococcal infections of the skin and pharynx. N Engl J Med 1977;297:311.

Powers GF, Boisvert PL. Age as a factor in streptococcosis. J Pediatr 1944;25:481.

Rotta J, Bednat B. Biological properties of streptococcal cell wall particles. J Exp Med 1969;130:31-45.

Smith TD, Wilkinson V, Kaplan EL. Group A streptococcus associated upper respiratory tract infections in a day-care center. Pediatrics 1989;83:380-384.

Stevens DL. Invasive group A streptococcal infections. Clin Infect Dis 1992;14:2-13.

Stevens DL. Streptococcal toxic-shock syndrome: spectrum of disease, pathogenesis, and new concepts in treatment. Emerg Infect Dis 1995;1:69-78.

Stevens DL, Tanner MH, Winship J, et al. Severe group A streptococcal infections associated with a toxic shock–like syndrome and scarlet fever toxin A. N Engl J Med 1989;321:1-7.

Stillerman M, Bernstein SH. Streptococcal pharyngitis; evaluation of clinical syndromes in diagnosis. Am J Dis Child 1961;101:476-480.

Wannamaker LW. Differences between streptococcal infections of the throat and of the skin. N Engl J Med 1970;282:23, 78.

Wannamaker LW. Perplexity and precision in the diagnosis of streptococcal pharyngitis. Am J Dis Child 1972;124:352-358.

Watson DW, Kim YB. Erythrogenic toxins. In Montic TC, Kadia S, Ajl Sj (eds). Microbial toxins. New York: Academic Press, 1970.

World Health Organization Study Group. Rheumatic fever and rheumatic heart disease. Tech Report Series No 764, Geneva, Switzerland: World Health Organization, 1988.

Zabriskie JB. The role of temperate bacteriophage in the production of erythogenic toxin by group A streptococci. J Exp Med 1964;119:761.

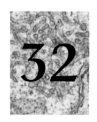

32 Tetanus (Lockjaw)

Catherine Wilfert and Peter Hotez

Clostridium tetani produces a potent, soluble exotoxin that is responsible for the clinical manifestations of tetanus. Tetanus, or "lockjaw," is an acute toxemia characterized by tonic spasms of voluntary muscles and a high fatality rate. *C. tetani* infection usually occurs at a break in the skin, which may be trivial or unrecognized, but the infection also can complicate burns; puerperal infections; infections of the umbilical stump (tetanus neonatorum); and certain surgical operations, in which the source of infection may be contaminated sutures, dressings, or plaster. The illness begins with tonic spasms of the skeletal muscles and is followed by paroxysmal contractions. The muscle stiffness involves the jaw (lockjaw) and neck first and later becomes generalized. Tetanus is a leading cause of death in childhood. The World Health Organization estimates that in 1992 there were over half a million infant deaths resulting from neonatal tetanus in developing countries.

ETIOLOGY

The tetanus bacillus is a long, thin (2 to 5 μm × 3 to 8 μm), motile, gram-positive anaerobic rod. Older cultures of these organisms and smears from wounds frequently stain as gram-negative microbes, and this result may be confusing to the uninitiated. These organisms may develop a terminal spore that does not take the Gram stain and gives the bacterium a drumstick appearance. The spores are very resistant to heat and the usual antiseptics, and they may persist in tissues for many months in a viable, although dormant, state. Under anaerobic conditions the organisms are easily isolated on blood agar or in cooked meat broth. The organism does not ferment carbohydrates, does not usually liquify gelatin, and produces little change in litmus milk.

The bacilli are widely distributed in soil; street dust; and the feces of some horses, sheep, cattle,

dogs, cats, rats, guinea pigs, and chickens. Consequently, manure-containing soil may be highly infectious. In agricultural areas a significant number of normal human adults may harbor the organisms, and agricultural workers have a higher incidence of infection. The spores have also been found in contaminated heroin.

Tetanus bacilli produce a potent neurotoxin that is one of the most toxic substances known; the mouse LD_{50} of highly purified preparations is between 0.1 and 1 ng/kg (Schiavo et al., 1995). Tetanus neurotoxin derives its potency by virtue of its absolute specificity for neuronal cells and its target intracellular catalytic activity. It resembles other clostridial neurotoxins in that the molecule is synthesized as a single inactive polypeptide chain of 150 kDa without a leader sequence: release of the neurotoxin occurs as a consequence of bacterial lysis in the host. Exposure and cleavage of a protease-sensitive loop within the molecule generates an active heterodimer composed of a 100-kDa heavy chain and a 50-kDa light chain joined by a disulfide bond. New evidence suggests that the light chain is catalytically active as a zinc metalloprotease. Once inside the host target cell the metalloprotease decreases specific protein components of the host neuroexocytosis apparatus. The major protease substrates are membrane proteins of synaptic vesicles, including synaptobrevin (also called VAMP), SNAP-25, and syntaxin.

PATHOGENESIS

The portal of entry is usually the site of a minor puncture wound or scratch, and the organism can proliferate only if the oxidation-reduction (Eh) potential is lower than that of normal living tissues. Deep puncture wounds, burns, and crush or other injuries that promote favorable conditions for the growth of anerobic organisms may be followed by tetanus. Occasionally, no apparent portal of entry

501

can be found. Under these circumstances the site of infection may have been the alimentary tract.

When conditions are favorable, the bacilli multiply at the site of primary inoculation and produce toxin. Toxin then travels centripetally in the axoplasm of the alpha motor fibers and accumulates in the motor neurons in the membrane-bound endoplasmic reticulum. Marie and Morax proposed this route of access of toxin to the central nervous system in 1902, as did Meyer and Ransome in 1903. It was shown experimentally that toxin was not lethal if the local motor nerves were severed. Toxin is neutralizable when it is free and is only partially neutralizable when it is on the cell surface. Pinocytosis, internalizing the toxin, renders it nonneutralizable. Thus fixation of toxin to nerves and its internalization result in irreversible effects. Cleavage of host neuronal cell membrane proteins by the catalytically active neurotoxin results in a persistent and sustained blockade of neuroexocytosis. The neuronal blockade then results in the uncontrolled spread of impulses, hyperreflexia, and constant muscle contraction. The strongest muscles, usually extensors, exert the greatest effects. The toxin also affects the sympathetic nervous system.

PATHOLOGY

There are no specific pathologic lesions caused by the infectious agent or toxin. Secondary effects of the muscular contractions may include vertebral fractures, pneumonia, and hemorrhages into the muscles.

CLINICAL MANIFESTATIONS

The incubation period is variable, with the usual range 5 to 14 days; however, it may be as short as 1 day or as long as 3 or more weeks. The appearance of the site of infection, if obvious, provides no clue to the impending toxemia. The disease begins insidiously, with progressively increasing stiffness of the voluntary muscles; generally, the muscles of the jaw and neck are involved first. Within 24 to 48 hours after the onset of the disease, rigidity may be fully developed and may spread rapidly to involve the trunk and extremities. With spasm of the jaw muscles, trismus (lockjaw) develops. The wrinkling of the forehead and distortion of the eyebrows, and the angles of the mouth produce a peculiar facial appearance called *risus sardonicus* (sardonic grin). The neck and back become stiff and arched (opisthotonos). The abdominal wall is boardlike, and the extremities are usually stiff and extended.

Painful paroxysmal spasms that persist for a few seconds or several minutes may be provoked by the most trivial kind of visual, auditory, or cutaneous stimuli, such as bright lights, sudden noises, and movement of the patient. Risus sardonicus and opisthotonos are most marked during these spasms. Initially the spasms occur at infrequent intervals, with complete relaxation between attacks. Later the spasms occur more often and are more prolonged and more painful. Involvement of the muscles of respiration, laryngeal obstruction caused by laryngospasm, or accumulation of secretions in the tracheobronchial tree may be followed by respiratory distress, asphyxia, coma, and death. Involvement of the bladder sphincter leads to urinary retention.

The manifestations of sympathetic nervous system involvement may include labile hypertension, tachycardia, peripheral vasoconstriction, cardiac arrhythmias, profuse sweating, hypercapnia, increased urinary excretion of catecholamines, and late-appearing hypotension.

During the illness the patient's sensorium is usually clear. The fever is generally low grade or absent. Patients who recover are usually afebrile. After a period of weeks the paroxysms decrease in frequency and severity and gradually disappear. Generally, the trismus is the last symptom to subside. Patients with fatal disease are usually febrile, with death occurring in most instances before the tenth day of illness.

The spinal fluid in patients with tetanus is normal. The peripheral white blood cell count may be normal or slightly elevated. Most patients with tetanus show the generalized manifestations described previously. Occasionally, however, generalized tetanus may be preceded by cephalic tetanus. In this case the incubation period is only 1 to 2 days; it follows a head injury or otitis media, and the patient has a poor prognosis (Bagratuni, 1952). This form of tetanus is characterized by involvement of various cranial nerves, especially the seventh, but the third, fourth, ninth, tenth, and twelfth may be affected also. Cephalic tetanus can occur without subsequent generalized disease.

Tetanus Neonatorum

The onset of tetanus neonatorum usually begins when the newborn infant is 3 to 10 days old and is manifested by difficulty in sucking and by excessive crying. Soon the infant's jaw becomes too stiff to suck, and the baby has difficulty swallowing. Shortly thereafter, stiffness of the body appears, and intermittent jerking spasms may begin. Variable degrees of trismus; sustained, tonic, or rigid states of muscle contraction; and spasms or convulsions occur. The spasms occur spontaneously or in response to stimuli with variable frequency. Deep-tendon reflex activity may be increased, or the deep tendons may show no response during testing because of constant generalized stiffness. Opisthotonos may be absent or so extreme that the head almost touches the heels. The cry varies from a repeated, short, mildly hoarse cry to a strangled-sounding voiceless noise. The patient's color may be normal, cyanotic, or pale from hypoxia and impending shock. Severe spasms may be followed by flaccidity, anoxia, and exhaustion.

■ **Case 1 F.F.,** a 13-day-old male infant, was brought to Children's Hospital of Los Angeles with respiratory arrest. The infant was born at another hospital to a gravida 5, para 5 mother. On the second day of life, the patient left the other hospital. On the tenth day the umbilical stump fell off and purulent drainage was observed at the site. On the thirteenth day the infant had trismus, was irritable, and refused feedings. On the morning of the fourteenth day, the day of admission to Children's Hospital, the infant was febrile, his body was rigid, his respirations were noisy, and he was drooling. He had frequent spasms of the extremities and the body triggered by external stimuli. The mouth was locked in an open position. Respirations were shallow, and an inspiratory rattle was heard that was suggestive of laryngospasm.

Gram-positive rods and spores were present in pus from the umbilicus. Treatment included tetanus antitoxin (human); surgical debridement of the umbilical stump; tracheostomy; reduction of environmental stimuli; and the use of diazepam (Valium), meprobamate, phenobarbital, thorazines, penicillin, and kanamycin. The infant received feedings by gavage, and the bladder was emptied by Credé's method.

The patient's condition improved steadily. Spasms decreased in frequency and stopped altogether after 4 weeks. The use of medications was also discontinued and the patient was discharged after 48 days in the hospital.

■ **Case 2 G.B.,** a 16-year-old white female, was admitted to Duke University Medical Center (DUMC), N.C. in March 1991 because of jaw tightness, tongue rolling, and neck stiffness of 1 day's duration. Approximately 3 weeks before admission a rusty fishhook had been caught in her scalp. She had received no immunizations for the past 10 years. The referring physician recognized trismus, opisthotonos, and risus sardonicus. He administered tetanus immune globulin, intubated her, and transported her to DUMC. Her temperature was 36.1° C (97° F); pulse, 35; respirations, 16; and blood pressure, 125/60.

She was sedated and paralyzed with pancuronium (Pavulon). She required respirator-assisted ventilation for 10 days, and she received parenteral penicillin, tetanus immune globulin, and tetanus toxoid. No bacterial pathogens were identified, and there was no wound to culture. She recovered completely and was discharged 17 days after admission.

DIAGNOSIS

The development of trismus, risus sardonicus, generalized tonic rigidity, and spasms in a patient with a clear sensorium and a recent history of trauma is highly suggestive of a diagnosis of tetanus. The recovery of *C. tetani* from the wound confirms the diagnosis; however, in most instances the organism is not detected.

DIFFERENTIAL DIAGNOSIS
Side Reaction to Phenothiazines

Among the extrapyramidal neurologic syndromes that may accompany the use of some phenothiazine drugs are acute dystonic reactions, with facial grimacing; torticollis; and muscle rigidity. They disappear with discontinuation of the drug.

Tetany

In patients with tetany, trismus is usually absent, but carpopedal spasms and laryngospasm may be present. A low blood calcium content confirms the diagnosis.

Peritonsillar Abscess

This febrile painful condition is usually accompanied by trismus. However, there are no generalized muscular spasms.

Encephalitis

Patients with viral and postinfectious encephalitides rarely have trismus, do not have clear minds as a rule, and usually have abnormal spinal fluid findings.

Rabies

Continuous tonic seizures are not present in patients with rabies; the seizures are usually intermittent and clonic. Trismus is rarely observed.

Strychnine Poisoning

Relaxation between convulsions is usually complete in patients with strychnine poisoning. When trismus occurs, it occurs late.

COMPLICATIONS

The interference with pulmonary ventilation by laryngospasm, respiratory muscle spasm, or accumulation of secretions may be followed by pneumonia and atelectasis. Vertebral compression fractures and lacerations of the tongue may follow a seizure.

PROGNOSIS

Tetanus remains a very serious disease. The declines in incidence (Fig. 32-1) and mortality rate of tetanus over the past two decades have been parallel, resulting in minor changes in the case fatality rate. In patients who survive, recovery is complete—without sequelae if supportive measures have provided adequate ventilation. The prognosis is significantly affected by the following factors.

Age

The highest mortality rate is found among patients in the extremes of life. For neonates the case fatality rate is 66%, and for persons 50 years of age or older it is 70%. In contrast, for patients 10 to 19 years old, the case fatality rate is 10% to 20%.

Incubation Period

The median incubation period of fatal and nonfatal tetanus cases with known wounds was 6.2 and 7.6 days, respectively, in 1968 and 1969. Christie (1969) believes that a more reliable guide to the prognosis is the length of the period of onset, defined as the interval between the first evidence of trismus and the first generalized convulsion. If this period is shorter than 48 hours, the attack probably will be severe; if the interval is longer, the illness will be milder. Nevertheless, the course of tetanus cannot be predicted until the severity and frequency of the convulsions have been made clear. It is easy to be misled in the first day or two.

Fever

In mild or moderately severe cases of tetanus, fever is not a common finding. In patients with involvement of the brain stem, fever or hyperpyrexia is often present. Afebrile patients have a better chance of recovery.

Extent of Involvement

In patients with local tetanus the symptoms are confined to the wound area, and the prognosis is usually good. Generalized involvement, however, is followed by a more serious outcome. The only manifestation of tetanus that correlates significantly with a poorer prognosis is convulsion, but this association applies only to patients less than 20 years old.

Antitoxin Therapy

In general, antitoxin therapy does not significantly affect the prognosis. Toxin usually has been fixed and is not available for neutralization. However, antitoxin may modify the disease if it is given during the incubation period or very early in the course of the illness.

EPIDEMIOLOGIC FACTORS

Tetanus is worldwide in distribution. Reported tetanus in the United States from 1955 to 1989 is shown in Fig. 32-1. The spores are widely disseminated in soil and in animal feces. Tetanus spores or toxin can contaminate a variety of biologic and surgical products, such as vaccines, sera, and catgut. Unimmunized persons of all ages and both sexes are equally susceptible. In spite of the ubiquity of *C. tetani*, tetanus is a relatively rare occurrence, but tetanus neonatorum is still a serious problem in de-

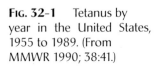

FIG. 32-1 Tetanus by year in the United States, 1955 to 1989. (From MMWR 1990; 38:41.)

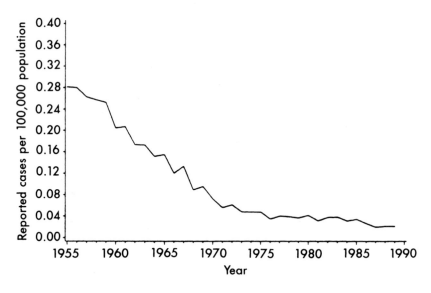

veloping countries, where it is the cause of between 8% and 69% of neonatal mortality. Southern Asia and sub-Saharan Africa are especially affected. In India, neonatal tetanus is, after septicemia, the leading cause of neonatal mortality. An estimated 1 million newborns contract tetanus each year, of which approximately 800,000 die. Community-based surveys have identified risk factors for neonatal tetanus, including the omission of maternal tetanus toxoid immunization during pregnancy, home delivery, unhygienic cutting of the umbilical cord, the application of an unhygienic dressing to the umbilical stump, and a history of neonatal tetanus after an earlier delivery (Galazka and Gasse, 1995). Thus the disease can be prevented in newborns by immunizing pregnant women and increasing the proportion of deliveries that are attended by trained individuals. In fact, with available tools of modern aseptic technique and active immunization, tetanus is a disease that could be eliminated. The World Health Organization estimates that in 1992 immunization and clean delivery practices prevented 686,000 neonatal deaths from tetanus (Glazka and Gasse, 1995). Many of these efforts were achieved through the Expanded Programme on Immunization (EPI).

IMMUNITY

It is estimated that 0.01 U of antibody to *C. tetani* toxin in serum is protective in humans. Maternal IgG antibodies, if present, are transmitted through the placenta. This passively acquired immunity is, however, of short duration, since maternal globulins are metabolized by the infant. The administration of tetanus toxoid to infants, children, and adults stimulates the production of antibodies that provide protection against the effects of toxin. This protective level can be maintained by periodic booster injections. Patients recovering from tetanus should be actively immunized because the extremely potent toxin may not stimulate an antibody response in the patient.

TREATMENT
Control of Muscular Spasms

The patient should be admitted to a quiet, darkened room where all possible auditory, visual, tactile, or other stimuli are reduced to a minimum. The first priority in the management of muscular spasms should be the administration of appropriate drugs to reduce the number and severity of spasms.

Diazepam is a valuable drug because it effectively controls spasms and hypertonicity without depressing the cortical centers. The recommended dosage for infants under 2 years of age is 8 mg per kilogram of body weight per day given in doses of 2 to 3 mg every 3 hours. Alternatively, an initial dose of 0.1 to 0.2 mg/kg, intravenously (IV), is used to relieve an acute spasm, followed by a continuous IV infusion of 15 to 40 mg/kg/day (Gerdes, 1995). As the patient improves, less drug is needed. The drug should be given orally when tolerated. Phenobarbital and morphine may also be used as an adjunctive therapy, with the understanding that it be administered only in a controlled, intensive setting because of the risk of apnea.

Antitoxin Therapy

After adequate sedation has been achieved, human tetanus immune globulin (TIG) should be given in a single dose (3000 to 6000 U, intramuscularly). Lower doses of 500 U may be appropriate for tetanus neonatorum. If human immune globulin is unavailable, equine tetanus antitoxin should be given if the sensitivity reactions to horse serum are negative. The antitoxin is given intravenously and intramuscularly, half the dose through each route. For neonates it may be necessary to delay active immunization with tetanus toxoid for 4 to 6 weeks following the administration of TIG.

Antimicrobial Therapy

It is recommended that aqueous penicillin G be given in a dosage of 100,000 U/kg/day, given at 4- to 6-hour intervals. Therapy for 10 to 14 days is recommended. Penicillin is effective against the vegetative form of the tetanus bacillus and kills growing bacteria, thus stopping toxin production. Penicillin does not alter the effects of existing toxin. Tetracycline (2 g daily [adult dose]) may be used if the patient is sensitive to penicillin.

Surgical Treatment

After the patient has been sedated and has received antitoxin, any wound should be thoroughly cleansed and débrided. Extensive surgical excision is usually not indicated.

Supportive Treatment

Good medical and nursing care must minimize stimuli that may precipitate a convulsion. Procedures such as catheterization or placement of indwelling lines should be carried out at a time when any sedative is exerting its maximal effect. Such procedures preferably are performed early in the course of clinical illness. In addition, care should be taken to anticipate and prevent complications such as aspiration pneumonia, lower-bowel obstruction resulting from fecal impaction, urinary retention, and decubitus ulcers. Adequate sedation may prevent a compression fracture of the vertebra. Respiratory support is essential, and intubation or tracheostomy with respirator ventilation may be required. High-quality intensive care during the first week (i.e., early intubation, mechanical ventilation, and neuromuscular blockade [pancuronium or its equivalent]) is an essential component of the management of a neonate with tetanus.

Tracheostomy

The combination of heavy sedation, difficulty in swallowing, laryngospasm, and accumulation of secretions leads to obstruction of the airway. A relatively low mortality rate of 10% was reported by Edmondson and Flowers (1979), who treated 100 patients with tetanus on an intensive care unit. Intubation can be lifesaving.

PREVENTIVE MEASURES
Active Immunization

Since many cases of tetanus follow minor abrasions and lacerations that are ignored, control of the disease can best be achieved by active immunization with toxoid before exposure. All infants should be immunized routinely with tetanus toxoid that is incorporated with diphtheria toxoid and pertussis vaccine. The usual basic series of the triple antigen is given at 8-week intervals for 3 doses, beginning at 2 to 4 months of age. A fourth dose, either of DTaP or DTP, is recommended 6 to 12 months after the third dose, usually at 15 to 18 months of age. A fifth dose of DTaP or DTP is given before school entry (elementary school) at 4 to 6 years of age, unless the fourth dose was given after the fourth birthday. After the initial immunization series is completed, a booster dose of tetanus toxoid should be given intramuscularly every 10 years. Since 1987 the World Health Organization has recommended active immunization for all women of childbearing age living in less developed countries.

In the event of an injury, administration of an additional booster dose of tetanus toxoid may be indicated; a protective antitoxin level is usually achieved within 1 week. It is common practice to use Td instead of tetanus toxoid alone in a child 7 years or older, so that adequate levels of diphtheria immunity are also maintained. Children younger than 7 years should receive either DTP or DTaP (unless pertussis vaccine is contraindicated). A

booster dose can provoke an adequate response after a 10-year lapse since the last injection. In severe, crush, and heavily contaminated wounds (particularly, compound skull fractures), human tetanus immune globulin (250 U) should be given intramuscularly in conjunction with the toxoid. This procedure should prevent a potential short–incubation period disease. Patients recovering from tetanus may not be immune; therefore they should be actively immunized with tetanus toxoid.

Passive Immunization

Persons who have not been actively immunized should be protected with human TIG in the event of an injury. Although the usual dose is 250 U given intramuscularly, patients with severe wounds may need 500 U.

Care of a Wound

A wound should be cleansed thoroughly, foreign bodies and necrotic tissues should be removed, and the area should be debrided when indicated.

BIBLIOGRAPHY

Adams JM, Kenny JD, Rudolph AJ. Modern management of tetanus neonatum. Pediatrics 1979;64:472.

Armitage P, Clifford R. Prognosis in tetanus: use of data from therapeutic trials. J Infect Dis 1978;138:1-8.

Bagratuni L. Cephalic tetanus: with report of a case. Br Med J 1952;1:461.

Bizzini B. Tetanus toxin. Microbiol Rev 1979;43:224-240.

Bjerregaard P, Steinglass R, Mutie DM, et al. Neonatal tetanus mortality in coastal Kenya: a community survey. Int J Epidemiol 1993;22:163-169.

Brand DA, Acampora D, Gottlieb ZD, et al. Adequacy of antitetanus prophylaxis in six hospital emergency rooms. N Engl J Med 1983;309:636-640.

Brooks VB, Asanuma H. Action of tetanus toxin in the cerebral cortex. Science 1962;137:674.

Brooks VB, Curtis DR, Eccles JC. Mode of action of tetanus toxin. Nature 1955;175:120.

Christie AB. Infectious diseases: epidemiology and clinical practice. Baltimore: Williams & Wilkins, 1969.

Corradin G, Watts C. Cellular immunology of tetanus toxoid. Curr Top Microbiol Immunol 1995;195:77-87.

Edmondson RS, Flowers MW. Intensive care in tetanus: management, complications, and mortality in 100 cases. Br Med J 1979;1:1401.

Edsall G. Specific prophylaxis of tetanus. JAMA 1959;171:417.

Edsall G. Passive immunization. Pediatrics 1963;32:599.

Eidels L, Proia RL, Hart DA. Membrane receptors for bacterial toxins. Microbiol Rev 1983;47:596-620.

Einterz EM, Bates ME. Caring for neonatal tetanus patients in a rural primary care setting in Nigeria: a review of 237 cases. J Trop Pediatr 1991;37:179-181.

Galazka A, Gasse F. The present status of tetanus and tetanus vaccination. Curr Top Microbiol Immunol 1995;195:31-53.

Gerdes JS. Tetanus neonatorum. In Burg FD, Ingelfinger JR, Wald ER, Polin RA (eds). Gellis & Kagan's Current Pediatric Therapy, ed 15. Philadelphia: W.B. Saunders, 1996.

Goyal RK, Neogy CN, Mathur GP. A controlled trial of anti-serum in the treatment of tetanus. Lancet 1966;2:1371.

Hlady WG, Bennett JV, Samadi AR, et al. Neonatal tetanus in rural Bangladesh: risk factors and toxoid efficacy. Am J Public Health 1992;82:1365-1369.

Kaeser HE, Sauer A. Tetanus toxin: a neuromuscular blocking agent. Nature 1969;223:842.

Kerr JH, et al. Involvement of the sympathetic nervous system in tetanus: studies on 82 cases. Lancet 1968;2:236.

Kessimer JG, Habig WH, Hardegree MC. Monoclonal antibodies as probes of tetanus toxin structure and function. Infect Immun 1983;42:942-948.

Laird WJ, Aronson W, Silver RP, et al. Plasmid-associated toxigenicity in *Clostridium tetani*. J Infect Dis 1980;142:623.

Levine L, Edsall G. Tetanus toxoid: what determines reaction proneness? J Infect Dis 1981;144:376.

Looney JM, Edsall G, Ispen J Jr, Chasen WH. Persistence of antitoxin levels after tetanus toxoid inoculation in adults and effects of a booster dose after intervals. N Engl J Med 1956;254:6.

Marie A, Morax V. Recherches sur l'absorption de la toxine tetanique. Ann Inst Pasteur 1902;16:818.

McCracken GH Jr, Dowell DL, Marshall FN. Double-blind trial of equine antitoxin and human immune globulin in tetanus neonatorum. Lancet 1971;1:1146.

Meyer H, Ransome F. Untersuchungen uber den Tetanus. Arch Exp Pathol Pharmakol 1903;49:369.

Pratt EL. Clinical tetanus: a study of 56 cases, with special reference to methods of prevention and a plan for evaluating treatment. JAMA 1945;129:1243.

Rubbo SD, Suri JC. Passive immunization against tetanus with human immune globulin. Br Med J 1962;2:79.

Rubinstein HM. Studies on human tetanus antitoxin. Am J Hyg 1962;76:276.

Schiavo G, Rossetto O, Tonello F, Montecucco C. Intracellular targets and metalloprotease activity of tetanus and botulism neurotoxins. Curr Top Microbiol Immunol 1995;195:257-274.

Smolens J, Vogt A, Crawford MN, Stokes J Jr. The persistence in the human circulation of horse and human tetanus antitoxins. J Pediatr 1961;59:899.

Stanfield JP, Gall D, Braden PM. Single dose-antenatal tetanus immunization. Lancet 1973;1:215.

Veronesi R. Clinical observations on 712 cases of tetanus subject to four different methods of treatment: 18.2 percent mortality rate under a new method of treatment. Am J Med Sci 1956;232:629.

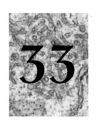

33   TICK–BORNE INFECTIONS

EUGENE D. SHAPIRO

Infections recognized as being transmitted by ticks in the United States have been increasing in both number and importance (Spach et al., 1993; Fishbein and Dennis, 1995). They include infections that have long been recognized, such as Rocky Mountain spotted fever and tick-borne relapsing fever, as well as "emerging" infections such as Lyme disease, ehrlichiosis, and babesiosis. A number of viruses—notably Powassan virus and the virus that causes Colorado tick fever in the United States, the virus that causes Congo-Crimean hemorrhagic fever in Africa, and the virus that causes tick-borne encephalitis in central Europe—also are transmitted by ticks. These viral illnesses are not covered in this chapter.

LYME DISEASE

Lyme disease is the most common vector-borne disease in the United States. Extensive publicity about the illness in the lay press, which at times has been accompanied by near-hysteria about its risks and its complications, has resulted in anxiety about the illness (among physicians, as well as patients and parents) that is out of proportion to the morbidity that it causes (Aronowitz, 1991). The clinical manifestations of Lyme borreliosis are protean. This fact, coupled with the practical difficulties of confirming the diagnosis in many patients, has led to many misconceptions about the symptoms of Lyme disease and the prognosis for patients who have it. These misconceptions are reinforced by a high frequency of misdiagnosis of Lyme disease in people with symptoms caused by other conditions.

Etiology and Epidemiology

Lyme disease is caused by the spirochete *Borrelia burgdorferi,* a fastidious, microaerophilic bacterium that replicates very slowly and requires special, complex media for in vitro growth (Burgdorfer et al., 1982; Benach et al., 1983; Steere et al.,

1983). *B. burgdorferi* is transmitted by ticks of the Ixodes species. In the United States the common vectors are *Ixodes scapularis* (the black-legged tick; commonly called the deer tick) in both the Northeast and the upper Midwest and *Ixodes pacificus* on the Pacific Coast (Steere et al., 1977). *Ixodes scapularis* was formerly known as *Ixodes dammini.* (Recent evidence indicated that *I. dammini* was actually identical to the previously described *I. scapularis.*)

The life cycle of *I. scapularis* consists of three stages—larva, nymph, and adult—that develop during a 2-year period (Lane et al., 1991). The adult female lays eggs in the spring. The larvae emerge in the early summer. Most larvae (98%) are born uninfected with *B. burgdorferi,* because transovarial transmission rarely occurs. The larvae feed on a wide variety of small mammals, such as *Peromyscus leucopus* (the white-footed mouse), which is a natural reservoir for *B. burgdorferi.* A deer tick may become infected with *B. burgdorferi* by feeding on a mouse or another small mammal that is infected with the spirochete. The tick emerges the following spring as a nymph. In this stage the tick (if it is infected with *B. burgdorferi*) may transmit the infection to humans. Alternatively, if the nymph is uninfected with *B. burgdorferi,* it may subsequently become infected if it feeds on an infected host. The nymphs molt in the late summer or fall and then reemerge as adults. If the adult is infected, it also may transmit *B. burgdorferi* to humans. The female spends the winter on an animal host, a favorite being white-tailed deer (hence its name, the deer tick). In the spring the females lay their eggs and die, thereby completing the 2-year life cycle.

There are a number of factors associated with the risk of transmission of *B. burgdorferi* from ticks to humans. First, a tick has to be infected to be able to transmit the organism. The proportion of infected ticks varies greatly both by geographic area and by the life-cycle stage of the tick. *I. pacificus* often feeds on lizards, which are not a competent reservoir for *B. burgdorferi*. Consequently, only 1% to 3% of these ticks, even in the nymphal and adult stages, are infected with *B. burgdorferi*. As a result, Lyme disease is rare in the Pacific states. In contrast, *I. scapularis* feeds on small mammals that are competent reservoirs for *B. burgdorferi*. As a result, in highly endemic areas the rates of infection for different stages of deer ticks are approximately 2% for larvae, 15% to 30% for nymphs, and 30% to 50% for adults.

B. burgdorferi is transmitted when an infected tick inoculates saliva into the blood vessels of the skin of its host. The risk of transmission of *B. burgdorferi* from infected deer ticks has been shown to be related to the duration of feeding. It takes hours for the mouth parts of ticks to implant fully in the host, and much longer (days) for the tick to become fully engorged. Experiments with animals have shown that infected nymphal-stage ticks must feed for 36 to 48 hours or longer and infected adult ticks must feed for 48 to 72 hours or longer before the risk of transmission of *B. burgdorferi* becomes substantial (Piesman et al., 1987, 1991; Piesman, 1993). Approximately 75% of persons who recognize that they have been bitten by a deer tick remove the tick <48 hours after it has begun to feed (Falco et al., 1996). This is an important part of the reason that only a small proportion of persons who recognize that they have been bitten by deer ticks subsequently develop Lyme disease.

There is substantial evidence that the risk of Lyme disease after a recognized deer tick bite, even in hyperendemic areas, does not exceed 1% to 2% (Shapiro et al., 1992). Although some argue in favor of antimicrobial prophylaxis for persons with bites associated with high risk (e.g., a nymphal-stage tick that has fed for >48 hours), estimates of the duration of feeding by patients are unreliable (Schwartz et al., 1993). Selective treatment of persons with "high-risk" tick bites assumes that the species, stage, and degree of engorgement of the ticks can be readily ascertained, which usually is not the case—special training and equipment are necessary. Many "ticks" are actually spiders, lice, scabs, or dirt, and thus they cannot transmit Lyme disease. Moreover, since only 20% to 30% of nymphal-stage ticks are likely to be infected even in areas with the highest incidence of Lyme disease, most bites will not result in Lyme disease,

even if the tick feeds to repletion. The risk may be higher for unrecognized bites since it is likely that, in this circumstance, the tick may feed for a longer time.

Ascertainment of whether the tick is infected using tests such as the polymerase chain reaction (PCR) is not useful. Although testing ticks with PCR may provide important epidemiologic information, the predictive values for infection of humans of either a positive or a negative PCR is unknown. The test may be positive even if only very few organisms are present, and it provides no information about the duration of feeding, both of which are key determinants of the risk of transmission. In addition, the test's validity is limited by problems of false-positive tests resulting from contamination with amplification products and false-negative tests resulting from inhibition of the PCR by substances (such as blood) in the sample.

Although Lyme disease occurs throughout the world, most cases occur in certain highly endemic areas. In the United States, most cases occur in southern New England, New York, New Jersey, Pennsylvania, Minnesota, and Wisconsin (see Fig. 33-1) (Centers for Disease Control, 1996). In Europe, most cases occur in the Scandinavian countries and in central Europe (especially in Germany, Austria, and Switzerland), although cases have been reported from throughout the region.

Although there has been an increase in frequency and an expansion of the geographic distribution of Lyme disease in the United States in recent years, the incidence of Lyme disease even in endemic areas varies substantially from region to region and within local areas (White et al., 1991; Dennis, 1991). Information about the incidence of the disease is complicated by reliance, in most instances, on passive reporting of cases, as well as by the high frequency of misdiagnosis of the disease. Furthermore, studies have indicated that 30% to 50% of patients who develop serologic evidence of recent infection with *B. burgdorferi* are asymptomatic (Hanrahan et al., 1984; Steere et al., 1986).

In 1995, 11,603 cases of Lyme disease were reported to the Centers for Disease Control by 43 states and the District of Columbia, which was the second highest number reported since surveillance began in 1982 (though it was an 11% decrease from the 13,043 cases reported in 1994) (see Fig. 33-2) (Centers for Disease Control, 1996). More than 75% of the reported cases occurred in just 63 counties (see Fig. 33-3).

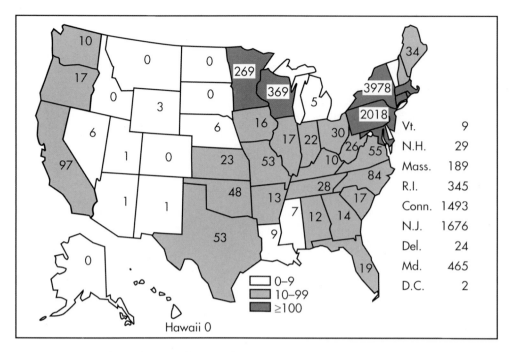

Fig. 33-1 Number of reported Lyme disease cases, by state—United States, 1995. (From MMWR 1996; 45[23]:483.)

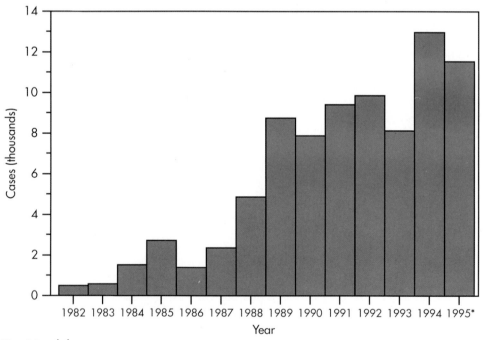

*Provisional data.

Fig. 33-2 Number of reported Lyme disease cases by year—United States, 1982-1995. (From MMWR 1996; 45[23]:482.)

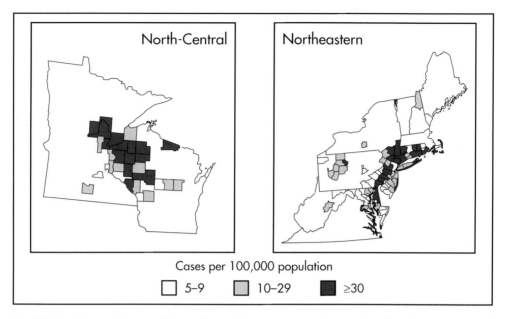

FIG. 33-3   Reported rates of Lyme disease, by county—north-central and northeastern United States, 1995. Excludes counties with fewer than five reported cases. (From MMWR 1996; 45[23]:483.)

Clinical Manifestations

Lyme disease generally is divided into three clinical stages: early localized disease, early disseminated disease, and late disease (Steere, 1989). The first clinical manifestation of Lyme disease is the typical annular rash at the site of the bite, erythema migrans (Fig. 33-4). Although it usually occurs 7 to 14 days after the bite, the onset of the rash has been reported from 3 to 32 days later. The initial lesion occurs at the site of the bite. The rash most often is uniformly erythematous, although it may appear as a target lesion with variable degrees of central clearing. Occasionally there may be a vesicular or necrotic center. The rash may be itchy, painful, or asymptomatic. There may or may not be associated systemic symptoms such as fever, myalgia, headache, or malaise. Untreated, the rash gradually expands to an average diameter of 15 cm, although lesions larger than 30 cm can occur. Without treatment it will remain present for 2 weeks or longer.

A substantial proportion of children with Lyme disease (about one third) develop early disseminated disease, the most common manifestation of which is multiple erythema migrans, which is a consequence of bacteremia with dissemination of organisms to multiple sites in the skin. Secondary lesions usually are smaller than the primary lesion and are often accompanied by fever, myalgia, headache, and fatigue; conjunctivitis and lymphadenopathy also may develop. Occasionally, when the erythema migrans rash resolves, new evanescent lesions, which usually are small (1 to 3 cm) erythematous annular lesions, appear transiently over a period of several weeks at different sites. Aseptic meningitis may occur (about 1% of patients). Carditis, usually marked by varying degrees of heart block, also may occur at this stage of Lyme disease, although it is rare (<1% of patients).

Focal neurologic involvement, particularly cranioneuropathy, also is a manifestation of this stage of the illness. Paralysis of the seventh cranial nerve is relatively common in children (3% to 5% of patients) and may be the only manifestation of Lyme disease. Paralysis usually lasts from 2 to 8 weeks before it resolves completely. Rarely, palsy resolves only partially or not at all. There is no evidence that the clinical course of the facial palsy is affected by antimicrobial treatment (the goal of treatment of affected children is to treat or to prevent other manifestations of Lyme disease). Radiculoneuritis, manifest as radicular pain with motor and sensory abnormalities of peripheral nerves, has been reported, although it is more common among adults and in Europe.

The usual manifestation of late Lyme disease (which occurs in about 7% of patients) is oligoarticular arthritis; it usually occurs months after the initial infection. The large joints, especially the knee (which is affected in more than 90% of cases), are usually involved (Eichenfield et al., 1986). Al-

Rocky Mountain Spotted Fever (RMSF)—by year, United States, 1965-1995

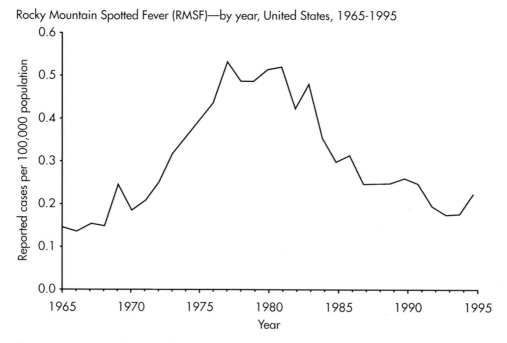

FIG. 33-4 Reported cases of Rocky Mountain spotted fever (RMSF) by year—United States, 1965-1995. (Centers for Disease Control. MMWR 1995; 44(53):52.)

though the affected joint is swollen and tender, the patient usually does not experience the exquisite pain that is typical of acute bacterial arthritis. Joint swelling usually resolves within 1 to 2 weeks (although it may last for several weeks) before recurring (in virtually all untreated patients), often in other joints. After treatment is begun, the arthritis usually abates over 4 to 7 days, although in some patients it may take 2 to 6 weeks before the symptoms completely resolve. Rarely, arthritis recurs in treated patients, but it usually resolves with retreatment. Chronic arthritis can occur, primarily among patients with DR-2, DR-3, or DR-4 HLA-types (Steere et al., 1990). The pathogenesis of this chronic, recurrent arthritis is most likely autoimmune (Nocton et al., 1994). Late manifestations of Lyme disease of the central nervous system rarely have been reported in children.

In the largest prospective study of children with Lyme disease that has been reported (a community-based study of 201 children with Lyme disease in Connecticut who were enrolled from April 1992 to November, 1993), the median age of the children was 7 years (Gerber et al., 1996). The initial (presenting) manifestations of Lyme disease in these children were single erythema migrans (66%), multiple erythema migrans (23%), arthritis (7%), facial palsy (3%), aseptic meningitis (1%), and

carditis (0.5%). Erythema migrans was more likely to occur on either the head or neck in younger children and on the extremities in older children, a finding similar to those reported from Europe. As in studies of primarily adults, only about one third of the children with a single erythema migrans rash had positive serologic results for *B. burgdorferi* at the time of presentation, whereas almost 90% of the children with multiple erythema migrans were seropositive. Of the patients with a single erythema migrans rash, 45% had had a recognized tick bite in the preceding month, but in only about half of these children was the recognized bite at the site of the rash (which indicates that the infection was transmitted by a different, unrecognized tick).

Congenital Lyme Disease

Because clinical syndromes caused by congenital infection have been recognized with other spirochetal infections such as syphilis, there has been concern about the possible transmission of *B. burgdorferi* from an infected pregnant woman to her fetus. Although case reports have been published in which *B. burgdorferi* has been identified from abortuses and from a few live-born children with congenital anomalies, the placentas, the abortuses, and the tissues from affected children in which the spirochete was identified did not show histologic evidence of inflammation. In addition, no consistent pattern of congenital malformations (as would be expected in a "syndrome" caused by congenital infection) has been identified. In two small longitudinal studies of pregnant women who developed Lyme disease that were conducted by the CDC, and in another conducted in the Czech Republic, the occasional adverse outcomes that occurred (such as spontaneous abortion) could not be attributed to infection with *B. burgdorferi*. In addition, two serosurveys conducted in endemic areas found no difference in the prevalence of congenital malformations between the offspring of women with serum antibodies against *B. burgdorferi* and the offspring of those without such antibodies (Williams et al., 1988; Nadal et al., 1989). In the most comprehensive study of Lyme disease in pregnancy, investigators prospectively studied 2,000 pregnant women in Westchester County, New York (Strobino et al., 1993). Although the number of exposed women was relatively small, no association was found between a mother's exposure to *B. burgdorferi* either before conception or during pregnancy and fetal death, prematurity, or congenital malformations.

To assess the frequency of clinically significant neurologic disorders attributable to congenital infection with *B. burgdorferi,* Gerber conducted a survey of all pediatric neurologists in areas of the country in which Lyme disease is endemic (Connecticut, Rhode Island, Massachusetts, New York, New Jersey, Wisconsin, and Minnesota) (Gerber and Zalneraitis, 1994). Of the 162 pediatric neurologists who responded to the survey (92%), none had seen a child with a clinically significant neurologic disorder that was attributed to congenital Lyme disease or whose mother had Lyme disease during her pregnancy. Thus there is no definite evidence that *B. burgdorferi* causes congenital disease. If it does occur, congenital Lyme disease is extremely rare. Transmission of Lyme disease through breast-feeding has not been documented.

Diagnosis

The diagnosis of Lyme disease, especially in the absence of the characteristic rash, may be difficult, since the other clinical manifestations of Lyme disease are not specific. Clinically, seventh-nerve palsy resulting from Lyme disease is indistinguishable from idiopathic Bell's palsy, and Lyme meningitis may mimic viral meningitis. The manifestations of Lyme arthritis may be indistinguishable from other causes of arthritis in children, such as

juvenile rheumatoid arthritis or HLA-B27 arthritis. Even the diagnosis of erythema migrans sometimes may be difficult, since the rash initially may be confused with nummular eczema, cellulitis, granuloma annulare, an insect bite, or tinea (ringworm). However, the relatively rapid expansion of erythema migrans helps to distinguish it from these other conditions.

Because the sensitivity of culture for *B. burgdorferi* is poor and it is necessary for patients to undergo an invasive procedure such as a biopsy or a lumbar puncture to obtain appropriate tissue or fluid for culture, such tests are indicated only in rare circumstances. Likewise, although preliminary studies in research laboratories suggest that the polymerase chain reaction (PCR) is a promising diagnostic test, its accuracy when used under nonexperimental conditions (especially in commercial laboratories rather than research laboratories) has not been established (Rosa and Schwan, 1989). Consequently, the confirmation of either early disseminated or late Lyme disease by the laboratory usually rests on the demonstration of antibodies to *B. burgdorferi* in the patient's serum. It is well documented that the sensitivity and specificity of antibody tests for Lyme disease vary substantially. The accuracy of prepackaged commercial kits is much poorer than that of tests performed by reference laboratories that maintain tight quality control and regularly prepare the materials that are used in the test (Bacterial Zoonoses Branch, CDC, 1991).

The use of Western immunoblots improves the specificity of serologic testing for Lyme disease (Dressler et al., 1993). Official recommendations from the Second National Conference on Serologic Diagnosis of Lyme Disease suggest that clinicians use a two-step procedure when ordering antibody tests for Lyme disease. First, a sensitive screening test, either an enzyme-linked immunosorbent assay (ELISA) or an immunofluorescent assay (IFA) and, if that result is positive or equivocal, a Western immunoblot to confirm the result (Centers for Disease Control, 1995). If the ELISA or the IFA is negative, an immunoblot is not necessary. Of course, antibody tests are not useful for the diagnosis of early localized Lyme disease, since only a minority of patients with single erythema migrans have a positive test.

As with any diagnostic test, the predictive value of antibody tests for Lyme disease (even of very accurate tests) is highly dependent on the prevalence of the infection among patients who are tested. Unfortunately, because many patients and many physicians have the erroneous impression that non-specific symptoms alone (e.g., headache, fatigue or arthralgia) may be manifestations of Lyme disease, parents of children with only nonspecific symptoms frequently demand that a child be tested for Lyme disease (and some physicians routinely order tests for Lyme disease on such patients). Lyme disease will be the cause of the nonspecific symptoms in very few such children, if any. However, because the specificity of even excellent antibody tests for Lyme disease rarely exceed 90% to 95%, some of the tests in children without specific signs or symptoms of Lyme disease will be positive; the vast majority of these (>90%) will be false-positive tests (Seltzer and Shapiro, 1996). Nevertheless, an erroneous diagnosis of Lyme disease, based on the results of these tests, frequently is made and such children often are treated unnecessarily with antimicrobials. In addition, even though a symptomatic patient has a positive serologic test for antibodies to *B. burgdorferi*, it is possible that Lyme disease may not be the cause of that patient's symptoms. In addition to the possibility that the positive test is falsely positive (by far the most common occurrence), the patient may have been infected with *B. burgdorferi* previously, and the patient's symptoms may be unrelated to that previous infection. In the latter instance, the positive test is accurate, but the test is "falsely positive" in terms of the cause of the patient's symptoms. Once serum antibodies to *B. burgdorferi* develop, they may persist for many years despite adequate treatment and clinical cure of the disease (Feder et al., 1992). In addition, because a substantial proportion of people who become infected with *B. burgdorferi* never develop symptoms, in endemic areas there will be a background rate of seropositivity among patients who have never had clinically apparent Lyme disease. When patients with previous Lyme disease (whether asymptomatic and untreated or clinically apparent and adequately treated) develop any kind of symptoms and are tested for antibodies against *B. burgdorferi*, their symptoms may erroneously be attributed to active Lyme disease. For all of these reasons, misdiagnosis is a common clinical problem (Steere et al., 1993; Sigel 1992, 1994, 1996).

Treatment

Recommendations for the treatment of children with Lyme disease have been extrapolated from studies of adults, since no clinical trials of treatment have been conducted among children (Rahn and Malawista, 1991; Shapiro, 1995). Either doxy-cycline or amoxicillin is used to treat most manifestations of Lyme disease; meningitis and severe carditis are treated with parenterally administered penicillin or ceftriaxone. Children <9 years of age should not be treated with doxycycline because it may cause permanent discoloration of their teeth. Jarisch-Herxheimer reactions occur infrequently.

Other antimicrobial agents, such as clarithromycin and azithromycin may be effective for the treatment of Lyme disease, although neither has been either adequately tested or licensed for such use. Preliminary results with azithromycin have been disappointing. Cefuroxime recently was licensed for the treatment of Lyme disease. There is little need for new agents because the results of treatment with standard therapy (e.g., amoxicillin or doxycycline) have been so good.

Symptoms such as fatigue, arthralgia, and myalgia sometimes persist for some time after completion of a course of treatment for Lyme disease. These nonspecific symptoms (which may either accompany or follow more specific symptoms and signs of Lyme disease but almost never are the sole presenting manifestations of Lyme disease) generally resolve over a period of weeks to months. There is little evidence that such symptoms are related to persistence of the organism. Likewise, there is no evidence that repeated courses of antimicrobials speed the resolution of such symptoms. Finally, antibodies against *B. burgdorferi* will persist after successful treatment of symptoms. There is no reason routinely to obtain follow-up tests of antibody concentrations against *B. burgdorferi*.

Prognosis

There is a widespread misconception that Lyme disease is difficult to treat successfully and that chronic symptoms and clinical recurrences are common. In fact, the most common reason for failure of treatment is misdiagnosis (i.e., the patient actually does not have Lyme disease). Likewise, Lyme disease does not require either multiple or prolonged treatment (although retreatment is recommended for the occasional patient with late disease who develops objective signs of relapse such as frank arthritis). Nonspecific symptoms such as arthralgia or fatigue that occur long after treatment should not be attributed to failure of treatment.

The prognosis for children treated for Lyme disease is excellent. In a review of 65 children who were treated for erythema migrans, at follow-up a mean of more than 3 years later, all of the children were well and none had developed symptoms of late Lyme disease (Salazaar et al., 1993). In a larger, prospective follow-up study of 201 children with newly diagnosed Lyme disease of all stages (though most had early-localized or early-disseminated disease), at follow-up a mean of 2.5 years later, all of the children were clinically cured (Gerber et al., 1996). The long-term prognosis for patients who are treated for late Lyme disease also is excellent. Although recurrences of arthritis do occur rarely, especially among patients with the DR-2, DR-3, or DR-4 HLA type, most children who are treated for Lyme arthritis are permanently cured (Zemel et al., 1995). One group of investigators performed neuropsychologic tests on children with Lyme disease up to 4 years after they were treated and found no evidence of any long-term sequelae of the infection (Adams et al., 1994; Rose et al., 1996). Other investigators who are conducting a community-based study of the long-term outcomes of persons with Lyme disease have also found no evidence of impairment of normal functioning in children 4 to 10 years after they were diagnosed with Lyme disease (Shapiro et al., 1996).

Prevention

In endemic areas it is very common for children to be bitten by deer ticks. Such bites often engender tremendous anxiety. However, the overall risk of acquiring Lyme disease is low (approximately 1% to 2%) even in areas where Lyme disease is endemic (Shapiro et al., 1992). Furthermore, treatment of the infection, if it develops, is highly effective. Consequently, the routine administration of antimicrobial prophylaxis (the efficacy of which is unproved) for persons who have been bitten by a deer tick is not recommended (Warshafsky et al., 1996). The routine testing of ticks that have been removed from humans for infection with *B. burgdorferi* also is not recommended, since the predictive value of a positive test for infection in the human host is unknown.

A more reasonable approach to preventing Lyme disease is to wear appropriate protective clothing (such as lightweight long pants) when entering tick-infested areas and to check for and to remove ticks after spending time in such areas. Insect repellants may provide temporary protection, but they may be absorbed from the skin and, if used frequently or in large doses, they may produce significant toxicity, especially in children.

There has been considerable effort to develop an effective vaccine against Lyme disease (Wormser, 1995). Antibodies against the outer surface A (OspA) protein protect against Lyme disease in animal models (Fikrig et al., 1990). Vaccines that use recombinant OspA proteins have been developed and are currently being tested in phase III trials in humans. Because the spirochete expresses OspA in ticks and in later stages of human illness but not at the time of initial infection in human skin, it is hypothesized that the vaccine works because the tick ingests human blood during feeding before inoculating the spirochete into humans. Presumably, antibody-dependent killing of *B. burgdorferi* occurs in the tick. Even if the vaccine is found to be efficacious, it is likely that it would be used selectively, since the risk of Lyme disease in most populations is low and poor outcome for persons with Lyme disease is rare. New vaccines that utilize other antigens are being developed.

RELAPSING FEVER

There are two different vectors, ticks and lice, that transmit the bacteria that cause relapsing fever to humans. Louse-borne relapsing fever, caused by *Borrelia recurrentis*, is transmitted by the body louse, *Pediculus humanus*. This section focuses on tick-borne recurrent fever.

Etiology and Epidemiology

The Borrelia that cause recurrent fever are fastidious, microaerophilic spirochetal bacteria that are characterized morphologically by coarse and irregularly shaped coils and were first identified in 1873 in the blood of a patient with recurrent fever. Tick-borne relapsing fever is caused by many different *Borrelia* species, including *B. duttoni*, *B. hermsii*, *B. parkerii*, and *B. mazzotti*. These bacteria are able to change the antigenic structure of their surface proteins by transposition of structural genes on a linear plasmid, which allows them temporarily to elude host defenses and results in "relapsing fever" in infected humans (Stoenner et al., 1982; Barbour et al., 1983; Plasterk et al., 1985). The resolution of symptomatic stages of the illness correlates with peaks in the concentrations of antibodies against the specific antigens of the circulating strain. The bacteria cause a vasculitis, with a predilection for capillaries and small arterioles of any organs, especially the reticuloendothelial system, the bone marrow, and the central nervous system.

Tick-borne relapsing fever is transmitted by various species of soft ticks of the genus *Ornitodoros*. Many small animals (chipmunks, rats, mice, squirrels, and others) serve both as reservoirs for these

Borrelia species and as hosts for *Ornitodoros* ticks (Felsenfeld, 1965). There is variable transovarial transmission of the bacteria to larval stages of the ticks, and there is a well-established enzootic cycle in certain areas of the United States. The ticks thrive in warm, humid environments and at altitudes of from 1500 to 6500 feet. Unlike the hard *Ixodes* ticks that transmit *B. burgdorferi* and *Babesia microti*, which feed for days, soft ticks feed for a much shorter time (5 to 30 minutes) yet are able to transmit the bacteria during this relatively brief period. Although there is some uncertainty as to the exact mode of transmission, it is generally believed that transmission occurs when either excrement or saliva from an infected tick comes into contact with the wound produced by the tick's bite. The ticks often feed at night. Although humans are the only hosts for *B. recurrentis* (the cause of louse-borne recurrent fever), humans are incidental hosts for the bacteria that cause tick-borne relapsing fever. Humans become infected when they enter or live in environments in which the ticks thrive, such as old cabins and caves. Tick-borne recurrent fever has a worldwide distribution. The disease is endemic in parts of East Africa, Asia, and South America. In the United States most cases occur in rural areas in the western states. Outbreaks have occurred among spelunkers and among tourists who stayed in log cabins at Grand Canyon National Park (Boyer et al., 1977; Edall et al., 1979).

Clinical Manifestations

Tick-borne and louse-borne relapsing fever are indistinguishable from each other clinically, although tick-borne disease tends to have more (though less severe) recurrences (Southern and Sanford, 1969; Le, 1980; Horton and Blaser, 1985). It is thought that the symptoms of relapsing fever begin 5 to 10 days after exposure. Symptoms begin with the sudden onset of fever and chills, usually accompanied by headache, myalgia, arthralgia, photophobia, and cough. Petechiae, purpura, conjunctivitis, nuchal rigidity, hepatosplenomegaly, and jaundice are common. This phase of the illness is associated with bacteremia, which usually lasts for 3 to 7 days, after which the fever rapidly resolves.

In the subsequent phase of the illness, patients are afebrile or have only low-grade fever and often have a diffuse maculopapular rash accompanied by diaphoresis, extreme fatigue, and occasionally hypotension. During this phase of the illness, cultures of the blood are sterile. It is presumed that or-ganisms multiply and develop antigenically different strains in the spleen or the liver. The relapse phase of the illness (which usually occurs 5 to 7 days after the primary bacteremia resolves) is again marked by the rapid onset of high fever and chills. In untreated patients, three to five relapses may occur.

Laboratory Findings and Diagnosis

Laboratory findings are nonspecific and usually include leukocytosis (with a shift to the left) and a markedly elevated erythrocyte sedimentation rate, as well as a mononuclear pleocytosis in the CSF. Awareness of the epidemiologic history is important. A history of recent visits to caves, old cabins, or other environments where rodents are common should make one consider relapsing fever in the differential diagnosis of patients with unexplained, persistent, or relapsing fever.

Routine cultures of the blood are not useful in making the diagnosis of relapsing fever because special media are required for the bacteria to grow. However, during the febrile phases of relapsing fever, the concentrations of the organism in the blood are very high, and the diagnosis often can be made by examining smears of the peripheral blood by dark-field microscopy or by examining smears stained with Wright's stain, Giemsa stain, or acridine orange.

Treatment and Prognosis

Tetracycline is the drug of choice for treating relapsing fever. In children younger than 8 years of age, erythromycin and penicillin are other options. Treatment is administered 4 times a day for 7 to 10 days. If vomiting is severe, the initial dose of the antimicrobial may be administered intravenously, although this may induce a severe Jarisch-Herxheimer reaction (the result of the release of toxins in association with lysis of the spirochetes).

Relapsing fever usually resolves even in untreated patients. Death is rare, although it does occasionally occur as a result of a ruptured spleen, severe hepatitis, myocarditis, or cerebral hemorrhage. Long-term sequelae are uncommon among those who survive. Iridocyclitis may result in scars and impaired vision. Pregnant women who become infected often abort, in most instances because of thrombocytopenia and retroplacental hemorrhage.

Prevention

The primary means of preventing tick-borne relapsing fever is the avoidance of the ticks that transmit this disease. The use of insecticides around the inner walls of old wooden buildings and huts (where ticks often are found) may help to prevent the disease.

TULAREMIA

Tularemia, the third most common tick-borne infection in the United States, is caused by *Francisella tularensis*, a small, fastidious, pleomorphic gram-negative coccobacillus. The bacterium was named after Edward Francis, who conducted early studies of tularemia, and can be acquired either from ticks or by direct contact with the organism (Francis, 1925).

Etiology and Epidemiology

There are two biovars of *F. tularensis*—type A and the less virulent type B. These strains are characterized on the basis of biologic rather than antigenic differences. Both biovars are prevalent in the United States. Biovar A, found only in North America, is found in rabbits and in ticks (primarily *Amblyomma americanum,* the Lone Star tick, in the Southern and Southeastern states; *Dermacentor variabilis,* the dog tick, in Eastern states; and *Dermacentor andersoni,* the wood tick, in Western states) (Hopla, 1974). The reservoir for biovar B is primarily water-dwelling rodents, such as beavers and muskrats. It is found throughout the world in temperate areas of the Northern hemisphere and often causes subclinical infections.

F. tularensis is highly infectious; exposure to as few as ten organisms can cause infection in humans. *F. tularensis* infects humans through either the skin (typically from the bite of an infected tick or through a wound) or the mucosa (e.g., via the conjunctivae or the upper respiratory tract). Transmission may occur from tick bites (about 50% of cases), through bites of or direct contact with tissues of infected animals, from inhalation of organisms, or by ingesting infected meat or contaminated water. From 100 to 300 cases of tularemia are reported to the CDC each year, most of which occur in the Southern states (Guerrant et al., 1976; Taylor et al., 1991).

Clinical Manifestations

The clinical manifestations of tularemia depend, in large part, on the route of inoculation (Jacobs and Narain, 1983; Jacobs et al., 1985). Ulceroglandular tularemia (the most common form of the illness) is a result of inoculation of the organism from an infected tick. The incubation period of tularemia

transmitted by ticks is 3 to 7 days (Evans et al., 1985). This form of the illness is characterized by an ulcer at the site of the bite, as well as local and regional lymph nodes that are tender and enlarged. Fever and other systemic symptoms may accompany the illness. Without treatment, the ulcer at the site of the bite may persist for weeks. Rarely, tick-borne disease may cause a flu-like illness without involvement of either the skin or the lymph nodes. Oculoglandular tularemia develops from primary infection of the conjunctivae (often from fingers that were contaminated from infected animals, usually rabbits). Ingestion of contaminated foods may cause oropharyngeal tularemia (which may simulate diphtheria), gastrointestinal tularemia (marked by diarrhea and abdominal pain), or a typhoidal form of tularemia that presents with fever and a sepsis-like picture. Pneumonia, which may rapidly be fatal, is due to inhalation of aerosolized organisms. Any form of the illness may be characterized by the sudden onset of fever, headache, chills, myalgia, and fatigue. However, the severity of tick-borne illness is highly variable and sometimes may be mild and self-limited (Markowitz et al., 1985).

Diagnosis

Because of the substantial risk to laboratory personnel, most laboratories will not culture the organism, although it may grow on media used for other bacteria. Consequently, the diagnosis of tularemia is usually based on the presence of agglutinating antibodies to *F. tularensis*. A fourfold increase in concentration of agglutinins between acute-phase and convalescent-phase sera is considered to be diagnostic of infection. A single titer of $\geq 1{:}160$ in a patient with a history and clinical symptoms compatible with tularemia strongly suggests the diagnosis. Tests that utilize PCR to detect the organisms in the blood are being developed (Long et al., 1993).

Treatment and Prognosis

Because agglutinins may not appear until near the end of the second week after infection begins, the patient should be treated empirically if tularemia is suspected. Streptomycin is the treatment of choice, although gentamicin or amikacin may be equally effective (Enderlin et al., 1994). Patients usually have a clinical response to treatment within 48 hours and should be treated for 7 to 10 days. Most patients who receive antimicrobial treatment have a complete recovery. The mortality rate of patients with tularemia is about 3%; fatalities occur primarily in patients with either pneumonia or the typhoidal form of the disease.

Prevention

Minimizing exposure to ticks, wearing gloves when handling game, and fully cooking meat should reduce the risk of developing tularemia. A live attenuated vaccine has proved useful for lowering the risk of infection of the respiratory tract in workers who are exposed in the laboratory, but it is not effective for tick-borne disease (Burke, 1977).

BABESIOSIS

Babesiosis, a zoonosis first described in humans in 1957, is caused by intraerythrocytic protozoa and has many clinical features in common with malaria.

Etiology and Epidemiology

Many different *Babesia* species infect a variety of domestic and wild animals throughout the world. In the United States, *B. microti*, a piroplasm of rodents, is the principal cause of human infection, which occurs primarily in the Northeastern and Midwestern states. The organism is transmitted by *Ixodes scapularis* (the deer tick), which also transmits *Borrelia burgdorferi*, the cause of Lyme disease. As with *B. burgdorferi*, rodents such as the white-footed mouse serve as reservoirs for *B. microti.* Consequently, coinfection with *B. microti* and *B. burgdorferi* (and sometimes with ehrlichia as well) occurs with some frequency (Magnarelli et al., 1995; Krause et al., 1996). Babesiosis has been transmitted via blood transfusion (Mintz et al., 1991). Serosurveys suggest that children may be infected more often than adults (Krause et al., 1992). In the Western United States there have been rare reports of human babesiosis caused by *B. gibsoni* (WA-1) or similar *Babesia* spp. (Persing et al., 1995). In Europe, *B. divergens*, a parasite of cattle, also infects people.

Babesia organisms have solid pyriform shapes and frequently are arranged in pairs. It is possible to infect a variety of animals experimentally; removal of the spleen often increases both the duration and the severity of infection. Microscopic study of an extensively parasitized patient during illness has shown that usually one to four of the basophilic parasites are seen in infected red blood cells, but as many as five to twelve parasites per cell are present. Different developmental stages of the parasite—including ring, ameboid, and other forms—can be seen even within a single cell. Extracellular merozoites are present singly or in a syncytial structure. Free ribosomes, endoplasmic reticulum, and small dense bodies may be seen in the cytoplasm of merozoites with a single, large, membrane-limited dense body (rhoptry). Trophozoites are surrounded by a single plasma membrane. Early in the course of illness, red blood cells show changes in their cell membranes, with protrusions and perforations.

Clinical Manifestations

Symptoms of babesiosis begin 1 to 9 weeks after the tick bite. Typical signs and symptoms include intermittent fever as high as 40° C and chills, sweats, myalgia, arthralgia, nausea, or vomiting (Sun et al., 1983; Reubush et al., 1977). The physical examination often is normal (except for fever) or reveals only mild splenomegaly or hepatomegaly. About half of the patients have abnormal liver function tests. Thrombocytopenia is also common. Invasion and subsequent lysis of erythrocytes by *B. microti* may result in mild to moderately severe hemolytic anemia with an elevated reticulocyte count. Unlike with malaria, the illness is not marked by periodicity of symptoms.

In most immunocompetent persons, the illness is indistinguishable from an acute viral infection, so the diagnosis rarely is made. However, immunocompromised patients, particularly those without a spleen, may have severe infection, with as many as 90% of the red blood cells parasitized. These patients may develop severe hemolysis, shock, thrombocytopenia, and disseminated intravascular coagulation.

Diagnosis

Babesiosis can be diagnosed by microscopic identification of the organism on either thick or thin smears of blood that are stained with either Giemsa or Wright's stains or by detection of antibodies to *Babesia* organisms. During the early stage of the illness, when most people seek medical attention, fewer than 1% of erythrocytes may be infected, so making the diagnosis may be difficult, and careful examination of multiple smears of blood is important. The polymerase chain reaction is a potentially useful new diagnostic technique that is both highly sensitive and highly specific in the setting of a research laboratory (Persing et al., 1992); its value as a commercially available test has not been assessed. Of the commonly used serologic tests the indirect immunofluorescent antibody assay is the most accurate and reliable (Krause et al., 1994). Titers greater than 1:64 are suggestive of recent infection, but paired sera with a fourfold or greater rise in concentration of antibody confirms the diagnosis.

Treatment and Prognosis

Most infections with *B. microti* are self-limited, and most patients recover without treatment. More severe infections that come to medical attention should be treated with both quinine and clindamycin. Patients who are extremely ill often require exchange transfusion to diminish the load of parasites. The infection may be fatal in asplenic patients. Untreated, the clinical illness usually lasts from a few weeks to several months. Parasitemia, which may persist for many months, may continue even after the patient's symptoms have resolved. Relapse is unusual but has occurred.

Prevention

There is no vaccine available. Preliminary evidence indicates that, as with transmission of *B. burgdorferi*, an infected tick must feed for at least 48 hours before the risk of transmission becomes substantial. Consequently, examination for and prompt removal of embedded ticks may decrease the risk of infection.

DISEASES CAUSED BY RICKETTSIAE

Rickettsiae are obligate intracellular gram-negative bacteria that are transmitted primarily by arthropod vectors. Humans are the incidental hosts for most rickettsial infections, except for epidemic typhus. The geographic distribution of most rickettsial diseases reflects that of their vectors. Diseases such as typhus have been recognized for centuries, but not until the early twentieth century was the causative group of agents recognized when Dr. Howard T. Ricketts produced disease by injecting blood from a patient with Rocky Mountain spotted fever into a guinea pig.

The taxonomy of the family Rickettsiaceae is shown in Fig. 33-5. All Rickettsiaceae organisms grow only within cells. The genus *Rickettsia* is a member of the tribe Rickettsieae (other members of which are Ehrlichieae and Wolbachleae) within the family Rickettsiaceae. Rickettsial diseases can be divided into three groups—typhus, spotted fever, and scrub typhus—with more than ten different species in these groups that cause human illness. The closely related genus *Coxiella* is composed of the species *Coxiella burnetti*, which, although similar to rickettsiae in morphology and intracellular growth, differs in major ways. This organism produces a sporelike small cell, has very

different DNA composition, and is transmitted to humans by aerosol rather than by ticks. As a result of molecular analyses of the bacteria, in 1993 the four members of the genus *Rochalimaea* (which had been in the Rickettsiaceae family), *Rochalimaea henselae*, *R. quintana*, *R. elizabethae*, and *R. vinsonii*, were renamed and moved to the genus *Bartonella* within the family Bartonellaceae.

The spectrum of clinical illnesses produced by the three genera of the Rickettsiaceae family include vasculitis (in Rocky Mountain spotted fever), pneumonia (in Q fever), febrile illness with infection of white blood cells (WBC) (in ehrlichiosis), recrudescent febrile infection (in Brill-Zinsser disease), and endocarditis (in Q fever) (Table 33-1). Endothelial damage and secondary inflammation are the hallmarks of these infections.

ETIOLOGY

Rickettsia are pleomorphic coccobacillary organisms that range from 0.3 to 0.6 μm in width and from 0.8 to 2.0 μm in length. They are gram-negative but stain poorly. The organisms are best visualized with a Gimenez modification of the

Table 30-1 Rickettsial diseases

Causative agent	Diseases
R. prowazekii	Epidemic typhus, Brill-Zinsser disease
R. typhi	Endemic or murine typhus
R. canada	?—disease similar to Rocky Mountain spotted fever
R. rickettsii	Rocky Mountain spotted fever
R. akari	Rickettsial pox
R. sibirica	North Asian tick typhus
R. australis	Queensland tick typhus
R. japonica	Japanese spotted fever
R. conorii	Boutonneuse fever
R. tsutsugamushi	Scrub typhus (chigger-borne typhus, mite-borne typhus, Japanese River fever, rural fever, tropical typhus)
Coxiella burnetti	Q fever
Ehrlichia sennetsu	Sennetsu fever
E. chaffeensis	Human monocytic ehrlichiosis
E. equi (a related ehrlichi-organism)	Human granulocytic ehrlichiosis

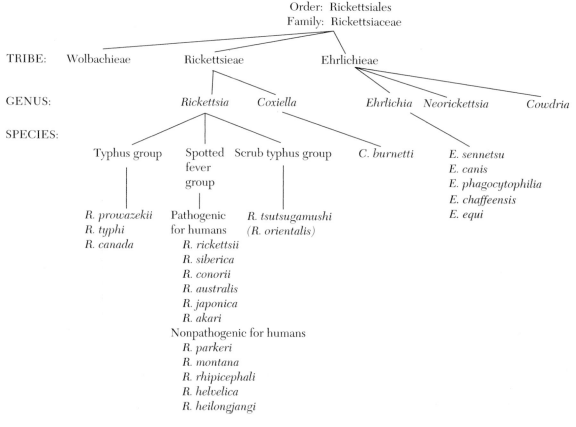

FIG. 33-5 Taxonomy of *Rickettsiales* spp.

Macchiavello method, which stains organisms red. These bacteria have a three-layered cell wall, trilaminar plasma membrane, ribosome-like particles, and intracellular organelles. They possess both RNA and DNA, and they divide by binary fission. The genome is large, varying from 1.0 to 1.5×10^9 daltons. They have developed carrier-mediated exchange transport systems for phosphorylated compounds (ADP and ATP) similar to those of mitochondria. The genome size, DNA-DNA hybridization, and guanosine-cytosine content are similar within species of a group, but significant differences exist between groups (e.g., between *C. burnetti* and *R. prowazekii*).

All members of the genus *Rickettsia* can obtain access to cytoplasm by traversing the membrane of the host cell and are unstable outside of the cell, whereas *Coxiella burnetti* is very resistant to both heating and drying. All members of the Rickettsiaceae family can be propagated in various tissue culture systems, embryonated eggs, laboratory animals, and certain arthropods. Generally, organisms in the typhus group grow in the cytoplasm, whereas organisms in the spotted fever group grow in both the cytoplasm and the nucleus.

THE SPOTTED FEVER GROUP
Rocky Mountain Spotted Fever (Tick-Borne Typhus)

Rickettsiae in the spotted fever group cause a diffuse vasculitis of the small vessels, which produces a rash that typically is petechial or purpuric. Any of the viscera may be involved with the clinical disease, which encompasses a spectrum of severity from unrecognized infection to fatal illness. Rocky Mountain spotted fever is the second most common reported tick-borne infection in the United States.

Etiology and Epidemiology. *R. rickettsii* is morphologically similar to other rickettsiae. *R. rickettsii* and *R. prowazekii* have a slime layer (glycocalix), probably composed of polysaccharide and external to the cell wall, which could be antigenically important or related to cell attachment (Silverman et al., 1978). *R. rickettsii* are labile and are

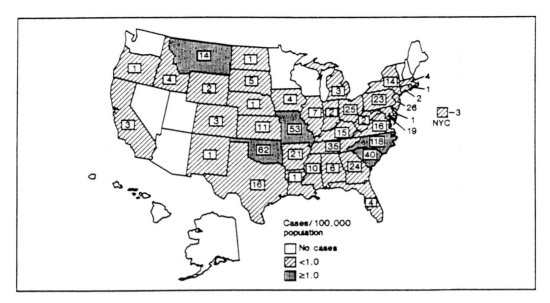

Fig. 33-6   Reported cases and rates of Rocky Mountain Spotted Fever, by state—United States, 1989. (From MMWR 1990;39:281.)

killed by drying at room temperature, by moist heat (≥50° C), and by formalin or phenol. *R. rickettsii* multiply in both the nucleus and the cytoplasm and produce demonstrable cytopathic effects. Studies with the scanning electron microscope have shown *R. rickettsii* exiting from cells on long cytoplasmic projections without causing lysis of the cell. Large numbers of cells become infected relatively quickly. These microorganisms live within ticks, in which they do not cause disease, and are transovarially transmitted from female ticks to their progeny. The ticks pass through three stages in their life cycle, and they can acquire infection at any stage by feeding on a rickettsemic animal. The infection is maintained by the tick through its sequential stages of development—egg to larvae to nymph to adult (i.e., transtadially). The arthropods are both reservoirs and vectors of infection.

Rocky Mountain spotted fever (tick-borne typhus) occurs only in the Western Hemisphere. The disease is most prevalent in the Piedmont region of the Southeastern United States and in Oklahoma. Small numbers of cases have been recognized over the years in almost every state. Approximately 650 cases of disease were reported to the Centers for Disease Control (CDC) in 1990 (Fig. 33-6). In the United States the reported incidence of Rocky Mountain spotted fever peaked at an annual incidence of approximately 0.5 cases/100,000 population in the late 1970s and early 1980s and subsequently declined (Fig. 33-4). Rocky Mountain

spotted fever is responsible for 95% of all reported rickettsial infections in the United States. Because the disease is transmitted by ticks, the incidence is seasonal, with most cases occurring during the peak period of exposure of humans to ticks—from April to September (D'Angelo et al., 1978; Wilfert et al., 1984). Persons who live in rural or suburban areas are more likely to acquire this disease than are persons who live in urban areas, though outbreaks have occurred in urban areas such as in New York City (Salgo et al., 1988). Very young infants (<2 years old) are rarely exposed, and illness in this age group is unusual. Persons who are outdoors in oak, hickory, and pine forests are most likely to be exposed and to acquire the disease.

Infection is transmitted to humans by ticks. Infection may be transmitted within the laboratory by aerosol (Oster et al., 1977), but aerosol transmission (which is associated with severe disease) is not known to occur in nature. Very rarely, transmission from human to human has occurred through a blood transfusion from a patient incubating disease or through an accidental stick by a needle contaminated with infected blood. The wood tick, *Dermacentor andersoni*, is the major vector of *R. rickettsii* in the Western United States. *D. variabilis*, the dog tick, is the major vector in both the Southeastern and the Northeastern United States. Ticks obtained from vegetation (not from dogs) harbor rickettsiae at varying frequencies (<1% to 10%); however, only 1 tick of 2,510 (0.03%) had *R. rickettsii* in one study conducted in North Carolina. The Lone Star tick *(Amblyomma americanum)* and the rabbit tick *(Haemaphysalis laporispalustris)* only occasionally transmit disease to humans, but they may be important in maintaining infection in animals. The infected tick must ingest a blood meal to "activate" the rickettsiae, which transmit the organism from their salivary glands during feeding. This phenomenon probably is related to increasing the temperature of the organism, which microscopically correlates with the presence of a microcapsular slime layer on the organism (Hayes and Burgdorfer, 1982).

Pathogenesis and Pathology. Rickettsiae initially enter the endothelial cells of small blood vessels (Silverman and Bond, 1979; Silverman, 1984). They are engulfed by the membrane of the host cell. Phospholipase may aid the organism in evading phagocytosis and may contribute to damage of the membrane of the host cell. In mammals, organisms multiply in the vascular endothelium and smooth muscle, producing endothelial damage and occlusion of small vessels, with extravasation of blood and fluid and attendant changes in serum electrolytes (especially hyponatremia). *R. rickettsii* stimulates endothelial cells and macrophages to secrete arachidonate-derived autocoids. Activation of the kallikrein-kinin system has been documented in humans, as has disseminated intravascular coagulation. Vasculitis is apparent in many tissues (Fig. 33-7), especially the skin, central nervous system (CNS), heart, lungs, liver, and kidney. Severe disease can cause occlusion of larger vessels as well as gangrene. In animal models the rickettsiae themselves cause cellular damage. Cell-mediated immunity to antigens of *R. rickettsii* has been demonstrated in vitro and may contribute to eradication of organisms in tissues. The immune response of the host may also contribute to the tissue damage (Teyssiere et al., 1992; Walker et al., 1993).

Clinical Manifestations. The clinical features of Rocky Mountain spotted fever have been well defined (Walker, 1995). The incubation period is usually 5 to 7 days, with a range of 3 to 12 days. The illness is characterized by a short prodromal period of headache, malaise, and myalgia. The abrupt onset of fever may be accompanied by chills, and the severity of myalgia and headache may increase. Usually a rash is noted 2 to 4 days after onset of illness, although there have been re-

ports of "spotless" and "almost spotless" fever (Sexton and Corey, 1992). It begins as a maculopapular eruption with a peripheral distribution. The skin lesions appear first on the thenar eminence and the flexor surfaces of the wrists and ankles. The rash spreads to involve the arms, legs, chest, and, finally, the abdomen. The palms and soles are nearly always affected. The lesions are at first discrete, macular, and maculopapular, and they blanch with pressure. Within 1 to 3 days the rash becomes hemorrhagic, and lesions may become confluent, with areas of necrosis at sites of maximal involvement. Gangrene of fingers, toes, genitalia, or the nose may develop (Kirkland et al., 1993). During the period of convalescence the rash becomes pigmented and evidence of desquamation appears over the more severely affected areas.

The illness varies in severity even without specific antimicrobial therapy. The case-fatality rate is 4%, which makes it the most common fatal tick-borne illness in the United States. Factors associated with higher mortality include increased age and an increased length of time from onset of the illness to initiation of therapy (Hattwick et al., 1978; Kirkland et al., 1995). The diffuse organ involvement of this infection results in protean manifestations. Myalgia and associated elevations of muscle enzymes are common. Hepatic involvement is frequent and may produce mild to severe hepatocellular dysfunction and jaundice. The gastrointestinal manifestations include abdominal pain, vomiting, and diarrhea. Myocardial involvement, with vasculitis and inflammation, is common (see Fig. 33-7). The patient may have an altered sensorium or may be comatose as a result of encephalitis, and there is frequently pleocytosis in the cerebrospinal fluid (CSF), although there usually are fewer than 100 to 200 WBC/mm^3 (Baganz et al., 1995). The peripheral WBC count is often normal, but there may be a shift to the left with prominent vacuolization of polymorphonuclear cells. Hyponatremia and mild peripheral edema are frequent consequences of the vasculitis. Increased antidiuretic hormone (ADH) levels have also been observed in patients with this disease.

Illness in the most severely affected patients may last from days to weeks. Prolonged fever of 10 days to several weeks and relapse after cessation of therapy may occur. It is likely that infections occur that either are asymptomatic or have relatively mild symptoms and thus are not recognized as Rocky Mountain spotted fever, since some persons with specific antibodies that indicate previous in-

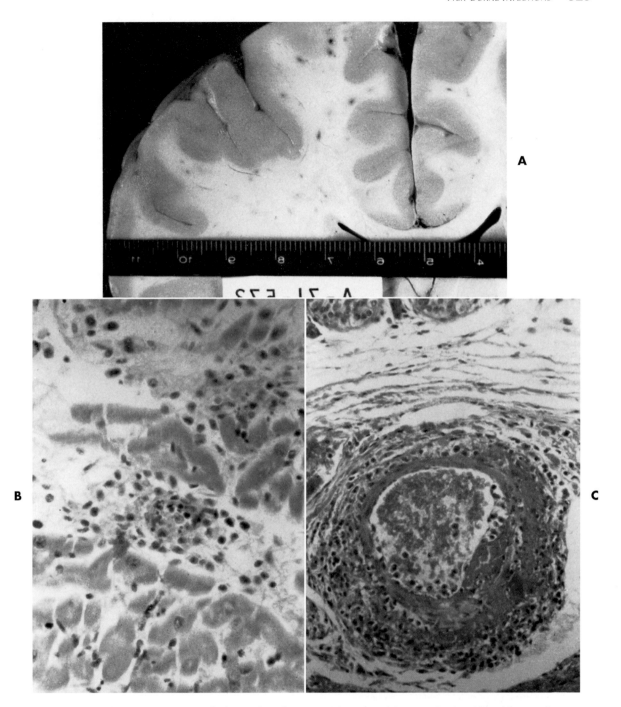

FIG. 33-7 Postmortem pathology of Rocky Mountain spotted fever. **A,** Brain with evidence of petechial hemorrhages. **B,** Tunica testes showing prominent vasculitis with endothelial thickening and fibrin deposition. **C,** Vasculitis of myocardium.

fection have had no known illness consistent with Rocky Mountain spotted fever.

Diagnosis. It is critical to consider the diagnosis of Rocky Mountain spotted fever in all patients in endemic areas who have symptoms that are com-

patible with this infection, especially during the months of peak exposure to ticks. In the absence of rash (e.g., early in the course of the illness or in the unusual patient in whom no rash develops) it is difficult to make a specific diagnosis. The differential diagnosis includes other diseases that cause similar rashes, such as meningococcemia, septic shock of any cause, erythema multiforme and other types of vasculitis, murine typhus, and enteroviral infections, as well as drug-induced rashes. A febrile illness with the characteristic rash often constitutes enough evidence to initiate therapy because of the poor outcomes of persons with this disease in whom treatment is delayed (Archibald and Sexton, 1995). Additional history such as a known tick bite, myalgia, headache, and hyponatremia constitute a compelling clinical constellation. Laboratory diagnosis has primarily depended on the demonstration of antibodies to *R. rickettsii*, which are rarely present during the first 3 to 5 days of illness. Accordingly, initiation of specific antimicrobial therapy should not await confirmation of diagnosis by serologic tests.

Isolation of *R. rickettsii* from the blood is expensive and time-consuming because it requires cell culture or inoculation of animals. It is done in only a few research laboratories. It takes several days for a culture to become positive, so culture cannot be used for early diagnosis of infection. Early diagnosis can be made by detection of intracellular *R. rickettsii* by fluorescein-conjugated antibody in biopsies of skin lesions (Woodward et al., 1976) (Fig. 33-8). *R. rickettsii* organisms are not present in areas of normal skin. This test may be negative in infected patients who received antibiotics for more than 24 hours before a specimen is obtained. It is also possible to demonstrate the presence of intracellular organisms in tissues obtained at autopsy.

Diagnosis generally is made by detection of antibodies that appear during convalescence. The Weil-Felix reaction is a test for nonspecific antibodies that often is positive in patients with Rocky Mountain spotted fever. Because of their O polysaccharide antigens, several strains of proteus (OX-19, OX-2, OX-K) are agglutinated by antibodies that are induced by rickettsial infections. Antibodies may be detected after the first week of illness, and a fourfold increase is suggestive of recent infection. The test is easy to perform and is inexpensive but both its specificity and its sensitivity are poor. Specific antibody to rickettsiae can be assessed by indirect hemagglutination (IHA), microimmunofluorescence (micro-IF), latex agglutination, ELISA, and complement-fixation (CF) tests. The sensitivity of the CF test is poor, and it is no longer in general use in the United States; antibodies detected by CF may develop late, and their development may be aborted by specific antibiotic therapy. The sensitivity and specificity of IHA, micro-IF, and latex ag-

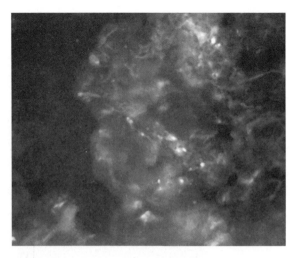

FIG. 33-8 Photomicrograph of a skin biopsy obtained from a 5-year-old child on the sixth day of illness. *R. rickettsii* are demonstrated by immunofluorescence. (×235.) (Courtesy Dr. David H. Walker, University of North Carolina at Chapel Hill.)

glutination tests are comparable (Philip et al., 1977). Recently developed ELISA tests that use a monoclonal antibody directed against specific antigens of *R. rickettsii* are more specific than earlier ELISA tests (Radulovic et al., 1993). An antibody rise of fourfold or greater in paired sera is diagnostic of acute infection. The presence of specific IgM antibody by immunofluorescence or ELISA suggests recent infection (Clements et al., 1983). Typical patterns of antibody titers over time in patients with Rocky Mountain spotted fever are shown in Fig. 33-9.

The polymerase chain reaction (PCR) also has been used successfully to diagnose Rocky Mountain fever in its early stages (Sexton et al., 1994; Dumler and Walker, 1994). However, as with other infections, the use of PCR as a diagnostic test is complicated by the possibility of false-positive tests caused by amplicon carryover, and the sensitivity of the test is not known. Additional experience is necessary before this technique becomes a standard method for making the diagnosis.

Immunity. A single infection with *R. rickettsii* probably confers long-term immunity. Persons who have been challenged twice with *R. rickettsii* develop clinical illness only after the first exposure (DuPont et al., 1973). A spectrum of antibodies develops in response to *R. rickettsii* (Anacker et al., 1983). Crossed immunoelectrophoresis demonstrates antibody responses to multiple different

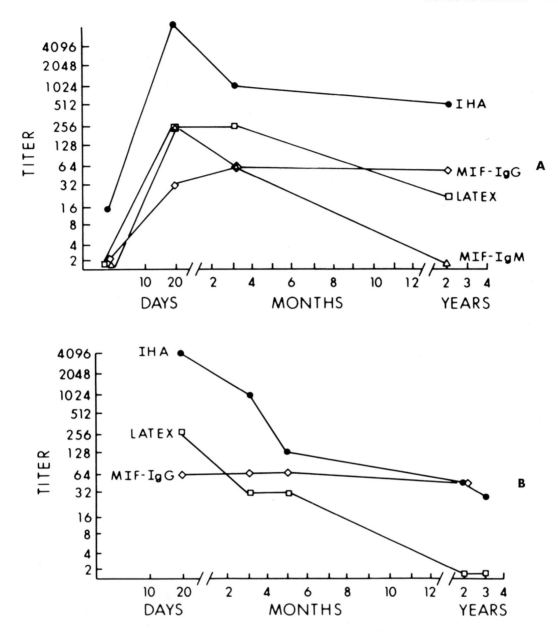

FIG. 33-9   Antibody titers to *R. rickettsii* measured by indirect hemagglutination *(IHA)*, microimmunofluorescence *(MIF)* for IgG and IgM, and latex agglutination. Titers are plotted by the time they were obtained in relation to onset of symptomatic illness. **A,** Titers obtained from serum of 62-year-old man with rash and fever hospitalized for 5 days and treated with tetracycline. **B,** Titers obtained from serum of 3-year-old boy who had a rash and fever; he was not hospitalized and did not receive specific therapy.

antigens of the organism; it is not known which antibodies confer protection against *R. rickettsii*. Antibody coating of *R. rickettsii* is necessary for phagocytosis and killing of the organism by guinea pig peritoneal macrophages in cell-culture systems. Lymphocytes from patients with prior infection have been shown in vitro to be sensitized to spotted fever group antigens. The relative importance in humans of antibody and of cell-mediated immunity in either response to infection or protection against subsequent infection is unknown.

Treatment and Prognosis.   Tetracycline, doxycycline, or chloramphenicol are the drugs of choice for treating Rocky Mountain spotted fever. Fluoroquinolone antimicrobials, which are rickettsiocidal, may also be effective, but there has not yet been enough experience with the use of these drugs in Rocky Mountain spotted fever to recommend them for routine use. For optimal effect it is critical to treat patients early in the course of the illness. Although tetracycline may permanently stain teeth of children <9 years of age, reports of poorer outcomes in persons treated with chloramphenicol have led some to suggest that tetracycline or doxycycline (the effect on teeth in relatively short courses of treatment are negligible) should be used even in young children. However, reports of poorer outcomes with chloramphenicol may be biased since it can be given parenterally; it is also possible that sicker patients were more likely to be treated with chloramphenicol. At this time, either approach can be supported. Patients should be treated for a minimum of 7 days.

Complications of Rocky Mountain spotted fever are more likely to occur in untreated patients and in patients in whom specific therapy is initiated after more than 4 days of clinical illness (Hattwick et al., 1978; Kirkland et al., 1995). CNS sequelae do occur in a small proportion of patients (Archibald and Sexton, 1995). Occasionally, amputation of fingers and toes or other tissues may be necessitated by gangrene (Kirkland et al., 1993). Arrhythmias have been observed as a manifestation of the myocardial involvement.

Prevention. Nonspecific measures to diminish exposure to ticks (such as use of long pants rather than shorts when walking in wooded areas) can be taken but have not been shown to be effective in preventing disease. Individuals who are exposed to ticks and tick-infested environments should inspect themselves for ticks and carefully remove any they find. A period of time is necessary for activation of *R. rickettsii* in infected ticks; therefore early removal of ticks could in theory prevent infection. Attached ticks should be removed with forceps and gentle traction. Care should be taken since tissues and feces of ticks are highly infectious if they contain *R. rickettsii*. Rocky Mountain spotted fever is not transmitted from human to human except for the unusual circumstance of blood transfusion or needle puncture. Therefore isolation of patients is unnecessary.

There is no vaccine available for prevention of Rocky Mountain spotted fever. A vaccine made from egg-grown rickettsiae was used until it was shown conclusively that it failed to prevent infection. An experimental vaccine grown in cell-culture systems also was tested in experimental trials in animals and humans. Although humoral antibodies and sensitization of lymphocytes could be demonstrated, it did not protect humans from infection; therefore studies of this vaccine have been stopped.

Rickettsialpox

Rickettsialpox is caused by *R. akari,* an organism of the spotted fever group that cross-reacts serologically with *R. rickettsii.* The disease is usually a mild febrile illness heralded by the development of a local eschar. Subsequently, a papulovesicular rash appears.

Etiology and Epidemiology. The common house mouse in the United States is infested with a mite (formerly known as *Allodermanyssus sanguineus* and now called *Lipryssoides anguineus*) that may be infected with *R. akari.* This organism may also be transmitted transovarially to the progeny of an infected mite. Humans enter the cycle of infection accidentally, often as the result of displacement of a rodent population by construction or during reduction of the rodent population by control programs. The mite attacks humans when its normal murine host is scarce. This rickettsia has also been found in a wild Korean rodent *(Microtus fortis).*

Persons of all ages are susceptible to rickettsialpox. The majority of cases have been reported in New York City, where the disease was originally described in the Kew Gardens area of the borough of Queens in 1946 (Sussman, 1946; Greenberg, 1948). It has also been identified in West Hartford, Connecticut; Boston; Philadelphia; Arkansas; Delaware; and Russia.

Clinical Manifestations. The incubation period is estimated to be 10 to 24 days. A triad of symptoms occur in sequence: the initial eschar, a febrile illness, and a generalized papulovesicular eruption. The primary lesion at the site of the original bite of the mite is a local erythematous papule that evolves into a vesicle over a period of days and, finally, into an eschar. Most patients are not aware of either the bite or the lesion. The eschar resolves over a period of 3 to 4 weeks, which is usually associated with enlarged regional lymph nodes.

Approximately 3 to 7 days after the appearance of the eschar, fever begins abruptly. Patients often have headache, malaise, and myalgia. Within 72 hours of the onset of fever, a rash develops. There is no characteristic distribution of this rash. It may occur on any part of the body, but it only rarely involves the palms or soles. The lesions are initially maculopapular and discrete, but small vesicles form on the summit of the papules. The lesions dry and may have tiny scabs that fall off without leaving scars. The entire course of illness is approximately 2 weeks. There usually is leukopenia with relative lymphocytosis.

Because there have been no reported deaths from this disease, only skin is usually available for histopathologic examination (Dolgopol, 1948). The initial lesion is a firm nodule approximately 1 cm in diameter. It consists of a vesicle or pustule covered with dry epithelium or crust. Histologically, the vesicle is situated subepidermally and may arise from vacuolar changes of the basal layer. Mononuclear infiltration of the epidermis is seen, with a mixed polymorphonuclear mononuclear cell infiltrate in the dermis. The capillaries of the stratum cornium are dilated and surrounded by mononuclear cells and the endothelial cells in blood vessels are swollen.

Diagnosis. Rickettsialpox may be confused with varicella (chickenpox) and is the only rickettsial disease characterized by the appearance of vesicular lesions. The presence of a primary eschar, however, differentiates it from varicella. In addition, the vesicular lesions in rickettsialpox are smaller than those in varicella and are usually situated on top of a papule. Rickettsialpox can affect persons of all ages, but varicella is more likely to occur in children. The typical crusting of varicella lesions may not be observed in many of the rickettsialpox lesions. The diffuse nature of the vesicular lesions is in contrast to the characteristic sequential eruption of varicella vesicles. This difference should also help to distinguish this illness from primary herpes simplex infection. The demonstration of multinuclear giant cells or isolation of either herpes simplex or varicella-zoster virus will easily distinguish these infections.

The diagnosis of rickettsialpox can be made clinically and confirmed by measurements of antibodies. Weil-Felix antibodies do not appear after infection with *R. akari.* However, more specific testing available at the Centers for Disease Control or at certain research laboratories can demonstrate an antibody response 1 to 2 months after the onset of illness. Because *R. rickettsii* and *R. akari* share some antigens, antibodies to *R. rickettsii* may be detected in some patients with rickettsialpox.

R. akari has been isolated from both the blood and the vesicular fluid of infected persons. To obtain diagnosis by culture it is necessary to use a research laboratory or one accustomed to diagnosis of this infection, since animals and embryonated eggs are used.

Treatment, Prognosis, and Prevention. Both tetracycline and chloramphenicol have been reported to shorten the course of the illness. Prevention is directed at control of the rodent host of the vector. Untreated rickettsialpox is a benign, self-limited, nonfatal disease. No complications have been reported. No vaccines are available, and there is little stimulus to develop additional preventive measures because of both the mild nature of and the rarity of this disease.

Other Tick-Borne Rickettsial Diseases

An illness similar to but milder than Rocky Mountain spotted fever has been ascribed to several other tick-borne rickettsiae. North Asian tick typhus, which occurs in Central Asia, Siberia, and Mongolia, is caused by *R. sibirica.* Queensland tick typhus is caused by *R. australis* and is found only in Australia. The illness known variously as South African tick bite fever, Kenya tick typhus, Indian tick typhus, and boutonneuse fever (Mediterranean region) is caused by *R. conorii. R. japonica* is the causative agent of Japanese spotted fever. All four of these rickettsiae infect different species of *Ixodes* ticks and their wild animal hosts. Humans are only incidentally infected and are not important as reservoirs for these illnesses. In contrast to Rocky Mountain spotted fever, these rickettsial illnesses are characterized by a local skin lesion at the site where the tick attaches and the formation of an eschar at the site of the bite, as with rickettsialpox. These illnesses are milder than Rocky Mountain spotted fever. Group-reactive complement-fixing antibodies have been demonstrated in response to infection with any of these four rickettsiae, but the Weil-Felix test is positive only occasionally. The diagnosis can be specific because the geographic distribution of the individual rickettsiae overlaps very little. These illness are also treated with chloramphenicol or tetracycline.

TYPHUS GROUP

The typhus group of rickettsiae causes epidemic typhus (including recrudescent disease) and murine typhus. These organisms share a common group-specific antigen and grow within the cytoplasm of cells.

Epidemic Typhus (Louse-Borne Typhus).

Epidemic typhus is an acute, potentially fatal infectious disease caused by *R. prowazekii* that has played an important role in history. For example, it has been estimated that in World War I more than 3 million Russians died as a result of this infection.

Etiology and epidemiology. *R. prowazekii* is similar to the previously described *Rickettsiae* species. The organisms multiply in cytoplasm much as do classic bacteria in liquid medium. The cells in which they grow exhibit few cytopathic effects. The organism is infectious for mice, guinea pigs, and embryonated eggs. Infectivity is maintained after either lyophilization or storage at −70° C. This organism can infect both the human body louse *(Pediculus humanus corporis)* and the head louse *(P. humanus capitis)*. *P. humanus corporis* feeds only on humans, and lice in all stages (egg, nymph, and adult) can be present on the same host. The louse becomes infected by taking a blood meal from a person with rickettsemia. *R. prowazekii* multiplies in the epithelial cells of the intestine of the louse. After 3 to 7 days, large numbers of rickettsiae are excreted in the feces. Fortunately, lice do not transmit the rickettsiae to their progeny, and infected lice die within several weeks. An infected louse transmits disease by moving to another person and excreting feces during the blood meal. The abrasions induced by scratching provide a portal of entry for rickettsiae deposited on the skin. Rarely, infections have been acquired by inhalation of dry infective feces of the louse. Humans are the primary reservoir of infection, although flying squirrels also may harbor the organism.

Epidemic typhus occurs throughout the world. All ages and both sexes are equally susceptible. It occurs chiefly in Asia, Africa, Europe, Central America, and South America. During World War II the disease was epidemic in Russia, Poland, Germany, Spain, and North Africa. Conditions that promote infestation with lice (including crowding, poor hygiene, and conditions under which the same clothing is worn for prolonged periods) favor the disease. The conditions favorable for proliferation of lice are associated with war, poverty, and famine. Lice apparently seek locations where the temperature is approximately 20° C; they abandon the host when the body temperature rises to ≥40° C.

The few sporadic cases of epidemic typhus in the United States have been associated with the flying squirrel *(Glaucomys volans);* its lice *(Neohaematopinus sciuropteri)* and fleas *(Orchopeas howardi)* are vectors that have been occasionally responsible for disease in Virginia, North Carolina, Florida, West Virginia, and other parts of the United States (Sonenshine et al., 1978; Duma et al., 1981).

Clinical manifestations. After an incubation period of 7 to 14 days, epidemic typhus begins abruptly with fever, chills, headache, malaise, and generalized aches and pains. The fever and constitutional symptoms increase in severity and are followed by a rash that erupts on the fourth to sixth day of illness. The maculopapular rash appears first on the trunk near the axillae and spreads to involve the extremities. The face, palms, and soles are usually not involved. Initially, the lesions are discrete pleomorphic macules that blanch on pressure. During the second week of illness, the skin lesions become petechial and purpuric, after which brownish pigmentation develops.

In the untreated patient, fever lasts for 2 weeks and then falls by lysis over a period of 2 to 3 days. Severe illness is characterized by stupor, delirium, hallucinations or excitability, marked weakness, prostration, and temporary deafness. By the second and third weeks the patient either recovers or progresses to coma and death. Early in the course of infection, relative bradycardia may be present; later, tachycardia and gallop rhythm may reflect inflammation of the myocardium. Splenomegaly, albuminuria, and elevated blood urea nitrogen (BUN) usually develop, and there may be leukopenia and anemia.

The primary insult is to the endothelial cells of the small blood vessels. Multiplication of the rickettsiae causes edema, deposition of both fibrin and platelets, and obstruction of the vessels, which may be followed by thrombosis; hemorrhage; and perivascular infiltration of neutrophils, macrophages, and lymphocytes. The vascular lesions are widely disseminated, but they are most numerous in the skin, myocardium, skeletal muscle, kidneys, and CNS.

Diagnosis. The diagnosis of epidemic typhus should be based on the clinical picture; appropriate therapy should not be withheld until there is laboratory confirmation of the diagnosis. Isolation of *R. prowazekii* can substantiate the clinical diagnosis, but doing so is both difficult and potentially dangerous and must be done with the use of special equipment by specially trained personnel. The organism also may be visualized in tissue and has been detected with the use of PCR (Carl et al., 1990). Primary isolation of *R. prowazekii* can be accomplished by inoculating blood into guinea pigs, adult white mice, or the yolk sac of embryonated eggs. Infection with *R. prowazekii* also induces the formation of antibodies that agglutinate the OX polysaccharide antigens of *Proteus vulgaris*. These agglutinins appear in the second week after onset of illness, and agglutination is usually maximal with OX-19 strains. A fourfold rise in agglutination titers is suggestive of recent infection. Complement-fixing antibodies can be detected in the third week after onset of the illness. However, as with Rocky Mountain spotted fever, immunofluorescence tests and microagglutination procedures (available in specialized laboratories) are more sensitive (Ormsbee, 1977).

Treatment and prognosis. Patients with epidemic typhus should be deloused, which can be accomplished by bathing with soap and water and with weekly dusting with 10% dichlorodiphenyltrichloroethane (DDT), 1% lindane, or another effective agent lethal to the lice. Tetracycline and chloramphenicol are the antimicrobials of choice for treatment. A therapeutic response usually occurs within 48 hours. Early treatment is more likely to induce a prompt clinical response.

Otitis media, parotitis, and bronchopneumonia may complicate epidemic typhus. Gangrene of portions of the extremities may also result from the vasculitis and thrombosis. Untreated epidemic typhus fever is a severe and potentially fatal infection. The mortality rate ranges from 10% to 40% and is higher in older individuals. The severe myocardial and CNS involvement is not usually followed by sequelae if the patient survives. If antimicrobial therapy is administered early in the course of the illness, death from the infection is rare.

Brill-Zinsser disease. Recrudescent infection sometimes occurs many years after an individual has had epidemic typhus. It was first suggested in 1934 that this recurrence was a relapse of a prior infection with *R. prowazekii*. Thus the disease may occur in an individual who lives in a louse-free environment. Brill-Zinsser disease most frequently occurs in immigrants from endemic areas. As the number of survivors of World War II who are alive diminishes, the frequency of Brill-Zinsser disease in the United States has decreased, since a majority of cases occurred in this group of patients. An additional aspect of recrudescent disease is that lice that feed on affected patients can become infected and subsequently initiate another cycle of transmission. Latent human infection therefore constitutes an interepidemic reservoir. Weil-Felix antibodies usually do not develop in patients with Brill-Zinsser

disease. However, specific IgG antibodies, detected by microimmunofluorescence, aid in making the diagnosis.

Prevention. After the patient and his or her clothing have been cleared of lice, no isolation is necessary because the patient will not transmit disease to other persons. Contacts known to have lice also should be deloused. After that, quarantine is not necessary. Specific protein antigens of *R. prowazekii* and of *R. typhi* have been characterized. Antibodies against these antigens are protective. These purified large polypeptides do not have significant endotoxin content. Both humoral and cellular immunity to these antigens does develop in humans after natural infection, and subunit vaccines that are composed of these antigens have been tested successfully for immunogenicity and efficacy in guinea pigs.

Murine Typhus (Endemic Typhus, Flea-Borne Typhus, Rat Typhus). Murine typhus fever is an acute, relatively mild infection caused by *R. typhi*. It is characterized clinically by headache, fever, malaise, and a maculopapular eruption with a centripetal distribution. Essentially it is a modified version of epidemic typhus fever.

Etiology and epidemiology. *R. typhi* is a natural infection of rodents that is spread to humans by the rat flea *(Xenopsylla cheopis)* and the rat louse *(Polyplax spinulosus)*. The vector, most frequently the rat flea, becomes infected with *R. typhi* by feeding on either a mouse or a rat that is infected. The rickettsiae multiply in cells of both the gut of the flea and in malpighian tubules. Thus infected, the flea may infect other susceptible rodents. Rickettsiae can be found in brains of infected rodents for up to several months. Fleas do not transmit *R. typhi* transovarially, so the murine hosts constitute the reservoir for the microorganisms. The infection is not transmitted by the bite of the flea. Transmission of *R. typhi* to humans occurs on occasions when the infected flea that is taking a blood meal is scratched by a human, thereby inoculating the infected feces of the flea into the excoriation. The feces of the flea are also infective if they happen to contact a mucosal surface such as the conjunctiva. *R. typhi* is very similar to *R. prowazekii* and is also infective for rats, mice, guinea pigs, and the yolk sac of embryonated eggs.

Murine typhus fever has a worldwide distribution and is endemic in many countries, including the United States. In the United States the largest number of cases has occurred in the Southern states along the Gulf of Mexico and the Atlantic seaboard and in California. In recent years the majority of reported cases in the United States have occurred in Texas. The disease occurs in areas that are infested with rats or mice; these animals tend to be present in large numbers where grains and feeds for animals are stored. The disease occurs most often during the summer months.

The incubation period of murine typhus ranges from 1 to 2 weeks. Clinically, murine typhus is indistinguishable from a mild case of epidemic typhus. The development of fever, headache, malaise, myalgia, and a maculopapular nonpruritic skin rash that becomes apparent on the third to the fifth day of the illness are typical. The rash is usually sparse, discrete, and rarely is hemorrhagic. In the untreated patient, fever seldom persists for more than 2 weeks.

Diagnosis. Murine typhus is clinically similar to but usually much milder than epidemic typhus, and the rash of murine typhus is less likely to be hemorrhagic. If a rickettsia is isolated and injected into guinea pigs, scrotal edema develops if the organism is *R. typhi* (the cause of murine typhus) but not if it is *R. prowazekii*. Specific antibody measurements establish the correct diagnosis. The distribution of the rash of murine typhus differs from that of Rocky Mountain spotted fever, since the former begins on the trunk and usually does not involve the palms and soles, whereas the latter is concentrated on the face and on the extremities (including the palms and soles). Specific antibody tests help distinguish these two illnesses. The patient with scrub typhus usually has a primary lesion that consists of a papule that progresses to become a vesicle and then a scab with an ulcer. The severe febrile illness and rash could be confused with epidemic typhus. Specific antibody tests can be used to distinguish between epidemic typhus and scrub typhus. Meningococcemia usually progresses more rapidly than typhus, a fact that may be helpful in making a clinical diagnosis. The symptoms of coryza, conjunctivitis, and fever that precede the maculopapular eruption often provide a useful way to distinguish between measles and typhus. The distribution of the rash of measles, with its initial appearance on the face and neck, is different from that of typhus. Hemorrhagic lesions are uncommon in patients with measles, and the fever usually subsides after the first week of illness.

Weil-Felix agglutinins to *Proteus OX-19* usually appear in the second week of infection. However, measurement of antibodies by micro-IF is both more sensitive and more specific. The CF assay is a standard method that is generally available, but it is less sensitive than micro-IF. Serologic cross-reactions among members of the typhus group occur frequently, but the concentrations to the homologous antigen usually is the greatest. Inoculation of organisms or of blood that contains organisms into the peritoneal cavity of a guinea pig produces severe vesicular lesions and scrotal swelling. *R. typhi* produces a much more severe disease in this animal than the disease caused by inoculation of *R. prowazekii*.

Treatment and prognosis. The treatment is the same as that for epidemic typhus. This disease is transmitted only by the infected vector and does not spread directly from person to person. The reported mortality rate is <2%. Cardiac, CNS, and renal manifestations occur less frequently in patients with murine typhus than in those with epidemic typhus.

Scrub Typhus. An additional group of rickettsiae, the scrub typhus group, is capable of producing a clinical illness in humans. These rickettsiae have different surface antigens, classified as Karp, Gilliam, or Kato; consequently persons can become infected and develop clinical illness caused by infection with these rickettsiae more than once. The different antigenic types are not associated with any differences in the clinical manifestations or infection.

Etiology and epidemiology. *R. tsutsugamushi* (or *R. orientalis*) causes scrub typhus. This rickettsia has been observed to form blebs from its outer membranes in cell culture just as do some other gram-negative organisms. The organism infects several species of trombiculid mites. The mites have a three-stage life cycle (i.e., larva, nymph, and adult). *R. tsutsugamushi* is transmitted transtadially. The larva, or chigger, is the only stage that feeds on vertebrates. After a blood meal the chigger detaches and matures into a nymph and, subsequently, into an adult. Both nymphs and adults are free living in the soil. Therefore trombiculid mites are the vectors, as well as the reservoirs, of the rickettsial infections they transmit. Normally the chiggers feed on small mammals or ground-feeding birds. Humans accidentally enter the natural cycle of infection in areas of secondary or scrub vegetation or on beaches and deserts and in rain forests. The disease is endemic in a geographic area of approximately 5 million square miles that includes Australia, Japan, Korea, India, and Vietnam. There was significant morbidity from scrub typhus during World War II among both American and Japanese soldiers. The disease usually occurs sporadically unless a group of people is brought into an endemic mite-infested area.

Clinical manifestations. The incubation period of scrub typhus ranges from 1 to 3 weeks. Clinical manifestations of scrub typhus are very similar to those of other rickettsial infections, with abrupt onset of fever, headache, vomiting, myalgia, and abdominal pain. A local cutaneous lesion evolves from a small indurated or vesicular lesion into an ulcerated area that is present at the time of onset of symptoms. An eschar is usually present as is local lymphadenopathy. Approximately 1 week after the onset of fever a macular or maculopapular rash appears and is apparent first on the trunk. Fatality rates in epidemics have varied from 0% to 50%. Antimicrobial therapy is effective and prevents fatal illness. Surface antigens of the causative organism vary, so infection with one strain of *R. tsutsugamushi* does not confer protection against other strains. Thus clinical disease may occur more than once in a single individual.

Diagnosis. Serologic diagnosis is difficult because different organisms express antigens that are not cross-reactive. Several antigens (usually the three strains cited earlier) must be used in a test such as a CF assay. A Weil-Felix reaction may be positive, with agglutinins to *Proteus* OX-K. The time course of the illness is similar to that of other rickettsial infections; antibodies become detectable in the second week of illness. Tests for agglutinins are less sensitive than is quantitation of antibodies by immunofluorescence.

Treatment and prognosis. Tetracycline and chloramphenicol are effective therapeutic agents that inhibit the growth of rickettsiae and usually produce prompt clinical improvement. If antibiotics are discontinued too early, relapse may occur.

Q Fever. *Coxiella burnetti* was isolated simultaneously from infected persons in Australia and from wood ticks in Montana and was identified as a rickettsia in 1939 (Burnet and Freeman, 1939). The name of the disease, Q fever, comes from the first initial of "query," which was the clinical designation for this unusual febrile illness.

Etiology and epidemiology. *C. burnetti* grows within cells in membrane-bound vesicles primarily in monocytes and macrophages. As an obligate intracellular organism, it parasitizes eukaryotic cells and goes through its developmental cycle in the phagolysosome. The metabolism of these organisms is active at a pH of 4.5, which is the intravacuolar pH, and is not active at a pH of 7.0. Thus this organism thrives in the usually hostile environment of the phagolysosome. Differences in surface antigens define phase I and phase II organisms, which are morphologically identical. Phase I organisms exist in nature, whereas phase II organisms develop with passage in embryonated eggs.

The ecology of *C. burnetti* is complex. One ecologic cycle involves arthropods, especially ticks, which infect a variety of vertebrates, including domestic animals but not humans. Another cycle is maintained among domestic animals (typically sheep). These animals may have inapparent infection and may shed large quantities of infectious organisms in urine, milk, and feces and from placentas. *C. burnetti* is resistant to drying, light, and extremes of temperature. Consequently, infectious material often becomes aerosolized. Humans and animals may become infected by inhaling the organism. Infection may also be acquired by ingestion of infected milk or by handling contaminated wool or hides. *C. burnetti* also can penetrate the skin (e.g., through a minor abrasion) and the mucous membranes. Rarely, human-to-human transmission has occurred. Q fever is an occupational risk in abattoir workers, farm workers, workers at tanneries and at plants that produce wool or felt, and workers in laboratories that use sheep and other livestock.

Clinical manifestations. The incubation period of Q fever is 2 to 3 weeks. Illness usually begins abruptly with fever, chills, headache, malaise, and weakness (Ruiz-Contreras et al., 1993). After 5 or 6 days of symptoms, cough and chest pain occur, and rales may be audible. Pneumonia usually is apparent on a radiograph of the chest by the third day of illness. The consolidation clears over a period of 1 to 2 weeks (Derrick, 1973). There are peribronchial and perivascular infiltrates of lymphocytes, plasma cells, and monocytes in the lungs. Fibrinous exudate fills the alveoli and bronchioles. Q fever is unique among the rickettsial diseases in that a rash is not a part of the clinical syndrome. Prolonged fever, endocarditis, and hepatitis may occur. There is a spectrum of illness; asymptomatic infection has been documented. Q fever endocarditis can occur months or years after the acute attack. Organisms isolated from persons with chronic illness contain a large plasmid (QpRS), whereas a smaller plasmid (QpH1) is present in organisms isolated from persons with acute illness.

Diagnosis. The compatible clinical picture, isolation of *C. burnetti* from the blood or sputum, and serologic tests establish the diagnosis. Unfortunately, isolation of the organism requires inoculation of blood or sputum into an animal such as a guinea pig, mouse, or hamster, or into embryonated eggs or cell culture. Because of the risk of transmission in the laboratory, this procedure is available only in research laboratories accustomed to dealing with the organism. Consequently, it is more reasonable to rely on serologic findings to confirm the diagnosis. Several state health departments perform the CF test using purified antigens. Since *C. burnetti* exists in two phases, tests have been devised that use either phase I or phase II antigens, which are useful in distinguishing acute from either chronic or past infection (antibodies to the phase II antigen are present in acute infection). Serosurveys with CF antibodies underestimate the prevalence of infection; intradermal skin tests are more sensitive. The use of ELISA for specific IgM antibody to *C. burnetti* may be helpful in diagnosing acute infection (Field et al., 1983). Weil-Felix agglutinins do not develop in response to infection with *C. burnetti.*

Treatment and prognosis. Q fever should be treated with either tetracycline or chloramphenicol; either drug should be administered for several days after the patient has become afebrile. The clinical response to treatment often is not as dramatic as that of patients with other rickettsial infections. The mortality rate of Q fever before antimicrobial therapy was available was approximately 1%. Fatalities are extraordinarily rare if patients are treated appropriately with an antimicrobial agent; the only exceptions are patients with endocarditis, for whom the mortality rate is higher. Replacement of an infected heart valve with a prosthetic valve combined with long-term antimicrobial therapy may improve the prognosis for patients with endocarditis.

Prevention. Transmission of *C. burnetti* via milk can be prevented by pasteurizing it; otherwise, it is difficult to interrupt the transmission of infection. Laboratory personnel who work with sheep or their tissues should do their research in a separate area away from other laboratories and areas where patients are treated. Use of seronegative flocks is another alternative; skin tests can be used to assess whether personnel have become infected previously or are at risk. Lymphocyte transformation studies and skin testing are better predictors of immunity than are measurements of antibodies because antibody-negative persons may be immune.

Human beings rarely transmit disease to one another; thus isolation of the infected patient is not indicated. A vaccine composed of inactivated phase II organisms was used effectively in Public Health Service and Army laboratories, but adverse reactions precluded widespread use of the vaccine. A formalin-inactivated vaccine against phase I *C. burnetti* has been effective in workers in Australian abbatoirs (Marmion et al., 1990).

Ehrlichiosis. Ehrlichieae is one of the three tribes of the family Rickettsiaceae (see Fig. 33-5). The genus *Ehrlichia* contains a number of species, at least three of which—*E. chaffeensis,* an unidentified species similar to *E. equi,* and *E. sennetsu*—cause human illness (McDade, 1989; Fishbein et al., 1994; Dumler and Bakken, 1995).

Etiology and epidemiology. *Ehrlichia* organisms are obligate intracellular bacteria nominally grouped with rickettsiae (see Fig. 33-5). Based on sequencing of their 16S rRNA genes, three different genogroups exist. The organisms of major importance in the first genogroup are *E. chaffeensis,* which causes human monocytic ehrlichiosis (HME), and *E. canis,* which causes ehrlichiosis in dogs. Another genogroup contains *E. phagocytophilia* and *E. equi,* which cause granulocytic ehrlichiosis in sheep, cattle, deer, and horses. The agent (which has yet to be identified) that causes human granulocytic ehrlichiosis (HGE) will be a member of this genogroup (Goodman et al., 1996). The final genogroup contains *E. sennetsu,* the cause of sennetsu fever in Japan.

These organisms replicate within the phagosome in the host cell and have a tropism for circulating leukocytes. Like chlamydiae, *Ehrlichia* organisms go through developmental stages of elementary bodies, initial bodies, and morulae. The individual organisms, called *elementary bodies,* are small, gram-negative rods that are about 0.5 μm in diameter. They are phagocytized either by monocytes (in HME) or by granulocytes (in HGE), and phagolysosomal fusion fails to occur. The elementary bodies divide by binary fission within the phagosome and form initial bodies, which are composed of many elementary bodies and can be seen as inclusions in the cells in 3 to 5 days. These initial bodies grow further and divide during the next 7 to 12 days so that by light microscopy the configuration resembles a mulberry, or morula. Each infected leukocyte can contain several morulae. Rupture of the infected cells releases individual elementary bodies from the broken morulae.

Ehrlichia organisms are transmitted by ticks. The primary vector for *E. chaffeensis* (which causes HME) is *Amblyomma americanum,* the Lone Star tick. Most cases occur in the Southern and South-Central United States. The vector for the agent that causes HGE is *Ixodes scapularis,* the deer tick. Most cases of HGE occur in the upper Midwestern states (Wisconsin and Minnesota), southern New England and the mid-Atlantic states (Pancholi et al., 1995; Bakken et al., 1996). It also has been reported in Europe (Brouqui et al., 1995). As with most tick-borne infections in temperate climates, the highest incidence of infection occurs during the peak months of human exposure to ticks—from April to September. The vector for *E. sennetsu* is unknown.

Clinical manifestations. In 1987 the first case of human ehrlichiosis in the United States was reported (Maeda et al., 1987). Since then, HME and HGE have been recognized with increasing frequency (Harkness et al., 1991; Barton et al., 1992). Despite differences in the cells that they infect, the clinical manifestations of HME and HGE are similar, and they resemble the clinical manifestations of Rocky Mountain spotted fever except that few patients have a rash (Bakken et al., 1996). Fever and headache are the most common manifestations of the illness, followed by myalgia, nausea, vomiting, and arthralgia. Leukopenia and thrombocytopenia occur in most patients in the first week of the illness. Fishbein et al. (1987, 1989) reported leukopenia in 57% of their patients and thrombocytopenia in 85% at the time of hospitalization. More than three quarters of the patients have elevated concentrations of either alanine or aspartate aminotransferase during the course of the illness, usually during the first week. During the acute illness, inclusion bodies may be seen in atypical lymphocytes, neutrophils, and monocytes. These inclusions are dark blue, round, and approximately 2 to 5 μm in diameter. Electron microscopy shows aggregates of organisms in membrane-lined vacuoles.

Sennetsu fever, described in the 1950s, is marked by the rapid onset of fever, lymphadenopathy, and atypical lymphocytosis. A rickettsia-like agent was isolated from the blood, lymph nodes, and bone marrow of an affected patient. The provisional name associated with the organism was *Rickettsia sennetsu;* however, the organism was reclassified as *E. sennetsu.* The disease rarely has been reported outside of Japan. One serologic survey from Malaysia suggested that a substantial number of patients with febrile illnesses had antibodies to this organism. The illness occurs predominately in the summer and fall. The incubation period is approximately 14 days, with sudden onset of illness and generalized adenopathy developing within the first week of illness. The untreated illness is benign, and no fatalities or serious complications have been described.

Diagnosis. Although examination of the peripheral smear for the presence of morulae may be helpful, the sensitivity of this method of diagnosis is poor. Culture of the organisms is possible, but it is difficult and not widely available (Goodman et al., 1996). Use of PCR to make the diagnosis also is promising but it is not yet suitable for general use (Everett et al., 1994). Consequently, the mainstay of diagnosis is serologic testing. To make a diagnosis of ehrlichiosis in a patient with a compatible clinical history, there should be a fourfold rise between acute-phase and convalescent-phase serum samples in the concentration of antibodies against *E. chaffeensis* (minimum titer, 1:64) for HME and, for HGE (until the causative agent is identified), a similar increase in antibody concentrations (or a single titer of $\geq$1:128) against *E. equi* (Dawson et al., 1990, 1991).

Treatment and prognosis. Tetracycline is the drug of choice to treat ehrlichiosis. Although chloramphenicol has been effective in many instances, there also are a considerable number of reports of failures of treatment with chloramphenicol. Consequently, even in young children many experts treat with tetracycline or doxycycline, since the risk of staining of the teeth from a short course of treatment is low and the potential benefit of the drug outweighs the small risk.

Ehrlichiosis sometimes (but rarely) is fatal. Serosurveys indicate that unrecognized infection is far more common than severe infection (some patients have either asymptomatic or unrecognized illness) (Magnarelli et al., 1995). The illness may be prolonged in some patients, but the ultimate prognosis is excellent.

Prevention. Measures that reduce the risk of exposure to ticks may be effective in limiting the opportunities for infection to occur. There is no effective vaccine.

BIBLIOGRAPHY

Fishbein DB, Dennis DT. Tick-borne diseases: a growing risk. N Engl J Med 1995;333:452-453.

Spach DH, Liles WC, Campbell GL, et al. Medical progress: Tick-borne diseases in the United States. N Engl J Med 1993;329:936-947.

Lyme disease

Adams WV, Rose CD, Eppes SC, et al. Cognitive effects of Lyme disease in children. Pediatrics 1994;94:185-189.

Aronowitz RA. Lyme disease: the social construction of a new disease and its social consequences. Milbank Q 1991;69:79-112.

Bacterial Zoonoses Branch, CDC. Evaluation of serologic tests for Lyme disease: report of a national evaluation. Lyme Disease Surveillance Summary 1991;2:1-3.

Benach JL, Bosler EM, Hanrahan JP, et al. Spirochetes isolated from the blood of two patients with Lyme disease. N Engl J Med 1983;308:740-742.

Burgdorfer W, Barbour AG, Hayes SF, et al. Lyme disease: a tick-born spirochetosis? Science 1982;216:1317-1319.

Centers for Disease Control. Recommendations for test performance and interpretation from the second national conference on serologic diagnosis of Lyme disease. MMWR 1995;44:590.

Centers for Disease Control. Lyme disease: United States, 1995. MMWR 1996;45:481-484.

Dennis DT. Lyme disease: tracking an epidemic. JAMA 1991;266:1269-1270.

Dressler F, Whalen JA, Reinhardt BN, et al. Western blotting in the serodiagnosis of Lyme disease. J Infect Dis 1993;167:392-400.

Eichenfield AH, Goldsmith DP, Benach JL, et al. Childhood lyme arthritis: experience in an endemic area. J Pediatr 1986;109:753-758.

Falco RC, Fish D, Piesman J. Duration of tick bites in a Lyme disease–endemic area. Am J Epidemiol 1996;143:187-192.

Feder HM Jr, Gerber MA, Luger SW, et al. Persistence of serum antibodies to *Borrelia burgdorferi* in patients treated for Lyme disease. Clin Infect Dis 1992;15:788-793.

Fikrig E, Barthold SW, Kantor FS, et al. Protection of mice against the Lyme disease agent by immunizing with recombinant OspA. Science 1990;250:553-556.

Gerber MA, Shapiro ED, Burke GS, et al. Lyme disease in children in Southeastern Connecticut. N Engl J Med 1996;335:1270-1274.

Gerber MA, Zalneraitis EL. Childhood neurologic disorders and Lyme disease during pregnancy. Pediatr Neurol 1994;11:41-43.

Hanrahan JP, Benach JL, Coleman JL, et al. Incidence and cumulative frequency of endemic Lyme disease in a community. J Infect Dis 1984;150:489-496.

Lane RS, Piesman J, Burgdorfer W. Lyme borreliosis: relation of its causative agent to its vectors and hosts in North America and Europe. Annu Rev Entomol 1991;36:587-609.

Nadal D, Hunziker UA, Bucher HU, et al. Infants born to mothers with antibodies against *Borrelia burgdorferi* at delivery. Eur J Pediatr 1989;148:426-427.

Nocton JJ, Dressler F, Rutledge BJ, et al. Detection of *Borrelia burgdorferi* DNA by polymerase chain reaction in synovial fluid from patients with Lyme arthritis. N Engl J Med 1994;330:229-234.

Piesman J. Dynamics of *Borrelia burgdorferi* transmission by nymphal *Ixodes dammini* ticks. J Infect Dis 1993;167:1082-1085.

Piesman J, Mather TN, Sinsky R. Duration of tick attachment and *Borrelia burgdorferi* transmission. J Clin Microbiol 1987;25:557-558.

Piesman J, Maupin GO, Campos EG, et al. Duration of adult female Ixodes dammini attachment and transmission of *Borrelia burgdorferi,* description of a needle aspiration isolation method. J Infect Dis 1991;163:895-897.

Rahn DW, Malawista SE. Lyme disease: recommendations for diagnosis and treatment. Ann Intern Med 1991;114:1472-1481.

Rosa PA, Schwan TG. A specific and sensitive assay for the lyme disease spirochete *Borrelia burgdorferi* using the polymerase chain reaction. J Infect Dis 1989;160:1018-1029.

Rose CD, Fawcett WV, Adams WV, et al. Cognitive effects of Lyme disease in children: A 4-year follow-up controlled study: 7th international congress on Lyme borreliosis, June 1996, San Francisco, abstract D656.

Salazaar JC, Gerber MA, Goff CW. Long-term outcome of Lyme disease in children given early treatment. J Pediatr 1993;122:591-593.

Schwartz B, Nadelman RB, Fish D, et al. Entomologic and demographic correlates of anti–tick saliva antibody in a prospective study of tick bite subjects in Westchester County, New York. Am J Trop Med Hyg 1993;48:50-57.

Seltzer EG, Shapiro ED. Misdiagnosis of Lyme disease: when not to order serologic tests. Pediatr Infect Dis J 1996;15:762-763.

Shapiro ED. Lyme disease. In Burg FD, Ingelfinger JR, Wald ER, Polin RA, (eds). Current pediatric therapy, vol 15. Philadelphia: WB Saunders, 1995.

Shapiro ED, Gerber MA, Holabird NB, et al. A controlled trial of antimicrobial prophylaxis for Lyme disease after deer-tick bites. N Engl J Med 1992;327:1769-73.

Shapiro ED, Seltzer EG, Gerber MA, et al. Long-term outcomes of children with Lyme disease. Pediatr Res 1996;39:185A (abstract 1094).

Sigal LH, Patella SJ. Lyme arthritis as the incorrect diagnosis in pediatric and adolescent fibromyalgia. Pediatrics 1992;90:523-528.

Sigel LH. Persisting complaints attributed to chronic Lyme disease: possible mechanisms and implications for management. Am J Med 1994;96:365-374.

Sigel LH. The Lyme disease controversy: social and financial costs of misdiagnosis and mismanagement. Arch Intern Med 1996;156:1493-1500.

Steere AC. Lyme disease. N Engl J Med 1989;321:586-596.

Steere C, Dwyer E, Winchester R. Association of chronic lyme arthritis with HLA-DR4 and HLA-DR2 alleles. N Engl J Med 1990;323:219-223.

Steere AC, Grodzicki RL, Kornblatt AN, et al. The spirochetal etiology of Lyme disease. N Engl J Med 1983;308:733-740.

Steere AC, Malawista SE, Snydman DR, et al. Lyme arthritis: an epidemic of oligoarticular arthritis in children and adults in three Connecticut communities. Arthritis Rheum 1977;20:7-17.

Steere AC, Taylor E, McHugh GL, et al. The overdiagnosis of Lyme disease. JAMA 1993;269:1812-1826.

Steere AC, Taylor E, Wilson ML, et al. Longitudinal assessment of the clinical and epidemiological features of Lyme disease in a defined population. J Infect Dis 1986;154:294-300.

Strobino BA, Williams CL, Abid S, et al. Lyme disease and pregnancy outcome: prospective study of two thousand prenatal patients. Am J Obstet Gynecol 1993;169:367-375.

Warshafsky S, Nowakowski J, Nadelman RB, et al. Efficacy of antibiotic prophylaxis for prevention of Lyme disease: a meta-analysis. J Gen Intern Med 1996;11:329-333.

White DJ, Chang H-G, Benach JL, et al. The geographic spread and temporal increase of the Lyme disease epidemic. JAMA 1991;266:1230-1236.

Williams CL, Benach JL, Curran AS, et al. Lyme disease during pregnancy: a cord blood serosurvey. Ann NY Acad Sci 1988;539:504-506.

Wormser GP. Prospects for a vaccine to prevent Lyme disease in humans. Clin Infect Dis 1995;21:1267-1274.

Zemel LS, Gerber MA, Shapiro ED. Lyme arthritis in children: clinical epidemiology and long-term outcomes. Pediatr Res 1995;37:191A (abstract 1131).

Relapsing fever

Barbour AG, Barrera O, Judd RC. Structural analysis of the variable major proteins of *Borrelia hermsii*. J Exp Med 1983;158:2127-2140.

Boyer KM, Munford RS, Maupin GO, et al. Tick-borne relapsing fever: an interstate outbreak originating at Grand Canyon National Park. Am J Epidemiol 1977;105:469-479.

Edall TA, Emerson JK, Maupin GO, et al. Tick-borne relapsing fever in Colorado: historical review and report of cases. JAMA 1979;241:2279-2282.

Felsenfeld O. Borrelia, human relapsing fever, and parasite-vector-host relationships. Bacteriol Rev 1965;29:46-74.

Horton JM, Blaser MJ. The spectrum of relapsing fever in the Rocky Mountains. Arch Intern Med 1985;145:871-875.

Le CT. Tick-borne relapsing fever in children. Pediatrics 1980;66:963-966.

Plasterk RHA, Simon MI, Barbour AG. Transposition of structural genes to an expression sequence on a linear plasmid causes antigenic variation in the bacterium *Borrelia hermsii*. Nature 1985;318:257-263.

Stoenner HG, Dodd T, Larsen C. Antigenic variation of *Borrelia hermsii*. J Exp Med 1982;156:1297-1311.

Southern PM, Sanford JP. Relapsing fever: a clinical and microbiological review. Medicine 1969;48:129-149.

Tularemia

Burke DS. Immunization against tularemia: analysis of the effectiveness of live *Francisella tularensis* vaccine in prevention of laboratory-acquired tularemia. J Infect Dis 1977;135:55-60.

Enderlin G, Morales L, Jacobs RF, et al. Streptomycin and alternative agents for the treatment of tularemia: review of the literature. Clin Infect Dis 1994;19:42-47.

Evans ME, Gregory DW, Schaffner W, et al. Tularemia: a 30-year experience with 88 cases. Medicine 1985;64:251-69.

Francis E. Tularemia. JAMA 1925;84:1243-1250.

Guerrant RL, Humphries MK Jr, Butler JE, et al. Tickborne oculoglandular tularemia: case report and review of seasonal and vectorial associations in 106 cases. Arch Intern Med 1976;136:811-813.

Hopla CE. The ecology of tularemia. Adv Vet Sci Compar Med 1974;18:25-53.

Jacobs RF, Condrey YM, Yamauchi T. Tularemia in adults and children: a changing presentation. Pediatrics 1985;76:818-822.

Jacobs RF, Narain JP. Tularemia in children. Pediatr Infect Dis 1983;2:487-491.

Long GW, Oprandy JJ, Narayanan RB, et al. Detection of *Francisella tularensis* in blood by polymerase chain reaction. J Clin Microbiol 1993;31:152-154.

Markowitz LE, Hynes NA, de la Cruz P, et al. Tick-borne tularemia: an outbreak of lymphadenopathy in children. JAMA 1985;254:2922-2925.

Taylor JP, Istre GR, McChesney TC, et al. Epidemiologic characteristics of human tularemia in the southwest-central states, 1981-1987. Am J Epidemiol 1991;133:1032-1038.

Babesiosis

Krause PJ, Telford SR III, Pollack RJ, et al. Babesiosis: an underdiagnosed disease of children. Pediatrics 1992;89:1045-1048.

Krause PJ, Telford SR III, Ryan R, et al. Diagnosis of babesiosis: evaluation of a serologic test for the detection of *Babesia microti* antibody. J Infect Dis 1994;69:923-926.

Krause PJ, Telford SR III, Spielman A, et al. Concurrent Lyme disease and babesiosis: evidence for increased severity and duration of illness. JAMA 1996;275:1657-1660.

Magnarelli LA, Dumler JS, Anderson JF, et al. Coexistence of antibodies to tick-borne pathogens of babesiosis, ehrlichiosis, and Lyme borreliosis in human sera. J Clin Microbiol 1995;33:3054-3057.

Meldrum SC, Birkhead GS, White DJ, et al. Human babesiosis in New York state: an epidemiological description of 136 cases. Clin Infect Dis 1992;15:1019-1023.

Mintz ED, Anderson JF, Cable RG, et al. Transfusion-transmitted babesiosis: a case report from a new endemic area. Transfusion 1991;31:365-368.

Persing DH, Herwaldt BL, Glaser C, et al. Infection with a babesia-like organism in northern California. N Engl J Med 1995;332:298-303.

Persing DH, Mathiesen D, Marshall WF, et al. Detection of *Babesia microti* by polymerase chain reaction. J Clin Microbiol 1992;30:2097-2103.

Reubush TK II, Cassaday PB, Marsh HJ, et al. Human babesiosis on Nantucket Island. Ann Intern Med 1977;86:6-9.

Sun T, Tenenbaum MJ, Greenspan J, et al. Morphologic and clinical observations in human infection with *Babesia microti*. J Infect Dis 1983;148:239-248.

Rocky Mountain spotted fever

Abramson JS, Givner LB. Should tetracycline be contraindicated for therapy of presumed Rocky Mountain spotted fever in children less than 9 years of age? Pediatrics 1990;86:123-124.

Anacker RL, Lissh RH, Mann RE, et al. Antigenic heterogeneity in high and low virulence strains of *Rickettsia rickettsii* revealed by monoclonal antibodies. Infect Immun 1986;51:653.

Anacker RL, Philip RN, Casper E, et al. Biological properties of rabbit antibodies to a surface antigen of *Rickettsia rickettsii*. Infect Immun 1983;40:292.

Anderson BE, Tzianabosj I. Comparative sequence analysis of a genus common rickettsial antigen gene. J Bacteria 1989;171:5199.

Archibald LK, Sexton DJ. Long-term sequelae of Rocky Mountain spotted fever. Clin Infect Dis 1995;20:1122-1125.

Baganz MD, Dross PE, Reinhardt JA. Rocky Mountain spotted fever encephalitis: MR findings. Am J Neuroradiol 1995;16(suppl):919-922.

Bradford WD, Croker BP, Tisher CC. Kidney lesions in Rocky Mountain spotted fever. Am J Pathol 1979;97:383.

Bradford WD, Hawkins HK. Rocky Mountain spotted fever in childhood. Am J Dis Child 1977;131:1228.

Clements ML, Dumler JS, Fiset P, et al. Serodiagnosis of Rocky Mountain spotted fever: comparison of IgM and IgG enzyme-linked immunosorbent assays and indirect fluorescent antibody test. J Infect Dis 1983;148:876.

D'Angelo LJ, Winkler WG, Bergman DJ. Rocky Mountain spotted fever in the United States, 1975-1977. J Infect Dis 1978;138:273.

Dumler JS, Walker DH. Diagnostic tests for Rocky Mountain spotted fever and other rickettsial diseases. Dermatol Clin 1994;12:25-36.

DuPont HL, Hornick RB, Dawkins AT, et al. Rocky Mountain spotted fever: a comparative study of the active immunity induced by inactivated and viable pathogenic *R. rickettsii*. J Infect Dis 1973;128:340.

Feng WC, Waner JL. Serological cross-reaction and cross-protection in guinea pigs infected with *Rickettsia rickettsii* and *Rickettsia montana*. Infect Immun 1980;28:627.

Hattwick MAW, Retailliau H, O'Brien RJ, et al. Fatal Rocky Mountain spotted fever. JAMA 1978;240:1499.

Hayes SF, Burgdorfer W. Reactivation of *Rickettsia rickettsii* in *Dermacentor andersoni* ticks: an ultrastructural analysis. Infect Immun 1982;37:779.

Hechemy KE, Michaelson EE, Anacker RL, et al. Evaluation of latex *Rickettsia rickettsii* test for Rocky Mountain spotted fever in 11 laboratories. J Clin Microbiol 1983;18:938.

King WV. Experimental transmission of Rocky Mountain spotted fever by means of the tick. Public Health Rep 1986;21:863.

Kirkland KB, Marcom PK, Sexton DJ, et al. Rocky Mountain spotted fever complicated by gangrene: report of six cases and review. Clin Infect Dis 1993;16:629-634.

Kirkland KB, Wilkinson WE, Sexton DJ. Therapeutic delay and mortality in cases of Rocky Mountain spotted fever. Clin Infect Dis 1995;20:1118-1121.

McDade JE, Newhouse VF. Natural history of *Rickettsia rickettsii*. Ann Rev Microbiol 1986;40:287.

McDonald GA, Anacker RL, Gargjian K. Cloned gene of *Rickettsia rickettsii* surface antigen: candidate vaccine for Rocky Mountain spotted fever. Science 1987;235:83.

Oster CN, Burke DS, Kenyon RH, et al. Laboratory-acquired Rocky Mountain spotted fever: the hazard of aerosol transmission. N Engl J Med 1977;297:859.

Philip RN, Casper EA, MacCormack JN, et al. A comparison of serologic methods for diagnosis of Rocky Mountain spotted fever. Am J Epidemiol 1977;105:56.

Radulovic S, Speed R, Feng HM, et al. EIA with species-specific monoclonal antibodies: a novel seroepidemiologic tool for determination of the etiologic agent of spotted fever rickettsiosis. J Infect Dis 1993;168:1292-1295.

Salgo MP, Telzak EE, Currie B, et al. A focus of Rocky Mountain spotted fever within New York City. N Engl J Med 1988;318:1345-1348.

Sexton DJ, Corey GR. Rocky Mountain "spotless" and "almost spotless" fever: a wolf in sheep's clothing. Clin Infect Dis 1992;15:439-448.

Sexton DJ, Kanj SS, Wilson K, et al. The use of a polymerase chain reaction as a diagnostic test for Rocky Mountain spotted fever. Am J Trop Med Hyg 1994;50:59-63.

Silverman DJ. *Rickettsia rickettsii*–induced cellular injury of human vascular endothelium in vitro. Infect Immun 1984;44:545.

Silverman DJ, Bond SB. Infection of human vascular endothelial cells by *Rickettsia rickettsii*. J Infect Dis 1979;26:714.

Silverman DJ, Wisseman CL. In vitro studies of rickettsia-host cell interactions: ultrastructural changes induced by *Rickettsia rickettsii* infection of chicken embryo fibroblasts. Infect Immun 1984;149:201.

Silverman DJ, Wisseman CL Jr, Waddell AD, Jones M. External layers of *Rickettsia prowazekii* and *Rickettsia rickettsii*: occurrence of a slime layer. Infect Immun 1978;22:233.

Teysseire N, Arnoux D, George F, et al. Von Willebrand factor release and thrombomodulin and tissue factor expression in *Rickettsia conorii*–infected endothelial cells. Infect Immun 1992;60:4388-4393.

Todd WJ, Burgdorfer W, Wray GP. Detection of fibrils associated with *Rickettsia rickettsii*. Infect Immun 1983;41:1252.

Walker DH. Rocky Mountain spotted fever: a seasonal alert. Clin Infect Dis 1995;20:1111-1117.

Walker DH, Firth WT, Edgell CJS. Human endothelial cell culture plaques induced by *Rickettsia rickettsii*. Infect Immun 1982;37:301.

Walker TS. Rickettsial interactions with human endothelial cells in vitro: adherence and entry. Infect Immun 1984;44:205.

Walker TS, Melott GE. Rickettsial stimulation of endothelial platelet-activating factor synthesis. Infect Immun 1993;61:2024-2029.

Wells GM, Woodward TE, Fiset P, Hornick RB. Rocky Mountain spotted fever caused by blood transfusion. JAMA 1978;239:2763.

Wilfert CM, MacCormack JN, Kleeman K, et al. Epidemiology of Rocky Mountain spotted fever as determined by active surveillance. J Infect Dis 1984;150:469-479.

Woodward TE, Pedersen SE, Oster CN, et al. Prompt confirmation of Rocky Mountain spotted fever: identification of rickettsiae in skin tissues. J Infect Dis 1976;134:297.

Rickettsialpox

Brettman LR, Lewin S, Holzman RS, et al. Rickettsialpox: report of an outbreak and a contemporary review. Medicine 1981;60:363.

Dolgopol VB. Histologic changes in rickettsialpox. Am J Pathol 1948;24:119.

Greenberg M. Rickettsialpox in New York City. Am J Med 1948;4:866.

Huebner RJ, Jellison WL, Pomerantz C. Rickettsialpox—a newly recognized disease. IV. Isolation of a rickettsia apparently identical with the causative agent of rickettsialpox from *Allodermanyssus sanguineus*, a rodent mite. Public Health Rep 1946;61:1677.

Sussman LN. Kew Gardens' spotted fever. NY Med J 1946;2:27.

Wong B, Singer C, Armstrong D, Millian SJ. Rickettsialpox. Case report and epidemiologic review. JAMA 1979;242:1998.

Typhus group

Berman SJ, Kundin WD. Scrub typhus in South Vietnam, a study of 87 cases. Ann Intern Med 1973;79:26.

Brown GW, Robinson DM, Huxsall DL, et al. Scrub typhus: a common cause of illness in indigenous populations. Trans R Soc Trop Med Hyg 1976;70:444.

Carl M, Tibbs CW, Dobson ME, et al. Diagnosis of acute typhus infection using the polymerase chain reaction. J Infect Dis 1990;161:791-793.

Dasch GA, Samms JR, Weiss E. Biochemical characteristics of typhus group rickettsiae with special attention to the *Rickettsia prowazekii* strains isolated from flying squirrels. Infect Immun 1978;19:676.

Duma RJ, Sonenshine DE, Bozeman FM, et al. Epidemic typhus in the United States associated with flying squirrels. JAMA 1981;245:2318.

Ormsbee RA. Serologic diagnosis of epidemic typhus fever. Am J Epidemiol 1977;105:261.

Osterman JV, Eisemann CS. Surface proteins of typhus and spotted fever group rickettsiae. Infect Immun 1978;21:866.

Samra Y, Shaked Y, Maier MK. Delayed neurologic display in murine typhus: report of two cases. Arch Intern Med 1989;149:949-951.

Silpapojakul K, Chupuppakarn S, Yuthasompob S, et al. Scrub and murine typhus in children with obscure fever in the tropics. Pediatr Infect Dis 1991;10:200-203.

Sonenshine DE, Bozeman M, Williams MS, et al. Epizootiology of epidemic typhus *(R. prowazekii)* in flying squirrels. Am J Trop Med Hyg 1978;27:339.

Traub R, Wisseman CL. The ecology of chigger-borne rickettsiosis (scrub typhus). J Med Entomol 1974;11:237.

Q fever

Amano KI, Williams JC. Sensitivity of *Coxiella burnetii* peptidoglycan to lysozyme hydrolysis and correlation of sacculus rigidity with peptidoglycan-associated proteins. J Bacteriol 1984;160:989.

Ascher MS, Berman MA, Ruppanner R. Initial clinical and immunologic evaluation of a new phase I Q fever vaccine and skin test in humans. J Infect Dis 1983;148:214.

Baca OG, Paretsky D. Q fever and *Coxiella burnetii:* a model for host-parasite interactions. Microbiol Rev 1983;47:127.

Burnet FM, Freeman M. A comparative study of rickettsial strains from an infection of ticks in Montana (United States of America) and from Q fever. Med J Aust 1939;2:887.

Derrick EH. The course of infection with *Coxiella burnetii.* Med J Aust 1973;1:1051.

Field PR, Hunt JG, Murphy AM. Detection and persistence of specific IgM antibody to *Coxiella burnetii* by enzyme-linked immunosorbent assay: a comparison with immunofluorescence and complement fixation tests. J Infect Dis 1983;148:477.

Hart RJC. The epidemiology of Q fever. Postgrad Med J 1973;49:535.

Marmion BP, Ormsbee RA, Kyrkou M, et al. Vaccine prophylaxis of abbatoir-associated Q fever: eight years' experience in Australian aborigines. Epidemiol Infect 1990;104:275-287.

Ruiz-Contreras J, Montero RG, Amador JTR, et al. Q fever in children. Am J Dis Child 1993;147:300-302.

Sawyer LA, Fishbein DB, McDade JE. Q fever: current concepts. 1987;9:935-946.

Williams JC, Peacock MG, McCaul TF. Immunological and biological characterization of *Coxiella burnetii,* phases I and II, separated from host components. Infect Immun 1981;32:840.

Ehrlichiosis

Bakken JS, Dumler JS, Chen S-M, et al. Human granulocytic ehrlichiosis in the upper midwest United States. JAMA 1994;272:212-218.

Bakken JS, Krueth J, Wilson-Nordskog C, et al. Clinical and laboratory characteristics of human granulocytic ehrlichiosis. JAMA 1996;275:199-205.

Barton LL, Rathore MH, Dawson JE. Infection with *Ehrlichia* in childhood. J Pediatr 1992;120:998-1001.

Brouqui P, Dumler JS, Liehnard R, et al. Human granulocytic ehrlichiosis in Europe. Lancet 1995;346:782-783.

Dawson JE, Fishbein DB, Eng TR, et al. Diagnosis of human ehrlichiosis with the indirect fluorescent antibody test: kinetics and specificity. J Infect Dis 1990;162:91-95.

Dawson JE, Rikihisa Y, Ewing SA, et al. Serologic diagnosis of human ehrlichiosis using two *Ehrlichia canis* isolates. J Infect Dis 1991;163:564-567.

Dumler JS, Bakken JS. Ehrlichial diseases of humans: emerging tick-borne infection. Clin Infect Dis 1995;20:1102-1110.

Dumler JS, Bakken JS. Human granulocytic ehrlichiosis in Wisconsin and Minnesota: a frequent infection with the potential for persistence. J Infect Dis 1996;173:1027-1030.

Everett ED, Evans KA, Henry RB, et al. Human ehrlichiosis in adults after tick exposure: diagnosis using polymerase chain reaction. Ann Intern Med 1994;120:730-735.

Fishbein DB, Kemp A, Dawson JE, et al. Human ehrlichiosis: prospective active surveillance in febrile hospitalized patients. J Infect Dis 1989;160:803-809.

Fishbein DB, Sawyer LA, Holland CJ, et al. Unexplained febrile illnesses after exposure to ticks. JAMA 1987; 257:3100-3104.

Fishbein DB, Dawson JE, Robinson LE. Human ehrlichiosis in the United States, 1985-1990. Ann Intern Med 1994;120:736-743.

Goodman JL, Nelson C, Vitale B, et al. Direct cultivation of the causative agent of human granulocytic ehrlichiosis 1996;334:209-215.

Harkness JR, Ewing SA, Brumit T, et al. Ehrlichiosis in children. Pediatrics 1991;87:199-203.

Maeda K, Markowitz N, Hawley RC, et al. Human infection with *Ehrlichia canis,* a leukocytic rickettsia. N Engl J Med 1987;316:853-856.

Magnarelli LA, Dumler JS, Anderson JF, et al. Coexistence of antibodies to tick-borne pathogens of babesiosis, ehrlichiosis, and Lyme borreliosis in human sera. J Clin Microbiol 1995;33:3054-3057.

McDade JE. Ehrlichiosis: a disease of animals and humans. J Infect Dis 1989;161:609-617.

Pancholi P, Kolbert CP, Mitchell PD, et al. *Ixodes dammini* as a potential vector of human granulocytic ehrlichiosis. J Infect Dis 1995;172:1007-1012.

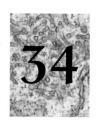

34   TOXOPLASMOSIS

FIONA ROBERTS, KENNETH BOYER, AND RIMA MCLEOD

Toxoplasmosis is disease caused by the ubiquitous, obligate intracellular protozoan *Toxoplasma gondii.* Infection is usually acquired orally or transplacentally, rarely by inoculation in a laboratory accident, by blood or leukocyte transfusion, or from a transplanted organ. Disease may also occur as the result of recrudescence of latent infection in immunocompromised individuals.

Clinical signs and symptoms depend in part on the host's immunologic status. In the immunologically healthy older child the acute infection may be asymptomatic, cause self-limited lymphadenopathy with or without fatigue and malaise, or occasionally cause significant organ damage. In the child who is immunocompromised by acquired immunodeficiency syndrome (AIDS), organ transplantation, cytotoxic therapy for malignancy or vasculitis, initial infection, or recrudescence of latent infection may cause severe illness. The most common presentation in immunocompromised individuals is that of neurologic disease.

Congenitally acquired toxoplasmosis almost always causes morbidity and occasionally causes mortality. Most congenital infections are not recognized at birth but are manifested in later infancy, childhood, or adulthood. When infection is acquired by a mother early in gestation, transmission of the infection to her fetus occurs less frequently than when her infection is acquired later in gestation. When infection is transmitted, however, neurologic and ophthalmologic impairment is often severe. Involvement is less severe at birth in infants born to mothers who acquired the disease later in gestation. Nonetheless, although these infants usually appear normal in initial newborn examinations, 80% to 90% of them have ophthalmologic lesions by adolescence. Because *T. gondii* is a major opportunistic pathogen for patients with AIDS, congenital transmission of human immunodeficiency virus (HIV) and *T. gondii* from such mothers is an emerging

problem, often causing extensive, fulminant, disseminated toxoplasmosis in the newborn infant.

Toxoplasmosis causes not only substantial morbidity and mortality for affected individuals, but also major expenditures for health care. For example, in 1975 Wilson and Remington (1980) estimated that the average lifetime cost of special care for each child with congenital toxoplasmosis was $67,000. Since the estimated incidence of congenital toxoplasmosis is 1.1 per 1,000 births, an estimated 3,300 infants are affected each year in the United States, resulting in a cost of $221,000,000 for lifetime care in 1975 dollars for infants born in just 1 year. Estimated productivity losses resulting from infection of children born in 1 year in the United States are $65 million to $1.6 billion, and estimated total preventable costs are $368 million to $8.7 billion dollars (Wilson and Remington, 1980; Roberts and Frenkel, 1990).

Congenital *Toxoplasma* infection in the fetus can be prevented by pregnant women if they avoid consumption of raw or undercooked meat and avoid accidental ingestion of material contaminated with cat feces. Serologic testing and antimicrobial therapy are important for prevention and treatment. Antimicrobial therapy given to an acutely infected mother can block transmission to her fetus (Desmonts and Couvreur, 1979). Such therapy can also cure signs of infection caused by proliferating tachyzoites in congenitally infected fetuses (Daffos et al., 1988; Hohlfeld et al., 1989); infants (McAuley et al., 1994; McGhee et al., 1992; McLeod et al., 1992; Mets et al., 1996; Patel et al., 1996; Roizen et al., 1995; Swisher et al., 1994); and immunocompromised individuals (McLeod et al., 1979). Development of vaccines that prevent toxoplasmosis in humans and in animal reservoirs is important for prevention of this disease. A commercial vaccine is available for sheep that reduces ovine abortion resulting from toxoplasmosis (Buxton and Innes,

1995). Vaccines to prevent oocyst shedding from cats (Frenkel et al., 1991) and vaccines that potentially could protect against initial infection or disease in humans (McLeod et al., 1988; Prince et al., 1989; Duquesne et al., 1990) are still experimental.

HISTORY

In 1908 Nicolle and Manceaux described tachyzoites in spleen and liver mononuclear cells from the North African rodent *Ctenodactylus gundi.* In 1923 *T. gondii* was implicated in human disease when Janku, an ophthalmologist in Prague, found cysts containing *T. gondii* in the retina of an 11-month-old child with congenital hydrocephalus. In 1937 Wolf and Cowen described an infant with granulomatous encephalitis. The protozoan parasite causing this infection was later identified by Sabin as *T. gondii.* In 1948 Sabin and Feldman developed the Sabin-Feldman dye test, which permitted serologic testing and provided another means, in addition to histopathologic testing, for detecting disease caused by *T. gondii.* In 1970 *T. gondii* was classified among the coccidia, and it was discovered that the domestic cat and other felines were the only hosts in which the sexual form develops. In the 1960s through the 1980s the full spectrum of clinical syndromes caused by *T. gondii* was defined, as were more rational approaches to antimicrobial therapy in different clinical settings.

Recent developments in immunology and molecular and cell biology and new developments in the care of pregnant women, children, and immunocompromised individuals have led to development of improved diagnostic tests and approaches to care for patients with toxoplasmosis. Recent studies also have further elucidated the pathogenesis of the infection, facilitated diagnostic testing, contributed to the development of effective antimicrobial agents, and provided the groundwork for development of vaccines.

THE ORGANISM

T. gondii, a coccidian parasite, exists in a number of forms: tachyzoites (the rapidly proliferative form, formerly referred to as "trophozoites"); bradyzoites (which replicate more slowly than tachyzoites and exist within tissue cysts); and oocysts (which contain highly infectious sporozoites).

Tachyzoites

Tachyzoites (Fig. 34-1, *A*) are crescent or oval in shape and are approximately 2 to 4 μm wide and 4 to 8 μm long. They stain well with either Wright's or Giemsa stain. Tachyzoites can invade and multiply in all mammalian cells. Their reproduction is by endodyogeny, a process of internal budding in which two daughter cells are formed within the parent cell. Daughter cells are released when the host cell wall is disrupted or lysed. Tachyzoites are fastidious and do not survive freezing, thawing, desiccation, or exposure to normal gastric secretions.

Bradyzoites

Bradyzoites (Fig. 34-1, *B*) in tissue cysts are crescent-shaped organisms that appear similar to tachyzoites but replicate more slowly. They have unique epitopes that are not expressed by tachyzoites or sporozoites. In electron micrographs, bradyzoites differ from tachyzoites in that they have amylopectin granules, more organelles called *micronemes,* and electron-dense rhoptry organelles. Tissue cysts vary in size and contain a few to approximately 10,000 bradyzoites. Tissue cysts can be stained with periodic acid–Schiff (PAS) stain. Primary human infection can also occur by ingestion of bradyzoites within cysts in raw or undercooked meat. After ingestion the cyst wall is disrupted by pepsin or trypsin. The liberated bradyzoites can remain viable for up to 2 hours in pepsin–hydrogen chloride or as long as 6 hours in trypsin. Bradyzoites then invade the digestive tract mucosa and can disseminate throughout the body. Tissue cysts have been found in virtually every organ but appear to have greatest predilection for the retina, brain, heart, and skeletal muscle. Cysts remain viable throughout the life of the host. These tissue cysts can be a source of local or disseminated infection if the host becomes immunocompromised. Freezing to −20° C (−4° F), heating to 60° C (140° F), desiccation, and irradiation destroy viability of encysted bradyzoites.

Oocysts and Sporozoites

Oocysts (see Fig. 34-1, *C*) are oval and approximately 10 to 12 μm in diameter. They complete the life cycle of *T. gondii* within the intestine of its definitive host, cats. They are found in the cat intestine only during primary infection or, rarely, in a chronically infected cat that acquires another coccidian parasite, *Isospora* spp. Oocysts can remain infectious in warm, moist soil for 1 year or more and easily resist the gastric acid barrier after ingestion. They can be killed by exposure to nearly boiling water for 5 minutes, by burning, or by

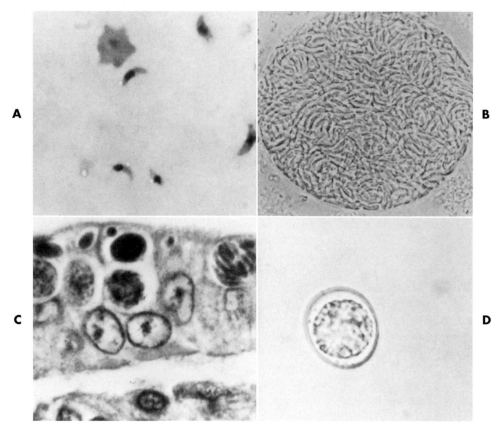

FIG. 34-1   Forms of *Toxoplasma gondii*. **A**, Tachyzoite. **B**, Bradyzoite in tissue cyst. **C**, Gametocytes in cat ileum. **D**, Unsporulated oocyst. (Adapted from Dubey JP, Beattie CP. Toxoplasmosis of animals and man. Boca Raton, Fla.: CRC Press, Inc, 1988, and Gardiner CH, Fayer R, Dubey JP. An atlas of protozoan parasites in animal tissues. Washington, D.C.: U.S. Department of Agriculture, Agriculture Handbook No. 651, 1988.)

contact with strong ammonia (7%) for 3 hours. Oocysts sporulate 1 to 5 days after excretion, and the sporozoites become highly infectious if they are ingested.

Life Cycle

There are two life cycles for *T. gondii*. The complete cycle—with schizogony (an asexual cycle) and gametogony (sporulating sexual cycle), which results in the formation of infectious oocysts— occurs only in members of the cat family. In all other animals only an incomplete cycle by schizogony occurs, forming tachyzoites or bradyzoites in tissue cysts. Toxoplasma are acquired by susceptible cats when they eat meat (e.g., mice) that contains tissue cysts or ingest oocysts excreted by other recently infected cats (Fig. 34-2). *T. gondii* then multiplies through both schizogonic and gametogonic cycles in the tips of villi in the cat's

distal ileum. The time of the first appearance of oocysts in cat feces depends on the form of *T. gondii* ingested: 3 to 5 days after ingestion of *T. gondii* tissue cysts; 7 to 10 days after ingestion of *T. gondii* tachyzoites; and 20 to 24 days after the ingestion of *T. gondii* oocysts. For a brief 1- to 3-week period, an acutely infected cat can excrete 10^7 to 10^9 oocysts per day.

EPIDEMIOLOGY

The prevalence of *Toxoplasma* infection in cats and in tissue cysts in meat used for human consumption varies widely, depending in part on locale. In early studies in the United States, 50% of domestic cats were seropositive. In a study in Costa Rica where the overall antibody prevalence in people was 60%, over 20% of 237 cats were shedding oocysts when examined, and 60% overall were infected as shown by either oocyst shedding or *T. gondii*–specific an-

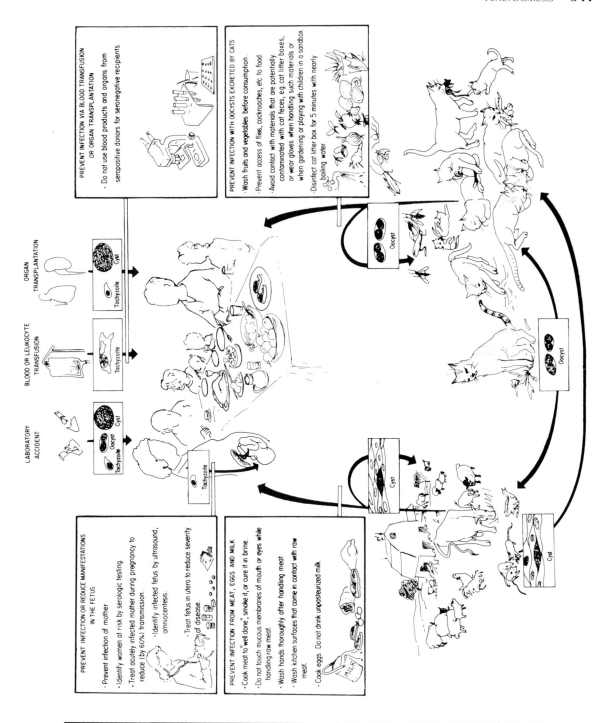

FIG. 34-2 Life cycle of *T. gondii* and prevention of acquisition by humans. Infection of older children and adults occurs primarily after ingestion of cysts in undercooked meat or oocysts excreted by cats or by the fetus transplacentally from an acutely infected mother. After ingestion, organisms invade the intestinal epithelium, either hematogenously or through lymphatics, are spread to other tissues, and when there is a normal immune response, they form cysts. Rarely, infection is acquired by blood or leukocyte transfusion, in a transplanted organ, or via a laboratory accident. (Adapted from McLeod and Remington. In Behrman RL, Vaughan VC III, Nelson WE [eds]. Nelson's textbook of pediatrics, ed 14. Philadelphia, WB Saunders, 1990.)

tibody (Ruiz and Frenkel, 1980). *T. gondii* has been isolated from the skeletal muscle of 23% of market pigs and 42% of breeder pigs in the United States. The prevalence in Czechoslovakia ranged from 43% to 73%. Sheep used for human consumption had a prevalence rate of 4% to 22% in California. Cattle apparently are infected less commonly than sheep or pigs in the United States, Europe, and New Zealand. The combined prevalence rates range from 1% to 33%. The prevalence of infection in humans is also highly variable, depending in part on locale and age. Highest rates of seropositivity occur in El Salvador, Tahiti, and France, where the prevalence of seropositivity is greater than 90% by the fourth decade of life. In the United Kingdom and in the United States approximately 10% of the population has IgG antibody at 10 years of age, 20% at 20 years, and 50% at 70 years. The prevalence of infection lessens in colder regions, in hot and arid climates, and at high elevations. There is no significant difference in prevalence between men and women.

There have been clusters of cases of toxoplasmosis or *T. gondii* infection (1) caused by common exposures in a riding stable or by exposure to water, (2) associated with eating similarly prepared meat, and (3) in families. Data in experimental animals demonstrate significant immunogenetic differences in the manifestations of infection in mice (Brown and McLeod, 1990). Recent work suggests that genetics also influences human toxoplasmosis (Mack et al., in press; McLeod et al., 1996; Suzuki et al., 1996). Congenital toxoplasmosis occurs when the mother acquires the infection for the first time during pregnancy. The risk of infection in an obstetric population depends on two factors: (1) the incidence of primary infection in the population as a whole, and (2) the proportion of women of childbearing age who have not been previously infected.

In the relatively few studies of prevalence of *Toxoplasma* antibodies in pregnant women, there is geographic variation. In the United States, 39% of 23,000 pregnant women in the Collaborative Perinatal Project had *T. gondii*–specific serum antibody. Other studies indicate a varying incidence of seropositivity in women of childbearing age in the United States: Denver, 3%; Palo Alto, California, 10%; Chicago, 12%; Boston, 14%; and Birmingham, Alabama, 30% (Remington et al., 1995). Seroprevalence studies of women of childbearing age from other nations or cities outside the United States also demonstrate variability in rates of seropositivity: Thailand, 3%; Australia, 4%; Japan, 6%; Scotland, 13%; London, 20%; Poland, 36%; Belgium, 53%; and Paris, 73%. Published estimates for the incidence of congenital toxoplasmosis range from 0.1 to 10 per 1,000 live births. Approximations per 1,000 births for individual cities are as follows: Birmingham, Alabama, 0.12; London, 0.07 to 0.25; Glasgow, Scotland, 0.46 to 0.93; Basel, Switzerland, 1; Brussels, 2; Melbourne, 2; and Vienna, 6 to 7. Sera from 330,000 newborns in Massachusetts and New Hampshire were tested using the double-sandwich (DS) IgM enzyme-linked immunosorbent assay (ELISA) of Remington and Naot, and the incidence of seropositivity using this test was 1 per 10,000 live births.

Acute maternal infection is transmitted to the fetus in approximately 40% of cases. Incidence and severity of congenital infection depend in part on the time of acquisition of infection during pregnancy (Table 34-1). By the last weeks of gestation the incidence of transmission to the fetus approaches 100%. The severity of manifestations of infection at birth decreases the later in gestation the infection is acquired. Approximately half of the infected infants detected in serologic screening programs who were initially believed normal based on routine newborn evaluations had one or more signs of infection apparent with more complete evaluations. Almost all infected infants have some evidence of infection (e.g., chorioretinitis) by adolescence if untreated or treated for only 1 month.

PATHOGENESIS

After acquisition by the older child or adult (usually through the gastrointestinal tract), organisms

Table 34-1 Inverse relationship between incidence of fetal infection and severity of fetal damage following acutely acquired maternal infection with *T. gondii* at different stages of gestation

Trimester of pregnancy	Fetuses infected (%)	Severity of illness
1	17	Most severe
2	25	Intermediate severity
3	65	Least severe or subclinical

Data from Remington JS, Desmonts G. In Remington JS, Klein JO (eds). Infectious diseases of the fetus and newborn infant, ed 3. Philadelphia: WB Saunders, 1990.

invade cells directly or are phagocytosed by leukocytes. Within these cells, organisms multiply, cause cell lysis, and are spread throughout the body hematogenously or through the lymphatics. Organisms can infect every mammalian cell. Proliferation of tachyzoites results in rupture of infected cells and eventually in areas of localized tissue necrosis surrounded by infiltrates of inflammatory cells. The eventual outcome of acute infection depends on the host's immune response. Cysts form in immunocompetent hosts, in whom both cellular and humoral immunity is intact. Cyst formation can be demonstrated as early as the seventh day after infection. Cysts can persist in many organs and tissues after immunity is acquired; thus T. gondii remains in tissues for the life of the host.

In immunodeficient individuals and in some apparently immunologically normal individuals the acute infection is not contained by an effective immune response; it may cause marked destruction of the host's tissues, leading to, for example, pneumonitis, myocarditis, or necrotizing encephalitis. Encysted organisms may also cause recrudescent disease in previously immunocompetent patients. Such previously latent infection is the major source of disease caused by T. gondii in patients with AIDS, transplant recipients, and older children who develop new or recrudescent chorioretinitis as a sequela of congenital T. gondii infection.

When a pregnant woman acquires T. gondii, tachyzoites are hematogenously spread to the placenta. The organism then can be transmitted transplacentally directly to the fetus during gestation or at birth. Overall, in approximately 60% of cases, maternal acute infection does not result in fetal infection. However, as stated previously, almost all infected infants have manifestations of infection (e.g., chorioretinitis) by adolescence if they are untreated. It has been suggested that the differences in rates of transmission during gestation depend on placental blood flow, virulence of the T. gondii strain, possibly genetic susceptibility of the patient, and the number of organisms hematogenously spread to the placenta. As in other congenital infections, the greater severity of toxoplasmic infection acquired early in gestation relates to the sensitivity of early fetal organs to damage by intracellular parasites, the placental barrier separating the fetus from the mother's humoral and cell-mediated immune responses, and the fetus's intrinsic immunologic immaturity. The most profoundly affected babies frequently exhibit specific immunologic tolerance in the perinatal period (McLeod et al., 1990).

PATHOLOGY

Information about pathologic changes observed in toxoplasmosis in humans is largely derived from lymph node biopsies, from autopsy data described in fatal congenital infections, and from immunodeficient individuals. Limited information is available on the pathologic changes in immunocompetent individuals since acute infection is usually asymptomatic or self-limited in such persons. Tachyzoites and tissue cysts are only rarely observed in conventionally stained sections. Tachyzoites may be observed with Wright's or Giemsa stain but are best demonstrated with the immunoperoxidase technique. Tissue cysts stain well with PAS stain, silver impregnation stains, and immunoperoxidase techniques.

Lymph Nodes

In acute acquired lymphadenopathic toxoplasmosis (Fig. 34-3) there is a characteristic triad of (1) reactive follicular hyperplasia, with (2) irregular clusters of epithelioid histiocytes, and (3) monocytoid B cells that distend the subcapsular and trabecular lymph node sinuses (Dorfman and Remington, 1973). Tachyzoites and tissue cysts are only very rarely demonstrable in affected nodes, but T. gondii DNA may be identified in tissue sections by the polymerase chain reaction.

Eye

Single or multiple foci of tissue necrosis in the retina and choroid are the earliest manifestations of T. gondii involvement of the eye. Secondary changes such as vitritis, iridocyclitis, and cataracts are complications of the chorioretinitis. Organisms first lodge in the capillaries of the inner layer of the retina, invade the endothelium, and extend to adjacent tissues. An intense local inflammatory reaction develops, with (1) edema, and (2) infiltration of lymphocytes, plasma cells, mononuclear cells, and occasionally eosinophils. Both intracellular and extracellular tachyzoites and tissue cysts may be seen. After resolution of the active infection, scarring is characterized by an area of gliosis with a hyperpigmented border resulting from disruption and proliferation of the pigmented retinal epithelium.

FIG. 34-3 Lymph node biopsy showing characteristic lymph node pathology in lymphadenitis caused by *Toxoplasma.* Epithelioid cells *(black arrow)* encroach upon and blur margins of germinal center *(white arrow).* There is focal distension of subcapsular and trabecular sinuses by "monocytoid" cells *(double black arrows).* Irregular clusters of epithelioid cells are scattered throughout paracortical lymphoid stroma. (Adapted from Dorfman RF, Remington JS: N Engl J Med 1973; 289-878.)

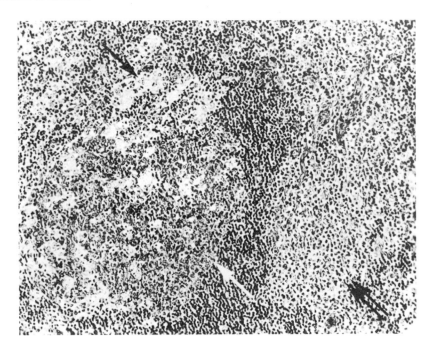

Central Nervous System

Along with involvement of the eye, congenital toxoplasmosis most often involves the central nervous system (CNS). In the CNS there may be acute and focal or multifocal diffuse meningoencephalitis, with cellular necrosis, microglial nodules, and perivascular mononuclear inflammation. In patients with congenital infection secondary vascular thrombosis may produce extensive areas of necrosis, often several centimeters in diameter. The basal ganglia are often severely involved, and scattered cortical lesions are often seen as well. Large areas of necrosis in congenital toxoplasmosis may lead to sloughing of periventricular tissue, which causes obstruction of the aqueduct of Sylvius or foramen of Monro and subsequent hydrocephalus. The protein count of such ventricular fluid is high (grams per deciliter) and contains large amounts of *T. gondii* antigen. Eventually, necrotic brain tissue may calcify, giving rise to the typical findings in conventional radiographs and computed tomography (CT) scans.

In cases of acute CNS infection acquired postnatally or with immunocompromise, there is focal or diffuse meningoencephalitis with necrosis and microglial nodules. In immunocompromised patients, such as infants and children with both congenital toxoplasmosis and AIDS, the major finding is necrotizing encephalitis in both acute and recrudescent disease.

Other Sites

Rarely, *T. gondii* infection gives rise to interstitial pneumonitis. The myocardium is a frequent site for necrosis, inflammation, and encysted organisms. Acute and chronic pericarditis have also been described. Infection of kidney (and antigen-antibody complex–mediated glomerulonephritis), spleen, liver, adrenals, pancreas, stomach, intestine, thyroid, thymus, testes, ovaries, and skin also have been described (reviewed in Remington et al., 1990).

CLINICAL MANIFESTATIONS
Acute Acquired Toxoplasmosis in Apparently Immunologically Normal Older Children and Adults

Infection acquired after birth is generally asymptomatic in 80% to 90% of immunologically normal persons, including pregnant women. Those with clinically apparent disease generally have lymphadenopathy with or without a "mononucleosis-like" illness. Rarely, severe systemic disease or specific organ involvement (e.g., encephalitis or chorioretinitis) occurs.

Lymphadenopathy is the most commonly recognized clinical manifestation of acute acquired toxoplasmosis (McCabe et al., 1987). Lymphadenitis can be generalized, but in approximately two thirds of patients only one area is affected. Cervical lymph nodes are the most frequently involved. However, axillary, inguinal, retroperitoneal, and mesenteric lymph nodes may also be involved. Lymph nodes generally measure 0.5 to 3.0 cm and can be tender or nontender. They are often firm, discrete, smooth, and mobile, but they do not suppurate or ulcerate. Although self-limited, lymphadenopathy can persist or recur for up to 1 year. Retroperitoneal or mesenteric node involvement with fever may mimic appendicitis. Toxoplasmic lymphadenopathy often raises concern about lymphoma or other malignancy. Appropriate serologic testing can differentiate this condition and avert the need for lymph node biopsy.

Occasionally, lymphadenopathy is accompanied by a constellation of symptoms suggestive of infectious mononucleosis, or these symptoms may occur alone. This infection also has a self-limited course; however, fatigue and lymphadenopathy may persist for months to a year. It usually ends with complete recovery.

Significant systemic disease can occur. Onset may be insidious, with weakness and malaise that persist for 6 to 10 days, followed by fever, rash, and symptoms of pneumonia or hepatitis. Temperature may be as high as 41° C (105.8° F). Abdominal pain may be present. A maculopapular, generalized rash may occur. It appears similar to that of Rocky Mountain spotted fever except that the palms of the hands and the soles of the feet are spared. These skin lesions are bright red to pale pink and may blanch with pressure. Signs of pneumonia may appear simultaneously with the rash or later. Roentgenographic examination of the chest may show irregular areas of increased density in the lower lobes or only accentuation of the hilar or lower-lobe markings.

Systemic toxoplasmosis in immunologically normal individuals has also been manifested as hepatitis, polymyositis, pericarditis with effusion, myocarditis, or meningoencephalitis. Toxoplasmic meningoencephalitis has been characterized by headache, vomiting, seizures, focal neurologic signs, and transitory confusion (Townsend et al., 1975). Temperature is not always elevated at the onset. Lymphadenopathy and splenomegaly are present in some cases. Cerebrospinal fluid (CSF) has increased numbers of white blood cells (WBCs), particularly mononuclear cells. Protein and glucose concentrations are normal or simulate those of bacterial meningitis. The patient's condition may steadily deteriorate, ending in death or survival with residual brain damage manifested by seizures or focal neurologic deficits. Complete recovery without residua has also been described.

Infection in the Immunocompromised Individual

Immunocompromised patients—such as those with AIDS, malignancy, autoimmune disease and its therapy, and solid organ or bone marrow transplants—are at risk for severe toxoplasmosis. In most cases, toxoplasmosis is caused by reactivation of latent infection rather than primary infection.

Approximately 50% of patients with AIDS who are chronically infected with *T. gondii* develop toxoplasmosis. Why the other 50% of such patients do not reactivate their infections is unknown. Pediatric AIDS and congenital *T. gondii* infections have been reported in the same infants. Such dual infections, including encephalitis and involvement of other organs (e.g., heart and lungs), usually have been fulminant and rapidly fatal. *T. gondii* infection has most often been diagnosed at postmortem examination. This infection is emerging as a particular problem in populations with a relatively high prevalence of both *T. gondii* and HIV infections.

Typical signs and symptoms of toxoplasmic encephalitis in adult AIDS patients include headache, fever, and focal neurologic deficits. Less commonly, meningitis, spinal cord involvement, and signs that reflect involvement of other organs are present. CNS lesions occur throughout the brain, with predilection for involvement of the basal ganglia and corticomedullary junction. Diffuse encephalitis diagnosed only at autopsy also has been reported (Leport, 1991), but most often there are focal lesions that enhance with contrast on brain CT scan or brain magnetic resonance imaging (MRI) scans. MRI scans almost always show multiple lesions (Fig. 34-4).

In a recent series of adult AIDS patients with toxoplasmosis (Leport, 1991) the most frequent clinical localization was in the brain, with focal abscesses (83%) and diffuse encephalitis (in the 17% with a normal CT scan). Fever occurred in 60% to 70%, 40% to 50% had headaches, 35% to 40% were confused, and 40% to 80% had focal neurologic signs. Specific IgG antibodies are detectable in most (>95%) adult patients with AIDS and toxoplasmosis. Of affected patients with toxoplasmic chorioretinitis, 65% had concomitant cerebral localization. With appropriate treatment there is usually an initial improvement within a few weeks and complete resolution of lesions seen on brain CT scan in 1 to 6 months. Delayed or absent response to this treatment is an indication for brain biopsy. Rupture of thrombosed vessels (secondary to intimal and perivascular inflammatory cell infiltrates) has

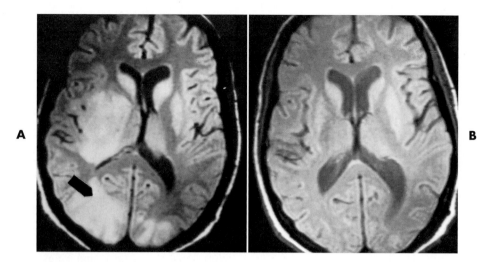

FIG. 34-4   MRI of the brain of a patient with AIDS and toxoplasmic encephalitis before
(**A**) and after (**B**) antimicrobial therapy. Note that large areas of necrosis and inflammation in
A *(arrow)* have resolved in **B**.

occurred. At autopsy, 40% to 70% of patients with AIDS and toxoplasmosis have involvement of the heart and lung. Involvement of pancreas, stomach, and intestine has been described.

In older immunocompromised children, toxoplasmosis generally occurs as a result of reactivation of latent infection. However, *T. gondii* may actually be transmitted through organ transplantation and leukocyte transfusion (see Fig. 34-2). Symptomatic toxoplasmosis has occurred when *T. gondii*–infected hearts or kidneys have been transplanted into seronegative recipients. In cardiac transplant recipients, toxoplasmosis may simulate rejection both clinically and in endomyocardial biopsies if the diagnosis is not suspected. The diagnosis of reactivated or primary toxoplasmosis in recipients of bone marrow transplants may be particularly difficult because *T. gondii*–specific antibody may be absent or may not increase in titer. Increase in antibody titer without overt disease has occurred when *T. gondii*–infected hearts have been transplanted into seropositive recipients.

Congenital Toxoplasmosis

Clinical Manifestations. Approximately 40% of untreated women who acquire the infection during pregnancy transmit *T. gondii* to their fetus. In an otherwise healthy woman, transmission to the fetus occurs only in the setting of primary (not recrudescent) infection. Only 10% to 40% of women who give birth to congenitally infected infants re-

call any signs or symptoms of acute infection. Rarely, cases of congenital transmission have been reported in women chronically infected with *T. gondii* and immunosuppressed from corticosteroid treatment or AIDS.

Manifestations of congenital infection are protean, varying from a mild or asymptomatic infection to a generalized infection dominated by signs of irreversible CNS damage. Disease may be seen initially in the neonatal period, in the first months of life, or at later ages—up to adulthood. Newborns and young infants are usually detected based on systemic, neurologic, or ophthalmologic signs (Table 34-2). Older children are seen with ophthalmologic and, less frequently, neurologic disease. Couvreur et al. (1984) reported data that indicate the spectrum and frequency of signs and symptoms noted in newborn infants born to mothers whose infections had been diagnosed in a systematic serologic screening program. Only 10% had substantial CNS, ocular, or systemic involvement; 34% had normal clinical examinations, with the exception of retinal scars or isolated calcifications; and 55% had no abnormalities detected. These prospective data from France likely underestimate the true proportion of severe infection because the most severe cases were not referred, therapeutic abortion often eliminated the most severely involved fetuses, and gestational spiramycin therapy may have reduced the severity of infection. Between 33% and 50% of the infants initially thought to have subclinical infection showed

Table 34-2 Numbers and percentages of 300 patients with congenital toxoplasmosis with various clinical manifestations at presentation

Clinical manifestations	Age when first diagnosed									Total
	1-5 mo	6-11 mo	12-23 mo	2-3 yr	4-7 yr	8-14 yr	15-29 yr	30 yr		
Neurologic disorders	42 (58)*	26 (81)	24 (57)	20 (42)	14 (42)	21 (54)	7 (29)	1		155 (52)
Hydrocephalus or microcephalus	40 (55)	12 (38)	14 (33)	6 (13)	—	4 (10)	1 (4)	1		78 (26)
Ocular disorders	52 (71)	27 (84)	32 (76)	26 (54)	31 (94)	35 (90)	24 (100)	1		228 (76)
Intracranial calcification	28 (38)	12 (38)	17 (40)	14 (29)	11 (33)	10 (26)	4 (17)	2		98 (33)
Jaundice	20 (27)	1 (32)	—	—	—	—	—	—		21
Hepatosplenomegaly	13 (18)	—	—	—	—	—	—	—		13
TOTALS	73	32	42	48	33	39	24	2		300

Modified from Couvreur J, Desmonts G: Dev Med Child Neurol 1962,4:519-530.

*Figure outside parentheses, number; figure inside parentheses, percentage of patients diagnosed at that age with this manifestation.

signs of infection (most commonly, abnormal CSF) with more detailed evaluation. At face value, however, these data imply that 90% of the infants with congenital toxoplasmosis would have been missed with a routine newborn physical examination.

In infants with generalized or primarily neuro-logic disease and with no or brief treatment, substantial long-term morbidity can be expected (Table 34-3). For example, of infants with neuro-logic disease who were reevaluated at 4 years of age (Eichenwald, 1960), 89% had IQs less than 70, 83% had convulsions, 76% had spasticity and

Table 34-3   Signs and symptoms occurring before diagnosis or during the course of untreated acute congenital toxoplasmosis in 152 infants and 101 of these same children when they had been followed 4 years or more

Signs and symptoms	Frequency of occurrence (%) in patients with	
	Neurologic disease*	**Generalized disease†**
	108 Patients	**44 Patients**
Infants		
Chorioretinitis	102 (94)‡	29 (66)
Abnormal spinal fluid	59 (55)	37 (84)
Anemia	55 (51)	34 (77)
Jaundice	31 (29)	35 (80)
Splenomegaly	23 (21)	40 (90)
Convulsions	54 (50)	8 (18)
Fever	27 (25)	34 (77)
Intracranial calcification	54 (50)	2 (4)
Hepatomegaly	18 (17)	34 (77)
Lymphadenopathy	18 (17)	30 (68)
Vomiting	17 (16)	21 (48)
Hydrocephalus	30 (28)	0 (0)
Diarrhea	7 (6)	11 (25)
Pneumonitis	0 (0)	18 (41)
Microcephalus	14 (13)	0 (0)
Eosinophilia	6 (4)	8 (18)
Rash	1 (1)	11 (25)
Abnormal bleeding	3 (3)	8 (18)
Hypothermia	2 (2)	9 (20)
Cataracts	5 (5)	0 (0)
Glaucoma	2 (2)	0 (0)
Optic atrophy	2 (2)	0 (0)
Microphthalmia	2 (2)	0 (0)
	70 Patients	**31 Patients**
Children 4 Years (or more) Old		
Mental retardation	62 (89)	25 (81)
Convulsions	58 (83)	24 (77)
Spasticity and palsies	53 (76)	18 (58)
Severely impaired vision	48 (69)	13 (42)
Hydrocephalus or microcephalus	31 (44)	2 (6)
Deafness	12 (17)	3 (10)
Normal	6 (9)	5 (16)

Modified from Eichenwald H. In Siim JC (ed). Human toxoplasmosis. Copenhagen: Munksgaard, 1960, pp 41-49. Study was performed in 1947. The most severely involved institutionalized patients were not included in the later study of 101 children.
*Patients with central nervous system disease in the first year of life.
†Patients with nonneurologic diseases during the first 2 months of life.
‡Figure outside parentheses, number; figure inside parentheses, percentage.

palsies, 69% had severely impaired vision, 20% were deaf, and only 9% were normal. Only 16% of the children who initially presented with generalized disease were normal at follow-up. In a study by Wilson et al. (1980) the outcome for infants who had "subclinical" infection at birth and who were evaluated when they were 9 to 10 years old also revealed substantial sequelae (Table 34-4). Sixteen percent were mentally retarded, 17% had seizures, 27% had unilateral blindness and 20% had bilateral blindness, 25% had hearing impairment, and 86% had sequentially lower IQ scores when tested at 5-year intervals. With 1 year of treatment, outcome apparently is substantially better for most (but not all) such infants (Rolzen et al., 1995).

Reported cutaneous manifestations in congenitally infected infants have included thrombocytopenia (e.g., petechiae, hemorrhage, ecchymoses) and rashes (fine punctate; diffuse maculopapular; lenticular deep blue-red; sharply defined and diffuse blue papules). The entire body, including palms and soles, has been involved with macular rashes. Jaundice, cyanosis, and edema secondary to hepatic, pulmonary, myocardial, and renal involvement have been reported.

General and systemic findings have included prematurity, low Apgar scores, intrauterine growth retardation, instability of temperature regulation with hypothermia, lymphadenopathy, hepatosplenomegaly, signs of myocarditis, pneumonitis, nephrotic syndrome, vomiting, diarrhea, and feeding problems. Endocrine abnormalities have also been reported and include hypothyroidism, diabetes insipidus, sexual precocity, and partial anterior hypopituitarism. Neurologic abnormalities have ranged from subtle findings to severe encephalitis. Hydrocephalus may be the only clinical manifestation of congenital toxoplasmosis and may be compensated or may require shunt placement. It may be seen in the perinatal period; later in infancy; or, rarely, up to adulthood. A variety of different seizure patterns may occur in the perinatal period and later in life. Central focal motor deficits have been noted, as have signs of spinal or bulbar involvement. Microcephaly in untreated infants is generally associated with diminished cognitive functioning. Mild and severe sensorineural hearing loss has been reported in approximately 20% of children with no or brief treatment, but this was not found in a recent study of treated infants and children (McGhee et al., 1992).

CSF is abnormal in at least one third of congenitally infected infants. Abnormalities include CSF

Table 34-4 Development of adverse sequelae in children born with subclinical congenital toxoplasma infection

	Group 1* (n = 13)	Group 2† (n = 11)
Ophthalmologic Finding		
No sequelae	2	0
Chorioretinitis		
Bilateral		
Bilateral blindness	0	5
Unilateral blindness	3	3
Moderate unilateral visual loss	0	1
Minimal or no visual loss	5	1
Unilateral		
Minimal or no visual loss	3	0
Mean age at onset (yr)	3.67	0.42
Range	0.08-9.33	0.25-1.00
Recurrences of active chorioretinitis	3	2
Neurologic Finding‡		
No sequelae	8	3
Major sequelae		
Hydrocephalus	0	1
Microcephaly	1	1
Seizures	1	3
Severe psychomotor retardation	1	2
Minor sequelae		
Mild cerebellar dysfunction	2	4
Transiently delayed psychomotor development	2	2
Other Abnormality		
Sensorineural hearing loss		
Moderate unilateral	1 of 10	1 of 9
Mild unilateral	1 of 10	0 of 9
Mild bilateral	1 of 10	1 of 9
Precocious puberty	2	0
Premature thelarche	0	1
Miscellaneous	3	1

Modified from Wilson et al. Pediatrics 1980;66:767-774.
*No abnormalities found on an extensive newborn evaluation based on awareness of a diagnosis of congenital toxoplasmosis.
†No abnormalities found on a routine newborn physical examination.
‡Eighty-six percent of eight children who were tested had sequentially lower intelligence quotient scores.

lymphocytic pleocytosis, hypoglycorrhachia, and elevated protein level. Remarkable elevations of CSF protein levels (with values of grams per deciliter when there is aqueductal obstruction and ventricular dilation) are characteristic of this congenital infection. Local production of *T. gondii*–specific antibodies may be present in CSF. Brain CT scan with contrast can determine ventricular size, detect calcifications, and define active inflammatory lesions and porencephalic cystic structures. Skull radiographs and ultrasonography are less sensitive than CT scan for detection of calcifications, but ultrasonography may be useful for following ventricular size. Brain MRI and radionuclide scans may be useful to detect active inflammation.

Case summaries that provide examples of infants with subclinical infection; generalized systemic, neurologic, and ophthalmologic disease; and severe neurologic and ophthalmologic disease follow.

■ **CASE 1: PATIENT WITH SUBCLINICAL DISEASE** The patient's family lived in a rural area, and two stray cats lived nearby. Although they had no known contact with these cats or with feces from the cats, the family did have a sandbox where the pregnant mother played in the sand with her older children. The mother also prepared a large number of hamburgers for a picnic 2 to 3 weeks before delivery of her son, but she did not recall sampling raw hamburger or eating raw or undercooked meat during her infant's gestation. She had no history of consuming raw milk or raw eggs.

The mother's pregnancy, labor, and delivery were uncomplicated. Her infant was born appropriate for gestational age (AGA) with Apgar scores of 9 and 9 and a birth weight of 3.9 kg, and he had no medical problems in the perinatal period. On the day after delivery the patient's mother noted that she had an enlarged posterior auricular lymph node. She had no other symptoms or signs and an otherwise normal physical examination, which included a retinal examination. The affected lymph node was excised, and microscopic studies of it revealed epithelioid histiocytes and monocytoid cells characteristic of toxoplasmic lymphadenopathy (similar to those shown in Fig. 34-3). Serologic tests for the mother and the child were obtained: the infant's serum Sabin-Feldman dye test titer was 1:8,000; his serum IgM ELISA level was 11; the IgM ISAGA level was 12; and the IgA ELISA level was 11 (see page 567 for definitions of terms). His mother's serum Sabin-Feldman dye test titer was 1:1,024 (300 IU), her IgM ELISA level was 11, and her AC/HS was 1600/>3200.

Results of general ophthalmologic and neurologic examinations, auditory brain stem response testing, and head CT scan with and without contrast were normal. CSF at 5 weeks of age had 30 WBCs/mm³, with 3%

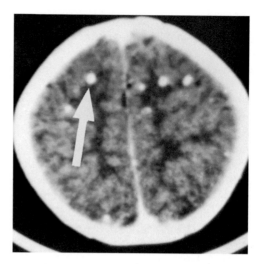

FIG. 34-5 Brain CT scan of an infant with congenital toxoplasmosis that demonstrates calcifications. This infant and other treated infants have developed normally in spite of calcifications *(arrow)* and even microcephaly.

PMNs, 91% lymphocytes, 3% monocytes, a protein level of 68 mg/dL, and a glucose level of 39 mg/dL.

The patient was treated with pyrimethamine, sulfadiazine, and leucovorin for 1 year and has had no clinical manifestations (other than slightly elevated CSF protein levels perinatally) of his third-trimester congenital infection.

■ **CASE 2: PATIENT WITH GENERALIZED SYSTEMIC, NEUROLOGIC, AND OPHTHALMOLOGIC DISEASE** This boy was the product of a first pregnancy and unremarkable gestation. During pregnancy his mother occasionally sampled raw hamburger, gardened, and had a pet cat but did not change the litter box.

An emergency cesarean section was performed after 30 hours of labor because of fetal distress (decreased fetal heart rate). The infant's Apgar scores were 2 at 1 minute and 3 at 5 minutes, leading to intubation and mechanical ventilation for his first 24 hours of life. During those 24 hours he had one episode that was considered to be a seizure, and administration of phenobarbital was begun. His birth weight was 3,450 g (fiftieth percentile); length, 19 inches (fiftieth percentile); and head circumference, 36 cm (fiftieth percentile). His platelet count on the first day of life was 44,000/mm³; thus a platelet transfusion was given and the platelet count subsequently returned to normal. Because of his asphyxial episode, a head CT scan was performed and revealed multiple discrete intracranial calcifications. Because of the presence of calcifications (similar to those in Fig. 34-5), the diagnosis of toxoplasmosis was suspected. An ophthalmologic examination revealed bilateral chorioretinitis, which was more prominent on the right side than on the left and involved the right macula. Hepatosplenomegaly was present, but the infant was considered normal otherwise. An examination of his CSF revealed 30 WBCs/mm^3, with a predominance of lymphocytes, a protein level of 215 mg/dL, and a glucose level of 86 mg/dL. Serologic test results included a serum dye test titer of 1:1,024; an IgM ELISA level of 2.0; and an IgA ELISA level of 2.5. The mother's serum on the same dates had a dye test titer of 1:8,000; DS IgM* ELISA level of 0.2; IgA ELISA level of 0.2; and AC/HS of 400/3,200. The infant was given pyrimethamine, sulfonamides, and leucovorin. His hepatosplenomegaly resolved. He is now 2 years old and has developed completely normally, with strabismus related to his macular scar as his only overt abnormality.

■ **CASE 3: PATIENT WITH SEVERE NEUROLOGIC AND OPHTHALMOLOGIC DISEASE** This boy's mother was a 21-year-old woman of Laotian descent with known hepatitis B surface antigenemia. She had minimal exposure to cats during the third trimester (i.e., she had visited in a house in which cats were present). She did not own a cat, nor did she clean a litter box or get scratched or bitten. She had no gardening or sandbox exposure. On one occasion she ate rare meat during the third trimester; however, she usually consumed well-cooked meat. She denied consumption of raw milk or raw eggs. In the eighth week of gestation a 1-week illness occurred, with swelling of her neck and face and with fever, lymphadenopathy, and night sweats. She was hospitalized, treated with antibiotics for presumed facial cellulitis, and had complete resolution of her symptoms. She also had intermittent headaches throughout her pregnancy. During the twenty-eighth week of gestation, at her request, a fetal ultrasound was performed that demonstrated a fetus with hydrocephalus. From that time on, she routinely underwent ultrasonography every 2 weeks until the thirty-fifth week of gestation.

A male infant was delivered at 35 weeks' gestation (34 weeks by Dubowitz) by cesarean section because of increasing ventriculomegaly. The infant's birth weight was 2,325 g (70%); head circumference, 34.5 cm (>90%); and length, 18 inches (70%). Apgar scores were 4 and 9 at 1 and 5 minutes of age, respectively. Hydrocephalus was prominent at birth as demonstrated by CT (similar to that in Fig. 34-6). The patient underwent ventriculoperitoneal shunting at 5 days of age, with resolution of increased intracranial pressure and appearance of thicker cortical mantle. Testing of ventricular fluid revealed 870 red blood cells; 43 WBCs; protein level of 1,155 mg/dL; and glucose level of 26 mg/dL. His serum Sabin-Feldman dye test titer was 1:4,096 and DS IgM ELISA level was 4. His IgA ELISA level was 3. His mother's serum Sabin-Feldman dye test titer was 1:2,048; IgM ELISA level was 4; IgA ELISA level was 12; and AC/HS was 800/3,200. Other complications noted during the infant's initial hospitalization included transient anemia, thrombocytopenia, transient hyperbilirubinemia, eleva-

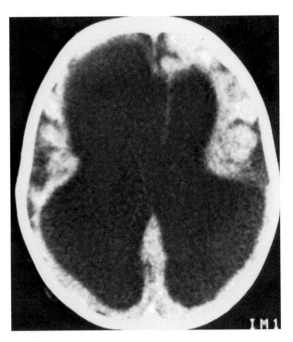

FIG. 34-6 Brain CT scan of an infant with congenital toxoplasmosis and hydrocephalus. Some (but not all) such treated infants with hydrocephalus from congenital toxoplasmosis have developed normally (with normal motor and cognitive function following prompt placement of ventriculoperitoneal shunts and with antimicrobial therapy). Poorer prognosis has been associated with delays in shunt placement or revisions or intercurrent complications such as prolonged hypoxia and hypoglycemia.

tion of liver transaminases, and diabetes insipidus. His examination also documented severe chorioretinitis, microophthalmia, hepatosplenomegaly, an umbilical hernia, and a hydrocele with micropenis. Administration of pyrimethamine, sulfadiazine, and folinic acid was begun at 18 days of age. At 24 days of age, prednisone was added and eventually tapered. He was started on vasopressin therapy. A repeat CT scan showed worsening hydrocephalus. Four months later, another repeat CT scan was performed and showed increased cerebral atrophy without clear indication of increased intracranial pressure. The infant is blind and has substantial development delay.

Ophthalmologic Disease

Clinical Manifestations. In the United States and in Western Europe, *T. gondii* is the most common cause of chorioretinitis, estimated to cause approximately 35% of cases. Toxoplasmic chorioretinitis is most frequently observed as an initial manifestation of or with reactivation of congenital infection. Almost all untreated congenitally infected individuals develop chorioretinal lesions (Koppe et al., 1986). Chorioretinitis is estimated to occur in 1% of immunologically normal individuals with acute acquired toxoplasmosis.

Chorioretinitis occurs early in gestation, and characteristic lesions have been described as early as 22 weeks gestation (Brezin et al., 1994). Infants with active congenital ocular toxoplasmosis may have microophthalmia, impaired vision, cataracts, chorioretinal scars, chorioretinitis, iritis, leukocoria, anisometropia, nystagmus, optic atrophy, microcornea, or strabismus (Mets et al., 1996). Older children may complain of blurred vision, photophobia, epiphora, loss of central vision, or "floaters." Recurrent symptoms occur at irregular intervals. Data from Couvreur et al. (1984) suggest that the appearance of recurrent or new retinal lesions during the first years of life may be prevented by therapy in alternate months with pyrimethamine and sulfadiazine and spiramycin. Longer follow-up is needed for definitive conclusions about whether such therapy reduces symptomatic, progressive ophthalmologic disease.

During an ophthalmoscopic examination, acute focal retinitis is seen as a fluffy white-yellow lesion with surrounding retinal edema and hyperemia (Fig. 34-7, *A*). Overlying vitritis may obscure the retina. Active lesions often are adjacent to old inactive lesions. Inactive lesions characteristically are atrophic, white to gray plaques, with distinct borders and choroidal black pigment (Fig. 34-7, *B*). The lesions may be single or multiple, large or small, unilateral or bilateral. They are often found at the posterior pole of the retina and commonly involve the macula, but also occur in the periphery. New lesions are often contiguous with older lesions, suggesting that the pathogenesis of new lesions is associated with cyst rupture and replication of the parasite in adjacent retinal cells. Papillitis (most often unilateral), optic atrophy, retinal detachment, and cortical blindness have also been observed. Other ophthalmologic findings include cells in the anterior chamber; neovascular formation on the iris's surface, sometimes with increased intraocular pressure; and glaucoma. The following case illustrates some of these findings.

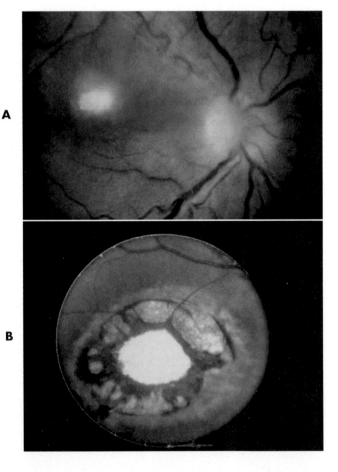

A

B

Fig. 34-7 Toxoplasmic chorioretinitis with acute lesion (**A**) and inactive macular scar (**B**). In **A** there is focal necrotizing retinitis with cottonlike patch in the fundus. Acute lesions (**A**) appear soft and white, have indistinct borders, and may have associated vitritis. Older lesions (**B**) are whitish gray and sharply demarcated and often have areas with choroidal pigment. (Adapted from McLeod R, Remington JS. In Behrman RL, Vaughan VC III, Nelson WE [eds]. Nelson's textbook of pediatrics, ed 14. Philadelphia: WB Saunders Co, 1990, and Remington JS, Desmonts G. In Remington JS, Klein JO [eds]: Infectious diseases of the fetus and newborn infant, ed 3. Philadelphia: WB Saunders, 1990.)

■ **CASE 4: PATIENT WITH TOXOPLASMIC CHORIORETINI-TIS** Her mother gardened and sampled uncooked hamburger during this child's gestation. The perinatal history was unremarkable except for the birth weight of 5 pounds, 9 ounces at a gestational age of 37 weeks. She had no medical problems identified in the newborn period and did not require hospitalization or treatment for any serious medical illness. Before entering nursery school when she was 4 years old, she had a routine ophthalmologic examination, which revealed decreased vision in her right eye and bilateral macular scars. Her visual acuity was 20/125 OD and 20/25 OS. There were cells in the anterior vitreous of the right eye and a few cells in the anterior vitreous of the left eye. The right vitreous had 1 to 2+ haze caused by the cells. In the right eye there was a one disc diameter foveal scar with a hyperpigmented center surrounded by a deeply pigmented area. A small, one-eighth disc diameter area of active retinitis was present between the disc and the macular scar. The left fundus had a trace of vitreous haze with macular scarring. The child's serum *Toxoplasma* IgG indirect fluorescent antibody (IFA) titer was 1:4,096, and her *Toxoplasma* IgM IFA titer was 0. The mother's serum contained *Toxoplasma*-specific IgG antibody. The child's active ocular toxoplasmosis was treated with prednisone, pyrimethamine, triple sulfonamides, and clindamycin. Signs of active retinal disease and vitritis resolved, and therapy was discontinued.

Three years later, her visual acuity was 20/50 OD and 20/30 OS. She had normal discs and vessels in both eyes, with bilateral macular scarring (similar to that shown in Fig. 34-7, *B*).

Holland et al. (1988) described eight patients with presumed toxoplasmic retinochoroiditis and AIDS. Their retinal lesions were frequently bilateral and multifocal. Hemorrhage was minimal, but prominent inflammatory reactions in the vitreous and anterior chamber were common. Histologic examination of two cases, however, showed scant retinal inflammation, which is similar to the lesions seen in toxoplasmic encephalitis in AIDS patients. In areas of necrosis there were numerous *T. gondii* tachyzoites and cysts. Preexisting retinal scars were rare, suggesting that most ocular lesions are the result of newly acquired disease or organisms newly disseminated to the eye from nonocular sites.

DIAGNOSIS

Multiple serologic tests may be needed to establish the diagnosis of acutely acquired or congenital *Toxoplasma* infection. Each laboratory must establish test values that are diagnostic of infection in particular clinical settings and must provide interpretation of the test results and appropriate quality control. If therapy is based on serologic test results, these results should be confirmed in a reference laboratory (e.g., Palo Alto Research Institute, Palo Alto, California, 415.326.8120). Diagnosis may also be established by microscopic demonstration of tachyzoites in smears prepared from body fluids (e.g., CSF) or tissue sections (e.g., brain biopsy) or by actual isolation of the organism from tissues such as placenta, fetal blood, amniotic fluid, or body fluids that are inoculated into tissue culture or mice. Characteristic histopathologic manifestations may also be noted in a lymph node biopsy.

Isolation

T. gondii can be isolated by inoculation of specimens (from body fluids, leukocytes, fetal blood clots, bone marrow, or homogenates of placenta) into the peritoneum of seronegative mice or into tissue culture. Ideally, material should be processed immediately, although *T. gondii* has been isolated from tissues and blood stored at 4° C overnight. Freezing or treatment of specimens with formalin kills the organism. Six to 10 days later, or earlier if the mice die, the peritoneal fluid of inoculated mice is examined microscopically for tachyzoites. If mice survive 4 to 6 weeks, their sera are then tested for IgG *Toxoplasma* antibody. If their sera contain specific antibody, definitive diagnosis is made by visualization of tissue cysts in the mouse brain. If no cysts are found, homogenates of mouse brain, liver, and spleen are subinoculated into other mice, and the process is repeated.

Tissue cultures (e.g., of fibroblasts) have also been used to isolate *T. gondii*. This apparently is a more convenient but less sensitive method than inoculation into mice. Tissue cultures are inoculated with clinical samples; if the result is positive, plaques generally form as early as 4 days after inoculation. Cultures are stained with Wright's or Giemsa stain and examined for plaques that contain necrotic cells and replicating tachyzoites. Isolation of *T. gondii* from placenta, blood, or body fluids (e.g., CSF or amniotic fluid) is diagnostic for both acute and congenital toxoplasmosis. In contrast, in suspected cases of reactivated disease, isolation of *T. gondii* from tissue homogenates may only reflect the presence of tissue cysts in a chronic, latent infection.

Histology

Tissue sections, smears from brain biopsy, bone marrow aspirates, or cytocentrifuge specimens of body fluids that demonstrate free or intracellular tachyzoites confirm the diagnosis of acute infection. Because tachyzoites are often difficult to see in ordinary stains, immunofluorescent antibody and immunoperoxidase techniques may be useful (Conley et al., 1981). The finding of tissue cysts is diagnostic of infection with *T. gondii* but does not differentiate between acute and chronic infection. Tissue cysts in the placenta or any tissue samples from a newborn do, however, indicate congenital transmission. Toxoplasmic lymphadenitis has characteristic histologic features (see Pathology), but tachyzoites are generally not demonstrable.

Serologic Testing

Clinical Use of Serologic Tests and Representative Results in Specific Clinical Settings. Serologic tests to detect *T. gondii*–specific IgG, IgM, or IgA antibodies include the Sabin-Feldman dye test, IFA tests, agglutination tests, and ELISAs. DNA probe methods (e.g., the polymerase chain reaction) have been described recently and have been used in France for prenatal diagnosis of congenital infection by amniocentesis. Tables 34-5 and 34-6 list specific tests that may be useful in particular clinical settings. Representative serologic test results from various clinical forms of infection are also listed in Table 34-6.

IgG Antibodies. The following serologic tests detect IgG antibodies to *T. gondii:* Sabin-Feldman dye test, IFA, IgG ELISA, direct agglutination, and complement fixation. The Sabin-Feldman dye test and the IgG IFA test measure the same antibodies, and titers are usually of approximately the same magnitude. The Sabin-Feldman dye test is both sensitive and specific. It is generally viewed as the "gold standard" for detection of *T. gondii*–specific IgG. In this test, live tachyzoites incubated with serum that contains antibodies to Toxoplasma and an exogenous source of complement will change in shape and no longer take up the vital stain, alkaline methylene blue dye, indicating cell death. The dye test titer is the serum dilution at which half of the tachyzoites are killed. The IgG IFA test measures Toxoplasma-specific IgG antibodies, using formalin-fixed tachyzoites, the patient's serum, and antibody to human IgG that is fluorescein conjugated. In both the IgG IFA test and the dye test, antibodies usually appear 1 to 2 weeks after infection and reach high titers (>1:1,000) after 6 to 8 weeks. Low titers of such IgG antibody usually persist for life. Results that demonstrate *T. gondii*-specific IgG using IgG ELISA also correlate well with results of the Sabin-Feldman dye and IgG IFA tests. The complement-fixation test, however, detects IgG antibody that is generated less rapidly than antibody detected by the dye test, IgG IFA test, or IgG ELISA. Antibody detected with the complement-fixation test appears in the serum 3 to 8 weeks after infection, rises over the next 2 to 8 months, and then declines to low levels within a year. This test is not useful for detection of acute infection because of high false-negative rates.

Agglutination tests to detect IgG antibody are available commercially in Europe. Formalin-preserved whole parasites are used to detect IgG. Interference of nonspecific IgM antibodies is a problem that can be eliminated with the use of 2-mercaptoethanol. This test is accurate, simple, and relatively inexpensive.

IgM Antibodies. Tests to detect IgM antibodies to *T. gondii* include the IgM IFA; double-sandwich enzyme-linked immunosorbent technique (DS IgM ELISA); and IgM ISAGA (an agglutination test). Since IgM antibodies usually appear within the first weeks of infection and disappear more rapidly than IgG antibodies, they are used to detect acute infection. IgM does not cross the placenta, so IgM antibodies detected in fetal or neonatal blood samples represent synthesis by an infected fetus or infant. IgM antibodies often are not present in sera of immunodeficient patients with active infection or in normal or immunodeficient patients during recrudescence in the eye. Specific IgM can be detected in sera of approximately 75% of newborns with congenital toxoplasmosis (when sera are tested using the DS IgM ELISA).

Although the IgM IFA is useful for the diagnosis of acute infection with *T. gondii* in the older child and adult, it is relatively insensitive and therefore not reliable in detection of infection in infants. It detects only 25% of congenital *T. gondii* infections. Moreover, sera containing antinuclear antibodies or rheumatoid factor may yield false-positive reactions in the IgM IFA test.

The DS IgM ELISA is more specific and sensitive for detecting anti–*T. gondii* IgM antibodies than the IgM IFA (Naot and Remington, 1980). It is useful for detection of both congenital toxoplasmosis in the infant and acute toxoplasmosis in the older child. Values indicative of infection must be determined by each laboratory. In one reference laboratory, levels of 1.7 (ELISA units) or greater usually indicate recently acquired infection in an older child or adult, although presence of specific

Table 34-5   Approach to serologic diagnosis of toxoplasmosis

Patient and specimen	T. gondii–specific IgG*				T. gondii–specific IgM†				T. gondii–specific IgA	T. gondii–specific IgE		Other tests		
	Dye test	IFA	IgG ELISA	Direct agglutination	DS-IgM ELISA	ISAGA	ELISA for IgM to P30	IFA	ELISA	ELISA	ISAGA	PCR	Isolation	AC/HS
Newborn congenital toxoplasmosis														
Serum	C	C	C	C	C	C	C	Do not use	C	C	C		C	
CSF	C				C	C						R	C	
Peripheral blood clot or peripheral blood cells (WBC)													C	
Placenta												R	C	
Pregnant woman														
Maternal serum	C	C	C	C	C	C	C	C	C	C	C			C
Amniotic fluid									C	C	C	C	C	
Immunologically normal child														
Serum	C	C	C	C	C	C	C	C	C	C	C			C
CSF	C	C	C	C	C	C	C	C	C	C	C			
Immunologically deficient child														
Serum	C	C	C	C	C‡	C‡	C‡	C‡	C	C	C			C
CSF	C	C	C	C	C‡	C‡	C‡	C‡	C	C	C	R	C	

IFA, Indirect fluorescent antibody; *ELISA*, enzyme immunoassay; *ISAGA*, immunosorbent test for IgM; *IgE*, immunoglobulin E; *PCR*, polymerase chain reaction; *AC/HS*, differential agglutination test; *C*, commercially available; *R*, research test at present in reference laboratories; *CSF*, cerebrospinal fluid; *WBC*, white blood cells.

*When properly standardized, any one of these tests is useful for demonstration of IgG antibody.

†ISAGA is usually most sensitive; IFA is least sensitive (do not use for congenital infection).

‡Rarely positive.

Table 34-6 Guidelines for interpretation of serologic tests for toxoplasmosis*

Test	Positive titer	Titer in congenital infection (infant); acute infection (older child, adult)	Titer in chronic infection	Duration of elevation of titer
IgG				
Sabin-Feldman dye test	Undiluted	NC, S; OCA, 1:4 to ≥1:1,000 (usual)	1:4 to 1:2,000	Years
Direct agglutination test	≥1:20	NC, S; OCA, rises slowly from negative to low to high titer (1:512)	Stable (≥1:1,000) or slowly decreasing titer	≥1 year
Indirect fluorescent IgG antibody	≥1:10	NC, S; OCA, ≥1:1,000	1:8 to 1:2,000	Years
Indirect hemagglutination test	≥1:16	NC, S; OCA, ≥1:1,000	1:16 to 1:256	Years
Complement fixation	≥1:4	NC, S; OCA, varies among laboratories	Negative to 1:8	Years
IgM				
Indirect fluorescent for IgM	≥1:10, adults	OCA, ≥1:80 (use only for OCA, not NC)	Negative to 1:20	Weeks to months, occasionally years
Double sandwich IgM ELISA	≥0.2, newborn, fetus ≥1.7, older children, adults	NC, ≥0.2; OCA, ≥1.7	Negative to 1.7 (OCA)	Can be ≥1 year
Immunosorbent test for IgM	≥3, infant; 8, adult	NC, ≥3; OCA, >8	Negative to 1	Unknown, can be ≥1 year
IgA				
IgA, ELISA	≥1.0, infants; ≥1.4, adults	NC, ≥1.0; OCA, >1.4	Negative to <1.0 Negative to ≤1.3	Weeks to months, occasionally longer
IgE				
IgE, ELISA	≥1.9 infants and adults	NC and OCA, ≥1.9	Negative	Weeks to months, occasionally longer
Immunosorbent test for IgE	≥4 infants and adults	NC and OCA, ≥4	Negative	Weeks to months, occasionally longer
AC/HS	See Table 286-10	See Table 286-10	See Table 286-10	Usually <9 months
PCR (amniotic fluid; CSF)	Positive	Positive	Negative	Only when *Toxoplasma* DNA present during active infection

NC, Titer in newborn with congenital infection; *OCA*, titer in older child or adult with acute, acquired infection; *S*, usually the same as the mother; *EIA*, enzyme immunosorbent; *AC/HS*, differential agglutinin test; *PCR*, polymerase chain reaction; *CSF*, cerebrospinal fluid.

*Values are those of one reference laboratory; each laboratory must provide its own standards and interpretation of results in each clinical setting.

serum IgM antibody can persist for up to 2 years. In that laboratory a value in serum of greater than 0.2 suggests congenital infection in a fetus or neonate. The DS IgM ELISA detects 75% of infants with congenital *Toxoplasma* infection compared to detection of 25% of such infants using the IgM IFA. If a fluorescent antibody (FAB) is used, the DS IgM ELISA avoids false-positive test results caused by rheumatoid factor or antinuclear antibody. The IgM ISAGA combines trapping of the patient's IgM to a solid surface and the use of formalin-fixed organisms or antigen-coated latex particles. It apparently is more sensitive than the DS IgM ELISA and, in the same manner, avoids false-positive results from rheumatoid factor or antinuclear antibodies.

IgA and IgE Antibodies and AC/HS. Other tests to detect antibody to *T. gondii* include the IgA ELISA; the enzyme-linked immunofiltration assay (for IgA and IgE); the immunosorbent agglutination assay for IgE; and a differential agglutination test, AC/HS (Dannemann et al., 1990). The IgA ELISA apparently is even more sensitive than the IgM ELISA for detection of congenital infection (Decoster et al., 1988; Stepick-Biek et al., 1990). Both *T. gondii*–specific IgM and IgA antibodies demonstrated in ELISA or ISAGA may remain elevated for prolonged times (i.e., many months to years in older children and adults) but more commonly are present only a short time. AC/HS (Dannemann et al., 1990) is useful in differentiating recent acquisition from remote acquisition of infection in older children and adults (Table 34-7). In this test, greater agglutination of acetone-fixed tachyzoites (relative to agglutination of formalin-fixed tachyzoites) is detected in patients with acute

infection. This test may be particularly helpful in differentiating recent infection from remote infection in a pregnant woman.

Local Antibody Production. The amount of *T. gondii*–specific antibody produced locally in CSF or aqueous humor has also been used to establish the presence of *T. gondii* infection. An organism-specific antibody index (OSAI), previously called "antibody coefficient (C)" or "*Toxoplasma*-specific index," is calculated as follows:

$$\text{OSAI} = \frac{\text{Reciprocal titer in body fluid} \div \text{Concentration of IgG in body fluid}}{\text{Reciprocal titer in serum} \div \text{Concentration of IgG in serum}}$$

An OSAI greater than or equal to 8 (in aqueous humor for ophthalmologic infection); greater than or equal to 4 (in CSF for congenital infection); or greater than or equal to 1 (in CSF for AIDS patients) indicates local antibody production. If the serum dye test titer is greater than or equal to 1,000, it is usually not possible to demonstrate local antibody production. IgM may also be present in CSF.

Antibody Load. In patients with congenital toxoplasmosis, serum *T. gondii*–specific IgG antibody (present at birth) usually reflects the level of passively transferred maternal IgG antibody. Synthesis of specific antibody by the infected infant often can be detected by serial measurement of the ratio of *T. gondii*–specific IgG to total IgG and comparison to the expected linear decline in this ratio in an uninfected infant (Remington et al., 1995). However, antimicrobial therapy may delay detection of the baby's specific antibody synthesis by this means.

Table 34-7   Interpretation of the AC/HS test

HS result (IU/ml)	AC result (IU/ml)							
	<50	50	100	200	400	800	1600	>1600
<100	NA	NA	A	A	A	A	A	A
100	NA	NA	A	A	A	A	A	A
200	NA	NA	A	A	A	A	A	A
400	NA	NA	A	A	A	A	A	A
800	NA	NA	NA	A	A	A	A	A
1600	NA	NA	NA	NA	A	A	A	A
3200	NA	NA	NA	NA	NA	A	A	A
>3200	NA	NA	NA	NA	NA	NA	A	A

Modified from Thulliez P, Remington JS. J Clin Microbiol 1990;28(9):1928-1933.
NA, Not acute; *A,* acute.

Polymerase Chain Reaction (PCR). This technique is promising for detection of *T. gondii* DNA in amniotic fluid and could potentially be useful for its detection in CSF or peripheral blood. PCR is used to amplify *T. gondii* DNA, which then is identified by hybridization with a labeled probe. A recent study in France (Hohlfeld et al., 1994) using PCR to test amniotic fluid for the *T. gondii* B1 gene gave only one false-negative result and no false-positive results, proving more sensitive and specific than conventional methods of testing. This technique, however, has not yet been fully evaluated in the United States.

Diagnosis In Utero

Amniocentesis and fetal ultrasound has been very useful in the diagnosis and treatment of congenital toxoplasmosis (Hohlfeld et al., 1994). These procedures should be performed only by physicians with considerable experience with the procedures and with the processing and interpretation of the data acquired. An example of the use of these techniques and of the need for experience and skill in interpretation of these results follows.

■ **Case 5** A 19-year-old woman had headaches, malaise, fatigue, and cervical lymphadenopathy 1 month before conception. She did not seek medical care, and her symptoms resolved over a 2-week period. She had cats and kittens that roamed outdoors, but she did not handle their litter box. She denied ingesting any raw or rare meat. On her first prenatal visit at 12 weeks' gestation by dates, serologic test results were as follows: Sabin-Feldman dye test, 1:2,048; IgA ELISA, 10; IgM ELISA, 6; and AC/HS, >1600/1600. Results from a fetal ultrasound at 14 weeks' gestation were normal. Spiramycin (3 g/day orally) was begun.

PCR to determine whether *T. gondii* DNA (the B1 gene) was present in the cell pellet from 10 ml amniotic fluid was negative. A cell pellet from 19 ml of amniotic fluid were inoculated into mice. Subinoculation studies were negative.

Spiramycin therapy was continued until delivery. Fetal ultrasound examinations were repeated every 2 weeks and were normal. The patient tolerated spiramycin therapy without any ill effects. She delivered a normal, uninfected infant, who was evaluated as described in Box 34-1.

Evaluation of the Infant at Birth

Diagnostic tests (in addition to *T. gondii*–specific serologic tests, attempts to isolate the organism, and histologic tests) that may be useful in evaluation of fetuses and infants with congenital toxoplasmosis are listed in Box 34-1.

BOX 34-1

EVALUATION OF NEONATE WHEN SEROLOGIC TESTS OF MOTHER OR THE ILLNESS OF THE NEONATE INDICATES THAT DIAGNOSIS OF CONGENITAL TOXOPLASMOSIS IS SUSPECTED OR LIKELY

In addition to a careful general examination, when congenital toxoplasmosis is a possible or likely diagnosis, the baby is examined by the following:

Clinical Evaluation and Nonspecific Tests
- By a pediatric ophthalmologist
- By a pediatric neurologist
- CT scan of the brain
- Blood tests
  Complete blood cell count with differential and platelet counts
  Serum total of IgM, IgG, IgA, and albumin
- Serum alanine aminotransferase total direct bilirubin
  Cerebrospinal fluid (CSF), cell count, glucose, protein, and total IgG

***T. gondii*–Specific Tests**
- Serum Sabin-Feldman dye test, IgM
  ELISA, IgM ISAGA, IgA ELISA, IgE ELISA/ISAGA (0.5 ml serum, sent to Serology Laboratory. Palo Alto Medical Foundation, 860 Bryant Street, Palo Alto, CA 94301)
- Lumbar puncture: cerebrospinal fluid (CSF) 0.5 ml CSF sent to Serology Laboratory (see above address) for dye test and IgM ELISA
- Sterile placental tissue (100 g in saline, no formalin from near insertion of cord from the fetal side) and newborn blood obtained for inoculation into mice (2 ml clotted whole blood in red topped tube)
- Maternal serum analyzed for antibody detected by dye test, IgM ELISA, IgA ELISA, IgE ELISA/ISAGA, and AC/HS

THERAPY

Pyrimethamine plus sulfadiazine or trisulfapyrimidines (triple sulfa) act synergistically against *T. gondii*. These antimicrobial agents (plus leucovorin) currently constitute the standard treatment for toxoplasmosis. In addition, spiramycin has been used extensively in France to prevent in utero transmission of infection to fetuses of acutely infected women

(Desmonts and Couvreur, 1974) and has been included in treatment regimens for congenital toxoplasmosis after birth (Remington et al., 1995). Clindamycin has been used in conjunction with pyrimethamine to treat toxoplasmosis in AIDS patients who have been unable to tolerate therapy with sulfadiazine. New antimicrobial agents that apparently are effective against encysted bradyzoites are promising.

Pyrimethamine

Pyrimethamine (Daraprim) inhibits dihydrofolate reductase. The plasma half-life is 90 hours in adults and 60 hours in infants (McLeod et al., 1992). Pyrimethamine has caused bone marrow suppression manifested by thrombocytopenia, granulocytopenia, and megaloblastic anemia. Reversible granulocytopenia is the most frequent adverse effect in treated infants. Seizures have also occurred with overdosage of pyrimethamine. Patients being treated with pyrimethamine should have their neutrophil counts monitored once weekly and their platelet counts and hematocrit level monitored once monthly. Folinic acid (leucovorin calcium) should always be administered with pyrimethamine to prevent bone marrow suppression. Folinic acid does not block the inhibitory effect of pyrimethamine and sulfadiazine on *Toxoplasma* replication at dosages used in the treatment of congenital toxoplasmosis.

Zidovudine, on the other hand, appears to antagonize the antitoxoplasmic effect of pyrimethamine and its synergy with sulfadiazine in vitro. Therapy with phenobarbital appears to reduce the half-life of pyrimethamine in infants (McLeod et al., 1992) probably by induction of hepatic enzymes, which degrade pyrimethamine. Pyrimethamine levels in fetal serum when mothers receive 50 mg pyrimethamine daily are in a relatively low, but potentially therapeutic, range (Dorangeon et al., 1990).

Sulfonamides

Sulfadiazine or trisulfapyrimidines (sulfadiazine, sulfamerazine, and sulfamethazine) should be used in combination with pyrimethamine for the treatment of toxoplasmosis. Other sulfonamides are less effective. Sulfadiazine and trisulfapyrimidines antagonize folic acid synthesis by inhibition of dihydrofolate synthetase. Sulfadiazine is rapidly absorbed from the gastrointestinal tract, and peak plasma concentrations are reached within 3 to 6 hours after ingestion of a single dose. Equilibration between maternal and fetal circulation is also established in this time. Sulfonamides readily pass through the placenta and reach the fetus in concentrations sufficient to exhibit both antimicrobial and toxic effects.

The side effects of sulfadiazine or trisulfapyrimidines include bone marrow suppression, diarrhea, rash, crystalluria with possible stone formation, and acute reversible renal failure. An increase in fluid intake, with maintenance of high urinary flow, is important in patients treated with sulfonamides. Hypersensitivity reactions can also occur, especially in patients with AIDS. Sulfadiazine interferes with the metabolism of hepatic microsomal enzymes and may inhibit metabolism of phenytoin, causing higher serum levels of this antiepileptic agent. Sulfonamides may also potentiate coumarin anticoagulants by displacing them from binding sites.

Spiramycin

Spiramycin is a macrolide and is available to physicians in the United States with individual permission of the Food and Drug Administration (phone 301.827.2335) and can be obtained from the drug manufacturer, Rhone Poulenc (phone 215.454.5399). It appears to reduce transmission of *T. gondii* from acutely infected pregnant women to their fetuses in utero by 60% (Desmonts and Couvreur, 1979). It is absorbed best without food. Side effects are usually minimal but have included gastrointestinal distress, local vasospasm, dysesthesias, dizziness, flushing, nausea, vomiting, tearing, diarrhea, anorexia, and allergy. There are no known deleterious effects on the fetus.

Clindamycin

Clindamycin is effective against murine toxoplasmosis. However, its effect in human infection is controversial. Despite its absent penetration into CSF and absent in vitro activity against *T. gondii* (presumably a metabolite is active in vivo), clindamycin has been used in combination with high dosages of pyrimethamine to treat successfully toxoplasmic encephalitis in patients with AIDS (with efficacy equal to treatment with pyrimethamine and sulfadiazine). It is recommended as an alternative therapy in conjunction with pyrimethamine if sulfonamide therapy cannot be tolerated. Uncontrolled studies have reported use of clindamycin to treat ocular toxoplasmosis.

Atovoquone (5-Hydroxy-Naphthoquinone) and Other Antimicrobial Agents

Reactivation of disease resulting from encysted organisms is an increasing problem because of the large numbers of patients with chronic latent infection with *T. gondii* and AIDS. Atovoquone, which appears to inhibit protozoan microbial electron transport enzyme cytochrome b, was felt to be promising as an agent effective against bradyzoites within cysts in vitro (Huskinson-Mark et al., 1991). However, in clinical trials, 40% of patients with AIDS developed relapse of their toxoplasmic encephalitis while being treated with this antimicrobial agent. Other antimicrobial agents with effect on *T. gondii* in vitro or in vivo include new macrolides (roxithromycin, clarithromycin, and azithromycin), cycloguanil, and artether (Holfels et al., 1994).

Therapy in Specific Clinical Settings

Summaries of currently used therapies for toxoplasmosis in specific clinical settings are in Tables 34-8 and 34-9.

Congenital Toxoplasmosis. Infected newborns should be treated whether or not they have overt clinical signs of infection.

In a study in France mothers received pyrimethamine and sulfonamide therapy to treat their infected fetuses in utero as outlined in Tables 34-8 and 34-9 (Daffos et al., 1988; Hohlfeld et al., 1989). The outcome was considerably better than was found for comparable historic controls who did not receive such treatment in utero. Forty-one treated children had subclinical infection, and twelve had only isolated asymptomatic signs (retinal scar with normal vision or cerebral calcifications with normal neurological status). Only one had signs of severe congenital infection.

The most extensive experience in treatment of congenital toxoplasmosis after birth has been with the regimen of Dr. Jacques Couvreur. It uses alternate courses of pyrimethamine, sulfadiazine, and spiramycin (see Table 34-9). Couvreur et al. (1984) reported a reduction in early ophthalmologic sequelae with this treatment.

In addition, a U.S. National Collaborative prospective, controlled treatment study with long-term follow-up to determine feasibility, safety, efficacy, and optimal dosage for treatment with pyrimethamine and sulfadiazine is ongoing (McGhee et al., 1992; McLeod et al., 1991a; Roizen et al., 1992; Mets et al., 1992). Preliminary results from this trial indicate that signs of active disease resolve with therapy and suggest that early outcome for most (but not all) treated infants is substantially better than the outcome reported for untreated infants or those treated for only 1 month, as described in the earlier literature (Eichenwald, 1960; Wilson et al., 1980). Neurologic, developmental, auditory, and ophthalmologic outcomes are evaluated. Study of the effect of newer antimicrobial agents that eliminate encysted organisms on ophthalmologic and neurologic sequelae is also planned. Infants can be referred to this National Collaborative study by telephoning 312.791.4152.

A method for preparation of pyrimethamine and sulfadiazine to facilitate their administration to infants, which currently is being used in this National Collaborative study, is shown in Fig. 34-8. Dosages of medications being evaluated are outlined in Table 34-9. Therapy with corticosteroids (prednisone, 1 mg/kg/day, divided into 2 doses) has been recommended when there is elevated CSF protein

Table 34-8 Management of pregnancies at risk for fetal infection according to time of maternal infection

Time of maternal infection	Pregnancies with fetal infection (%)	Prenatal diagnostic tests	Management
Periconception	1 with treatment	Ultrasound every 2 wk; fetal blood sampling plus amniocentesis	Spiramycin; if fetal infection, termination or possibly antiparasitic treatment
5 to 16 wk	4 with treatment; 12 without treatment	Ultrasound every 2 wk; amniocentesis	Spiramycin; if fetal infection, termination or possibly antiparasitic treatment*
16 wk to term	20 to 30, between 16 and 28 wks, increasing incidence closer to term with treatment	Ultrasound every 2 wk; amniocentesis	Spiramycin; if fetal infection, discontinue spiramycin, use antiparasitic treatment* or possibly termination

Modified from Daffos F, et al.: N Engl J Med 1988;318:271.
*Treatment of the fetus or infant is with pyrimethamine, sulfadiazine, and folinic acid without spiramycin.

Table 34-9   Treatment of toxoplasmosis

Manifestation of disease	Therapy	Dosage (oral unless specified)	Duration
Congenital toxoplasmosis*	Pyrimethamine*	Loading dose: 2 mg/kg per day for 2 days, then 1 mg/kg/day for 2 or 6 months, then this dose on each Monday, Wednesday, and Friday	1 yr
	and		
	Sulfadiazine*	100 mg/kg/day in two daily divided doses	1 yr
	and		
	Leucovorin (folinic acid)*	5-10 mg three times weekly†	1 yr
	Corticosteroids (prednisone)§	1 mg/kg/day in two daily divided doses	Until resolution of elevated (≥1 g/dl) cerebrospinal fluid protein level or active chorioretinitis that threatens vision
In immunologically normal children			
Lymphadenopathy	No therapy	—	—
Significant organ damage that is life threatening	Pyrimethamine	A = Loading dose: 2 mg/kg/day (maximum, 50 mg) for 2 days, then maintenance, 1 mg/kg/day (maximum, 25 mg)	D = Usually 4-6 wk or 2 wk beyond time that signs and symptoms have resolved
	and		
	Sulfadiazine	B = Loading dose: 75 mg/kg, then maintenance, 50 mg/kg q 12 hr	Same as D
	and		
	Leucovorin	C = 5-20 mg three times weekly†	Same as D
Active chorioretinitis in older children	Pyrimethamine	Same as A	Same as D
	and		
	Sulfadiazine	Same as B	
	and		
	Leucovorin	Same as C	
	Corticosteroid§	Same as for congenital toxoplasmosis	Same as for congenital toxoplasmosis
In immunocompromised children			
Non-AIDS	Pyrimethamine	Same as A	E = 4-6 wk beyond complete resolution of symptoms and signs
	and		
	Sulfadiazine	Same as B	Same as E
	and		
	Leucovorin	Same as C	Same as E

*Optimal dosage, feasibility, toxicity currently being evaluated or planned in ongoing National Collaborative Treatment Trial (773.834.4152).

†Adjusted for megaloblastic anemia, granulocytopenia, or thrombocytopenia; blood counts, including platelets, should be monitored as described in text.

‡Available only on request from the Food and Drug Administration (301.827.2335).

§Corticosteroids should be continued until signs of inflammation (high CSF protein ≥1 g.dl) or active chorioretinitis that threatens vision have subsided, dosage then can be tapered and discontinued; use only in conjunction with pyrimethamine, sulfadiazine, and leucovorin.   *Continued*

Table 34-9   Treatment of toxoplasmosis—cont'd

Manifestation of disease	Therapy	Dosage (oral unless specified)	Duration
In immunocompromised children—cont'd			
AIDS	Pyrimethamine and	Same as A	Lifetime
	Sulfadiazine and	Same as B	Lifetime
	Leucovorin	Same as C	Lifetime
	Clindamycin may be used instead of sulfadiazine	Reported trials for adults but not infants and children	Lifetime
In pregnant women with acute toxoplasmosis			
First 21 wk of gestation or until term if fetus not infected	Spiramycin‡	1 g every 8 hr without food	F = Until fetal infection documented or excluded at 21 weeks; if documented, treat with pyrimethamine, leucovorin, and sulfadiazine until term
If fetal infection confirmed after 17th wk of gestation or if infection acquired in last few weeks of gestation (after amniocentesis and PCR to determine if fetus is infected with *T. gondii*)	Pyrimethamine	Loading dose: 100 mg/day in divided doses for 2 days followed by 50 mg daily	Same as F
	and Sulfadiazine	Loading dose: 75 mg/kg/day in two divided doses (maximum, 4 g/day) for 2 days, then 100 mg/kg/day in two divided doses (maximum, 4 g/day)	Same as F
	and Leucovorin†	5-20 mg daily	Same as F

(≥1 g/dL) or active chorioretinitis that threatens vision (Remington et al., 1995).

Immunologically Normal Children with Lymphadenopathy, Severe Symptoms, or Damage to Vital Organs. Children with lymphadenopathy alone do not need specific treatment. If severe or persistent symptoms occur or there is evidence of organ damage, therapy with a combination of pyrimethamine, sulfadiazine, and leucovorin is indicated. Patients who are immunologically normal but have severe symptoms or damage to vital organs (e.g., chorioretinitis, myocarditis, or pneumonitis) should be treated until all symptoms and signs resolve, followed by an additional 2 weeks of therapy. The usual course of therapy is approximately 4 to 6 weeks; dosages of medications are in Table 34-9. A loading dose of pyrimethamine (2 mg/kg body weight, maximum of 50 mg) is given daily for 2 days, followed by a maintenance dose (1 mg/kg body weight, maximum of 25 mg) daily. The loading dose of sulfadiazine is 75 mg/kg body weight, followed by a maintenance dose of 50 mg/kg body weight every 12 hours. Folinic acid (calcium leucovorin) is administered orally whenever pyrimethamine is given. Dosage is 5 to 20 mg given 3 to 7 times weekly, depending on the results of blood and platelet counts.

Active Chorioretinitis in Older Children. Chorioretinitis is the most frequent manifestation of congenital disease, and relapse may occur throughout childhood and adult life. Although active chorioretinitis may remit spontaneously without specific therapy, treatment with pyrimethamine, sulfadiazine, and leucovorin appears to

WEIGH BABY <u>EACH</u> WEEK.
INCREASE MEDICATIONS ACCORDINGLY.

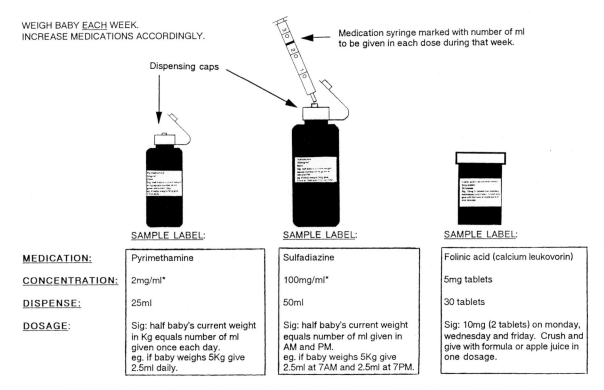

Medication syringe marked with number of ml
to be given in each dose during that week.

Dispensing caps

SAMPLE LABEL: SAMPLE LABEL: SAMPLE LABEL:

	SAMPLE LABEL:	SAMPLE LABEL:	SAMPLE LABEL:
MEDICATION:	Pyrimethamine	Sulfadiazine	Folinic acid (calcium leukovorin)
CONCENTRATION:	2mg/ml*	100mg/ml*	5mg tablets
DISPENSE:	25ml	50ml	30 tablets
DOSAGE:	Sig: half baby's current weight in Kg equals number of ml given once each day. eg. if baby weighs 5Kg give 2.5ml daily.	Sig: half baby's current weight equals number of ml given in AM and PM. eg. if baby weighs 5Kg give 2.5ml at 7AM and 2.5ml at 7PM.	Sig: 10mg (2 tablets) on monday, wednesday and friday. Crush and give with formula or apple juice in one dosage.

Fɪɢ. 34-8   Preparation and administration of medications used to treat congenital toxoplasmosis in a National Collaborative Study. (Adapted from McAuley et al., in preparation.)

reduce signs and symptoms. Therapy for active chorioretinitis is outlined in Table 34-9. Therapy should be given in conjunction with care by an ophthalmologist. With treatment, borders of retinal lesions sharpen, and vitreous haze should disappear within approximately 10 days. Corticosteroids should be added if lesions involve the macula, optic nerve head, or papillomacular bundle. Use of clindamycin has been described extensively in the ophthalmologic literature and has been recommended as an alternative to the sulfonamide-pyrimethamine combination. However, definitive studies demonstrating efficacy have not been performed. In some severe cases, vitrectomy and/or removal of the lens has been used to improve visual acuity. Retinal detachment (which is potentially surgically correctable) has been reported.

Immunocompromised Patients. Toxoplasmosis in patients who are immunocompromised by underlying disease (e.g., lymphoma, AIDS) or by therapy (e.g., corticosteroids, cytotoxic drugs) should be treated. Serologic evidence of active infection in an immunocompromised patient, regardless of clinical signs and symptoms, or documentation of the presence of tachyzoites in tissue is an indication for treatment. In patients with AIDS, clinical symptoms with radiologic findings (CT or MRI) that are suggestive of infection may in themselves be indications for treatment. If there is no response to a therapeutic trial of pyrimethamine and sulfadiazine within approximately 10 to 14 days, brain biopsy to exclude other diagnoses should be considered. In 80% of patients with AIDS in whom the diagnosis was made antemortem, there was clear and rapid (<1 month) improvement with antimicrobial treatment. In the same group of patients, more than half of those responding showed complete resolution of clinical and brain CT scan abnormalities. For immunosuppressed individuals it is imperative to suspect and establish the diagnosis quickly and to begin treatment as soon as possible.

For children whose immunosuppression can be reduced (by discontinuation of chemotherapy or corticosteroids), treatment with sulfadiazine, pyrimethamine, and leucovorin should be continued for 4 to 6 weeks beyond complete resolution of all signs and symptoms of active disease.

In immunocompromised adults with AIDS relapse is frequent if therapy is discontinued. Until agents that can eliminate encysted organisms have demonstrated efficacy in humans, suppressive therapy with pyrimethamine and sulfadiazine should be continued for the remainder of such patients' lives. There are no reported results from studies to examine relative effects of different suppressive regimens, but some that have been recommended are included in Table 34-9. In a recent controlled study the combination of pyrimethamine and sulfadozine, one tablet biweekly, was reported to reduce the occurrence of toxoplasmic encephalitis (Ruf et al., 1991). In this study the incidence of subsequent encephalitis was reduced to four (11%) out of thirty-seven with prophylaxis and to eight (67%) out of twelve without prophylaxis. When used as primary prophylaxis in seropositive individuals without overt disease, the incidence of subsequent encephalitis was reduced to two (5%) out of thirty-eight with sulfadoxine and pyrimethamine (Fansidar) and seven out of twenty-eight (25%) without it. It is not known whether suppressive doses of pyrimethamine and sulfonamides are either necessary or effective in preventing relapse in infants with congenital or acute acquired toxoplasmosis and AIDS. Based on data in adults, it is reasonable to treat children with AIDS and toxoplasmic encephalitis with pyrimethamine and sulfadiazine for the remainder of their lives.

Pregnant Women with Acute Acquired T. Gondii Infection or Chronic T. Gondii Infection and Immunocompromise.

In general, if *T. gondii* infection is acquired by an immunologically normal mother before conception, the fetus is not at risk for congenital toxoplasmosis. There have been only two reports of a normal woman who acquired *T. gondii* 2 months before conception who transmitted the infection to her fetus in utero (Remington et al., 1995; Vogel et al., 1996). Treatment with spiramycin of an immunologically normal pregnant woman who acquires an acute infection during pregnancy reduces the chance of congenital infection in her infant by 60% (Desmonts and Couvreur, 1974). Spiramycin (1.5 g every 12 hours without food) is continued throughout pregnancy unless fetal infection is demonstrated by ultrasound or analysis of amniotic fluid (see Table 34-8). If evidence of infection is present in the fetus, pyrimethamine, sulfadiazine, and leucovorin therapy (dosages are listed in Table 34-9) have been substituted in alternate months for spiramycin. If no fetal involvement is found, spiramycin alone is continued until term. Such treatment reduces the ability to isolate *T. gondii* from the placenta. In one study, *T. gondii* was isolated from placentas of untreated infected infants 95% of the time, but only 80% of the time from placentas of infected infants whose mothers were treated with spiramycin and only 50% of the time from placentas of infants whose mothers were treated with pyrimethamine and sulfadiazine and spiramycin in alternate months (Couvreur et al., 1988).

Chronically infected women who become immunosuppressed by cytotoxic drugs, corticosteroids, or HIV infection have also transmitted *T. gondii* to the fetus. Most of these women develop toxoplasmosis by recrudescence of latent *T. gondii* rather than from newly acquired infection. Such women, who do not have overt toxoplasmosis, should at least receive spiramycin throughout pregnancy.

PROGNOSIS

Toxoplasmic lymphadenopathy in the immunologically normal individual is self-limited and resolves without antimicrobial therapy. Treatment with pyrimethamine, sulfadiazine, and leucovorin results in resolution of active signs of *T. gondii* infection in most immunologically normal, immunocompromised, and congenitally infected individuals.* The prognosis for infants with congenital toxoplasmosis that is untreated or is treated with 1 month of pyrimethamine and sulfadiazine is poor for those who have neurologic or generalized infection at presentation in their first year of life (see Table 34-3). The prognosis also is guarded for those with subclinical infection at birth (see Table 34-4). The outcome is substantially better for most (but not all) infants who are treated in utero and/or for 1 year with pyrimethamine and sulfadiazine (Tables 34-10 and 34-11). Favorable outcomes have been associated with prompt diagnosis and initiation of antimicrobial therapy and with prompt attention to the need for shunting of patients with hydrocephalus or revision of malfunctioning ventriculoperitoneal shunts (McAuley et al., 1994).

PREVENTION

At present, the major component of primary prevention is educating susceptible patients, especially seronegative pregnant or immunodeficient individuals. Given the morbidity, mortality, and expense of the disease in terms of care of affected

---

*McAuley et al., 1994; McGhee et al., 1992; McLeod et al., 1979; McLeod et al., 1992; Mets et al., 1996; Patel et al, 1996; Roizen et al, 1995; Swisher et al, 1994.

Table 34-10 Contrasts of neurologic and developmental outcomes in Eichenwald, Wilson, and Chicago studies

		% With outcome			
Signs neonatally	Study	Seizures	Abnormal motor/tone	IQ <70	Sequentially lower IQ
Generalized neurologic	Eichenwald, 1960 (n = 101)	81	70	86	n/a
	Chicago, 1991a (n = 33)	11	24	32	Not significant*,†
Subclinical	Wilson et al., 1980 (n = 33)	17	21	17	86*
	Chicago, 1991a (n = 3)	0	0	0	0*

Adapted from Boyer KM, McLeod RL, In Long SS, Prober CG, Pickering LK (eds). Principles and practice of infectious diseases. New York: Churchill Livingstone, 1996, pp 645-672. With permission.
*In Chicago study: generalized/neurologic n = 27; subclinical n = 2; In Wilson study: n = 7.
†Three increased, three decreased; thus no significant differences for group; ³/₁₁ (27%).

Table 34-11 Fetal toxoplasmosis: outcome of pregnancy and infant follow-up after in utero treatment*

	Trimester										
	First				Second				Third		
	1972-1981		1982-1988		1972-1981		1982-1988		1972-1981		1982-1988
Outcome	Number	%	Number	%	Number	%	Number	%	Number	%	Number
Subclinical	1	10	6	67	23	37	33	77	74	68	2
Benign	5	50	2	22	28	45	10	23	31	29	0
Severe	4	40	1	11	11	18	0		3	3	0
TOTAL	10		9		62		43		108		2

Modified from Hohlfeld P, et al. J Pediatr 1989;115:765.
*Infants were not treated in utero 1972-1981 and were treated in utero 1982-1988. Trimester indicates time of acquisition of acute infection by the mother. Note in utero treatment was associated with marked diminution of clinical signs or severity of infection.

patients, major attempts to define and initiate better forms of prevention are needed. All physicians responsible for the care of pregnant women, those attempting to conceive, or immunosuppressed patients should inform them of simple measures for prevention. Provision of informational material to pregnant women in France reduced the incidence of congenital infection by 50%. An educational pamphlet and videotape (phone 800.323.9100), as well as information on the Internet at http:\\ www.iit.edu\~toxo\pamphlet, are also available.

The goal of primary prevention is to avoid ingestion of cysts or contact with sporulated oocysts. Methods of prevention are outlined in Fig. 34-2. Tissue cysts can be rendered noninfectious by heating meat or eggs to 66° C (150.8° F) or by smoking, curing, or freezing meat to −22° C (−7.6° F). Most home freezers do not become this cold. Hands should be washed thoroughly after handling raw meat and vegetables. Steak tartare or other foods featuring uncooked meat should be avoided. Eggs should not be ingested raw, and unpasteurized milk (particularly from goats) should not be consumed. Any kitchen surfaces that come in contact with raw meat or vegetables should be washed thoroughly. Patients should also be warned not to touch mucous membranes or eyes while handling raw meat.

To prevent infection with the oocyst, cat feces should be avoided. Cat feces should be disposed of daily (because sporulation occurs 1 to 5 days after excretion) either by incineration or by flushing down the toilet. Cat litter pans should be used with liners and changed by someone other than the pregnant or immunosuppressed individual. The pan can then be rendered free of viable oocysts by pouring boiling water into the pans and letting the water remain for at least 5 minutes before rinsing. Ammonia (7%) can also kill oocysts but requires 3 hours of exposure. Chlorine bleach, dilute ammonia, quater-

Approach to prenatal prevention, diagnosis and treatment

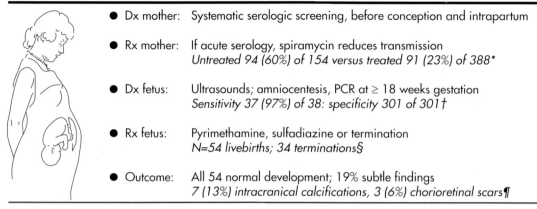

●	Dx mother:	Systematic serologic screening, before conception and intrapartum
●	Rx mother:	If acute serology, spiramycin reduces transmission *Untreated 94 (60%) of 154 versus treated 91 (23%) of 388**
●	Dx fetus:	Ultrasounds; amniocentesis, PCR at ≥ 18 weeks gestation *Sensitivity 37 (97%) of 38: specificity 301 of 301†*
●	Rx fetus:	Pyrimethamine, sulfadiazine or termination *N=54 livebirths; 34 terminations§*
●	Outcome:	All 54 normal development; 19% subtle findings *7 (13%) intracranical calcifications, 3 (6%) chorioretinal scars¶*

*Desmonts and Couvreur, 1974.
†Hohlfeld et al, 1994.
§Daffos et al, 1988.
¶Hohlfeld et al, 1989.

FIG. 34-9 Prevention, diagnosis, and treatment of toxoplasmosis.

nary ammonia compounds, or other household detergents are not sufficient to destroy oocysts. When working in sand or soil possibly contaminated with cat feces, gloves should be worn. Hands should be thoroughly washed before handling any items that would be ingested or come in contact with mucous membranes. Since the cat is the only animal that is known to produce oocysts, efforts should also be directed toward preventing infection in cats. Feeding cats commercially dried, canned, or cooked food rather than allowing them to hunt possibly infected prey will reduce the likelihood of their infection. These general precautionary measures, rather than serologic testing of cats, are recommended.

Although primary prevention theoretically can be achieved by education about hygienic measures as described previously, secondary prevention consists of identification of acutely infected individuals in high-risk populations and the early institution of specific therapy to prevent or minimize complications. Since approximately 90% of women infected during pregnancy have no clinical illness, sequential serologic testing of seronegative pregnant women is the only way to identify the fetus at risk of congenital infection. Standardized screening, followed by sequential testing, is routinely performed in areas of high incidence, such as France and Austria. However, there is no universally adopted policy for screening or sequential testing of pregnant women for congenital toxoplasmosis in the United

States. Cost-effectiveness has been suggested but not proven (McCabe and Remington, 1988). Problems with the reliability of some commercially available serologic tests have in the past dissuaded certain authors from recommending widespread serologic screening. Before the initiation of therapy in any setting, positive serologic test results should be confirmed in a reference laboratory (e.g., Palo Alto Research Institute; phone 415.326.8120). Some serologic screening programs have involved all women in their childbearing years before and during pregnancy to determine prior exposure (e.g., France), and some have involved screening of all newborns (e.g., the model of the Massachusetts State Screening Program). If women are seronegative, systematic serologic screening at specific intervals during pregnancy is used (Fig. 34-9). This is a reasonable approach because it is possible to prevent or modify illness caused by congenital *T. gondii* infection by treatment during gestation and because reliable serologic tests are now commercially available in the United States. The individual suffering and the cost to families and society of caring for children born with congenital toxoplasmosis make increased use of screening tests potentially important (Featherstone, 1981).

THE FUTURE

Major future advances in prevention and treatment of toxoplasmosis are likely. Development of a vac-

BOX 34-2
PERTINENT PHONE NUMBERS

Reference laboratory for serology, isolation, and PCR	415.326.8120
FDA for IND number to obtain spiramycin for treatment of a pregnant woman	301.827.2335
Spiramycin (Rhone Poulence) for treatment of a pregnant woman	215.454.5399
Congenital toxoplasmosis study	312.791.4152
Educational pamphlet	312.435.4007
Information concerning AIDS and congenital toxoplasmosis	305.547.6676
Educational information on Internet	http:\\www.iit.edu\~toxo\pamphlet

cine to prevent infection in humans and cats remains at an experimental stage, but a number of lines of investigation are promising. Use of educational programs for pregnant and immunocompromised individuals should further reduce infection rates. Paradigms for prevention of congenital infection or its sequelae are being developed and tested. More sensitive and specific serologic and direct (e.g., PCR) tests are being evaluated. Additional reference laboratories to perform serologic testing reliably are needed. Studies to determine optimal means to treat congenital toxoplasmosis and toxoplasmosis in patients with AIDS are in progress. Ongoing development and testing of new antimicrobial agents that eliminate encysted organisms that are the source of recrudescent disease in congenital, ophthalmologic, and disseminated or neurologic toxoplasmosis in immunocompromised individuals are promising.

RESOURCES

A variety of resources are available to assist in the prevention and treatment of toxoplasmosis. These resources (with phone numbers) are shown in Box 34-2.

GLOSSARY

AC/HS: Differential agglutination test using acetone (AC) and formalin (HS) fixed tachyzoites; useful in determining whether infection was acquired in the 6 months before the serum sample was obtained.

Chronic infection with *T. gondii:* Condition of asymptomatic parasite latency that follows primary infection or successful treatment of recrudescence.

Cyst: Contains bradyzoites and is present in chronic infection.

Double sandwich (DS) IgA ELISA: Measures *T. gondii*–specific IgA; possibly more sensitive than the DS IgM ELISA for diagnosis of congenital infection.

Double sandwich (DS) IgE ELISA: Measures *T. gondii*–specific IgE; possibly more sensitive than the IgM ELISA for diagnosis of congenital infection.

Double sandwich (DS) IgM ELISA: Measures *T. gondii*–specific IgM; positive at birth in approximately 75% of congenitally infected infants.

IgE ISAGA: Measures *T. gondii*–specific IgE; probably more sensitive than the DS IgM ELISA.

IgM ISAGA: Measures *T. gondii*–specific IgM; usually more sensitive than the DS IgM ELISA.

Mouse inoculation: Inoculation of body fluid or placental tissue intraperitoneally into mice; mice then are observed for proliferating tachyzoites in their ascitic fluid, brain cyst development, and *T. gondii*–specific serum antibodies.

Oocyst: Contains sporozoites and is excreted by cats.

Sabin-Feldman dye test: "Gold standard" test for measurement of IgG antibody that damages the surface membrane of live tachyzoites in the presence of complement, rendering the tachyzoite unstained by the vital dye methylene blue; performed by reference laboratories.

***Toxoplasma gondii* bradyzoite:** Slowly proliferative form present within tissue cysts in chronic, latent infection; source of infection ingested in undercooked meat.

***Toxoplasma gondii* sporozoite:** Highly infectious form in oocyst, which sporulates after fecal excretion by cats.

***Toxoplasma gondii* tachyzoite:** Rapidly prolifera-
tive form present in acute and active infection.

Toxoplasmosis: Disease caused by *T. gondii;* may
be primary or recrudescent.

BIBLIOGRAPHY

Aspock P. Prevention of congenital toxoplasmosis by serological surveillance during pregnancy: current strategies and future perspectives. In Marget W, Lang W, Gabler-Sandberger
E (eds). Parasitic infections, immunology, mycotic infections,
general topics, vol 3. Munich: MMV Medizin Verlag, 1986.

Boyer KM, McLeod RL. *Toxoplasma gondii* (toxoplasmosis).
In Long SS, Prober CG, Pickering LK (eds). Principles and
practice of infectious diseases. New York: Churchill Livingstone, 1996.

Brézin AP, Kasner L, Thulliez P, et al. Ocular toxoplasmosis in
the fetus: immunohistochemistry analysis and DNA amplification. Retina 1994;14.1:19-26.

Brown C, McLeod R. Class I MHC genes and CD8+ T cells determine cyst number in *Toxoplasma gondii* infection. J Immunol 1990;145:3438-3441.

Burg JL, Grover CM, Pouletty P, Boothroyd JC. Direct and sensitive detection of a pathogenic protozoan, *Toxoplasma
gondii,* by polymerase chain reaction. J Clin Microbiol
1989;27:1787.

Buxton D. Toxoplasmosis: the first commercial vaccine. Parisi-
tol Today 1993;9:335-337.

Buxton D, Innes EA. A commercial vaccine for ovine toxoplasmosis. Parasitology 1995;110(suppl):S11-S16.

Conley JK, Jenkins KA, Remington JS. *Toxoplasma gondii* infection of the central nervous system: use of the peroxidase-
antiperoxidase method to demonstrate *Toxoplasma* in formalin-fixed, paraffin-embedded tissue sections. Hum Pathol
1981;12:690.

Couvreur J, Desmonts G. Congenital and maternal toxoplasmosis: a review of 300 congenital cases. Dev Med Child Neurol
1962;4:519-530.

Couvreur J, Desmonts G, Aron-Rosa D. Le pronostic oculaire
de la toxoplasmose congenitale: role du traitement. Ann Pediatr 1984;31:855-858.

Couvreur J, Desmonts G, Thulliez P. Prophylaxis of congenital
toxoplasmosis: effect of spiramycin on placental infection. J
Antimicrob Chemother 1988;22:193-200.

Daffos F, Forestier F, Capella-Pavlovsky M, et al. Prenatal management of 746 pregnancies at risk for congenital toxoplasmosis. N Engl J Med 1988;318:271.

Dannemann BR, Vaughan WC, Thulliez P, et al. The differential
agglutination test for diagnosis of recently acquired infection
with *Toxoplasma gondii.* J Clin Microbiol 1990; 28:1928.

Decoster A, Darcy F, Caron A, et al. IgA antibodies against P30
as markers of congenital and acute toxoplasmosis. Lancet
1988;2:1104.

Derouin F, Devergie A, Auber P. Toxoplasmosis in bone-mar-
row transplant recipients: report of seven cases and review.
Clin Infect Dis 1992;15:267-270.

Desmonts G, Couvreur J. Congenital toxoplasmosis: a prospective study of 378 pregnancies. N Engl J Med 1974;290:
1110-1116.

Desmonts G, Couvreur J. Congenital toxoplasmosis: a prospective study of the offspring of 542 women who acquired toxoplasmosis during pregnancy: pathophysiology of congenital
disease. In Thalhammer O, Baumgarten K, Pollak A (eds).
Perinatal medicine: sixth European Congress. Stuttgart, Germany: Georg Thieme, 1979.

Desmonts G, Couvreur J. Natural history of congenital toxoplasmosis. Ann Pediatr 1984;31:799.

Desmonts G, Remington JS. Direct agglutination test for diagnosis of *Toxoplasma* infection. Method for increasing sensitivity and specificity. J Clin Microbiol 1980;11:562.

Dorangeon PH, Fay R, Marx-Chemla C, et al. Passage transpla-
centaire de l'association pyrimethamine-sulfadoxine hors du
traitement antenatal de la toxoplasmose congenital. Presse
Med 1990;2036:22-29.

Dorfman RF, Remington JS. Value of lymph node biopsy in the
diagnosis of acute acquired toxoplasmosis. N Engl J Med
1973;289:878.

Duquesne V, Auriault C, Darcy F, et al. Protection of nude rats
against *Toxoplasma* infection by excreted-secreted antigen-
specific helper T cells. Infect Immunol 1990;58:2120.

Eichenwald HF. A study of congenital toxoplasmosis, with particular emphasis on clinical manifestations, sequelae, and
therapy. In Siim JC (ed). Human toxoplasmosis. Copenhagen:
Munksgaard, 1960.

Featherstone H. A difference in the family. New York: Penguin,
1981.

Forestier F, Daffos F, Rainant M, Cox WC. The assessment of
fetal blood samples. Am J Obstet Gynecol 1988;158:1184-
1188.

Frenkel JK, Pfefferkorn ER, Smith DD, Fishback JL. Prospective vaccine prepared from a new mutant of *Toxoplasma
gondii* for use in cats. Am J Vet Res 1991;52:759-763.

Grover CM, Thulliez P, Remington JS, et al. Rapid prenatal diagnosis of congenital *Toxoplasma* infection by using polymerase chain reaction and amniotic fluid. J Clin Microbiol
1990;28:2297.

Guerina NG, Hsu Ho-Wen, Meissner HC, et al. Neonatal serologic screening and early treatment for congenital *Toxoplasma gondii* infection. N Engl J Med 1994;33:1858-1863.

Hoff R, Weiblen BJ, Reardon LA, Maguire JH. Screening for
congenital toxoplasma infection. In Transplacental disorders:
perinatal detection, treatment, and management (including
pediatric AIDS). New York: Alan R Liss, 1990.

Hohlfeld P, Daffos T, Costa JM et al. Prenatal diagnosis of congenital toxoplasmosis with a polymerase-chain reaction test
on amniotic fluid. N Engl J Med 1994;331:695-699.

Hohlfeld P, Daffos F, Thulliez P, et al. Fetal toxoplasmosis: outcome of pregnancy and infant follow-up after in utero treatment. J Pediatr 1989;115:765-769.

Holfels E, McAuley J, Mack D, et al. In vitro effects of
artemisinin ether, cycloguanil hydrochloride (alone and in
combination with sulfadiazine), quinine sulfate, mefloquine,
primaquine phosphate, trifluoperazine hydrochloride, and
verapamil on *Toxoplasma gondii.* Antimicrob Agents
Chemother 1994;38:1392-1396.

Holland GN, Engstrom RE Jr, Glasgow BJ, et al. Ocular toxoplasmosis in patients with the acquired immunodeficiency
syndrome. Am J Ophthalmol 1988;106:653-667.

Huskinson-Mark J, Araujo FG, Remington JS. Evaluation of the
effect of drugs on the cyst form of *Toxoplasma gondii.* J Infect Dis 1991;164:170-177.

Israelski DM, Remington JS. Toxoplasmic encephalitis in patients with AIDS. In Sande MA, Volberding PA (eds). The medical management of AIDS. Philadelphia: WB Saunders, 1988.

Israelski DM, Tom C, Remington JS. Zidovudine antagonizes the action of pyrimethamine in experimental infection with *Toxoplasma gondii.* Antimicrob Agents Chemother 1989; 33:30.

Khan A, Ely K, Kasper L. A purified parasite antigen (p30) mediates CD8 T-cell immunity against fatal *Toxoplasma gondii* infection in mice. J Immunol 1991;147:3501-3506.

Koppe JG, Kloosterman GJ, deRoever-Bonnet H, et al. Toxoplasmosis and pregnancy, with a long-term follow-up of the children. Europ J Obstet Gynecol Reprod Biol 1974;413:101-110.

Koppe JG, Loewer-Sieger DH, deRoever-Bonnet H. Results of 20-year follow-up of congenital toxoplasmosis. Lancet 1986;1:254-256.

Labadie MD, Hazeman JJ. Apport des bilans de sante de l'efant pour le depistage et l'etude epidemiologiquede la toxoplasmose congenitale. Ann Pediatr 1984;31:823-828.

Leport C. Toxoplasmosis in AIDS. 17th International Congress of Chemotherapy, June 28, 1991, Berlin, Germany.

Luft BJ, Naot Y, Araujo FG, et al. Primary and reactivated *Toxoplasma* infection in patients with cardiac transplants: clinical spectrum and problems in diagnosis in a defined population. Ann Intern Med 1983;99:27-31.

Luft BJ, Remington JS. Acute *Toxoplasma* infection among family members of patients with acute lymphadenopathic toxoplasmosis. Arch Intern Med 1984;144:53-56.

Mack D, Johnson J, Roberts F, et al. Murine and human MHC class II genes determine susceptibility to toxoplasmosis. (In press).

McAuley JB, Boyer KM, Patel D, et al. Early and longitudinal evaluations of treated infants and children and untreated historical patients with congenital toxoplasmosis: the Chicago Collaborative Treatment Trial. Clin Infect Dis 1994; 18:38-72.

McAuley J, Roizen N, Beckman J, et al. Early evaluations and treatment of 43 infants and children with congenital toxoplasmosis. Clin Inf Dis 1994; 18:38-72.

McCabe RE, Brooks RG, Dorfman RF, Remington JS. Clinical spectrum in 107 cases of toxoplasmic lymphadenopathy. Rev Infect Dis 1987;9:754.

McCabe RE, Remington JS. Toxoplasmosis: the time has come. N Engl J Med 1988;318:313-315.

McGhee T, Wolters C, Stein L, et al. Absence of sensorineural hearing loss in treated infants and children with congenital toxoplasmosis. Otolaryngol Head Neck Surg 1992;106(1): 75-80.

McLeod R, Berry PF, Marshall WH, et al. Toxoplasmosis presenting as brain abscesses: diagnosis by computerized tomography and cytology of aspirated purulent material. Am J Med 1979;67:711-714.

McLeod R, Boyer K, Roizen N, et al. Treatment of congenital toxoplasmosis. 17th International Congress of Chemotherapy, June 18, 1991a, Berlin.

McLeod R, Frenkel JK, Estes RG, et al. Subcutaneous and intestinal vaccination with tachyzoites of *Toxoplasma gondii* and acquisition of immunity to peroral and congenital *Toxoplasma* challenge. J Immunol 1988;140:1632-1637.

McLeod R, Johnson J, Estes R, Mack D. Immunogenetics in pathogenesis of and protection against toxoplasmosis. In U. Gross (ed). *Toxoplasma gondii.* Berlin: Springer-Verlag, 1996.

McLeod R, Mack DG, Boyer KM, et al. Phenotypes and functions of lymphocytes in congenital toxoplasmosis. J Lab Clin Med 1990;116:623-635.

McLeod R, Mack D, Brown C. *Toxoplasma gondii:* new advances in cellular and molecular biology. Exp Parasitol 1991b;72:109-121.

McLeod R, Mack D, Foss R, et al. Levels of pyrimethamine in sera and cerebrospinal and ventricular fluids from infants treated for congenital toxoplasmosis. Antimicrob Agents Chemother 1992;36(5):1040-1048.

McLeod R, Remington JS. Toxoplasmosis. In Behrman RL, Vaughan VC III, Nelson WE (eds). Nelson's textbook of pediatrics, ed 14. Philadelphia: WB Saunders, 1990.

Mets MB, Holfels E, Boyer KM, et al. Eye manifestations of congenital toxoplasmosis. Am J Ophthalmol 1996;122(3): 309-324.

Mets M et al. Ophthalmic findings in congenital toxoplasmosis. Sarasota, FL: Association for Research and Vision in Ophthalmology, 1992.

Mitchell CD, Erlich SS, Mastrucci MT, et al. Congenital toxoplasmosis occurring in infants perinatally infected with human immunodeficiency virus 1. Pediatr Infect Dis 1990;9:512.

Naot Y, Remington JS. An enzyme-linked immunosorbent assay for detection of IgM antibodies to *Toxoplasma gondii:* use for diagnosis of acute acquired toxoplasmosis. J Infect Dis 1980;142:757.

O'Connor GR. Manifestations and management of ocular toxoplasmosis. Bull NY Acad Med 1974;30:192.

Patel DV, Holfels EM, Vogel NP, et al. Resolution of intracerebral calcifications in children with treated congenital toxoplasmosis. Radiology 1996;199:433-440.

Polis MA. Differential diagnosis of retinal lesions in persons with HIV infection. Opportun Infect Interact 1994;3:1-3.

Prince JB, Araujo FG, Remington JS, et al. Cloning of cDNAs encoding a 28 kilodalton antigen of *Toxoplasma gondii.* Mole Biochem Parasitol 1989;34:3-14.

Remington JS, McLeod R, Desmonts G. In Remington JS, Klein J (eds). Infectious diseases of the fetus and newborn infant, ed 4. Philadelphia: WB Saunders, 1995.

Roberts T, Frenkel JK. Estimating income losses and other preventable costs caused by congenital toxoplasmosis in people in the United States. J Am Vet Med Assoc, 1990; 196:249-256.

Roizen N, Swisher C, Stein M, et al. Neurologic and developmental outcome in treated congenital toxoplasmosis. Pediatrics 1995;95:11-20.

Roizen N et al. Developmental and neurologic function in treated congenital toxoplasmosis. Baltimore: Society for Pediatric Research, 1992.

Roux C, Desmonts G, Molliez N, et al. Toxoplasmose et grossesse. Bilan deux ans de phropylaxie de la toxoplasmose congenitale à la maternité de l'hôpital Saint Antoine (1973-1974). J Gynecol Obstet Biol Reprod 1976;5(2):249-264.

Ruf B, Schurmann D, Pohle HD. The efficacy of Fansidar in preventing AIDS-associated neurotoxoplasmosis and *Pneumocystis carinii* pneumonia. 17th International Congress of Chemotherapy, June 28, 1991, Berlin.

Ruiz A, Frenkel JK. *Toxoplasma gondii* in Costa Rican cats. Am J Trop Med Hyg 1980;29:1150.

Stepick-Biek P, Thulliez P, Araujo FG, Remington JS. IgA antibodies for diagnosis of acute congenital and acquired toxoplasmosis. J Infect Dis 1990;162:270-273.

Suzuki Y, Wong S-Y, Grumet FC, et al. Evidence for genetic regulation of susceptibility to toxoplasmic encephalitis in AIDS patients. J Infect Dis 1996;173:265-268.

Swisher CN, Boyer K, McLeod R. Clinical toxoplasmosis. Semin Pediatr Neurol 1994;1(1):4-25.

Townsend JJ et al. Acquired toxoplasmosis. Arch Neurol 1975;32:335.

Vogel NP, Patel D, Roizen N, et al. Congenital transmission of *Toxoplasma gondii* from an immunologically normal mother infected prior to pregnancy. Clin Inf Dis. 1996; 23:1055-1060.

Wilson CB, Remington JS. What can be done to prevent congenital toxoplasmosis? Am J Obstet Gynecol 1980;138: 357-363.

Wilson CB, Remington JS, Stagno S, Reynolds DW. Development of adverse sequelae in children born with subclinical congenital *Toxoplasma* infection. Pediatrics 1980;66: 767-774.

Wong S-Y, Hajdu MP, Ramirez R, et al. The role of specific immunoglobulin E in the diagnosis of acute *Toxoplasma* infection and toxoplasmosis. J Clin Microbiol 1993;31:2952-2959.

Wong S-Y, Remington JS. Toxoplasmosis in pregnancy. Clin Infect Dis 1994;18:853-861.

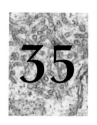

35 TUBERCULOSIS

JEFFREY R. STARKE

Although tuberculosis is an ancient disease that is known to have existed in prehistoric times, it remains the most important infectious disease in the world in terms of morbidity, mortality, and economic impact. Tuberculosis was recognized as a clinical entity in the early nineteenth century but was not determined to be an infectious disease until 1882 when Koch identified *Mycobacterium tuberculosis.* The recognized spread of tuberculosis became a concern of public health authorities, and efforts to control tuberculosis became the cornerstone of modern public health.

Although the cause of tuberculosis is the bacillus *Mycobacterium tuberculosis,* it has long been recognized that stresses within populations—famine, war, adverse working conditions, population displacements, and crowded living conditions—favor the spread of tuberculosis in human beings and the development of disease from asymptomatic infection. In the mid-1800s the death rate from tuberculosis in large cities in the United States was approximately 400 per 100,000 per year, making it the leading cause of death. Over the next 100 years, despite the lack of specific chemotherapy, the incidence of both disease and death from tuberculosis dropped dramatically as a result of improved health care and living and working conditions, as well as genetic selection within the population.

Tuberculosis currently is in a rapidly shifting position worldwide. After years of steady decline in its incidence in the United States, the Centers for Disease Control and Prevention (CDC) in 1989 developed a plan to eliminate tuberculosis by the year 2010. Unfortunately, the onset of the epidemic as a result of the human immunodeficiency virus (HIV), changes in immigration patterns, and increased transmission of *M. tuberculosis* in congregate settings in urban areas provoked the resurgence of tuberculosis in the United States from the mid-1980s to the mid-1990s. Worldwide, 10 million people

develop tuberculosis annually and one third of the world's population is infected with *M. tuberculosis.* The World Health Organization (WHO) has declared tuberculosis to be a "global health emergency," the first infectious disease to receive this designation (Kochi, 1991). To put it simply, in the mid 1990s there is more tuberculosis in the world than at any time in the history of mankind.

TERMINOLOGY

The pathophysiology of tuberculosis is complicated and the time delay between infection and disease makes certain events less distinct. Many experts now divide tuberculosis into three major stages: exposure, infection, and disease (Table 35-1).

Exposure means that the child has had significant contact with an adult or adolescent with suspected or proven infectious pulmonary tuberculosis. The contact investigation—examining those individuals close to a suspected case of tuberculosis with a tuberculin skin test, chest radiograph, and physical examination—is the most important activity to prevent cases of tuberculosis in children (Hsu, 1963). The most frequent setting for exposure of a child is the household, but it can occur in a school, day-care center, or other closed settings (Hoge et al., 1994; Lincoln, 1965). In the exposure stage the tuberculin skin test is negative, the chest radiograph is normal, and the child lacks signs or symptoms of disease. Because development of a reactive tuberculin skin test may take up to 3 months after the child has inhaled droplet nuclei infected with *M. tuberculosis,* some exposed children may be infected but no test can confirm it. Young children in the exposure stage usually are treated to prevent the rapid development of disseminated or meningeal tuberculosis, which can occur even before the skin test becomes reactive.

Infection occurs when the individual inhales droplet nuclei containing *M. tuberculosis,* which

Table 35-1   The stages of tuberculosis in children

	Stage		
	Exposure	Infection	Disease
Skin test	Negative	Positive	Positive (90%)
Physical exam	Normal	Normal	Usually abnormal*
Chest radiograph	Normal	Usually normal†	Usually abnormal‡
Treatment	If <5 years old	Always	Always
Number of drugs	One	One	Three or four

*Up to 50% of older children with pulmonary tuberculosis have a normal physical exam.
†Calcification or a small granuloma are considered infection, not disease.
‡Some children with extrapulmonary tuberculosis have a normal chest radiograph.

become established intracellularly within the lung and associated lymphoid tissue. The hallmark of tuberculosis infection is a reactive skin test. The child has no signs or symptoms of disease and the chest radiograph is either normal or reveals only calcifications or granuloma in the lung parenchyma and/or regional lymph nodes. In industrial countries all children with tuberculosis infection should receive treatment, usually with isoniazid, to prevent the development of tuberculosis disease in the near or distant future.

Disease occurs when signs or symptoms or radiographic manifestations caused by *M. tuberculosis* become apparent. Not all infected individuals have the same risk of developing disease. An immunocompetent adult with untreated tuberculosis infection has a 5% to 10% lifetime risk of developing disease. One half of the risk occurs in the first 2 to 3 years after infection. Adults with tuberculosis infection who become infected with HIV have a 5% to 10% annual risk of developing tuberculosis disease. Historic studies show that up to 40% of immunocompetent infants with untreated tuberculosis infection develop disease—often serious, life threatening forms—within 1 to 2 years.

ETIOLOGY

Mycobacterium tuberculosis, commonly referred to as the tubercle bacillus, is a member of the genus *Mycobacterium.* Mycobacteria are nonmotile, nonspore forming, pleomorphic, weakly gram-positive rods, 1 to 5 μm long, typically slender, and slightly bent. Some appear beaded and some are clumped under the microscope. The cell wall constituents of mycobacteria determine their most striking biologic properties. The cell walls contain 20% to 60% lipids, largely bound to proteins and carbohydrates. Their growth is slow with a generation time of 14 to 24 hours on solid media, perhaps because of the slow metabolic exchange through the waxy capsule. Their hydrophobic properties make them difficult to study.

Acid-fastness is the capacity to perform stable mycolate complexes with certain aryl methane dyes—specifically carbolfuchsin, crystal violet, auramine, and rhodamine—which are not removed readily even by rinsing with 90% ethanol plus hydrochloric acid. The cells appear red when stained with fuchsin (as with the Ziehl-Neelsen or Kinyoun stains), appear purple with crystal violet, or exhibit yellow-green fluorescence under ultraviolet light when stained with auramine and rhodamine, as in Truant stain. Truant stain is considered the best for specimens expected to contain small numbers of organisms.

Identification of various mycobacteria depends on their staining properties and their biochemical and metabolic characteristics. All mycobacteria are obligate aerobes. Their growth requirements are simple. Isolation of *M. tuberculosis* on solid media often takes 3 to 6 weeks followed by another 2 to 4 weeks for drug susceptibility testing. Identification of specific mycobacterial species often requires a complex set of biochemical tests. Recent improvements in laboratory methods now permit more rapid culture, identification, and drug susceptibility testing of mycobacteria by an automatic radiometric method known as *BACTEC,* in which a decontaminated, concentrated specimen is inoculated into a bottle of medium containing carbon 14–labeled palmitic acid as the substrate. As mycobacteria metabolize the labeled acid, carbon dioxide-14 accumulates in the bottle where radioactivity can be measured. The addition of appropriate dillusions of antituberculosis drugs permits the evaluation of drug susceptibility. The time for isolation and drug susceptibility testing of mycobacteria can be reduced to 1 to 3 weeks using the radiometric system.

The recent use of high-pressure liquid chromatography allows for rapid speciation of isolated organisms, usually within 24 hours.

EPIDEMIOLOGY
Incidence and Prevalence

The WHO estimates that during the 1990s there will be 90 million new cases of tuberculosis worldwide with 30 million deaths caused by the disease (Raviglione et al., 1995). About 13 million new cases and 5 million deaths will occur among children younger than 15 years of age. More than 40% of the world's population is infected with *M. tuberculosis.* Over the past decade the number of tuberculosis cases has increased in every region of the world except Western Europe. Without the development of a truly effective vaccine against tuberculosis, it is unlikely that the world's tuberculosis situation will improve in the near future.

The incidence and mortality attributable to tuberculosis in the United States declined steadily during the twentieth century until the year 1985, when the overall case rate was approximately 10 per 100,000, for a total of 22,201 new active cases. Unfortunately, a resurgence of the disease led to the recognition of 26,673 cases in 1992. Although total tuberculosis case numbers rose 20% in the United States from 1985 to 1992, the number of pediatric tuberculosis cases rose 40% (Cantwell et al., 1994; Starke et al., 1992). Most experts site four causes for these increases: (1) the coepidemic of HIV infection, because immunosuppression from HIV is the most potent risk factor for development of tuberculosis disease in a previously infected adult (Barnes et al., 1991; Selwyn et al., 1989; Whalen et al., 1995); (2) increasing rates of tuberculosis in foreign-born individuals in the United States caused by an increased number of infected individuals entering the country and more persons developing tuberculosis after arrival (McKenna et al., 1995); (3) increased transmission of *M. tuberculosis* in congregate settings, especially jails and prisons; nursing homes; homeless shelters; HIV treatment facilities; certain hospitals; and, rarely, schools (Alland et al., 1994; Bellin et al., 1993; Leggiadro et al., 1989; Small et al., 1994); and (4) a decline in the tuberculosis public health infrastructure in many regions and cities (Brudney and Dobkin, 1991). Fortunately, after much attention and increase in tuberculosis-related budgets, the number of tuberculosis cases in the United States declined again to 21,327 in 1996.

Decades ago, when tuberculosis was more prevalent in the United States, the risk of exposure

---

BOX 35-1

HIGH RISK GROUPS FOR TUBERCULOSIS IN NORTH AMERICA

Increased Risk of Infection

Foreign-born (or traveled) persons from high-prevalence countries

Users of illicit drugs

Residents of jails, prisons, long-term care facilities

Homeless persons

Health-care workers who care for high-risk patients

Children exposed to adults in high-risk groups (except health-care workers)

Increased Rate of Progression of Infection to Disease

Coinfection with HIV

Other immunocompromising diseases

Immunosuppressive therapies

Malnutrition

Age less than 4 years

---

to an adult with infectious tuberculosis was high and fairly uniform across the entire population. In most industrialized countries, tuberculosis rates are now highest in some fairly well-defined groups of high-risk persons (Box 35-1). Risk factors can be divided into those that increase the risk of initial infection with *M. tuberculosis* and those that increase the risk of progression from asymptomatic infection to disease. The risk factors for children becoming infected are usually defined by the risk factors of the adults in their environment for developing contagious tuberculosis. When obtaining a history about tuberculosis for a child, the clinician must delve into the risk factors of the adults in frequent contact with the child.

Among young adults in the United States, tuberculosis is predominantly a disease of racial and ethnic minorities. Although some studies have indicated that genetic factors may partly control an individual's susceptibility to tuberculosis infection and disease, extrinsic differences in socioeconomic status, nutrition, access to health care, and crowded living conditions undoubtedly contribute heavily to the increased tuberculosis case rates among minority groups. Approximately 85% of childhood tuberculosis cases in the United States occur among African-American, Hispanic, Asian and Native American children (Ussery et al., 1996).

In 1996 37% of persons with tuberculosis in the United States were foreign born. About 20% of tuberculosis cases in children less than 5 years of age and almost 50% of cases among adolescents occur among the foreign born. Children immigrating through established channels to the United States receive neither a chest radiograph nor a tuberculin skin test per normal immigration procedures (Lange et al., 1989). In several skin-testing programs in urban areas, between 60% and 90% of the positive tuberculin skin tests occur among foreign-born children (Barry et al., 1990). It is from this pool of infected children that many cases of tuberculosis among adults will arise in the future.

The recent epidemic of HIV infection has had a profound effect on the epidemiology of tuberculosis among children by two major mechanisms (Gutman et al., 1994): (1) HIV-infected adults with tuberculosis may transmit *M. tuberculosis* to children, some of whom will develop tuberculosis disease; and (2) children with HIV infection may be at increased risk of progressing from tuberculosis infection to disease (Hoffman et al., 1996). Several studies of childhood tuberculosis have demonstrated that increased case rates have been associated with a simultaneous increase among HIV-infected adults in the community (Jones et al., 1992). Relatively little is known about HIV-infected children because relatively few cases have been reported. In general, HIV-infected children may be more likely to have contact with HIV-infected adults who are at high risk for tuberculosis. Tuberculosis may be underdiagnosed among HIV-infected children because of the similarity of its clinical presentation to other opportunistic infections and AIDS-related conditions, and because of the difficulty in confirming the diagnosis with positive cultures. All children with tuberculosis disease should have HIV serotesting because the two infections are linked epidemiologically and recommended treatment for tuberculosis is prolonged for HIV-infected patients.

One of the most important factors determining whether tuberculosis infection will progress to disease is the age of the child. In the United States about 60% to 70% of pediatric cases occur in infants and children less than 5 years of age. The ages between 5 and 14 years have often been called the "favored age"; children of this age may develop infection but are much less likely to progress immediately to disease. The gender ratio for tuberculosis disease in children is usually about 1:1, but during adolescence there may be a female predominance. This is in contrast to tuberculosis in adults, where there is a 3:1 male predominance.

Although data on tuberculosis disease in children are readily available, information concerning the incidence and prevalence of tuberculosis infection without disease is lacking. Tuberculosis infection is a reportable condition in only five states, and national surveys were discontinued in 1971. Few other countries have any tuberculin skin test surveillance at all. However, the increased incidence of tuberculosis disease among children in the United States, the results of some skin tests surveys, and the influx of foreign-born children into the United States over the past decade indicate that the pool of infected children and young adults in the United States is probably growing.

Transmission

Transmission of *M. tuberculosis* is from person to person, usually by droplet nuclei that become airborne when the ill individual coughs, sneezes, laughs, sings, or even breathes heavily. These droplet nuclei may remain suspended in the air for hours, long after the infectious person has left the environment. Certain environmental factors such as poor air circulation can enhance transmission. Only particles less than 10 μm in diameter can reach alveoli and establish infection. Rarely, transmission can occur by direct contact with infected body fluids such as urine or purulent sinus tract drainage. Cases of tuberculosis transmitted via a lung transplant have been reported. Several patient-related factors are associated with an increased chance of transmission (Blumberg et al., 1995). The most important is a positive acid-fast smear of the sputum, which most closely correlates with the infectivity of the patient. Extensive epidemiologic studies have shown that children with primary tuberculosis rarely, if ever, infect other children or adults (Wallgren, 1937). Tubercle bacilli are relatively sparse in the endobronchial secretions of children with pulmonary tuberculosis, and significant cough is usually lacking. When young children with tuberculosis do cough, they rarely produce sputum, and they lack the tussive force necessary to suspend infectious particles of the correct size. Children with tuberculosis often have been cared for by their families or in hospitals and other institutions without infecting their contacts. When transmission of *M. tuberculosis* has been documented in children's hospitals, it almost invariably has come from an adult with undiagnosed pulmonary tuberculosis (Aznar et al., 1995; George et al., 1986; Weinstein et al., 1995).

Infectivity must be considered in several clinical situations in pediatrics. Adolescents with the reactivation form of pulmonary tuberculosis, having cavities or extensive infiltrates in the lungs, should be considered potentially infectious to others. The CDC has issued guidelines for when children and adolescents with tuberculosis should be considered potentially infectious (Centers for Disease Control, 1994). Within a hospital, a child or adolescent with suspected tuberculosis should be isolated if the chest radiograph shows a cavity or extensive infiltrate, if the child has a productive cough, or if a high-risk procedure such as bronchoscopy is being performed. Most experts feel that other children with tuberculosis do not need to be isolated, especially if the adults accompanying the child have received proper evaluation for infectious tuberculosis.

It is difficult to determine when a potentially infectious patient with pulmonary tuberculosis is no longer infectious after therapy has begun. The decision must be based on improvement in symptoms, decreased number of acid-fast bacilli in the sputum smear, initial chest radiograph findings, and adherence to treatment. Studies of transmission to animals and retrospective human epidemiology have indicated that most initially infectious patients become noninfectious within 2 weeks or less of starting treatment. However, occasional patients remain infectious from weeks to months after beginning ultimately effective treatment. Many investigations have shown that the vast majority of close contacts to infectious cases are infected before diagnosis and treatment, and that continued exposure to the case after diagnosis leads to little or no incremental risk of infection.

PATHOGENESIS
Initial Infection

The lung is the most common portal of entry for tubercle bacilli. If the bacilli are ingested, infection in the upper respiratory or intestinal tract may result. This was more common in previous decades when bovine tuberculosis, which can be transmitted in unpasteurized milk, was more frequent. Contamination of superficial skin or mucous membrane lesions—such as an abrasion of the sole of the foot or the elbow, an insect bite, or a ritual circumcision—may lead to infection. Infection by inoculation with a sputum-contaminated syringe has been reported. True congenital infection, although rare, occurs either when the mother suffers from lymphohematogenous spread during pregnancy or has smoldering endometritis.

At the site of entry the bacilli multiply and create an area of inflammatory exudate. The bacteria multiply most readily within nonsensitized alveolar macrophages. Almost as soon as the infection occurs, bacilli are carried through the local lymphatic system to the nearest group of lymph nodes that drain the area in which the focus is situated. When the portal of entry is the lung, the bronchopulmonary nodes—either hilar or mediastinal nodes—usually form the complex. Until delayed hypersensitivity develops, the area of infection may expand and remains unencapsulated. These events usually occur at the microscopic level; the patient has no signs or symptoms and the chest radiograph reveals no lesions. However, occasionally children experience low-grade fever and cough early in the infection, and the chest radiograph may show a localized, nonspecific infiltrate that resolves spontaneously. With the onset of delayed hypersensitivity, the microscopic infiltrate generally increases in size, the regional lymph nodes may enlarge, and the initial lesion may become caseous and walled-off. Many caseous lesions eventually calcify; most experts estimate at least 6 months are required for calcification to occur. Living tubercle bacilli persist within these walled-off foci for years, perhaps for the life of the individual.

The most common location for the initial infection is subpleural. It appears that virtually any part of the lung has an equal chance of receiving the initial infection. About 70% to 85% of initial infections are initiated by one focus. However, multiple foci are frequent in children.

Intrathoracic Tuberculosis

In most children the initial infection is walled off, clinical signs and symptoms and radiographic manifestations are absent, and the only manifestation of the initial infection is a reactive tuberculin skin test that develops after the onset of delayed hypersensitivity. The initial lymphadenitis cannot be detected clinically and rarely on the chest radiograph. However, in some children, particularly infants, the regional lymph nodes increase in size to the point where they cause partial or complete obstruction of the associated bronchus. Acid-fast studies of smears and sections of these enlarged lymph nodes have confirmed that the caseum has few tubercle bacilli; propensity for enlargement of lymph nodes is probably as much a result of the host's immune response as it is of the burden of organisms. At first, the lymph nodes may impinge on the bronchus, compressing it from outside and causing diffuse inflammation of its wall. Eventually, complete obstruction may occur, rarely as a result of external compression, but more often as a result of invasion of the bronchial wall by the caseous lesion, resulting in endobronchial tuberculosis. Other causes of obstruction include (1) damage to the bronchial cartilage that leads to gradual perforation of the bronchus, and (2) formation of plugs of toothpaste-like caseum that partially or completely occlude the bronchus.

There are three possible outcomes of bronchial obstruction. The first is sudden death by asphyxia, which, fortunately, is an extremely rare event. The second is obstructive hyperaeration of a lobar segment, an entire lobe, or even an entire lung. This reaction is most common in children younger than 2 years of age. In most cases the obstruction ultimately resolves by itself; however, treatment with corticosteroids and antituberculosis medications may hasten radiographic and clinical recovery. The third possible result is the appearance of a segmental lesion, often appearing fan-shaped on the radiograph, and almost always involving the segment occupied by the primary pulmonary focus. The radiographic opacity results from a combination of the primary pulmonary focus, the caseous material from an eroded bronchus, the inflammatory response elicited by the caseum, and atelectasis. In some cases, acute secondary bacterial infection plays a part. The younger the child is, the more common the segmental (also known as a *collapse-consolidation*) lesion is. This lesion is likely to form during the first 3 to 6 months after infection. Multiple segmental lesions can occur simultaneously; up to 25% of children with pulmonary tuberculosis have involvement of more than one lobe.

Other complications may be caused by enlarging thoracic lymph nodes, including stridor and respiratory distress (peritracheal nodes); difficulty swallowing (subcarinal nodes); and bronchoesophageal fistula (subcarinal nodes). Rarely, enlarging nodes may compress the subclavian vein, producing edema of hand and arm, or may erode into major blood vessels including the aorta. Finally, lymph nodes may rupture into the pericardial sac, resulting in pericardial tuberculosis.

Late results of bronchial obstruction include (Morrison, 1973): (1) complete reexpansion of the lung and resolution of the radiographic findings; (2) disappearance of the segmental lesion with residual calcification of the primary focus or regional lymph nodes; or (3) scarring and progressive contraction of the lobe or segment, often associated with bronchiectasis. Permanent anatomic sequelae result from untreated segmental lesions in about 60% of cases, even though the abnormality may not be apparent on radiographs. Stenosis of the bronchus and cylindrical bronchiectasis are most common. Fortunately, most of these abnormalities are asymptomatic in the upper lobes. However, secondary infection may occur in the middle and lower lobes, leading to progressive lung damage. Occasionally the chronic vascularity that accompanies bronchiectasis leads to poor oxygen saturation during exercise and to restricted body growth.

Calcification of the primary complex is common, particularly in untreated infection. Calcium usually is deposited as fine particles creating a stippled effect. However, it may be deposited in large, even enormous masses. Calcification may persist without change or may be reabsorbed within 5 years and eventually disappear completely.

Reactivation pulmonary tuberculosis is the type of disease seen in pulmonary tissue sensitized and immunized by an earlier tuberculosis infection. The source of this type of disease is organisms inhaled years or even decades earlier, that have remained dormant within the lung tissue and then become reactivated. Often the stimulus for reactivation (usually involving an insult to the immune system) can be identified, but sometimes there is no obvious predisposing etiology. This type of tuberculosis occurs most commonly in the superior segments of the upper lobes. The disease often arises from Assmann and Simon foci, which result from organisms that seeded the upper lobes during the lymphohematogenous spread at the time of initial infection.

Lymphohematogenous Spread

Tubercle bacilli from the lymphadenitis of the primary complex probably are disseminated during the incubation period in all cases of tuberculosis infection. The organisms reach the blood stream either directly from the initial focus or by way of the regional nodes and the thoracic duct. The sporadic dissemination ceases after delayed hypersensitivity develops. Many extrapulmonary lesions regress and heal completely, but some may progress immediately or remain quiescent but contain viable tubercle bacilli. There are three potential clinical outcomes from this dissemination:

1. The lymphohematogenous dissemination may be occult, in which case it produces no signs or symptoms. Again, this is the inciting

event for future cases of extrapulmonary tuberculosis and reactivation pulmonary tuberculosis in adolescents and adults.

2. Protracted hematogenous tuberculosis, rarely seen today, is characterized by high spiking fever; hepatomegaly and splenomegaly; and general glandular enlargement sometimes with repeated evidence of metastatic seeding of the eyes, kidney, and skin. Although this type of tuberculosis in past years often ended tragically in tuberculous meningitis, today it is completely treatable if diagnosed in time.

3. The third form of lymphohematogenous spread is miliary tuberculosis. This arises from a discharge of a caseous focus, often a lymph node, into a blood vessel such as a pulmonary vein. It may be self-propagating, with repeated discharge arising at various sites. It occurs most commonly during the first 2 to 6 months after infection in infancy but can also arise in older children or adults months to years after the initial infection.

RESISTANCE AND IMMUNITY

Natural resistance to tuberculosis infection varies greatly among animal species. The differences between resistant and susceptible animals appears to lie in the ability of the former to produce an effective immune response; this ability may be controlled genetically. Identical twins have shown some concordance in the propensity to develop tuberculosis disease after infection.

Young age appears to predispose to development of tuberculosis disease. However, it is possible that the apparent increased susceptibility is due to genetic factors or to a larger infecting dose of bacteria caused by the more intimate contact between the very young child and the adult source case. Many viral infections depress tuberculin reactivity, but only measles and perhaps influenza have been incriminated in lowering resistance to tuberculosis.

The exact mechanisms by which *M. tuberculosis* evades host defenses and persists are poorly understood. It appears that a state of intracellular parasitism is established by which the bacilli survive and grow within human cells. The means by which *M. tuberculosis* resists killing by macrophages has been studied extensively. Viable mycobacteria appear to prevent fusion of phagosomes with lysosomes that contain the toxic substances for killing ingested microbes.

Cell-mediated immunity is regarded as most important in host defense against *M. tuberculosis*

(Dannenberg, 1991). The T cell–mediated immune response involves a variety of cell subsets that are involved in numerous functions, including protection, delayed hypersensitivity, cytolysis, and establishing memory immunity. The functions also involve an array of cytokines, several of which direct cells of the monocyte-macrophage axis to contain and destroy the invading bacilli. The exact role of the individual cytokines is not clear, but an emerging concept is that much of the clinical response to the presence of *M. tuberculosis* is determined by the balance of the cellular-cytokine response, which, to some degree, is under genetic influence (Dannenberg, 1991; Orme et al., 1993). Factors that compromise cell-mediated immunity—such as HIV infection or therapy with corticosteroids or other immunosuppressing agents—often permit the spread or reactivation of infection leading to tuberculosis disease.

CLINICAL FORMS OF TUBERCULOSIS
Pulmonary

Primary. The primary complex includes three elements: the primary pulmonary focus, lymphangitis, and regional lymphadenitis. The hallmark of the initial disease is the relatively large size and importance of the adenitis compared with the relatively insignificant size of the initial focus in the lung. Because lymphatic drainage within the chest occurs predominately from left to right, the nodes in the right upper paratracheal area appear to be the ones most often affected.

Although interpretation of the size of intrathoracic lymph nodes in radiographs can be difficult, they are usually readily apparent when there is adenopathy resulting from tuberculosis (Fig. 35-1) (Delacourt et al., 1993). As the lymph nodes continue to enlarge, partial obstruction of the regional bronchus may lead to hyperinflation and, eventually, to atelectasis (Daly et al., 1952). Fig. 35-2 shows an early segmental lesion with hilar adenopathy and atelectasis and, possibly, some infiltrate. The radiographic findings in this type of disease are similar to those caused by aspiration of a foreign body; in essence, the lymph node is acting as the foreign body. Segmental atelectasis and hyperinflation lesions may occur together.

Other radiographic findings occur in some patients (Pineda et al., 1993; Schaaf et al., 1995; Stransberry, 1990). Occasionally children have a picture of lobar pneumonia without adenopathy being readily apparent. In smaller children the radiographic appearance can be that of exudative pneu-

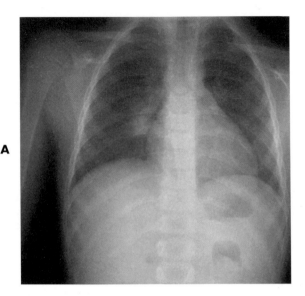

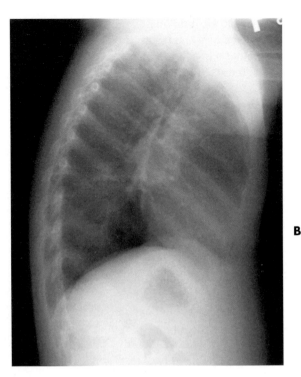

FIG. 35-1   A posteroanterior (**A**) and lateral (**B**) chest radiograph of a child with hilar adenopathy caused by *Mycobacterium tuberculosis.*

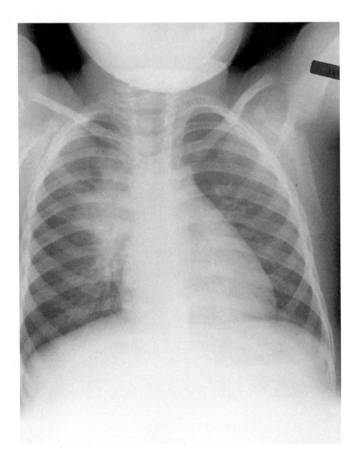

FIG. 35-2   Hilar and mediastinal adenopathy, and a partial segmental lesion in a child with tuberculosis.

monia with bowing of the fissure (Fig. 35-3). The radiographic picture is similar to that seen with pyogenic pneumonia, particularly when caused by *Klebsiella pneumoniae.* Indeed, secondary bacterial infection of tuberculosis may contribute to this appearance.

The symptoms and physical signs of pulmonary tuberculosis in children are surprisingly meager considering the degree of radiographic changes often seen; the roentgenogram is sicker than the patient (Lincoln et al., 1958). The physical manifestations of disease tend to differ by the age of onset. Young infants and adolescents are more likely to have significant signs or symptoms, whereas school-age children usually have clinically silent disease (Schaaf et al., 1993; Vallejo et al., 1994).

About one half of infants and children with radiographically moderate to severe pulmonary tuberculosis have no physical findings and are discovered only via contact tracing of an adult with suspected tuberculosis. Infants are more likely to experience signs and symptoms because of their small airway diameters relative to the parenchymal lymph node changes. Nonproductive cough and mild dyspnea are the most common symptoms. Systemic complaints such as fever, night sweats, anorexia, and de-

creased activity occur less often. Some infants have difficulty gaining weight or develop a true failure-to-thrive presentation. Pulmonary signs are even less common. Some infants and young children with bronchial obstruction show signs of air trapping, such as localized wheezing or decreased breath sounds that may be accompanied by tachypnea or frank respiratory distress. Occasionally these nonspecific symptoms and signs are alleviated by antibiotics, suggesting that bacterial superinfection distal to the focus of tuberculous bronchial obstruction has contributed to the clinical presentation of disease.

Progressive. Progressive pulmonary tuberculosis is a serious complication of the primary complex in which the original pulmonary focus, instead of resolving or calcifying, enlarges steadily and develops a large caseous center. The center then liquifies and empties into an adjacent bronchus, creating a primary cavity (Harris et al., 1977; Teeratkulpisarn et al., 1994). This liquefaction is associated with particularly large numbers of tubercle bacilli, and this may be the young child who is capable of transmitting *M. tuberculosis* to other individuals. Further dissemination of tubercle bacilli to other parts of the

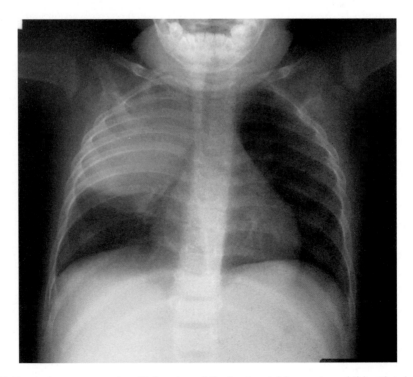

FIG. 35-3   Lobar pneumonia with bowing of the horizontal fissure in a child with tuberculosis. Many of this child's initial symptoms improved after several days of cefuroxime therapy, implying that a secondary bacterial pneumonia may have been present.

lobe and to the entire lung may occur. On rare occasions, an enlarging primary focus ruptures into the pleural cavity, creating a pneumothorax, bronchopleural fistula, or caseous pyopneumothorax, or into the pericardial sac or mediastinum.

The radiographic and clinical picture of progressive primary tuberculosis is that of bronchial pneumonia with high fever, moderate to severe cough, night sweats, dullness to percussion, rales, and decreased breath sounds. Before chemotherapy the inability to contain the primary focus was associated with a grave outlook; up to 65% of patients died. With appropriate treatment the prognosis is excellent. It may be difficult to distinguish between progressive pulmonary tuberculosis and a simple tuberculous focus with a superimposed acute bacterial pneumonia. Antimicrobial agents effective against common pathogens such as *Staphylococcus* spp., *Klebsiella* spp., and anaerobes may be indicated in addition to appropriate antituberculosis drugs. During convalescence from pulmonary tuberculosis, bullous lesions may develop and persist for several months (Matsaniotis et al., 1967). These lesions may be due to bacterial superinfection or to the tuberculosis itself.

Chronic (Reactivation). Even before the discovery of antituberculosis drugs, chronic pulmonary tuberculosis was rare in children. It appears more frequently among children in the lower socioeconomic strata of society, in girls more than boys, and when there is significant delay in diagnosis. It has been noted that children who survive with a healed, untreated tuberculosis infection acquired before 2 years of age rarely develop chronic pulmonary tuberculosis, but it is a much more frequent complication among children who acquire their initial infection near puberty. In some children, progressive pulmonary tuberculosis cannot be differentiated from chronic tuberculosis unless the approximate date of acquiring the infection is known.

Chronic pulmonary tuberculosis is more common in adolescents than younger children (Lincoln et al., 1960). The radiographic features are typical of those seen in adults—mostly upper lobe infiltrates and, eventually, cavitation (Fig. 35-4). Children and adolescents with this type of disease are more likely to experience fever, anorexia, malaise, weight loss, night sweats, productive cough, chest pain, and hemoptysis than children with primary pulmonary tuberculosis. However, findings on physical examination are usually minor or absent

even when cavities or large infiltrates are present. Most signs and symptoms improve within several weeks of starting effective treatment, although cough may last for several months. This form of disease usually remains localized in the lungs because the presensitization of tissue to tuberculin evokes an immune response that prevents further hematogenous spread.

Pleural

Pleural effusion caused by tuberculosis can be localized or generalized, unilateral or bilateral. Localized pleural effusion so frequently accompanies the primary pulmonary focus that it is practically a component of the primary complex. All tuberculous effusions probably originate as a discharge of bacilli into the pleural space from an adjacent lesion, often a subpleural pulmonary focus. The breakthrough may be small and the pleuritis localized and asymptomatic, or it may occur in the form of a generalized effusion, usually 3 to 6 months after infection (Fig. 35-5). Effusions are bilateral in only 5% of cases and probably arise from bilateral primary infections. Tuberculous pleural effusion is rare in children younger than 2 years of age and uncommon in children younger than 5 years of age. It is more common in boys than in girls but is almost never associated with a segmental lesion.

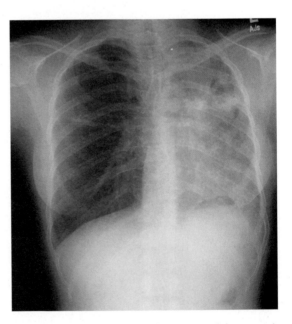

FIG. 35-4 Severe tuberculosis caused by a multidrug resistant strain of *M. tuberculosis* in a 15-year-old from Nigeria. There is evidence of early bronchogenic spread from the left to right side.

The onset of pleurisy usually is abrupt, resembling bacterial pneumonia with fever; chest pain; shortness of breath; and, on physical examination, dullness to percussion and diminished breath sounds (Lincoln et al., 1958). Fever may be high and, in untreated cases, last for several weeks.

Thoracentesis is the essential diagnostic procedure. The puncture should be made in the area shown on the radiograph to have the greatest fluid accumulation. The fluid is often a greenish yellow color, occasionally blood-tinged, with a high protein count and often a low glucose level. There are usually several hundred white cells per mm^3, with a predominance of leukocytes or lymphocytes, depending on the age of the effusion. Tubercle bacilli usually are present in such small numbers that results from direct smears and cultures are disappointing; smears are almost always negative and pleural fluid cultures are positive in less than 30% of cases. Pleural punch biopsy is a useful diagnostic procedure because the finding of either the typical tubercles on histologic study or culture of the tiny plug from the trocar is more likely to establish the diagnosis. The prognosis for children with tuberculous effusion is generally excellent. Rarely, permanent impairment of pulmonary function occurs secondary to the development of scoliosis.

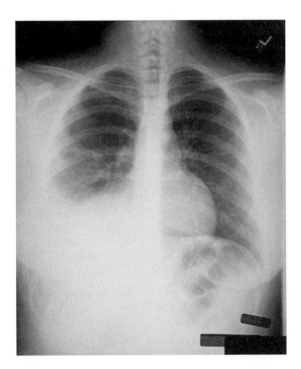

FIG. 35-5 Tuberculous pleural effusion in a teenage girl. The pleural biopsy had caseating granulomas.

Pericardial

Tuberculous pericarditis complicates only 0.4% of untreated tuberculosis infections in children. It usually arises by direct invasion or lymphatic drainage from caseous subcarinal nodes, with resulting exudation of hemorrhagic fluids and development of granulation tissue on the visceral and parietal surfaces of the pericardium. The pericardial fluid may be serofibrinous (forming strands upon standing, which may also be seen by echocardiography) or hemorrhagic. However, direct acid-fast smear is usually negative. Extensive fibrosis may led to obliteration of the pericardial space, with resulting constrictive pericarditis.

The presenting symptoms usually are nonspecific: low-grade fever; malaise; anorexia; and, more rarely, chest pain (Hugo-Hamman et al., 1994). A pericardial friction rub may be heard or—if a large effusion is present—tachycardia, distant heart sounds, and a narrow pulse pressure may suggest the diagnosis. The diagnosis is confirmed by radiography; echocardiography; the tuberculin skin test; aspiration of fluid for culture; and, when necessary, biopsy of the pericardium. With appropriate chemotherapy and possibly use of corticosteroids to acutely reduce the size of the effusion, as well as occasional pericardectomy, the prognosis is very good.

Lymphohematogenous

The initial lymphohematogenous spread of tubercle bacilli during the primary infection is usually asymptomatic. Rarely patients experience protracted hematogenous tuberculosis caused by intermittent release of tubercle bacilli as a caseous focus erodes through the wall of a blood vessel. Although the clinical picture may be acute, it is usually indolent and prolonged, with spiking fever accompanying the release of organisms. Multiple organ involvement is common, often leading to hepatosplenomegaly, lymphadenitis in superficial or deep nodes, or papulonecrotic tuberculids appearing in crops on the skin. Other organs are involved less commonly. Meningitis, which occurs only late in the course of the disease, may be the cause of death when the disease goes untreated. Early pulmonary involvement is surprisingly mild, but diffuse lung involvement becomes apparent if treatment is not provided promptly.

The most common clinically significant form of disseminated tuberculosis is miliary disease, which occurs when massive numbers of tubercle bacilli are released into the bloodstream, causing disease in two or more organs. This type of disease usually occurs within 2 to 6 months of the primary infection. Although this form of disease is most common in infants and young children, it is also found in older adults as a result of the breakdown of a previously healed or calcified pulmonary lesion that formed years earlier.

The clinical manifestations of miliary tuberculosis are protean and depend on the load of organisms that disseminate and where they lodge (Schuit, 1979). Tissues have different susceptibility to infection; lesions are usually larger and more numerous in the lungs, spleen, liver, and bone marrow than other organs.

The onset of clinical miliary disease is sometimes explosive, with the patient becoming gravely ill in several days. More often the onset is insidious (Hussey et al., 1991). The patient may not be able to pinpoint the exact time of initial symptoms accurately. Early systemic signs include malaise, anorexia, weight loss, and low-grade fever. At this time, abnormal physical signs are usually absent. Within several weeks, hepatosplenomegaly and generalized lymphadenopathy develop in about one half of cases. About this time the fever may become higher and more sustained, although the chest radiograph usually is normal and respiratory symptoms are rare (Optican et al., 1992). Within several more weeks, the lungs become filled with tubercles, and dyspnea, cough, rales, or wheezing occur. As the pulmonary disease progresses, alveolar-

air block syndrome may result in frank respiratory distress, hypoxia, pneumothorax, or pneumomediastinum. Signs and symptoms of meningitis are found in only 20% to 40% of patients with advanced disease. Chronic or recurrent headache in a patient with miliary tuberculosis usually indicates the presence of meningitis, whereas the onset of abdominal pain or tenderness is usually a sign of tuberculous peritonitis. Cutaneous lesions such as tuberculids, nodules, or purpura may appear in crops. Up to 75% of patients develop choroid tubercles, which are highly specific for miliary tuberculosis.

The diagnosis of miliary tuberculosis is usually established by finding a consistent clinical picture and the typical chest radiograph findings of millet seed–like lesions (Fig. 35-6). The tuberculin skin test is nonreactive in up to 50% of patients. Culture confirmation of disease can be extremely difficult and may require a liver, lung, bone marrow, or skin biopsy. In some cases, *M. tuberculosis* can be isolated from sputum, gastric aspirate, or urine.

Central Nervous System

Tubercle bacilli distribute into all parts of the central nervous system (CNS) during lymphohematogenous spread. They do not multiply as well in nervous tissue as in some other tissues. Tuberculous meningitis rises from caseous foci, often very small ones, situated in the brain or meninges. The caseous foci discharge bacilli directly into the sub-

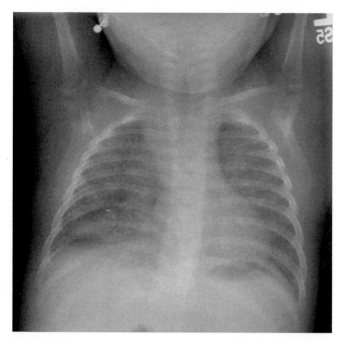

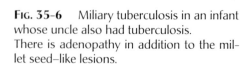

FIG. 35-6   Miliary tuberculosis in an infant whose uncle also had tuberculosis.
There is adenopathy in addition to the millet seed–like lesions.

arachnoid space, resulting in a thick gelatinous exudate that lies in the meshes of the pia-arachnoid, where it infiltrates the walls of meningeal arteries and veins. Inflammation, caseation, and obstruction are produced and extend along small vessels into the cortex, occluding blood vessels and producing infarcts (Leiguarda et al., 1988). The same exudate interferes with the normal flow of the cerebrospinal fluid (CSF) in and out of the ventricular system (Palur et al., 1991). The predilection of the exudate for the base of the brain accounts for the frequent involvement of the third, sixth, and seventh cranial nerves and the optic chiasm. The combination of vascular lesions producing infarcts, interference with cerebrospinal fluid flow resulting in hydrocephalus, and direct cranial nerve involvement cause the devastating damage that all too often results from tuberculous meningitis. Profound abnormalities in electrolyte metabolism, especially hyponatremia, also contribute to the pathophysiology. The syndrome of inappropriate antidiuretic hormone secretion is common and may last for weeks after appropriate therapy is started. Salt wasting may make correction of the electrolyte disturbances difficult.

Tuberculous meningitis complicates about 0.3% of untreated tuberculosis infections in children. Meningitis is extremely rare in infants less than 4 months of age because pathologic events usually need this time to develop. It is most common in children between 6 months and 4 years of age. Because tuberculous meningitis is an early manifestation of the initial infection, occurring within 2 to 6 months after infection, the adult whom the child got the infection from usually can be identified (Doerr et al., 1995).

Although the onset of tuberculous meningitis may be explosive, it is more often gradual, occurring over a period of several weeks (Curless and Mitchell, 1991; Waeker and Connor, 1990). Rapid progression tends to occur more often in infants and small children, who may experience symptoms for only several days before the onset of acute hydrocephalus, seizures, or cerebral edema. The disease is often divided into three stages. The first stage, which typically lasts 1 to 2 weeks, is characterized by nonspecific symptoms such as fever, headache, irritability, drowsiness, and malaise. Focal neurologic signs are absent, but infants may experience a stagnation or loss of developmental milestones. The second stage usually begins abruptly and includes lethargy, nuchal rigidity and Kernig's or Brudzinski's signs, seizures, hyperto-

nia, vomiting, cranial nerve palsies, or other focal neurologic signs. Although some children have no evidence of meningeal irritation at this time, they may have signs of encephalitis such as disorientation, abnormal movements, or speech impairment. The third stage is marked by coma; hemiplegia or paraplegia; hypotension; posturing; deterioration in vital signs; and, eventually, death. Papilledema is noted only late in the clinical course.

One important aid in diagnosis is a history of contact with an adult with tuberculosis; however, the family history for tuberculosis often is falsely negative because the incubation period of meningitis is short and the contagious adult has not yet been discovered (Doerr et al., 1995). The tuberculin skin test is positive in only 50% of cases of tuberculous meningitis. The chest radiograph is often abnormal in children with tuberculous meningitis and reveals changes typical of primary tuberculosis. The most important laboratory test is the evaluation of the CSF. The lumbar spinal fluid usually is clear but under substantially increased pressure. It contains 50 to 500 WBC/mm^3, with polymorphonuclear leukocytes predominant early and lymphocytes predominant later. The spinal fluid glucose level may be at the lower limits of normal if the patient is examined early in the course, but by the third stage the levels are low. The protein content may be normal at the time of the first spinal tap but rises steadily to very high concentrations. Acid-fast stain of the pellicle of the CSF can be helpful but is positive in less than 10% of cases. Unfortunately, *M. tuberculosis* can be isolated from the CSF in only 50% of cases of tuberculous meningitis in children. Results of culture are more likely to be positive if a larger volume of fluid is obtained. Often the culture confirmation comes from other clinical samples, especially gastric washings in a child who also has pulmonary tuberculosis. Computed tomography (CT) (Wallace et al., 1991) or magnetic resonance imaging (MRI) (Offenbacher et al., 1991) of the brain of patients with tuberculous meningitis may be normal during early stages of disease. With progression, basilar enhancement and communicating hydrocephalus with signs of cerebral edema or early focal ischemia is the most common finding. The findings of basilar meningitis, hydrocephalus, or infarct accompanying clinical meningitis in a child should immediately raise the question of tuberculosis as the cause of the meningitis. In most cases, empiric therapy for tuberculosis should be started while further epidemiologic and laboratory investigations are undertaken.

The prognosis of tuberculous meningitis correlates most closely with the clinical stage at the time chemotherapy has started (Humphries et al., 1990). The vast majority of patients in the first stage have an excellent outcome, whereas most patients in the third stage who survive have permanent disabilities including blindness, deafness, paraplegia, diabetes insipidus, or mental retardation. The prognosis for young infants is also worse.

Tuberculoma is manifested clinically as a brain tumor (Fig. 35-7). Tuberculomas account for up to 40% of brain tumors in some areas of the world but are rare in North America. Tuberculomas are more common in children less than 10 years of age. They are usually singular but may be multiple. In adults, lesions are most often supratentorial, but in children they are often infratentorial, located at the base of the brain near the cerebellum. A well-recognized phenomenon is the development of symptomatic intracranial tuberculomas when the child is undergoing therapy for meningeal, miliary, or even pulmonary tuberculosis (Doerr et al., 1995; Shepard et al., 1986; Teoh et al., 1987). This phenomenon appears to be mediated immunologically; it usually responds to corticosteroids and does not necessitate a change in antituberculosis chemotherapy. CT or

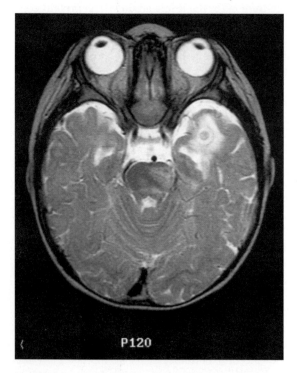

Fig. 35-7   A magnetic resonance image of tuberuloma in a child with culture-positive tuberculous meningitis. The child presented with fever, altered mental status, and hemiparesis.

MRI of the head should be obtained when neurologic signs or symptoms accompany any form of tuberculosis. The most common signs or symptoms accompanying tuberculomas are headaches, convulsions, fever, and other signs and symptoms usually associated with brain abscess or tumor. A tuberculin skin test is usually positive but the chest radiograph is often normal, since the tuberculoma has developed some time after the initial infection. The major determinant of the specific signs and symptoms is the anatomic location of the tuberculoma.

Cutaneous

Cutaneous tuberculosis, which was more common decades ago, arises as an extension of disease from the primary focus, from hematogenous dissemination, or from hypersensitivity to the tubercle bacillus. Skin lesions associated with the primary complex may be caused by direct inoculation of bacilli into a traumatized area such as a lesion on the sole of the child's foot or an insect bite. The initial skin focus usually is a small, painless nodule with tiny satellite lesions that turn into indolent ulcers without surrounding information. The most striking feature is regional lymphadenitis, which is what often convinces the patient to see a physician. Fever and other systemic reactions are minimal. A strongly positive tuberculin skin test usually is present. Scrofuloderma represents tuberculosis of the skin overlying a caseous lymph node—most often in the cervical area—that has ruptured to the outside, leaving either a shallow ulcer or a deep sinus tract, sometimes surrounded by nodules.

Manifestations that arise from hematogenous dissemination are papulonecrotic tuberculids and tuberculosis verrucosa cutis. Tuberculids are miliary tubercles in the skin that usually appear as tiny papules with "apple-jelly" centers, most commonly on the trunk, thighs, and face. They are similar to papular urticaria or early varicella lesions. Lupus vulgaris is a rare form of chronic indulent tuberculosis on the face that often seems to evolve from tuberculids. Tuberculosis verrucosa cutis is a condition characterized by a large skin lesion, which usually appears on the arms, legs, or buttocks, suggesting that trauma may play some part in its causation. The lesions often have a warty appearance but there is no associated regional lymphadenitis. Biopsy and culture of the lesions are often required for correct diagnosis.

Erythema nodosum is a hypersensitivity manifestation of tuberculosis. It occurs most often in young teenage girls. It usually begins with fever and systemic toxicity soon after the initial infection and is characterized by large, deep, and painful indurated nodules on the shins and sometimes on the thighs, elbows, and forearms. The nodules gradually change from a light pink to a bruiselike color. Tuberculin hypersensitivity is pronounced in children with tuberculosis underlying erythema nodosum, and tuberculin skin testing should be performed with extreme caution.

Skeletal

Skeletal tuberculosis usually results from lymphohematogenous seeding of bacilli during the primary infection. The disease also might originate as the result of direct extension from a caseous regional lymph node or by extension from a neighboring infected bone. The time interval between infection and disease can be as short as 1 month in cases of tuberculosis dactylitis, or several years or longer for tuberculosis of the hip. The infection usually begins in the metaphysis of the bone. Granulation tissue and caseation—which destroy bone both by direct infection and pressure necrosis—are common. Soft tissue abscess and extension of the infection through the epiphysis into the nearby joint often complicate bone infection. The infection frequently becomes apparent clinically only after joint involvement progresses.

Weight-bearing bones and joints are affected most commonly by tuberculosis (Bavadekan, 1982; Haygood and Williamson, 1994). Most cases occur in the vertebrae, causing tuberculosis of the spine or Pott's disease. Although any vertebral body can be involved, there is a predilection for the lower thoracic and upper lumbar vertebrae. Involvement of two or more vertebrae is common; these vertebrae are usually contiguous but there may be skip areas between the lesions. The infection is in the body of the vertebra, leading to bone destruction and collapse. Tuberculous spondylitis progresses from initial narrowing of one or more disk spaces to collapse and wedging of the vertebral body, with subsequent angulation of the spine causing either gibbus or kyphosis. The infection usually extends out from the bone causing a paraspinal (Pott's), psoas, or retropharyngeal abscess.

The most common clinical signs and symptoms of Pott's disease in children are low-grade fever, irritability, and restlessness especially at night; back pain without significant tenderness; and abnormal positioning and gait or refusal to walk. Spinal rigidity may be caused by profound muscle spasm, which results from the patient's involuntary effort to immobilize the spine. Neurologic complications most often arise from cervical and lumbar vertebral

lesions and comprise various degrees of neuroplegia, paraplegia, or quadriplegia. The complications are caused by inflammation of the spinal cord secondary to a neighboring cold abscess, caseum, or granuloma in the extradural area, or by spinal vessel thrombosis. Although surgery for spinal tuberculosis was long considered an important adjunct to therapy, most cases are now treated primarily with chemotherapy, surgery being undertaken only if stabilization of the spine is necessary. A surgical procedure may be necessary to obtain clinical material and establish the diagnosis by culture.

Other sites of skeletal tuberculosis, in approximate order of frequency, are the knee, hip, elbow, and ankle. The involvement can range from joint effusion without bone destruction to frank destruction of bone and restriction of the joint caused by chronic fibrosis of the synovial membrane (Vallejo et al., 1994). This more severe type of bone tuberculosis, which usually evolves over months or years, most commonly causes mild pain, stiffness, limp, and restricted joint motion. With tuberculosis of the hip, if the disease is limited at the time of discovery to the acetabulum or the head of the femur, good mobility of the joint usually can be preserved by effective chemotherapy.

The diagnosis of skeletal tuberculosis should be considered in any child who is known to be infected with *M. tuberculosis* and in whom a bone or joint lesion develops, and in any child with a persistent, unexplained bone or joint lesion. The tuberculin skin test is positive in up to 90% of cases. Culture of the joint fluid or bone biopsy usually yields the organism; synovial biopsy often reveals granulomas.

Superficial Lymph Nodes

Tuberculosis of the superficial lymph nodes, often referred to as *scrofula,* is the most common form of extrapulmonary tuberculosis in children (Dandapat et al., 1990). Historically, scrofula was often caused by drinking unpasteurized cow's milk laden with *Mycobacterium bovis.* Most current cases occur within 6 to 9 months of the initial infection with *M. tuberculosis,* although some cases appear years later. The tonsillar, anterior cervical, and submandibular nodes become involved secondary to extension of the initial lesion from the upper lung field or abdomen. Infected nodes in the inguinal, epitrochlear, or axillary regions result from regional lymphadenitis associated with tuberculosis of the skin or skeletal system.

In the early stages the nodes enlarge gradually. The nodes are firm but not hard, discrete, and nontender. They often feel fixed to underlying or overlying tissues. Disease is most often unilateral, but bilateral involvement may occur because of crossover drainage patterns of lymphatic vessels in the chest and lower neck. As infection progresses, multiple nodes are affected, often resulting in a mass of matted nodes. Systemic signs and symptoms other than low-grade fever are usually absent. The tuberculin skin test is usually reactive. Although a primary pulmonary focus is virtually always present, it is visible radiographically in less than 50% of cases. Occasionally the onset of illness is more acute with rapid enlargement of nodes, high fever, tenderness, and fluctuance simulating pyogenic adenitis. The initial presentation is rarely a fluctuant mass with overlying cellulitis or skin discoloration.

If left untreated, lymph node tuberculosis may resolve, but more often it progresses to caseation and necrosis of the lymph node. The capsule of the node breaks down, resulting in the spread of infection to adjacent nodes and other structures. Rupture results in a draining sinus tract that may require surgical removal.

Infection with pyogenic bacteria may enhance mycobacterial adenitis; it is frequently wise to begin conventional antibacterial therapy while awaiting the results of the tuberculin skin test and other diagnostic maneuvers. Surgical excision of nodes infected with *M. tuberculosis* is usually not necessary; however, since distinguishing between tuberculosis and adenitis caused by nontuberculous mycobacteria can be difficult, and the treatment of choice for lymph node disease caused by other mycobacteria is complete excision of the nodes, surgical procedures may be undertaken for tuberculous adenitis (Schuit and Powell, 1978). Even with complete surgical removal of the lymph node, however, tuberculous lymphadenitis requires chemotherapy because it is just one part of a systemic infection.

Eye and Ear

Ocular tuberculosis is uncommon in children. When it does occur, the conjunctiva and cornea are the areas most often involved. Unilateral redness and lacrimation are usually associated with the enlargement of the preauricular, submandibular, or cervical lymph nodes. Tuberculosis of the ciliar body, iris, and tuberculosis uveitis are exceedingly rare in children. These forms of tuberculosis are very hard to diagnose because there is no material available for culture, the chest radiograph is usually normal, and the adult source of infection often cannot be traced.

Tuberculosis of the middle ear is a relatively rare manifestation (MacAdam and Rubio, 1977). It occurs as a primary focus in the area of the eustachian tube in neonates who have aspirated infected amniotic fluid or older infants who have ingested tuberculous material (Mumtaz et al., 1983). It can occur as a metastatic lesion in older children who have a primary focus elsewhere. Otorrhea is common and painless and may become foul smelling because of the bacterial contamination with enteric organisms. The disease is almost always unilateral. Older patients may complain of tinnitus and "funny noises." The eardrum often is damaged extensively. A large central perforation or several smaller perforations are characteristic. Diagnosis can be difficult for two reasons: (1) stains and cultures are frequently negative, and (2) histology of the affected tissue often shows acute and chronic inflammation without granuloma formation.

Abdominal

Abdominal tuberculosis may occur after ingestion of tubercle bacili or as part of generalized lymphohematogenous spread (Bhansali, 1977). Tuberculous enteritis always has been uncommon. Tubercle bacilli penetrate the gut wall via the Peyer's patches or the appendix, giving rise to local ulcers followed by mesenteric lymphadenitis and sometimes peritonitis. Occasionally in older children, tuberculosis enteritis accompanies extensive pulmonary cavitation as a result of the swallowing of infected secretions. Symptoms and signs include vague abdominal pain, blood in the stools, and sinus formation after a seemingly routine appendectomy. Tuberculous enteritis should be suspected in any child with chronic gastrointestinal complaints and a reactive tuberculin skin test. Biopsy, stain, and culture of the lesions are often necessary to confirm the diagnosis.

Tuberculous peritonitis, which occurs most often in young men, is uncommon in adolescents and rare in young children (Chavalittamvong and Talalak, 1982). It arises from direct extension of a primary intestinal focus or from a tuberculous salpingitis. Generalized peritonitis may result from subclinical or miliary hematogenous dissemination. Initially pain and tenderness are often mild. Rarely the lymph nodes, omentum, and peritoneum become matted in children; they can be palpated as a doughy, irregular, nontender mass. Ascites and low-grade fever occur commonly. The tuberculin skin test is usually reactive. The diagnosis usually can be confirmed by paracentesis with appropriate stains and cultures, but this procedure must be performed extremely carefully to avoid bowel intertwined with the matted omentum. Laparoscopy with fine-needle aspiration also may be helpful.

Renal

Renal tuberculosis is an uncommon complication of pulmonary tuberculosis in children, rarely occurring in less than 4 or 5 years after the initial infection (Smith and Lattimer, 1973). However, tubercle bacilli can be recovered from the urine in many cases of miliary tuberculosis and some cases of pulmonary tuberculosis in young children (Ehrlich, 1971). Hematogenous dissemination can give rise to tubercles in the glomeruli, with resultant caseating, sloughing lesions that discharge tubercle bacilli into the tubules. Occasionally, in the zone between the renal pyramid and cortex, an encapsulated caseous mass develops that calcifies or discharges into the pelvis of the kidney, forming a cavity quite analogous to a pulmonary cavity. Infection can be unilateral or bilateral and can spread downward to involve the bladder. Frequently dysuria, hematuria, and sterile pyuria are the presenting findings in the urine. They may occur grossly but usually not until late in the course of disease that has strikingly few specific symptoms. Appropriate examination and culture of early morning urine specimens usually reveal tubercle bacilli. A tuberculin skin test is positive in most cases. It should be remembered that urine from patients with renal tuberculosis may be highly infectious and such children should be isolated until their urine is sterile.

Genitourinary

Tuberculosis of the genital tract is rare in both males and females before puberty. The condition originates from lymphohematogenous spread, although it can complicate direct spread from the intestinal tract or bone. Sexual transmission of *M. tuberculosis* has been postulated but never proven. Genital tuberculosis is a particular hazard for adolescent girls with tuberculosis infection. The fallopian tubes are most often involved, followed in incidence by the endometrium, ovaries, and cervix. The usual symptoms are lower abdominal pain and dysmenorrhea or amenorrhea. Systemic manifestations are often absent, and the chest radiograph is normal in the majority of cases. However, some patients have accompanying pulmonary or pleural tuberculosis. Chronic genital tract infection in women leads to infertility.

Genital tuberculosis in adolescent males can cause epididymitis or orchitis. This condition occurs as a unilateral nodular, painless swelling of the scrotum. Involvement of the glans penis is extremely rare.

Perinatal

Transmission of tuberculosis infection from mother to infant via the placenta or amniotic fluid has been reported in only about 300 patients. Perinatal tuberculosis can be acquired by the infant via one of several routes. First, transplacental spread via the umbilical vein from a mother with primary hematogenous tuberculosis may occur at the end stages of pregnancy, resulting in true congenital tuberculosis. In these infants the primary infection often is in the liver, although the liver may be bypassed, with the primary infection occurring in the lung. Second, aspiration in utero of amniotic fluid infected from endometritis in the mother or from the placenta occurs rarely; this is also a form of true congenital tuberculosis. Third, the infant may ingest infected amniotic fluid or secretions during delivery. Finally, the most common mode of transmission to newborns is inhalation of tubercle bacilli at or soon after birth that originated from the mother or other relatives with infectious pulmonary tuberculosis. It is not always possible to be sure of the type of infection in a particular neonate since only clear-cut evidence of a primary infection in the liver establishes a definite diagnosis of true congenital tuberculosis. However, the presence of early forms of tuberculosis or documentation of endometrial tuberculosis in the mother after delivery is strong evidence of congenital tuberculosis in the infant. When an infant is suspected of having congenital tuberculosis, endometrial biopsy of the mother is an integral part of the evaluation (Vallejo and Starke, 1992).

Diagnosis of perinatal tuberculosis is usually difficult and often delayed. At least one half of the reported cases have been diagnosed only at autopsy of the baby. Disease in the mother is often overlooked; the mother may have nonspecific symptoms of pulmonary infection or lingering endometritis that are not recognized to be due to tuberculosis. The early symptoms and signs in the neonate also may be overlooked and may be similar to those caused by other congenital infections. Once the diagnosis is suspected, treatment should be started immediately and diagnostic procedures carried out as rapidly and as aggressively as possible. Tuberculosis in the neonate should be suspected when signs and symptoms consistent with it are present and other causes, especially other congenital infections, have been ruled out.

The clinical manifestations of perinatal tuberculosis vary according to the size of the infecting dose of bacilli, as well as the site and size of the caseous lesions (Hageman et al., 1980; Nemir and O'Hare, 1985). Symptoms usually appear during the second week of life and include loss of appetite and failure to gain weight, fever, nasal or ear discharge, cough, bronchopneumonia, jaundice, hepatosplenomegaly, and lymph node enlargement (Cantwell et al., 1994). Respiratory embarrassment may be a late symptom of the disease. Many infants have an initially normal chest radiograph that later becomes abnormal, most often having a miliary pattern. Hilar and mediastinal lymphadenopathy and lung infiltrates also are common. The most important clue for rapid diagnosis of perinatal tuberculosis is the maternal and family history for tuberculosis. Frequently, however, the mother's disease is discovered only after the neonate's condition is suspected or diagnosed. The tuberculin skin test on the infant is essentially always negative initially, but it may become positive in 1 to 3 months. A positive acid-fast stain of an early morning gastric washing from a newborn usually indicates tuberculosis. Direct acid-fast stains of middle ear fluid, bone marrow, tracheal aspirates, or biopsy tissue can be useful and should be performed. The cerebrospinal fluid should be examined and cultured, although the yield for isolating *M. tuberculosis* is low, since less than 25% of infected infants have meningitis.

HIV-Related

In adults infected with both HIV and *M. tuberculosis,* the rate of progression from tuberculosis infection to disease is greatly increased. The clinical manifestations of tuberculosis in HIV-infected patients are typical when the CD4+ cell count is more than 500 per mm^3. Extrapulmonary foci occur in up to 60% of profoundly immunocompromised patients. Pulmonary cavities are rare; lower lobe infiltrates or nodules often accompanied by thoracic adenopathy are common, especially if the patient's tuberculosis infection is recent. Of course, many patients have a nonreactive tuberculin skin test. Sputum is less likely to be produced or to contain visible acid-fast organisms.

When HIV-infected children develop tuberculosis, the clinical features tend to be fairly typical of childhood tuberculosis in immunocompetent patients, although the disease often progresses more rapidly and clinical manifestations are more severe (Chan et al., 1996; Khouri et al., 1992). There may be an increased tendency for extrapulmonary disease, especially disseminated disease and meningitis. Diagnosis can be very difficult because the yield for cultures is so low in children. A diligent search for an infectious adult in the child's environment may yield the best clue to the correct diagnosis.

DIAGNOSIS
Tuberculin Skin Test

Two major techniques are used for tuberculin skin testing: the multiple-puncture test and the Mantoux test. The multiple-puncture tests have been used widely because of the speed by which they can be administered by even relatively unskilled personnel. However, these tests are even less accurate than the Mantoux tuberculin skin test. Virtually all experts, the CDC, and the American Academy of Pediatrics (AAP) agree that there is no place in practice for multiple-puncture skin testing. These tests magnify the inherent problems with the Mantoux test and make a relatively inaccurate test even less accurate.

The Mantoux tuberculin skin test using five tuberculin units (TU) of purified protein derivative (PPD) is the "gold standard" skin test. When administered properly, a wheal 6 to 10 mm in diameter should be raised. It is helpful for the person administering the test to anchor the side of his or her hand against the side of the child's arm and inject the solution in a transverse direction (Fig. 35-8). With this technique one can maintain a firm grasp, anticipate the child's tendency to move, and create a fulcrum to guide proper entry of the needle. The amount of induration caused by the test should be measured as accurately as possible by a trained health-care worker (not the parent) 48 to 72 hours after administration (Cheng et al., 1996; Howard and Soloman, 1988; Graziani and MacGregor, 1995). The test should not be interpreted before 48 hours because false-positive results can occur as a result of different immunologic mechanisms. The size of induration should be recorded in the medical record in millimeters even if there is no induration; use of the words *negative* and *positive* should be avoided because interpretation can change as more epidemiologic information becomes available. An occasional patient will have a reaction later than 72 hours after administration; this late induration should be considered the test result (Hsu, 1983).

The tuberculin skin test is subject to a variety of factors that can cause false-negative and false-

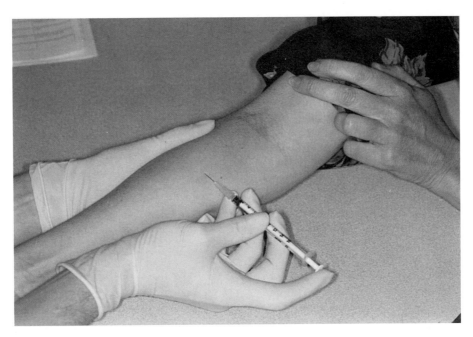

Fig. 35-8   An excellent technique to control placement of the Mantoux tuberculin skin test on an infant or child.

positive results (Huebner et al., 1993). The most common causes of false-negative results are incubation of viral infections such as influenza and varicella; incubation of bacterial infections; overwhelming tuberculosis; recent administration of live viral vaccines; severe malnutrition; diseases and drugs causing anergy; extremes of age (newborns and the elderly); and factors related to the administration of the test. It is acceptable to place the tuberculin skin test at the same time that a live viral vaccine is given or corticosteroids are started, since the test suppression takes several days to weeks to start (Schick and Dolgin, 1963). Approximately 10% of immunocompetent children with culture-documented tuberculosis do not react initially to the tuberculin skin test (Starke and Taylor-Watts, 1989; Steiner et al., 1980). Most become reactive after several months of treatment, suggesting that the disease has caused the anergy. The lack of skin reactivity can be global or specific for tuberculin. Children with tuberculosis and HIV infection more often experience widespread anergy to a variety of skin test antigens, including tuberculin. A negative tuberculin skin test never rules out tuberculosis in a child.

False-positive reactions to the tuberculin skin test most often are attributed to asymptomatic infection by nontuberculous mycobacteria. These cross-reactions are usually small (10 mm) but often are larger. Previous receipt of a bacille Calmette-Guérin (BCG) vaccination can cause increased reactivity to a subsequent tuberculin skin test, but the association is weaker than many clinicians suspect (Comstock et al., 1971; Menzies and Vissandjee, 1992). Many studies have shown that fewer than 50% of infants given a BCG vaccination shortly after birth have a reactive tuberculin skin test at 6 to 12 months of age, and virtually all vaccinated infants have a nonreactive skin test by 5 years of age. Older children and adults who receive a BCG vaccination have a higher likelihood of developing a reactive skin test and maintaining it longer, but by 10 to 15 years after vaccination most individuals have lost tuberculin skin test reactivity (Comstock et al., 1971). Many foreign-born individuals who have had BCG vaccination have a reactive tuberculin skin test because they also have been infected with *M. tuberculosis* and are at risk of developing tuberculosis disease in the near or distant future (Lindgren, 1965). In general, the tuberculin skin test reaction should be interpreted in the same manner for persons who had BCG in the past as they are for those who have not been vaccinated (Nemir and Teichner, 1983). Repeated or serial skin testing can cause boosting, an increased response to subsequent tuberculin skin tests in individuals with a waned sensitivity to mycobacterial antigens (Thompson et al., 1979). Children who previously received a BCG vaccine may have a boostable reaction because of the BCG, not tuberculosis infection (Sepulveda et al., 1988).

There have been several important and significant changes in recommendations by the CDC and AAP for the interpretation of a Mantoux tuberculin skin test (American Academy of Pediatrics, 1994, 1996). The reason for these changes is the adherent difficulty in interpreting a test that has a sensitivity and specificity of only about 90% (Huebner et al., 1993). When a test with these characteristics is applied to a population with a 90% prevalence of tuberculosis infection, the positive predictive value of the skin test is 99%, an excellent result. That is, 99% of the people with positive reactions have true tuberculosis infection. However, if the same test is applied to a population that has only a 1% prevalence of tuberculosis infection, the positive predictive value drops to 8%; 92% of the positive results are false-positive, mostly caused by biologic variability and infection by nontuberculous mycobacteria. Because the skin test is not only the screening test but also the definitive test, true-positives cannot be differentiated from false-positives by further testing. All persons who test positive must therefore be evaluated and treated in the same manner, even though in certain groups the vast majority of those with positive results do not have tuberculosis infection. These false-positive test results lead to unnecessary treatment, cost, and anxiety for the family and clinician. In short, the relatively low sensitivity and specificity of the tuberculin skin test makes it useful for persons in high-prevalence groups (at high risk for tuberculosis infection) but undesirable for use in persons from low-prevalence groups.

In recent years the CDC and AAP have recommended varying the size of induration considered positive for different groups and individuals (Box 35-2). This is an attempt to alter the sensitivity and specificity of the test to make it more accurate in very high, high, and low prevalence groups. It is crucial to minimize the false-negative results in very-high-risk individuals who are at the highest risk of developing tuberculosis disease in the near future. Similarly, there is great desire to minimize the false-positive results in truly low-risk individuals. For children at the highest risk for tuberculosis infection progressing to disease, a reactive area of 5 mm or more is classified as positive, probably indicating infection by *M. tuberculosis.* For other high-risk groups a reactive area of 10 mm or more is a positive result. For individuals with no risk fac-

---

BOX 35-2

AMOUNT OF INDURATION TO A MANTOUX TUBERCULIN SKIN TEST CONSIDERED POSITIVE

≥5 mm	Contacts to infectious cases
	HIV-infected or otherwise immunosuppressed
	Abnormal chest radiograph or suspicion of tuberculosis disease
≥10 mm	High-risk individuals listed in Box 35-1
≥15 mm	Individuals without risk factors

---

tors a reaction of 15 mm or more is a positive result. However, even at the 15-mm cut point, the majority of "positive" reactions in truly low-risk individuals is still a false-positive result.

Diagnostic Mycobacteriology

Acid-Fast Stain and Culture. The demonstration of acid-fast bacilli in stained smears of sputum or other body fluids is presumptive evidence of pulmonary tuberculosis in most cases. However, in children, tubercle bacilli usually are relatively few in number, and sputum cannot be obtained in children younger than 10 years of age (Khan and Starke, 1995). Gastric washings are often obtained in lieu of sputum, although they can be contaminated with acid-fast organisms from the mouth. Fluorescence microscopy of gastric washings has been found useful in settings where malnutrition and tuberculin-negative tuberculosis are rampant. Tubercle bacilli in cerebrospinal fluid, pleural fluid, lymph node aspirates, and urine are sparse and only rarely detected on smears. Cultures for tubercle bacilli are of greater importance, not only to confirm the diagnosis but increasingly to permit testing for drug susceptibility. However, if culture and drug susceptibility data are available from the associated adult case and the child has a classic clinical and radiographic presentation of tuberculosis, obtaining cultures from the child adds little to the management because the susceptibilities are known and the child will be treated even if his or her cultures are negative.

Painstaking collection of specimens is essential for diagnosis of tuberculosis in children, since fewer organisms are present than in adults. Gastric lavage should be performed in the very early morning, before peristalsis has moved the overnight swallowed respiratory secretions that remain in the stomach. The gastric acidity should be neutralized immediately because acid conditions are poorly tolerated by *M. tuberculosis*. Unfortunately, even with optimal, in-hospital collection of three early morning gastric aspirate samples, *M. tuberculosis* can be isolated from only 30% to 40% of children and 70% of infants with pulmonary tuberculosis. The yield from random outpatient gastric aspirate samples is exceedingly low, and this practice cannot be recommended. If bronchial secretions can be obtained from a child with suspected tuberculosis by stimulating cough with an aerosol solution, this practice may increase the yield of the culture. Bronchoscopy also can be an adjunct to culture diagnosis, but, in most studies, the yield of *M. tuberculosis* from bronchoscopy specimens has been lower than from properly obtained gastric washings (Abadco and Steiner, 1992; Chan et al., 1994; de Blic et al., 1991).

Nucleic Acid Amplification, Serologic Testing, Antigen Detection. The main form of nucleic acid amplification studied in children with tuberculosis is the polymerase chain reaction (PCR), which uses specific DNA sequences as markers for the presence of microorganisms. Various PCR techniques, most using the mycobacterial insertion element IS6110 as the DNA marker for *M. tuberculosis* complex organisms, have a sensitivity and specificity of more than 90% compared with sputum culture for detecting pulmonary tuberculosis in adults (Eisenach et al., 1991). However, test performance varies even among reference laboratories, with both false-positive and false-negative results being fairly common. The test is relatively expensive, requires fairly sophisticated equipment and requires scrupulous technique to avoid cross-contamination of specimens (Dunlap et al., 1995).

Use of PCR in childhood tuberculosis has been limited. Compared with a clinical diagnosis of tuberculosis in children, the sensitivity of PCR has varied from 25% to 83% and the specificity has varied from 80% to 100% (Delacourt et al., 1995; Pierre and Lecossier, 1993; Smith et al., 1996). The PCR of gastric aspirates may be positive in a recently infected child even when the chest radiograph is normal, demonstrating the occasional arbitrariness of the distinction between tuberculosis infection and disease in children. PCR may have a useful but limited role in evaluating children with suspected tuberculosis. A negative PCR never

eliminates tuberculosis as a diagnostic possibility and a positive result does not confirm it. The major use of PCR will be in evaluation of children with significant pulmonary disease when the diagnosis is not established readily by clinical or epidemiologic rounds. PCR may be particularly helpful in evaluating immunocompromised children with pulmonary disease, especially children with HIV infection, although published reports of performance in such children are lacking. PCR also may aid in confirming the diagnosis of extrapulmonary tuberculosis, although only a few case reports involving samples other than sputum or gastric washings have been published (Mancao et al., 1994). Currently PCR is approved for use only on acid-fast smear–positive specimens.

Despite hundreds of published studies, serologic testing has found no place in the routine diagnosis of tuberculosis in children (Daniel and Debanne, 1987). Recent studies using a variety of mycobacterial antigens have yielded conflicting results (Delacourt et al., 1993; Turneer et al., 1994). In general, the sensitivity and specificity of the tests are unacceptably low to be of use. Mycobacterial antigen detection has been evaluated in clinical samples from adults, but rarely from children (Sada et al., 1992). These techniques generally require sophisticated and expensive equipment not available where tuberculosis in children is common.

History and Clinical Scoring

In the developing world the only way children with tuberculosis disease are discovered is when they present with a profound illness that is consistent with one presentation of tuberculosis. Having an ill adult contact is a obvious clue to the correct diagnosis. The only available laboratory test usually is an acid-fast smear of the sputum, which the child rarely produces. In many regions, chest radiographs are not available. To aid in diagnosis, a variety of scoring systems have been devised based on available tests; clinical signs and symptoms; and, most importantly, known exposures to adult cases (Migliori et al., 1992). However, the sensitivity and specificity of these systems can be very low, leading to both overdiagnosis and underdiagnosis.

Even in industrialized countries, epidemiology remains extremely important for the diagnosis of tuberculosis. Cases can be culture-confirmed only in 40% of children; it is usually the combination of uncovering risk factors for recent tuberculosis infection, a positive tuberculin skin test, and radiographic or clinical evidence of tuberculosis disease that leads to the correct diagnosis. Children with tuberculosis in industrialized countries usually are discovered in one of two ways. One way is the consideration of tuberculosis being the cause of a symptomatic illness. The second way—which may be the method by which half the children are discovered—is during contact investigation of an adult with suspected tuberculosis. Typically, affected children have few signs or symptoms, but investigation reveals a positive tuberculin skin test and an abnormal chest radiograph. In industrialized countries it is rare to find tuberculosis disease in a child as a result of a community or school-based testing program.

TREATMENT
Antituberculosis Drugs

Over a dozen drugs are used for the treatment of tuberculosis in industrialized countries. Five drugs are used commonly for drug-susceptible tuberculosis (Table 35-2) and eight drugs are used only in cases of drug-resistant tuberculosis (Table 35-3).

Isoniazid is the mainstay of treatment of tuberculosis in children. It is inexpensive, readily dif-

fuses into all tissues and body fluids, and produces a very low rate of adverse reactions. It can be administered either orally or intramuscularly. At the usual daily dose of 10 mg/kg, serum concentrations greatly exceed the minimum inhibitory concentration for *M. tuberculosis*. Peak concentrations in blood, sputum, and cerebrospinal fluid are reached within a few hours and persist for at least 6 to 8 hours.

Isoniazid is metabolized by acetylation in the liver. Rapid acetylation is more frequent among blacks and Asians than among whites. However, in children there is no correlation between acetylation rate and efficacy or rate of adverse reactions (Martinez-Roig et al., 1986).

Isoniazid has two principle toxic effects, both of which are rare in children. Peripheral neuritis results from competitive inhibition of pyridoxine utilization. Pyridoxine levels are decreased in children taking isoniazid, but clinical manifestations are rare (Pellock et al., 1985). Pyridoxine administration is not recommended except for teenagers with inadequate diets, children from groups with

Table 35-2 Commonly used drugs for the treatment of tuberculosis in children

Drug	Dosage forms	Daily dosage (mg/kg/day)	Twice-weekly dosage (mg/kg/dose)	Maximum daily dose
Ethambutol	Tablets 100 mg 400 mg	15-25	50	2.5 g
Isoniazid*	Scored tablets 100 mg 300 mg Syrup† 10 mg/ml	10-15‡	20-30	Daily, 300 mg; twice weekly, 900 mg
Pyrazinamide	Scored tablets 500 mg	20-40	50	2 g
Rifampin*	Capsules 150 mg 300 mg Syrup Formulated in syrup from capsules	10-20	10-20	Daily, 600 mg; twice weekly, 900 mg
Streptomycin (IM administration)	Vials 1 g 4 g	20-40	20-40	1 g

*Rifamate is a capsule containing 150 mg of isoniazid and 300 mg of rifampin. Two capsules provide the usual adult (>50 kg body weight) daily doses of each drug.
†Most experts advise against the use of isoniazid syrup because of its instability and a high rate of gastrointestinal adverse reaction (diarrhea, cramps).
‡When isoniazid is used in combination with rifampin, the incidence of hepatoxicity increases if the isoniazid dose exceeds 10 mg/kg/day.

low levels of milk and meat intake, pregnant teenagers and women, and breast-feeding babies (McKenzie et al., 1976). The most common physical manifestation of peripheral neuritis is numbness and tingling in the hands or feet. Central nervous system toxicity from isoniazid is rare, occurring usually when there is significant overdose. Seizures are the most common manifestations (McKenzie et al., 1976; Parish and Brownstein, 1986; Shah et al., 1995).

The major and most feared toxic effect of isoniazid is hepatotoxocity, which is also rare in children but increases with age (Beaudry et al., 1974). Three to ten percent of children taking isoniazid experience transient elevated serum transaminase levels. Clinically significant hepatotoxicity is very rare and is more likely to occur in adolescents or children with severe forms of tuberculosis, or those who have underlying liver disease or are taking other hepatotoxic medications (Snider and Caras, 1992; Vanderhoof and Ament, 1976). Simultaneous administration of rifampin increases the likelihood of hepatotoxicity, especially if the isoniazid daily dose exceeds 10 mg/kg (Kumar et al., 1991; O'Brien et al., 1983). The possible occurrence of hepatitis raises the question of routine monitoring of liver enzyme levels in children receiving isoniazid. The advantage of doing so has to be weighed against the expense and the difficulty of ensuring regular physician or clinic visits if the patient and parents know that every clinic visit requires a venipuncture. Most experts prefer to substitute routine questions about appetite and well-being, determination of weight, a check of the appearance of the sclera, and examination of the abdomen for frequent blood drawing. Patients should be counseled to stop the isoniazid and contact the clinician immediately if significant nausea, vomiting, abdominal pain, or jaundice occurs during the use of isoniazid.

Allergic manifestations or hypersensitivity caused by isoniazid are very rare. Isoniazid increases phenytoin levels, which can lead to toxicity by blocking its metabolism level. Occasionally isoniazid reacts with theophylline, requiring modification of its dosage. Rare side effects of isoniazid include pellagra, hemolytic anemia, and a lupuslike reaction with skin rash and arthritis.

Rifampin is a semisynthetic drug that is an important part of the modern management of tuberculosis. It is well absorbed from the gastrointestinal tract during fasting, with peak serum levels occurring within two hours. Oral and intravenous forms are

Table 35-3   Drugs for treatment of drug-resistant tuberculosis in children

Drug	Dosage forms	Daily dosage (mg/kg/day)	Maximum daily dose
Capreomycin	Vials 1 g	15-30 (IM)	1 g
Ciprofloxacin	Tablets 250 mg 500 mg 750 mg	Adults 500-1500 mg in 2 divided doses	1.5 g
Clofazamine	Capsules 50 mg 100 mg	50-100 mg/day	200 mg
Cycloserine	Capsules 250 mg	10-20	1 g
Ethionamide	Tablets 250 mg	15-20, given in 2 or 3 divided doses	1 g
Kanamycin	Vials 75 mg/2 ml 500 mg/2 ml 1 g/3 ml	15-30 (IM)	1 g
Ofloxacin	Tablets 200 mg 300 mg 400 mg	Adults 400-800 mg total/day	800 mg
Para-aminosalicylic acid	Packets 4 g	200-300, given in 2 to 4 divided doses	10 g

now available. Like isoniazid, rifampin is distributed widely in tissue and body fluids, including the CSF. Although excretion is mainly via the biliary tract, effective levels are reached in the kidneys and urine. Side effects are more common than with isoniazid and include orange discoloration of urine and tears (with permanent staining of contact lenses); gastrointestinal disturbances; and hepatotoxicity, usually manifested as asymptomatic elevation of serum transaminase levels. Intermittent administration of rifampin over weeks has been associated with thrombocytopenia and an influenza-like syndrome consisting of fever, headache, and malaise. Rifampin can render oral contraceptives ineffective and interacts with several other drugs, including quinidine, warfarin sodium, and corticosteroids.

Pyrazinamide was developed in 1949 but fell into disuse because of hepatotoxicity observed at the then standard dosage of 50 mg/kg/day. In adults a once-daily dosage of 30 mg/kg/day produces adequate serum levels and little liver toxicity. The optimal dosage in children is unknown, but this dosage causes high CSF levels (Donald and Seifart, 1988), is well tolerated by children, and correlates with clinical success in treatment trials of tuberculosis in children. Extensive experience with pyrazinamide in children has verified its safety. Although 10% of adults treated with pyrazinamide develop arthralgias or arthritis resulting from hyperuricemia, and uric acid levels are elevated in children taking pyrazinamide, clinical manifestations of hyperuricemia in children are extremely rare. Hepatotoxicity occurs at high doses but is very rare in children.

Rifamate is a capsule with fixed doses of isoniazid (150 mg) and rifampin (300 mg). Rifater is a pill containing fixed doses of isoniazid, rifampin, and pyrazinamide. These fixed-dose combination capsules and pills should be used whenever possible to be sure that patients on self-supervised therapy are taking all of their tuberculosis medications together.

Streptomycin is used less frequently than in the past for the treatment of childhood tuberculosis but is important for the treatment of drug-resistant disease. It must be given intramuscularly or intravenously. Streptomycin penetrates inflamed meninges fairly well but does not cross uninflamed meninges. Its major current use is in cases where initial isoniazid resistance is suspected or when the child has life-threatening tuberculosis, such as meningitis or disseminated disease. The major toxicity of streptomycin is through the vestibular and auditory portions of the eighth cranial nerve. Renal toxicity is much less frequent. However, streptomycin is contraindicated in pregnant women because up to 30% of their infants will suffer severe hearing loss (Snider and Johnson, 1984).

Ethambutol has received little attention in children because of its toxicity to the eye. At a dosage of 15 mg/kg/day it is primarily bacteriostatic, and its historic purpose has been to prevent emergence of resistance to other drugs. It is well tolerated by adults and children when given orally once or twice a day. The major potential toxicity is optic neuritis. Review of the world's literature has shown there has been no report of optic toxicity in children, but the drug has not been used widely because of the inability to routinely test visual fields and acuity in children. Ethambutol is not recommended for general use in young children for whom vision cannot be adequately examined, but it can be used safely in children with drug-resistant tuberculosis or who may have been infected with a strain of drug-resistant *M. tuberculosis* when other agents are not available or cannot be used.

Ethionamide is a bacteriostatic drug whose major purpose is treatment of drug-resistant tuberculosis. It penetrates into the CSF very well and may be particularly useful in cases of tuberculous meningitis (Donald and Seifart, 1989). It is generally well tolerated by children but often must be given in 2 or 3 divided daily doses because of gastrointestinal disturbance. Ethionamide is chemically similar to isoniazid and can cause significant hepatitis.

Other antituberculosis drugs may be needed for patients with organisms that are resistant to the standard drugs. The aminoglycosides kanamycin, amikacin, and capreomycin have a spectrum of activity that differs from that of streptomycin with respect to individual mycobacterial strains. Cycloserine is an effective antituberculosis drug in adults but has been used infrequently in children because of its major side effects of impairment of thought processes and tendency to cause depression and other psychiatric abnormalities. The drug is usually given in 1 or 2 divided doses, and most experts recommend monitoring serum levels during its administration. Pyridoxine supplementation should be given when cycloserine is used. Ciprofloxacin and ofloxacin are fluoroquinolones with significant antituberculosis activity that are used commonly for drug-resistant tuberculosis in adults (Kennedy et al., 1993). These drugs are generally contraindicated for long-term administration in children because they can cause destruction of growing carti-lage in some animal models. However, they have been used effectively in some cases of drug-resis-tant tuberculosis in children when other effective agents were not available (Hussey et al., 1992). Para-aminosalicyclic acid is an old tuberculosis drug that had been extremely difficult to take be-cause of the need to administer a large number of pills. The drug is now available as granules pro-vided in packets. The major side effect is gastroin-testinal intolerance, which is extremely common and necessitates the drug being given in 3 or 4 di-vided doses. Clofazamine is used to treat leprosy, but many strains of *M. tuberculosis* also are suscep-tible (Jagannath et al., 1995).

Rationale For Therapy

The tubercle bacillus can be killed only during replication, which occurs among organisms that are metabolically active. Environmental conditions for growth are best within lung cavities, leading to a huge bacterial population—up to 10^9 organisms. The caseous lesions that are most common in pedi-atric tuberculosis contain much smaller numbers of organisms—10^4 to 10^6—than cavitary lesions. Naturally occurring, drug-resistant mutant organ-isms occur within large populations of tubercle bacilli even before chemotherapy is started. All known genetic loci for drug resistance in *M. tuber-culosis* are located on the chromosome; no plas-mid-mediated resistance is known. The rate of re-sistance within large populations of organisms is related to the rate of mutations at these genetic loci. Although a large population of bacilli as a whole may be considered drug-susceptible, a subpopula-tion of drug-resistant organisms occurs at fairly predictable rates. The estimated frequency of these drug-resistant mutations is about 10^{-6}, but it varies among drugs. Therefore a cavity that contains 10^9 bacilli has thousands of single drug-resistant or-ganisms, whereas a closed caseous lesion contains few, if any, resistant mutants (Swanson and Starke, 1995).

The two microbiologic properties of population size and drug-resistant mutations explain why sin-gle antituberculosis drugs cannot cure cavitary tu-berculosis in adults (Mitchison and Nunn, 1986). When a single drug is given to these patients, they have some initial improvement in signs and symp-toms, but they relapse with organisms that are now completely resistant to the administered medica-tion. Fortunately, the occurrence of resistance to one drug is independent of resistance to any other drug because the resistance loci are not linked (Te-lenti et al., 1993; Zhang, 1993). The chance of hav-ing even one organism with mutations causing re-sistance to two drugs before the start of chemotherapy is on the order of 10^{-13}. Populations of this size are extremely rare in patients, and or-ganisms naturally resistant to two drugs are essen-tially nonexistent.

The population size of tubercle bacilli within a patient determines the appropriate therapy (Starke, 1992). For patients with large bacterial population (adults with cavities or extensive infiltrates), many single drug-resistant organisms are present, and at least two antituberculosis drugs must be used. Con-versely, for patients with tuberculosis infection but no disease, the bacterial population is very small (about 10^3 to 10^4 organisms), drug-resistant organ-isms are rare, and a single drug can be used. Chil-dren with pulmonary tuberculosis and patients of all ages with extrapulmonary tuberculosis have medium-size populations where drug-resistant mu-tants may or may not be present. In general, these patients are treated with at least two drugs (Bid-dulph, 1990).

Exposure

In the United States, children exposed to poten-tially infectious adults with pulmonary tuberculosis are started on treatment, usually isoniazid, if the child is younger than 5 years of age or has other risk factors for the rapid development of tuberculo-sis disease, such as immunocompromise (Starke and Correa, 1995). Failure to do this may result in development of severe tuberculosis disease even before the tuberculin skin test becomes reactive; the "incubation" period of disease may be shorter than the time it takes for the skin test to become re-active. The child is treated for a minimum of 3 months after contact with the infectious case has been broken by physical separation or effective treatment. After 3 months the tuberculin skin test is repeated. If the second test is positive, infection is documented and isoniazid should be continued for total duration of 9 months; if the second skin test is negative, the treatment can be stopped. If the expo-sure was to a case with an isoniazid-resistant but ri-fampin-susceptible isolate, rifampin is the recom-mended treatment.

Two special circumstances of exposure deserve attention. A difficult situation arises when exposed children are anergic because of HIV infection. These children are particularly vulnerable to rapid progression of tuberculosis, and it will not be possible to tell if infection has occurred. In general, these children should be treated as if they have tuberculosis infection. The second situation is potential exposure to a newborn by a mother or other adult with a positive tuberculin skin test (Dormer et al., 1959; Steiner and Rao, 1993). The management is based on further evaluation of the adult (Kendig and Rodgers, 1958; Light et al., 1974). If the adult has a normal chest radiograph, no separation of the child from the adult is required. However, the adult should receive treatment for tuberculosis infection and other household members should be evaluated for tuberculosis infection or disease. The infant requires no specific evaluation or treatment unless a case of disease is found. If the mother or other adult has an abnormal chest radiograph, the child should be separated from her until evaluation has occurred. If the radiograph, medical and social history, physical examination, and analysis of sputum reveal no evidence of active pulmonary tuberculosis, it is reasonable to assume the infant is at low risk of infection. However, if the adult remains untreated, he or she may develop contagious tuberculosis and expose the infant. If the radiograph and clinical history are suggestive of pulmonary tuberculosis, the child and adult should remain separated until both have begun appropriate chemotherapy. The infant should be evaluated for congenital tuberculosis. The placenta should be examined if at all possible. The infant should receive isoniazid and close follow-up care. The infant should have a tuberculin skin test 3 or 4 months after the adult is judged to no longer be contagious; evaluation of this infant then follows the guidelines for other exposures of children. If no infection is documented during follow-up, it is prudent to repeat a tuberculin skin test in 6 to 12 months.

Infection

Isoniazid is effective in preventing progression of tuberculosis infection in children (Ferrebee, 1969). Before its discovery (Brailey, 1958), Brailey reported a mortality rate of 16% for black children and 8% for white children who were infected with *M. tuberculosis* before 3 years of age. In contrast, recent reports have documented no death and no disease in similar children who received isoniazid for 9 to 12 months (Hsu, 1984). Other studies of children of all ages with tuberculosis infection have shown that isoniazid treatment produces a 90% to 100% reduction in tuberculosis disease during the first year after treatment, and the protective effect can last at least 30 years (Comstock et al.,

1979; Hsu, 1983). Although many adults are treated with a 6-month course of isoniazid for tuberculosis infection (International Union Against Tuberculosis Committee on Prophylaxis, 1982; Snider et al., 1986), the CDC and AAP recommend a 9-month duration of isoniazid treatment for children with tuberculosis infection (American Academy of Pediatrics, 1996; American Thoracic Society, 1994). Children with HIV infection and tuberculosis infection should receive therapy for 1 year. If infection is with an isoniazid-resistant but rifampin-susceptible organism, rifampin should be used. In general, isoniazid is given on a daily basis. However, patient adherence to treatment is notoriously low, especially if the child's reactive skin test was discovered through a screening program. In situations in which the risk of progression to disease is high and family adherence to taking medication is difficult, isoniazid can be administered twice a week under the direct observation of a third party such as a public health worker or school nurse. This is called *directly observed therapy* (DOT). Although no studies have been published that document the effectiveness of twice-weekly DOT for tuberculosis infection, there are numerous studies that show its effectiveness in treating tuberculosis disease.

Treatment of tuberculosis infection in children with isoniazid has proved to be very safe (Byrd et al., 1979). Routine testing of blood chemistries and serum liver enzymes is unnecessary unless the child has hepatic disease or dysfunction or is taking other hepatotoxic drugs. It is recommended that the child be evaluated by a clinician every 4 to 6 weeks and that no more than a 6-week supply of medicine be given to avoid the possibility of massive overdose.

Disease

The major importance of the distinction between tuberculosis infection and disease in children is that the treatment regimens for them are different. The bacterial population is much larger in disease and there is an increased propensity for the emergence of drug resistance with larger mycobacterial populations (British Thoracic Society, 1984). The simple adage to remember is "more bugs, more drugs." Because antituberculosis medications are so well tolerated by children and inadequate treatment can have devastating effects, most experts feel it is safer to overestimate rather than underestimate the extent of disease, particularly in a young child known to be at high risk with recent infection by *M. tuberculosis.* In general, any radiographic or clinical manifestations that are attributed to the presence of *M. tuberculosis* (except for single granulomas in the lung) are considered disease, and the child is treated with more than one medication. The AAP and CDC currently recommend that standard treatment for pulmonary tuberculosis in children should be a 6-month course of isoniazid and rifampin supplemented during the first 2 months with pyrazinamide (American Academy of Pediatrics, 1992; American Thoracic Society, 1994). If the risk for initial isoniazid resistance is significant—particularly if the probable adult source case for infection has risk factors for drug-resistant tuberculosis—a fourth drug, usually ethambutol, should be given until drug susceptibility information is known (Centers for Disease Control, 1993). As soon as isoniazid and rifampin susceptibility is established or considered likely, the ethambutol can be discontinued. In many published studies, the overall success rate of this regimen has been greater than 98%, and the incidence of clinically important adverse reactions has been less than 2% (Abernathy et al., 1983; Hong Kong Chest Service/British Medical Research Council, 1991; Tsakalidis et al., 1992). Because of the slow replication time of *M. tuberculosis* and the fairly long half-lives of most antituberculosis medications, they can be administered twice weekly under directly observed therapy after the first 2 to 4 weeks of daily administration (Cohn et al., 1990). Studies using twice-weekly therapy have shown results equivalent to those using daily therapy throughout the full 6 months (Kumar et al., 1990).

Controlled treatment trials for various forms of extrapulmonary tuberculosis are rare. In most reports, extrapulmonary cases have been combined with pulmonary cases and may not be analyzed separately. Several of the 6-month, three- or four-drug trials in children included extrapulmonary cases. Most non–life threatening forms of drug-susceptible extrapulmonary tuberculosis can be treated with a 6-month regimen of isoniazid, rifampin, and pyrazinamide (Dutt et al., 1986; Jawahar et al., 1990). One exception may be bone and joint tuberculosis, which has a higher failure rate when 6-month chemotherapy regimens are used, especially when surgical intervention has not occurred (Medical Research Council Working Party on Tuberculosis of the Spine, 1993). Most experts recommend 9 to 12 months of therapy for bone and joint tuberculosis. Tuberculous meningitis usually is not included in trials of extrapulmonary tuberculosis therapy because of its serious nature and low incidence. Recent studies have shown that inclusion of pyrazinamide in the regimen for tuberculous meningitis is extremely important (Jacobs et al., 1992). The AAP and CDC currently recommend treating tuberculous meningitis for 9 to 12 months, starting with four drugs to guard against initial drug resistance.

Corticosteroids have a place in the treatment of some patients with tuberculosis (Smith, 1958). They never should be used except under the cover of effective antituberculosis drugs. Corticosteroids would be expected to be beneficial in situations when the host inflammatory reaction contributes to tissue damage or impairs function. They should be used in all cases of suspected tuberculous meningitis, especially when increased intracranial pressure is present. Their major actions are to reduce vasculitis; inflammation; and, ultimately, intracranial pressure. Several studies have demonstrated lower rates of mortality and long-term neurologic sequelae among patients with tuberculous meningitis treated with corticosteroids compared with non–steroid treated control patients (Excobar et al., 1975; Girgis et al., 1991). Corticosteroid treatment also may be considered (1) in cases of acute pericardial effusion when tamponade is occurring; (2) in cases of pleural effusion when there is shift of the mediastinum and acute respiratory embarrassment (Lee et al., 1988); (3) in patients with miliary tuberculosis if the inflammatory reaction is so severe as to produce alveolocapilliary block syndrome; and (4) in patients with enlarged mediastinal lymph nodes that are causing respiratory difficulty or a severe collapse-consolidation lesion, particularly in the lower lobe, where bronchiectasis is likely to be a troublesome sequela (Nemir et al., 1967). The dosage of corticosteroids should be in the antiinflammatory range—that is, prednisone, 1 to 2 mg/kg every 24 hours for 4 to 6 weeks, with gradual withdrawal. There is no evidence that one corticosteroid is preferable to another.

The major problem with treatment of tuberculosis infection and disease is nonadherence to the drug regimen by patients over the long-term therapy (Beyers et al., 1994; Cuneo and Snider, 1989; Snider et al., 1984). In the United States it is almost the standard of care that all patients with tuberculosis disease be treated with directly observed therapy (Iseman et al., 1990; Kohn et al., 1996; Weis et al., 1994). Direct observation means that a healthcare worker or nonrelated third party (such as a teacher, school nurse, or social worker) is physically present when the patient ingests the medication. Up to 50% of patients taking long-term tuberculosis medications have significant nonadherence without direct observation, and its occurrence is not predictable even by experienced clinicians (Chaulk et al., 1995; Sumartojo, 1993).

Drug Resistance

The incidence of drug-resistant tuberculosis is increasing in the United States and the world as a result of poor adherence by the patient, the availability of some antituberculosis drugs in over-the-counter formulations, and poor management of patients by physicians and tuberculosis control programs (Mahmoudi and Iseman, 1993). In the United States about 10% of *M. tuberculosis* isolates are resistant to at least one drug (Bloch et al., 1994; Frieden et al., 1993). The initial drug resistance rate is as high as 80% in adults with pulmonary tuberculosis in some countries, and rates of 20% to 30% are common. The resistance is most common to streptomycin and isoniazid and is still relatively rare for rifampin. Certain epidemiologic factors—such as disease in an Asian or Hispanic immigrant to the United States, homelessness in some communities, and history of prior antituberculosis therapy—correlate with drug resistance in adult patients (Barnes, 1987; Small et al., 1993). Patterns of drug resistance in children tend to mirror what is found in adult patients in the population (Snider et al., 1985; Steiner et al., 1985). The key to determining drug resistance in childhood tuberculosis usually comes from the drug susceptibility profile of the infectious adult contact case's isolate.

Therapy for drug-resistant tuberculosis is successful only when at least two bactericidal drugs to which the infecting strain of *M. tuberculosis* is susceptible are given (Passannante et al., 1994). If only one effective drug is given, secondary resistance will develop to it. When isoniazid resistance is considered a possibility on the basis of epidemiologic risk factors or the identification of an isoniazid-resistant source case isolate, a fourth drug, usually ethambutol or streptomycin, should be given initially to the child with tuberculosis disease until the exact susceptibility pattern of the isolate is determined and a more specific regimen can be designed. The exact treatment regimens of drug-resistant tuberculosis must be tailored to the specific pattern of resistance (Goble et al., 1993; Iseman, 1993). Duration of therapy usually is extended to at least 9 to 12 months if either isoniazid or rifampin can be used and to at least 18 to 24 months if resis-

tance to both drugs is present (Park et al., 1996; Telzak et al., 1995). Occasionally, surgical resection of a diseased segment or lobe is required (Iseman et al., 1990). An expert in tuberculosis always should be involved in the management of children with drug-resistant tuberculosis infection and disease (Steiner and Rao, 1993).

PREVENTION
Public Health Measures

Prevention of tuberculosis may involve (1) protection against exposure to the organism; (2) use of antituberculosis drugs in tuberculin-negative individuals with high risk of infection; and (3) immunization of tuberculin-negative individuals. Protection against exposure to disease is the ideal form of prevention. It presupposes thorough preemployment and ongoing case-finding programs among all who come in contact with children, such as daycare center and school personnel, teachers, healthcare workers, babysitters, household workers, and others. The best way to protect a child from acquiring tuberculosis infection is to be sure that the adults in his environment do not have active tuberculosis.

It is obvious that the control of tuberculosis—for a community and for individuals—depends on close cooperation between the clinician and the health department. It is critically important that clinicians report *suspected* cases of tuberculosis to the Public Health Department as soon as possible. The clinician should not wait for microbiologic confirmation of the diagnosis, because it is the reporting of suspicion that leads to the initiation of the contact investigation that may find exposed or infected children and allow them to be treated before disease develops. If the clinician waits for confirmatory laboratory results from the suspected adult case, the child may progress from infection to disease before intervention occurs (Mehta and Bentley, 1992; Nolan, 1986).

Since the advent of isoniazid treatment in the 1950s, screening children for tuberculosis infection often has been an integral part of local tuberculosis control programs. The major purpose of finding and treating infected individuals is to prevent future cases of tuberculosis disease (Centers for Disease Control and Prevention, 1994). However, frequent or periodic skin testing of children will prevent very few cases of pediatric tuberculosis, especially if the screening is centered on school-age children (American Academy of Pediatrics, 1994, 1996; Mohle-Boetani et al., 1995). The majority of cases of tuberculosis disease among children occur in preschool-age children, and school-based screenings thus have little benefit. The major purpose of testing school-age children is to prevent future cases of tuberculosis in adults. Clearly, the best way to prevent tuberculosis disease among children is through prompt contact investigation centered on adults with suspected contagious tuberculosis. These contact investigations not only have the highest yield, because 30% to 50% of household contacts have a positive tuberculin skin test, but they also find the most important individuals—those most recently infected who are in the period of their lives when they are most likely to develop tuberculosis disease. The most important activity in a community to prevent cases of pediatric tuberculosis is the contact investigation performed by the Public Health Department (Kimmerling et al., 1995; Perry and Starke, 1993).

Bacille Calmette-Gúerin Vaccination

Immunization against tuberculosis would be a tremendous advance for medicine, but in practice it has been fraught with enormous difficulties. The only available vaccines against tuberculosis are the bacille Calmette-Gúerin (BCG) vaccines, named for the two French investigators responsible for their development. The original vaccine organism was a strain of *Mycobacterium bovis* attenuated by subculture every 3 weeks for 13 years. The strain was then distributed to dozens of laboratories, each of which continued to subculture the organism under various conditions. The result has been production of many daughter BCG strains that differ widely in morphology, growth characteristics, sensitizing potency, and animal virulence.

The route of administration and dosing schedule for the BCG vaccines are important for determining vaccine efficacies. The preferred route of administration is intradermal injection with a syringe and needle because it is the only method that permits accurate measurement of an individual dose. The use of this route is relatively expensive, however, and, in developing countries, needles and syringes may be reused, with the resulting danger of transmission of HIV and hepatitis viruses. There are no reported trials comparing various methods of administration, although the complication rates generally are lower with multipuncture devices.

The BCG vaccines are extremely safe in immunocompetent hosts (Gonzalez et al., 1989). Local ulceration and regional suppurative lymphadenitis occur in 0.1% to 1% of vaccine recipients.

Local lesions do not suggest underlying immune defects and appear not to affect the level of protection. Rarely, surgical incision of a suppurative draining lymph node is necessary, but this should be avoided if possible. Although osteomyelitis near the inoculation site of BCG has been reported, this effect appears to be related only to certain strains of the vaccine that are no longer in wide use. Systemic complaints such as fever, convulsions, loss of appetite, and irritability are extremely rare after BCG vaccination. There has been great concern recently about the effects of BCG vaccination in HIV-infected children. Currently the World Health Organization recommends BCG vaccination for asymptomatic HIV-infected children (Ryder et al., 1993). However, there is some evidence that local BCG reactions may be more common in HIV-infected children (O'Brien et al., 1995); that disseminated BCG-osis occurs (although rarely); and that complications may occur even decades after the BCG vaccination. In the United States, HIV infection is considered a contraindication to BCG vaccination (Centers for Disease Control, 1994).

Accurate assessment of the effectiveness of BCG vaccines is extremely difficult. Recommended vaccine schedules vary widely among countries. The official WHO recommendation is a single dose administered during infancy. However, in some countries, multiple doses are given with or without a reactive tuberculin skin test, or a single dose may be administered later in childhood or during adolescence. The optimal age for administration is completely unknown, since adequate comparative trials never have been performed.

Although dozens of BCG trials on many varied human populations have been reported, the most useful data have come from several controlled trials and several case-control studies. The results of these studies are disparate; some demonstrated a great deal of protection from BCG, but others showed no efficacy at all. A recent metaanalysis of these studies showed the average effectiveness of BCG in preventing pulmonary disease to be about 50% (Colditz et al., 1994); effectiveness was higher for protection against life-threatening forms of tuberculosis in children (Colditz et al., 1995). A variety of explanations for the different apparent responses to BCG vaccines have been proposed, including methodologic and statistical variations among populations, interactions with nontuberculous mycobacteria that either enhance or decrease the protection afforded by BCG, different potencies among the various BCG vaccines, and genetic factors for reaction to BCG within the various study populations. It is apparent that BCG vaccination during infancy has little effect on the ultimate incidence of tuberculosis within a population. However, many experts believe that BCG may be more effective in preventing tuberculosis among infants and young children, particularly the serious forms of tuberculous meningitis and disseminated disease.

In summary, BCG vaccination has worked well in some situations but poorly in others. Clearly, BCG vaccination has had essentially no effect on the control of tuberculosis throughout the world. It does not substantially influence the rate of transmission, because those cases of contagious pulmonary tuberculosis in adults that can be prevented by BCG vaccination constitute a very small fraction of the sources of infection in a population. Any protective effect created by BCG probably wanes over time. The best use of BCG appears to be for prevention of life-threatening forms of tuberculosis in infants and young children.

BCG vaccination never has been adopted as part of the strategy for the control of tuberculosis in the United States. BCG vaccination in the United States is recommended only for tuberculin skin test–negative infants and children who are at high risk of intimate and prolonged exposure to untreated or ineffectively treated patients or to patients with tubercle bacilli that are resistant to both isoniazid and rifampin when other control measures cannot be used (Centers for Disease Control, 1996; Kendig, 1969). The only strain of BCG vaccine currently licensed in the United States is the Tice strain, which must be administered with a clumsy multipuncture device.

BIBLIOGRAPHY

Abadco D, Steiner P. Gastric lavage is better than bronchoalveolar lavage for isolation of *Mycobacterium tuberculosis* in childhood pulmonary tuberculosis. Pediatr Infect Dis J. 1992;11:735-738.

Abernathy RS, Dutt AK, Stead WW, et al. Short-course chemotherapy for tuberculosis in children. Pediatrics 1983; 72:801-806.

Alland D, Kolkut GE, Moss A, et al. Transmission of tuberculosis in New York City: an analysis by DNA fingerprinting and conventional epidemiologic methods. N Engl J Med 1994; 330:1710-1716.

American Academy of Pediatrics, Committee on Infectious Diseases. Chemotherapy for tuberculosis in infants and children. Pediatrics 1992;89:161-165.

American Academy of Pediatrics, Committee on Infectious Diseases. Screening for tuberculosis in infants and children. Pediatrics 1994;93:131-134.

American Academy of Pediatrics, Committee on Infectious Diseases. Update on tuberculosis skin testing of children. Pediatrics 1996;97:282-284.

American Thoracic Society. Treatment of tuberculosis and tuberculosis infection in adults and children. Am J Respir Crit Care Med 1994;144:1359-1374.

Aznar J, Safi H, Romero J, et al. Nosocomial transmission of tuberculosis infection in pediatric wards. Pediatr Infect Dis J 1995;14:44-48.

Barnes PF. The influence of epidemiologic factors on drug resistance rates in tuberculosis. Am Rev Respir Dis 1987;136: 325-328.

Barnes PF, Bloch AB, Davidson PT, et al. Tuberculosis in patients with human immunodeficiency virus infection. N Engl J Med 1991;324:1644-1650.

Barry MA, Shirley L, Grady MT, et al. Tuberculosis infection in urban adolescents: results of a school-based testing program. Am J Public Health 1990;80:439-441.

Bavadekan AV. Osteoarticular tuberculosis in children. Prog Pediatr Surg 1982;15:131-151.

Beaudry PH, Brickman HF, Wise MB. Liver enzyme disturbances during isoniazid chemophylaxis in children. Am Rev Respir Dis 1974;110:581-584.

Bellin EY, Fletcher DD, Safyer SM. Association of tuberculosis infection with increased time in or admission to the New York City jail system. JAMA 1993;269:2228-2231.

Beyers N, Gie R, Schaaf H, et al. Delay in the diagnosis, notification, and initiation of treatment and compliance in children with tuberculosis. Tubercle Lung Dis 1994;75:260-265.

Bhansali SK. Abdominal tuberculosis: experience with 300 cases. Am J Gastroenterol 1977;67:324-337.

Biddulph J. Short-course chemotherapy for childhood tuberculosis. Pediatr Infect Dis J 1990;9:794-801.

Bloch A, Cauthen G, Onorato I, et al. Nationwide survey of drug-resistant tuberculosis in the United States. JAMA 1994;271:665-671.

Blumberg HM, Watkins DL, Berschling JD, et al. Preventing the nosocomial transmission of tuberculosis. Ann Intern Med 1995;122:658-663.

Brailey ME. Tuberculosis in white and negro children. II. The epidemiologic aspects of the Harriet Lane study. Cambridge, Mass: Harvard University Press, 1958.

British Thoracic Society. A controlled trial of 6 months' therapy in pulmonary tuberculosis, final report: results during the 36 months after the end of chemotherapy and beyond. Br J Dis Chest 1984;78:330-336.

Brudney K, Dobkin J. Resurgent tuberculosis in New York City: human immunodeficiency virus, homelessness, and the decline of tuberculosis control programs. Am Rev Respir Dis 1991;144:745-749.

Byrd RB, Horn BR, Solomon DA, et al. Toxic effects of isoniazid in tuberculous chemoprophylaxis: role of biochemical monitoring in 1000 patients. JAMA 1979;241:1239-1241.

Cantwell M, Shehab Z, Costello A, et al. Brief report: congenital tuberculosis. N Engl J Med 1994;330:1051-1054.

Cantwell M, Snider DE Jr, Cauthern G, et al. Epidemiology of tuberculosis in the United States, 1985 through 1992. JAMA 1994;272:535-539.

Centers for Disease Control. Initial therapy for tuberculosis in the era of multidrug resistance. MMWR 1993;42(RR-7):1-8.

Centers for Disease Control. Guidelines for preventing the transmission of *Mycobacterium tuberculosis* in health-care facilities, 1994. MMWR 1994;43(RR-13):1-133.

Centers for Disease Control. Screening for tuberculosis and tuberculosis infection in high-risk populations. MMWR 1995;44(RR-11):19-34.

Centers for Disease Control. The role of BCG vaccine in the prevention and control of tuberculosis in the United States: a joint statement by the Advisory Council for the Elimination of Tuberculosis and the Advisory Committee on Immunization Practices. MMWR 1996;45(RR-4):1-18.

Chan S, Abadco D, Steiner P. Role of flexible fiberoptic bronchoscopy in the diagnosis of childhood endobronchial tuberculosis. Pediatr Infect Dis J 1994;13:506-509.

Chan SP, Birnbaum J, Rao M. Clinical manifestation and outcome of tuberculosis in children with acquired immunodeficiency syndrome. Pediatr Infect Dis J 1996;15:443-447.

Chaulk CP, Moore-Rice K, Rizzo R, et al. Eleven years of community-based directly observed therapy for tuberculosis. JAMA 1995;274:945-951.

Chavalittamvong B, Talalak P. Tuberculosis peritonitis in children. Prog Pediatr Surg 1982;15:161-167.

Cheng TL, Ottolin M, Getson P, et al. Poor validity of parent reading of skin test induration in a high-risk population. Pediatr Infect Dis J 1996;15:90-91.

Cohn DL, Catlin BJ, Peterson KC, et al. A 62-dose, 6-month therapy for pulmonary and extrapulmonary tuberculosis. Ann Intern Med 1990;112:407-415.

Colditz G, Berkey CS, Mosteller F, et al. The efficacy of bacillus Calmette-Gúerin vaccination of newborns and infants in the prevention of tuberculosis: meta-analysis of the published literature. Pediatrics 1995;96:29-35.

Colditz G, Brewer T, Berkey C, et al. Efficacy of BCG vaccine in the prevention of tuberculosis: meta-analysis of the published literature. JAMA 1994;271:698-702.

Comstock GW, Baum C, Snider DE Jr. Isoniazid prophylaxis among Alaskan Eskimos: final report of the Bethel isoniazid studies. Am Rev Respir Dis 1979;119:827-830.

Comstock GW, Edwards LB, Nabangxang H. Tuberculin sensitivity eight to fifteen years after BCG vaccination. Am Rev Respir Dis 1971;103:572-575.

Cuneo WD, Snider DE Jr. Enhancing patient compliance with tuberculosis therapy. Clin Chest Med 1989;10:375-380.

Curless RG, Mitchell CD. Central nervous system tuberculosis in children. Pediatr Neurol 1991;7:270-274.

Daly JF, Brown DS, Lincoln EM, et al. Endobronchial tuberculosis in children. Dis Chest 1952;22:380-398.

Dandapat MC, Mishra BM, Dash SP, et al. Peripheral lymph node tuberculosis: review of 80 cases. Br J Surg 1990;77:911-912.

Daniel T, Debanne S. The serodiagnosis of tuberculosis and other mycobacterial diseases by enzyme-linked immunosorbent assay. Am Rev Respir Dis 1987;135:1137-1151.

Dannenberg AM Jr. Delayed-type hypersensitivity and cell-mediated immunity in the pathogenesis of tuberculosis. Immunol Today 1991;12:228-234.

de Blic J, Azevedo I, Burren C, et al. The value of flexible bronchoscopy in childhood pulmonary tuberculosis. Chest 1991; 100:188-192.

Delacourt C, Gobin J, Gaillard J, et al. Value of ELISA using antigen 60 for the diagnosis of tuberculosis in children. Chest 1993;104:393-398.

Delacourt C, Mani TM, Bonnerot V, et al. Computed tomography with normal chest radiograph in tuberculous infection. Arch Dis Child 1993;69:430-432.

Delacourt C, Poveda JD, Chur̀ean C, et al. Use of polymerase chain reaction for improved diagnosis of tuberculosis in children. J Pediatr 1995;126:703-709.

Doerr CA, Starke JR, Ong LT. Clinical and public health aspects of tuberculous meningitis in children. J Pediatr 1995;127:27-33.

Donald PR, Seifart H. Cerebrospinal fluid pyrazinamide concentrations in children with tuberculous meningitis. Pediatr Infect Dis J 1988;7:469-471.

Donald PR, Seifart HI. Cerebrospinal fluid concentrations of ethionamide in children with tuberculous meningitis. J Pediatr 1989;115:483-486.

Dormer BA, Harrison I, Swart JA, et al. Prophylactic isoniazid protection of infants in a tuberculosis hospital. Lancet 1959; 2:902-903.

Dunlap NE, Harris RH, Benjamin WH Jr, et al. Laboratory contamination of *Mycobacterium tuberculosis* cultures. Am J Respir Crit Care Med 1995;152:1702-1704.

Dutt AK, Moers D, Stead WW. Short-course chemotherapy for extrapulmonary tuberculosis. Ann Intern Med 1986;107:7-12.

Ehrlich RM, Lattimer J. Urogenital tuberculosis in children. J Urol 1971;105:461-465.

Eisenach KD, Sifford MD, Cave MD, et al. Detection of *Mycobacterium tuberculosis* in sputum samples using a polymerase chain reaction. Am Rev Respir Dis 1991;144:1160-1163.

Excobar JA, Belsey MA, Dueñas A, et al. Mortality from tuberculous meningitis reduced by steroid therapy. Pediatrics 1975;56:1050-1055.

Ferrebee SH. Controlled chemoprophylaxis trials in tuberculosis: a general review. Adv Tuberc Res 1969;17:28-106.

Frieden TR, Sterling T, Pablos-Mendez A, et al. The emergence of drug-resistant tuberculosis in New York City. N Engl J Med 1993;328:521-526.

George RH, Gully PR, Gill ON, et al. An outbreak of tuberculosis in a children's hospital. J Hosp Infect 1986;8:129-142.

Girgis NI, Fariz Z, Kilpatrick ME, et al. Dexamethasone adjunctive treatment for tuberculous meningitis. Pediatr Infect Dis J 1991;10:179-182.

Goble M, Iseman MD, Madsen LA, et al. Treatment of 171 patients with pulmonary tuberculosis resistant to isoniazid and rifampin. N Engl J Med 1993;328:527-532.

Gonzalez B, Moreno S, Burdach R, et al. Clinical presentation of bacillus Calmette-Gúerin infections in patients with immunodeficiency syndromes. Pediatr Infect Dis J 1989;8:201-206.

Graziani AL, MacGregor RR. Self-reading of tuberculin testing vs physician reading. Infect Dis Clin Pract 1995;4:72-74.

Gutman L, Moye J, Zimmer B, et al. Tuberculosis in human immunodeficiency virus-exposed or -infected United States children. Pediatr Infect Dis J 1994;13:963-968.

Hageman J, Shulman S, Schreiber M, et al. Congenital tuberculosis: critical reappraisal of clinical findings and diagnostic procedures. Pediatrics 1980;66:980-984.

Harris VJ, Dida F, Landers SS, et al. Cavitary tuberculosis in children. J Pediatr 1977;90:660-661.

Haygood T, Williamson S. Radiographic findings of extremity tuberculosis in childhood: back to the future? Radiographics 1994;14:561-570.

Hoffman ND, Kelly C, Futterman D. Tuberculosis infection in human immunodeficiency virus–positive adolescents and young adults: a New York City cohort. Pediatrics 1996; 97:198-203.

Hoge C, Fisher L, Donnell D, et al. Risk factors for transmission of *Mycobacterium tuberculosis* in a primary school outbreak: lack of racial difference in susceptibility to infection. Am J Epidemiol 1994;139:520-530.

Hong Kong Chest Service/British Medical Research Council. Controlled trial of 2, 4, and 6 months of pyrazinamide in 6-month, three-times-weekly regimens for smear-positive pulmonary tuberculosis, including an assessment of a combined preparation of isoniazid, rifampin, and pyrazinamide: results at 30 months. Am Rev Respir Dis 1991;143:700-706.

Howard TP, Soloman DA. Reading the tuberculin skin test: who, when, and how? Arch Intern Med 1988;148:2457-2459.

Hsu KHK. Contact investigation: a practical approach to tuberculosis eradication. Am J Public Health 1963;53:1761-769.

Hsu KHK. Tuberculin reaction in children treated with isoniazid. Am J Dis Child 1983;137:1090-1092.

Hsu KHK. Thirty years after isoniazid: its impact on tuberculosis in children and adolescents. JAMA 1984;251:1283-1285.

Huebner RE, Schein MF, Bass JB. The tuberculin skin test. Clin Infect Dis 1993;17:968-975.

Hugo-Hamman CT, Scher H, DeMoor MMA. Tuberculous pericarditis in children: a review of 44 cases. Pediatr Infect Dis J 1994;13:13-18.

Humphries MJ, Teoh R, Lau J, et al. Factors of prognostic significance in Chinese children with tuberculous meningitis. Tubercle 1990;71:161-168.

Hussey G, Chisolm T, Kibel M. Miliary tuberculosis in children: a review of 94 cases. Pediatr Infect Dis J 1991;10:832-836.

Hussey G, Kibel M, Parker N. Ciprofloxacin treatment of multiply drug-resistant extrapulmonary tuberculosis in a child. Pediatr Infect Dis J 1992;11:408-409.

International Union Against Tuberculosis Committee on Prophylaxis. Efficacy of various durations of isoniazid preventive therapy for tuberculosis: five years of follow-up in the IUAT trial. Bull World Health Organ 1982;160:555-564.

Iseman MD. Treatment of multidrug-resistant tuberculosis. N Engl J Med 1993;329:784-791.

Iseman MD, Cohn DL, Sbarbaro JA. Directly observed treatment of tuberculosis: we can't afford not to try it. N Engl J Med 1993;328:576-578.

Iseman MD, Madsen L, Goble M, et al. Surgical intervention in the treatment of pulmonary disease caused by drug-resistant *Mycobacterium tuberculosis.* Am Rev Respir Dis 1990; 141: 623-625.

Jacobs RF, Sunakorn P, Chotpitayasunonah T, et al. Intensive short-course chemotherapy for tuberculous meningitis. Pediatr Infect Dis J 1992;11:194-198.

Jagannath C, Reddy MV, Kailasam S, et al. Chemotherapeutic activity of clofazamine and its analogues against *Mycobacterium tuberculosis.* Am J Respir Crit Care Med 1995; 151:1083-1086.

Jawahar MS, Sivasubramanian S, Vijayan VK, et al. Short-course chemotherapy for tuberculous lymphadenitis in children. Br Med J 1990;301:359-362.

Jones D, Malecki J, Bigler W, et al. Pediatric tuberculosis and human immunodeficiency virus infection in Palm Beach County, Florida. Am J Dis Child 1992;146:1166-1170.

Kendig EL Jr. The place of BCG vaccine in the management of infants born to tuberculous mothers. N Engl J Med 1969; 281:520-523.

Kendig EL Jr, Rodgers WL. Tuberculosis in the neonatal period. Am Rev Tuberc Pulm Dis 1958;77:418-422.

Kennedy N, Fox R, Kisyombe GM, et al. Early bactericidal and sterilizing activities of ciprofloxacin in pulmonary tuberculosis. Am Rev Respir Dis 1993;148:1547-1551.

Khan EA, Starke JR. Diagnosis of tuberculosis in children: increased need for better methods. Emerg Infect Dis 1995; 1:115-123.

Khouri Y, Mastrucci M, Hutto C, et al. *Mycobacterium tuberculosis* in children with human immunodeficiency virus type 1 infection. Pediatr Infect Dis J 1992;11:950-955.

Kimmerling ME, Vaughn ES, Dunlap NE. Childhood tuberculosis in Alabama: epidemiology of disease and indicators of program effectiveness, 1983 to 1993. Pediatr Infect Dis J 1995;14:678-684.

Kochi A. The global tuberculosis situation and the new control strategy of the World Health Organization. Tubercle Lung Dis 1991;72:1-6.

Kohn MR, Arden MR, Vasilakis J, et al. Directly observed preventive therapy: turning the tide against tuberculosis. Arch Pediatr Adolesc Med 1996;150:727-729.

Kumar L, Dhand R, Singhi PD, et al. A randomized trial of fully intermittent vs daily followed by intermittent short-course chemotherapy for childhood tuberculosis. Pediatr Infect Dis J 1990;9:802-806.

Kumar A, Misra PK, Mehotra R, et al. Hepatotoxicity of rifampin and isoniazid: is it all drug-induced hepatitis? Am Rev Respir Dis 1991;143:1350-1352.

Lange WR, Warnock-Eckhart E, Bean ME. *Mycobacterium tuberculosis* infection in foreign-born adoptees. Pediatr Infect Dis J 1989;8:625-629.

Lee C, Wang W, Lan R, et al. Corticosteroids in the treatment of tuberculous pleurisy: a double-blind, placebo-controlled randomized study. Chest 1988;94:1256-1259.

Leggiadro RJ, Collery B, Dowdy S. Outbreak of tuberculosis in a family day-care home. Pediatr Infect Dis J 1989;8:52-54.

Leiguarda R, Berthier M, Starkstein S, et al. Ischemic infarction in 25 children with tuberculous meningitis. Stroke 1988;19:200-204.

Light IJ, Saidleman M, Sutherland JM. Management of newborns after nursery exposure to tuberculosis. Am Rev Respir Dis 1974;109:415-419.

Lincoln EM. Epidemics of tuberculosis. Adv Tuberc Res 1965;14:159-197.

Lincoln EM, Davies PA, Bovornkitti S. Tuberculous pleurisy with effusion in children. Am Rev Tuberc 1958;77:271-289.

Lincoln EM, Gilbert L, Morales SM. Chronic pulmonary tuberculosis in individuals with known previous primary tuberculosis. Dis Chest 1960;38:473-482.

Lincoln EM, Harris LC, Bovornkitti S, et al. Endobronchial tuberculosis in children. Am Rev Tuberc Pulm Dis 1958;77: 39-61.

Lindgren I. Pathology of tuberculous infection in BCG-vaccinated humans. Adv Tuberc Res 1965;14:203-231.

MacAdam AM, Rubio T. Tuberculous otomastoiditis in children. Am J Dis Child 1977;131:152-156.

Mahmoudi A, Iseman M. Pitfalls in the care of patients with tuberculosis: common errors and their association with the acquisition of drug resistance. JAMA 1993;270:65-68.

Mancao MY, Nolte FS, Nahmias AJ, et al. Use of polymerase chain reaction for diagnosis of tuberculous meningitis. Pediatr Infect Dis J 1994;13:154-155.

Martinez-Roig A, Cami J, Llorens-Terol J, et al. Acetylation phenotype and hepatotoxicity in the treatment of tuberculosis in children. Pediatrics 1986;77:912-915.

Matsaniotis N, Kattanis C, Economou-Mavrou C, et al. Bullous emphysema in childhood tuberculosis. J Pediatr 1967; 71:703-708.

McKenna MT, McCray E, Onorato IM. The epidemiology of tuberculosis among foreign-born persons in the United States, 1986 to 1993. N Engl J Med 1995;332:1071-1076.

McKenzie SA, McNab AJ, Katz G. Neonatal pyridoxine responsive convulsions due to isoniazid therapy. Arch Dis Child 1976;51:567-568.

Medical Research Council Working Party on Tuberculosis of the Spine. Twelfth report: controlled trial of short-course regimens of chemotherapy in the ambulatory treatment of spinal tuberculosis. J Bone Joint Surg 1993;75(B):240-248.

Mehta JB, Bentley S. Prevention of tuberculosis in children: missed opportunities. Am J Prev Med 1992;8:283-286.

Menzies R, Vissandjee B. Effect of bacille Calmette-Gúerin vaccination on tuberculin reactivity. Am Rev Respir Dis 1992;141:621-625.

Migliori GB, Borghesi A, Rossanigo P, et al. Proposal of an improved score method for the diagnosis of pulmonary tuberculosis in childhood in developing countries. Tubercle Lung Dis 1992;73:145-149.

Mitchison DA, Nunn AJ. Influence of initial drug resistance on the response to short-course chemotherapy of pulmonary tuberculosis. Am Rev Respir Dis 1986;133:423-428.

Mohle-Boetani JC, Miller B, Halpern M, et al. School-based screening for tuberculous infection: a cost benefit analysis. JAMA 1995;274:613-619.

Morrison JB. Natural history of segmental lesions in primary pulmonary tuberculosis. Arch Dis Child 1973;48:90-98.

Mumtaz MA, Schwartz RH, Grundfast KM, et al. Tuberculosis of the middle ear and mastoid. Pediatr Infect Dis 1983;2:234-236.

Nemir RL, Cardona J, Vaziri F, et al. Prednisone as an adjunct in the chemotherapy of lymph node–bronchial tuberculosis in childhood: a double-blind study. II. Further term observation. Am Rev Respir Dis 1967;95:402-410.

Nemir RL, O'Hare D. Congenital tuberculosis. Am J Dis Child 1985;139:284-287.

Nemir RL, Teichner A. Management of tuberculin reactors in children and adolescents previously vaccinated with BCG. Pediatr Infect Dis 1983;2:446-451.

Nolan R Jr. Childhood tuberculosis in North Carolina: a study of the opportunities for intervention in the transmis-sion of tuberculosis in children. Am J Public Health 1986;76:26-30.

O'Brien K, Ruff A, Louis M, et al. Bacillus Calmette-Gúerin complications in children born to HIV-1–infected women with a review of the literature. Pediatrics 1995;95:414-418.

O'Brien RJ, Long MW, Cross FS, et al. Hepatotoxicity from isoniazid and rifampin among children treated for tuberculosis. Pediatrics 1983;72:491-499.

Offenbacher H, Fazekas F, Schmidt R, et al. MRI in tuberculous meningoencephalitis: report of four cases and review of the neuroimaging literature. J Neurol 1991;238:340-344.

Optican RJ, Ost A, Ravin CE. High-resolution computed tomography in the diagnosis of miliary tuberculosis. Chest 1992;102:941-943.

Orme IM, Anderson P, Boom WH. T-cell response to *Mycobacterium tuberculosis*. J Infect Dis 1993;167:1481-1497.

Palur R, Rajohekhar V, Chandy MJ, et al. Shunt surgery for hydrocephalus in tuberculous meningitis: a long-term follow-up study. J Neurosurg 1991;74:64-69.

Parish RE, Brownstein D. Emergency department management of children with acute isoniazid poisoning. Pediatr Emerg Care 1986;2:88-90.

Park MM, Davis AL, Schluger NW, et al. Outcome of MDR-TB patients, 1983-1993: prolonged survival with appropriate therapy. Am J Respir Crit Care Med 1996;153:317-324.

Passannante M, Gallagher C, Reichman L. Preventive therapy for contacts of multidrug-resistant tuberculosis: a Delphi study. Chest 1994;106:431-434.

Pellock JM, Howell J, Kendig EL Jr, et al. Pyridoxine deficiency in children treated with isoniazid. Chest 1985;87:658-661.

Peloquin CA, MacPhee AA, Berning SE. Malabsorption of antimycobacterial medications. N Engl J Med 1993;329:1122-1123.

Perry S, Starke JR. Adherence to prescribed treatment and public health aspects of tuberculosis in children. Semin Pediatr Infect Dis 1993;4:291-298.

Pierre C, Olivier C, Lecossier D, et al. Diagnosis of primary tuberculosis in children by amplification and detection of mycobacterial DNA. Am Rev Respir Dis 1993;147:420-424.

Pineda P, Leung A, Muller N, et al. Intrathoracic pediatric tuberculosis: a report of 202 cases. Tubercle Lung Dis 1993;74:261-266.

Raviglione MC, Snider D Jr, Kochi A. Global epidemiology of tuberculosis: morbidity and mortality of a worldwide epidemic. JAMA 1995;273:220-226.

Reynes J, Perez C, Lamaury I, et al. Bacille Calmette-Gúerin adenitis 30 years after immunization in a patient with AIDS. J Infect Dis 1989;160:727.

Ryder RW, Oxtoby MJ, Mvula M, et al. Safety and immunogenicity of bacille Calmette-Gúerin, diptheria-tetanus-pertussis, and oral polio vaccines in newborn children in Zaire infected with human immunodeficiency virus type 1. J Pediatr 1993;122:697-702.

Sada E, Aguilar D, Torres M, et al. Detection of lipoarabinomannan as a diagnostic test for tuberculosis. J Clin Microbiol 1992;30:2415-2418.

Schaaf HS, Beyers N, Gie RP, et al. Respiratory tuberculosis in childhood: the diagnostic value of clinical features and special investigations. Pediatr Infect Dis J 1995;14:189-194.

Schaaf HS, Gie RP, Beyers N, et al. Tuberculosis in infants less than 3 months of age. Arch Dis Child 1993;69:371-374.

Schick B, Dolgin J. The influence of prednisone on the Mantoux reaction in children. Pediatrics 1963;31:856-859.

Schuit KE. Miliary tuberculosis in children. Am J Dis Child 1979;133:583-585.

Schuit KE, Powell DA. Mycobacterial lymphadenitis in childhood. Am J Dis Child 1978;132:675-677.

Selwyn P, Hartel D, Lewis V, et al. A prospective study of the risk of tuberculosis among intravenous drug users with human immunodeficiency virus infection. N Engl J Med 1989;320:545-550.

Sepulveda RL, Burr C, Ferrer X, et al. Booster effect of tuberculosis testing in healthy 6-year-old schoolchildren vaccinated with bacille Calmette-Gúerin at birth in Santiago, Chile. Pediatr Infect Dis J 1988;7:578-582.

Shah BR, Santucci K, Sinert R, et al. Acute isoniazid neurotoxicity in an urban hospital. Pediatrics 1995;95:700-704.

Shepard WE, Field ML, James DH, et al. Transient appearance of intracranial tuberculomas during treatment of tuberculous meningitis. Pediatr Infect Dis J 1986;5:599-601.

Small P, Hopewell P, Singh S, et al. The epidemiology of tuberculosis in San Francisco: a population-based study using conventional and molecular methods. N Engl J Med 1994;330:1703-1709.

Small PM, Shafer RW, Hopewell PC, et al. Exogenous reinfection with multidrug-resistant *Mycobacterium tuberculosis* in patients with advanced HIV infection. N Engl J Med 1993;328:1137-1144.

Smith AM, Lattimer JK. Genitourinary tract involvement in children with tuberculosis. NY State J Med 1973;73:2325-2328.

Smith KC, Starke JR, Eisenach K, et al. Detection of *Mycobacterium tuberculosis* in clinical specimens from children using a polymerase chain reaction. Pediatrics 1996;97:155-160.

Smith MHD. The role of adrenal steroids in the treatment of tuberculosis. Pediatrics 1958;22:774-776.

Snider DE Jr, Caras GJ. Isoniazid-associated hepatitis deaths: a review of available information. Am Rev Respir Dis 1992; 145:494-497.

Snider DE Jr, Caras GJ, Kaplan JP. Preventive therapy with isoniazid: cost-effectiveness of different durations of therapy. JAMA 1986;255:1579-1583.

Snider DE, Graczyk J, Bek E, et al. Supervised six-months treatment of newly diagnosed pulmonary tuberculosis using isoniazid, rifampin, and pyrazinamide with and without streptomycin. Am Rev Respir Dis 1984;130:1091-1094.

Snider DE Jr, Johnson KE. Should women taking antituberculosis drugs breastfeed? Arch Intern Med 1984;144:589-590.

Snider DE Jr, Kelly GD, Cauthen GM, et al. Infection and disease among contacts of tuberculosis cases with drug-resistant and drug-susceptible bacilli. Am Rev Respir Dis 1985; 132:125-128.

Starke JR. Current chemotherapy for tuberculosis in children. Infect Dis Clin N Amer 1992;6:215-238.

Starke JR, Correa AG. Management of mycobacterial infection and disease in children. Pediatr Infect Dis J 1995;14:455-470.

Starke JR, Jacobs R, Jereb J. Resurgence of tuberculosis in children. J Pediatr 1992;120:839-855.

Starke JR, Taylor-Watts KT. Tuberculosis in the pediatric population of Houston, Texas. Pediatrics 1989;84:28-35.

Steiner P, Rao M. Drug-resistant tuberculosis in children. Semin Pediatr Infect Dis 1993;4:275-282.

Steiner P, Rao M, Mitchell M. Primary drug-resistant tuberculosis in children: correlation of drug-susceptibility patterns of matched patient and source-case strains of *Mycobacterium tuberculosis*. Am J Dis Child 1985;139:780-782.

Steiner P, Rao M, Victoria MS, et al. Miliary tuberculosis in two infants after nursery exposure: epidemiologic, clinical, and laboratory findings. Am Rev Respir Dis 1976;113:267-271.

Steiner P, Rao M, Victoria MS, et al. Persistently negative tuberculin reactions: their presence among children culture-positive for *Mycobacterium tuberculosis*. Am J Dis Child 1980; 134:747-750.

Stransberry SD. Tuberculosis in infants and children. J Thorac Imag 1990;5:17-27.

Sumartojo E. When tuberculosis treatment fails: a social behavior account of patient adherence. Am Rev Respir Dis 1993;147:1311-1320.

Swanson DS, Starke JR. Drug-resistant tuberculosis in pediatrics. Pediatr Clin North Am 1995;42:553-581.

Teeratkulpisarn J, Lumbigagnon P, Pairojkul S, et al. Cavitary tuberculosis in a young infant. Pediatr Infect Dis J 1994; 13:545-546.

Telenti A, Imboden P, Marchesi F, et al. Detection of rifampin-resistance mutations in *Mycobacterium tuberculosis*. Lancet 1993;341:647-650.

Telzak EE, Sepkowitz K, Alpert P, et al. Multidrug-resistant tuberculosis in patients without HIV infection. N Engl J Med 1995;333:907-911.

Teoh R, Humphries MJ, O'Mahony G. Symptomatic intracranial tuberculoma developing during treatment of tuberculosis: report of 10 patients and review of the literature. QJM 1987;63:449-460.

Thompson WJ, Glassroth JL, Snider DE Jr, et al. The booster phenomenon in serial tuberculin testing. Am Rev Respir Dis 1979;119:587-597.

Tsakalidis D, Pratsidou P, Hitoglou-Makedou A, et al. Intensive short-course chemotherapy for treatment of Greek children with tuberculosis. Pediatr Infect Dis J 1992;11:1036-1042.

Turneer M, VanNerom E, Nyabenda J, et al. Determination of humoral immunoglobulins M and G directed against mycobacterial antigen 60 failed to diagnose primary tuberculosis and mycobacterial adenitis in children. Am J Respir Crit Care Med 1994;150;1508-1512.

Ussery XT, Valway SE, McKenna M, et al. Epidemiology of tuberculosis among children in the United States. Pediatr Infect Dis J 1996;15:697-704.

Vallejo J, Ong L, Starke JR. Clinical features, diagnosis, and treatment of tuberculosis in infants. Pediatrics 1994;94:1-7.

Vallejo J, Ong L, Starke JR. Tuberculous osteomyelitis of the long bones in children. Pediatr Infect Dis J 1995;14:542-546.

Vallejo JG, Starke JR. Tuberculosis and pregnancy. Clin Chest Med 1992;13:693-707.

Vanderhoof JA, Ament ME. Fatal hepatic necrosis due to isoniazid chemoprophylaxis in a 15-year-old girl. J Pediatr 1976;88:867-868.

Waeker NJ Jr, Connor JD. Central nervous system tuberculosis in children: a review of 30 cases. Pediatr Infect Dis J 1990;9:539-543.

Wallace RC, Burton EM, Barrett FF, et al. Intracranial tuberculosis in children: CT appearance and clinical outcome. Pediatr Radiol 1991;21:241-246.

Wallgren A. On contagiousness of childhood tuberculosis. Acta Paediatr 1937;22:229-234.

Weinstein J, Barrett C, Baltimore R, et al. Nosocomial transmission of tuberculosis from a hospital visitor on a pediatrics ward. Pediatr Infect Dis J 1995;14:232-234.

Weis S, Slocum P, Blais F, et al. The effects of directly observed therapy on the rates of drug resistance and relapse in tuberculosis. N Engl J Med 1994;330:1179-1184.

Whalen C, Horsburgh C, Hom D, et al. Accelerated course of human immunodeficiency virus infection after tuberculosis. Am J Respir Crit Care Med 1995;151:129-135.

Zhang Y. Genetic basis of isoniazid resistance of *Mycobacterium tuberculosis*. Rev Microbiol 1993;144:143-150.

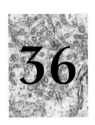

36 URINARY TRACT INFECTIONS

KEITH M. KRASINSKI

The term *urinary tract infection* (UTI) refers to a clinical entity that may involve the urethra; bladder (lower urinary tract); and the ureters, renal pelvis, calyces, and renal parenchyma (upper urinary tract). Urethritis as a clinical entity is discussed in Chapter 28.

Because it is often impossible to localize the infection to either the lower tract or the upper tract, UTI is a convenient designation. Most bacterial UTIs are characterized by the presence of significant numbers of bacteria in the urine.

The designation *significant bacteriuria* refers to the number of bacteria in excess of the usual bacterial contamination of the anterior urethra. The presence of more than 100,000 bacteria per milliliter of urine in a clean voided specimen probably is the result of infection, not contamination at the time of voiding. Asymptomatic bacteriuria is defined as significant bacteriuria in a patient who has no clinical evidence of active infection.

Lower UTI is usually characterized by dysuria, frequency, urgency, and possibly suprapubic tenderness. The clinical manifestations of acute pyelonephritis may include fever, lumbar pain and tenderness, dysuria, urgency, and frequency associated with significant bacteriuria.

Recurrence of a UTI may be caused by a relapse or a reinfection. A relapse is a recurrence of the infection with the same infecting microorganism, perhaps indicating inadequate therapy. A reinfection is a new infection caused by a bacterium that is different from the one responsible for the previous episode. Specific identification may require serotyping, pyocin typing, phage typing, or antibiotic typing of the bacterium (e.g., *Escherichia coli*), procedures that are not uniformly available to the clinician. These identification techniques may also be useful for associating individual incidents with hospital outbreaks of infection. The term *chronic infection* is sometimes used to describe (1) persistence of the UTI associated with the same organism for many months or years, or (2) frequent recurrences over many months or years.

ETIOLOGY

Some of the microorganisms that cause UTIs include the following:
Gram-negative bacteria
    E. coli
    Klebsiella pneumoniae
    Proteus mirabilis
    Enterobacter aerogenes
    Pseudomonas aeruginosa
    Serratia marcescens
    Salmonella species
    Haemophilus influenzae
    Gardnerella vaginalis
Gram-positive bacteria
    Staphylococcus epidermidis
    Enterococcus spp.
    Staphylococcus aureus
    Staphylococcus saprophyticus
    Streptococcus pneumoniae
Other agents
    Adenovirus types 11 and 21
    BK virus
    Candida albicans
    Mycoplasma hominis
    Ureaplasma urealyticum
    Mycobacterium tuberculosis
    Schistosoma hematobium

The most common pathogens are the gram-negative bacilli. Of this group, *E. coli* is responsible for most acute infections. The other gram-negative bacteria—such as *Proteus, Pseudomonas, Klebsiella,* and *Enterobacter* species—are more likely to be associated with chronic or recurrent infections. *Salmonella bacteriuria* is usually associated with salmonellal sepsis.

Gram-positive bacteria such as *S. epidermidis, S. saprophyticus,* and *S. aureus* have been identified as causes of UTIs. Coagulase-negative staphylococci have been detected as urinary tract pathogens in sexually active young women (Bailey, 1973; Vosti, 1975) and newborns (Khan et al., 1975). Coagulase-positive staphylococci may invade the urinary tract through the hematogenous route.

Adenovirus types 11 and 21 and the human papovavirus BK have been reported as causes of acute hemorrhagic cystitis (Hashida et al., 1976; Mufson and Belshe, 1976; Padgett et al., 1987; Rice et al., 1985). Symptomatic and asymptomatic BK viruria is associated with bone marrow transplantation. Fungi such as *C. albicans* may be responsible for UTIs (1) in patients with indwelling catheters during the course of their treatment with antibiotics; (2) in patients immunocompromised as a result of disease, steroids, or cytotoxic chemotherapy; and (3) as a result of renal seeding during fungemia.

PATHOGENESIS

The ascending route is the most common pathway of urinary tract infection. Bacteria that colonize the perineum and distal urethra may eventually spread to the bladder. Massage of the urethra such as occurs during masturbation and sexual intercourse forces bacteria into the bladder (Bran et al., 1972; Buckley et al., 1978). Hematogenous spread may occur during the course of neonatal sepsis; however, even in infants, ascending infection leading to bacteremia is more common. Lymphatic spread has been suggested, but it has not been proved (Murphy et al., 1960).

In older children and adolescents with staphylococcal sepsis or endocarditis, hematogenous spread to the kidney may result in abscess formation. Abscesses also result from infection ascending via the collecting system, followed by renal seeding and localized liquefaction. This condition has been termed *lobar nephronia*. Intrarenal suppurative necrosis is most evident in the cortex when it occurs; however, abscesses also occur in the medulla. The natural methods of extension include rupture into the renal pelvis and extension through the renal capsule, producing a perinephric (perirenal) abscess.

The pathogenesis of a UTI is dependent in great part on factors associated with both the microorganism and the host. The following virulence factors of microorganisms are associated with UTIs:

1. Size of inoculum
2. Pili (mucosal cell adherence)
   a. Mannose-sensitive type 1, common
   b. P pili
   c. X pili
3. Surface antigens
4. Motility
5. Urease production

Microorganism

Experimental studies in mice have revealed that the greater the number of organisms delivered to the kidney the greater the chance of inducing pyelonephritis (Gorrill and De Navasquez, 1964). Thus the size of the inoculum is an important factor. Evidence accumulated during the course of studies by Gruneberg et al. (1968) and by Kaijser (1973) indicates that certain organisms apparently are particularly virulent for the urinary tract. Of the 150 or more *E. coli* O serogroups, only a few (01, 02, 04, 06, 07, 075) have been responsible for most UTIs, and these especially include those that possess large quantities of K antigen. *E. coli* K antigen types 11, 24, 36, and 37 account for the majority of isolates from children with pyelonephritis (Kaijser et al., 1977).

E. coli O antigens are cell-wall lipopolysaccharides that are immunogenic and induce local and systemic antibody responses in patients with pyelonephritis. Strains most often associated with pyelonephritis are representatives of eighty antigen groups. The specific O antigens appear to confer the ability to resist agglutination and bactericidal effects of serum, in contrast to the O serotypes of organisms causing cystitis (Lindberg et al., 1975; Smith et al., 1977).

A primary pathogenic factor is the presence of carbohydrate-binding proteins (adhesions, lectins, or hemagglutinins) often localized to pili. Pili are important for the attachment of *E. coli* and *P. mirabilis* to the urinary tract epithelium (Silverblatt, 1974). Almost all *E. coli* contain type 1 common pili that bind to (Ofek et al., 1977) mannose-containing receptors on epithelial cells of the urethra and vagina and are thought to be of primary importance in colonizing the lower urinary tract (Iwahi et al., 1983; Svanborg-Eden et al., 1983). *E. coli* isolates from patients with cystitis have a greater avidity and adhere in higher numbers to uroepithelial cells than do *E. coli* fecal isolates (Svanborg-Eden et al., 1976, 1981). Uropathogenic *E. coli* and *P. mirabilis* are capable of altering their surface composition (phase variation) and tend to lose their type 1 pili on arrival in the kidney (Silverblatt, 1974; Ofek et al., 1981). This ability to adapt to the microenvironment constitutes a selective advantage by promoting renal cell attachment and especially because variation of mannose receptors of type 1 pili allows escape from phagocytosis by polymorphonuclear leukocytes (Perry et al., 1983).

P pili bear an adhesin called *PapG* that causes mannose-resistant hemagglutination and binds to specific Galα 1-4 Gal glycolipid receptor sites on human epithelial cells (Kallenivs et al., 1981; Leffler and Svanborg-Eden, 1981; Svanborg-Eden et al., 1981, 1983; Stromberg et al., 1990). *E. coli* with P pili have their favored site of attachment on the uroepithelium of the kidneys, where receptors are distributed with greatest density (Svanborg-Eden et al., 1976, 1983). UTIs are more likely to occur in persons who express the P blood group antigen (Lindberg et al., 1983).

A third type of pili, X pili, are also capable of binding to uroepithelium. Their receptor sites have not been identified; however, they also have an affinity for the upper urinary tract.

Motility probably also is an important pathogenic factor. Weyrauch and Bassett (1951) have shown that motile bacteria can ascend in the ureter against the flow of the urine. Moreover, the ascent of these bacteria may be facilitated by the decreased ureteral peristalsis attributed to the endotoxin of gram-negative bacilli.

The production of urease by the infecting bacteria may affect their capacity to cause pyelonephritis. When UTI was induced in experimental animals by the retrograde administration of *P. mirabilis,* a urease-producing organism, there was a high degree of correlation between the number of bacteria in the kidney and the extent of renal damage. However, treatment with a urease inhibitor reduced the extent of renal damage and the number of bacteria in the kidney without a significant decrease in the number of bacteria in the urine (Musher et al., 1975).

Host

The known host defense mechanisms of the urinary tract are as follows:

Antibacterial activity of urine
Prostatic secretions of postpubescent males
Flushing mechanisms of the bladder
Low vaginal pH
Estrogen
Antiadherence effect of uromucoid
Antiadherence effect of mucopolysaccharide
Humoral immunity
Local secretory immunity, IgA
Lack of P blood group antigen
Normal flora

The long male urethra, in contrast to the short female urethra, has been implicated as a reason for the disproportionately high female predilection for UTI.

Antibacterial activity of urine against certain bacteria has been described. Kaye (1968) has reported that extremes of osmolality, high urea concentration, low pH, and high concentration of organic acids may inhibit the growth of some bacteria that cause UTIs. However, with the usual range of pH (5.5 to 7.0) and osmolality (300 to 1,200), the rate of growth of *E. coli* has been reported as unaffected (Asscher et al., 1966).

The flushing mechanism of the bladder enhances the spontaneous clearance of bacteria. Voiding and dilution probably play an important role. However, when considering antimicrobial therapy, overhydration can have the negative effect of diluting and washing out the active antimicrobial substances.

In adolescents and adults prostatic fluid may inhibit bacterial growth (Stamey et al., 1968). The role of prostatic secretions in prepubescent males is unknown. The presence of estrogen may enhance the growth of some strains of *E. coli* (Harles et al., 1920). Glucose makes urine a better culture medium, and it inhibits the migrating, adhering, aggregating, and killing functions of polymorphonuclear leukocytes. In addition, the intact mucosal surfaces of animal bladders are resistant to bacterial invasion (Cobbs and Kaye, 1967).

Low vaginal pH apparently is an important factor responsible for lack of colonization (Stamey and Timothy, 1975). For example, serogroups of *E. coli* that usually cause UTIs are more resistant to low pH than serogroups that are less common causes of infection (Stamey and Kaufman, 1975). Similarly, low pH has an inhibitory effect on *P. mirabilis* and *P. aeruginosa* (Stamey and Mihara, 1976). This phenomenon may possibly account for the higher incidence of *E. coli* infection.

Tamm-Horsfall protein is secreted by renal tubular cells and is present in the urine as uromucoid (Orskov et al., 1980). Since uromucoid is rich in mannose residues, it may serve as decoy oligosaccharides that bind, prevent attachment, and allow adequate flushing out of bacteria. This hypothesis has been supported by an animal model in which mannose can prevent colonization (Aronson et al., 1979). Parsons et al. (1975) have demonstrated that an antiadherence mechanism of the bladder (in rabbits) exists by pretreatment of the bladder with dilute hydrochloric acid. Acid-treated bladders had twentyfold to fiftyfold increases of bacterial adherence over controls. Adherence was enhanced by ablation of mucopolysaccharide and glycosaminoglycan from the surface of bladder epithelium (Parsons et al., 1975, 1978). This could result from exposure of additional binding sites. The rapid recovery of protection suggests a secretory component that inhibits binding. Increased adherence apparently is species-specific (Sobel and Vardi, 1982).

It is possible that antibacterial mechanisms are responsible for the rapid disappearance of bacteria applied to bladder mucosa in an experimental model (Vivaldi et al., 1965; Cobbs and Kaye, 1967; Norden et al., 1968); however, the nature of these mechanisms has not been established. Secretory IgA does decrease adherence and colonization of perineal cells by *E. coli* (Stamey et al., 1978) and is increased in children with UTIs (Uehling and Stiehm, 1971).

The role of humoral immunity as a mechanism of the host's defense against UTI has not been satisfactorily clarified. Hanson et al. (1977) reported that acute *E. coli* pyelonephritis induced serum antibodies to O antigens but rarely to K antigens. In contrast, increased levels of O antibodies were not detected in sera from patients with cystitis or asymptomatic bacteriuria. Using the sensitive enzyme-linked immunosorbent assay (ELISA), Hanson et al. (1977) found high levels of *E. coli* O antibody in the urine of most patients with acute pyelonephritis, lower levels in those with asymptomatic bacteriuria and cystitis, and minimal or no detectable levels in the urine of healthy children. Serum antibodies to O antigen, K antigen, and type 1 pili have been found in patients with pyelonephritis (Hanson et al., 1977; Mattsby-Baltzer et al., 1982; Rene and Silverblatt, 1982), and IgM is the predominant species detected during acute infections. IgG antibody to the lipid A component of gram-negative rods is also detectable and may be a measure of the severity of renal disease and tissue destruction (Mattsby-Baltzer et al., 1981). A secretory IgA response can also be detected in the urine in both upper- and lower-tract disease (Hopkins et al., 1987).

Animal studies suggest that humoral antibody is protective against ascending infection with organisms expressing P pili and O and K antigens (Mattsby-Baltzer et al., 1982; Kaijser et al., 1983; O'Hanley et al., 1983). The protective effect is mediated by blocking attachment to the uroepithelium of the upper urinary tract (Svanborg-Eden and Svennerholm, 1978). The role of the host's normal perineal flora—lactobacilli, *Staphylococcus epidermidis,* corynebacteria, streptococci, and anaerobes—in preventing colonization with uropathogens is not understood.

A number of factors intrinsic and extrinsic to the host combine to predispose to UTI. They include the following:

Intrinsic
  Obstruction
  Stasis
  Reflux
  Pregnancy
  Sexual intercourse (in females)
  Hyperosmolality of renal medulla
  Host cell receptor sites for attachment
  Immunologic cross-reactivity of bacterial antigen and human protein
  Chronic prostatitis
  B or AB blood type
  Genetic predisposition
  Immunodeficiency
Extrinsic
  Instrumentation (catheters)
  Antimicrobial agents

Probably the single most important host factor affecting the occurrence of UTIs is urinary stasis resulting from obstruction of urinary flow or bladder dysfunction. This predisposing host condition is more frequently observed in the younger patient and should prompt a more timely roentgenographic investigation of the urinary system. The most common causes of stasis include:

  Congenital anomalies of ureter or urethra (valves, stenosis, bands)
  Calculi
  Dysfunctional or incomplete voiding
  Extrinsic ureteral or bladder compression
  Neurogenic bladder (functional obstruction)

Stasis is associated with increased susceptibility to infection.

There is a striking correlation between vesicoureteral reflux and the occurrence of UTIs. Reflux, the retrograde flow of urine into the ureter and kidney, is caused by the incompetence of the normal valvular action of the ureterovesicular junction. It may occur when this area is affected by congenital anatomic defects, disease, or distal obstruction. Reflux tends to perpetuate infection by maintaining a residual pool of infected urine in the bladder after voiding. Children with reflux may develop upper UTIs and renal scarring. Smellie and Normand (1975) have reported that reflux can be detected in 30% to 50% of children with symptomatic or asymptomatic bacteriuria and that the scarred kidney associated with reflux is more susceptible to reinfection.

Physiologic alterations of the urinary tract that increase the likelihood of UTI occur as a result of pregnancy. These changes include decreased bladder and ureteral tone, decreased ureteral peristalsis, hydroureter, and increased residual bladder urine, all of which serve to cause or aggravate obstruction, stasis, and reflux.

Sexual intercourse in females produces transient bacteriuria and is associated with an increased risk of UTI. This is substantiated by the studies of Nicolle et al. (1982) and Pfau et al. (1983), which showed that 80% of UTIs begin within 24 hours of intercourse in sexually active women.

Hyperosmolality of the renal medulla inhibits the migration of polymorphonuclear leukocytes to damaged medullary tissue and decreases phagocytosis of bacteria (Rocha and Fekety, 1964).

Several facts suggest a genetic predisposition to UTI, including the association of blood group P antigen (Lindberg et al., 1983) with blood groups B and AB, that is, those lacking anti-B isohemagglutinin (Kinane et al., 1982). Studies on the occurrence of periurethral or vaginal defects in host defenses have been inconclusive. Women with recurrent UTIs who are ABO nonsecretors have vaginal epithelial cells that have substantially more receptors allowing attachment of uropathogenic *E. coli* (Stapleton et al., 1982). Vesicoureteral reflux can also be an inherited trait; therefore, family history is important.

Adult males with chronic prostatitis are at risk for recurrent urinary tract infections because of intermittent seeding of their urinary bladders.

Finally, there is evidence that chronic interactions of the host's immune system with retained bacterial antigens or mimicking host antigens is responsible for chronic progressive renal damage. Bacterial antigen may not be eradicated and may trigger formation of antigen-antibody complexes (Hanson et al., 1977). Tamm-Horsfall protein antigen can permeate the renal interstitial spaces and evoke an aggressive humoral and cellular immune response (Work and Andriole, 1980; Mayrer et al., 1983). The most aggressive response occurs in persons with vesicoureteral reflux independent of bacteriuria. Furthermore, Tamm-Horsfall protein cross-reacts with gram-negative bacilli (Fasth et al., 1980).

Two important extrinsic host factors, instrumentation and antimicrobial agents, predispose to UTI. This is particularly true in hospitalized patients with indwelling catheters and patients with chronic bladder dysfunction. Catheters produce their damage by eroding the slime layer of the urethra and bladder and by serving as a nidus for intraluminal concretions and bacterial colonization (Rubin, 1980). The pericannular space is not subject to mechanical washing out of bacteria, as is the un-catheterized urethra. Suction ulcers of the bladder mucosa develop at the site of the bladder portal when urinary drainage systems are not properly vented (Monson et al., 1977). Antimicrobial agents apparently have the effect of altering the host's normal perineal flora, allowing easier colonization with uropathogens. In patients with urinary catheters, antibiotics have the effect of shifting colonization to antibiotic-resistant strains (Britt et al., 1977; Butler and Kunin, 1968; Warren et al., 1982, 1983).

PATHOLOGY

Mucosal and submucosal edema and infiltration of the tissue with leukocytes are the prominent histopathologic changes of cystitis. In patients with acute pyelonephritis and upper UTIs the kidney is usually enlarged; its capsular surface is smooth, and the pelvic mucosa may also be involved. The microscopic findings include edema, congestion, polymorphonuclear infiltration of the interstitium, and abscess formation. Tubules may be distended by exudate consisting of leukocytes, bacteria, and debris, occasionally causing necrosis. The medulla is involved to a greater degree than the cortex.

In patients with chronic pyelonephritis the kidney is usually contracted; its surface is scarred, and its capsule is thickened. The calyces and pelvis are fibrotic, and the thickness of the parenchyma is decreased. The glomeruli show evidence of proliferation, crescents, and hyalinization, and they are surrounded by pericapsular fibrosis. The renal architecture is disrupted by fibrotic bands and collections of lymphocytes, eosinophils, and plasma cells. Tubules are atrophied and dilated.

CLINICAL MANIFESTATIONS

The clinical manifestations of UTIs are dependent on the age of the patient, as well as the anatomic location and severity of the infection. The following symptoms in newborn infants and in those less than 2 years of age are characteristically nonspecific and apparently are related to the gastrointestinal tract rather than the urinary tract: failure to thrive, feeding problems, vomiting, diarrhea, abdominal distention, and late-onset jaundice. Infants may have signs of balanitis, prostatitis, and orchitis or overt manifestations of sepsis.

The infection in children more than 2 years of age may be characterized by fever, frequency, and dysuria. Classic signs of cystitis in adults more often result from other causes of urethral irritation in children, such as bubble bath, vaginitis, pinworms, masturbation, or sexual abuse. Abdominal pain, flank pain, and hematuria may be present. The occurrence of enuresis in a child who has been toilet trained could also be a manifestation of a UTI. Young infants and boys may have an obstructive uropathy characterized by dribbling of urine, straining with urination, or a decrease in the force and size of the urinary stream. These findings of obstruction can be aggravated by infection. Other historic elements that should be sought include infrequent voiding, incomplete voiding, and a weak urinary stream.

The manifestations of UTIs in adolescents and adults are fairly specific. Lower–urinary tract symptoms include frequency, urgency, dysuria, and painful urination of a small amount of turbid urine that occasionally may be grossly bloody. Fever is usually absent. The differential diagnosis of cystitis includes vaginitis, urethritis, and chemically induced irritation from female hygiene products. In contrast, upper UTI may be characterized by fever, chills, and flank pain or abdominal pain. Upper- and lower-tract symptoms and signs may coexist. Occasionally the lower-tract symptoms may appear 1 to 2 days before the upper-tract symptoms. The clinical manifestations in some patients may be so atypical that they resemble gallbladder disease or acute appendicitis.

Given the appropriate clinical setting, the diagnosis is suggested by the detection of white blood cells (WBCs) and bacteria in the urine. The diagnosis of UTI requires confirmation by quantitative culture of urine and localization of the site of infection.

DIAGNOSIS

Normal urine is a sterile acellular glomerular filtrate influenced by tubular secretion and absorption.

Presumptive Tests

Pyuria. Pyuria is usually defined as the presence of more than 5 to 8 WBCs per cubic millimeter of uncentrifuged urine. This usually represents more than 1 WBC per high-power field. In centrifuged urine the measurement would be 50 to 100 WBCs/mm^3, that is, more than 5 WBCs per high-power field.

A standardized approach to urinalysis is valuable. Generally, 5 ml of urine is centrifuged at 3,000 rpm for 3 minutes, followed by resuspension of the sediment. The occurrence of more than 20 WBCs per high-power field usually correlates with significant bacteriuria of 100,000 colonies in a clean-catch sample. However, pyuria does not necessarily indicate the presence of a UTI. Patients of all ages with or without pyuria may or may not have an infection. Unfortunately, false-positive results of approximately 30% have been reported (Brumfitt, 1965) and may be caused by vaginal washout, chemical irritation, fever, viral infection, or glomerulonephritis. It is likely that most patients with symptomatic UTIs will have pyuria.

Microscopic Examination of Urine for Bacteria. A Gram stain of uncentrifuged urine is a useful test for the presumptive diagnosis of UTI. Infection is suggested by the presence of at least 1 bacterium per oil-immersion field in a midstream clean-catch urine specimen, equivalent to approximately 100,000 bacteria per milliliter. On examination of centrifuged sediment, approximately 10 to 100 bacteria per high-power field correlate with significant bacteriuria.

Chemical Tests. Nitrite detection in urine is based on the observation that many urinary pathogens convert nitrate to nitrite in the bladder. The nitrite strip for detection of UTI rarely yields false-positive results. False-negative results are more common (25% to 30%) as a result of inadequate dietary nitrates; diuresis; an inadequate time for bacterial proliferation; or infections caused by nitrite negative organisms, including *Staphylococcus saprophyticus, Acinetobacter* species, enterococci, and pseudomonads. The test is best used on concentrated or first-morning samples and may have an important role for outpatient and home monitoring following diagnosis and treatment of a UTI (Todd, 1977).

Leukocyte esterase testing detects enzymes generated by inflammatory cells. This test is neither more sensitive nor more specific than the detection of the cells themselves, but it may be easier to perform in some clinical settings. As with pyuria, a positive test does not establish the diagnosis of UTI.

Bioluminescence. The quantitative detection of bacterial production of ATP is another sensitive and specific screening test for UTI and detects both gram-positive and gram-negative organisms (Hanna, 1986).

Molecular detection of nucleic acids of prokaryotic cells in urine is being developed as a screening test for UTI. Although this strategy probably will be highly sensitive, it is also relatively expensive and labor-intensive; thus its role in clinical-laboratory diagnosis of UTI remains to be determined.

Specific Tests

Culture of carefully collected fresh (less than 30 minutes old, refrigerated or held on ice) urine, minimizing the likelihood of contamination is the cornerstone of diagnosis of UTI. Overdiagnosis carries the risks of unnecessary treatment, diagnostic work-up, and their attendant visits and costs, as well as unnecessary worry. Underdiagnosis carries the risks of continued symptoms and chronic progressive renal disease.

Quantitative Culture of Urine. Urine for culture may be obtained (1) as a midstream clean-catch specimen in adults, adolescents, and older children; (2) by catheterization; or (3) by suprapubic aspiration in young children and infants. Suprapubic aspiration is accomplished by introduction of a needle in the midline 2 to 4 cm above the symphysis pubis, after appropriate disinfection of the skin, with gentle traction applied to the syringe plunger. The needle is advanced through the bladder wall until urine flows into the syringe. Success with this procedure is maximized by ensuring that the patient has not recently voided; by palpating, percussing, or transilluminating the bladder; and by digital compression of the urethra to prevent reflex voiding. Strait catheterization follows gentle cleansing of the anterior urethra with soap and water. The catheter is advanced through the urethra into the bladder until urine flows into the catheter. Because the urethra cannot be sterilized, the first aliquot of urine that flows should be discarded to avoid collecting bacteria that have been pushed into the bladder. A later aliquot should be sent for culture (Todd, 1995). Unfortunately, there are no direct comparative studies of the sensitivity and specificity of these methods in children. A negative culture of a clean-catch specimen would obviate the need for catheterization or suprapubic aspiration. Urine collected as a bag specimen should not be submitted for bacterial culture. Screening for asymptomatic bacteriuria is not recommended.

Organisms, in any number, are considered significant when obtained by suprapubic aspiration. When urine is collected by catheterization, a colony count greater than 1,000 per milliliter of urine is usually considered diagnostic. However, for infants, counts of 10,000 cfu/ml or greater have been obtained from catheterized specimens in the absence of other findings of UTI. Hoberman et al. (1994) propose that for urine obtained by catheter, infections should be defined by a colony count greater than 50,000 cfu/ml and pyuria of at least 10 leukocytes/mm^3. If the quantitative culture from a midstream sample reveals 100,000 bacteria or more per milliliter of urine, it also indicates the presence of significant bacteriuria. A count of less than 10,000 bacteria per milliliter suggests probable contamination. The specificity of this technique is enhanced from 80% to 95% if significant bacteriuria is demonstrated on repeat testing. In the presence of pyuria and symptoms, a single culture indicating significant bacteriuria is considered diagnostic in adolescents and adults.

A false-positive test may be due to contamination or prolonged incubation of urine before culture. False-negative results may reflect the following: prior antimicrobial therapy, the presence of a fastidious organism that grows slowly or is difficult to culture, rapid flow of urine, inactivation of bacteria by an extremely acid pH, or a break in technique such as spilling soap or other cleansing agents into the urine. Therefore there are clinical situations in which colony counts of less than 100,000 may indicate significant bacteriuria.

Convenient, accurate, inexpensive culture techniques have become available for clinic or office practice and are most useful for screening for asymptomatic bacteriuria. They include the filter-strip, dip-slide, dip-strip, pad culture, and roll tube techniques. Of these techniques the dip-slide apparently is the most sensitive and specific (Eichenwald, 1986). The filter-strip technique does not differentiate gram-negative and gram-positive bacteria. The dip-slide and dip-strip techniques do use discriminating agars that allow differentiation of gram-negative and gram-positive organisms.

The specific bacterium recovered by culture should be identified as a guide to appropriate therapy. Quantitative urine cultures should be performed. Commonly this is done using a 0.001-ml calibrated loop inoculated onto blood agar and MacConkey's agar for gram-negative rods and onto chocolate agar for *H. influenzae*. The culture is incubated overnight, counted, and multiplied by 1,000. In certain circumstances, special media (e.g., Sabouraud's dextrose agar for fungi and human embryonic kidney, HeLa, or Hep-2 tissue culture for viral isolation) are required. When suprapubic aspiration is performed, 0.1 ml of urine should be spread over the plate, incubated overnight, and counted.

In uncomplicated disease the best test of antibiotic susceptibility is the test of cure. Successful treatment is followed by negative culture results within 24 to 72 hours after institution of therapy. If positive cultures are obtained, susceptibility results should be sought so that treatment can be tailored to the specific pathogen in neonates and in those with systemic illness, recurrent symptoms, or persistently positive follow-up cultures. Laboratory evaluation of response to therapy in children is required. For complicated disease, renal parenchymal disease, and nosocomially acquired organisms, antibiotic susceptibilities on the diagnostic urine specimen are useful in guiding therapy.

Localization of Site of Infection. It is important to determine if the infection involves the lower tract (probably cystitis) or the upper tract (probably pyelonephritis). Although pyelonephritis is classically associated with fever, flank pain or tenderness, decreased renal concentrating ability, and an elevated erythrocyte sedimentation rate (ESR), the absence of these findings does not reliably exclude upper-tract disease. Collection of urine by ureteral catheterization for quantitative culture is the most reliable method of localizing the site of infection; however, it is an invasive test and may require general anesthesia. Therefore its role in children is limited to research applications. Stamey et al. (1965) evaluated ninety-five females and twenty-six males by this method. Their observation that the site of infection was limited to the bladder in 50% of this group could not be predicted by history and physical examination. Localization by bladder washout (Fairley technique) is less invasive and does not require anesthesia; however, this is a cumbersome test and is not routinely performed.

The use of technetium (Tc 99m) dimercaptosuccinic acid (DMSA) or glucoheptonate scanning has gained favor in the early diagnosis of upper–urinary tract infections. DMSA scanning appears to be more sensitive than other easily available methods of localization (Buyan et al., 1993; Majid and Rushton, 1992; Rosenberg et al., 1992). In experimental studies the sensitivity and specificity of scanning was 91% and 99%, respectively, with overall 97% agreement with histopathologic findings (Majid and Rushton, 1992). The detection of antibody coating of bacteria is a sensitive, reliable, noninvasive indicator of renal bacteriuria in adults (Jones et al., 1974; Thomas et al., 1974). After addition of fluorescein-conjugated anti–human globulin to urine, the demonstration of fluorescence of the antibody-coated bacteria indicates upper-tract involvement. Unfortunately, when this immunofluorescence technique has been applied to children with bacteriuria, it has been neither sensitive nor specific (Hellerstein

et al., 1978; McCracken et al., 1981). Urinary lactic dehydrogenase (LDH) isoenzyme 5 is more accurate for localizing the site of infection in infants and children. Lorentz and Resnick (1979) have reported that elevations of urinary LDH greater than 150 U/L and elevations of fractions 4 and 5 are good indicators of acute pyelonephritis.

C-reactive protein (CRP) is also useful for distinguishing upper from lower UTI and has a sensitivity and specificity of approximately 90% when compared to bladder washout (McCracken et al., 1981). A CRP value greater than 30 μg/ml suggests upper-tract disease.

Finally, response to therapy is a clinical indication of the site of infection in adults. Studies in women indicate that more than 90% of patients with lower UTI but less than 50% of those with upper UTI are cured by a single dose of antibiotic if the organism is susceptible (Ronald et al., 1976; Fang et al., 1978). In children, however, recurrences of infection after short-duration therapy occur in approximately 30% of those treated (McCracken, 1982). This does not differ from the frequency of recurrences following conventional therapy.

Attention to other evaluations is also important when considering UTIs. Blood pressure should be measured because hypertension may be caused by chronic renal failure. Abdominal examination may reveal a mass, tenderness, or organomegaly. Genital examination should be conducted to investigate vaginitis and labial adhesions in girls; phimosis in boys; and evidence of irritation, sexual activity, or sexual abuse. Rectal examination allows assessment for lax sphincter tone, which may be associated with neurogenic bladder. Similarly, examination of the back may reveal a dimple or other defect associated with neurogenic bladder as a result of spinal cord involvement.

DIFFERENTIAL DIAGNOSIS

The differential diagnosis of UTI is dependent in great part on the age of the patient. The clinical manifestations in newborn infants and in infants under 2 years of age are nonspecific. The findings of irritability, failure to thrive, vomiting, diarrhea, and jaundice suggest the possibility of bacterial sepsis, acute gastroenteritis, or hepatitis. The appropriate blood, stool, and urine cultures should provide a clue to the correct diagnosis. In older children and adults the various conditions that may simulate cystitis or pyelonephritis should be considered. For example, the symptoms of gonorrheal or chlamydial urethritis may suggest a lower UTI. A right-sided pyelonephritis could be confused with acute appendicitis, gallbladder disease, or hepatitis. When the presenting complaint is hematuria and bacterial cultures are negative, viral cultures may reveal the diagnosis. Again, the appropriate cultures and serologic tests should help identify the true diagnosis.

COMPLICATIONS

Failure to recognize and to treat acute UTIs may result in recurrent infections and progression to chronic pyelonephritis. Children with chronic pyelonephritis associated with ureteral reflux and obstructive uropathy may develop consequences of chronic renal failure such as anemia, hypertension, growth failure, and metabolic abnormalities. Nephrolithiasis and stricture formation may also develop and further complicate management. A rare complication is that of renal abscess, which may rupture into the perirenal space.

PROGNOSIS

The prognosis depends on the site of involvement, the presence or absence of obstructive uropathy, and vesicoureteral reflux and is therefore related to the age of the patient. Young patients with obstructive uropathy and infection are much more likely to have serious long-term sequelae. Most single, uncomplicated episodes of infection respond to specific antimicrobial therapy. However, approximately one third of these patients may relapse within 1 year. Relapses decrease in frequency beyond this time; however, 1% of patients may relapse up to 6 years after initial infection. The prognosis is less favorable for patients with obstructive lesions and for those with chronic pyelonephritis. In spite of specific antimicrobial therapy, most of these patients have repeated recurrences, and those with bilateral renal involvement may progress to chronic renal insufficiency.

Reflux can be detected in up to 50% of children with bacteriuria (Boineau and Levy, 1975; Smellie and Normand, 1975). The confluence of infection and reflux is associated with renal scarring in a subset of these children (McCracken and Eichenwald, 1978; Huland and Busch, 1984; Smellie and Normand, 1975).

EPIDEMIOLOGY

UTIs involve all age groups from neonates to geriatric patients. Studies involving routine suprapubic puncture in over 1,000 infants revealed the presence of bacteriuria in 0.1% to more than 1% (Wiswell and Geschke, 1989; Wiswell and Roscelli, 1986; Wiswell et al., 1987). UTI was more common in males, with the majority of these infections occurring in uncircumcised infants. However, circumcision to prevent UTI is not warranted by the low frequency and usually mild nature of the disease. Premature infants have 2 to 3 times this rate of UTI. During preschool years, UTI is more common in girls (4.5%) than in boys (0.5%).

Long-term surveillance studies by Kunin et al. (1962) and Kunin (1970, 1976) of school children revealed persistent bacteriuria in 1.2% of girls and in 0.4% of boys. Each year an additional 0.4% of girls developed bacteriuria. Thus the overall prevalence in school girls was 5%. These studies indicated that the peak incidence of UTI in children occurred between 2 and 6 years of age. White girls tended to have more frequent reinfections than black girls. The incidence of UTI in females of high school and college age is approximately 2%.

TREATMENT

The objectives of treatment of children with UTIs are fourfold: (1) to eliminate the infection, (2) to detect and correct functional or anatomic abnormalities, (3) to prevent recurrences, and (4) to preserve renal function. The achievement of these goals requires successful identification of the causative microorganism, selection of optimal antimicrobial drugs and patient compliance in their use, roentgenographic evaluation of the urinary tract, screening for recurrent infections with periodic urine cultures, and use of general hygienic measures to prevent reinfections. Surgery may be required to correct severe reflux in children with UTIs and especially to correct obstructive lesions.

Antimicrobial Therapy

Newborn infants with UTIs and children suspected of having pyelonephritis should be treated empirically at the time of diagnosis because of the frequency of associated bacteremia. Empiric therapy for newborn infants with UTI and suspected sepsis should include ampicillin (100 to 200 mg/kg/day) and gentamicin (5 mg/kg/day for infants <1 week of age and 7.5 mg/kg/day for infants >1 week of age) or another aminoglycoside. Table 36-1 provides recommendations for initial therapy of newborn infants without sepsis or meningitis when a specific organism can be predicted or when an organism has been isolated and susceptibilities are

Table 36-1 Initial therapy for predicted cause of acute urinary tract infections in newborn infants while awaiting susceptibility results

Gram stain	Cause	Initial therapy
Gram-negative rods	Coliforms (*Escherichia coli, Klebsiella pneumoniae, Enterobacter aerogenes*)	Gentamicin 3 mg/kg/day or amikacin 10 mg/kg/day
	Proteus mirabilis	Ampicillin 50-75 mg/kg/day
	Pseudomonas aeruginosa	Mezlocillin or ticarcillin 75-100 mg/kg/day or ceftazidime 100-150 mg/kg/day
Gram-positive cocci in chains	*Streptococcus faecalis,* Enterococci	Ampicillin 30 mg/kg/day IM or 50 mg/kg/day PO; add an aminoglycoside if synergy is needed
Gram-positive cocci in clusters	*Staphylococcus aureus,* methicillin-resistant (MRSA)	Methicillin or oxacillin 50-75 mg/kg/day Vancomycin 30 mg/kg/day
	Staphylococcus epidermidis	As for *S. aureus*

not yet available. Alternatively, cefotaxime alone is satisfactory for treatment of enteric gram-negative bacillary urinary tract infection.

Older children with suspected pyelonephritis can be treated empirically with gentamicin (5 to 7.5 mg per kilogram of body weight per day), possibly with the addition of ampicillin. Table 36-2 contains recommendations for initial therapy of older children when a specific organism can be predicted or when an organism has been isolated and susceptibilities are not yet available. Parenterally administered cephalosporin drugs are also used for this indication. Recent data indicate that orally administered cephalosporin drugs with activity against gram-negative rods are as effective in the time to defeverescence (approximately 25 hours), ability to eradicate the organism from the urine, prevention of recurrences, and prevention of renal scarring at 6 months (Hoberman et al., 1996). Children with mild symptoms and those with lower UTIs may not require antimicrobial therapy until the results of urine culture are available. If therapy is indicated before the results of culture become available, oral sulfisoxazole or triple sulfonamides are suggested because *E. coli* and other gram-negative bacilli are the most common pathogens. Ampicillin or amoxicillin (30 mg per kilogram of body weight per day in 3 doses) may be used as an alternative to sulfonamides. In selecting antibiotic therapy the history of first-versus-recurrent infection, the prior use of antibiotics, and any history of drug allergy should be considered. When the results of urine culture and antibiotic sensitivities are known, the antimicrobial therapy can be changed if necessary. If a repeat urine culture 48 hours after initiation of therapy is negative, the treatment should be continued, regardless of the results of in vitro sensitivity studies. For

those treated parenterally a switch to oral therapy can be considered if symptoms have abated and an oral agent to which the pathogen is susceptible is available. If the repeat culture is still positive and the colony count has not decreased, the results of the sensitivity tests should be used as a basis for changing the antimicrobial therapy.

In adolescents with acute obstructive, persistent, or frequently recurrent UTIs and for those with nosocomially acquired organisms, fluoroquinolones, imipenem-cilastatin, ticarcillin-clavulanate, or extended spectrum cephalosporins are acceptable alternative drugs.

For children in whom clinical and laboratory measurements indicate lower-tract infection, the use of single-dose or short-term regimens should be restricted to those beyond the newborn period with their first UTI. However, it may be more cost-effective to complete 10 days of therapy than to risk the need to reevaluate and treat a recurrence. Reexamination of the patient and reculture of the urine after short-term therapy is mandatory. Amoxicillin, cefadroxil, nitrofurantoin, and trimethoprim-sulfamethoxazole have all been used as short-term regimens.

A "cure" is determined by the demonstration of several negative cultures after cessation of therapy. Therapeutic failures after short-course or conventional antibiotic treatment of susceptible organisms suggest upper-tract disease. Consideration should be given to a 6-week regimen in patients who do not respond to conventional therapy. Follow-up should continue for at least 2 years with a routine culture schema such as monthly urine culture for the first 3 months followed by three cultures 3 months apart and two semiannual cultures. If reinfection occurs, the susceptibility of the organism

Table 36-2 Initial therapy for predicted cause of urinary tract infection in older children while awaiting susceptibility results

Clinical condition	Cause	Initial therapy*
Acute nonobstructive gram-negative rods	Coliforms	Sulfisoxazole 120-150 mg/kg/day or amoxicillin 30 mg/kg/day or trimethoprim (TMP)–sulfamethoxazole (SMX), TMP 8 mg/kg/day, SMX 40 mg/kg/day
	Pseudomonas species	Carbenicillin 30-50 mg/kg/day PO or parenteral or mezlocillin 100 mg/kg/day or ceftazidine 100-150 mg/kg/day
Gram-positive cocci in chains	Enterococci	Ampicillin 50-100 mg/kg/day; aminoglycoside if necessary for synergy
Gram-positive cocci in clusters	*Staphylococcus aureus, Staphylococcus epidermidis*	Nafcillin 100 mg/kg/day; or vancomycin 40 mg/kg/day or cephalexin 25-50 mg/kg/day
	Staphylococcus aureus, methicillin-resistant (MRSA)	Vancomycin 40 mg/kg/day
Acute nonobstructive with suspected sepsis	Coliforms	Gentamicin 5 to 7.5 mg/day or TMP 8 mg/kg with SMX 40 mg/kg/day
Acute obstructive	Coliforms	TMP 8 mg with SMX 40 mg/kg/day or nitrofurantoin 5 to 7 mg/kg/day for 3 weeks or gentamicin 3 mg/kg/day
Persistent, recurrent, or hospital acquired (acute therapy)	Coliforms	Amikacin 15 to 22 mg/kg/day or carbenicillin indanyl 10 to 30 mg/kg/day or TMP 30 mg with SMX, 6 mg/kg/day
Persistent, recurrent, or hospital acquired with sepsis	Coliforms	Amikacin 15-22 mg/kg/day or cefuroxime 75-150 mg/kg/day or mezlocillin 200 to 300 mg/kg/day or piperacillin 200-300 mg/kg/day or ceftriaxone 50-100 mg/kg/day or ceftazidime 100-150 mg/kg/day
Prophylaxis for chronic or recurrent infection		TMP 2 mg with SMX 10 mg/kg/day or nitrofurantoin 1-2 mg/kg PO q12d at bedtime

*Alterations and subsequent therapy should be based on culture and sensitivity reports. The usual duration of therapy for acute infec-

should be determined, and the appropriate therapy should be instituted. Reinfection is differentiated from recurrence by typing the causative agent.

Radiologic Evaluation

After initial infection in all infants, in boys of any age, and girls less than 3 years, radiologic evaluation is indicated. In girls more than 3 years of age, imaging is also indicated in the presence of symptomatic infection, physical examination findings suggestive of possible renal or collecting system abnormalities, abnormal voiding, hypertension, or poor physical development (Eichenwald, 1986).

Information developed by these radiographic studies affects management. Children with no reflux or grade I reflux require only follow-up examination. Children with grade II or III reflux may be candidates for suppressive therapy. Children with grade IV reflux are also candidates for suppressive therapy, and urologic consultation should be obtained.

If radiographic studies are not performed in older girls after the primary infection, they are indicated if there is a recurrence. Radiographic studies are usually performed 6 weeks or longer after acute infection to avoid detection of grade I or II reflux caused by irritation of the vesicoureteral junction. Children with clinical signs of upper-tract disease who fail to respond promptly to antibiotic therapy warrant evaluation with ultrasound or intravenous pyelography during their acute infection to investigate the role of obstruction. If grade III or IV reflux is detected, it probably will be persistent and not be the result of acute infection.

Levitt et al. (1977) found that cystograms frequently revealed abnormalities in girls with dysuria and frequency (41%) but pyelograms rarely did

(2%). However, if upper-tract disease was suspected, pyelograms detected abnormalities in 40%, and findings included obstruction and hydronephrosis. This usually was true even if a first episode of UTI was being studied. In cases diagnosed as upper-tract disease based on elevations of CRP and ESR and abnormal renal concentrating ability, 7% of children studied by intravenous pyelogram developed renal scarring (Pylkkanen et al., 1981). When diagnostic findings were expanded to include reflux and fever, fever alone had a positive predictive value of 45%, and reflux had a positive predictive value of 40% for children, less than 5 years, likely to have radiographically demonstrable abnormalities (Johnson et al., 1985). In addition to radionuclide techntium Tc 99m DMSA or glucoheptonate scanning for localization, radionuclide scanning appears to have increased sensitivity in detecting renal scars following acute pyelonephritis. Serial observations indicate that approximately two thirds of abnormalities demonstrated acutely resolve over time (Jakabsson et al., 1994; Rosenberg et al., 1992). In the experience of Rushton et al. (1992) all new scarring occurred at sites corresponding to the localization of acute inflammation and appears to be unrelated to vesicoureteral reflux. The long-term clinical consequences of scarring in children with anatomically normal urinary tracts are unknown. Similarly, the clinical importance of the increased sensitivity of DMSA scanning is unknown (Rushton et al., 1992).

Ultrasonography is a rapid, noninvasive method for evaluating the renal parenchyma and renal collecting system and is capable of imaging the surrounding retroperitoneum without radiation exposure. In the hands of experienced individuals, ultrasound has supplanted the intravenous pyelogram and voiding cystourethrogram. However, ultrasound may not be able to detect significant reflux or to determine reliably the degree of renal scarring. In one study (Rosenberg et al., 1992), the use of DMSA and ultrasound detected all reflux detected by cystourethrography.

When detailed anatomic information is required, computed tomography or magnetic resonance imaging should be performed. Radionuclide cystography may be most useful in older children in whom reflux is considered unlikely, as well as for screening families and follow-up of surgical, as well as nonsurgical, interventions (Lebowitz, 1992). When imaging studies reveal reflux, they should be repeated in 6 months to follow the course

of the finding. When no abnormality is detected, they ordinarily need not be repeated. Urologic referrals are appropriate for patients with obstruction, urethral valves, renal scarring, anatomic abnormalities, and dysfunctional voiding.

PROPHYLAXIS

Patients with frequent recurrences and those with persistent infections may require suppressive therapy for many years. As indicated in Table 36-2, the use of trimethoprim-sulfamethoxazole should be considered. No therapy with any prophylactic agent is completely safe because drug-related toxicities can occur.

Several regimens are available when breakthrough infections occur. Although low-dose ampicillin interferes with adherence of E. coli to bladder mucosa (Redjeb et al., 1982), the clinical relevance of this finding has not been determined. Postcoital UTI may also be reduced by prophylaxis and by voiding after intercourse.

Various other nonspecific general measures may be helpful in preventing recurrences of UTIs. They include adequate fluid intake; frequent voiding, especially before bedtime; proper perineal hygiene, particularly after defecation; and avoidance of chronic constipation, which could produce rectal distention that might distort the bladder. Uncircumcised males with phimosis may benefit from circumcision. Physical and chemical irritants of the urethra should be identified and minimized or eliminated. Persons with functional abnormalities of the bladder benefit from intermittent catheterization programs. Acidification programs and long-term treatment with methenamine are occasionally effective; however, they are difficult to maintain.

BIBLIOGRAPHY

Aronson M, Medalia O, Schori L, et al. Prevention of colonization of the urinary tract of mice with Escherichia coli by blocking of bacterial adherence with methyl-a-D-mannopyanoside. J Infect Dis 1979;139:329-332.

Asscher AW, et al. Urine as a medium for bacterial growth. Lancet 1966;2:1037.

Bailey RR. Significance of coagulase-negative Staphylococcus in urine. J Infect Dis 1973;127:179.

Boineau FG, Lewy JE. Urinary tract infections in children: an overview. Pediatr Ann 1975;4:515-526.

Bran JL, Levison ME, Kaye D. Entrance of bacteria into the female urinary bladder. N Engl J Med 1972;286:626.

Britt MR, Garibaldi RA, Miller WA, et al. Antimicrobial prophylaxis for catheter-associated bacteriuria. Antimicrob Agents Chemother 1977;11:240-243.

Brumfitt W. Urinary cell counts and their value. J Clin Pathol 1965;18:550.

Buckley RM, McGuckin M, MacGregor RR. Urine bacterial counts following sexual intercourse. N Engl J Med 1978;298:321.

Butler HK, Kunin CM. Evaluation of specific systemic antimicrobial therapy in patients while on closed catheter drainage. J Urol 1968;100:567-572.

Buyan N, Bircan ZE, Asanoglu E, et al. The importance of 99m Tc DMSA scanning in the localization of childhood urinary tract infections. Int Urol Nephrol 1993;25:11-17.

Cobbs CG, Kaye D. Antibacterial mechanisms in the urinary bladder. Yale J Biol Med 1967;40:93.

Eichenwald HF. Some aspects of the diagnosis and management of urinary tract infection in children and adolescents. Pediatr Infect Dis J 1986;5:760-765.

Fang LST, Tolkoff-Rubin NE, Rubin R. Efficacy of single-dose and conventional amoxicillin therapy in urinary tract infection localized by the antibody-coated bacteria technique. N Engl J Med 1978;298:413-416.

Fasth A, Ahlstedt S, Hanson LA, et al. Cross-reaction between Tamm-Horsfall glycoprotein and Escherichia coli. Int Arch Allergy Appl Immunol 1980;63:303-311.

Gorrill RH, De Navasquez SJ. Experimental pyelonephritis in the mouse produced by Escherichia coli, Pseudomonas aeruginosa, and Proteus mirabilis. J Pathol Bacteriol 1964;87:79.

Gruneberg RN, Leigh DA, Brumfitt W. Escherichia coli serotypes in urinary tract infection: studies in domiciliary, antenatal, and hospital practice. In O'Grady F, Brumfitt W (ed). Urinary tract infection. London: Oxford University Press, 1968.

Hanna BA. The detection of bacteriuria by bioluminescence. Methods Enzymol 1986;311:22-27.

Hanson LA, et al. Antigens of Escherichia coli, human immune response, and the pathogenesis of urinary tract infections. J Infect Dis 1977;136:S144.

Hanson LA, Fasth A, Jodal U, et al. Biology and pathology of urinary tract infection. J Clin Pathol 1981;34:695-700.

Harles EMJ, Bullen JJ, Thompson DA. Influence of estrogen on experimental pyelonephritis caused by Escherichia coli. Lancet 1975;2:283-286.

Hashida Y, Gaffney PC, Yunis EJ. Acute hemorrhagic cystitis of childhood and papovavirus-like particles. J Pediatr 1976;89:85-87.

Hellerstein S, Kennedy E, Nussbaum L, et al. Localization of the site of urinary tract infections by means of antibody-coated bacteria in the urinary sediments. J Pediatr 1978;92:188-193.

Hoberman A, Wald ER, Reynolds EA, et al. Pyuria and bacteriuria in urine specimens obtained by catheter from young children with fever. J Pediatr 1994;124:513-519.

Hoberman A, Wald ER, Reynolds EA, Chanon M. Oral vs. intravenous therapy for acute pyelonephritis in children 1-24 months. Pediatric Research 1996;39:134A (abstract 787).

Hopkins WJ, Uehling DT, Balish E. Local and systemic antibody responses accompanying spontaneous resolution of experimental cystitis in cynomolgus monkeys. Infect Immunol 1987;55:1951-1956.

Huland H, Busch R. Pyelonephritic scarring in 213 patients with upper and lower urinary tract infections: long-term follow-up. J Urol 1984;132:936-939.

Iwahi T, Abe Y, Nakao M, et al. Role of type I fimbriae in the pathogenesis of ascending urinary tract infection induced by Escherichia coli in mice. Infect Immun 1983;39:1307-1315.

Jakobsson B, Berg U, Svensson L. Renal scarring after acute pyelonephritis. Arch Dis Child 1994;70:111-115.

Johnson CE, Shurin P, Marchant C, et al. Identification of children requiring radiologic evaluation for urinary infection. Pediatr Infect Dis 1985;4:656-663.

Jones SR, Smith JW, Sanford JP. Localization of urinary tract infections by detection of antibody-coated bacteria in urine sediment. N Engl J Med 1974;290:591.

Kaijser B. Immunology of Escherichia coli: K antigen and its relation to urinary-tract infection. J Infect Dis 1973;127:670.

Kaijser B, Hanson LA, Jodal U, et al. Frequency of E. coli K antigens in urinary tract infections in children. Lancet 1977;1:663-666.

Kaijser B, Larsson P, Olling S, et al. Protection against acute ascending pyelonephritis caused by Escherichia coli in rats, using isolated capsular antigen conjugated to bovine serum albumin. Infect Immunol 1983;39:142-146.

Kaijser B, Olling S. Experimental hematogenous pyelonephritis due to Escherichia coli in rabbits: the antibody response and its protective capacity. J Infect Dis 1973;128:41.

Kallenius G, Mollby R, Svensson SB, et al. Occurrence of P-fimbriated Escherichia coli in urinary tract infection. Lancet 1981;2:1369-1372.

Kaye D. Antibacterial activity of human urine. J Clin Invest 1968;47:2374.

Khan AJ, Evans HE, Bombeck E, et al. Coagulase-negative staphylococcal bacteriuria: a rarity in infants and children. J Pediatr 1975;86:309-313.

Kinane DF, Blackwell CC, Brettle RP, et al. ABO blood group, secretor state and susceptibility to recurrent urinary tract infection in women. Br Med J 1982;285:7-9.

Kunin CM. The natural history of recurrent bacteriuria in school girls. N Engl J Med 1970;282:1443.

Kunin CM. Urinary tract infections in children. Hosp Pract 1976;113:91.

Kunin CM, Zacha E, Paquin AJ. Urinary tract infections in school children. I. Prevalence of bacteriuria and associated urologic findings. N Engl J Med 1962;206:1287.

Lebowitz RL. The detection and characterization of vesicoureteral reflux in the child. J Urol 1992;148:1640-1642.

Leffler H, Svanborg-Eden C. Glycolipid receptors for uropathogenic Escherichia coli on human erythrocytes and uroepithelial cells. Infect Immunol 1981;34:920-929.

Levitt SB, Bekirov HM, Kogan SJ, et al. Proposed selective approach to radiographic evaluation of children with urinary tract infections. In Birth defects: original article series, vol 13, no 5. New York: The National Foundation—March of Dimes, 1977.

Lindberg H, Hanson LA, Jacobsson B, et al. Correlation of P blood group, vesiculoureteral reflux, and bacterial attachment in patients with recurrent pyelonephritis. New Engl J Med 1983;308:1189-1192.

Lindberg U, Hanson LA, Jodal U, et al. Asymptomatic bacteriuria in school girls. II. Differences in E. coli causing symptomatic and asymptomatic bacteriuria. Acta Pediatr Scand 1975;64:432-436.

Lorentz WB, Resnick MI. Comparison of urinary lactic dehydrogenase with antibody-coated bacteria in the urine sediment as a means of localizing the site of urinary tract infection. Pediatrics 1979;64:672.

Majid M, Rushton HG. Renal cortical cintigraphy in the diagnosis of acute UTI. Sem Nuclear Med 1992;22:98-111.

Mattsby-Baltzer I, Claesson I, Hanson LA, et al. Antibodies to lipid A during urinary tract infection. J Infect Dis 1981;144:319-328.

Mattsby-Baltzer I, Hanson LA, Kaijser B, et al. Experimental *Escherichia coli* ascending pyelonephritis in rats: changes in bacterial properties and the immune response to surface antigens. Infect Immunol 1982;35:639-646.

Maybeck CE. Significance of coagulase-negative staphylococcal bacteriuria. Lancet 1969;2:1150-1152.

Mayrer AR, Miniter P, Andriole VT. Immunopathogenesis of chronic pyelonephritis. Am J Med 1983;75:59-70.

McCracken G, Eichenwald H. Antimicrobial therapy: therapeutic recommendations and a review of new drugs. J Pediatr 1978;93:366.

McCracken GH Jr. Management of urinary tract infections in children. Pediatr Infect Dis 1982;1(suppl):52-56.

McCracken GH Jr, Ginsburg CM, Namasanthi V, et al. Evaluation of short-term antibiotic therapy in children with uncomplicated urinary tract infections. Pediatrics 1981;67:796-801.

Miller TE, North JD. Host response in urinary tract infections. Kidney Int 1974;5:179.

Monson TP, Macalalad FV, Hamman JW, et al. Evaluation of a vented drainage system in prevention of bacteriuria. J Urol 1977;177:216-219.

Mufson MA, Belshe RB. A review of adenoviruses in the etiology of acute hemorrhagic cystitis. J Urol 1976;115:191.

Murphy JJ et al. The role of the lymphatic system in pyelonephritis. Surg Forum 1960;10:880.

Musher DM et al. Role of urease in pyelonephritis resulting from urinary tract infection with *Proteus*. J Infect Dis 1975;131:177.

Nelson JD. Pocketbook of pediatric antimicrobial therapy, ed 10. Baltimore: Williams & Wilkins, 1993.

Nicolle L, Harding GKM, Preiksaitis J, et al. The association of urinary tract infection with sexual intercourse. J Infect Dis 1982;278:635-642.

Norden CW, Green GM, Kass EH. Antibacterial mechanisms of the urinary bladder. J Clin Invest 1968;47:2689-2700.

Ofek I, Mirelman D, Sharon N. Adherence of *Escherichia coli* to human mucosal cells mediated by mannose receptors. Nature 1977;265:623-625.

Ofek I, Mosek A, Sharon N. Mannose-specific adherence of *Escherichia coli* freshly extracted in the urine of patients with urinary tract infections and of isolates subcultured from the infected urine. Infect Immunol 1981;34:708-711.

O'Hanley PD, Lark D, Falkow S, et al. A globaside-binding *Escherichia coli* pilus vaccine prevents pyelonephritis. Clin Res 1983;31:372A (abstract).

Orskov I, Ferenez A, Orskov F. Tamm-Horsfall protein or uromucoid is the normal urinary slime that traps type I fimbriated *Escherichia coli*. Lancet 1980;1:887.

Padgett BL, Walker DL, Desquitado MM, et al. BK virus and non-hemorrhagic cystitis in a child. Lancet 1987;1:770.

Parsons CL, Greenspan C, Mulholland SG. The primary antibacterial defense mechanism of the bladder. Invest Urol 1975;13:72-76.

Parsons CL, Schrom SH, Hanno P, et al. Bladder surface mucin: examination of possible mechanisms for its antibacterial effect. Invest Urol 1978;6:196-200.

Perry A, Ofek I, Silverblatt JF. Enhancement of mannose-mediated stimulation of human granulocytes by type I fimbriae aggregated with antibodies on *Escherichia coli* surfaces. Infect Immunol 1983;39:1334-1335.

Pfau A, Sacks T, Engtestein D. Recurrent urinary tract infections in premenopausal women: prophylaxis based on an understanding of the pathogenesis. J Urol 1983;129:1152-1157.

Pylkkanen J, Vilska J, Koskimies O. The value of level diagnosis of childhood urinary tract infection in predicting renal injury. Acta Paediatr Scand 1981;70:879-883.

Redjeb SB, Slim A, Horchani A, et al. Effects of ten milligrams of ampicillin per day on urinary tract infections. Antimicrob Agents Chemother 1982;22:1084-1086.

Rene P, Silverblatt FJ. Serological response to *Escherichia coli* pili in pyelonephritis. Infect Immunol 1982;37:749-754.

Rice SJ, Bishop JA, Apperly J, et al. BK virus as a case of hemorrhagic cystitis after bone marrow transplant. Lancet 1985;2:844-845.

Rocha H, Fekety FR. Acute inflammation in the renal cortex and medulla following thermal injury. J Exp Med 1964;119:131-138.

Ronald AR, Boutros P, Mourtada H. Bacteriuria localization and response to single-dose therapy in women. JAMA 1976;235:1854-1856.

Rosenberg AR, Rossleigh MA, Brydon MP, et al. Evaluation of acute urinary tract infection in children by dimercaptosuccinic acid scintigraphy: a prospective study. J Urol 1992;148:1746-1749.

Rubin M. Effect of catheter replacement on bacterial counts in urine aspirated from indwelling catheters. J Infect Dis 1980;142:291.

Rushton HG, Majid M, Jantausch B, et al. Renal scanning following reflux and nonreflux pyelonephritis in children: evaluation with 99mTechnetium dimercaptosuccinic acid scintigraphy. J Urol 1992;148:898.

Silverblatt FS. Host-parasite interaction in the rat renal pelvis: a possible role of pili in the pathogenesis of pyelonephritis. J Exp Med 1974;140:1696-1711.

Smellie JM, Normand ICS. Bacteriuria, reflux, and renal scarring. Arch Dis Child 1975;50:581.

Smith JW, Jones SR, Kaijser B. Significance of antibody-coated bacteria in urinary sediment in experimental pyelonephritis. J Infect Dis 1977;135:577-581.

Sobel JD, Vardi Y. Scanning electron microscopy study of *Pseudomonas aeruginosa* in vivo adherence to rat bladder epithelium. J Urol 1982;128:414-417.

Stamey TA, Govan DE, Palmer JM. The localization and treatment of urinary tract infections: the role of bactericidal urine levels as opposed to serum levels. Medicine 1965;44:1.

Stamey TA, Kaufman MF. Studies of introital colonization in women with recurrent urinary infections. II. A comparison of growth in normal vaginal fluid of common versus uncommon serogroups of *E. coli*. J Urol 1975;114:264.

Stamey TA, Mihara G. Studies of introital colonization in women with recurrent urinary infections. V. The inhibitory activity of normal vaginal fluid on *Proteus mirabilis* and *Pseudomonas aeruginosa*. J Urol 1976;115:416.

Stamey TA, Timothy MM. Studies of introital colonization in women with recurrent urinary infections. I. The role of vaginal pH. J Urol 1975;114:261.

Stamey TA, Wehner N, Mihara G, et al. The immunologic basis of recurrent bacteriuria: role of cervicovaginal antibody in enterobacterial colonization of the introital mucosa. Medicine 1978;57:47-56.

Stamey TA et al. Antibacterial nature of prostatic fluid. Nature 1968;218:444.

Stapleton A, Nudelman E, Clausen H, et al. Binding of uropathogenic *Escherichia coli* R45 to glycolipids extracted from vaginal epithelial cells is dependent on histo–blood group secretor status. J Clin Invest 1992;90:965-972.

Stromberg N, Marklund B-I, Lund B, et al. Host-specificity of uropathogenic *Escherichia coli* depends on differences in binding specificity to gal 1-4 gal-containing isoreceptors. EMBO J 1990;9:2001-2010.

Svanborg-Eden C, Hagberg L, Hanson LA, et al. Adhesion of *Escherichia coli* in urinary tract infection. CIBA Found Symp 1981;80:161-187.

Svanborg-Eden C, Hanson LA, Jodol U, et al. Variable adherence to normal human urinary tract epithelial cells of *Escherichia coli* strains associated with various forms of urinary tract infection. Lancet 1976;2:490-492.

Svanborg-Eden C, Gotschlich EC, Korhonan TK, et al. Aspects of structure and function of pili of uropathogenic *E. coli*. Prog Allergy 1983;33:189-202.

Svanborg-Eden C, Svennerholm AM. Secretory immunoglobulin A and G antibodies prevent adhesion of *Escherichia coli* to human urinary tract epithelial cells. Infect Immun 1978;22:790-797.

Thomas V, Shelokov A, Forland M. Antibody-coated bacteria in the urine and the site of urinary tract infection. N Engl J Med 1974;290:588.

Todd JK. Management of urinary tract infections: children are different. Pediatr Rev. 1995;16:190-196.

Todd JK. Have follow-up of urinary tract infection: comparison of two non-culture techniques. Am J Dis Child. 1977;131:860-861.

Uehling DT, Stiehm ER. Elevated urinary secretory IgA in children with urinary tract infection. Pediatrics 1971;47:40-46.

Vivaldi E, Munoz J, Cotran R, et al. Factors affecting the clearance of bacteria within the urinary tract. In Kass EH (ed). Progress in pyelonephritis. Philadelphia: FA Davis, 1965, pp 531-535.

Vosti CL. Recurrent urinary tract infections: prevention by prophylactic antibiotics after sexual intercourse. JAMA 1975;231-934.

Warren JW, Anthony WC, Hoopes JM, et al. Cephalexin for susceptible bacteriuria in afebrile, long-term catheterized patients. JAMA 1982;248:454-458.

Warren JW, Hoopes JM, Muncie HL, et al. Ineffectiveness of cephalexin in treatment of cephalexin-resistant bacteriuria in patients with chronic indwelling urethral catheters. J Urol 1983;129:71-73.

Weyrauch HM, Bassett JB. Ascending infection in an artificial urinary tract. An experimental study. Stanford Med Bull 1951;9:25.

Wiswell TE, Geschke DW. Risks from circumcision during the first month of life compared with those for uncircumcised boys. Pediatrics 1989;83:1011-1015.

Wiswell TE, Roscelli JD. Corroborative evidence for the decreased incidence of urinary tract infections in circumcised male infants. Pediatrics 1986;78:96-99.

Wiswell TE, Enzenauer RW, Holton ME, et al. Declining frequency of circumcision: implications for changes in the absolute incidence and male to female sex ratio of urinary tract infections in early infancy. Pediatrics 1987;79:338-342.

Work J, Andriole VT. Tamm-Horsfall protein antibody in patients with end-stage kidney disease. Yale J Biol Med 1980;53:133-148.

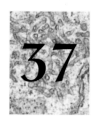

37 VARICELLA–ZOSTER VIRUS INFECTIONS

ANNE A. GERSHON AND PHILIP LaRUSSA

Varicella (chickenpox) is a common contagious disease usually of childhood, which is the result of primary infection with varicella-zoster virus (VZV). Varicella in children is characterized by a short or absent prodromal period and by a pruritic rash consisting of crops of papules, vesicles, pustules, and eventual crusting, although many skin lesions do not progress to the vesicular stage. In normal children the systemic symptoms are usually mild. Serious complications are the exception but can occur in adults and in children with deficiencies in cell-mediated immunity (CMI), where the disease may be manifested by an extensive eruption, severe constitutional symptoms, and pneumonia, possibly with a fatal outcome if no antiviral therapy is given.

Zoster, which is caused by reactivation of latent VZV acquired during varicella, is characterized by a localized unilateral rash consisting of varicella-like lesions in the distribution of a sensory nerve. Occasionally more than one nerve is involved, and in some patients hematogenous dissemination of virus occurs, leading to a generalized rash developing after the localized eruption. Zoster occurs most often in immunocompromised individuals; it is also more common in the elderly than in the young, and it is more likely to be accompanied by dermatomal pain in adults compared to children.

ETIOLOGY

A member of the herpesvirus group, VZV is composed of an inner core containing nucleoprotein and DNA, an icosahedral capsid surrounded by a tegument, and an outer lipid-containing envelope. Enveloped VZV particles range in size from 150 to 200 nm (Fig. 37-1).

Weller et al. (1954, 1958) were the first to propagate VZV in vitro and to show that one virus causes both diseases. He and his colleagues successfully infected cell cultures of human embryonic lung fibroblasts with vesicular fluid from patients with chickenpox and with zoster; demonstrated the presence of eosinophilic intranuclear inclusion bodies and multinucleated cells typical of VZV in culture; and passed the agent in series, using the cellular components of infected tissue cultures (Weller and Witton, 1958). Using these cultures as the antigen, Weller et al. demonstrated a rise in antibody titer to the agent in convalescent-phase serum from patients with varicella and patients with zoster.

The following body of evidence indicates that the agents that cause varicella and zoster are identical:

1. Varicella was transmitted to susceptible children by inoculating them with vesicular fluid from patients with zoster. The experimental disease was contagious, and it produced chickenpox in other children (Bruusgaard, 1932; Kundratitz, 1925).
2. The cytopathic effect of varicella virus in tissue cultures is neutralized not only by varicella immune serum but also by zoster immune serum. Both sera also neutralize virus obtained from patients with zoster (Weller and Coons, 1954).
3. Morphologically identical particles are seen in electron microscopic studies of vesicular fluid from patients with varicella and patients with zoster. Biopsies of skin lesions in both diseases reveal the same type of eosinophilic inclusion bodies, and smears of varicella and zoster lesions show the same type of multinucleated giant cells. Viruses from both clinical entities are indistinguishable by immunofluorescence assays (Weller and Witton, 1958).
4. Virus obtained from varicella and zoster lesions from the same patient have identical DNA restriction endonuclease digest patterns (Straus et al., 1984; Hayakawa et al., 1984; Williams et al., 1985; Gelb et al., 1987).

Glycoproteins specified by VZV are present both on the membranes of infected cells and on the

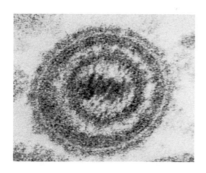

FIG. 37-1 Electron micrograph of varicella-zoster virus. This specimen was obtained from vesicular fluid of a child 1 day after the onset of varicella. The structural elements of the virion are the central DNA core, the protein capsid, the tegument, and the envelope. The last structure contains glycoproteins and is important for infectivity of the virion. (×175,000.) (Courtesy Michael D. Gershon, M.D.)

envelope of the virus. At least six glycoproteins, designated I through VI, have been identified for VZV; they are homologues of glycoproteins E, B, H, I, C, and L, respectively, of herpes simplex virus (HSV) (reviewed in Arvin and Gershon, 1996). These glycoproteins play important roles in viral pathogenesis and in the generation of cellular and humoral immunity in the infected host. For example, glycoproteins B and H are required to facilitate transmission of VZV from one cell to another (Edson et al., 1985; Arvin and Gershon, 1996). In addition to glycoprotein antigens, VZV DNA also encodes for other structural and nonstructural proteins including enzymes and proteins that regulate viral development (Grose, 1987; Straus et al., 1988). VZV DNA is synthesized in a cascade of immediate early (IE) or α regulatory genes, followed by early (E) or β regulatory and structural genes, followed by late (L) or γ structural genes. Interruption of the cascade, particularly at the IE stage, results in failure to synthesize infectious virus (Hay and Ruyechan, 1994). The linear double-stranded DNA genome of VZV has been fully sequenced (Davison and Scott, 1986). The genome is quite stable, as evidenced by the comparison of viral isolates obtained from patients during primary infection and during subsequent reactivation infection (Gelb et al., 1987; Hayakawa et al., 1984; Straus et al., 1984; Williams et al., 1985). Genome differences do exist, however, enabling differentiation of vaccine strains of VZV from wild-type strains (Martin et al., 1982; Gelb et al., 1987; LaRussa et al., 1992; Hayakawa et al. 1984).

VZV does not cause clinical disease in common laboratory animals, although simian forms of varicella have been described. Newborn hairless guinea pigs may be infected with VZV that has been adapted in vitro to guinea pig tissue (Myers et al., 1980, 1985, 1991).

PATHOLOGY

The following sequence of events is believed to occur when a varicella-susceptible person is infected (Fig. 37-2). The virus gains entry at the respiratory mucosa and presumably multiplies in the regional lymphatic tissue. Four to six days after infection a low-level primary viremia is believed to occur, allowing the virus to infect and multiply in the liver, spleen, and possibly other organs. Approximately 10 to 12 days after infection a secondary viremia of greater magnitude occurs, at which time the virus reaches the skin (Grose, 1981). The rash results, on the average, 14 days after infection. Viremia, which has been demonstrated during the early stage of clinical varicella, is more difficult to demonstrate in normal than in immunocompromised children (Asano et al., 1985a, 1990; Feldman and Epp, 1976, 1979; Myers, 1979; Ozaki et al., 1986). Viremia has also been reported in some patients with zoster (Feldman et al., 1977; Gershon et al., 1978). The skin lesions of varicella begin as macules, the majority of which progress to papules, vesicles, pustules, and crusts over a few days. Some lesions regress after the macular and papular stages. Vesicles are located primarily in the epidermis; the roof is formed by the stratum corneum and stratum lucidum and the floor by the deeper prickle cell layer. Ballooning degeneration of epidermal cells is followed by formation of multinucleated giant cells, many of which contain typical type A intranuclear inclusion bodies. Inclusion bodies are also present in vascular endothelial cells, presumably indicating the mode of spread of virus from the blood to the tissues. Vesicles are formed by accumulation of fluid derived from dermal capillaries, which fills in the space created by degenerating epidermal cells.

As the skin lesions progress, polymorphonuclear leukocytes invade the corium and vesicular fluid (Stevens et al., 1975), and the fluid changes from clear to cloudy. Interferon has been demonstrated in vesicular fluid and is believed to reflect the CMI response to the virus by the host (Merigan et al., 1978). The resolution of skin lesions leads to the formation of a scab, which is at first adherent but later becomes detached. Mucous membrane lesions

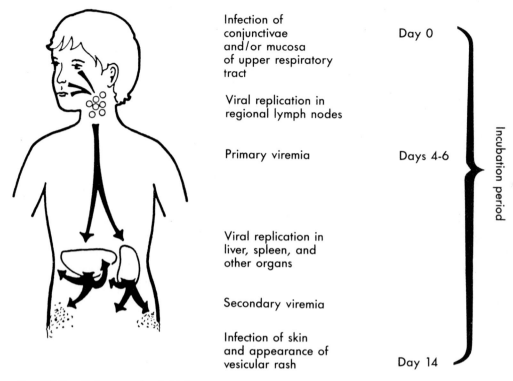

Infection of conjunctivae and/or mucosa of upper respiratory tract — Day 0

Viral replication in regional lymph nodes

Primary viremia — Days 4-6

Viral replication in liver, spleen, and other organs

Secondary viremia

Infection of skin and appearance of vesicular rash — Day 14

Incubation period

Fig. 37-2   Pathogenesis of chickenpox. (From Grose C. Varicella-zoster virus. Boca Raton, Fla: CRC, 1987.)

develop in the same way but do not progress to scab formation. The vesicles usually rupture and form shallow ulcers, which heal rapidly. Although the most obvious target organ of the virus is the skin, children with benign cases of varicella and transiently elevated aspartate aminotransferase (AST) levels (>50 IU/L) have been described (Myers, 1982; Pitel et al., 1980).

Postmortem examination of infants and adults who died of varicella reveals evidence of involvement of many organs. Areas of focal necrosis and acidophilic inclusion bodies may be present in the esophagus, liver, pancreas, kidney, gastrointestinal tract, ureter, bladder, uterus, and adrenal glands. The lungs show evidence of widely disseminated interstitial pneumonia, with numerous hemorrhagic areas of nodular consolidation. Histologically, the exudate consists chiefly of red blood cells, fibrin, and many mononuclear cells, some containing intranuclear inclusion bodies (Fig. 37-3). Encephalitis complicating varicella is pathologically similar to that with measles and to other types of postinfectious encephalitis showing perivascular demyelination in the white matter.

Latent infection with VZV is believed to develop when sensory nerve endings in the epidermis are invaded by the virus during varicella when the virus is present on the skin. Virions presumably are transported up the sensory nerves to the ganglia where latency is established. Alternatively, latent infection may result from seeding of nerve tissue during viremia. During latency, several viral genes are expressed in sensory ganglia; these are mostly IE genes, although some E genes are also expressed. However, L genes are not expressed, and infectious particles are not formed or released (Croen et al., 1988; Straus et al., 1988; Hay and Ruyechan, 1994). At least one protein encoded by an IE gene expressed during latency has been identified in ganglia latently infected with VZV (Mahalingham et al., 1996). Reactivation of VZV in human neurons in dorsal root ganglia has been demonstrated using in situ hybridization in autopsy specimens (Lungu et al., 1995). As shown in Fig. 37-4, when viral reactivation occurs, infectious virions are produced, and virions are transported down the sensory nerve to the skin where vesicles appear (Hope-Simpson, 1965; Lungu et al., 1995). Patients with impaired CMI have the highest rate of zoster, which is consistent with the hypothesis that at least some aspects of VZV latency are under immunologic control (Arvin et al., 1978, 1980; Hardy

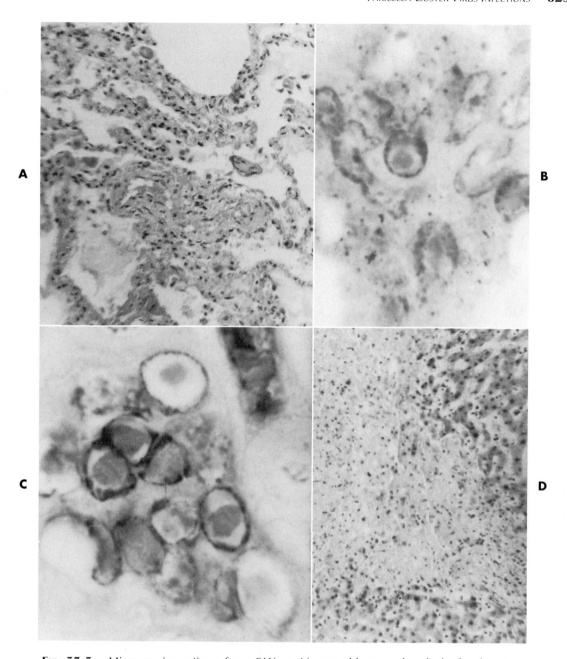

FIG. 37-3   Microscopic sections from E.W., a 44-year-old man who died of pulmonary edema after 5 days of hemorrhagic varicella associated with severe right upper quadrant abdominal pain, cough, dyspnea, tachypnea, cyanosis, and hemoptysis. **A,** Interstitial mononuclear cell infiltration and fibrinous exudate in the alveoli of the lung. **B,** Intranuclear inclusion bodies in the lung. **C,** Multinucleated cell with intranuclear inclusions in the skin. **D,** Typical focus of necrosis in the liver. (From Krugman S et al. N Engl J Med 1957;257:843.)

et al., 1991). The incidence of zoster probably increases in the elderly because CMI responses to VZV diminish with advancing age (Burke et al., 1982; Miller, 1980). An increased incidence of zoster with a short latency period has also been observed in children who experienced varicella in prenatal life or early infancy, presumably because of immaturity of the CMI response to VZV during primary infection (Baba et al., 1986; Brunell and Kotchmar, 1981; Dworsky et al., 1980; Guess et al., 1985; Terada et al., 1994). Brunell and Kotchmar (1981) described five infants with zoster, all of whose mothers had varicella between 3 and 7 months' gestation. These infants had no evidence of varicella after birth. Presumably all had varicella in utero, since they developed zoster after an average latent period of only 21 months (range, 3 to 41 months). Usually the latent period between varicella and zoster lasts for decades.

Efforts to culture infectious virus from such ganglia have been not been successful. Using in situ hybridization and polymerase chain reaction (PCR), however, VZV DNA and RNA and viral proteins have been demonstrated in human sensory ganglia obtained from autopsy material (Mahalingham et al., 1990; Hyman et al., 1983; Croen et al., 1988). These data indicate that the site of VZV latency is in sensory ganglia.

CLINICAL MANIFESTATIONS OF VARICELLA

After an incubation period of 14 to 16 days, with outside limits of 10 to 21 days, the disease begins with low-grade fever, malaise, and the appearance of rash. In children the exanthem and constitutional symptoms usually occur simultaneously. In adolescents and adults the rash may be preceded by a 1- to 2-day prodromal period of fever, headache, malaise, and anorexia. The typical clinical course of varicella is illustrated in Fig. 37-5.

Rash

The typical vesicle of chickenpox is superficially located in the skin. It has thin, fragile walls that rupture easily. A vesicle resembles a dewdrop in appearance; it is usually elliptical in shape, 2 to 3 mm in diameter, and surrounded by an erythematous area. This red areola is most distinct when the vesicle is fully formed and becomes pustular; it fades as the lesion begins to dry. The drying process, which begins in the center of the vesicle or pustule, produces an umbilicated appearance and eventually a crust. After a variable interval of 5 to 20 days, depending on the depth of skin involvement, the scab falls off, leaving a shallow pink depression. The site of the lesion becomes white, usually with no scar formation. Secondarily infected lesions and prematurely removed scabs may be followed by scarring.

Skin lesions appear in crops that generally involve the trunk, scalp, face, and extremities. The distribution is typically central, with the greatest concentration of lesions on the trunk and face (Fig. 37-6). The rash is more profuse on the proximal parts of the extremities (upper arms and thighs) than on the distal parts (forearms and legs). A distinctive manifestation of the eruption is the presence of lesions in all stages in any one general anatomic area; macules, papules, vesicles, pustules, and crusts are usually located in proximity to each other (Fig. 37-7). Many maculopapular lesions progress to the vesicular stage and resolve without crusting.

In the typical case of chickenpox, three successive crops of lesions appear over a 3-day period in the characteristic central distribution just described.

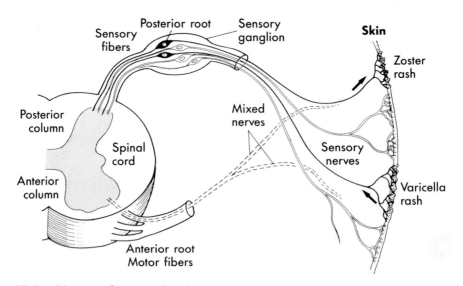

FIG. 37-4   Diagram of proposed pathogenesis of zoster. Latent VZV infection in dorsal root ganglia develops during the rash of varicella. Reactivation of VZV in ganglia may subsequently occur, resulting in zoster. Affected neurons and affected sensory nerves are in black. (Modified from Hope-Simpson RE. Proc R Soc Med 1965;58:9-20.)

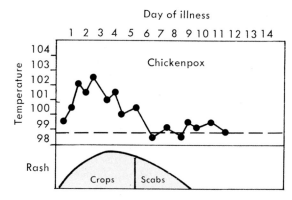

FIG. 37-5 Schematic diagram illustrating clinical course of typical case of chickenpox. Crops of lesions appear, with rapid progression from macules to papules to vesicles to scabs.

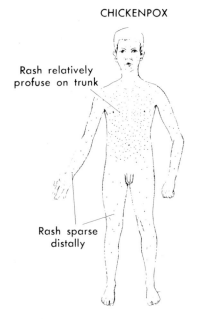

FIG. 37-6 Schematic drawing illustrating typical distribution of rash of chickenpox.

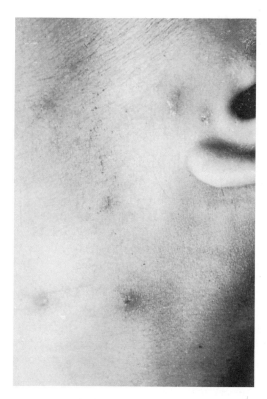

FIG. 37-7 Chickenpox lesions in various stages.

The extremes of this picture may range from (1) a single crop of a few scattered lesions to; (2) a series of five or more crops developing over a week, with an uncountable number of lesions covering the entire skin surface of the body. In a study of over 750 cases of chickenpox in otherwise healthy children, the average child developed approximately 300 skin vesicles (Ross et al., 1962). In secondary cases in a household the rash is usually more extensive than in the primary case (Ross et al., 1962).

Vesicles may develop on the mucous membranes of the mouth in addition to the skin. They occur most commonly over the palate and usually rupture so rapidly that the vesicular stage may be missed. They resemble the shallow, white, 2- to 3-mm ulcers of herpetic stomatitis. The palpebral conjunctiva, pharynx, larynx, trachea, and rectal and vaginal mucosa may also be involved. Areas of local inflammation such as ammoniacal dermatitis in the diaper area or sunburned skin may have a significant increase in the number of lesions. These vesicles are generally smaller than usual, are usually in the same stage of development, and may become confluent.

In summary, the rash of chickenpox is characterized by (1) a rapid evolution of macule to papule to vesicle to pustule to crust, (2) a central distribution of lesions that appear in crops, (3) intense itching, and (4) the presence of lesions in all stages in any one anatomic area.

Fever

The temperature curve of a typical case of chickenpox is illustrated in Fig. 37-5. The height of the fever usually parallels the severity of the rash. When the eruption is sparse, the temperature is usually normal or slightly elevated; an extensive rash more likely will be associated with high and more prolonged fevers. Temperatures up to 40.6° C (105° F) are not unusual in severe cases of chickenpox with involvement of almost the entire skin surface.

Other Symptoms

Headache, malaise, and anorexia usually accompany the fever. In many cases the most distressing symptom is pruritus, which is present during the vesicular stage of the disease.

CLINICAL MANIFESTATIONS OF ZOSTER

A previous clinical or subclinical episode of varicella is a prerequisite. The incubation period of zoster is unknown because it is impossible to determine the time of reactivation of latent VZV. The predilection of the virus for the posterior nerve root areas accounts for the severe pain and tenderness along the involved nerves and the corresponding areas of skin seen in elderly patients. Fever may not be present, especially in children in whom the disease is often mild.

Zoster occurs only when CMI to VZV is decreased. This depression may be transient such as when otherwise healthy young persons develop the illness, progressive with increasing age, or it may be secondary to severe immunosuppression induced by diseases such as malignancy, by anticancer chemotherapy or radiotherapy, or after immunosuppression for organ transplantation. Following development of zoster, there is a rapid increase in specific CMI in most patients (Berger et al., 1981; Burke et al., 1982).

Zoster is usually characterized by a unilateral rash with a dermatomal distribution. The lesions begin as macules and papules and progress through the same stages similar to those of varicella. The regional lymph nodes may be enlarged and tender. The rash may appear on the face (involvement of the trigeminal ganglia), the trunk (thoracic ganglia), the shoulders, arms, and neck (cervical ganglia), or the perineal area and lower extremities (lumbar or sacral ganglia). When the trigeminal nerve is involved, infection of the maxillary division is associated with lesions of the uvula and tonsillar area; the mandibular division, with lesions of the buccal mucosa, the floor of the mouth, or anterior part of the tongue; and the ophthalmic division, with scleral and corneal lesions. Infection of the geniculate ganglion of the facial nerve can result in pain, a vesicular eruption in the auditory canal, and facial paralysis, which usually subsides but may be permanent (Ramsay Hunt syndrome). Severe neuralgia, which may persist for many months after convalescence, is much more common in elderly adults than in children. It is also thought that in immunologically normal, as well as in immunocompromised, hosts viral reactivation can occur without development of skin lesions; this phenomenon has been termed *zoster sine herpete* (Luby et al., 1977; Gershon et al., 1982; Ljungman et al., 1986; Wilson et al., 1991). VZV DNA, RNA, and some proteins moreover have also been found in the circulating peripheral white blood cells in elderly patients with and without postherpetic neuralgia (Vafai et al., 1988; Devlin et al., 1992), suggesting that subclinical reactivation can occur. Viremia caused by VZV has been demonstrated in asymptomatic patients following bone marrow transplantation, indicating subclinical reactivation of VZV (Wilson et al., 1992).

DIAGNOSIS OF VARICELLA
Confirmatory Clinical Factors

The typical case of chickenpox can be recognized clinically with ease. The characteristic diagnostic features include (1) development of a pruritic papulovesicular eruption concentrated on the face, scalp, and trunk associated with fever and mild constitutional symptoms; (2) the rapid progression of macules to papules, vesicles, pustules, and crusts; (3) the appearance of these lesions in crops; (4) the presence of shallow white ulcers on the mucous membranes of the mouth; and (5) the eventual crusting of the skin lesions. The knowledge of an exposure to a person with either varicella or zoster is always helpful when present.

Detection of the Causative Agent

Laboratory diagnosis by methods such as demonstration of VZV antigens or DNA in, or viral isolation from, skin lesions are indicated for identification of atypical or unusual types of chickenpox. VZV antigens may readily be detected in vesicles by various immunologic means, including direct immunofluorescence with commercially available monoclonal antibodies. Such assays can be performed within an hour's time and can distinguish between VZV and HSV (Rawlinson et al., 1989; Gleaves et al., 1988; Zeigler and Halonen: 1985; Zeigler, 1984). PCR has proven useful for diagnosis of VZV infection using swabs of lesions or vesicular fluid (La Russa et al., 1993). VZV may be isolated from vesicular fluid obtained within the first 1 to 3 days of rash by employing cell cultures such as human embryonic lung fibroblasts, although these assays may not be available in all laboratories and the virus is rather labile.

Detection of the presence of VZV DNA by PCR in cerebrospinal fluid (CSF) has also been used to implicate VZV as causing encephalitis (Puchhammer-Stockl et al., 1991; LaRussa et al., 1995).

Serologic Tests

Antibody can be detected in serum within days after onset of varicella and can be expected to increase in titer over the next 1 to 2 weeks. Consequently, a retrospective diagnosis is possible if acute- and convalescent-phase serum specimens are available. The first sample of blood should be collected as soon as possible after the onset of disease; the second should be obtained approximately 10 days later. Enzyme-linked immunosorbent assay (ELISA), which is commercially marketed, is the most frequently used serologic test (Demmler et al., 1988; Forghani et al., 1978; Gershon et al., 1981; Shanley et al., 1982; Shehab and Brunell, 1983). ELISA may also be used to determine immune status to varicella; if a significant amount of antibody is present in serum, it indicates a prior episode of varicella even in the absence of a history of the illness. The fluorescent antibody to membrane antigen (FAMA) assay, anticomplement immunofluorescence, and radioimmunoassay (RIA) are extremely sensitive but are not commercially available (Campbell-Benzie et al., 1983; Presissner et al., 1982; Richman et al., 1981; Williams et al., 1974; Zaia and Oxman, 1977). These tests are more sensitive for identification of immunity to varicella than ELISA but are not necessarily any better than ELISA for making a serologic diagnosis of the disease. A latex agglutination (LA) test, utilizing latex particles coated with VZV antigen, has shown great promise as a sensitive and specific VZV serologic test, especially to document immune status to varicella (Steinberg and Gershon, 1991; Gershon et al., 1994).

A skin test using VZV antigen was developed and used to identify individuals who lack CMI to VZV and may be susceptible to varicella (Florman et al., 1985; Kamiya et al., 1977; LaRussa et al., 1985). This test is most accurate in persons under age 40, when there is a good correlation between the presence of specific antibodies and CMI to VZV; however, it is currently not available.

Ancillary Laboratory Findings

The white blood cell count is not consistently abnormal, and in most cases it is within the normal range. It is not unusual for adults with primary varicella pneumonia to have leukocytosis with a predominance of polymorphonuclear leukocytes.

DIAGNOSIS OF ZOSTER

Identification of VZV is essential for a definitive diagnosis of zoster. Characteristic zosteriform skin lesions have on occasion been observed in HSV infections; in a study of forty-seven adults with clinical signs and symptoms compatible with zoster, six (13%) yielded HSV from cultures of skin lesions (Kalman and Laskin, 1986). Laboratory diagnosis is made best by demonstration of the virus or viral antigens in vesicular fluid. A fourfold rise in VZV antibody titer 2 to 4 weeks after appearance of lesions provides confirmation of the diagnosis, although increases in VZV antibody titer have been described in HSV infections because of shared antigens between these viruses (Schmidt, 1982; Vafai et al., 1990).

DIFFERENTIAL DIAGNOSIS OF VARICELLA

The differential diagnosis of varicella is also discussed in Chapter 40. Varicella may resemble the following conditions.

Impetigo

The skin lesions of impetigo are vesicular at first but rapidly progress to honey-colored crusts. They differ from chickenpox in appearance and distribution. They do not appear in crops, do not involve the mucous membranes of the mouth, and are not accompanied by constitutional symptoms. The lesions commonly involve the nasolabial area because of the tendency for a child to scratch this area with contaminated fingers. Other areas that are easily scratched also become involved.

Insect Bites, Papular Urticaria, and Urticaria

Insect bites, papular urticaria, and urticaria are not accompanied by constitutional symptoms. They are papular and pruritic but do not have the typical vesicular appearance and distribution. Vesicles, if present, are pinpoint in size. The scalp and mouth are devoid of lesions.

Scabies

The differential points of scabies are the same as those of insect bites. In addition, the observation of burrows between the fingers and toes and the microscopic identification of *Sarcoptes scabiei* help confirm the diagnosis.

Rickettsialpox

Rickettsialpox has the classic triad of signs and symptoms in the following order: (1) the appearance of a primary lesion or eschar on some part of the body, (2) the development of an influenza-like syndrome, and (3) the occurrence of a generalized papulovesicular eruption. The rash of rickettsialpox differs from that of varicella in that the vesicles are much smaller and are superimposed on a firm papule. Crusts do not develop regularly; if they do, they are very small. The diagnosis is confirmed by a specific antibody test.

Eczema Herpeticum and Other Forms of HSV Infection

A patient with eczema herpeticum may have a history of contact with a person who had a fever blister; the rash is caused by either primary or reactivated HSV infection. The vesicular and pustular lesions are most profuse over the sites of eczema. The different type of distribution is the most useful differential point. At times it may be necessary to perform laboratory examinations (e.g., direct immunofluorescence, described previously) to identify the causative agent. Eczema vaccinatum could also be confused with varicella, but since smallpox vaccine is no longer used, this diagnosis is highly unlikely.

In the newborn infant, HSV and varicella may be confused when only a few vesicular skin lesions are present and there is no history of exposure to either virus. In this instance, direct immunofluorescence of skin lesions is extremely helpful. Zosteriform lesions in the neonate caused by HSV infection have been reported (Music et al., 1971; Rabalais et al., 1991).

Stevens-Johnson Syndrome

With this syndrome there may be a prior history of use of medications and allergy. Annular skin lesions and extensive involvement of mucous membranes suggest Stevens-Johnson syndrome.

COMPLICATIONS OF VZV INFECTION

Complications of varicella are not common; uneventful recovery is the rule except in immunocompromised persons. The following incidence of serious complications in children aged 1 to 14 years per 100,000 cases of varicella has been recorded: encephalitis, 1.7; Reye's syndrome, 3.2; hospitalization, 1.7; and death, 2.0 (Preblud et al., 1984). More recently, however, Choo et al. (1995) noted in a retrospective study of varicella in a large health maintenance organization (HMO) with 250,000 members that the rate of hospitalization ranged from 4 to 11 times higher in children than previously estimated.

Secondary Bacterial Infection

The secondary infection of skin lesions is not common enough to warrant the use of prophylactic antimicrobials. Staphylococci or group A β-hemolytic streptococci may gain entry into the lesions and produce impetigo, furuncles, cellulitis, and erysipelas. Scalded skin syndrome (Melish, 1973; Wald et al., 1973) and toxic shock–like syndrome (Bradley et al., 1991) have both been reported as complications of chickenpox. Although bacterial superinfections can result in septicemia, pneumonia, suppurative arthritis, osteomyelitis, or local gangrene, there has been a low incidence of these complications, even in the era before antibiotics were available. Bullous impetigo caused by exfoliative toxigenic *S. aureus,* phage type II, may be considered a secondary bacterial infection. Neutropenia that occasionally follows varicella may predispose to secondary bacterial infections (Koumbourlis, 1988).

There is evidence that the incidence of infection with highly virulent group A β-hemolytic streptococci may be increasing in recent years. Following varicella, these infections may be superficial or highly invasive, resulting in deep-seated infections such as pneumonia, necrotizing fasciitis, and osteomyelitis (Brogan et al., 1995; Davies et al., 1996; Gonzalez-Ruiz et al., 1995; Mills et al., 1996; Peterson et al, 1995; Peterson et al., 1996; Vugia et al., 1996; Wilson et al., 1995). Fatalities have been reported. In one epidemiologic study of streptococcal infection, varicella was the most significant risk factor for this infection in children less than 10 years of age, with an attack rate of 4.4 per 100,000 cases and a relative risk of 39 during the 2 weeks following varicella (Davies et al., 1996).

Bullous Varicella. Bullous varicella is an unusual manifestation characterized by the simultaneous occurrence of typical varicelliform lesions and bullae. Published reports indicate that the bullous lesions are caused by phage group II staphylococci (Melish, 1973; Wald et al., 1973). These staphylococci produce epidermolytic toxin, the cause of staphylococcal scalded skin syndrome. In this complication, VZV is not present in the bullous fluid.

Second Attacks of Varicella. It was once generally accepted that varicella occurs only once in a lifetime. Second attacks of clinical illness are difficult to confirm by laboratory means because most first attacks are diagnosed only clinically. There is a growing body of evidence, however, suggesting that second attacks of varicella may occur. Varicella has been observed in persons shown to have specific antibodies before onset of illness (Weller, 1983; Gershon et al., 1984a, 1988, 1989; Zaia et al., 1983; Junker et al., 1991; Junker and Tilley, 1994). Serologic evidence of subclinical infection of varicella-immune individuals closely exposed to VZV has also been reported (Arvin, et al, 1983; Gershon et al., 1982, 1984b, 1988, 1989; Luby et al., 1977). Many second attacks are mild. Second attacks are most common in immunocompromised persons, in those who originally had subclinical infections, and in children who had varicella in early infancy.

Central Nervous System Involvement.
Central nervous system involvement is rare but may complicate a mild or a severe infection. Guess et al. (1986) reported an incidence of acute cerebellar ataxia of 1 in 4000 cases of varicella and of other forms of varicella encephalitis (excluding Reye's syndrome) of 1 in 33,000 cases. According to Peters et al. (1978), cerebellar involvement with ataxia is also the most common form of encephalitis following varicella. If cerebellar ataxia occurs as an isolated phenomenon, the prognosis is excellent. The symptoms usually develop between the third and eighth days after the onset of rash, but at times they may precede the exanthem. It is not yet clear whether CNS involvement represents the direct effect of viral replication or the immune response to the presence of VZV in the CNS. Although VZV is rarely cultured from the spinal fluid in these cases, both VZV specific antibody and DNA have been shown to be present (LaRussa et al., 1995).

The signs of cerebral involvement include those of meningoencephalitis, with fever; headache; stiff neck; change in sensorium; and, occasionally, convulsions, stupor, coma, and paralysis. The cerebral form of encephalitis carries a more guarded prognosis. At one time it was difficult to differentiate between varicella encephalitis and Reye's syndrome. In a survey of fifty-nine cases of varicella encephalitis, Applebaum et al. (1953) reported complete recovery in 80%, evidence of brain damage in 15%, and death in 5%. Of 302 cases of varicella encephalitis reported in the United States during 3 years (1963 to 1965), 82 (27.1%) were fatal (McCormick et al., 1969). Other rare CNS complications include transverse myelitis, peripheral neu-

ritis, and optic neuritis (Jemsek et al., 1983). In both cerebellar and cerebral types, CSF changes include pleocytosis with a predominance of lymphocytes, an elevated protein value, and a normal glucose value.

Encephalitis ranging from mild to severe, either accompanying or following zoster, is not uncommon. Other neurologic complications of zoster include motor and autonomic nerve involvement with paralysis, and cerebral angiitis. These complications of zoster are much more frequent in older adults than in children. Encephalopathy resulting from reactivation of VZV in the CNS in the absence of rash has been reported in immunocompromised patients (Dueland et al., 1991; Silliman et al., 1993). This form of encephalopathy may be disabling and eventually prove fatal.

Reye's Syndrome. Elevations of liver enzyme levels are not infrequent in otherwise healthy children during varicella (Ey and Fulginiti, 1981; Myers, 1982; Pitel et al., 1980). Pitel et al. studied thirty-nine children with varicella; transaminase elevations were greater than normal in 77%. Jaundice is rare, and the condition is almost always self-limited. Until these studies were reported, it was not realized that the liver can be involved in uncomplicated varicella. The relationship, if any, between this asymptomatic form of varicella hepatitis and Reye's syndrome is not known, although some children have experienced severe vomiting episodes during the period of abnormal liver enzyme activity. Lichtenstein et al. (1983) obtained liver biopsies from nineteen children who had marked elevation of aminotransferase activity with minimal neurologic symptoms (lethargy) after varicella (eight children) or an upper respiratory tract infection (eleven children). Microscopic evidence suggesting Reye's syndrome was found in fourteen (74%). Reye's syndrome as a complication of varicella has become significantly more rare since the administration of aspirin became contraindicated during chickenpox.

Varicella in the Adult. Varicella, like many other viral infections, is more likely to be severe in adults than in children. The risk of dying from varicella in persons more than 20 years of age is 25 times greater than it is in children (Preblud et al., 1984). In general, the fever is higher and more prolonged, the constitutional symptoms are more severe, the rash is more profuse, and complications are more frequent in adults than in children. Primary varicella pneumonia is a significant complication in adults. A prospective evaluation of 114 military personnel with varicella revealed roentgenographic evidence of pulmonary involvement in 16%, although clinical signs were present in only 4% (Weber and Pellecchia, 1965). The severity of varicella in adults may be related to the impaired ability of adults to mount a CMI response to VZV in comparison to children (Gershon, 1995; Nader et al., 1995).

Varicella Pneumonia. Varicella pneumonia has been recognized chiefly in otherwise healthy adults and immunocompromised patients of all ages. It is rare in normal children, but it has been seen in some infants with neonatal varicella (see the following section). One to five days after chickenpox begins, there is an onset of cough; chest pain; dyspnea; tachypnea; and, possibly, cyanosis and hemoptysis. Rales are usually heard over both lung fields. The roentgenogram shows characteristic nodular densities throughout both lung fields (Fig. 37-8). The bilateral nodular infiltrates vary in size and occasionally coalesce to form larger areas of consolidation. The leukocyte count may be either normal or slightly elevated.

The course of the pneumonia is variable. It may be extremely mild with little or no cough and no respiratory distress, and roentgenographic evidence of the disease may subside within 1 week. On the other hand, respiratory problems may be severe, with chest pain, hemoptysis, cyanosis, a stormy course of 7 to 10 days, and roentenographic findings that persist for as long as 4 to 6 weeks. Occasionally there is a fatal outcome despite antiviral therapy. Varicella pneumonia may be further complicated by pleural effusion, subcutaneous emphysema, pulmonary edema, and adult respiratory distress syndrome (ARDS). Some patients with varicella pneumonia show evidence of other visceral involvement such as hepatitis. Mackay and Cairney (1960) reported roentgenographic evidence of widespread, evenly distributed 1- to 3-mm nodules of calcific density in seven adults who had severe varicella after the age of 19 years. The roentgenograms were taken 3 to 32 years after onset of varicella. A summary of the epidemiologic and clinical manifestations of primary varicella pneumonia in the pre–antiviral drug era is given in Table 37-1.

Congenital Varicella Syndrome. The congenital varicella syndrome is rare. Since the 1940s when it was first recognized, approximately fifty

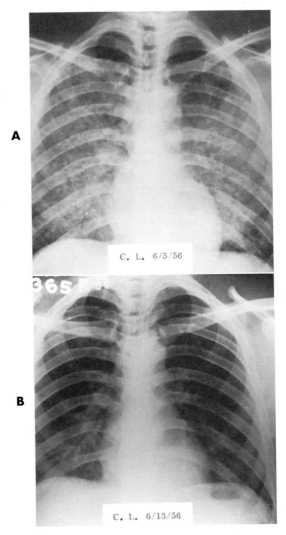

A

B

FIG. 37-8 Roentgenograms of the chest of C.L., a 24-year-old man with varicella, characterized on the third day by severe cough, dyspnea, tachypnea, cyanosis, and hemoptysis. **A,** Roentgenogram taken on the fourth day of pneumonia, showing extensive nodular infiltrates throughout both lung fields. **B,** Appearance 8 days later; there was considerable clearing. (From Krugman S et al. N Engl J Med 1957;257:843.)

cases have been recorded in the world literature (Alkalay et al., 1987; Gershon, 1994; Paryani and Arvin, 1986). Frequent manifestations of the syndrome include a hypoplastic extremity, zosteriform skin scarring, microphthalmia, cataracts, chorioretinitis, and abnormalities of the CNS (Table 37-2 and Fig. 37-9). There is a spectrum of disease, with most children severely affected but some with only a few stigmata, such as chorioretinitis or vocal cord paralysis (Randel et al., 1996).

Table 37-1 Summary of epidemiologic and clinical manifestations of 30 cases of primary varicella pneumonia in the pre–antiviral drug era

Age	Range: 4 to 82 yr			Mean average: 33 yr
	(only two children, 4 and 6 years of age, both with leukemia)			
Sex	Male: 22			Female: 8
Season	January to March: 15 cases	April to June: 14 cases		October to December: 1 case
Day of onset of cough	First: 5	Second: 15	Third: 7	Fourth and fifth: 3
Clinical manifestation	*Severe*	*Moderate*	*Mild*	*None*
Cough	11	8	11	—
Dyspnea	11	7	1	11
Cyanosis	10	0	0	19
Hemoptysis	10	3	1	15
Rales	11	8	1	10
Roentgenographic findings	11	8	11	—
White blood count	Range: 4,000 to 16,200			Mean: 8,600
Complications	Hepatitis (4)			
	Pleural effusion (3)			
	Pulmonary abscesses (2)			
	Subcutaneous emphysema (1)			
	Gastric ulcers (1)			
Deaths	Pulmonary edema (1)			
	Pulmonary abscesses and gastric ulcers (1)			
	Hepatitis (3)			
	Pulmonary abscesses and Hodgkin's disease (1)			
	Leukemia (1)			

Table 37-2 Clinical and laboratory data of 39 infants with the congenital varicella syndrome

Occurrence	(%)
After maternal varicella	87
After maternal zoster	13
Time (weeks) of maternal infection	
Median	12
Range	8-28

Major Malformations Described	(%)
Cicatricial skin lesions	72
Ocular abnormalities: cataract, chorioretinitis, Horner's syndrome, microphthalmia, nystagmus	62
Hypoplastic limb	46
Cortical atrophy and/or mental retardation	31
Early death	24

Modified from Gershon A. Chickenpox, measles, and mumps. In Remington JS, Klein JO (eds). Infections of the fetus and newborn infant, ed 3. Philadelphia: WB Saunders, 1990.

The incidence of this syndrome following gestational varicella in the first trimester is approximately 2% (Preblud et al., 1986). There have been six studies, four of which were prospective, of pregnant women with varicella and their offspring, (Manson et al., 1960; Siegel, 1973; Enders, 1984; Paryani and Arvin 1986; Balducci et al., 1992; Pastuszak et al., 1994) in which 288 pregnancies (maternal varicella in the first trimester in 220) were followed and 4 affected infants resulted (2%). Women whose infants were affected had varicella ranging from the seventh to the twenty-eighth week of pregnancy, with most cases occurring at about week 13. Fortunately, the syndrome is very rare, since there is no practical way to diagnose it in utero. There is one reported instance in which congenital defects were identified by fetal ultrasound (Essex-Cater and Heggarty, 1983) and another in which defects could not be identified by ultrasound (DaSilva et al., 1990). There is a high correlation (>50%) between a hypoplastic extremity and severe brain damage and/or early death (Gershon, 1994).

The pathogenesis is not understood, but the rarity of the illness and the pattern of cicatricial skin lesions with damage to the nervous system suggest that the fetus may have experienced varicella secondary to maternal viremia, followed by reactivation resulting in zoster in utero. Interestingly, infants with the syndrome have also been reported to develop clinical zoster with a short period of viral latency in postnatal life (Kotchmar et al., 1984). This is ascribed to the immature CMI response to

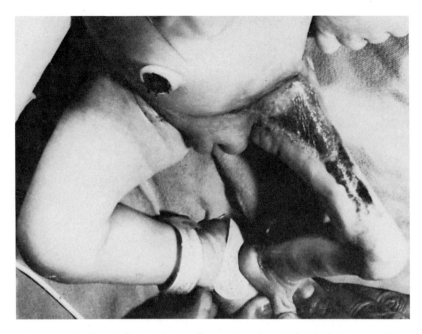

FIG. 37-9   Congenital varicella syndrome illustrating cicatricial skin lesions and hypotrophic left lower limb. (From Srabstein JC et al. J Pediatr 1974;84:239.)

VZV in fetal life (Terada et al., 1994). Maternal varicella itself may also be severe during pregnancy, and fatalities have been reported (Paryani and Arvin, 1986).

Severe disseminated and fatal varicella in 5- to 10-day-old infants, resembling that in leukemic children, may occur in offspring whose mothers have varicella 5 days or less before delivery. This phenomenon may be related to several factors. In infants who develop the illness between 5 and 10 days of age (an incubation period of approximately 10 days), the cellular immune response to VZV is still immature. In addition, the size of the inoculum introduced into the infant by the mother's viremia may be large, which might account for the shorter incubation period. Furthermore, when the mother has had varicella for less than 5 days before delivery, she has not made or transferred VZV antibody to her baby; maternally derived antibody may act as a form of passive immunization for the infant born to women who develop varicella a week or longer before delivery. The clinical attack rate of varicella in newborn infants born to women with onset of varicella 5 days or less before delivery has been reported to range from 20% to 50% (Meyers, 1974; Hanngren et al., 1985; Preblud et al., 1986). In infected infants who have been neither passively immunized with varicella-zoster immune globulin (VZIG) nor treated with an antiviral drug, the mortality rate is approximately 35% (Meyers,

Table 37-3   Maternal varicella near term: effect on the newborn infant (50 cases)

Onset	Effect
Maternal varicella, 5 or more days before delivery; baby's varicella, age 0-4 days	27 of 27 survived
Maternal varicella, 4 days or less before delivery; baby's varicella, age 5-10 days	16 of 23 survived (7 died of disseminated varicella, 2 had severe disease with survival)

From Gershon AA. In Krugman S, Gershon AA (eds). Infections of the fetus and newborn infant. New York: Alan R Liss, 1975.

1974). In the United States, administration of passive immunization has made severe varicella of the newborn a rarity (Bakshi et al., 1986).

Disseminated varicella infection in a newborn infant is characterized by hemorrhagic lesions and involvement of the lungs and the liver. Effects on the newborn infant when maternal varicella occurs near term are shown in Table 37-3.

Hemorrhagic, Progressive, and Disseminated Varicella. Varicella in an immunocompromised host may be characterized by a hemorrhagic, progressive, or disseminated infection with a potentially fatal outcome. Feldman et al. (1975) observed seventy-seven children with cancer at St. Jude Children's Research Hospital who contracted varicella in the pre–antiviral therapy era. No complications were observed among the seventeen children no longer receiving anticancer chemotherapy. In contrast, of the sixty children still receiving anticancer chemotherapy, nineteen (32%) had evidence of visceral dissemination and four (7%) died. Deaths were associated with varicella pneumonia (all four patients) and encephalitis (two of the four patients). Disseminated varicella occurred more frequently in children with absolute lymphopenia who had fewer than 500 lymphocytes/mm^3.

In a more recent assessment of children with underlying cancer and varicella at the same institution, Feldman and Lott (1987) reported 127 patients observed between 1962 and 1986. They found that despite passive immunization and antiviral therapy, fatalities caused by varicella still occurred. Children with leukemia fared more poorly than children with other malignancies, although the incidence of varicella pneumonia was high in each group—32% and 19%, respectively. In children with leukemia who had received passive immunization with VZIG, the incidence of primary viral pneumonia was 15%. Cessation of anticancer chemotherapy during the incubation period did not significantly decrease the incidence of varicella pneumonia.

There are two possible courses of severe varicella in immunocompromised children. In some a fulminant disease with hemorrhagic lesions, pneumonia, and disseminated intravascular coagulation occurs; death usually ensues within a few days, often despite antiviral therapy. In other children a more protracted illness develops, with new crops of vesicles occurring for as long as 2 weeks. At first these children may appear to have mild disease, but, as new lesions continue to develop, accompanied by fever, toxicity, abdominal and back pain, and pneumonia, the serious nature of the illness becomes apparent, usually during the second week after onset.

Severe, progressive, fatal varicella infection has also been observed in children treated with high doses of corticosteroids for conditions other than cancer. Gershon et al. (1972) described the development of fulminant varicella in two boys treated with corticosteroids for rheumatic fever; deaths occurred 2 and 4 days after onset of rash. Although

children with asthma treated with low doses of steroids apparently are not at risk to develop severe varicella, fatalities have been reported in those receiving high doses (Kasper and Howe, 1991; Silk et al., 1988). Whether children receiving inhaled steroids for prophylaxis against asthma are predisposed to varicella is unclear; these children are not considered to be immunocompromised. One anecdotal report of two patients using daily inhaled steroids to control asthma who developed severe varicella may represent coincidence rather than cause and effect (Choong et al., 1995).

Severe varicella has been described in patients who have undergone renal (Feldhoff et al., 1981; Lynfield et al., 1992) and bone marrow (Locksley et al., 1985) transplantation, and in children with acquired immunodeficiency syndrome (AIDS) (Acheson et al., 1988; Jura et al., 1989; Pahwa et al., 1988). They and other immunocompromised patients are also at high risk to develop varicella or zoster that may be recurrent or chronic, although the frequency of this occurrence is unknown (Acheson et al., 1988; Feldhoff et al., 1981; Gershon et al., 1984a; Morens et al., 1980; Patterson et al., 1989). Development of zoster in young adults is a sentinel for subsequent development of AIDS (Colebunders et al., 1988; Melbye et al., 1987). Development of zoster at a rate as high as 70% has been reported in children infected with HIV with CD4+ lymphocyte counts under 15% at onset of varicella (Gershon et al., 1996).

It has long been thought that immunocompromised children are predisposed to develop severe varicella because their CMI response to VZV is deficient. In immunocompromised patients the in vitro lymphocyte response to VZV antigen has been reported to develop more slowly in those with severe disease than in those with an uncomplicated illness (Arvin et al., 1986). Furthermore, lymphocytes from leukemic children with prior varicella show decreased in vitro responses to VZV antigen in comparison to lymphocytes from healthy controls (Giller et al., 1986). This phenomenon is attributed to decreased numbers of circulating lymphocytes rather than to impaired antigen presentation. Studies of lymphoid cells from patients with fatal varicella indicate the inability of these cells to inactivate VZV in vitro in contrast to lymphoid cells from control individuals (Gershon and Steinberg, 1979). There is no apparent correlation of poor antibody responses after vaccination with severe varicella in immunocompromised patients.

Severe and fatal cases of varicella have been observed in children with underlying AIDS, in whom a new syndrome of chronic VZV infection has also been described. After recovery from varicella these children may develop scattered, sparse, wartlike lesions from which VZV can be isolated (Jura et al., 1989; Pahwa et al., 1988). Although the natural history of this form of varicella is not yet fully understood, VZV infections seem to smolder in some HIV-infected patients and may eventually result in chronic progressive encephalitis, with a potentially fatal outcome even if treated (Gilden et al., 1988; Pahwa et al., 1988; Silliman et al., 1993). VZV resistant to acyclovir (ACV) has developed in some of these patients who were treated for many months (Jacobson et al., 1990; Linnemann et al., 1990; Pahwa et al., 1988).

Disseminated Zoster. Disseminated zoster is not uncommon; it is usually seen in children and adults with marked persistent depression of CMI to VZV. In contrast to what usually appears to occur in the normal host, a viremia develops following the localized dermatomal rash, resulting in an additional generalized rash. Fever is more likely to be present than in localized zoster. The number of skin lesions outside the dermatomal area ranges from a few to thousands; the extent of the rash reflects the seriousness of the infection. Fatalities may occur when there is extensive visceral involvement if no antiviral therapy is given (Feldman et al., 1973; Shepp et al., 1986; Whitley et al., 1982).

Patients who have undergone bone marrow transplantation are not only at increased risk to develop zoster, but also to develop severe symptoms. In a study of 1394 adults who underwent bone marrow transplantation, the incidence of zoster after 1 year was approximately 17% (Locksley et al., 1985). Of these adults, 45% developed disseminated disease, and the overall fatality rate in the group was 6% despite antiviral therapy. There was also a high incidence of postherpetic neuralgia, skin scarring, and bacterial superinfections.

Rare Complications

Retinitis caused by VZV may be a manifestation of the congenital varicella syndrome, and it may be a complication of zoster in HIV-infected patients (Chambers et al., 1989; Friedman et al., 1994; Kuppermann et al., 1994). Acute glomerulonephritis has been described in patients either with or without evidence of associated streptococcal infection (Yuceoglu et al., 1967). Myocarditis has also been recorded (Kirk et al., 1987; Lorber et al., 1988; Waagoner and Murphy, 1990), as has orchitis (Wesselhoft and Pearson, 1950; Liu et al, 1994).

Varicella arthritis is a rare complication that is usually self-limited. The arthritis is usually monoarticular, with swelling, tenderness, pain, and joint effusion, but with no erythema. The synovial fluid contains a predominance of lymphocytes and is free of bacteria (Mulhern et al., 1971; Priest et al., 1978; Ward and Bishop, 1970; Baird et al., 1991). Isolation of VZV from joint fluid obtained from a patient with varicella arthritis has been reported (Priest et al., 1978), and the diagnosis has also been established by PCR (Baird et al., 1991).

A very rare complication of purpura fulminans and gangrene of the extremities and face has been described following varicella (deKoning et al., 1972; Smith, 1967). Another very rare complication of varicella, as well as zoster, is vasculitis and thrombosis leading to neurologic symptoms (Fikrig and Barg, 1989; Liu and Holmes, 1990; Caekebeke et al., 1990; Bodensteiner et al., 1991; Amlie-Lefond et al., 1995).

PROGNOSIS

Varicella is usually a benign disease of childhood, although recent evidence suggests that it may be potentially more serious than previously thought (Choo et al., 1995). The typical case usually clears spontaneously without sequelae or skin scarring. Lesions that are secondarily infected are likely to be followed by permanent scars if the deep layers of the skin are involved. The rare case of sepsis, bacterial pneumonia, or osteomyelitis usually responds to appropriate antibacterial therapy. Preblud et al. (1985) estimated that there are fewer than 10 annual deaths caused by varicella in infants under 1 year of age in the United States per year, primarily as a result of pneumonia or encephalitis. Although this represents a risk of death of 8 per 100,000 cases—4 times greater than that of older infants and children with varicella—the risk is obviously very small (Preblud et al., 1985). There are an estimated 100 deaths annually in the United States from varicella and 9000 hospitalizations (Gershon et al., 1995). Since zoster is a secondary infection, the risk of fatalities associated with zoster is lower than that for varicella.

IMMUNITY

An attack of chickenpox usually confers lasting immunity; second attacks are unusual (Gershon et al., 1984a; Weller, 1983; Junker et al., 1989, 1991,

1994). Varicella-zoster antibody persists for many years after chickenpox. Most immune adults have antibodies detectable by ELISA, FAMA, LA, or RIA.

Transplacental immunity has been examined. In one study 200 mother-infant (cord) serum specimens for VZV antibody were tested by FAMA; 10% of the pairs in this group were seronegative (Gershon et al., 1976). The maternal and cord blood antibody titers were essentially the same. Women born in the United States were more likely to be immune than those born in Latin American countries. Only 5% of U.S.-born women were seronegative, compared to 16% of those born in Latin America. A high incidence of susceptibility to varicella in adults from tropical areas also has been noted (Nassar and Touma, 1986). The disappearance of passively acquired antibody in the first year of life is shown in Fig. 37-10. By 6 months of age, most infants no longer have detectable VZV antibody. Transplacentally acquired VZV antibody has been detected in the blood of low birth weight infants, even those weighing less than 1500 g (Raker et al., 1978), but not in infants less than 1000 g at birth (Wang et al., 1983). Development of mild varicella in young infants despite the presence of transplacental maternal antibody has been reported (Baba et al., 1982).

The immune correlates of VZV infection remain incompletely understood. During the course of vaccine trials with the live attenuated varicella vaccine, it was recognized that the presence of specific serum antibody at the time of exposure to the virus does not necessarily guarantee protection from clinical varicella, especially in immunocompromised patients. A minority of recipients of varicella vaccine who had underlying leukemia devel-

oped mild clinical varicella after an exposure several months after immunization despite serum VZV antibody titers that were predicted as protective (Gershon et al., 1984b, 1989). In addition, varicella has been reported in persons having detectable VZV antibody after natural infection (Zaia et al., 1983; Gershon et al., 1984a). These observations led to reexamination of the mechanism by which immunity to varicella is mediated. Serum antibody may not be fully protective; either CMI or secretory immunity may also be important in protection. (Bogger-Goren et al., 1984; Cooper et al., 1988; Diaz et al., 1989; Gershon and Steinberg, 1980; Giller et al., Hayward et al., 1986; Ihara et al., 1986; Rand et al., 1977; Arvin and Gershon, 1996).

It was recognized many years ago that the prognosis of varicella in children with isolated defects in humoral immunity was excellent. In contrast, children with congenital defects in CMI were recognized to be at high risk to develop severe infections. Specific CMI to VZV develops after an attack of varicella. Failure to develop a positive cellular immune response correlates with death from varicella (Arvin et al., 1986; Gershon and Steinberg, 1979; Patel et al., 1979). Various types of CMI to VZV have been described, including T-cell and macrophage cytotoxicity, antibody dependent cellular cytotoxicity (ADCC), and natural killer (NK) cells. (Cooper et al., 1988; Diaz et al., 1989; Gershon and Steinberg, 1980; Giller et al., 1989; Hayward et al., 1986; Ihara et al., 1986; Patel et al., 1979; Rand et al., 1977; Arvin and Gershon, 1996).

The exact roles of humoral and cellular immunity in protection against VZV infection are under continued investigation and are summarized as follows (reviewed in Arvin and Gershon, 1996). Structural and regulatory proteins of VZV are recognized by T lymphocytes during varicella and play the major role in protection of the host from further VZV infection. This is consistent with the observation that patients with agammaglobulinemia are not subject to bouts of recurrent varicella. Memory immunity mediated by both CD4+ and CD8+ T lymphocytes is maintained for decades and can be demonstrated by in vitro proliferation and cytokine assays. Memory responses may normally persist because of periodic exogenous reexposure to others with either varicella or zoster. Immunity may also be maintained by endogenous reexposure to the virus as a result of subclinical reactivation of latent VZV. Sensitized T lymphocytes

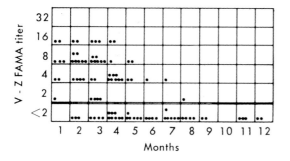

FIG. 37-10 Detection of varicella–zoster antibody in the first year of life in 67 infants. The sensitive fluorescent antibody against membrane antigen (FAMA) test was used for the assay. (From Gershon AA, et al. Pediatrics 1976;58:692.)

that are exposed to VZV antigens produce cytokines of the TH1 type, such as interleukin-2 (IL-2) and interferon-γ (IFN-γ); these potentiate the clonal expansion of virus-specific T cells (Arvin and Gershon, 1996). That CMI rather than humoral immunity is required to maintain the balance between the host and latent VZV is demonstrated by the correlation between diminished CMI and the increased risk of zoster in immunocompromised and in elderly individuals. Patients who develop zoster, however, usually have a rapid increase in VZV CMI because of endogenous exposure to viral antigens. This enhanced CMI is usually persistent, which may explain why second episodes of zoster are uncommon. Susceptibility of individuals to VZV reactivation, in contrast, is not related to levels of VZV antibodies. A diagram depicting the summary of the dynamic natural history of VZV infections is shown in Fig. 37-11.

EPIDEMIOLOGIC FACTORS

Chickenpox is worldwide in distribution, being endemic in all large cities. Epidemics do not have the periodicity of measles; they occur at irregular intervals determined chiefly by the size and concentration of new groups of susceptible children. All races and both sexes are equally susceptible. In countries with tropical climates there is decreased spread of VZV among children, and varicella in adults is a common occurrence. Seasonable distribution varies with the particular geographic zone; in temperate areas the incidence rises during the late autumn, winter, and spring. In contrast to varicella, zoster occurs with equal frequency throughout the year.

Varicella is predominantly a disease of childhood, with the highest age incidence between 2 and 10 years. Its occurrence is unusual in adults who have lived in heavily populated urban areas but not uncommon in those who have come from isolated rural areas. Ross et al. (1962) observed a group of 641 adults and 501 children who had intimate household exposures to varicella. The overall attack rates were 1.4% for adults and 78% for children. Of 79 adults with a negative history of varicella, only 8% acquired the disease. In contrast, 87% of 441 children with no history of varicella acquired the disease.

Studies in New York City have indicated that of ninety-two consecutive adults with no history of varicella, twenty-three (25%) were actually susceptible (LaRussa et al., 1985). Others have noted a similar percentage of susceptibility in adults from throughout the United States (Alter et al., 1986; Steele et al., 1982). In the continental United States the overall rate of susceptibility to varicella in adults is less than 5%.

Nosocomial varicella is a significant problem, not only because some patients may be at risk to develop a severe infection, but also because of the expense and administrative problems associated with management of a potential hospital outbreak (Krasinski et al., 1986; Weber et al., 1988). Often physicians, nurses, and other personnel susceptible to varicella must be furloughed after an exposure until the potential incubation period ends. In a study of Weber et al. the cost per year at a university hospital was $56,000 for passive immunization of high-risk susceptibles and furloughs of susceptible

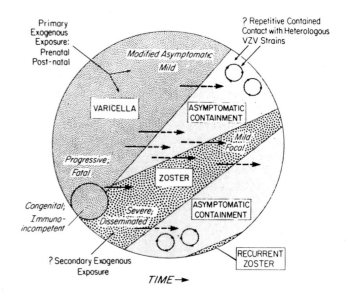

FIG. 37-11 Diagrammatic summary of the natural history of infection with varicella-zoster virus. Two variables are depicted: time and clinical severity. In the competent host the containment period is on the order of decades; however, in the immunocompromised person the two clinical processes may merge without an intervening asymptomatic interval. The containment period after congenital varicella is typically of short duration. During the asymptomatic containment period, episodes of endogenous viral replication probably occur, and contact with heterologous exogenous strains may stimulate host defenses, usually in the absence of overt disease. (From Weller TH. N Engl J Med 1983;309:1362–1368,1434–1440.)

staff personnel. Similar hospital costs for a year's time were recorded by Krasinski et al. (1986). Transmission of varicella is rare, however, in the setting of the newborn nursery. Only three instances of such nosocomial spread have been recorded (Gershon et al., 1976; Gustafson et al., 1984; Friedman et al., 1994a).

Although apparent hospital outbreaks of zoster have been described (Schimpff et al., 1972), in many instances they are probably coincidental occurrences, since they involve a high proportion of immunocompromised patients. Some apparent cases of zoster are probably second attacks of varicella (Morens et al., 1980).

Zoster is predominantly a disease of adults, in contrast to varicella. A study of 108 zoster patients revealed that 69% were 50 years of age or older and less than 10% were children (Miller and Brunell, 1970). In a study of 192 cases the annual incidence of zoster per 1000 persons was 0.74 in children under 10 years, 2.5 in persons aged 20 to 50, and 10 in those over age 80 (Hope-Simpson, 1965).

Immunocompromised children are at increased risk to develop zoster compared to healthy children. In a study of children with malignant disease the overall rate of zoster was 9% (Feldman et al., 1973). This study involved 1132 patients over a 10-year period. The rate of zoster in patients with Hodgkin's disease was 22%; it was 10% in children with acute lymphoblastic leukemia, and 5% in children with solid tumors. No specific chemotherapy was associated with increased risk of infection. A similar high rate of zoster of about 15% in leukemic children was observed in more recent studies (Brunell et al., 1986; Lawrence et al., 1988; Hardy et al., 1991). Children with HIV infection who develop varicella when they have CD4+ levels of less than 15% have been reported to have a rate of zoster as high as 70% (Gershon et al., 1996).

Chickenpox is one of the most highly contagious diseases, comparable to measles and smallpox in this respect. The infection is spread chiefly by direct contact with a patient with active varicella or zoster. The major source of the virus may be from skin lesions, although respiratory spread can also occur in varicella (Brunell, 1989; Tsolia et al., 1990). It is virtually impossible to culture VZV from the throat even in the early stages of varicella, but viral isolation from skin can be easily accomplished. The chances of viral transmission are directly related to the number of skin lesions (Tsolia

et al., 1990). Patients are probably most contagious in the early stages of illness, when they have the greatest numbers of moist vesicular skin lesions. That the virus is spread by the airborne route has been determined in hospital outbreak studies in which airflow patterns from patient rooms have been examined (Gustafson et al., 1982; Josephson and Gombert, 1988; Leclair et al., 1980). Presumably as a result of scratching of the pruritic skin lesions, VZV gains access to the air. Under hospital conditions, indirect contact through the medium of a third person has not been documented, and it is not likely that medical personnel carry the infection from one place or patient to another.

A patient with chickenpox can transmit the disease to other susceptible persons from 1 or 2 days before onset of rash until all the vesicles have become dry. A mild case will show complete crusting within 5 days and a severe case within 10 days. Dry scabs do not contain infectious virus, although VZV DNA may still be demonstrable by PCR. Patients with zoster remain infectious to others who have not had varicella as long as new lesions continue to develop and the existing ones remain moist. This may be longer than the interval of contagion for varicella.

TREATMENT

Chickenpox in otherwise healthy children is normally a self-limited disease. Symptomatic therapy includes acetaminophen for high fever and constitutional symptoms. A comparison of the course of varicella in children who did or did not receive acetaminophen revealed minimal differences in the course of the illness, with the children who were treated having a slightly longer course (Doran et al., 1989). It seems unlikely that the differences in the course of illness are clinically significant, however, and the relief of fever afforded by acetaminophen therapy seems worth the theoretical minimal risk. Aspirin should not be given, since it may lead to development of Reye's syndrome (Mortimer and Lepow, 1962; Starko et al., 1980). Although some reports suggest an association of use of with nonsteroidal antiinflammatory drugs with severe streptococcal disease in children with varicella, this has not been proven (Peterson et al., 1996). Since it is unclear whether treatment with nonsteroidal antiinflammatory drugs predisposes to bacterial superinfection, for theoretical reasons these medications should be avoided in varicella until the issue is clarified. Oral antihistamines and local applications of calamine lotion may help control the itching of varicella. Fingernails should be kept short and clean in an attempt to minimize secondary skin infections. For the same reason, daily bathing is also recommended during chickenpox.

Treatment of Complications

Bacterial Infections. Bacterial infections complicating chickenpox are most often caused by *S. aureus* or group A β-hemolytic streptococci. Infection of local lesion usually responds to simple measures such as warm compresses. Antimicrobial therapy is indicated for cellulitis, sepsis, or pneumonia. The treatment of severe streptococcal and staphylococcal infections are discussed in detail in Chapters 30 and 31, respectively.

Encephalitis. Patients in coma require careful observation and supportive treatment such as parenteral and tube feedings for the maintenance of hydration and adequate nutrition. Corticosteroids have not provided effective therapy for varicella encephalitis. Antiviral therapy may be used but is of no proven value. Cerebellar ataxia is usually a self-limited complication for which specific treatment is unnecessary.

Specific Antiviral Therapy for Varicella and Zoster

The antiviral drug ACV (9,2-hydroxyethoxy-methylguanine) has become the drug of choice for specific therapy of VZV infections, but the drug does not prevent or cure latent VZV. ACV is available in topical, oral, and intravenous formulations, but only the latter two are useful against VZV. Only approximately 15% to 20% of orally administered ACV is absorbed.

ACV is relatively nontoxic because it interferes mainly with synthesis of viral rather than host DNA; it is not antiviral itself. To interfere with DNA synthesis, ACV must be phosphorylated by a virus-induced enzyme, thymidine kinase. This enzyme is present almost exclusively in infected cells; therefore the effect of ACV on uninfected cells is minimal. Since the enzyme is not required for viral synthesis, strains of VZV can become resistant to ACV either (1) by ceasing to produce thymidine kinase, or (2) by producing a truncated or altered enzyme or altered viral DNA polymerase that will not bind the phosphorylated ACV. A few thymidine kinase–negative, ACV-resistant strains of VZV have been reported in AIDS patients (Jacobson et al., 1990; Linnemann et al., 1990; Pahwa et al., 1988). The clinical relevance of these ACV-resistant viruses remains unknown since resistant strains are less invasive than sensitive strains, and transmission to non-AIDS patients has not been observed. ACV-resistant strains are generally also resistant to drugs such as famciclovir and valacyclovir, which have mechanisms of action similar to those of ACV. Foscarnet, a pyrophosphate analogue, which exerts its antiviral effect by inhibition of the viral DNA polymerase, has been useful in the treatment of these ACV-resistant strains. Renal toxicity has limited more widespread use of foscarnet.

The dose of ACV used to treat VZV infections is higher than that used to treat HSV infections, since VZV is less sensitive to this drug than is HSV. Usual plasma concentrations necessary for inhibition of VZV are 1 to 2 mcg/ml, with a range of roughly 0.5 to 11 mcg/ml. Commonly used doses of intravenous ACV almost always result in plasma levels significantly above maximal inhibitory concentrations for VZV isolates. In contrast, orally administered ACV leads to drug levels (1 to 1.5 mcg/ml) that will inhibit most but not all VZV strains. Toxicity of ACV includes nausea, vomiting, skin rash, phlebitis (if given intravenously), and precipitation of the drug in the renal tubules in poorly hydrated patients. Since ACV is excreted by the kidney, lower doses should be used for patients with abnormalities in renal function (Arvin, 1986; Balfour et al., 1983).

In a double-blind, placebo-controlled study of its efficacy, ACV was administered orally at high dosage in otherwise healthy children (Balfour et al., 1990). An oral dose of 20 mg/kg of ACV 4 times daily for 5 days was given to 50 children within 24 hours of onset of the skin rash. A similar group received placebo. The duration of the disease was shortened by approximately 1 day as evidenced by defervescence and healing of rash, but treated children did not return to school any sooner than placebo recipients, and the rate of complications of varicella was not altered by therapy. These studies were confirmed in a larger collaborative controlled study involving about a thousand children (Dunkel et al., 1991). Treatment with ACV does not appear to interfere with development of immunity to VZV (Englund et al., 1990; Levin et al., 1995). Since varicella is statistically but not significantly clinically altered by ACV, whether or not to routinely treat children with varicella with ACV is problematic. The drug is expensive and whether there are long-term adverse effects of ACV is not known for certain. Moreover, the possibility that drug resistance of VZV to ACV may increase with widespread use of this drug must be considered. One possible approach is to give ACV to adolescents, who are at greater risk to develop more significant clinical manifestations of varicella, and to secondary cases of varicella in the household, since secondary cases usually are more severe than index cases. Early therapy administered within the first day of onset of rash is also important and is potentially easier to implement in secondary cases in a household in which the disease can be quickly recognized. There is positive anecdotal experience in administration of ACV to adults with varicella (Feder, 1990; Haake et al., 1990). However, a small double-blind study did not indicate clear efficacy (Wallace et al., 1993).

Orally administered ACV has been used with success to decrease the morbidity of otherwise healthy adults with zoster by relieving acute pain and promoting healing of the skin lesions (Cobo, 1988; Huff et al., 1988; McKendrick et al., 1986; Wood et al., 1988, 1996). A dosage of 4 g per day (800 mg 5 times a day by mouth for 7 days) is used. Since otherwise healthy children who develop zoster usually have only a mild illness, ACV is not often given to children with zoster. Newer drugs, valacyclovir and famciclovir, are recommended for treatment of zoster but have neither been tested in children nor tested for treatment of varicella. These drugs, referred to as *prodrugs,* are converted in the liver after oral administration to the parent compound. They are well absorbed by the oral route and therefore result in higher drug levels than administration of the parent compound itself, thus requiring less frequent dosing intervals. The parent compound of valacyclovir is ACV; for famciclovir the parent is penciclovir (Spring et al., 1994). These drugs are used at dosages of 500 (famciclovir) and 1000 (valacyclovir) mg tid orally for 1 week for treatment of zoster in adolescents and adults.

Severe Varicella and Zoster. ACV administered intravenously (IV), is the drug of choice for treatment of severe varicella or zoster and for varicella that is potentially life threatening. When administered IV to immunocompromised children within 3 days of onset of rash, this drug decreases mortality from varicella (Balfour, 1984; Prober et al., 1982) and prevents viral dissemination (Berger et al., 1981; Feldman et al., 1986; Nyerges et al., 1988). Administering intravenous ACV also results in more rapid healing of zoster in normal and immunocompromised patients, ameliorates acute pain, and decreases the likelihood of viral dissemi-

nation (Balfour, 1984; Balfour et al., 1983; Peterslund, 1988; Shepp et al., 1988). In uncontrolled studies, ACV has been used to treat varicella pneumonia in adults, including pregnant women, with apparent success (Eder et al., 1988; Landsberger et al., 1986; Schlossberg and Littman, 1988). ACV is superior to vidarabine for treatment of VZV infections, mainly because of its lower toxicity (Feldman et al., 1986; Shepp et al., 1988).

For treatment of immunocompromised patients with varicella or zoster, ACV should be administered IV at a dose of 1500 mg/m^2 of body surface area per day, divided q8 hours, for 7 to 10 days. Reduced dosages should be used for patients with impaired renal function. For adolescents a dosage of 10 mg/kg of body weight every 8 hours may be used.

Because the dosage for newborn infants with severe varicella is not known, use of a dosage of 750 mg/m^2/day is suggested. Some investigators have recommended that all infants who develop neonatal varicella, even those who have been passively immunized with VZIG, be treated with ACV (Haddad et al., 1987; Holland et al., 1986; Sills et al., 1987). Another possible approach is to initiate therapy with oral medication, reserving intravenous ACV for those whose infection is progressing. In the United States most can be expected to recover without antiviral therapy (Hanngren et al., 1985; Preblud et al., 1986). Very rare fatalities caused by varicella have been recorded in infants who contracted varicella from their mothers near the time of delivery despite administration of VZIG at an appropriate time and dosage (Bakshi et al., 1986; King et al., 1986). The case reported by King et al. is of special interest because the mother developed the rash of varicella on the second postpartum day.

It is recommended that immunocompromised children who have not been actively or passively immunized be treated with intravenous ACV as soon as possible after the diagnosis of varicella has been made, although most patients so treated would recover on their own. Even if the disease appears mild at first, it is impossible to predict which children will develop severe infections. Once varicella has become severe, ACV may not be effective. There is no consensus as to whether it is preferable to withhold anticancer chemotherapy (including steroids) after an exposure to varicella and/or after the onset of varicella, with the exception that in steroid-dependent children this medication should not be abruptly withdrawn. Decisions about treatment of these patients should be individualized and made in consultation with the oncologist following the child.

It may seem more compelling to treat all immunosuppressed patients with varicella, since the mortality rate approaches 10%, than to treat all such patients with zoster, which has a lower mortality rate of perhaps 1% to 2%. Among zoster patients, adults with lymphoproliferative cancers and those who have had bone marrow transplantation are at greatest risk for severe disease (Whitley et al., 1982). Since ACV is relatively nontoxic, however, an argument can be made to treat most immunocompromised patients with zoster, including children, to decrease morbidity from the illness. In zoster patients who are not especially ill, an attempt to treat with orally administered ACV may be made, using, for children, the dosages administered for varicella. The use of antiviral therapy in patients with CNS complications of varicella or zoster is controversial because the underlying pathology is not well understood. Many physicians elect to treat immunocompromised patients—but not those who are immunologically normal—with antiviral drugs.

Alternative secondary drugs, vidarabine and interferon, are also effective in treatment of varicella and zoster but have significant toxicity and are rarely used (Arvin et al., 1982; Merigan et al., 1978; Whitley et al., 1982). VZIG is not useful for therapy of VZV infection. Until more information on the long-term persistence of immunity becomes available, prophylactic ACV is not recommended for exposed varicella-susceptibles (Asano et al., 1993; Huang et al, 1995).

PREVENTIVE MEASURES
Passive Immunization

Preventive measures are not usually recommended for healthy varicella-susceptible children who have been exposed to VZV. On the other hand, exposed susceptible immunocompromised children, as well as adults proven susceptible, should be passively immunized with VZIG (Centers for Disease Control, 1996). Infants whose mothers have the onset of the rash of varicella within 5 days before and 2 days after delivery should be protected with passive immunization. Indications for the use of VZIG—based on the recommendations of the Committee on Infectious Diseases of the American Academy of Pediatrics and the Advisory Committee on Immunization Practices of the Centers for Disease Control in Atlanta, Georgia—are shown in Box 37-1.

Successful passive immunization against varicella was first accomplished with zoster immune globulin (ZIG). ZIG was prepared from plasma of patients convalescing from zoster. A dose of 5 ml of ZIG, given within 72 hours of a household exposure to children with underlying leukemia, modified chickenpox (Brunell et al., 1969; Gershon et al., 1974; Judelsohn et al., 1974; Orenstein et al., 1981).

ZIG has now been supplanted by VZIG, which is prepared from plasma of healthy donors with high antibody titers against VZV. VZIG is similar to ZIG in its ability to modify varicella in high-risk children (Zaia et al., 1983). The dosage of VZIG is 1.25 ml/10 kg of body weight, administered intramuscularly within 3 days of exposure. VZIG may also be effective up to 5 days after exposure, but it is probably not worthwhile to administer it after that interval following exposure.

BOX 37-1

INDICATIONS FOR USE OF VZIG

1. **No previous history of clinical varicella**
   and
2. **Underlying condition**

Leukemia, lymphoma

Congenital or acquired deficiency of cellular immunity *or*

Immunosuppressive therapy (including prednisone) *or*

Newborn infant of mother with onset of varicella within 5 days before delivery and 2 days after delivery *or*

Premature infant more than 28 weeks' gestation whose mother has no prior history of varicella *or*

Premature infant less than 28 weeks' gestation and/or birth weight under 1,000 g, regardless of maternal history of varicella
   and
3. **Significant exposure**

Continuous household contact *or*

Playmate contact greater than 1 hour indoors *or*

Hospital contact: in same two- or four-bed room or in adjacent beds in large ward; face-to-face contact with an infectious employee or patient *or*

Newborn contact with infected mother
   and

Within 3 days of contact (preferably given sooner; in some cases may give up to 5 days after exposure)

Modified from MMWR 1984;33:84-100.

VZIG has been used successfully to modify varicella in approximately 100 newborn infants whose mothers had varicella at delivery (Hanngren et al., 1985; Preblud et al., 1986). In both studies the attack rate of varicella was approximately 50%, not indicative of a decrease in the attack rate after passive immunization. However, as in immunocompromised children, the illness was clearly modified, with most infants developing mild disease and no fatalities clearly caused by varicella. An alternative to VZIG is intravenous globulin (Paryani et al., 1984). Neither VZIG nor globulin can be expected to prevent or modify zoster in high-risk patients (Groth et al., 1978; Merigan et al., 1978).

Active Immunization

A live attenuated varicella vaccine developed in Japan by Takahashi et al. (1974), the Oka strain, was licensed for routine use in susceptible children and adults in the United States in 1995. This vaccine was prepared by serial passage of wild-type VZV isolated from an otherwise healthy 3-year-old Japanese boy (whose last name was Oka) with varicella. After approximately thirty-five passages in various cell cultures of guinea pig and human origin, the agent remained immunogenic but rarely caused symptoms on administration by injection.

In clinical trials in the United States in healthy children (Arbeter et al., 1982, 1984, 1986a, 1986b; Brunell et al., 1988; Englund et al., 1989; Johnson et al., 1988); healthy adults (Alter et al., 1985; Arbeter et al., 1986; Gershon et al., 1988; Hardy and Gershon, 1990); and children with underlying leukemia (Gershon et al., 1984b, 1989), the vaccine was demonstrated to be safe and highly effective in preventing severe varicella.

Immunization against varicella in healthy children is associated with minimal adverse effects—mainly a mild rash of about five lesions in about 5%, and transient redness, swelling, and rash at the injection site in about 20%. Transmission of vaccine type VZV from healthy vaccinees with a rash to other varicella-susceptible contacts has been recorded on rare occasions. Contact cases are mild, indicating the attenuation of the vaccine strain (Tsolia et al., 1989). The vaccine provides approximately 90% protection in prevention of varicella. The few children who develop breakthrough varicella almost always have very mild disease with few skin lesions and little systemic toxicity. In research studies, administering varicella vaccine in combination with measles-mumps-rubella (MMR) vaccine has resulted in excellent antigenic responses to all four viruses (Arbeter et al., 1986; Brunell et al., 1988; Englund et al., 1989), but the final formulation of this product has not been determined and this combination vaccine is not yet available. However, varicella vaccine and MMR vaccine can be administered simultaneously using separate sites and syringes.

Varicella vaccine is recommended for healthy varicella-susceptible children and adults. Children between the ages of 12 months and 12 years should be given 1 dose of vaccine. Adults and children who have reached their thirteenth birthday should be given 2 doses of vaccine at 4 to 8 week intervals. Individuals receiving low or moderate doses of steroids (less than the equivalent of 2 mg/kg/day of prednisone) may be immunized (Centers for Disease Control, 1996; Committee on Infectious Diseases, 1996). Contraindications to immunization include severe allergy to any vaccine component, significant immunosuppression, and pregnancy. Because of the association of natural varicella, aspirin use, and Reye's syndrome, the package insert recommends as a precautionary measure that children receiving chronic aspirin therapy not be vaccinated.

Varicella vaccine has not yet been approved for use in high-risk immunocompromised children in the United States (except for leukemic children who can be immunized on a "compassionate use" mechanism), despite the demonstrated efficacy of this approach in published studies. Approximately 85% of leukemic children were protected against chickenpox after vaccination, and all were protected from severe disease in studies involving over 500 children. Although 50% of leukemics may develop a vaccine-associated rash in the month after immunization, serious rashes can be prevented by administration of high-dose oral ACV (Gershon et al., 1984b, 1989; Gershon, 1990). Immunocompromised children such as leukemics who develop a vaccine-associated rash have greater potential to spread vaccine-type VZV to others than healthy individuals. Contact cases, however, are extremely mild, indicating that the vaccine virus is attenuated (Gershon et al., 1984b; Tsolia et al., 1990). "Breakthrough" cases of wild-type chickenpox in leukemic vaccinees after exposure to natural VZV have been mild (Gershon et al., 1989). Children with chronic renal insufficiency were successfully immunized against chickenpox with few adverse effects except for a mild rash in 5% to 10% (Broyer and Boudailliez, 1985a, 1985b).

The incidence of zoster was initially reported not to be increased after vaccination of leukemic children who are ordinarily at high risk to develop reactivation of VZV (Brunell et al., 1986; Lawrence et al., 1988; Sakurai et al., 1982). It is now clear from controlled studies that the incidence of zoster is lower after vaccination than after the natural disease in leukemic children (Hardy et al., 1991). There is also no evidence of an increased incidence of zoster in healthy children or adults (Gershon et al., 1990; Plotkin et al., 1989). With time, it is anticipated that the incidence of zoster after vaccination will be found to be lower than after natural infection in healthy vaccinees.

Studies thus far indicate that varicella vaccine will provide long-lasting protection from chickenpox, based on persistence of antibodies to VZV after vaccination. A 10-year follow-up study by Asano et al. (1985b) and a small 20-year follow-up in Japan (Asano et al., 1995) indicated that positive antibody titers and protective immunity were maintained in healthy children for this period. Studies in the United States involving approximately 100 children have indicated persistence of antibodies for as long as 6 years in close to 100% of children (Kuter et al., 1991; Clements et al., 1995; Krause et al., 1995; Watson et al., 1995).

Antiviral Prophylaxis

A number of small studies (Asano et al., 1993; Huang et al., 1995) suggested the efficacy of giving ACV on exposure to VZV, but this approach is not generally accepted.

ISOLATION AND QUARANTINE

Unless there are specific local regulations, isolation and quarantine procedures should be individualized. Most authorities agree that (1) the patient with chickenpox or zoster should be kept at home until all the vesicles have dried, (2) contacts should

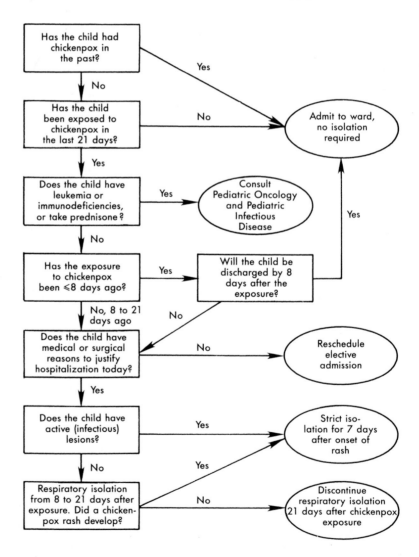

FIG. 37-12 Algorithm for chickenpox exposure. (From Brawley RL, Wenzel RP. Pediatr Infect Dis 1984;3:502-504.)

not be quarantined but merely observed, and (3) efforts to institute isolation precautions within the home to protect siblings are useless and should not be attempted.

On the other hand, rigid isolation precautions should be used for the prevention of chickenpox in high-risk children. Appropriate measures should be instituted to prevent contact with a definite or potential case of chickenpox. If exposure has occurred or is inevitable, use of the preventive measures already described would be indicated. Widespread use of varicella vaccine may decrease the necessity of isolation of cases in the future. An algorithm for the management of hospital exposures to varicella is shown in Fig. 37-12.

BIBLIOGRAPHY

Acheson DWK, Leen CL, Tariq WU, Mandal B. Severe and recurrent varicella-zoster virus infection in a patient with the acquired immune deficiency syndrome. J Infect Dis 1988; 16:193-197.

Alkalay AL, Pomerance JJ, Yamamura JM, et al. Congenital anomalies associated with maternal varicella infections during early pregnancy. J Perinatol 1987;7:69-71.

Alter SJ, Hammond JA, McVey CJ, Myers M. Susceptibility to varicella-zoster virus among adults at high risk for exposure. Infect Contr 1986;7:448-451.

Alter SJ, McVey CJ, Jenski L, Myers M. Varicella live virus vaccine in normal susceptible adults at high risk for exposure. Interscience Conference on Antimicrobial Agents and Chemotherapy, 1985 (abstract 457).

Amlie-Lefond C, Kleinschmidt-DeMasters BK, Mahlingham R, et al. The vasculopathy of varicella-zoster virus encephalitis. Ann Neurol 1995;37:784-790.

Applebaum E, Rachelson MH, Dolgopol VB. Varicella encephalitis. Am J Med 1953;15:523.

Arbeter A, Starr S, Weibel RE, Plotkin SA. Live attenuated varicella vaccine: immunization of healthy children with the Oka strain. J Pediatr 1982;100:886-893.

Arbeter AM, Baker L, Starr SE, et al. Combination measles, mumps, rubella, and varicella vaccine. Pediatrics 1986a; 78:742-742.

Arbeter A, Starr SE, Plotkin SA. Varicella vaccine studies in healthy children and adults. Pediatrics 1986b; 78(suppl): 748-756.

Arbeter AM, Starr SE, Preblud S, et al. Varicella vaccine trials in healthy children: a summary of comparative follow-up studies. Am J Dis Child 1984;138:434-438.

Arvin A. Oral therapy with acyclovir in infants and children. Pediatr Infect Dis 1986;6:56-58.

Arvin A, Gershon A. Live attenuated varicella vaccine. Ann Rev Microbiol 1996;50:59-100.

Arvin AM, Koropchak CM, Williams BR, et al. Early immune response in healthy and immunocompromised subjects with primary varicella-zoster virus infection. J Infect Dis 1986; 154:422-429.

Arvin A, Koropchak CM, Wittek AC. Immunologic evidence of reinfection with varicella-zoster virus. J Infect Dis 1983; 148:200-205.

Arvin AM, Kushner JH, Feldman S, et al. Human leukocyte interferon for the treatment of varicella in children with cancer. N Engl J Med 1982;306:761-765.

Arvin AM, Pollard RB, Rasmussen L, Merigan T. Selective impairment in lymphocyte reactivity to varicella-zoster antigen among untreated lymphoma patients. J Infect Dis 1978; 137:531-540.

Arvin AM, Pollard RB, Rasmussen L, Merigan T. Cellular and humoral immunity in the pathogenesis of recurrent herpes viral infections in patients with lymphoma. J Clin Invest 1980;65:869-878.

Asano Y, Itakura N, Hiroishi Y, et al. Viremia is present in incubation period in nonimmunocompromised children with varicella. J Pediatr 1985a;106:69-71.

Asano Y, Itakura N, Kajita Y, et al. Severity of viremia and clinical findings in children with varicella. J Infect Dis 1990; 161:1095-1098.

Asano Y, Nagai T, Miyata T, et al. Long-term protective immunity of recipients of the Oka strain of live varicella vaccine. Pediatrics 1985b;75:667-671.

Asano Y, Yoshikawa T, Suga S, et al. Postexposure prophylaxis of varicella in family contact by oral acyclovir. Pediatrics 1993;92:219-222.

Baba K, Yabuuchi H, Takahashi M, Ogra P. Immunologic and epidemiologic aspects of varicella infection acquired during infancy and early childhood. J Pediatr 1982;100:881-885.

Baba K, Yabuuchi H, Takahashi M, Ogra P. Increased incidence of herpes zoster in normal children infected with varicella-zoster virus during infancy: community-based follow-up study. J Pediatr 1986;108:372-377.

Baird RE, Daly P, Sawyer M. Varicella arthritis diagnosed by polymerase chain reaction. Ped Infect Dis J 1991; 12:950-951.

Bakshi S, Miller TC, Kaplan M, et al. Failure of VZIG in modification of severe congenital varicella. Ped Infect Dis 1986;5:699-702.

Balducci J, Rodis JF, Rosengren S, et al. Pregnancy outcome following first-trimester varicella infection. Obstet Gynecol 1992;79:5-6.

Balfour H. Intravenous therapy for varicella in immunocompromised children. J Pediatr 1984;104:134-140.

Balfour H, Bean B, Laskin O, et al. Burroughs-Wellcome Collaborative Acyclovir Study Group. Acyclovir halts progression of herpes zoster in immunocompromised patients. N Engl J Med 1983;308:1448-1453.

Balfour H, McMonigal K, Bean B. Acyclovir therapy of varicella-zoster virus infection in immunocompromised patients. J Antimicrob Chemo 1983;12(suppl B):169-179.

Balfour HH, Kelly JM, Suarez CS, et al. Acyclovir treatment of varicella in otherwise healthy children. J Pediatr 1990; 116:633-639.

Berger R, Florent G, Just M. Decrease of the lympho-proliferative response to varicella-zoster virus antigen in the aged. Infect Immunol 1981;32:24-27.

Bodensteiner JB, Hille MR, Riggs JE. Clinical features of vascular thrombosis following varicella. Amer J Dis Child 1991; 146:100-102.

Bogger-Goren S, Bernstein JM, Gershon A, Ogra PL. Mucosal cell-mediated immunity to varicella-zoster virus: role in protection against disease. J Pediatr 1984;105:195-199.

Bradley JS, Schlievert PM, Sample TG. Streptococcal toxic shock–like syndrome as a complication of varicella. Pediatr Infect Dis 1991;10:77-78.

Brogan TV, Niozet V, Waldhausen JHT, et al. Group A streptococcal necrotizing fasciitis complicating primary varicella: a series of fourteen patients. Ped Infect Dis J 1995;14:588-594.

Broyer M, Boudailliez B. Prevention of varicella infection in renal transplanted children by previous immunization with a live attenuated varicella vaccine. Transplant Proc 1985a; 17:151-152.

Broyer M, Boudailliez B. Varicella vaccine in children with chronic renal insufficiency. Postgrad Med J 1985b; 61(S4):103-106.

Brunell PA. Transmission of chickenpox in a school setting prior to the observed exanthem. Am J Dis Child 1989; 143:1451-1452.

Brunell PA, Kotchmar GSJ. Zoster in infancy: failure to maintain virus latency following intrauterine infection. J Pediatr 1981;98:71-73.

Brunell PA, Miller L, Lovejoy F. Zoster in children. Am J Dis Child 1968;115:432.

Brunell PA, Novelli VM, Lipton SV, Pollock B. Combined vaccine against measles, mumps, rubella, and varicella. Pediatrics 1988;81:779-784.

Brunell P, Ross A, Miller L, Kuo B. Prevention of varicella by zoster immune globulin. J Engl J Med 1969;280:1191-1194.

Brunell PA, Taylor-Wiedeman J, Geiser CF. Risk of herpes zoster in children with leukemia: varicella vaccine compared with history of chickenpox. Pediatrics 1986;77:53-56.

Bruusgaard E. The mutual relation between zoster and varicella. Br J Dermatol Syph 1932;44:1-24.

Burke BL, Steele RW, Beard OW, et al. Immune responses to varicella-zoster in the aged. Arch Intern Med 1982;142: 291-293.

Caekebeke JFV, Boudewyn P, Peters AC, et al. Cerebral vasculopathy, associated with primary varicella infection. Arch Neurol 1990;47:1033-1035.

Campbell-Benzie A, Heath RB, Ridehalgh M, Craddock-Wilson JE. A comparison of indirect immunofluorescence and radioimmunoassay for detecting antibody to varicella-zoster virus. J Virol Meth 1983;6:135-140.

Centers for Disease Control. Prevention of varicella: recommendations of the Advisory Committee on Immunization Practices (ACIP). 1996;45:1-36.

Chambers RB, Derick RJ, Davidorf FH, et al. Varicella-zoster retinitis in human immunodeficiency virus infection. Arch Ophthalmol 1989;107:960-961.

Choo PW, Donahue JG, Manson JE, Platt R. The epidemiology of varicella and its complications. J Infect Dis 1995;172: 706-712.

Choong K, Zwaignebaum L, Onyett H. Severe varicella after low dose inhaled corticoids. Ped Infect Dis J 1995;14:809-811.

Clements DA, Armstrong CB, Ursano AM, et al. Over five-year follow-up of Oka/Merck varicella vaccine recipients in 465 infants and adolescents. Ped Infect Dis J 1995;14:874-879.

Cobo M. Reduction of the ocular complications of herpes zoster ophthalmicus by oral acyclovir. Am J Med 1988;85(S2A): 90-93.

Colebunders R, Mann J, Francis H, et al. Herpes zoster in African patients: a clinical predictor of human immunodeficiency virus infection. J Infect Dis 1988;157:314-319.

Committee on Infectious Diseases. Live attenuated varicella vaccine. Pediatrics 1995;95:791-796.

Cooper E, Vujcic L, Quinnan G. Varicella-zoster virus-specific HLA-restricted cytotoxicity of normal immune adult lympho-cytes after in vitro stimulation. J Infect Dis 1988;158: 780-788.

Croen K, Ostrove J, Dragovic L, Straus S. Patterns of gene expression and sites of latency in human ganglia are different for varicella-zoster and herpes simplex viruses. Proc Soc Natl Acad Sci USA 1988;85:9773-9777.

DaSilva O, Hammerberg O, Chance GW. Fetal varicella syndrome. Pediatr Infect Dis 1990;9:854-855.

Davies HD, McGeer A, Schwarts B, et al. Invasive group A streptococcal infections in Ontario, Canada. N Engl J Med 1996;335:547-553.

Davison AJ, Scott JE. The complete DNA sequence of varicella-zoster virus. J Gen Virol 1986;67:1759-1816.

Demmler G, Steinberg S, Blum G, Gershon A. Rapid enzyme-linked immunosorbent assay for detecting antibody to varicella-zoster virus. J Infect Dis 1988;157:211-212.

Devlin ME, Gilden DH, Mahlingham R, et al. Peripheral blood mononuclear cells of the elderly contain varicella-zoster virus DNA. J Infect Dis 1992;165:619-622.

Diaz P, Smith S, Hunter E, Arvin A. T-lymphocyte cytotoxicity with natural varicella-zoster virus infection and after immunization with live attenuated varicella vaccine. J Immunol 1989;142:636-641.

Doran TF, DeAngelis C, Baumgardner RA, Mellits ED. Acetaminophen: more harm than good for chickenpox? J Pediatr 1989;114:1045-1048.

Dueland AN, Devlin M, Martin JR, et al. Fatal varicella-zoster virus meningoradiculitis without skin involvement. Annal Neurol 1991;29:569-572.

deKoning J, Frederiks E, Kerkhoven P. Purpura fulminans following varicella. Helv Paediatr Acta 1972;27:177.

Dunkel et al. A controlled trial of acyclovir for chickenpox in normal children. N Engl J Med 1991;325:1539-1544.

Dworsky M, Whitely R, Alford C. Herpes zoster in early infancy. Am J Dis Child 1980;134:618-619.

Eder SE, Appuzzio JJ, Weiss G. Varicella pneumonia during pregnancy. Am J Perinatol 1988;5:16-18.

Edson CM, Hosler BA, Poodry CA, et al. Varicella-zoster virus envelope glycoproteins: biochemical characterization and identification in clinical material. Virology 1985;145:62-71.

Enders G. Varicella-zoster virus infection in pregnancy. Progr Med Virol 1984;29:166-196.

Englund JA, Arvine A, Balfour H. Acyclovir treatment for varicella does not lower gpI and IE-62 (p170) antibody responses to varicella-zoster virus in normal children. J Clin Virol 1990;28:2327-2330.

Englund JA, Suarez CS, Kelly J, et al. Placebo-controlled trial of varicella vaccine given with or after measles-mumps-rubella vaccine. J Pediatr 1989;114:37-44.

Essex-Cater A, Heggarty H. Fatal congenital varicella syndrome. J Infect Dis 1983;7:77-78.

Ey JL, Fulginiti VA. Varicella hepatitis without neurologic symptoms or visceral involvement. Pediatrics 1981;67: 285-287.

Feder H. Treatment of adult chickenpox with oral acyclovir. Arch Intern Med 1990;150:2061-2065.

Feldhoff C, Balfour H, Simmons SR, et al. Varicella in children with renal transplants. J Pediatr 1981;98:25-31.

Feldman S, Chaudhary S, Ossi M, Epp E. A viremic phase for herpes zoster in children with cancer. J Pediatr 1977;91: 597-600.

Feldman S, Epp E. Isolation of varicella-zoster virus from blood. J Pediatr 1976;88:265-267.

Feldman S, Epp E. Detection of viremia during incubation period of varicella. J Pediatr 1979;94:746-748.

Feldman S, Hughes W, Daniel C. Varicella in children with cancer: 77 cases. Pediatrics 1975;80:388-397.

Feldman S, Hughes WT, Kim HY. Herpes zoster in children with cancer. Am J Dis Child 1973;126:178-184.

Feldman S, Robertson PK, Lott L, Thornton D. Neurotoxicity due to adenine arabinoside therapy during varicella-zoster virus infections in immunocompromised children. J Infect Dis 1986;154:889-893.

Feldman S, Lott L. Varicella in children with cancer: impact of antiviral therapy and prophylaxis. Pediatrics 1987;80:465-472.

Fikrig E, Barg NL. Varicella associated intracerebral hemorrhage in the absence of thrombocytopenia. Diagn Micro Infect 1989;12:357-359.

Florman A, Umland E, Ballou D, et al. Evaluation of a skin test for chickenpox. Inf Cont 1985;6:314-316.

Forghani B, Schmidt N, Dennis J. Antibody assays for varicella-zoster virus: comparison of enzyme immunoassay with neutralization, immune adherence hemagglutination, and complement fixation. J Clin Microbiol 1978;8:545.

Frey H, Steinberg S, Gershon A. Varicella-zoster infections: rapid diagnosis by countercurrent immunoelectrophoresis. J Infect Dis 1981;143:274-280.

Friedman SM, Margo CE, Connelly BL. Varicella-zoster virus retinitis as the initial manifestation of the acquired immunodeficiency syndrome. Am J Ophthalmol 1994;117:536-538.

Friedman CA, Temple DM, Robbins KK, et al. Outbreak and control of varicella in a neonatal intensive care unit. Ped Infect Dis J 1994a;13:152-154.

Gelb LD, Dohner DE, Gershon AA, et al. Molecular epidemiology of live attenuated varicella virus vaccine in children and in normal adults. J Infect Dis 1987;155:633-640.

Gershon A. Varicella in mother and infant: problems old and new. In Krugman S, Gershon A (eds). Infection of the fetus and newborn infant. New York: Alan R Liss, 1975.

Gershon A. Commentary on VZIG in infants. Pediatr Infect Dis 1987;6:469.

Gershon A. Chickenpox, measles, and mumps. In Remington J, Klein J (eds). Infections of the fetus and newborn infant, ed 4. Philadelphia: WB Saunders, 1994.

Gershon A. Varicella-zoster virus: prospects for control. Adv. Ped. Infect. Dis. 1995;10:93-124.

Gershon A, Brunell P, Doyle EF, Claps A. Steroid therapy and varicella. J Pediatr 1972;81:1034.

Gershon A, Frey H, Steinberg S, et al. Enzyme-linked immunosorbent assay for measurement of antibody to varicella-zoster virus. Arch Virol 1981;70:169-172.

Gershon A, LaRussa P, Steinberg S. Varicella vaccine: use in immunocompromised patients. In: J. White RE, ed. Infectious Disease Clinics of North America. Philadelphia: Saunders, 1996.

Gershon A, Mervish N, et al. VZV in HIV, IDSA, New Orleans, 1996. Vol. Sept 1996.

Gershon A, Raker R, Steinberg S, et al. Antibody to varicella-zoster virus in parturient women and their offspring during the first year of life. Pediatrics 1976;58:692-696.

Gershon A, Steinberg S. Cellular and humoral immune responses to VZV in immunocompromised patients during and after VZV infections. Infect Immun 1979;25:828.

Gershon A, Steinberg S. Antibody-dependent cellular cytotoxicity inactivates varicella-zoster virus in vitro: 11th ICC and 19th ICAAC. Curr Chem Infect Dis 1980;1322 (abstract).

Gershon A, Steinberg S, Borkowsky W, et al. IgM to varicella-zoster virus: demonstration in patients with and without clinical zoster. Pediatr Infect Dis 1982;1:164-167.

Gershon A, Steinberg S, Brunell P. Zoster immune globulin: a further assessment. N Engl J Med 1974;290:243-245.

Gershon AA, Steinberg S, Gelb L, NIAID Collaborative Varicella Vaccine Study Group. Clinical reinfection with varicella-zoster virus. J Infect Dis 1984a;149:137-142.

Gershon AA, Steinberg S, Gelb L, NIAID Collaborative Varicella Vaccine Study Group. Live attenuated varicella vaccine: efficacy for children with leukemia in remission. JAMA 1984b;252:355-362.

Gershon AA, Steinberg S, LaRussa P, et al., NIAID Collaborative Varicella Vaccine Study Group. Immunization of healthy adults with live attenuated varicella vaccine. J Infect Dis 1988;158:132-137.

Gershon A, Steinberg S, LaRussa P. Measurement of antibodies to VZV by latex agglutination. Anaheim, Calif: Society for Pediatric Research, 1992.

Gershon A, Steinberg S, LaRussa P. Detection of antibodies to varicella-zoster virus by latex agglutination. Clinical and Diagnostic Virology 1994;2:271-277.

Gershon AA, Steinberg S, NIAID Collaborative Varicella Vaccine Study Group. Persistence of immunity to varicella in children with leukemia immunized with live attenuated varicella vaccine. N Engl J Med 1989;320:892-897.

Gershon AA, Steinberg S, NIAID Collaborative Varicella Vaccine Study Group. Live attenuated varicella vaccine: protection in healthy adults in comparison to leukemic children. J Infect Dis 1990;161:661-666.

Gershon A, Steinberg S, Silber R. Varicella-zoster viremia. J Pediatr 1978;92:1033-1034.

Gilden D, Rozenman Y, Murray R, et al. Detection of varicella-zoster virus nucleic acid in neurons of normal human thoracic ganglia. Ann Neurol 1987;22:337-380.

Gilden DH, Murray RS, Wellish M, et al. Chronic progressive varicella-zoster virus encephalitis in and AIDS patient. Neurology 1988;38:1150-1153.

Gilden DH, Wright R, Schneck S, et al. Zoster sine herpete, a clinical variant. Ann Neurol 1994;35:530-533.

Giller RH, Bowden RA, Levin M, et al. Reduced cellular immunity to varicella-zoster virus during treatment for acute lymphoblastic leukemia of childhood: in vitro studies of possible mechanisms. J Clin Immunol 1986;6:472-480.

Giller RH, Winistorfer S, Grose C. Cellular and humoral immunity to varicella-zoster virus glycoproteins in immune and susceptible human subjects. J Infect Dis 1989;160:919-928.

Gleaves C, Lee C, Bustamante C, Meyers J. Use of murine monoclonal antibodies for laboratory diagnosis of varicella-zoster virus infection. J Clin Microbiol 1988;26:1623-1625.

Gonzalez-Ruiz A, Ridgway GL, Cohen SL, et al. Varicella gangrenosa with toxic shock–like syndrome due to group A streptococcus infection in an adult. Clin Infect Dis 1995;20:1058-1060.

Grose C. Varicella-zoster virus: pathogenesis of human diseases, the virus and viral replication, and the major glycoproteins and proteins. Boca Raton, Fla: CRC Press, 1987.

Grose CH. Variation on a theme by Fenner. Pediatrics 1981;68:735-737.

Groth KE, McCullough J, Marker S, et al. Evaluation of zoster immune plasma: treatment of herpes zoster in patients with cancer. JAMA 1978;239:1877-1879.

Guess H, Broughton DD, Melton LJ, Kurland L. Epidemiology of herpes zoster in children and adolescents: a population-based study. Pediatrics 1985; 76:512-517.

Guess H, Broughton DD, Melton LJ, Kurland L. Population-based studies of varicella complications. Pediatrics 1986; 78:723-727.

Gustafson TL, Lavely GB, Brauner ER, et al. An outbreak of nosocomial varicella. Pediatrics 1982;70:550-556.

Gustafson TL, Shehab Z, Brunell P. Outbreak of varicella in a newborn intensive care nursery. Am J Dis Child 1984; 138:548-550.

Haake D, Zakowski PC, Haake DL, Bryson YJ. Early treatment with acyclovir for varicella pneumonia in otherwise healthy adults: retrospective controlled study and review. Rev Infect Dis 1990;12:788-798.

Haddad J, Simeoni U, Messer J, Willard D. Acyclovir in prophylaxis and perinatal varicella. Lancet 1987;1:161.

Hanngren K, Grandien M, Granstrom G. Effect of zoster immunoglobulin for varicella prophylaxis in the newborn. Scand J Infect Dis 1985;17:343-347.

Hardy I, Gershon A. Prospects for use of a varicella vaccine in adults. Infect Dis Clin North Am 1990;4:160-173.

Hardy IB, Gershon A, Steinberg S, et al. The incidence of zoster after immunization with live attenuated varicella vaccine: a study in children with leukemia. N Engl J Med 1991; 325:1545-1550.

Hay J, Ruyechan WT. Varicella-zoster virus: a different kind of herpesvirus latency? Semin Virol 1994;5:241-248.

Hayakawa Y, Torigoe S, Shiraki K, et al. Biologic and biophysical markers of a live varicella vaccine strain (Oka): identification of clinical isolates from vaccine recipients. J Infect Dis 1984;149:956-963.

Hayward AR, Herberger M, Lazlo M. Cellular interactions in the lysis of varicella-zoster virus–infected human fibroblasts. Clin Exp Immunol 1986;63:141-146.

Holland P, Isaacs D, Moxon ER. Fatal neonatal varicella infection. Lancet 1986;2:1156.

Hope-Simpson RE. The nature of herpes zoster: a long-term study and a new hypothesis. Proc R Soc Med 1965;58:9-20.

Huang Y-C, Lin T-Y, Chiu C-H. Acyclovir prophylaxis of varicella after household exposure. Pediatr Infect Dis J 1995; 14:152-154.

Huff C, Bean B, Balfour H, et al. Therapy of herpes zoster with oral acyclovir. Am J Med 1988;85(A2A):84-89.

Hurwitz ES, Goodman RA. A cluster of cases of Reye syndrome associated with chickenpox. Pediatrics 1982;70:901-906.

Hyman RW, Ecker JR, Tenser RB. Varicella-zoster virus RNA in human trigeminal ganglia. Lancet 1983;2:814-816.

Ihara T, Ito M, Starr SE. Human lymphocyte, monocyte, and polymorphonuclear leukocyte-mediated antibody-dependent cellular cytotoxicity against varicella-zoster virus–infected targets. Clin Exp Immunol 1986;63:179-187.

Jacobson MA, Berger TG, Fikrig S. Acyclovir-resistant varicella-zoster virus infection after chronic oral acyclovir therapy in patients with the acquired immunodeficiency syndrome. Ann Intern Med 1990;112:187-191.

Jemsek J, Greenberg SB, Taber L, et al. Herpes zoster–associated encephalitis: clinicopathologic report of 12 cases and review of the literature. Medicine 1983;62:81-97.

Johnson CE, Shurin PA, Fattlar D, et al. Live attenuated varicella vaccine in healthy 12- to 24-month-old children. Pediatrics 1988;81:512-518.

Josephson A, Gombert ME. Airborne transmission of nosocomial varicella from localized zoster. J Infect Dis 1988; 158:238-241.

Judelsohn RG, Meyers JD, Ellis RJ, Thomas EK. Efficacy of zoster immune globulin. Pediatrics 1974;53:476.

Junker K, Avnstorp C, Nielson C, Hansen N. Reinfection with varicella-zoster virus in immunocompromised patients. Curr Probl Derm 1989;18:152-157.

Junker AK, Angus E, Thomas E. Recurrent varicella-zoster virus infections in apparently immunocompetent children. Ped Infect Dis J 1991;10:569-575.

Junker AK, Tilley P. Varicella-zoster virus antibody avidity and IgG-subclass patterns in children with recurrent chickenpox. J Med Virol 1994;43:119-124.

Jura E, Chadwick S, Joseph SH, Steinberg S, et al. Varicella-zoster virus infections in children infected with human immunodeficiency virus. Pediatr Infect Dis 1989;8:586-590.

Kalman CM, Laskin OL. Herpes zoster and zosteriform herpes simplex virus infections in immunocompetent adults. Am J Med 1986;81:775-778.

Kamiya H, Ihara T, Hattori A, et al. Diagnostic skin test reactions with varicella virus antigen and clinical application of the test. J Infect Dis 1977;136:784-788.

Kasper WJ, Howe P. Fatal varicella after a single course of corticosteroids. Pediatr Infect Dis 1991;9:729-732.

King S, Gorensek M, Ford-Jones EL, Read S. Fatal varicella-zoster infection in a newborn treated with varicella-zoster immunoglobulin. Pediatr Infect Dis 1986;5:588-589.

Kirk S, Marlow N, Quershi S. Cardiac tamponade following varicella. Int J Cardiol 1987;17:221-224.

Kotchmar G, Grose C, Brunell P. Complete spectrum of the varicella congenital defects syndrome in 5-year-old child. Pediatr Infect Dis 1984;3:142-145.

Koumbourlis AC. Varicella infection with profound neutropenia, multisystem involvement, and no sequelae. Pediatr Infect Dis 1988;3:142-145.

Krasinski K, Holzman R, LaCoutre R, Florman A. Hospital experience with varicella-zoster virus. Infect Contr 1986;7:312-316.

Krause P, Klinman DM. Efficacy, immunogenicity, safety, and use of live attenuated chickenpox vaccine. J Pediatr 1995; 127:518-525.

Kundratitz K. Experimentelle Ubertragung von Herpes Zoster auf den Mensschen und die Beziehungen von Herpes Zoster zu Varicellen. Monatssbl Kinderheilled 1925;29:516-523.

Kuppermann BD, Quiceno JI, Wiley C, et al. Clinical and histopathological study of varicella-zoster virus retinitis in patients with the acquired immunodeficiency syndrome. Am J Ophthalmol 1994;118:589-600.

Kuter BJ, Weibel RE, Guess HA, et al. Oka/Merck varicella vaccine in healthy children: final report of a 2-year efficacy study and 7-year follow-up studies. Vaccine 1991;9:643-647.

Landsberger EJ, Hager WD, Grossman JH. Successful management of varicella pneumonia complicating pregnancy: a report of 3 cases. J Reprod Med 1986;31:311.

LaRussa P, Lungu O, Hardy I, et al. Restriction fragment length polymorphism of polymerase chain reaction products from vaccine and wild-type varicella-zoster virus isolates. J Virol 1992;66:1016-1020.

LaRussa P, Gershon A, Steinberg S, et al. Diagnosis of VZV by PCR, Society for Pediatric Research annual meeting, 1993.

LaRussa P, Steinberg S, Gershon A. Amplification of VZV DNA in CSF by PCR. Presented at 35th ICAAC, Sept 1995, San Francisco, Calif, (abstract 1817).

LaRussa P, Steinberg S, Seeman MD, Gershon AA. Determination of immunity to varicella by means of an intradermal skin test. J Infect Dis 1985;152:869.

Lawrence R, Gershon A, Holzman R, Steinberg S, NIAID Varicella Vaccine Collaborative Study Group. The risk of zoster in leukemic children who received live attenuated varicella vaccine. N Engl J Med 1988;318:543-548.

Leclair JM, Zaia J, Levin MJ, et al. Airborne transmission of chickenpox in a hospital. N Engl J Med 1980;302:450-453.

Levin MJ, Rotbart HA, Hayward AR. Immune response to varicella-zoster virus 5 years after acyclovir therapy of childhood varicella. J Infect Dis 1995;171:1383-1384.

Lichtenstein PK, Heubi JE, Daugherty CC, et al. Grade I Reye's syndrome: a frequent cause of vomiting and live dysfunction after varicella and upper respiratory tract infection. N Engl J Med 1983;309:133-139.

Linnemann CC, Biron KK, Hoppenjans WG, Solinger AM. Emergence of acyclovir-resistant varicella zoster virus in an AIDS patient on prolonged acyclovir therapy. AIDS 1990;4:577-579.

Liu H-C, Tsai T-C, Chang P-Y, Shih B-F. Varicella orchitis: report of two cases and review of the literature. Ped Infect Dis J 1994;13:748-750.

Liu GT, Holmes GL. Varicella with delayed contralateral hemiparesis detected by MRI. Ped Neurol 1990;6:131-134.

Ljungman P, Lonnqvist B, Gahrton G, et al. Clinical and subclinical reactivations of varicella-zoster virus in immunocompromised patients. J Infect Dis 1986;153:840-847.

Locksley RM, Fluornoy N, Sullivan KM, Meyers J. Infection with varicella-zoster virus after marrow transplantation. J Infect Dis 1985;152:1172-1181.

Lorber A, Zonis Z, Maisuls E, et al. The scale of myocardial involvement in varicella myocarditis. Int J Cardiol 1988;20:257-262.

Luby J, Ramirez-Ronda C, Rinner S, et al. A longitudinal study of varicella-zoster virus infections in renal transplant recipients. J Infect Dis 1977;135:659-663.

Lungu O, Annunziato P, Gershon A, et al. Reactivated and latent varicella-zoster virus in human dorsal root ganglia. Proc Nat Acad Sci USA 1995;92:10980-10984.

Lynfield R, Herrin JT, Rubin RH. Varicella in Pediatric renal transplant patients. Pediatrics 1992;90:216-220.

Mackay JB, Cairney P. Pulmonary calcification following varicella. N Z Med J 1960;59:453.

Mahalingham R, Wellish M, Cohrs R, et al. Expression of protein encoded by varicella-zoster virus open reading frame 63 in latently infected human ganglionic neurons. Proc Nat Acad Sci 1996;93:2122-2124.

Mahalingham R, Wellish M, Wolf W, et al. Latent varicella-zoster viral DNA in human trigeminal and thoracic ganglia. N Engl J Med 1990;323:627-631.

Manson MM, Logan WPD, Loy RM. Rubella and other virus infections during pregnancy: reports on public health and medical subjects. London: Her Majesty's Stationery Office, 1960.

Martin JH, Dohner D, Wellinghoff WJ, Gelb LD. Restriction endonuclease analysis of varicella-zoster vaccine virus and wild type DNAs. J Med Virol 1982;9:69-76.

McCormick WF, Rodnitzky RL, Schochet SSJ, McKee AP. Varicella-zoster encephalomyelitis: a morphologic and virologic study. Arch Neurol 1969;9:251-266.

McKendrick M, McGill J, White J, Woos M. Oral acyclovir in acute herpes zoster. Br Med J 1986;293:1529-1532.

Melbye M, Grossman R, Goedert J, et al. Risk of AIDS after herpes zoster. Lancet 1987;1:728-730.

Melish ME. Bullous varicella: its association with the staphylococcal scalded skin syndrome. J Pediatr 1973;83:1019.

Merigan TC, Rand K, Pollard R, et al. Human leukocyte interferon for the treatment of herpes zoster in patients with cancer. N Engl J Med 1978;298:981-987.

Meyers J. Congenital varicella in term infants: risk reconsidered. J Infect Dis 1974;129:215-217.

Miller AE. Selective decline in cellular immune response to varicella-zoster in elderly. Neurology 1980;30:582-587.

Miller L, Brunell PA. Zoster, reinfection, or activation of latent virus? Am J Med 1970;49:480.

Mills WJ, et al. Invasive group A streptococcal infections complicating primary varicella. J Pediatr Orthoped 1996;16:522-528.

Morens DM, Bregman DJ, West M, et al. An outbreak of varicella-zoster virus infection among cancer patients. Ann Intern Med 1980;93:414-419.

Mortimer EA, Lepow ML. Varicella with hypoglycemia possibly due to salicylates. Am J Dis Child 1962;103:583.

Mulhern LM, Friday GA, Perri JA. Arthritis complicating varicella infection. Pediatrics 1971;48:827.

Music SI, Fine EM, Togo Y. Zoster-like disease in the newborn due to herpes-simplex virus. N Engl J Med 1971;284:24-26.

Myers MG. Viremia caused by varicella-zoster virus: association with malignant progressive varicella. J Infect Dis 1979;140:229-233.

Myers MG. Hepatic cellular injury during varicella. Arch Dis Child 1982;57:317-319.

Myers MG, Connelly B, Stanberry LR. Varicella in hairless guinea pigs. J Infect Dis 1991;163:746-751.

Myers M, Duer HL, Haulser CK. Experimental infection of guinea pigs with varicella-zoster virus. J Infect Dis 1980;142:414-420.

Myers M, Stanberry L, Edmond B. Varicella-zoster virus infection of strain 2 guinea pigs. J Infect Dis 1985;151:106-113.

Nader S, Bergen R, Sharp M, Arvin A. Comparison of cell-mediated immunity (CMI) to varicella-zoster virus (VZV) in children and adults immunized with live attenuated varicella vaccine. J Infect Dis 1995;171:13-17.

Nassar NT, Touma HC. Brief report: susceptibility of Filipino nurses to the varicella-zoster virus. Infect Contr 1986;7:71-72.

Nyerges G, Meszner Z, Gyrmati E, Kerpel-Fronius S. Acyclovir prevents dissemination of varicella in immunocompromised children. J Infect Dis 1988;157:309-313.

Olding-Stenkvist E, Grandien M. Early diagnosis of virus-caused vesicular rashes by immunofluorescence on skin biopsies. I. Varicella, zoster, and herpes simplex. Scand J Infect Dis 1976;8:27-35.

Orenstein W, Heymann D, Ellis R, et al. Prophylaxis of varicella in high-risk children: response effect of zoster immune globulin. J Pediatr 1981;98:368-373.

Ozaki T, Ichikawa T, Matsui Y, et al. Lymphocyte-associated viremia in varicella. J Med Virol 1986;19:249.

Pahwa S, Biron K, Lim W, et al. Continuous varicella-zoster infection associated with acyclovir resistance in a child with AIDS. JAMA 1988;260:2879-2882.

Palmer SR, Caul EO, Donald DE, et al. An outbreak of shingles? Lancet 1985;2:1108-1111.

Paryani SG, Arvin AM. Intrauterine infection with varicella-zoster virus after maternal varicella. N Engl J Med 1986;314:1542-1546.

Paryani SG, Arvin AM, Koropchak C, et al. Do varicella-zoster antibody titers alter the administration of intravenous immune serum globulin or varicella-zoster immune globulin. Am J Med 1984;76:124-127.

Pastuszak AL, Levy M, Schick B, et al. Outcome after maternal varicella infection in the first 20 weeks of pregnancy. N Engl J Med 1994;330:901-905.

Patel PA, Yoonessi S, O'Malley J, et al. Cell-mediated immunity to varicella-zoster virus in subjects with lymphoma or leukemia. J Pediatr 1979;94:223-230.

Patterson L, Butler K, Edwards M. Clinical herpes zoster shortly following primary varicella in two HIV-infected children. Clin Pediatr 1989;28:854.

Peters ACB, Versteeg J, Lindenman J, et al. Varicella and acute cerebellar ataxia. Arch Neurol 1978;35:769.

Peterslund NA. Management of varicella-zoster infections in immunocompetent hosts. Am J Med 1988;85(2A):74-78.

Peterson C, Vugia D, Meyers H, et al. Group A streptococcal infections in children with varicella: results of a case-control study. 35th Interscience Conference on Antimicrobia Agents and Chemotherapy, San Francisco, Calif, 1995.

Peterson CL, Vugia D, Meyers H, et al. Risk factors for invasive group A streptococcal infections in children with varicella: a case-control study. Ped Infect Dis J 1996;15:151-156.

Pitel PA, McCormick KL, Fitzgerald E, Orson JM. Subclinical hepatic changes in varicella infection. Pediatrics 1980; 65:631-633.

Plotkin SA, Starr S, Connor K, Morton D. Zoster in normal children after varicella vaccine. J Infect Dis 1989;159: 1000-1001.

Preblud S, Bregman DJ, Vernon LL. Deaths from varicella in infants. Pediatr Infect Dis 1985;4:503-507.

Preblud S, Cochi S, Orenstein W. Varicella-zoster infection in pregnancy. N Engl J Med 1986;315:1416-1417.

Preblud S, Orenstein W, Bart K. Varicella: clinical manifestations, epidemiology, and health impact on children. Pediatr Infect Dis 1984;3:505-509.

Presissner C, Steinberg S, Gershon A, Smith TF. Evaluation of the anticomplement immunofluorescence test for detection of antibody to varicella-zoster virus. J Clin Microbiol 1982;16:373-376.

Priest JR, Groth KE, Balfour HH. Varicella arthritis documented by isolation of virus from joint fluid. J Pediatr 1978;93:990.

Prober C, Kirk LE, Keeney RE. Acyclovir therapy of chickenpox in immunocompromised children—a collaborative study. J Pediatr 1982;101:622-625.

Puchhammer-Stockl E, Popow-Kraupp T, Heinz F, et al. Detection of varicella-zoster virus DNA by polymerase chain reaction in the cerebrospinal fluid of patients suffering from neurological complications associated with chickenpox or herpes zoster. J Clin Microbiol 1991;29:1513-1516.

Rabalais GP, Adams G, Yusk J, Wilkerson SA. Zosteriform denuded skin caused by intrauterine herpes simplex virus infection. Pediatr Infect Dis 1991;10:79-80.

Raker R, Steinberg S, Drusin L, Gershon A. Antibody to varicella-zoster virus in low birth weight infants. J Pediatr 1978;93:505-506.

Rand KH, Rasmussen LE, Pollard RB, et al. Cellular immunity and herpesvirus infections in cardiac transplant patients. N Engl J Med 1977;296:1372-1377.

Randel R, Kearns DB, Sawyer MH. Vocal cord paralysis as a presentation of intrauterine infection with varicella-zoster virus. Pediatrics 1996;97:127-128.

Rawlinson WD, Dwyer DE, Gibbons V, Cunningham A. Rapid diagnosis of varicella-zoster virus infection with a monoclonal antibody-based direct immunofluorescence technique. J Virol Meth 1989;23:13-18.

Richman DD, Cleveland PH, Oxman MN, Zaia JA. A rapid radioimmunoassay using 125-I–labeled staphylococcal protein A for antibody to varicella-zoster virus. J Infect Dis 1981; 143:693-699.

Ross AH, Lencher E, Reitman G. Modification of chickenpox in family contacts by administration of gamma globulin. N Engl J Med 1962;267:369-376.

Sakurai N, Ihara T, Ito M, et al. Application of a live varicella vaccine in children with acute leukemia. Amsterdam: Exerpta Medica, 1982.

Schimpff S, Serpick A, Stoler B, et al. Varicella-zoster infection in patients with cancer. Ann Intern Med 1972;76:241-254.

Schlossberg D, Littman M. Varicella pneumonia. Arch Intern Med 1988;148:1630-1632.

Schmidt NJ. Further evidence for common antigens in herpes simplex and varicella-zoster virus. J Med Virol 1982;9:27-36.

Shanley J, Myers M, Edmond B, Steele R. Enzyme-linked immunosorbent assay for detection of antibody to varicella-zoster virus. J Clin Microbiol 1982;15:208-211.

Shehab Z, Brunell PA. Enzyme-linked immunosorbent assay for susceptibility to varicella. J Infect Dis 1983;148:472-476.

Shepp D, Dandliker P, Meyers J. Current therapy of varicella-zoster virus infection in immunocompromised patients. Am J Med 1988;85(S2A):96-98.

Shepp DH, Dandliker PS, Meyers JD. Treatment of varicella-zoster virus infection in severely immunocompromised patients: a randomized comparison of acyclovir and vidarabine. N Engl J Med 1986;314:208-212.

Siegel M. Congenital malformations following chickenpox, measles, mumps, and hepatitis. Results of a cohort study. JAMA 1973;226:1521-1524.

Silk H, Guay-Woodford L, Perez-Atayde A, et al. Fatal varicella in steroid-dependent asthma. J Allerg Clin Immunol 1988;81:47-51.

Silliman CC, Tedder D, Ogle JW, et al. Unsuspected varicella-zoster virus encephalitis in a child with acquired immunodeficiency syndrome. J Pediatr 1993;123:418-422.

Sills J, Galloway A, Amegavie L, et al. Acyclovir in prophylaxis and perinatal varicella. Lancet 1987;1:161.

Smith H. Purpura fulminans complicating varicella: recovery with low molecular weight dextran and steroids. Med J Aust 1967;2:685.

Spring S, Laughlin C, Arvin A, et al. Varicella-zoster virus infection and postherpetic neuralgia: new insights into pathogenesis and pain management. J Neurol 1994;35:S2-S3.

Starko KM, Ray CG, Dominguez BS, et al. Reye's syndrome and salicylate use. Pediatrics 1980;66:859-864.

Steele R, Coleman MA, Fiser M, et al. Varicella-zoster in hospital personnel: skin test reactivity to monitor susceptibility. Pediatrics 1982;70:604.

Stevens D, Ferrington R, Jordan G, Merigan T. Cellular events in zoster vesicles: relation to clinical course and immune parameters. J Infect Dis 1975;131:509-515.

Straus S, Ostrove J, Inchauspe G, et al. Varicella-zoster virus infections: biology, natural history, treatment, and prevention. Ann Intern Med 1988;108:221-237.

Straus SE, Reinhold W, Smith HA, et al. Endonuclease analysis of viral DNA from varicella and subsequent zoster infections in the same patient. N Engl J Med 1984;311: 1362-1364.

Takahashi M, Otsuka T, Okuno Y, et al. Live vaccine used to prevent the spread of varicella in children in hospital. Lancet 1974;2:1288-1290.

Terada K, Kawano S, Yoshihiro K, Morita T. Varicella-zoster virus (VZV) reactivation is related to the low response of VZV-specific immunity after chickenpox in infancy. J Infect Dis 1994;169:650-652.

Tsolia M, Gershon A, Steinberg S, Gelb L. Live attenuated varicella vaccine: evidence that the virus is attenuated and the importance of skin lesions in transmission. J Pediatr 1990; 116:184-189.

Vafai A, Murray R, Wellish W, et al. Expression of varicella-zoster virus and herpes simplex virus in normal human trigeminal ganglia. Proc Soc Natl Acad Sci USA 1988; 85:2362-2366.

Vafai A, Wellish M, Gilden D. Expression of varicella-zoster virus in blood mononuclear cells of patients with postherpetic neuralgia. Proc Natl Acad Sci USA 1988;85:2767-2770.

Vafai A, Wroblewska Z, Graf L. Antigenic cross-reaction between a varicella-zoster virus nucleocapsid protein encoded by gene 40 and a herpes simplex virus nucleocapsid protein. Virus Res 1990;15:163-174.

Vugia DJ, Peterson CL, Meyers HB, et al. Invasive group A streptococcal infections in children with varicella in Southern California. Ped Infect Dis J 1996;15:146-150.

Waagoner DC, Murphy T. Varicella myocarditis. Pediatr Infect Dis 1990;9:360-363.

Wald EL, Levine MM, Togo Y. Concomitant varicella and staphylococcal scalded skin syndrome. J Pediatr 1973; 83:1017.

Wallace MR, Bowler WA, Oldfield EC. Treatment of varicella in the immunocompetent adult. J Med Virol 1993; suppl 1:90-92.

Wang E, Prober C, Arvin AM. Varicella-zoster virus antibody titers before and after administration of zoster immune globulin to neonates in an intensive care nursery. J Pediatr 1983; 103:113-114.

Ward JR, Bishop B. Varicella arthritis. JAMA 1970;212:1954.

Watson B, Boardman C, Laufer D, et al. Humoral and cell-mediated immune responses in healthy children after one or two doses of varicella vaccine. Clin Infect Dis 1995;20:316-319.

Weber DJ, Rotala WA, Parham C. Impact and costs of varicella prevention in a university hospital. Am J Public Health 1988;78:19-23.

Weber DM, Pellecchia JA. Varicella pneumonia: study of prevalence in adult men. JAMA 1965;192:572.

Weller TH. Varicella and herpes zoster: changing concepts of the natural history, control, and importance of a not-so-benign virus. N Engl J Med 1983;309:1362-1368,1434-1440.

Weller TH, Coons AH. Fluorescent antibody studies with agents of varicella and herpes zoster propagated in vitro. Proc Soc Exp Biol Med 1954;86:789.

Weller TH, Witton HM. The etiologic agents of varicella and herpes zoster: serologic studies and the viruses as propagated in vitro. J Exp Med 1958;108:869-890.

Wesselhoft C, Pearson CM. Orchitis in the course of severe chickenpox with pneumonitis, followed by testicular atrophy. N Engl J Med 1950;242:651.

Whitley R, Soong S, Dolin R, et al., NIAID Collaborative Study Group. Early vidarabine to control the complications of herpes zoster in immunosuppressed patients. N Engl J Med 1982;307:971-975.

Williams DL, Gershon A, Gelb LD, et al. Herpes zoster following varicella vaccine in a child with acute lymphocytic leukemia. J Pediatr 1985;106:259-261.

Williams V, Gershon A, Brunell P. Serologic response to varicella-zoster membrane antigens measured by indirect immunofluorescence. J Infect Dis 1974;130:669-672.

Wilson A, Sharp M, Koropchak C, et al. Subclinical varicella-zoster virus viremia, herpes zoster, and T-lymphocyte immunity to varicella-zoster viral antigens after bone marrow transplantation. J Infect Dis 1992;165:119-126.

Wilson G, Talkington D, Gruber W, et al. Group A streptococcal necrotizing fasciitis following varicella in children: case reports and review. Clin Infect Dis 1995;20:1333-1338.

Wood MJ, Kay R, Dworkin RH, et al. Oral Acyclovir therapy accelerates pain resolution in patients with herpes zoster: a metaanalysis of placebo-controlled trials. Clin Infect Dis 1996;22:341-347.

Wood MJ, Ogan P, McKendrick MW, et al. Efficacy of oral acyclovir treatment of acute herpes zoster. Am J Med 1988; 85(S2A):79-83.

Yuceoglu AM, Berkovich S, Minkowitz S. Acute glomerular nephritis as a complication of varicella. JAMA 1967;202:113.

Zaia J, Levin M, Preblud S, et al. Evaluation of varicella-zoster immune globulin: protection of immunosuppressed children after household exposure to varicella. J Infect Dis 1983; 147:737-743.

Zaia J, Oxman M. Antibody to varicella-zoster virus–induced membrane antigen: immunofluorescence assay using monodisperse glutaraldehyde-fixed target cells. J Infect Dis 1977; 136:519-530.

Zeigler T. Detection of varicella-zoster viral antigens in clinical specimens by solid-phase enzyme immunoassay. J Infect Dis 1984;150:149-154.

Zeigler T, Halonen PE. Rapid detection of herpes simplex and varicella-zoster virus antigens from clinical specimens by enzyme immunoassay. Antiviral Res 1985; suppl 1:107-110.

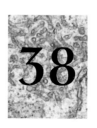

38 VIRAL INFECTIONS OF THE CENTRAL NERVOUS SYSTEM

Although they occur with far less frequency than infections of the respiratory, gastrointestinal, or genitourinary tracts, central nervous system (CNS) viral infections are often the cause of greater anxiety because of an awareness of the possible morbidity, serious sequelae, or mortality. The infrequent examples of severe or fatal illness and the possibility of lifelong residual disability caused by failure of recovery or regeneration of damaged neurons provoke heightened concern in each case. However, the majority of CNS viral infections are relatively benign, self-limited, and without lasting functional compromise.

The varied sites of involvement include the meninges, spinal cord, and brain parenchyma. The clinical syndromes are somewhat arbitrarily divided depending on the principal clinical manifestations. The benign syndrome of headache, fever, nuchal rigidity, vomiting, and other meningeal signs with a cerebrospinal fluid (CSF) pleocytosis fits the aseptic meningitis syndrome. The more virulent clinical picture of obtundation, delirium, agitation, somnolence, seizures, and coma with associated neurologic dysfunction and abnormality reflects inflammation of the brain parenchyma and produces illness far more severe than that of viral meningitis. To a varying degree there may be meningeal involvement with encephalitis or mild parenchymal involvement with meningitis, so the term *meningoencephalitis* is used when there is such overlap. Other less frequent neurologic manifestations of viral infection include myelitis, transverse myelitis, cranial nerve palsies, radiculitis, neuritis, Guillain-Barré syndrome, and chronic persistent encephalitis of immunocompromised patients. In this last group are CNS lymphomas, which have been attributed to EB virus activation of lymphocytes in patients with AIDS or with marked immunosuppression for organ or bone marrow transplantation (see Chapters 1, 8).

This chapter focuses principally on viral meningitis and viral encephalitis because they are by far the most common results of viral CNS infection. Although there is some continuing uncertainty regarding pathogenesis, at least two forms of encephalitis can be attributed to viral infection.

The first is the result of direct viral invasion of the CNS, with resultant inflammatory changes and neuronal damage. This is often spoken of as primary or acute viral encephalitis. In contrast, postinfectious encephalitis follows an acute viral illness and has a sudden onset of neurologic symptoms after a latent phase of varying duration. This is thought by some to be an autoimmune disorder and, before the widespread use of measles vaccines, was most frequently seen after measles virus infections. However, a variety of other respiratory viruses, as well as varicella, have been noted to precede it. The pathology of postinfectious encephalitis is distinct from that of acute infection, with demyelination as its hallmark (Johnson et al., 1984; Johnson and Mims, 1968).

VIRAL ENCEPHALITIS

Viral encephalitis may be characterized by (1) a mild abortive infection, (2) a type of illness barely distinguishable from aseptic meningitis, or (3) a severe involvement of the CNS. The last is often characterized by sudden onset, high fever, meningeal signs, stupor, disorientation, tremors, convulsions, spasticity, coma, and death. Case fatality rates vary widely. Sequelae are more common in infants.

Etiology

For a number of reasons the establishment of definite etiologic diagnoses for patients with clinical encephalitis has been difficult. Many cases are never assigned a specific causative agent. The diagnostic techniques may be complex, time consuming, and expensive, requiring the inoculation of a variety of cell culture systems and laboratory animals. The responsible virus may be detectable solely in the brain itself and may not be present, or only very transiently found, in the blood, cerebrospinal fluid (CSF), or other usually available samples. The beginning application of newer highly sensitive molecular techniques such as PCR has greatly enhanced the diagnostic capability of those laboratories employing this technology. Amplification and identification of viral nucleic acid in CSF has proven sensitive and specific for a number of etiologic agents (Chapters 7, 12, 13, and 37), but availability of the tests is limited at present (Jeffery et al., 1997; Sawyer et al., 1994). The multiplicity of possible causative agents makes serologic diagnosis difficult unless there are epidemiologic or clinical clues that enable the laboratory in search of an antibody rise to focus on a limited number of antigens. The increasing availability of virus-specific IgM antibody determinations by ELISA has facilitated etiologic diagnoses based on a single serum specimen obtained early in the acute phase of illness.

Because the diagnostic tests to establish the etiology of an individual case of viral encephalitis are available only in selected laboratories, and because specimens are frequently not submitted early in the onset of disease, the rates and numbers of cases reported annually are very rough estimates with considerable variation. In an attempt to provide specific diagnoses for all cases of CNS infection, Nicolosi and colleagues (1986) studied all reported CNS infections in Olmstead County, Minnesota, from 1950 to 1981. Their data revealed incidence rates several times higher than those reported annually through the passive system of the Centers for Disease Control (Table 38-1). This was true also for aseptic meningitis.

Because of the availability of specific antiviral chemotherapy, vigorous approaches (including brain biopsy) are pursued if herpes simplex virus is suspected (Chapter 12). However, only a relatively small number of sporadic cases are caused by this agent, perhaps 10% of all encephalitis cases reported (Whitley, 1990).

The common causes of acute viral encephalitis in the United States and among U.S. travelers abroad are as follows:

Togaviruses
  Alphaviruses
    Eastern equine encephalitis (EEE)
    Western equine encephalitis (WEE)
    Venezuelan equine encephalitis (VEE)
  Flaviviruses
    St. Louis encephalitis (SLE)
    Japanese encephalitis (JE)
    Tick-borne complex (TBC)
    Powassan
    Murray Valley
    West Nile fever
Bunyaviruses
  California group
    LaCrosse
    California encephalitis
    Jamestown Canyon
  Phlebovirus
    Rift valley fever
Arenaviruses
  Lymphocytic choriomeningitis (LCM)
  Argentinian hemorrhagic fever (Junin virus)
  Bolivian hemorrhagic fever (Machupo virus)
  Tacaribe
  Sabia
Reoviruses (Orbivirus)
  Colorado tick fever
Rabies (Chapter 24)
Herpes simplex 1 and 2 (Chapter 12)
Human herpes virus 6 (Chap 13)
Enteroviruses (Chapter 7)
  Coxsackievirus A and B
  Echovirus
Varicella-zoster (Chapter 37)
Infectious mononucleosis (Epstein-Barr virus)
  (Chapter 8)
Cytomegalovirus (Chapter 4)
Human immunodeficiency virus (HIV-1) (Chapter 1)
Postinfectious agents
  Measles (Chapter 16)
  Mumps (Chapter 18)
  Rubella (Chapter 26)

Table 38-1 Reported cases of CNS viral infections in the United States, 1990–1994

Type of infection	1990	1991	1992	1993	1994
Aseptic meningitis	11,852	14,526	12,223	12,848	8,932
Encephalitis, primary	1,341	1,021	774	919	717
Encephalitis, postinfections	105	82	129	170	143

Data from CDC, 1996.

Chickenpox (varicella-zoster) (Chapter 37)
Influenza (Chapter 25)

Probably the most precise study of etiologies for suspected acute viral encephalitis was that conducted by the NIAID Collaborative Antiviral Study Group. This involved the use of selected diagnostic brain biopsy for cases of presumptive herpes simplex virus (HSV) encephalitis. Of 432 patients suspected of HSV encephalitis, 193 were confirmed by the biopsy; 239 were negative and were carefully evaluated for other causes. Among those discovered, in addition to other nonherpes viral infections were brain tumor, subdural hematoma, systemic lupus erythematosus, brain abscess, vascular disease, and a variety of bacterial and fungal infections (Soong et al., 1991).

In a separate study, Rantala and Uhari (1989) examined the occurrence of encephalitis among children in Finland in an area where no arbovirus infections occur. They found an annual incidence of 8.8 per 100,000 children less than 16 years of age and listed the most common responsible viruses as varicella, mumps, herpes simplex, and measles. Additionally, there were a number of individual cases caused by respiratory and enteric viruses. Reports from other areas of the world would add an even greater number of those viruses involved with arthropod vectors (togaviruses and bunyaviruses) and those associated with hemorrhagic fevers (arenaviruses, filoviruses, Haantan viruses). Although the term *arbovirus* is still used to indicate those agents whose transmission involves the bite of an insect vector, the term retains epidemiologic and ecologic importance but does not apply to viral taxonomy and classification.

On the basis of differing pathology and the temporal association of the second group with a recent acute infection, encephalitis reporting is usually divided into two categories (Table 38-1). The first includes all those infections where direct viral invasion of the CNS is thought to occur; the second, those that are "postinfectious" after a common acute non-CNS infection followed by an immune-reactive demyelinating process. This second category may then include many of the usual childhood infections, the stereotype of which was measles before its control by vaccination. The etiology of more than half of the annual reported cases of encephalitis is never determined.

The togaviruses include many of the agents formerly called arboviruses. They possess single-stranded RNA genomes and are enveloped with surface projections or spikes. The genus alphavirus has 37 members, agents with particles 40 to 65 nm in diameter. The flavivirus genus contains 68 members of both Old and New World prevalence with particle size 40 to 60 nm. Most agents pathogenic for humans and detected in the United States are mosquito borne, but Powassan virus, which is found principally along the United States-Canadian border, is carried by *Ixodes* ticks.

The bunyaviruses are enveloped RNA agents possessing a segmented genome within a lipid envelope. Their diameter ranges from 80 to 120 nm. The four members of the California group listed are all carried by *Aedes* mosquitoes. Rift Valley fever virus is of special interest because of its epizootics in south and east Africa and its spread into Egypt; thus it also poses a risk to American tourists in those areas. Rift Valley fever virus has been detected in West Africa as well, with an outbreak in Mauritania and Senegal involving more than 1264 cases with 224 deaths (Walsh, 1988). In addition to a unique late-onset retinal vasculitis, it is an occasional cause of encephalitis. Transmission is either by mosquito vector or via aerosol from infected domestic animals.

The arenaviruses include at least six human pathogens. They are RNA viruses with round pleomorphic particles ranging from 60 to 300 (average 100) nm, budding from the cytoplasmic membranes of infected cells. Transmission from infected animal to human occurs through contamination of food by saliva, urine, or feces from infected rodents; aerosolization of rodents' excreta; or, rarely, animal bite. Lymphocytic choriomeningitis is the arenavirus most commonly encountered within the United States and has been the source of research laboratory outbreaks from contaminated hamster tissues.

All of the remaining viruses listed are discussed in greater detail in other chapters, with the exception of Colorado tick fever virus. It is an unusual member of the Reoviridae family, which chronically infects rodents and may be transmitted to humans by wood ticks, inciting a dengue-like illness. When children are infected they occasionally develop a fatal encephalitis.

Reservoirs of infection for the togaviruses, bunyaviruses, and arenaviruses are found in birds and various animals. The persistence of these agents in nature involves a complicated, fascinating ecosystem. Some of the responsible elements include transovarial viral transmission in the insect, lengthy months of viremia in apparently healthy water birds, and feeding and migratory patterns of insect vectors and of natural bird and mammalian reservoirs.

The properties of the other viruses causing encephalitis and the associated CNS manifestations are described in the chapters noted in parentheses on p. 651.

Pathology and Pathogenesis

Virus reaches the CNS following introduction at a distant portal of entry, local replication, and subsequent viremia. The interval between initial infection and eventual CNS involvement may be days or weeks. A number of routes are available but the most likely are (1) extension of virus into neuronal and glial cells adjacent to infected endothelial cells of small capillaries, or (2) directly into CSF from the vessels of the choroid plexus via the ependyma. Rabies virus (Chapter 24) in its passage centrally via peripheral nerve pathways is an exception, and some of the herpesviruses may also use similar direct neural transmission under some circumstances (Johnson and Mims, 1968).

In general, invading viruses give rise to similar pathologic changes in the CNS. It is usually impossible to distinguish between them on the basis of pathologic examination alone. Gross examination of the brain and cord reveals edema and congestion. There may be small hemorrhages. Microscopic examination shows perivascular cellular infiltration and infiltration of the meninges, chiefly with lymphocytes. The principal lesion in the parenchyma consists of neuronal necrosis and degeneration accompanied by neuronophagocytosis. Perivascular cuffing and glial proliferation are common. Destruction of the ground substance of the gray or white matter may be severe. Multiple acellular plaques of necrosis may be seen. The spinal cord may be involved in some types of encephalitis. In general, neuronal lesions and foci of cellular infiltration are widely distributed throughout the brain and spinal cord.

The detection in brain biopsy or autopsy specimens of inclusions within the nucleus or cytoplasm of neuronal or glial cells permits the consideration of a more restricted array of possible causes. Herpes simplex, cytomegalovirus, measles, and rabies are those agents most likely to induce inclusion-bearing cells. A few viruses have predilections to localize in selected anatomic sites. Neonatal cytomegalovirus infection may be most marked in the periventricular subependymal matrix; herpes simplex encephalitis in the older infant or child often

affects the frontotemporal lobes. Rabies shows a predisposition for the brain stem and cortical gray matter.

Attempts have been made to divide the encephalitides listed on p. 651 and tabulated in Table 38-1 into two groups: (1) those with evidence of direct invasion of the CNS by virus; and (2) those considered to involve a postinfectious, autoimmune process. Recent evidence indicates that these are not always necessarily separate and distinct forms, as suggested by their pathologic changes; rather, the differences between the two groups may hinge on timing of the onset of encephalitis in relation to the systemic manifestations and differences in the degree of immune response of the host. The demonstration of measles virus antigens and incomplete virions in the brains of patients with subacute measles encephalitis (SME) and subacute sclerosing panencephalitis (SSPE) confirmed the participation of active viral replication in the pathogenesis of these rare complications (Chapter 16). The sequence of events in acute postinfectious measles encephalitis is less certain, resembling in many ways experimental allergic encephalomyelitis. A study of nineteen patients in Peru from 1980 to 1983 (Johnson et al., 1984) revealed myelin basic protein in their CSF and proliferative lymphocytic responses to this protein, strengthening the conclusion that this is an autoimmune process.

Clinical Manifestations

There are many types of viral encephalitides, varying from benign forms of meningoencephalitis that last a few days and are followed by complete recovery to fulminating encephalitis with the clinical manifestations of paresis, sensory changes, convulsions, increased intracranial pressure, coma, and death. Mumps meningoencephalitis is a good example of the usually benign form. Encephalitis caused by herpes simplex virus, on the other hand, is a devastating infection with a high case fatality rate (Chapter 12).

The onset of viral encephalitis may be sudden or gradual and is marked by fever, headache, dizziness, vomiting, apathy, and stiffness of the neck. Ataxia, tremors, mental confusion, speech difficulties, stupor or hyperexcitability, delirium, convulsions, coma, and death may follow. Papilledema may be detected as a sign of increased intracranial pressure, along with palsies of cranial nerves III and VI. In some cases there may be a prodromal period of 1 to 4 days manifested by chills and fever, headache, malaise, sore throat, conjunctivitis, and pains in the extremities and abdomen followed by encephalitic signs just mentioned. Abortive forms with headache and fever only or a syndrome resembling aseptic meningitis may occur. Lymphocytic choriomeningitis virus infection may be accompanied by arthritis, orchitis, and parotitis.

The many variations in the clinical patterns of encephalitis depend on the distribution, location, and concentration of neuronal lesions. Ocular palsies and ptosis are uncommon. Cerebellar incoordination is seen. Flaccid paralysis of the extremities resembling that of poliomyelitis is sometimes encountered. Paralysis of the shoulder girdle muscles is described as a singular feature of a tick-borne encephalitis.

The CSF is clear, and manometric readings of pressure vary from normal to markedly elevated. As a rule, pleocytosis of 10 to 1000 cells, chiefly mononuclear, is found. The protein and glucose values may be slightly elevated or normal. In eastern equine encephalitis, the CSF may contain 1000 or more cells per cubic millimeter. In the early stages the cells are predominantly polymorphonuclear leukocytes, shifting later to mononuclear elements. In this form of encephalitis the peripheral white blood cell count may be as high as 66,000, with 90% polymorphonuclear leukocytes; in the other types it is lower, ranging from 10,000 to 20,000, predominantly neutrophils. A general, diffuse, bilateral slowing of background activity is the most usual EEG finding. With accompanying seizures, epileptiform patterns may also be seen. The delineation of virus infections of the brain has been significantly aided by contrast-enhanced computed tomography (CT) and magnetic resonance imaging (MRI). MRI provides better delineation of parenchymal alterations and has greater sensitivity for detection of the demyelinating lesions seen with postinfectious encephalitis rather than acute viral infection (Smith, 1992; Shaw and Cohen, 1993). Masden et al. (1995) emphasized the increased sensitivity of perfusion single-photon emission CT (SPECT).

The course of encephalitis varies from that of the fulminating type, ending in death in 2 to 4 days, to that of a mild form in which the illness subsides in 1 or 2 weeks with complete recovery.

Diagnosis

A diagnosis of acute encephalitis is indicated by the clinical findings. The circumstances in which the disease occurs are important. The age and geographic distribution are described later in the discussion of epidemiologic factors. The specific type of encephalitis can be determined only by isolation or identification of the virus or by demonstration of the formation of or rise of level of antibody in convalescence. Togaviruses are rarely detected in the CSF, blood, or other materials during life.

On the other hand, enteroviruses, mumps virus, adenoviruses, varicella-zoster virus, and cytomegalovirus may be detected in the CSF and other appropriate materials (see chapters on specific viruses). A serologic diagnosis may be reached by means of various antibody tests. Paired serum specimens may be necessary. The first should be drawn as soon after onset as possible and the second, 2 or 3 weeks later.

A number of diagnostic tests under study and in varying stages of development exploit techniques for the detection of specific viral antigens or early antibodies in CSF. These tests are available in a limited number of laboratories. Tests employing immunoglobulin M capture, enzyme-linked immunosorbent assays for a variety of causative agents have permitted a specific diagnosis on a single acute phase serum or CSF by the arbovirus reference laboratories of the Centers for Disease Control. Tsai (1991) and Calisher (1994) have published extensive reviews of the arthropod-borne virus infections seen most often in the United States.

Differential Diagnosis

Other diseases of the CNS may be confused with viral encephalitis. Although human rabies is extremely rare in the United States, it should be considered (Chapter 24). Several cases of rabies in recent years have been labeled "viral" encephalitis during the patient's illness, and the diagnosis of rabies was appreciated only on postmortem examination with the discovery of Negri bodies in the hippocampus or cerebellum.

Tuberculous meningitis or *pyogenic meningitis* may present the clinical picture of encephalitis. In this circumstance, the key lies in the CSF, which may be cloudy, shows greater pleocytosis, has low glucose and high protein levels, and usually has microorganisms that are evident on smear or culture (Chapter 35). In the case of tuberculous meningitis or tuberculoma, a chest roentgenogram and skin tests with tuberculin may provide additional clues.

Reye's syndrome played a significant role in the diagnosis of acute childhood encephalopathic states following its description in 1963 by the Australian pathologist, Kenneth Reye. Affected children had an acute encephalopathy with hepatic dysfunction that occurred within a few days of a preceding infection, usually influenza virus or varicella. Epidemiologic studies in the early 1980s disclosed the close association of ingestion of aspirin during the preceding chickenpox or influenza illness and the metabolic aspects of the syndrome. With widespread public education to the hazards of aspirin administered to children with acute respiratory infections and chickenpox, there has been a resultant marked decrease in the numbers of reported cases of Reye's syndrome in the United States (Centers for Disease Control, 1991b; Hurwitz, et al., 1987).

Tumor, trauma, and *abscess* of the brain may be mistaken for encephalitis and are often difficult to differentiate. Roentgenograms of the skull, electroencephalograms, radioisotopic scans, arteriography, and computed tomography may help in the solution of the problem. *Lead encephalopathy* is distinguished from viral encephalitis (1) by the CSF findings, which consist mainly of increased level of protein, often quite marked, and by no increase or only a slight increase in number of cells; (2) by chemical detection of abnormal amounts of lead in the blood or CSF; (3) by roentgenographic evidence of lead line in the bone; (4) by lead line in the gums if teeth are present; (5) by basophilic stippling and anemia; and (6) by urinary coproporphyrins.

Alcohol, drugs, and other toxins must also be considered in a review of possible causes.

Prognosis

Once viruses reach the CNS, a number of host features render the brain more vulnerable. There is no lymphatic drainage and no secondary immune organs (lymph nodes) within the CNS. The blood-brain barrier normally impedes the entry of both humoral and cellular immune components. Although the CNS possesses some immunologic defenses, they are significantly different from those of other tissues and organs, and their extent has not yet been fully elucidated. It is also important to realize that specific receptor sites or other related membrane functions permit the attachment of given viruses to selected susceptible cells.

The specific virus, the inoculum size, the clinical type of illness, and the age of the patient are some of the factors influencing the outcome of the disease. The decrease in the postchildhood infection category stems mainly from the striking drop in measles in the United States.

Mumps encephalitis carries the lowest mortality, only 1% to 2%. The majority of patients with mumps have CNS involvement, but this is nearly always a benign meningitis. A few patients undergo frank encephalitis, which may result in occasional deaths, but of greater concern is a 25% incidence of CNS sequelae among the survivors (Koskiniemi et al., 1983).

Mortality also varies from epidemic to epidemic. Eastern equine, Japanese, and tick-borne encephalitides are generally associated with higher fatality rates (30% to 50%) than the St. Louis, Western equine, and California types. The overall mortality from St. Louis encephalitis is 5% to 7% and, from Western equine, 7% to 10%. Recovery from either, when it occurs, is usually complete. In young infants with St. Louis or Western equine encephalitis, however, permanent injury to the CNS may occur. Seizures, hydrocephalus, and mental retardation have been seen in outbreaks of the St. Louis type, affecting 10% to 40% of infants below the age of 6 months. Similar permanent brain damage was observed in two thirds of the patients surviving Eastern equine encephalitis in the Massachusetts epidemic of 1938. The fatality rate is high in Japanese encephalitis.

The fatality rate for measles encephalitis was 12%; for varicella encephalitis it was 28%. The prognosis in general for herpes simplex encephalitis is poor. Death occurs in about one third and serious sequelae occur in about half of the survivors, even in those who received antiviral therapy. The cases of encephalitis caused by enteroviruses are few, so it is difficult to estimate the prognosis, although from the available data it appears to be similar to that of mumps. A focal encephalitis with seizures and full recovery was reported in four pediatric patients described by Modlin et al. (1991). Acute onset of hemiparesis or hemiplegia was seen in three other children, who were left with significant sequelae.

Long-term follow-up studies of patients recovering from encephalitis to determine the incidence and severity of sequelae have been limited to small, selected groups of patients. Because so much of CNS development occurs in the early postnatal years, it has always been assumed that adverse events would be recognized more frequently in children. Rantala and colleagues (1991) reviewed the records of 73 children seen at a hospital in Finland between 1973 and 1983 whose diagnostic criteria fit acute encephalitis. Follow-up examinations revealed that 61 of the youngsters had lowered performance and IQs lower than randomly selected age-matched controls, but these differences were less severe than anticipated. They concluded that the prognosis for childhood encephalitis, with the exception of that caused by herpes simplex virus, was more optimistic than previously considered. Unfortunately, they did not list the specific viruses responsible. In contrast, significant neurologic sequelae following Japanese encephalitis virus infection have been reported in as many as 80% of survivors, especially among children. These involved intellectual, motor, and emotional impairment (Monath, 1988).

Epidemiologic Factors

The distribution of viral encephalitis varies according to season. Arbovirus encephalitis is a warm weather disease. Epidemics and sporadic cases of the North American forms (St. Louis, California, and the two equine encephalitides) and of Japanese encephalitis begin during the hot summer months and subside during the autumn. Tick-borne encephalitides, unlike the others, attack chiefly forest workers, beginning most frequently in May and June and diminishing over the summer months. Heightened interest in Japanese encephalitis has arisen with increased tourism and commercial travel to areas where epidemics have recently occurred (People's Republic of China, Thailand, India, Nepal, Vietnam, Japan, Korea, and Taiwan).

Enteroviral encephalitis occurs predominantly during the summer and fall months. Mumps encephalitis occurs year-round, with periodic increases in incidence during the winter and early spring months. The incidence of varicella encephalitis begins to rise in the winter months, peaks in the spring, and declines slowly to lowest levels in the summer and fall.

The extensive use of MMR vaccine has markedly reduced the annual numbers of reported mumps cases (658 in 1996) and correspondingly those with any CNS involvement. It is anticipated that the use of varicella-zoster virus vaccine—initiated in 1995 in the United States (Chapter 37)—will have a similar impact over the next years on the occurrence of chickenpox and its encephalitis.

Cases of encephalitis of unknown cause show consistent peaks during the summer months corresponding with those of arbovirus encephalitis. This suggests that some of the undiagnosed cases may be caused by arboviruses, although enteroviruses are also prevalent during the same months.

The age distribution shows that St. Louis, Japanese, and Western equine encephalitides all have a predilection for people in the extremes of life. The incidence of St. Louis encephalitis is high in infants and older people and lowest in children from 5 to 12 years of age. Similarly, about 60% of those attacked by Japanese encephalitis are over 50 years of age. In Okinawa and Taiwan, however, the largest proportion of cases has occurred in children. The highest attack rates of Western equine encephalitis are likely to be found among male outdoor workers 20 to 50 years old. High attack rates have also been found in infants. Eastern equine encephalitis attacks primarily the young. In the Massachusetts outbreak of 1938, 70% were under 10 years of age, 25% were below 1 year of age, and only 15% were over 21 years of age.

In general, the incidence is higher in males than in females. There may be an occupational factor in the sex differences observed in western equine and tick-borne encephalitides. The sex ratio in Japanese encephalitis is 124 males to 100 females. Both sexes are equally attacked by Eastern equine encephalitis.

Although many of the names of the viruses are derived from their initial geographic sites of detection, surveillance in ensuing years has revealed more variable distribution than was originally appreciated. Western equine encephalitis is found throughout the entire United States and Canada. St. Louis encephalitis has a similar widespread distribution. Eastern equine encephalitis is still confined mainly to the Eastern seaboard. Powassan virus, a tick-borne agent, is found mainly along the United States–Canadian border. California group viruses, as exemplified by LaCrosse virus, are annually the most prevalent mosquito-borne infection detected in the United States and have been isolated in many states other than California and Wisconsin (first patient with LaCrosse virus), ranging from Utah to North Carolina and from Minnesota to Arkansas. In 1993, fifty-five cases of California encephalitis were reported from 11 different states. Only eighteen patients with SLE were detected in five states. The last nationwide epidemic of SLE was in 1975 and 1976, when 2194 cases were identified in thirty-five states.

Small outbreaks of Eastern equine encephalitis have occurred in Massachusetts (1938, 1955, 1956, 1971, and 1983) and in Louisiana (1947). During the summer of 1959, New Jersey was struck by a sharp outbreak associated with a high mortality. Cases have occurred sporadically in human beings in Texas, Georgia, Florida, Rhode Island, and Tennessee. The disease in horses and mules is widespread over eastern United States and Canada and areas in Central and South America.

Recent arboviral experiences in the United States have included California serogroup viruses in the upper Midwest, St. Louis encephalitis virus in Texas and Louisiana communities bordering the Gulf of Mexico, and Eastern equine encephalitis in Florida. Of sixty-two confirmed cases of LaCrosse infection in 1986, forty-four were in children under 18 years of age. In contrast, an outbreak of St. Louis encephalitis in Harris County, Texas, involved twenty-eight cases with five fatalities, all of whom were older than 55 years. Of seven patients with Western equine encephalitis virus, four were infants under 6 months of age. In 1991 an outbreak in Arkansas involved twenty-four cases of St. Louis encephalitis in late July and early August associated with an increase in the population of infected Culex mosquitoes. (Centers for Disease Control, 1984, 1986, 1990, 1991a, 1991c). The accuracy and completeness of detection and reporting of arbovirus infections vary greatly according to the extent of surveillance activities in individual states. Approximately one half of U.S. states pursue arbovirus surveillance including virus isolation; serologic assays; or antigen detection involving mosquitoes, birds, and humans.

The ecologic and epidemiologic features of these infections are complex, with transmission cycles that may include primary and secondary vertebrate hosts and vectors.

The mode of transmission of St. Louis, Japanese, and Eastern and Western equine encephalitides is the bite of the mosquito. Mosquitoes become infected by biting wild birds or occasionally certain mammals. Human-to-human transmission does not occur under natural conditions. St. Louis encephalitis and Western equine encephalitis are very much alike in respect to ecologic and epidemiologic factors. Both infect horses in nature, and reservoirs of silent infection have been found in domestic animals and birds. Both are found in wild caught mosquitoes (*Culex tarsalis* and *Culex pipiens*) and can be transferred in the laboratory by the bite of such mosquitoes. Both viruses have been acquired by mosquitoes feeding on birds with occult infection (viremia). The Midwestern and Western states are seeded with both viruses, which give rise to infection in humans during the summer.

St. Louis encephalitis virus has also been detected in chicken mites (*Dermanyssus gallinae*) during a nonepidemic period. Since transovarian infection has been shown to take place in the mite, the latter may play an important role in maintaining the virus in nature.

Japanese encephalitis virus has been detected in naturally infected mosquitoes (*Culex tritaeniorhynchus*) in Japan, and experimental transmission of infection by mosquitoes has been established. Many animals and wading birds have been suspected of maintaining reservoirs of infection. There is evidence of widespread infection among farm animals, especially pigs.

Eastern equine encephalitis virus has been isolated from naturally infected mosquitoes and birds. Pheasants seem particularly prone to epizootics. The virus has been isolated from chicken mites and chicken lice in an epidemic area. The factors involved in transmission are apparently similar to those found in Western equine and St. Louis encephalitides.

The vector for Colorado tick fever is *Dermacentor andersoni,* and the principal host reservoirs are ground squirrels and chipmunks. Powassan virus apparently is transmitted by *Ixodes* ticks, and squirrels and chipmunks may provide the reservoir.

Treatment

It is recommended that all patients suspected of having encephalitis be evaluated promptly to confirm the diagnosis and to rule out other diseases such as partially treated bacterial meningitis, tuberculous meningitis, brain abscess, drug overdosage, toxins, metabolic encephalopathy, or brain tumor. Diagnostic evaluation may include CSF examination; electroencephalogram; CT scan; ultrasound; MRI; and chemical analyses for toxins, drugs, and metabolic aberrations.

Although there was little to offer in the way of specific treatment for viral encephalitis in the past, acyclovir may be lifesaving in patients with encephalitis caused by herpes simplex virus (Chapter 12). Treatment is most beneficial when given early in the course of the disease, before brain damage occurs from necrotic infection or increased intracranial pressure.

The patient with depressed consciousness will be best monitored and managed in a critical care unit where aggressive supporting therapy is available. Increased intracranial pressure, seizures, hyperpyrexia, fluid and electrolyte imbalance, respiratory decompensation, hypotension, and selected organ failures may develop, necessitating prompt awareness and interventions. The wide range of individual patients' variations in course will determine specific interventions, such as fluid restriction, anticonvulsant drugs, ventilatory support, treatment of secondary infections (at sites of catheters, indwelling venous or venous or arterial lines, endotracheal tubes), and parenteral nutrition. The use of corticosteroids to reduce intracranial pressure or decrease toxic effects of inflammatory cytokines is a controversial issue (Hoke et al., 1992).

Control Measures

Active Immunization. Effective means of control of postinfectious encephalitis caused by measles, mumps, and rubella viruses have been available for some time. Widespread use of vaccines has significantly reduced the incidence of encephalitis associated with these diseases. On the other hand, the control of arbovirus infections presents many problems. Since man is not part of the infection chain but most often represents an accidental, "dead-end" infection and since outbreaks are unpredictable, a rational basis for mass immunization is hard to demonstrate. In any event, with the exception of Japanese encephalitis, no vaccine suitable for human use is available for the arbovirus infections listed on p. 651. Japanese encephalitis (JE) vaccine, prepared from infected suckling mouse brains, is produced in Japan (Biken JE vaccine) and has been made available to U.S. travelers before departure for endemic areas. It requires three doses subcutaneously at days 0, 7, and 30. Serologic studies suggest that the neutralizing antibodies produced are effective in vitro against strains of Japanese encephalitis from both India and Japan.

Arthropod Control. Attempts to control the arbovirus encephalitides should be directed against the arthropod vector and reservoirs of infection in order to interrupt the natural cycle of transmission.

In the Western states, where outbreaks are rural, the intensive use of agricultural insecticides has been followed by reduction in mosquitoes and in human infection rates. In the central states, where outbreaks of St. Louis encephalitis occur in urban-suburban areas, the main vectors are *C. pipiens* and *C. quinquefasciatus* mosquitoes, which are known to multiply in dirty water and in places where there is inadequate drainage. The characteristic pattern observed in many epidemics is a period of heavy rainfall followed by drought, resulting in many pools of stagnant water yielding vast numbers of mosquitoes. Prompt drainage of these areas and application of insecticides (larvicides and adulticides) should interrupt the infection chain and thereby reduce the incidence of human infection.

This discussion has been limited to encephalitis, the major acute manifestation of viral infection of

the brain, but it is important to remember that slow viral infections of the CNS have been demonstrated and that the entire field of chronic degenerative disease of the CNS caused by viruses or related transmissible agents ("prions") remains to be elaborated further.

Slow Infections. Caused by conventional viruses, slow infections include subacute sclerosing panencephalitis (SSPE), caused by measles (Chapter 16), and chronic meningoencephalitis of immunodeficiency, caused by enteroviruses (Chapter 7). Progressive multifocal leukoencephalopathy (PMI), caused by a papovavirus (JC) of the polyoma group, nearly always is associated with immune compromise such as that caused by leukemia or AIDS (Chapter 1). JC virus is ubiquitous and benign among normal children (Box 38-1). Current concerns regarding bovine spongiform encephalopathy (BSE) (Anderson et al., 1996) and its possible relationship to a new variant of Creutzfeldt-Jakob disease (nvCJD) (Will et al., 1996) have led to augmented interest in a number of similar transmissible CNS disorders (Brown et al., 1994). The agents responsible do not meet the criteria for viruses, since they lack a demonstrable RNA or DNA genome, but consist of protease-resistant proteins (*prions,* or PrP) (Prusiner, 1991, 1994). Clarification of their role and replication remains controversial. The common denominators of these CNS diseases are their transmissibility via brain, spinal cord, or lymphoid tissues; their lengthy incubation periods (months or years); degenerative neurologic disease; and a neuropathologic picture of spongiform encephalopathy with widespread marked vacuolation, loss of neurons, glial proliferation and

---

BOX 38-1

SLOW VIRUS CNS INFECTIONS

Conventional Viruses

Subacute sclerosing panencephalitis (SSPE)	Measles
Progressive multifocal leukoencephalopathy (PML)	Papova
Chronic meningoencephalitis of immunodeficiency	Enteros

Unconventional Agents

Spongiform encephalopathies	Prions

absence of inflammation. In contrast to those slow virus CNS infections caused by conventional viruses, these disorders remain the subject of continued debate and research regarding their etiology.

The initial linkages between these unusual disorders of animals and humans emerged with the appreciation of marked similarities in the histology of kuru and scrapie. Subsequently, a uniformity of course, pathogenesis, and neuropathology led to inoculation experiments in nonhuman primates that further demonstrated their relatedness. Box 38-2 lists the recognized examples of alleged prion-induced spongiform encephalopathies. CJD, an unusual dementia of older adults, is recognized in both sporadic and occasional familial (genetic) patterns. Transmission has been documented via transplantation of tissues (cornea, dura mater) from CJD patients, as well as from contaminated neurosurgical instruments and cortical electrodes. Before the availability of recombinant human growth hormone (HGH) a cluster of cases appeared among young recipients of HGH prepared from pooled cadaveric pituitary glands. GSS, a familial encephalopathy, resembles CJD but includes prominent cerebellar ataxia. An even rarer adult disorder, FFI, involves severe insomnia and progressive autonomic insufficiency. The epidemic of bovine spongiform encephalopathy (BSE) (known popularly as "mad cow disease") in the United Kingdom, led to the slaughter of nearly 200,000 cows; an embargo on British beef; and, most alarmingly, the suspicion that a cluster of cases of early onset "new variant" nvCJD (Will et al., 1996) in English patients represents a crossing of species barriers and transmission to humans by direct contact with or ingestion of BSE-contaminated materials (Anderson et al., 1996; Lanchester, 1996).

VIRAL MENINGITIS

Viral meningitis is usually a benign syndrome of multiple etiology characterized by headache, fever, vomiting, and meningeal signs. The CSF shows an increase in mononuclear cells, and it yields no bacterial or fungal growth on culture. Recovery occurs in about 3 to 10 days and is nearly always complete. Wallgren (1925), a Swedish pediatrician, recognized and described the meningitis syndrome in the 1920s, delineating its clinical features and differentiating it from bacterial meningitis.

The viruses responsible for the viral meningitis syndrome may also give rise to a more severe involvement of the CNS, such as meningoencephalitis, encephalitis, and encephalomyelitis. The boundary line between viral meningitis and encephalitis is often indistinct and is drawn arbitrarily on clinical grounds. The clinical picture may not always reveal the full extent of CNS involvement. An estimated 30,000 to 50,000 cases of aseptic meningitis are thought to occur annually in the United States (Centers for Disease Control, 1997).

Etiology and Epidemiology

Viral meningitis may be associated with a wide variety of viral agents. Many of these are as follows:

Mumps
Echovirus
Poliovirus
Coxsackievirus
Adenoviruses
Lymphocytic choriomeningitis
Herpes 1, 2, 6
Herpes zoster
Epstein-Barr virus (EBV)
Human immunodeficiency virus (HIV-I)
Encephalitis: St. Louis, California, Eastern equine, and Western equine
Parainfluenza type 3

In spite of improved methods of recognizing these agents, the cause of a large proportion of cases of viral meningitis remains unknown.

Enteroviruses (Chapter 7) have been recognized as significant agents in CNS infections ever since the polioviruses were first known to cause both paralytic and nonparalytic disease. With the marked decrease in circulation of polioviruses, the Coxsackieviruses and echoviruses continue to be important causes of viral meningitis. They are probably responsible for approximately three fourths of

---

BOX 38-2

TRANSMISSIBLE SPONGIFORM ENCEPHALOPATHIES

Animals

Scrapie of sheep and goats
Transmissible mink encephalopathy (TME)
Chronic wasting disease of mule deer and elk
Bovine spongiform encephalopathy (BSE)

Human

Kuru
Creutzfeldt-Jakob disease (CJD)
Gerstmann-Straussler-Scheinker syndrome (GSS)
Fatal familial insomnia (FFI)

the cases of viral meningitis reported in the United States (Table 38-1). The characteristics of the enteroviruses and the clinical manifestations produced by them are described in detail in Chapter 7.

In the first 36 weeks of 1991, Echovirus type 30 was the most common isolate encountered in laboratories throughout New England and the middle and south Atlantic states. In 1990 more than 20% of isolates referred to the Centers for Disease Control were identified as Echovirus 30 (Centers for Disease Control, 1991). Some of the epidemiology was familiar, with a cluster of cases in a middle school football team involving the coach, the student manager, and several of the players during an 8-day period in September (Centers for Disease Control, 1981; Baron et al., 1982).

In attempting to focus on one or another of the many, varied causes of viral meningitis, the physician may be greatly assisted by a careful epidemiologic history. Occupational exposure to mouse colonies or a new pet hamster in the home raises the question of lymphocytic choriomeningitis (LCM) virus. Recent travel to endemic or epidemic areas and a history of insect bites may stimulate more careful investigation of current arbovirus infections.

Mumps virus was also a common cause of viral meningitis. It should be considered in unimmunized patients. Mumps meningitis may occur in the absence of parotitis or other manifestations of mumps infection (see Fig. 18-3). The diagnosis of mumps and other features of the disease are discussed in Chapter 18. Widespread use of the trivalent measles-mumps-rubella (MMR) vaccine has markedly reduced the numbers of cases of mumps virus infections in the United States in the past decades.

In a 5-year investigation of the causes of certain syndromes of the CNS, Meyer et al. (1960) determined the cause in 305 cases of viral meningitis. In their study the enteroviruses, excluding polioviruses, accounted for 30% of the cases and mumps virus for about 16%. Lymphocytic choriomeningitis (LCM) and herpes simplex virus are less commonly detected as causes of viral meningitis.

It is difficult to assess the overall contribution of the arboviruses, but in epidemics of arbovirus encephalitis a sizable number of patients, especially children, will acquire a benign illness with neurologic manifestations, predominantly those of viral meningitis, accompanied by no significant change in the sensorium. For example, in the epidemic of St. Louis encephalitis in Houston in 1964, fifteen of a total of twenty-six patients had the mild illness that was confirmed serologically as St. Louis encephalitis virus infection (Barrett et al., 1965). The seasonal distribution of agents associated with viral meningitis is an important clue to their recognition. The enteroviruses and arboviruses predominate during the warm months, whereas mumps virus was present chiefly during the winter and spring months. Because mumps has been reduced greatly as a result of vaccine, and meningitis is now rarely seen.

Lymphocytic choriomeningitis may be established by the detection of virus in CSF or blood and by a rise in the level of either complement-fixing or neutralizing antibody. The diagnosis of herpes simplex is described in Chapter 12, of herpes zoster in Chapter 37, and of infectious mononucleosis in Chapter 8. The recognition of the remaining causes of viral meningitis depends on the distinctive clinical picture of the various diseases, the etiologic agent, or the demonstration of an increase in the level of antibody.

Bacterial meningitis may sometimes be a confusing factor. Tuberculous meningitis in the early stages and pyogenic meningitis, either early or modified by antibiotic treatment, may resemble aseptic meningitis. The CSF in such cases may show an increase in cells, predominantly lymphocytes. The glucose value is not invariably low and cultures may be sterile (see Chapter 17 and 35).

Some drugs, especially nonsteroidal antiinflammatory agents, have induced aseptic meningitis in patients who have apparently developed an immediate hypersensitivity to the components. Derbes (1984) reported a woman who underwent four separate episodes of viral meningitis after ingestion of trimethoprim-sulfamethoxizole and a fifth attack after trimethoprim alone.

Kawasaki's syndrome, for which an etiology has yet to be determined, is often accompanied by a viral meningitis that may be responsible in part for the irritability and misery displayed by many of these patients (Chapter 15). Viral meningitis has also complicated Lyme disease, a disorder now attributed to a spirochete (Chapter 33). Mollaret's syndrome is a recurrent viral meningitis of unknown etiology with repeated episodes of fever and sterile meningitis lasting 4 or 5 days, occurring as frequently as monthly over a 3- or 4-year period.

The introduction into the subarachnoid space of foreign materials such as contrast media (for myelography) or medications (for CNS tumor therapy) may initiate a brisk meningeal pleocytosis with an accompanying clinical syndrome indistinguishable from infectious meningitis. The human diploid cell rabies vaccine (Chapter 24) is far less likely to provoke CNS reactions than were its predecessors, duck embryo or rabbit nervous tissue vaccines.

Usually the attack rates of infection and viral meningitis during enterovirus outbreaks are highest in infants and young children. In the 10-year period from 1970 to 1979, 64% of enterovirus isolates were from children under 10 years of age, 50% from those under 4 years, and 29% from those under 1 year (Moore, 1981). Clusters of enterovirus meningitis have been reported among high school football players (Baron et al., 1982; Moore et al., 1983). They experience higher attack rates, suffer greater morbidity, and more frequently require hospitalization than their classmates. The agents most frequently isolated from clinical specimens in a 7-year period (1978 to 1984) are listed in Table 38-2 from data published by CDC. Regrettably, such numbers are no longer regularly reported, and only occasional descriptions of outbreaks are published (Centers for Disease Control, 1997).

Pathology

Since most patients with viral meningitis recover completely, few postmortem studies have been reported. A leptomeningitis with inflammatory cell infiltration, polymorphonuclear cells in perivascular sheaths, and mononuclear cells in the choroid plexus has been described.

Clinical Manifestations

The onset may be abrupt or gradual. The initial features are headache, fever, malaise, gastrointestinal symptoms, and signs of meningeal irritation. Abdominal pain is a common complaint. Some patients have ill-defined chest pain or generalized muscular pains or aches. Sore throat is occasionally encountered. Nausea and vomiting are common.

Table 38-2 Reported cases of viral meningitis, United States, 1978–1984

Year	No. cases	Most common agents
1978	6,573	Echovirus 4, 9
1979	8,754	Echovirus 7, 11
1980	8,028	Echovirus 11, Coxsackievirus B5
1981	9,547	Echovirus 9, 30
1982	9,680	Echovirus 11, 30
1983	11,740	Coxsackievirus B5, Echovirus 30, 11, 24
1984	8,036	Echovirus 9, 30, Coxsackievirus B5, A9

Stiffness of the neck or back may develop a day or so after the onset. The deep tendon reflexes are normal or show hyperactivity. Muscle power is normal, as a rule, but there may be slight or transitory weakness. A maculopapular rash may accompany the viral meningitis syndrome, especially in association with certain types of Echovirus and Coxsackievirus infections. The CSF shows pleocytosis with a predominance of lymphocytes. The symptoms and signs usually subside spontaneously and rapidly. The patient is well in 3 to 10 days.

Headache. Headache is one of the most common manifestations and often the initial complaint. It is likely to be severe. Characteristically frontal in location, it may be retrobulbar, occipital, or generalized.

Fever. The temperature ranges from 37.8° C (100° F) to as high as 40° to 40.6° C (104° or 105° F). The fever lasts from 3 to 9 days, with a mean of about 5 days. Sometimes it is biphasic, and this should make one alert for enteroviral infection.

Gastrointestinal Symptoms. Gastrointestinal symptoms, including nausea and abdominal pain, are frequent early manifestations. Vomiting may occur at the onset or a day or two later. Diarrhea is more common than constipation.

Pain. Pain occurs in the epigastric or periumbilical areas fairly often. Thoracic pain suggests pleurodynia and Coxsackievirus infection, but mild chest pain may occur in aseptic meningitis caused by echovirus type 6 and other agents. Generalized muscular pain in the back and extremities is more likely to appear in enteroviral infections than in mumps meningitis.

Meningeal Signs. Signs consisting of stiff neck, stiff back, and tightness of the hamstring muscles are present in the majority of patients. Brudzinski's sign is usually present.

Neuromuscular Changes. Deep tendon reflexes are normal or show hyperactivity. Signs of muscle weakness are usually absent or equivocal, but myalgia may be prominent. Slight or transitory weakness along with muscle pain and tenderness and abnormal tendon or superficial reflexes point toward the possibility of enterovirus infections. Definite paresis or paralysis has been noted with certain of the enteroviruses (especially echovirus 2,

4, 6, 16; Coxsackievirus A4, B2, B3; and the newer enterovirus types 70 and 71). This weakness usually recedes more rapidly than with classic poliomyelitis and rarely, if ever, leaves residual paralysis beyond 30 to 60 days from onset. Transitory weakness seldom occurs in other forms of aseptic meningitis. In any patient showing definite or persistent motor weakness or encephalitic signs, a more extensive involvement of the CNS should be considered.

Rash. A macular, maculopapular, or tiny vesicular rash accompanies certain enteroviral infections, particularly echovirus types 4, 6, 9, and 16 and Coxsackievirus types A9 and A16. Petechial eruptions have accompanied echovirus type 9 infection. The details are described in Chapter 7.

Seizures. Seizures are rarely observed in viral meningitis except in younger patients with high fevers where they may represent febrile convulsions. Their infrequency, however, necessitates a careful consideration of other possible causes. Early bacterial meningitis, a parameningeal inflammatory focus, brain tumor, vascular malformations, local cerebritis, and septic emboli with endocarditis are among the conditions to be considered. Careful observation of the patient's course will be helpful in setting the priority of any further investigative studies.

Laboratory Findings. Except for changes in the CSF, the usual clinical laboratory tests are seldom helpful. The CSF shows a leukocyte count ranging from 10 to 1000 cells per mm^3. The cell count is usually low, the average being under 150 cells. A total cell count over 1500 is not likely but has been seen in echovirus and coxsackievirus infections. Studies of CSF from patients in an epidemic setting have revealed positive cultures for enterovirus even with cell counts less than 10 per mm^3 (Dagan et al., 1988). In mumps meningitis the cells usually number less than 1000, but counts between 1500 and 4000 have been observed. Mononuclear cells as a rule predominate in all forms of viral meningitis. However, CSF obtained early in the course of illness will frequently display a polymorphonuclear cell preponderance. This will shift rapidly over the next 6 to 8 hours so that a repeat lumbar puncture will yield CSF with more than 50% mononuclear cells.

The shift of CSF polymorphonuclear nuclear cells was shown in most children with viral meningitis caused by enteroviruses to fall below 50% after 24 hours of clinical illness (Amir et al., 1991).

The presence of a CSF eosinophilia suggests a helminthic infestation, lymphocytic choriomeningitis virus, or a number of noninfectious disorders such as Hodgkin's disease (Chesney et al., 1979). In mumps the cells are almost entirely lymphocytes. The total protein content varies from normal to values as high as 100 mg/dl. It may rise even higher in lymphogranuloma venereum and lead poisoning. The glucose content is usually normal or slightly elevated. It is characteristically low in lymphogranuloma venereum and meningitides caused by the tubercle bacillus and other bacteria. Cultures for bacteria and fungi are negative, and the other constituents of the CSF are normal.

Diagnosis

Recognition of the syndrome of viral meningitis is straightforward but can be troublesome (Singer et al., 1980). Headache, fever, vomiting, and signs of meningeal irritation call for a lumbar puncture. The CSF shows characteristic pleocytosis, with predominantly mononuclear elements. The varying causes of this syndrome have been discussed previously. The clinical and epidemiologic circumstances often give clues leading to the underlying cause. Since viral infections are the most common causes of aseptic meningitis, a search should be made for the etiologic agent in the CSF, throat, and stool specimens. Serum specimens from the acute and convalescent phases tested for rise in the level of antibody may help in the diagnosis.

■ **Case Report** B.C., a $3^{8/12}$-year-old boy, was brought by his parents to the emergency room of Duke Hospital in July with a history of fever, malaise, drowsiness, irritability, and headache of 3 days' duration. The headache had increased markedly in the past 12 hours. He had vomited after each of several small meals that day and complained of photophobia. Temperature was 39.5° C. There was no rash or conjunctivitis. He had marked nuchal rigidity and positive Kernig's and Brudzinski's signs. Lumbar puncture disclosed turbid CSF under slightly increased pressure. CSF cell count was 460 WBC/mm^3, 75% of which were polymorphonuclear. Gram stain and coagglutination of CSF were negative for bacteria and bacterial antigens, respectively. CSF protein was 48 mg/100 ml; glucose was 75 mg/100 ml (blood glucose 110 mg/100 ml). Chloramphenicol and ampicillin were administered intravenously and he was admitted to the hospital.

A second lumbar puncture, performed 8 hours after the initial one, disclosed a white blood cell count of 375/mm^3, 35% of which were polymorphonuclear and

65% mononuclear. CSF glucose and protein were essentially unchanged. By the next morning, 18 hours after hospital admission, he was markedly improved, smiling, comfortable, and active. The emergency room CSF culture revealed no bacterial growth and his antibiotic therapy was discontinued. Although his temperature rose again during the second hospital day to 39° C, he remained alert and increasingly active. The next morning he was discharged home with instructions to his parents to bring him promptly back to the emergency room if his improvement failed to continue. Two days after his discharge, both the CSF and an admission stool specimen submitted to the virology laboratory were positive for enterovirus.

In the case report, the most compelling evidence for a viral, rather than bacterial, etiology was the rapid shift of the CSF distribution of white blood cells in 8 hours from an initial polymorphonuclear to a mononuclear cell preponderance. Even with early antibiotic therapy of pyogenic bacterial meningitis, 48 hours or more will elapse before such a cellular shift occurs. With suspected viral meningitis patients, a prompt second CSF examination after 6 to 8 hours may be of great help in resolving the differential diagnosis between bacterium and virus.

Rotbart (1990, 1995) has developed a number of more rapid diagnostic approaches to viral meningitis, particularly that caused by enteroviruses. Earlier studies with nucleic acid hybridization assays were unhelpful because of low virus titers in CSF. Using a modified polymerase chain reaction (PCR) assay, he was able to detect enterovirus RNA in CSF of thirteen patients whose clinical diagnoses were consistent with enteroviral meningitis. Virus cultures were positive in only nine of the thirteen. If this approach can be extended to diagnostic microbiology laboratories, the confirmation of enterovirus meningitis diagnoses could be far more rapid and sensitive than current systems permit (Chapter 7). Also, it could be extended to agents other than the enteroviruses.

Differential Diagnosis

The various conditions that may be confused with aseptic meningitis are considered in Chapter 17 in the discussion of the differential diagnosis of acute bacterial meningitis. In certain cases of the latter, the CSF may be sterile and contain a predominance of mononuclear cells. This is particularly true of patients with pyogenic meningitis who have previously received antibacterial treatment.

Dagan and colleagues (1988) demonstrated that meningitis, although unsuspected, was frequently present in young infants who were hospitalized with other manifestations of enterovirus infection. When CSF was examined, most of these infants had a pleocytosis, but 9% did not. The most frequent isolates in their series were echoviruses 30 and 11 and several Coxsackie B viruses.

Complications

As a rule there are no complications in normal hosts. When they do arise, they are those of the underlying disease.

Prognosis

The prognosis is generally excellent. Recovery is rapid and complete. Few fatalities have been reported. There have been few longitudinal follow-up studies of patients with viral meningitis and it is exceedingly difficult without histologic confirmation to be certain whether an element of encephalitis supervened.

In two groups of patients, very young infants, and children of any age with agammaglobulinemia, viral meningitis may not be a benign illness. The enteroviruses have produced severe infections and some fatalities in newborns and infants in the first months of life (Bacon and Sims, 1976; Modlin et al., 1991). Longitudinal studies of survivors suggest that language difficulties and smaller head circumference were more common among these infants than among uninfected controls or patients with enterovirus meningitis after the first year of life (Sells et al., 1975; Lepow, 1978; Wilfert et al., 1980). Wilfert et al. (1977) have reported chronic persistent echovirus meningitis in patients whose immunologic deficit was characterized by absence of surface-immunoglobulin-bearing B lymphocytes. Types 9, 19, 30, and 33 echoviruses were recovered repeatedly from CSF for periods from 2 months to 3 years after onset of viral meningitis, and several of these children developed a dermatomyositis-like syndrome. Their CNS manifestations ranged at various times from asymptomatic to meningitic to encephalitic.

Treatment

The main practical problem confronting the clinician is whether to treat the patient with antimicrobial agents. The diagnosis of viral meningitis is seldom confirmed by the laboratory in the first days of the patient's illness. Nevertheless, a strong indication of viral cause may be gained from the circumstances in which the disease occurs—that is, in the midst of an outbreak of viral meningitis in the community during the summer or fall months; in the presence of a rash, enanthem, or other features of enteroviral infection; or with exposure to mumps or in the presence of parotitis in the patient. These conditions may suffice to justify withholding antimicrobial treatment. On the other hand, in those situations in which the patient has already received antimicrobial agents in either adequate or inadequate amounts, the physician may choose to continue therapy, observe the patient carefully, and follow laboratory developments until a diagnosis of bacterial meningitis has been excluded (see Chapter 17).

The characteristics of the CSF are not always completely helpful in the decision of whether to treat with antimicrobial agents. Early in viral meningitis, polymorphonuclear leukocytes may predominate; conversely, in the early stages of bacterial meningitis the pleocytosis may consist predominantly of lymphocytes. Rapid tests such as coagglutination or latex agglutination may assist in early bacterial diagnosis in the absence of a positive Gram stain before a culture report is available.

The importance of repeated examination of the CSF cannot be overstressed. In as short a time as 8 hours the CSF may markedly change its cellular content (Amir et al., 1991; Harrison and Risser, 1988). Antimicrobial treatment may be started in cases in which the cause is uncertain and be discontinued if the bacterial cultures of the CSF taken *before* treatment prove to be sterile.

Supportive and symptomatic treatment may require analgesics for headaches and pains and antiemetics for vomiting. When the patient is afebrile and asymptomatic, it is important to evaluate muscle power to detect the rare instance of residual weakness that may require continuing physiotherapy. Aside from antiviral agents available for cytomegalovirus (Chapter 4), herpes simplex (Chapter 12) and varicella-zoster (Chapter 37), there are no specific therapies for the remainder of the causative viruses. An investigational drug for treatment of enterovirus CNS infections is undergoing early trials (Chapter 7).

BIBLIOGRAPHY

Adair CV, Ross LG, Smadel JE. Aseptic meningitis, a disease of diverse etiology: clinical and etiologic studies on 854 cases. Ann Intern Med 1953;39:675.

Anderson RM, Donnelly CA, Ferguson NM, et al. Transmission dynamics and epidemiology of BSE in British cattle. Nature 1996;382:779-88.

Amir J, Harel L, Frydman E, et al. Shift of cerebrospinal polymorphonuclear cell percentage in the early stage of aseptic meningitis. J Pediatr 1991;119:938-941.

Bacon CJ, Sims DG. Echovirus 19 infection in infants under 6 months. Arch Dis Child 1976;51:631.

Baron RC, Hatch MH, Kleeman K, et al. Aseptic meningitis among members of a high school football team: an outbreak associated with echovirus 16 infection. JAMA 1982; 284:1724.

Barrett FF, Yow MD, Phillips CA. St. Louis encephalitis in children during the 1964 epidemic. JAMA 1965;193:381.

Bergman I, Painter MJ, Wald ER, et al. Outcome of children with enterovirus meningitis during the first year of life. J Pediatr 1987;110:705-709.

Berlin LE, Rorabaugh ML, Heldrich F, et al. Aseptic meningitis in infants <2 years of age: diagnosis and etiology. J Infect Dis 1993;168:888-892.

Brown P, Gibbs CJ, Rodgers-Johnson P, et al. Human spongiform encephalopathy: The National Institutes of Health series of 300 cases of experimentally transmitted disease. Ann Neurol 1994;35:513-529.

Calisher CH. Medically important arboviruses of the United States and Canada. Clin Microbiol Rev 1994;7:89-116.

Centers for Disease Control. Aseptic meningitis surveillance. U.S. Department of Health, Education, and Welfare, Public Health Service, Jan. 1979.

Centers for Disease Control. Aseptic meningitis in a high school football team. MMWR 1981;29:631.

Centers for Disease Control. Human arboviral encephalitis—United States 1983. MMWR 1984;33:339.

Centers for Disease Control. St. Louis encephalitis—Baytown and Houston, Texas. MMWR 1986;35:693-695.

Centers for Disease Control. Update: St. Louis encephalitis—Florida and Texas, 1990. MMWR 1990;39:756-759.

Centers for Disease Control. Eastern equine encephalitis—Florida, eastern United States, 1991. MMWR 1991a;40: 533-535.

Centers for Disease Control. Reye syndrome surveillance—United States, 1989. MMWR 1991b;89:88-90.

Centers for Disease Control. St. Louis encephalitis outbreak—Arkansas 1991. MMWR 1991c;40:605-607.

Centers for Disease Control. Summary of notifiable diseases, United States 1995. MMWR 1996;44:1-87.

Centers for Disease Control. Outbreak of aseptic meningitis—Whiteside County, Illinois, 1995. MMWR 1997;46:221-224.

Chesney PJ, Katcher ML, Nelson DB, Horowitz SD. CSF eosinophilia and chronic lymphocytic choriomeningitis virus meningitis. J Pediatr 1979;94:750.

Cramblett HG, Stegmiller H, Spencer C. California encephalitis virus infections in children. JAMA 1966;198:128.

Dagan R, Jenista JA, Menegus MA. Association of clinical presentation, laboratory findings, and virus serotypes with the presence of meningitis in hospitalized infants with enterovirus infection. J Pediatr 1988;113:975-978.

Derbes SJ. Trimethoprim-induced aseptic meningitis. JAMA 1984;252:2865.

Eglin RP, Swann RA, Isaacs D, Moxon ER. Simultaneous bacterial and viral meningitis. Lancet 1984;2:984.

Ehrenkrantz NJ, Sinclair NC, Buff E, Lyman DO. The natural occurrence of Venezuelan equine encephalitis in the United States. N Engl J Med 1970;282:298.

Goddard J. Viruses transmitted by mosquitoes: St. Louis encephalitis. Infect Med 1996;13:747-751.

Harrison SA, Risser WL. Repeated lumbar puncture in the differential diagnosis of meningitis. Pediatr Infect Dis 1988; 7:143-145.

Haymaker W, Smadel JE. The pathology of viral encephalitis. Washington D.C. Army Medical Museum, 1943.

Hoke CH Jr, Vaughn DW, Nisalak, et al. Effect of high-dose dexamethasone on the outcome of acute encephalitis due to Japanese encephalitis virus. J Infect Dis 1992;165:631-7.

Hurwitz ES, Barrett MJ, Bregman D, et al. Public Health Service study of Reye's syndrome and medications: report of the main study. JAMA 1987;257:1905-1911.

Jarvis WR, Tucker G. Echovirus type 7 meningitis in young children. Am J Dis Child 1981;135:1009.

Jeffrey KJM, Read SJ, Peto TEA, et al. Diagnosis of viral infections of the central nervous system: clinical interpretation of PCR results. Lancet 1997;349:313-317.

Johnson RT. The pathogenesis of acute viral encephalitis and postinfectious encephalomyelitis. J Infect Dis 1987;155:359-364.

Johnson RT. Slow infections of the central nervous system caused by conventional viruses. Annals NY Acad Sci 1994; 724:6-13.

Johnson RT. Acute encephalitis. Clin Infect Dis 1996;23: 219-226.

Johnson RT, Griffin DE, Hirsch RL, et al. Measles encephalomyelitis—clinical and immunologic studies. N Engl J Med 1984;310:137.

Johnson RT, Mims CA. Pathogenesis of viral infections of the nervous system. N Engl J Med 1968;278:23.

Kappus KD, Calisher CH, Baron RC, et al. La Crosse virus infection and disease in western North Carolina. Am J Trop Med Hyg 1982;31:556.

Kelsey DS. Adenovirus meningoencephalitis. Pediatrics 1978;61:291.

Kono R, Miyamura K, Tajiri E, et al. Virological and serological studies of neurological complications of acute hemorrhagic conjunctivitis in Thailand. J Infect Dis 1977;135:706.

Koskiniemi M, Donner M, Pettay O. Clinical appearance and outcome in mumps encephalitis in children. Acta Pediatr Scand 1983;72:603.

Lanchester J. A new kind of contagion. New Yorker 1996;Dec 2:70-81.

Lennette EH, Magoffin RL, Knouf EG. Viral central nervous system disease: an etiologic study conducted at the Los Angeles General Hospital. JAMA 1962;179:687.

Lepow ML. Enteroviral meningitis: a reappraisal. Pediatrics 1978;62:267.

Lepow ML, et al. A clinical, epidemiologic, and laboratory investigation of aseptic meningitis during the four-year period, 1955-1958. I. Observations concerning etiology and epidemiology. N Engl J Med 1962a;266:1181.

Lepow ML, et al. A clinical, epidemiologic and laboratory investigation of aseptic meningitis during the four-year period, 1955-1958. II. The clinical disease and its sequelae. N Engl J Med 1962b;266:1188.

Levitt LP, Lovejoy FH Jr, Daniels JB. Eastern equine encephalitis in Massachusetts: first human case in 14 years. N Engl J Med 1971;284:540.

Luby JP. St. Louis encephalitis. Epidemiol Rev 1979;1:55.

Marier R, et al. Coxsackievirus B5 infection and aseptic meningitis in neonates and children. Am J Dis Child 1975;129:321.

Masden JC, Van Heertum RL, Abdel-Dayem H. Viral infections of the brain. J Neuroimaging 1995;5(suppl 1):S40-S44.

McKinney RE, Katz SL, Wilfert CM. Chronic enteroviral meningoencephalitis in agammaglobulinemic patients. Rev Infect Dis 1987;9:334-356.

Medovy H. Western equine encephalomyelitis in infants. J Pediatr 1943;22:308.

Meyer HM Jr, et al. Central nervous system syndromes of viral etiology: study of 713 cases. Am J Med 1960;29:334.

Modlin JF, Dagan R, Berlin LE, et al. Focal encephalitis with enterovirus infections. Pediatr 1991;88:841-845.

Monath TP. Japanese encephalitis—a plague of the Orient. N Engl J Med 1988;319:641-643.

Moore M. Enterovirus surveillance report, 1970-1979. Atlanta: Centers for Disease Control, 1981.

Moore M, Baron RC, Filstein MR, et al. Aseptic meningitis and high school football players. JAMA 1983;249:2039.

Nicolosi A, Hauser A, Beghi E, et al. Epidemiology of central nervous system infections in Olmsted County, Minnesota, 1950-1981. J Infect Dis 1986;154:399-408.

Powell KE, Blakey DL. St. Louis encephalitis, the 1975 epidemic in Mississippi. JAMA 1977;237:2294.

Prusiner SB. Molecular biology of prion diseases. Science 1991;252:1515-1522.

Prusiner SB. Biology and genetics of prion diseases. Ann Rev Microbiol 1994;48:655.

Rantakallio P, Lapinheimu K, Mantyharvi R. Coxsackie B5 outbreak in a newborn nursery with 17 cases of serous meningitis. Scand J Infect Dis 1970;2:17.

Rantala H, Uhari M. Occurrence of childhood encephalitis: a population-based study. Pediatr Infect Dis 1989;8:426-430.

Rantala H, Uhari M, Saukkonen AL, et al. Outcome after childhood encephalitis. Devel Med Child Neurol 1991;33:858-867.

Reye RDK, Morgan G, Baral J. Encephalopathy and fatty degeneration of the viscera: disease entity in childhood. Lancet 1963;2:749.

Rorabaugh ML, Berlin LE, Heldrich F, et al. Aseptic meningitis in infants younger than 2 years of age: acute illness and neurologic complications. Pediatr 1993;92:206.

Rotbart H. Diagnosis of enteroviral meningitis with the polymerase chain reaction. J Pediatr 1990;117:85-89.

Rotbart HA. Enteroviral infections of the central nervous system. Clin Infect Dis 1995;20:971-981.

Sawyer MH, Holland D, Aintablian N, et al. Diagnosis of enteroviral central nervous system infection by polymerase chain reaction during a large community outbreak. Pediatr Infect Dis J 1994;13:177.

Sells CJ, Carpenter RL, Ray CG. Sequelae of central nervous system enterovirus infection. N Engl J Med 1975;293:1.

Shaw DW, Cohen WA. Viral infections of the CNS in children: imaging features. Amer J Roentgen 1993;160:125-33.

Singer JL, Maur PR, Riley JP, Smith PB. Management of central nervous system infections during an epedemic of enteroviral aseptic meningitis. J Pediatr 1980;96:559.

Smith RR. Neuroradiology of intracranial infection. Pediatr Neurosurg 1992;18:92.

Swender PT, Shott RJ, Williams ML. A community and intensive care nursery outbreak of coxsackievirus B5 meningitis. Am J Dis Child 1974;127:42.

Tsai TF. Arboviral infections in the United States. Infect Dis Clin North Am 1991;5:73-102.

Vianna N, et al. California encephalitis in New York State, Am J Epidemiol 1971;94:50.

Wallgren A. Une nouvelle maladie infectieuse du systeme nerveux central. Acta Paediatr. 1925;4:158.

Whitley RJ. Viral encephalitis. N Engl J Med 1990;323: 242-250.

Wilfert CM, Buckley RH, Mohanakumar T et al. Persistent and fatal central nervous system echovirus infections in patients with agammaglobulinemia. N Engl J Med 1977;296:1485.

Wilfert CM, Lehrmann SN, Katz SL. Enteroviruses and meningitis, Pediatr Infect Dis 1983;2:333.

Wilfert CM, Thompson RJ Jr, Sunder TR, et al. Longitudinal assessment of children with enteroviral meningitis during the first 3 months of life. Pediatrics 1980;67:811.

Will RG, Ironside JW, Zeidler M, et al. A new variant of Creutzfeldt-Jakob disease in the UK. Lancet 1996;347:921-925.

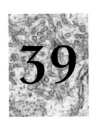

39 WOUNDS, ABSCESSES, AND OTHER INFECTIONS CAUSED BY ANAEROBIC BACTERIA

SHIRLEY JANKELEVICH

GENERAL PRINCIPLES OF ANAEROBIC INFECTIONS

Infections caused by anaerobic bacteria are an important cause of morbidity and mortality in the pediatric population, although the incidence of these infections is lower in the pediatric than the adult population (Citron et al., 1995). Anaerobic bacteria predominate bacteria at all mucosal sites, and although many different anaerobic bacteria exist in each site, only a subset is responsible for causing disease. Anaerobes may be present in pure culture or as part of a mixed infection with other anaerobic and aerobic bacteria and may cause serious and life-threatening infection at any site in the body, from the intracranium to muscle and bone. The ability of certain anaerobes to cause disease is determined by factors at the site of infection, inoculum size, virulence factors of the organisms, and the health of the individual.

Identification of anaerobic bacteria from an infected site is dependent on an understanding of the normal distribution of anaerobic bacterial species that are normally present at sites involved in infection, as well as proper handling techniques of clinical specimens for anaerobic bacteriology. Knowledge of antimicrobial susceptibility of anaerobic and aerobic bacteria in mixed infections is necessary in making appropriate treatment choices. Finally, the importance of surgical drainage and débridement in the treatment of many anaerobic infections cannot be overemphasized.

Epidemiology

The incidence of anaerobic infections in children is lower than that in adults, most likely because of the lower frequency of debilitating diseases in children that predispose to anaerobic infections, such as lung abscesses and gynecologic infections. However, certain children may be at higher risk of anaerobic infection. These include neonates and children with neurologic impairments, chronic renal insufficiency, leukemia and other malignant neoplasms, and immunologically comprising conditions (Dunkle et al., 1976; Thirmuoothi et al., 1976; Brook et al., 1979; Brook, 1995; Citron et al., 1995). Anaerobic bacteria isolated from children revealed that the abdomen was the source of >50% of anaerobic isolates. Sources from the head and neck, soft tissue below the waist, blood, respiratory, cerebrospinal fluid (CSF), and unknown accounted for the remaining isolates, respectively (Citron et al., 1995).

Etiology

Anaerobic bacteria are defined as those bacteria that do not require oxygen for growth and replication. For simplicity, anaerobic bacteria can be classified into two groups based on tolerance to oxygen, the aerotolerant and the strict (obligate) anaerobic bacteria (Loesche, 1969). Aerotolerant bacteria, such as *Prevotella* (formerly *Bacteroides*) *melaninogenicus* and *Fusobacterium nucleatum,* can grow in the presence of low concentration of oxygen (0.1% to 4%), depending on the isolate. Although strict anaerobes, such as *Clostridium haemolyticum* and some *Treponema* spp., generally cannot grow in the presence of greater than 0.5% oxygen and will die after a brief exposure to air, most anaerobic bacterial pathogens are aerotolerant and will remain viable if exposed to air for several hours.

Anaerobic pathogens may be from an endogenous or exogenous source. Most pathogens are from an endogenous origin. These bacteria normally colonize mucosal surfaces and cause disease after damage to the mucosal barrier or skin, allowing bacterial invasion. A few examples of endogenous pathogenic bacteria are *Bacteroides* spp., *Fusobacterium* spp., and *P. melaninogenicus.* The most common exogenous anaerobic bacterial pathogens are *Clostridium botulinum* and *Clostridium tetani*. These spore-forming bacteria are found in soil or contaminated food. The spores gain entry through the gastrointestinal (GI) tract or through soil-contaminated wounds, germinate, multiply, and elaborate a variety toxins with different pathogenic effects.

Pathogenesis

Every surface of our body, including skin; mouth; and gastrointestinal, respiratory, and genitourinary tracts, has numerous microenvironments that provide ideal growth conditions (i.e., decreased oxygen tension and low oxidation-reduction potential) for indigenous aerobic and anaerobic microflora.

A balanced ecologic system found in each microenvironment is relatively stable over time but can be changed by factors such as antibiotics, chemotherapeutic agents, obstruction, and various diseases. Undesirable consequences may occur when the balance is changed, leading to proliferation of indigenous anaerobes that are normally kept in check. Alteration in the normal gastrointestinal flora with administration of antibiotics can allow unrestrained growth of *Clostridium difficile*, resulting in sufficient toxin to cause pseudomembranous colitis. Obstruction, stasis, tissue destruction, aerobic infection, and decreases in normal blood flow may allow aerobic and anaerobic bacteria to gain access into normally sterile sites and act synergistically to produce infection. Examples of pathogenic conditions that promote anaerobic infections are gastrointestinal obstruction, trauma or surgery, aspiration of vomitus into lungs, human and animal bites, and wounds that become contaminated with soil containing clostridial spores. These pathogenic processes result in lowered oxygen tension and accumulation of reducing products, leading to conditions that favor infection with indigenous anaerobes, usually in combination with facultative aerobic bacteria. In addition, numerous virulence factors produced by anaerobes, such as toxins and enzymes capable of destroying components of not only host tissue but also neutrophils and macrophages, polysaccharide capsules that promote formation of abscesses and protect bacteria from phagocytosis, and adherence factors may promote the invasion and growth of anaerobes, resulting in abscess formation. Once infection is established and an abscess is formed, the microenvironment within the abscess sustains the infectious processes. Continued growth of bacteria and destruction of tissue maintain a favorable reducing environment for anaerobic bacteria and abscess enlargement.

Immunity

Experiment evidence suggests that several arms of the immune system may function in the control of anaerobic infections. Cellular immunity may play a role in protection against abscess formation by *Bacteroides fragilis* (Onderdonk et al., 1982; Powell et al., 1985). Phagocytic activity may also be important in controlling anaerobic infections (Klempner, 1984). However, the phagocytic response may be compromised in mixed or pure anaerobic infections (Styrt and Gorbach, 1989). *B. fragilis* and *P. melaninogenicus* may be protected from opsonophagocytosis by capsule formation (Zaleznik and Kasper, 1982). Neutrophilic chemotaxis may be suppressed by *Bacteroides* spp. (Styrt and Gorbach, 1989). Factors produced by anaerobes may protect other bacteria from host defenses, as exemplified by the inhibition of phagocytosis of *Proteus mirabilis* and *Escherichia coli* by *B. fragilis* and *P. melaninogenicus* (Rotstein, 1993). In addition, virulence factors may directly destroy host leukocytes. Although there is extensive experimental evidence demonstrating a role for phagocytosis and host humoral and cellular immunity in controlling anaerobic infections, the contribution of each host defense in vivo is not yet known (Lorber, 1995).

Diagnosis

An important part of the diagnosis of anaerobic infection is an understanding of the pathogenic processes that lead to anaerobic infection and proper collection, transport, and culture of the organisms from the infected site. Anaerobes are the predominant bacterial species on mucosal surfaces. Therefore both anaerobic and aerobic infection should be suspected when infections occur near oral, gastrointestinal, or genital mucosa. The presence of gas and foul odor may point to an anaerobic infection but may also occur with infections caused by aerobic bacteria. It is imperative that samples of blood, infected fluid, and tissue be collected properly and handled carefully to permit the growth and identification of anaerobes. All specimens should be kept in a low-oxygen, moist, warm environment and should be transported to the microbiology laboratory soon after collection. Blood should be collected in both anaerobic (unvented) and aerobic (vented) bottles. Aspirates should be collected, whenever possible, by needle and syringe. Air should be expelled from the syringe, and the contents of the syringe should be injected into an anaerobic transport tube or vial containing, if possible, a prereduced transport medium. If a specimen must be collected with a swab, an oxygen-free swab obtained from the microbiology laboratory should be used. The oxygen-free swab should then be transported to the microbiology laboratory in an oxygen-free transport container. Clinical specimens obtained by swab from superficial lesions; from vaginal, cervical, and urethral sites; from the respiratory tract that have contacted the oral mucosa; and from stool or rectal area will be contaminated with the normal anaerobes that colonize those sites. Such specimens should not be sent for anaerobic culture. Tissue from the infected site should be should be placed in oxygen-free transport tubes or vials containing a prereduced transport medium. Consultation with the microbiology laboratory before sample collection will provide guidance on the proper collection and transport of these specimens.

Treatment

Properties of the anaerobic environment within the abscess and enzymes produced by anaerobic bacteria may decrease or eliminate antibiotic activity. Tissue necrosis with resultant decreased blood flow to the site of infection may prevent many antibiotics from gaining entry into an abscess. Aminoglycosides are not active against anaerobes, because they require oxygen transport to penetrate the bacterial cell envelope (Bryan and Van Den Elzen, 1976). In addition, aminoglycosides become inactivated by purulent material and have decreased activity at the low pH found in abscesses. Bacteria within abscesses that contain large numbers of organisms are usually in the stationary phase of growth. Therefore, β-lactam antibiotics, which work by preventing cell wall formation in actively growing bacteria, cannot kill the bacteria. β-lactam antibiotics may also be inactivated by the production of β-lactamases produced by anaerobic organisms such as *B. fragilis.* Therefore, in a mixed anaerobic/aerobic infection, a β-lactam antibiotic determined to be active in vitro against a bacterial isolate from the infected site may be inactive against the isolate within the abscess (O'Keefe et al., 1978).

Although antibiotics are essential in the treatment of anaerobic infection, the difficulty in eradicating anaerobes from an infected site with antibiotics alone most often necessitates the use of surgical débridement of necrotic tissue and removal of infected material from an abscess. Fortunately, drainage of certain abscesses may be effected percutaneously with ultrasound or computed tomography (CT) guidance.

Box 39-1 and Table 39-1 provide antibiotic regimens and dosages for infections associated with anaerobic bacteria.

WOUND AND SOFT TISSUE INFECTIONS

Wound and soft tissue infections include superficial infections of the skin and skin structures, subcutaneous infections, and deeper infections of the fascia or muscle. They are generally classified by the type of bacteria infecting the wound, the level of tissue infected, and the absence or presence of tissue necrosis. The categorization of some soft tissue infections, however, is complicated by the variable involvement of several layers of tissue.

The most common superficial infections that may involve anaerobes include furuncles, paronychia, infected ulcers and cysts, infected gastrostomy tube sites wound (Brook, 1995), infected tracheostomy site wound (Brook, 1995), and hidradenitis suppurativa. Subcutaneous tissue infections include cutaneous and subcutaneous abscesses (Brook and Frazier, 1990), pilonidal abscess and sinus (Sondenaa et al., 1995), infected decubitus ulcers (Brook, 1995), infected bite wounds (Griego et al., 1995), and the superficial necrotizing soft tissue infections (nonclostridial anaerobic cellulitis, clostridial anaerobic cellulitis, bacterial synergistic gangrene). The deeper necrotizing soft tissue infections are necrotizing fasciitis and clostridial and nonclostridial myonecrosis.

Pathogenesis

Soft tissue infections most often occur after introduction of endogenous or exogenous bacteria into soft tissue during minor or major trauma, surgery, ischemia, obstruction of drainage, presence of foreign body or blood, and vascular stasis. Once infection is established, virulence factors elaborated by the infecting pathogens and bacterial synergy often determine the extent and severity of infection.

Necrotizing soft tissue infections deserve special mention because of their life-threatening nature. They are caused by growth of bacteria, most often anaerobes, which elaborate various toxins that result in tissue necrosis. Liquefaction necrosis of the infected tissues is common to all of these infections. Elaboration of enzymes by the infecting bacteria

BOX 39-1

TREATMENT OF INFECTIONS ASSOCIATED WITH ANAEROBES

Wounds and Soft Tissue Infections

Furuncles and carbuncles

Dicloxacillin

or

Clindamycin (if the lesion is present in an area
   associated with anaerobic bacteria)

Infected cysts

Amoxicillin/clavulanate (ampicillin/sulbactam)

Hidradenitis suppurativa

Amoxicillin/clavulanate (ampicillin/sulbactam)

Infected gastrostomy tube sites wound

Clindamycin, cefotaxime (or ceftriaxone) plus an
   aminoglycoside

or

Metronidazole, oxacillin, and cefotaxime (or
   ceftriaxone) plus an aminoglycoside

or

Ampicillin/sulbactam plus an aminoglycoside

or

Imipenem/cilastin

Pilonidal abscess

Clindamycin, cefotaxime (or ceftriaxone) plus an
   aminoglycoside

or

Metronidazole, oxacillin, and cefotaxime (or
   ceftriaxone) plus an aminoglycoside

or

Ampicillin/sulbactam

or

Imipenem/cilastin

Infected decubitus ulcer

Clindamycin, cefotaxime (or ceftriaxone) plus an
   aminoglycoside

or

Metronidazole, oxacillin, and cefotaxime (or
   ceftriaxone) plus an aminoglycoside

or

Ampicillin/sulbactam

or

Imipenem/cilastin

Human bite or clenched fist injury

(Assess patient's tetanus status)

Amoxicillin/clavulanate or ampicillin/sulbactam

or

Cefoxitin

or

Clindamycin and penicillin G

Superficially infected animal bite wounds

(Assess patient's tetanus status)

(Consider rabies immune globulin and
   immunization)

Amoxicillin-clavulanate

or

Cefuroxime axetil

or

Penicillin V plus dicloxacillin or cephalexin

or

Tetracycline (for penicillin-allergic patient)

Severely infected animal bite wounds

(Assess patient's tetanus status)

(Consider rabies immune globulin and
   immunization)

Ampicillin/sulbactam

or

Penicillin G plus oxacillin or cefazolin

Bacterial synergistic gangrene

Oxacillin plus gentamicin or a third-generation
   cephalosporin

or

Vancomycin plus gentamicin or a third-generation
   cephalosporin

Anaerobic cellulitis

Penicillin plus clindamycin plus an aminoglycoside
   or a third-generation cephalosporin

Necrotizing fasciitis

Penicillin plus clindamycin plus an aminoglycoside

or

Chloramphenicol plus aminoglycoside (penicillin-
   allergic patient)

Synergistic nonclostridial anaerobic myonecrosis

Clindamycin plus ceftriaxone or cefotaxime and an
   aminoglycoside

Clostridial myonecrosis

Penicillin (sodium salt)

or

Chloramphenicol (penicillin-allergic patient)

Anaerobic bacteremia

Metronidazole plus PCN G plus coverage of
   aerobic organisms isolated

or

Imipenem/cilastin

or

Ampicillin/sulbactam

Intracranial Abscesses

Metronidazole plus oxacillin (or nafcillin) plus
   cefotaxime (or ceftriaxone)

or

PCN G plus metronidazole plus oxacillin (or
   nafcillin)

BOX 39-1

TREATMENT OF INFECTIONS ASSOCIATED WITH ANAEROBES—cont'd

or
PCN G plus chloramphenicol
or
Vancomycin plus metronidazole plus aztreonam or
   gentamicin (penicillin-allergic patient)

Intraperitoneal Abscesses

Clindamycin or metronidazole plus
   aminoglycoside or third-generation
   cephalosporin or monobactam
or
Imipenem/cilastin plus an aminoglycoside
or
Ampicillin/sulbactam plus an aminoglycoside
or
Cefoxitin plus an aminoglycoside

Peritonitis

Primary (immunocompetent)
Oxacillin and gentamicin or a third-generation
   cephalosporin
Primary (immunocompromised)
Clindamycin plus ampicillin plus gentamicin or a
   third-generation cephalosporin
Secondary to intraabdominal source
Clindamycin or metronidazole plus
   aminoglycoside or third-generation
   cephalosporin or monobactam
***Secondary to intraabdominal source (in neonate
with necrotizing enterocolitis)***
Clindamycin plus vancomycin plus gentamicin and
   clindamycin
Secondary to intraperitoneal dialysis
Ampicillin plus gentamicin or a third-generation
   cephalosporin plus vancomycin

Acute Appendicitis

Ruptured or appendiceal abscess
Clindamycin, gentamicin, and ampicillin
Unruptured (perioperative prophylaxis)
Clindamycin or metronidazole plus an
   aminoglycoside or third-generation
   cephalosporin
or
Cefoxitin

Splenic Abscess

Secondary to an intraabdominal abscess
Clindamycin or metronidazole plus an
   aminoglycoside or third-generation
   cephalosporin
Secondary to trauma or bacterial endocarditis
Metronidazole plus oxacillin plus a third-
   generation cephalosporin

Retroperitoneal Abscess

Clindamycin or metronidazole plus oxacillin plus
   gentamicin or third-generation cephalosporin

Psoas Abscess

Clindamycin or metronidazole plus oxacillin plus
   gentamicin or third-generation cephalosporin

Anorectal Abscess

Clindamycin plus an aminoglycoside
or
Metronidazole plus oxacillin plus an
   aminoglycoside

---

results in tissue destruction. *Staphylococcus aureus, Clostridial* spp., and streptococci can elaborate hyaluronidase, an enzyme that digests hyaluronic acid, the ground substance of connective tissue, whereas *Clostridium perfringens* produces collagenase, a proteolytic enzyme that digests collagen. Synergism between different species of bacteria that coexist in an infected site permits increased growth and greater tissue destruction, increasing the severity of necrotizing soft tissue infections. Bacteria that often exhibit this phenomenon are *Bacteroides* spp.; anaerobic streptococci; and *Clostridial* spp., in combination with such aerobic bacteria as coliforms, streptococci, and staphylococci.

Inoculation of these bacteria into a reducing environment with low oxygen content provides favorable conditions for growth of these anaerobic bacteria. A wound that contains necrotic debris, old hematoma, or foreign material such as sutures or that is already infected with aerobic or facultative bacteria or has had its blood supply disrupted due to the surgical procedure provides such an environment. Pathogenic anaerobes associated with necrotizing infections are, to varying degrees, tolerant of low amounts of oxygen. Thus, these bacteria, once introduced into the wound, can remain viable until conditions result in decreased oxygen tension and exponential growth. The proliferation of these

Table 39-1 Antibiotics useful in the treatment of anaerobic infections

Antibiotic/tissue distribution	Anaerobic bacteria covered*	Anaerobic bacteria not covered	Precautions and comments†	Dose	Conditions requiring dose adjustment
Ampicillin Wide distribution including liver; lung; gallbladder; kidney; muscle; pleural, joint, and peritoneal fluids; bile in varying amounts; CSF if inflammation present	Clostridium sp. Peptostreptococcus sp. Propionibacterium sp.	(±) B. fragilis B. fragilis group, other Prevotella sp. Porphyromonas sp.	Contraindicated if hypersensitivity to penicillins	**Adults:** 500-2000 gm/day ÷ q4-6h (IV) (max dose 12 gm/24hr) **Children:** Mild-moderate infection: 50-100 mg/kg/day ÷ q6h (IV/IM) Severe infection: 200-400 mg/kg/day ÷ q4-6h (IV/IM) (max dose 12gm/24hr) **Neonates:** ≤1 week old: ≤2 kg: 25-50 mg/kg q12h (IV/IM) >2 kg: 25-50 mg/kg q8h (IV/IM) >1 week old: ≤2 kg: 25-50 mg/kg q8h (IV/IM) >2 kg: 25-50 mg/kgq6h (IV/IM) (Use higher doses to treat meningitis)	Renal insufficiency
Ampicillin/ sulbactam (IV) Wide distribution including urine, tissue fluid, peritoneal fluid, gallbladder, other; CSF if inflammation present	B. fragilis B. fragilis group, other Prevotella sp. Porphyromonas sp. Clostridium sp. Peptostreptococcus sp. Propionibacterium sp.		Contraindicated if hypersensitivity to penicillins MRSA resistant to A/S; sulbactam inhibits a wide range of β-lactamases produced by bacteria resistant to penicillins and cephalosporins	**Adults:** 1.5-3.0 gm (2:1 ratio ampicillin: sulbactam) q6h (IV) **Children:** Safety and efficacy not established for children <12 years old but has been used in children >3 months old: 200 mg/kg/day ÷ q6h (IV) (2:1 ratio ampicillin: sulbactam)	Renal insufficiency
Cefoperazone Wide distribution including ascitic, bile, sputum, endometrium, myometrium, tonsils, low concentration in CSF (slightly higher if meningeal inflammation)	Clostridium sp. Peptococcus sp. Peptostreptococcus sp. Propionibacterium sp. Fusobacterium sp.	(±) B. fragilis B. fragilis group, other	Contraindicated if hypersensitivity to cephalosporins Rarely, vitamin K deficiency— monitor PT and replace vitamin K as needed	**Adults:** 1-2 gm q12h (IV) **Children:** Safety and efficacy not established for children <12 years old but has been used in neonates and children: 25-100 mg/kg q12h (IV)	

Drug / Distribution	Spectrum	Adverse effects / Contraindications	Dosage	Notes
Cefoxitin Wide distribution including urine, pleural, joint, bile; little in CSF even if meningeal inflammation present	B. fragilis B. fragilis group, other Prevotella sp. Porphyromonas sp. Peptostreptococcus sp. Propionibacterium sp. (±) Clostridium sp.	Contraindicated if hypersensitivity to cephalosporins	**Adults:** 1-2 gm q4-8h (IV) (depending on severity of infection) **Children** (>3 months old): 80-160 mg/kg/day ÷ q4-6h (IV)	Renal insufficiency
Chloramphenicol Wide distribution including liver; kidney; pleural fluid, ascitic fluid; CSF (even in the absence of meningeal inflammation); brain	B. fragilis B. fragilis group, other Prevotella sp. Porphyromonas sp. Clostridium sp. Peptostreptococcus sp. Propionibacterium sp.	Serious and fatal blood dyscrasias (aplastic anemia, hypoplastic anemia, thrombocytopenia); gray baby occur in neonates (also seen in neonate born to mother receiving chloramphenicol) MUST measure serum levels for all patients	For all patients, dose must be adjusted to maintain serum concentration between 10-25 µg/ml **Adults‡:** 50-100 mg/kg/day ÷ q6h; max dose: 4 gm/24 hr (IV or PO) **Infants and Children‡:** 50-100 mg/kg/day ÷ q6h; max dose: 4 gm/24 hr (IV or PO) **Neonates‡:** <2 kg or <2 weeks old: 25 mg/kg/day ÷ q24h (IV) ≥2 weeks old: 50 mg/kg/day ÷ q24h or q12h (IV)	Hepatic insufficiency
Clindamycin Wide distribution including ascites, pleural and synovial fluid, bone, bile; little in CSF even if meningeal inflammation present	(±) B. fragilis Prevotella sp. Porphyromonas sp. (±) Clostridium sp. (±) Peptostreptococcus sp. (±) B. fragilis group, other	May be associated with pseudomembranous colitis	**Adults:** Serious infections: 600-1200 mg/day ÷ q12h or q8h or q6h (IV/IM) Severe infections: 1200-4800 mg/day ÷ q12h or q8h or q6h (IV/IM)	

*C. difficile not included in evaluation.

†Consult appropriate pharmaceuticals resources for further discussion of other precautions, as well as drug interactions.

‡Use high dose only as required to inhibit moderately resistant bacteria—decrease dose to 50 mg/kg/day as soon as possible.

Continued

Table 39-1 Antibiotics useful in the treatment of anaerobic infections—cont'd

Antibiotic/tissue distribution	Anaerobic bacteria covered*	Anaerobic bacteria not covered	Precautions and comments†	Dose	Conditions requiring dose adjustment
	Propionibacterium sp.			**Children:** >4 weeks old: 20-40 mg/kg/day ÷ q8h or q6h (IV/IM) 8-25 mg/kg/day ÷ q8h or q6h (PO) **Neonates:** Premature or <1 week old: 15 mg/kg/day ÷ q8h (IV/IM) ≥1 week old: 15-20 mg/kg/day ÷ q6-8h (IV/IM)	
Imipenem/cilastin Widely distributed including pleural, bone, bile, intestine, peritoneal, pleural, interstitial, and wound fluids; low concentration in CSF	*B. fragilis* *B. fragilis* group, other *Prevotella* sp. *Porphyromonas* sp. *Clostridium* sp. *Peptostreptococcus* sp. *Fusobacterium* sp. *Propionibacterium* sp. *Actinomyces*		Decreases seizure threshold Increased seizures when used in children if meningitis present	**Adults:** 250-1000 mg/dose q6-8h (not to exceed 4 gm/day [IV]) **Children:** Safety and efficacy not been established for children <12 years old but has been used in limited number children 3 months old to 12 years old: 15-25 mg/kg q6h (IV)	Renal insufficiency
Metronidazole Distributed widely into all tissues and fluids	*B. fragilis* *B. fragilis* group, other *Prevotella* sp. *Porphyromonas* sp. *Clostridium* sp. *Fusobacterium* sp.	*Peptostreptococcus* sp. *Propionibacterium* sp.		**Adults:** 15 mg/kg loading dose then 30 mg/kg/day ÷ q6h (IV) Max dose: 4gm/24hr **Children:** Safety and efficacy not established for children <12 years old but has been used in clinical practice in doses of: Infants and children: 15 mg/kg loading dose: then 30 mg/kg/day ÷ q6h (IV) (max dose: 4gm/24hr)	Use with caution if severe hepatic or renal disease

Drug / Distribution	Organisms	Contraindications	Dose	Adjustment
Mezlocillin Wide distribution including ascitic, pleural, peritoneal and wound fluid, bile, heart, prostatic tissue, bronchial secretions, tonsils, muscle, gallbladder, adipose tissue, bone, gynecologic tissue; low concentration in CSF (slightly higher if inflammation present)	*B. fragilis* *B. fragilis* group, other *Peptostreptococcus* sp. *Peptococcus* sp. *Fusobacterium* sp. *Clostridium* sp.	Contraindicated if hypersensitivity to penicillins	**Adults:** 3 gm q4h or 4 gm q6h (IV) Max dose: 24gm/24hr **Children:** Infants >1 month old and children: 50-75 mg/kg q4h (IV) **Neonates:** ≤1 week old: 75 mg/kg q12h (IV) >1 week old: <2 kg: 75 mg/kg q8h (IV) >2 kg: 75 mg/kg q6h (IV)	Renal or marked hepatic insufficiency
Penicillin G Wide distribution including urine, tissue fluid, peritoneal fluid, gallbladder, other; CSF if inflammation present	*Peptostreptococcus* sp. *Fusobacterium* sp. *Clostridium* sp. *Actinomyces* sp. *Propionibacterium* sp.	*B. fragilis* (±) *Prevotella* sp.	Contraindicated if hypersensitivity to penicillins	**Adults:** 2-24 million U/day ÷ q4-6h (IV/IM) **Children:** 100,000-400,000 U/kg/day ÷ q4-6h (IV/IM) Max dose: 24 million U/q24h **Neonates:** ≤1 week old: ≤2 kg: 50,000-100,000 U/kg/day ÷ q12h (IV/IM) >2 kg: 75,000-225,000 U/kg/day ÷ q8h (IV/IM) >1 week old: ≤2 kg: 75,000-225,000 U/kg/day ÷ q8h (IV/IM) >2 kg: 100,000-200,000 U/kg/day ÷ q6h (IV/IM)	Renal insufficiency

C. difficile not included in evaluation.

†Consult appropriate pharmaceuticals resources for further discussion of other precautions, as well as drug interactions.

‡Use high dose only as required to inhibit moderately resistant bacteria—decrease dose to 50 mg/kg/day as soon as possible.

anaerobes results in the production of by-products of anaerobic metabolism, which further reduces the local environment, enhancing bacterial growth and extension of the infection. As the infection persists, thrombosis of the blood vessels in the dermis occurs, resulting in necrosis of the skin, which now becomes obvious on physical exam.

Necrotizing soft tissue infections may remain localized to the dermis or may extend to the fascia or underlying muscle. Initially, edema and pain are the only local symptoms around the surgical wound. The physician may not attribute these signs to the life-threatening process occurring within the deeper tissues. Only after the infection spreads through the soft tissue, causing thrombosis of the blood vessels in the dermis, does the overlying skin become necrotic. In addition, pressure caused by edema and exudation into the infected underlying soft tissue causes the formation of large bullae in the skin. The bullae rupture, releasing the foul-smelling serosanguineous exudate. The mortality of this disease at this point is extremely high, even with aggressive treatment. Certain *Clostridial* spp. may also produce early severe systemic disease because of absorption of some of the bacterial toxins.

Etiology

Infections of soft tissue may be caused by either aerobic or anaerobic bacteria, and both may be present simultaneously. Synergism may occur between anaerobic and aerobic bacteria within a wound, causing more severe infection than that caused by either organism alone. The type of pathogens found are in part determined by the method of wound acquisition and the site of infection. For example, in postsurgical wound infections, bacteria from exogenous sources include hospital-acquired organisms, such as methicillin-resistant *S. aureus* and various gram-negative bacteria, especially *Pseudomonas aeruginosa*, whereas those from endogenous sources of bacteria are *S. aureus,* group A beta-hemolytic streptococci, and aerobic and anaerobic bacteria normally found in the gut.

Epidemiology

A variety of conditions lead to wound infection. Surgical wounds may become infected during or after an operative procedure. Wounds acquired from an animal or human bite may become infected, depending on the source, type, and location of the bite. Traumatic wounds are more likely to become infected if either exogenous or endogenous bacteria are introduced into the wound. In addition,

certain children, such as those with neurologic impairment, are at increased risk of certain types of wound infections.

Postoperative wound infections are a major cause of soft tissue infections in children. Several factors appear to increase the incidence of these infections (Dineen, 1961; Leigh et al., 1974; Cruse and Foord, 1976; Finland and McGowan, 1976; Nichols, 1980). Length of stay in the hospital before surgery increases the incidence of wound infection. Neonates have a higher rate of wound infection than older children. Contaminated wounds become infected more often than clean wounds. Surgery of greater duration is associated with a higher incidence of wound infection. Administration of perioperative antibiotics also influences the incidence of postoperative infections (Gorbach, 1991). A higher incidence of abdominal wound infections was noted for patients given perioperative antibiotics for clean (uncontaminated) surgery, whereas infection was decreased with administration of perioperative antibiotics for contaminated surgery. An increased risk of postsurgical infections is also present in penetrating trauma (Nichols et al., 1984), emergent surgery, and repeat surgical procedures. In children, appendicitis was the condition most frequently associated with postsurgical abdominal infection, probably because of the frequency of this surgical condition in this age population. The risk of developing a wound infection after removal of a normal or an inflamed appendix without suppuration (clean-contaminated surgery) is approximately 10% in patients without preoperative or perioperative antibiotic prophylaxis (Forster et al., 1986), whereas the presence of a gangrenous or perforated appendix (dirty surgery) resulted in an infection rate of about 35%.

Children with increased risk of decubitus ulcers, gastrostomy, and tracheostomy wound site infections (Brook, 1995) are those with neurologic impairments. Paronychia is more common in children who nail bite or finger suck. Pilonidal abscesses are more common in pubescent children, possibly because of plugging and secondary infection of hair follicles in the pilonidal sinus (Sondenaa et al., 1995).

Animal and human bites account for approximately 1% of emergency department visits (Goldstein, 1992). The three most common types of bites are dog, cat, and human. Although the majority of these bites are caused by dogs, cat bites more often become infected. Location of bites may alter the risk of infection. Bites located on the hands are twice as likely to become infected as those located elsewhere.

Superficial Soft Tissue Infections

Furuncles and Carbuncles. Furuncles are localized pyogenic infections that originate from hair follicles. Carbuncles result from the coalescence of several furuncles. They usually occur in areas exposed to friction and perspiration. Although *S. aureus* is most commonly found in these lesions, less commonly, anaerobic bacteria, such as *Peptococcus, Peptostreptococcus,* and *Bacteroides* spp. have been associated with furuncles that develop in the groin area. Therapy requires drainage, either by application of moist heat locally, or, if unsuccessful, by surgical incision. If surrounding cellulitis is present, systemic antibiotics with an antistaphylococcal antibiotic such as dicloxacillin are required. If the lesion is present in an area associated with anaerobic bacteria, clindamycin can be used.

Infected Cysts. Epidermal cysts may become infected with aerobic and/or anaerobic bacteria. Isolates most frequently encountered are *S. aureus,* streptococci, *Peptostreptococcus,* and *Bacteroides* spp. These cysts can be found about the head, trunk, extremities, perineum, vulvovaginal, and scrotal areas. Surgical drainage and antimicrobial agents directed at the organisms isolated are required (Brook, 1989a).

Hidradenitis Suppurativa. Hidradenitis suppurativa is a chronic, recurrent infection of apocrine glands that become plugged with keratinous material (Olafsson and Khan, 1992). Lesions usually develop in plugged, inflamed glands in the axilla, groin, and buttocks. This condition is more common in adults but may occur at the time of puberty as well. Bacteria associated with these lesions are staphylococci, nonhemolytic streptococci, gram-negative bacilli, *Bacteroides* spp., and anaerobic gram-positive cocci. Antibiotic treatment may not be successful, because the precipitating condition is chronic plugging of apocrine gland ducts, inflammation, formation of sinus tracts, and scarring, creating conditions that may not allow entry of antibiotics to the sites of infection. Local care to promote drainage and antibiotic therapy directed at the bacteria isolated from the lesion should be instituted initially. Occasionally, in very severe disease, radical excision of the area with skin grafting is required.

Infected Gastrostomy Tube Sites Wound. Gastrostomy site infection may occur in patients who require prolonged gastrostomy tube feeding (Brook, 1995). The infection presents as an area of induration and erythema, with exudate formation in and around the gastrostomy wound site. Leakage of gastric contents from the wounds may be present and may contribute to the presence of anaerobes in the wound. A mixed bacterial population is usually found with anaerobes predominating. The most common isolates found in these wounds are *Peptostreptococcus* spp., *B. fragilis* group, *E. coli,* and *Enterococcus* spp. (Brook, 1995), although other aerobic bacteria, such as *S. aureus,* and anaerobic bacterial species may be present. Bacteremia may be present in a minority of patients. After wound cultures are obtained, local wound care should be instituted. In cases of more severe infection, blood cultures should be obtained and empiric systemic therapy should be directed against the most frequent isolates, as well as *S. aureus.* Clindamycin, cefotaxime (or ceftriaxone) plus an aminoglycoside or metronidazole, oxacillin, and cefotaxime (or ceftriaxone) plus an aminoglycoside are two possible treatment combinations. Imipenem/cilastin or ampicillin/sulbactam plus an aminoglycoside may be used in children over 12 years of age, although imipenem/cilastin should not be used in children who are seizure prone, because this drug lowers the seizure threshold. The therapy should then be directed at the organisms isolated from wound and blood.

Subcutaneous Tissue Infections

Pilonidal Abscess. Pilonidal abscesses occur when a pilonidal sinus, a midline closure defect in the sacral region, becomes infected, probably after the sinus becomes plugged with debris (Sondenaa et al., 1995). Occasionally, infection may be chronic, resulting in chronic pilonidal sinus disease. Infection is usually caused predominantly by anaerobes and enteric gram-negative bacilli. *S. aureus* is less commonly isolated. Treatment consists of incision and drainage and may be followed by systemic antibiotics directed at anaerobes and enteric gram-negative bacilli. Postoperative wound infections and recurrence of disease are not uncommon in this condition.

Infected Decubitus Ulcers. Decubitus ulcers may develop in immobilized or bedridden children (Brook, 1995). Pressure on tissue that exceeds vascular perfusion pressure results in tissue ischemia. Tissue breakdown is further aggravated by moisture and friction, resulting in tissue maceration. Endogenous bacteria, aerobic and anaerobic, find easy entrance into the wound and can penetrate layers of tissues, resulting in further necrosis of the ulcer, bacteremia, sepsis, osteomyelitis, and infection of joints. Regions most often affected by decubitus ulcers are those that overly bony prominences such as the sacrum, greater trochanter, and heels. Ulcers located in regions such as the sacrum are more likely to become infected with fecal flora.

Polymicrobial infection of these ulcers is most common. *S. aureus, Peptostreptococcus* spp., *Bacteroides* spp., and gram-negative enteric bacteria are most commonly isolated. Cultures should be obtained from decubitus ulcers by collecting material from deep within the wound.

Treatment consists of surgical débridement of necrotic tissue, antimicrobial treatment, and local wound care. If the ulcer is deep and wide, skin grafting is sometimes necessary. Two treatment regimens are clindamycin, cefotaxime (or ceftriaxone), and an aminoglycoside or metronidazole, oxacillin, cefotaxime (or ceftriaxone), and an aminoglycoside. Imipenem/cilastin or ampicillin/sulbactam alone may be used in children over 12 years of age, although imipenem/cilastin should not be used in children who are seizure prone, because this drug lowers the seizure threshold.

Infected Bite Wounds. The risk of infection of bite wounds is determined by the source of the bite, the type of injury, and the bite location. Even though infection of bite wounds is most often polymicrobial, certain infecting microorganisms are often unique to the source of the bite. Anaerobic bacteria are present in about 40% to 75% of dog, cat, and human bites. The three most common bite wounds are those caused by dog, cat, and human, in order of decreasing frequency. However, bites caused by cats become infected at a rate of about 30% to 50%, twice that of dog and human bites.

Dog bites often cause crush injury but may also result in punctures avulsions, tears, and abrasions (Zook et al., 1980; Goldstein, 1992). However, with cat bites, small diameter puncture wounds occur, allowing bacteria to enter deep into tissue in an anaerobic environment. Often three to four bacteria will be cultured from an infected bite. The most common anaerobic bacteria isolated are *B. fragilis, Prevotella, Porphyromonas, Peptostreptococcus,* and *Fusobacterium* spp. Most commonly encountered aerobes are *Pasteurella multocida, Staphylococcus* spp., streptococci, *Corynebacterium* spp., gram-negative enteric bacteria, and *Eikenella corrodens.*

Most anaerobes from animals do not produce β-lactamases. A much less commonly encountered bacteria from infected wound bites is *Capnocytophaga canimorsus* (formerly DF-2). Infection with this organism has been reported to result in fatal infections in patients with certain predisposing conditions such as splenectomy and steroid therapy.

Human bites that occur as a clenched fist injury can result in a very serious infection with major complications. This is an injury that usually results to a hand that has made forceful contact with another individual's mouth. A puncture or laceration of the skin may occur, inoculating bacteria into the deep tissue of the hand. If injury occurs over the metacarpophalangeal joint, infection can enter the joint, resulting in inoculation of human oral bacteria into the tendon sheath. Complications of this injury include septic arthritis, osteomyelitis, spread of infection into the compartments of the hand, and tendon and nerve laceration and fractures of the phalangeal or metacarpal bones. Often, multiple bacterial isolates are found in infected human bites, usually with a predominance of anaerobic bacteria. The most common anaerobic isolates seen are *B. fragilis, Prevotella, Porphyromonas, Peptostreptococcus, Fusobacterium,* and *Clostridium* spp. The most frequently encountered aerobes are streptococci, *S. aureus, Staphylococcus epidermidis, Corynebacterium* spp., and *E. corrodens.* Anaerobes found in human bites often produce β-lactamases, unlike those found in animal bites.

Other infectious agents can also be transmitted through bites. Cat bites may transmit *Bartonella henselae* (cat scratch bacillus), whereas either may introduce *C. tetani* or rabies virus into the bite. Human bites may be associated with transmission of herpesvirus type 1 and 2, hepatitis B and C, *Actinomyces* spp., *C. tetani, Mycobacterium tuberculosis,* and *Treponema pallidum.* The transmission of human immunodeficiency virus (HIV) through human bites appears unlikely although not improbable.

Treatment of a bite wound includes extensive irrigation. Although débridement should be performed to remove devitalized or crushed tissue and contaminating material, puncture wounds usually cannot be débrided without causing more extensive trauma. If signs of infection are present, aerobic and anaerobic cultures should be obtained before irrigation and débridement. Care must be taken so that cultures represent bacteria within the wound. Primary closure of bite wounds is controversial. Primary closure should not be performed on deep puncture wounds, wounds present for greater than 24 hours, infected wounds, and bites to the hands. Superficially infected animal bite wounds can be treated initially with amoxicillin/clavulanate or with tetracycline in penicillin-allergic patients. Cefuroxime axetil or combination penicillin V plus dicloxacillin or cephalexin are two other alternative regimens. For more severely infected wounds, penicillin G plus oxacillin or cefazolin, or ampicillin/sulbactam can be used.

The risk of tetanus and rabies needs to be considered when treating a bite wound. Information of the patient's last tetanus immunization should be obtained. A fully immunized child with a minor bite wound that is carefully irrigated needs no further tetanus prophylaxis. The need for administration of tetanus immunization and immunoglobulin for complicated wound bites is determined by the patient's immunization status. Rabies immune globulin and rabies immunization may be required for certain animal bites.

Necrotizing Soft Tissue Infections

Anatomy and Pathogenesis. An understanding of the structure of the skin provides an understanding of the pathophysiology of wound infections. The skin consists of two layers, the stratified squamous keratinizing epithelium and the deeper layer of connective tissue called the dermis. The epithelial layer contains no blood vessels and is therefore dependent on the diffusion of interstitial fluid from the well-vascularized dermis. The dermis rests on the superficial fascia, a layer of subcutaneous tissue that is superficial to the abdominal wall musculature. The blood supply to both the overlying skin and the underlying adipose tissue is derived from arteries that lie in the superficial fascia. Therefore the blood supply to the skin can be disrupted by an infectious process deep to the skin, resulting in skin necrosis indirectly. For example, an established anaerobic infection within the dermis causes thrombosis of these vessels late in the disease process. The overlying skin initially may only show mild signs of pathology, such as edema. The soft tissue may not exhibit the classic signs of local tissue inflammation (Finegold et al., 1985). Because of the paucity of symptoms, early diagnosis of such processes may be very difficult. As the underlying disease progresses and the deep tissues become necrotic, the overlying skin also becomes necrotic. However, by the time this occurs, the infectious process is already life threatening.

Superficial Necrotizing Soft Tissue Infections

Bacterial Synergistic Gangrene. Bacterial synergistic gangrene (progressive bacterial synergistic gangrene) is a slowly progressing infection involving the dermis and, less commonly, the fascia (Meleny, 1933; Baxter, 1972). Coinfection of tissue with *S. aureus* or gram-negative bacilli and microaerophilic or anaerobic streptococci results in a synergistic infection. Local tissue destruction and lowered oxidation-reduction potential resulting from infection with aerobic bacteria enable entry of anaerobic or microaerophilic streptococci into the tissue. Infection can then extend beyond the site of initial wound. Although any area can be affected, abdominal wounds and tissue around ileostomies or colostomies, surgical drains, or retention sutures may be more likely to develop such an infection because of contamination with the offending bacteria during or after abdominal surgery.

Predominant early signs of infection are local exquisite pain, tenderness, edema, and erythema. Subsequently, the central portion of the wound develops a purplish coloration surrounded by a margin of erythema and eventually ulcerates and becomes undermined. If left untreated, the infection spreads as the zone of gangrenous skin at periphery of the lesion to involve the fascia. Because fever and signs of systemic illness often appear later in the course of infection, the serious nature of infection may not be realized early in the disease course.

Once the diagnosis is entertained, the infecting bacteria should be identified by culturing two separate sites. One sample should be taken from the central portion of the wound to identify aerobic bacteria. A second specimen obtained from the undermined margins should be cultured anaerobically. This infection has a poor response to antibiotic therapy alone because of the presence of extensive necrosis, and wide surgical excision of the lesion is often required. Empiric intravenous antibiotics, directed against anaerobic/microaerophilic streptococci, *S. aureus,* and a wide range of gram-negative enteric organisms should be instituted promptly. Oxacillin or vancomycin and gentamicin or a third-generation cephalosporin is an effective regimen. Once bacterial isolates are identified, antibiotic therapy should then be directed against bacteria isolated from the wound. Full recovery can be achieved with early treatment. Treatment delays may necessitate wide excision of the infected area, leading to prolonged hospital stay and skin grafting.

Anaerobic Cellulitis (Clostridial and Nonclostridial Anaerobic Cellulitis)

Anaerobic cellulitis is a necrotizing infection of de-vitalized subcutaneous tissue. The infection is usu-ally superficial to the fascia (MacLennan, 1962; Bornstein et al., 1964; Bessman and Wagner, 1975).

Clostridium spp. is the usual cause of these in-fections, although other non–spore-forming anaer-obes in combination with gram-negative enterics have also been implicated. Anaerobic cellulitis de-velops within 3 days after bacterial contamination of subcutaneous tissue and spreads rapidly through adjacent tissue. Initially, mild pain, erythema, and edema of the skin around the wound are present early in the course. As the infection progresses, the skin overlying the infected area becomes erythem-atous and tender, and skin necrosis and small flat blebs that discharge a serous, foul-smelling liquid may be present. Crepitance is often present because of subcutaneous gas. The patient is usually not sys-temically ill. Aerobic and anaerobic blood culture, as well as Gram stain and aerobic and anaerobic cultures of the exudate from either the wound or from the blebs on the skin. Plain radiographs will reveal abundant gas in the superficial soft tissues of the abdominal wall. A frozen-section biopsy may reveal the level of soft tissue affected by the necrotic process. Anaerobic cellulitis is treated by antibiotic therapy and local débridement to remove the infected necrotic tissue. Empiric antibiotic treatment should have activity against *Clostridium* spp., *Bacteroides* spp., anaerobic streptococci, and gram-negative enteric organisms. A combination such as an aminoglycoside or third-generation cephalosporin, penicillin, and clindamycin will provide coverage for these organisms. Full recov-ery is expected with early treatment.

Infections that Extend to the Fascia

Necrotizing Fasciitis. Necrotizing fasciitis, also known as hospital gangrene and hemolytic streptococcal gangrene, is a life-threatening infec-tion, a rapidly progressive necrotizing disease that has been, fortunately, relatively uncommon in the pediatric population. Most cases of pediatric necro-tizing fasciitis occur in neonates after infection of the umbilical stump.

Necrotizing fasciitis may involve any area of the body, including the perineum, scrotum, and penis (Fournier's gangrene) in children (Adams et al., 1990). It often presents within 1 to 4 days after trauma, contamination of a surgical wound, infec-tion of umbilical stump (omphalitis) in neonates

(Mason et al., 1989), or infection of skin vesicles following chickenpox (Falcone et al., 1988), but it may also occur without known antecedent trauma in patients with neutropenia or diabetes mellitus. As the infection extends along the fascial planes, edema and necrosis of the superficial fascia and the deeper layer of the dermis occur. Compression or destruction of the nerves innervating the skin and thrombosis of the small blood vessels result in anesthesia and necrosis of the overlying dermis and epidermis. Undermining of the overlying skin oc-curs, a key to the diagnosis of this infection.

The infection is frequently polymicrobial, usu-ally involving enteric gram-negative bacilli and anaerobic bacteria, including *Bacteroides, Pep-tostreptococcus,* and *Clostridium* spp. However, *Staphylococcus pyogenes* or *S. aureus* may alone be isolated (Guiliano et al., 1977; Barker et al., 1987).

Pain and swelling around the site of infection are the initial symptoms. Induration and erythema oc-cur within 24 hours. A purple discoloration and hy-pesthesia of the overlying skin develop, along with extensive tissue edema. Within 3 to 5 days after ini-tial infection, skin necrosis occurs and bullae elab-orating thick, foul-smelling purple fluid appear. Crepitance may be present over the affected area. Severe systemic toxicity with decreased myocar-dial contractility, oliguria, adult respiratory distress syndrome, and extensive extravasation of intravas-cular fluid into tissue and multiple laboratory ab-normalities may occur, including electrolyte abnor-malities, bone marrow suppression and hemolysis, and saponification secondary to necrosis of the subcutaneous fat in extensive infections resulting in hypocalcemia.

Because there is a paucity of external signs in the first 24 hours, the diagnosis may be difficult to make. Frozen-section biopsy, a procedure that al-lows rapid evaluation of the pathology and organ-isms underlying the intact skin, is a rapid and very helpful test that can be done by the surgeons to make an early diagnosis of necrotizing fasciitis (Stamenkovic and Lew, 1984). The diagnosis can be confirmed by the ability to pass a sterile instru-ment along a plane superficial to the deep fascia without resistance. Aerobic and anaerobic cultures of blood and wound exudate should be obtained, although bacteremia is uncommon. Radiographs may show subcutaneous gas.

Because of the systemic toxicity that results from this infection, the patients often require correction of fluid, electrolyte, hematologic, renal, cardiac, and pulmonary abnormalities. Empiric therapy with an aminoglycoside, penicillin, and clindamycin or an aminoglycoside and chloramphenicol should be started to cover gram-negative enterics, anaerobes, *S. aureus,* and beta-hemolytic streptococci. Emergent widespread surgical débridement of all necrotic tissue must be performed to decrease mortality from this disease. Repeat débridement within 24 to 48 hours may be necessary because of continued dissection of the infection into surrounding tissue. Antibiotic treatment can be tailored to cover the organisms isolated from blood and surgical specimens.

Patients who survive the infection often require an extensive hospital stay. Disfigurement often results from the radical débridement required to treat this disease. Untreated, this infection has a high mortality. With appropriate and early surgical débridement, the mortality can be reduced to less than 30%.

Synergistic Nonclostridial Anaerobic Myonecrosis.
Synergistic nonclostridial anaerobic myonecrosis (Baxter, 1972), also called synergistic necrotizing cellulitis, cutaneous gangrene, necrotizing cutaneous myositis, and gram-negative anaerobic cutaneous gangrene, is an uncommon, aggressive, life-threatening necrotizing infection that affects the skin, dermis, fascia, and muscle. It is a polymicrobial infection. Anaerobic streptococci, *Bacteroides* spp., and several species of gram-negative enteric bacilli are most frequently isolated.

The infection occurs within 3 to 14 days after contamination of a wound. Exquisite tenderness around the wound that is out of proportion to the physical findings is often the first symptom. The area around the wound is initially only erythematous. Unfortunately, by the time edema and a characteristic blue-gray discoloration occur, there is already extensive muscle necrosis. Bullae form in the overlying skin and drain a foul-smelling liquid described as "dishwater pus," and occasionally crepitance can be felt. Systemic toxicity develops rapidly.

Aerobic and anaerobic blood cultures and cultures of the exudate, present only in the later stages of this disease, should be obtained. Frozen-section biopsy may be helpful in determining the presence of tissue necrosis underlying the relatively normal appearing skin early in the disease course and will provide material for bacterial culture. Biopsy will also help distinguish myonecrosis from necrotizing fasciitis, which leaves the underlying muscle intact.

Hypovolemia, acidosis, clotting disturbances, anemia, septic shock, renal failure, disorientation, and adult respiratory distress syndrome can occur early in this infection. Correction of these disturbances and intensive cardiovascular support must be provided in preparation for the emergent radical surgical débridement that is required to treat this disease. Débridement may need to be repeated to ensure removal of all necrotic tissue. Antibiotics can control the extension of infection only if removal of all necrotic and infected tissue is complete. Empiric antibiotics should cover anaerobic and gram-negative enteric organisms. Because this disease may be clinically indistinguishable from clostridial myonecrosis, an antibiotic active against *Clostridium* spp. should initially be used. A combination such as clindamycin, ceftriaxone, or cefotaxime and an aminoglycoside may be used.

Radical débridement, necessary for the treatment of this disease, is associated with severe disfigurement. Irreversible multisystem organ failure may occur. Untreated, the mortality of this disease is about 75%. Treated early, the mortality still reaches 10%.

Clostridial Myonecrosis (Gas Gangrene).
Clostridial myonecrosis is an uncommon but virulent, life-threatening necrotizing infection of all the soft tissues, including the muscle (Fromm and Silen, 1969; Darke et al., 1977; Hart et al., 1983). It may occur in any tissue that has been devitalized by trauma, surgery, or the normal process of umbilical cord necrosis after delivery. Once devitalized tissue is infected with *Clostridium* spp., elaboration of clostridial exotoxins and enzymes that cause necrosis of adjacent muscle allows the infection to spread extensively and rapidly into healthy, untraumatized muscle. *C. perfringens,* the most virulent of these organisms, is most often responsible for this disease. Released toxins from this organism are absorbed into the systemic circulation and cause massive hemolysis, cardiotoxicity, renal failure, and CNS dysfunction. The massive hemolysis, in turn, leads to hemoglobinuria, jaundice, and renal failure.

Aside from sudden and severe pain in the wound, which spreads along the path of the infection, there is a paucity of physical findings initially. With progression of disease, skin overlying the affected area becomes pale and tense because of the underlying edema caused by massive myonecrosis. Occasionally the underlying muscle may be so edematous that herniation through an incision site may occur.

Anaerobic metabolism by *Clostridium* spp. results in gas accumulation within the infected tissues. Serous, nonpurulent exudate, described as having a sickly sweet odor, emanates from the wound, and the skin overlying the affected area takes on a bronze or purple coloration. The disease is so rapidly progressive that these changes in the skin can occasionally progress over a period of hours. Changes in mental status and rapid onset of severe systemic toxicity occur, notably with tachycardia out of proportion to the moderate rise in temperature. Within a short time, hypotension and renal failure occur, and, if untreated, this infection will rapidly lead to death, sometimes within 12 hours.

As soon as this disease is suspected, anaerobic and aerobic cultures from blood should be obtained and wound and skin bullae should be Gram stained immediately. If gram-positive bacilli are seen, surgical débridement should be planned immediately. In the early stages of infection, it may be very difficult to distinguish clostridial myonecrosis from anaerobic cellulitis and necrotizing fasciitis. Although CT may be helpful in detecting gas in muscle, surgery examination of the wound may be the only way to distinguish clostridial myonecrosis from the other necrotizing infections. The dermis, fascia, and muscle must be carefully examined for signs of necrosis and for the presence and types of bacteria. Once the diagnosis is entertained, surgery should never be delayed while awaiting scheduling of CT scan or results of wound culture. Full critical care support is required before and during immediate surgical débridement of all compromised subcutaneous tissue and muscle, as well as necrotic debris and hematomata. Although treatment with antibiotics alone will not alter the course of this disease, it may play a role in limiting infection once full débridement is achieved. The antibiotic choice for *Clostridium* spp. is penicillin, given intravenously in high doses as the sodium salt (hyperkalemia caused by renal failure and muscle and erythrocyte destruction are often present). A patient who has a penicillin allergy can be treated with chloramphenicol or clindamycin, although some strains of clostridia have become resistant to clindamycin. If other bacterial species are seen on Gram stain, additional antibiotic coverage may be needed. Hyperbaric oxygen therapy, in combination with surgical débridement and antibiotic therapy, may decrease mortality from this disease (Hart et al., 1983). Children who survive have prolonged hospital courses with slow recovery and required reconstructive surgery because of the extensive surgical débridement that is required to arrest the infection. Mortality for clostridial myonecrosis is about 60%.

ANAEROBIC BACTEREMIA
Etiology

The most common isolates found in anaerobic bacteremia are *B. fragilis,* other *Bacteroides* spp., *Clostridium, Peptostreptococcus* and *Fusobacterium* spp., and *Propionibacterium acnes* (Brook, 1980a; Brook, 1989b; Citron et al., 1995). The species of bacteria isolated from the blood often reflects the primary portal of entry and gives clues that may help identify the source of infection. In many cases, infection is polymicrobial and aerobic bacteria are often isolated. The isolation of fecal anaerobes such as *B. fragilis* and *Clostridium* spp. suggests a gastrointestinal source of infection, whereas *Peptostreptococcus* spp. and *Fusobacterium* spp. are often associated with sinusitis, oropharyngeal infection, and chronic otitis media (Brook, 1980a). Bacteremia with *P. acnes* may indicate that a CSF or cardiovascular shunt is infected (Brook, 1980a). In all cases of bacteremia, a careful search for the source of infection should be made.

Epidemiology

Anaerobes are a minor contributor to bacteremia in children (Thirmuoothi et al., 1976; Brook, 1989b). Neonates and children with chronic diseases, cancer, neurologic impairment, and immunodeficiencies may have a higher incidence of anaerobic bacteremia (Brook, 1989b; Brook, 1995; Citron et al., 1995).

Clinical Manifestations

Entry of anaerobes into the bloodstream occurs after a breach in either the protective mucosal layer or skin. Bacteremia caused by anaerobic bacteria shows a clinical picture reflective of the original site of infection. The clinical picture of anaerobic bacteremia includes fever, chills, and leukocytosis. Leukocytosis will not be seen in children with neutropenia caused by chemotherapeutic therapies and acquired immunodeficiency syndrome (AIDS). Bacteremia with *Clostridium septicum* may result in a devastating and fatal clinical course that is caused not only by the patient's underlying condition but also by the elaboration of bacterial toxins that cause severe hemolysis, shock, and sepsis.

Diagnosis

A high degree of clinical suspicion is often needed initially to make the diagnosis of anaerobic bacteremia. The diagnosis of anaerobic bacteremia is often made empirically, because isolation of anaerobic bacteria takes a week or longer due to their slow growth. The presence of a pathologic process or condition that predisposes the child to infection with anaerobic bacteria often suggests the primary source of infection, although secondary sites of infection may occur. The secondary sites may be adjacent to the original site (meningitis or subdural abscess after direct extension of infection in sinuses) (Brook, 1989b) or distant from the primary source (osteomyelitis after hematogenous spread of bacteria from an oropharyngeal source). Therefore appropriate diagnostic procedures such as plain radiographs, radionuclide scans, ultrasound, CT scan, or magnetic resonance imaging (MRI) must be undertaken to identify these sites. A definitive diagnosis can be made after identification of anaerobic bacteria from blood cultures.

Complications

The mortality rate for anaerobic bacteremia in children is variable, with rates between 18% (Brook, 1980a) and 37% (Dunkle et al., 1976). The mortality often reflects the severity of the child's underlying disease, the location of primary and secondary sites of infection, the pathogen, rapidity of diagnosis, and institution of appropriate antibacterial agents.

Treatment

Anaerobic bacteremia is often polymicrobial, and identification of anaerobic organisms requires considerable time. Therefore initial treatment is often empirical and should cover suspected anaerobic and aerobic bacteria. The antibiotics chosen should be based on the source of infection, if one has been identified (e.g., abdominal, oropharyngeal process) and the prevalence of bacterial resistance in the geographic locale (e.g., recent increase in incidence of resistance of *B. fragilis* to clindamycin in Children's Hospital in Los Angeles) (Citron et al., 1995). Once identification and susceptibility of pathogens are made, the narrowest spectrum antibiotic(s) that covers the isolated organisms should be used. The source of infection, if not obvious, should be identified and surgical débridement or drainage should be performed if a collection of pus is found.

INTRACRANIAL ABSCESSES
Epidemiology

Brain abscesses are most frequently caused by (Wispelwey and Scheld, 1995) (1) local extension of an infection in the head and neck, most often from the frontal sinuses, and less frequently, mastoid, dental, and pulmonary; (2) hematogenous

spread from a distant focus, seen more frequently in children with cyanotic congenital heart disease (CCHD) or children with pulmonary arteriovenous fistulas; and (3) less commonly, intracranial trauma or neurosurgical procedure that allows access of bacteria into the brain parenchyma. In 15% to 20% of cases, no source is identified (Garfield, 1969; Nielse and Harmsen, 1982).

Two percent to 6% of children with CCHD develop brain abscesses because of the presence of right-to-left intracardiac shunts (Fischbein et al., 1981; Spires et al., 1985; Theophilo et al., 1985). Children with Fallot's tetralogy, dextroposition of the great arteries, complete atrioventricular canal, tricuspid atresia, double outlet right ventricle, and truncus arteriosis are at increased risk of developing brain abscesses.

Subdural and extradural empyema and septic thrombophlebitis are most often caused by extension of infection located in the head. A well-reported phenomenon that occurs predominantly in adolescent males is the development of subdural empyema after frontal sinusitis without history of chronicity (Kaufman et al., 1983).

Pathogenesis

Intracranial infections can occur after penetration of bacteria through the cranium from a contiguous site of infection or through hematogenous spread from a distant site. Direct extension of infection intracranially can occur through the cranial bones or via the valveless diploic or emissary veins. Infection in the frontal sinuses can readily spread intracranially through the thin frontal bones and via the diploic veins to cause subdural and extradural empyemas, frontal brain abscess, subgaleal abscess, and septic thrombophlebitis of cortical veins and intracranial venous sinuses (Fairbanks and Milmoe, 1985). Subdural and extradural empyemas can be present simultaneously (Hlavin et al., 1994). Ethmoid sinus infection can also result in subdural empyema. Abscesses from infected mastoids are most likely spread contiguously to the temporal lobe or cerebellum, possibly through the internal auditory canal, cochlear and vestibular aqueducts, or between temporal suture lines (Gower and McGuirt, 1983; Spires et al., 1985). Sphenoid sinusitis, although relatively uncommon, can spread to the temporal lobe or sella turcica (Lew et al., 1983). Dental abscesses, especially those involving the molar teeth, can lead to brain abscesses (usually in the frontal but occasionally in the temporal lobes) (Hollin et al., 1967), as well as subdural empyema (Brook, 1992).

Brain abscesses from a distant infected site often occur when pathologic conditions that may cause decreased brain capillary blood flow, leading to "microinfarction and reduced tissue oxygenation," are present. Such conditions may occur in patients with CCHD because of increased blood viscosity secondary to polycythemia or in patients with septic emboli released from a distal infected site (endocarditis, osteomyelitis) (Wispelwey and Scheld, 1995). Hematogenously spread abscesses usually occur along the distribution of the middle cerebral artery in the frontal and parietal lobes. Occasionally, subdural empyema can occur via hematogenous spread (Wispelwey and Scheld, 1995).

Penetrating head trauma may result in the formation of brain abscess or subdural empyema after introduction of bacteria through a break in the dura (Foy and Skarr, 1980; Tay and Garland, 1987).

Pathology

Brain abscesses are thought to evolve through several stages that can be distinguished by differences in contrast enhancement on pre- and postcontrast CT scan (Britt et al., 1981; Britt and Enzmann, 1983). In the early stages, referred to as *cerebritis,* the site of infection is localized but unencapsulated, whereas in the later stage the mature abscess has a fibrous, collagenized capsule encasing the necrotic center. In all stages, edema may surrounds the abscess. The significance in distinguishing the stages of the abscess is the possible difference in response to antibiotic therapy without surgical drainage. Abscesses in very early stages may respond to prolonged antibiotic therapy alone, whereas those with established capsule formation require either aspiration/drainage or excision of the abscess (Britt and Enzmann, 1983; Keren, 1984; Wispelwey and Scheld, 1995).

Subdural empyema is a collection of pus within the potential space between the dura and arachnoid, the two outer layers of the meninges (Smith and Hendrick, 1983; Greenlee, 1995b). The cranial subdural space is subdivided into several large compartments that confine large infection areas over the brain. Subdural empyemas may be bilateral. The most common locations over the convexity of the brain are the base of the brain or along the falx cerebri. As the empyema enlarges within its confined space, a large mass effect causing brain compression may result. Septic thrombosis of bridging veins crossing the subdural space may result, causing hemorrhagic infarction. Life-threatening transtentorial herniation caused by subdural mass effect and

cerebral edema may eventually occur (LeBeau et al., 1973; Greenlee, 1995b).

Intracranial epidural (extradural) abscesses are located between the cranial bone and dura, which forms the innermost layer of the cranial periosteum (Smith and Hendrick, 1983; Greenlee, 1995a). They occur most often as a complication of frontal sinusitis but can also be secondary to mastoiditis, craniotomy, or head trauma (Greenlee, 1995a). After extension of bacteria within the frontal sinus through the frontal bone, the pus collects between the osteomyelitic bone and dura and remains relatively confined within this space. Infection may also spread via bridging veins into the subdural space.

Etiology

Intracranial abscesses/empyemas may be caused by anaerobic and aerobic bacteria (Jadavji, 1985; Chun et al., 1986; Wispelwey and Scheld, 1995). The role of anaerobic bacteria in these infections has probably been underestimated (Brook, 1992), especially in those patients who have developed abscesses/empyemas secondary to spread from a contiguous focus of infection (i.e., paranasal sinusitis, mastoiditis, or odontogenic infection). The pathogens found in these intracranial infections are usually a subset of those found in the primary source of infection.

Subdural empyema and brain abscesses in the older child are most often associated with paranasal sinusitis and have the same spectrum of anaerobic and aerobic bacteria found in brain abscesses secondary to paranasal sinusitis. A recent study of 39 pediatric patients with either brain abscess or subdural empyema demonstrated the anaerobic bacteria in 32 patients, with anaerobes alone in 22 patients and in mixed infection with aerobes in 10 patients (Brook, 1992). Only 7 patients in this study had aerobic pathogens only. Predominant anaerobic organisms in intracranial abscesses are *Peptostreptococcus* spp., *Fusobacterium* spp., *Bacteroides* spp., (including *B. fragilis*) and *Prevotella* spp. Aerobic bacteria associated intracranial abscesses are *S. aureus,* Enterobacteriaceae, alpha- and beta-hemolytic streptococci, and *Haemophilus* spp.

Hematogenous brain abscesses, most often seen in children with CCHD, are often caused by anaerobic and microaerophilic streptococci and streptococci viridans (Brook, 1989b). Subdural empyemas are most often secondary to meningitis in children younger than 5 years (Farmer and Wise, 1973). Gram-negative bacillary meningitis can be complicated by subdural empyema, as well as brain abscess, in neonates. In toddlers, *Haemophilus influenzae* meningitis is often associated with subdural effusion or subdural empyema. Fortunately this disease is much less commonly seen because of the widespread use of *H. influenzae* vaccine. Posttraumatic brain abscesses are most often caused by *S. aureus,* whereas *S. aureus* and *P. acnes* may be associated with abscess after neurosurgical procedures.

Clinical Manifestations

Brain abscesses are space-occupying lesions. Headache and fever are often present. Depending on the location, there may be progressive focal neurologic deficits, as well as general signs of increased intracranial pressure. Nausea, vomiting, seizures, meningismus, and papilledema are variably present. The primary focus of infection may be apparent by history and physical examination.

Patients with subdural empyema are usually acutely ill with fever, headache, and meningismus. If enlargement occurs, signs of an intracranial mass lesion will be present. Signs and symptoms attributable to the primary source of infection may be noted. Epidural abscess often has an indolent course, unless accompanied by subdural. If the abscess is secondary to frontal sinusitis, frontal bone osteomyelitis (Pott's puffy tumor) may be seen.

Intracranial abscess or empyema may be associated with venous sinus thrombosis. In addition to clinical findings caused by abscess or empyema, characteristic presentations are associated with thrombosis of each different venous sinus (Greenlee, 1995a).

Diagnosis

An intracranial lesion should be suspected in a child with fever and focal neurologic signs. A lumbar puncture (LP) is contraindicated in these cases because of the risk of herniation until studies determine that an intracranial mass lesion is not present. In addition, LP results are often not helpful in making the diagnosis. A radiologic imaging procedure should be performed as rapidly as possible. CT scan with contrast is extremely sensitive in showing the presence of an established brain abscess but may be less sensitive in the detection of a subdural empyema and epidural abscess. In addition, a distinction cannot be made between brain abscess and neoplasms, granulomas, cerebral infarction, and resolving hematoma with contrast-enhanced CT scanning (Wispelwey and Scheld, 1995). CT is also less helpful in the early stages of abscess formation or if abscess rupture into the ventricles has oc-

curred. Contrast-enhanced MRI scan is superior to contrast-enhanced CT for the diagnosis of brain abscess, especially in the early stage of abscess formation, subdural empyema, and epidural abscess (Haimes et al., 1989; Wispelwey and Scheld, 1995). MRI also permits the diagnosis of venous sinus thrombosis. Both MRI and CT scans show the presence of sinusitis, otitis, or mastoiditis. Technetium brain scan is also a very sensitive test in the diagnosis of brain abscess, but it will not distinguish abscess from necrotic tumor or infarction. In neonates, ultrasonography is often useful in the diagnosis of brain abscess. If there is a delay in obtaining a CT or MRI and a distinction between bacterial meningitis and a mass lesion cannot be made, blood cultures and antibiotics should be started while awaiting scheduling and results of the imaging procedure.

Differential Diagnosis

Although the etiologies of an intracranial lesion are extensive, the differential diagnosis can be narrowed by the history, physical exam, and presence of factors that may predispose the patient to different types of intracranial lesions. The presence of sinusitis, otitis, mastoiditis, recent periodontal or neurosurgical procedures, head trauma, CCHD, or meningitis should alert the physician to the possibility of an intracranial abscess. A history of travel may suggest parasitic lesion. Other central nervous system (CNS) lesions that must be considered in the diagnosis are herpes simplex encephalitis, CNS vasculitis, cerebral infarction, and tumor. In children with AIDS, other intracranial lesions that must be considered include toxoplasmosis, CNS lymphoma, and cryptococcal and other fungal lesions.

Treatment

Treatment of intracranial abscesses most often consists of medical and surgical treatment. In addition to supportive care that includes control of intracranial pressure and seizures, empiric antibiotics that have been shown to penetrate into intracranial sites of infection must be used (Kramer et al., 1969). Until the microbial agents are identified, an antibiotic regimen such as oxacillin, metronidazole, and ceftriaxone, which will provide coverage of streptococci, staphylococci, anaerobes, and gram-negative bacilli (Donald, 1990; Sjoln et al., 1993), should be used. The initial regimen may be altered once the primary source and bacteria are identified.

For brain abscess, surgical aspiration through a burr hole or by stereotatic CT guidance (Lunsford and Nelson, 1984; Wispelwey and Scheld, 1995) or craniotomy with complete abscess excision is often required (Stepanov, 1988; Wispelwey and Scheld, 1995). In early stages of abscess development, it may be possible to treat unencapsulated abscesses (cerebritis) with prolonged antibiotic treatment (Wispelwey and Scheld, 1995). Although the appropriate length of antibiotic is unknown, a generally accepted course of therapy is 6 to 8 weeks, with at least 3 weeks of therapy administered intravenously. Early abscesses not drained may require a longer duration of therapy.

Treatment of subdural empyema and epidural abscess includes prompt institution of empiric antibiotic therapy and urgent surgical drainage. For all intracranial infections, the primary source of infection should be identified and corrected.

Complications and Prognosis

Brain abscesses and subdural empyemas can result in a mass effect, causing midline shifts, necrosis, and herniation, all of which can result in permanent and severe neurologic impairment, seizure disorder, and/or death. Brain abscesses can also rupture into ventricles, resulting in ventriculitis, meningitis, and septic thrombosis. Because subdural empyemas can enlarge rapidly and extend over a large area of the brain, severe neurologic sequelae can result if rapid intervention does not occur. Because of the often insidious nature of epidural abscesses, neurologic sequelae and a mass lesion effect may not be seen until the abscess becomes sufficiently large or until it extends into the subdural space.

Mortality of brain abscesses has improved considerably from 40% to 60% before the use of antibiotics to between 0% and 24%. The advent of antibiotics and the use of radio imaging that now allow early intervention have resulted in improved survival and decreased complications. Mortality associated with subdural empyema ranges from 4% to 18%. Early diagnosis and intervention markedly decrease the mortality and improve the outcome.

INTRAABDOMINAL INFECTIONS
Introduction to Intraabdominal Infections

Intraabdominal infections are a major cause of morbidity and mortality in the pediatric population. They can occur in a variety of locations and may be localized or diffuse. Within the intraperitoneal cavity, infection may be localized, occurring as single or multiple abscesses, or it may be diffuse, result-

ing in peritonitis. Abscesses may occur in multiple anatomic spaces or may occur within solid viscera, such as liver and spleen. Although many infections remain localized, infection can become generalized as microorganisms are carried to various intraperitoneal locations by the flow of peritoneal fluid within the intraabdominal cavity (Meyers, 1987).

Microorganisms indigenous to the gastrointestinal tract are responsible for most intraabdominal infections, which escape their normal anatomic confines when bowel wall integrity is altered by a variety of pathologic conditions. Microorganisms can then seed areas that are adjacent or are accessible by continuity of the blood supply.

Infection of the intraabdominal cavity is most often caused by spread of microorganisms indigenous to the gastrointestinal tract that have escaped their normal anatomic confines when bowel wall integrity is altered by a variety of pathologic conditions. Microorganisms can also enter the intraabdominal cavity through the bloodstream during episodes of bacteremia, or they can be spread from adjacent infected organs such as the uterine cavity and fallopian tubes in the female.

The difficulty in diagnosing localized intraabdominal infections in the infant and toddler may lead to a delay in treatment that may be associated with extension of infection throughout the peritoneal cavity, resulting in peritonitis. In the older child the history and physical examination often enable the physician to determine the location and extent of infection. Diagnostic radiologic studies are often necessary to ascertain the site and extent of infection. A decision, in consultation with the surgical service, must be made about the need and method of surgical drainage. Microbiologic specimens, aerobic and anaerobic, should be obtained whenever possible. The patient's medical history and age, the location of the infection, and the results of microbiologic specimens should guide the physician in the use of antimicrobial agents and other appropriate medical management.

Anatomy. The relationships between the spaces and organs within the abdomen dictate the localization or spread of intraabdominal infections (Meyers, 1987). The abdomen is anatomically divided into three compartments, the peritoneal cavity, the retroperitoneum, and the abdominal wall, and infection can spread between these compartments.

The peritoneal cavity is enclosed by a serous membrane, the peritoneum, which forms a sac within the abdominal cavity and covers most of the abdominal organs. During embryogenesis, the abdominal viscera undergo complex rotation and the simple peritoneal sac becomes compartmentalized. Recesses and pathways develop within the peritoneal cavity that have the potential to collect and sequester infected fluid or allow movement of infected fluid from one area of the abdomen to another.

The intraperitoneal organs are suspended within the peritoneal sac by folds of peritoneum, called *mesenteries* and *ligaments*. Several abdominal structures are only partially encased by peritoneum. These are the liver, spleen, ascending and descending colon, and rectum. The bare area of the liver comes in direct contact with the diaphragm. The pancreas and duodenum are overlaid with peritoneum but are located within the retroperitoneal area. In the male, the peritoneum is a closed sac. However, in the female, the peritoneum has continuity with the mucous membranes of the fallopian tubes. This communication allows the spread of infection of the female genital tract to the intraperitoneal cavity.

The lesser peritoneal sac, the largest recess of the peritoneal cavity, is separated from the greater peritoneal cavity by the lesser omentum. These two peritoneal cavities communicate through a small opening called the epiploic foramen (Winslow's). A collection of infected material in the lesser sac lies between the stomach and pancreas and may be present with little involvement of the remainder of the peritoneal cavity. Infected fluid in the lesser sac can enter the right subhepatic space through Winslow's foramen, resulting in an abscess that overlies the right kidney or can become sequestered if Winslow's foramen closes because of inflammation.

The normal flow of peritoneal fluid via distinct pathways within the peritoneal cavity determines the spread of infection within the peritoneal space (Meyers, 1987). Infected fluid collections originating from distal intraperitoneal foci can form in areas where fluid normally collects. Fluid in the left upper peritoneal space collects in the left subphrenic space and does not travel caudally, because flow is limited anatomically. However, the right paracolic gutter provides a freely communicating pathway between right subhepatic and subphrenic spaces and the pelvis, making these three spaces the most common sites of abscess formation within the intraperitoneal cavity. Fluid in the right upper peritoneal cavity moves into Morrison's pouch, a recess of the right subhepatic space, located between the liver and the right kidney, to the right subphrenic space and then caudally into the pelvis via the right paracolic gutter. This pathway also allows infected fluid from the pelvic recess to travel cephalad to the right subhepatic space, often collecting in Morrison's pouch and then traveling around the lateral border of the liver to the right subphrenic space.

Intraperitoneal Abscesses

Epidemiology. In children, intraperitoneal abscesses are most commonly caused by appendicitis with perforation (Janik and Firor, 1979). Abscesses also result from abdominal surgical procedures and trauma, especially those involving the colon.

Pathogenesis. An abscess is a collection of bacteria, pus, and necrotic material that has been localized but not resolved by the body's defense system. Viable bacteria within the abscess cavity may continue multiplying, resulting in increased abscess size. In early stages of abscess formation or in the neutropenic host, localization of infection may not occur, resulting in a phlegmon, or inflammatory mass, that can serve as a continued source of infection with seeding of other areas of the body. It is important to make a distinction between a phlegmon and an abscess, because drainage is required for abscess resolution, whereas a phlegmon cannot be drained but will respond to appropriate antibiotic therapy.

Abscesses form within the abdomen when bacteria enter the normally sterile peritoneal space and cannot be cleared by the defense mechanisms of the peritoneum. An essential ingredient for abscess formation is the presence of necrotic debris or other foreign material such as meconium, barium, gastric contents, and sutures, in addition to the bacterial contamination. These ingredients encourage the growth of anaerobes by establishing a microenvironment with low oxygen concentration, and the foreign material may interfere with phagocytosis and chemotaxis. Within the growing abscess cavity, host defenses are diminished.

Intraabdominal abscesses in children result from altered bowel wall integrity caused by bowel wall ischemia or necrosis as in necrotizing enterocolitis, intussusception, volvulus, incarcerated hernia, perforation of the bowel as in rupture of an inflamed appendix or Meckel's diverticulum, Crohn's disease and ulcerative colitis, trauma to the bowel, or after surgery on the GI tract with resulting contamination of the peritoneal cavity with bowel flora (Brook, 1989b). Abscesses occur after incomplete resolution of diffuse peritonitis or may originate from a perforation that was successfully localized but not cleared by the peritoneal defenses. An abscess can also occur after contamination of a hematoma with bacteria. Pelvic abscess may also occur after rupture of a tuboovarian abscess.

The location of abscess formation is dependent on the source of the contaminating bacteria and flow of peritoneal fluid (Wilson, 1982a; Levison and Bush, 1995). Most abscesses from appendiceal rupture remain in the right lower quadrant, although the infecting material may be distributed within the peritoneal cavity to the pelvic area and to the subphrenic and subhepatic spaces via the right paracolic gutter (Mackenzie and Young, 1975). Abscesses can form in the spaces between the loops and mesentery of the small bowel or paracolic gutters (Wilson, 1982a). Abscesses secondary to direct spread from the liver and spleen will be located in the subphrenic space. Many left-sided subphrenic abscesses occur after colonic surgery (Wang and Wilson, 1977). Abscesses in the lesser peritoneal sac occur infrequently but are very important clinically because of the difficulty in diagnosing them. Although many abscesses are solitary, multiple abscesses are found in approximately 15% of cases of intraabdominal abscesses.

Etiology. The microorganisms found within an intraabdominal abscess are determined by the age of the child and source of the abscess. Intraabdominal abscesses in neonates after perforation of the bowel reflect normal bowel colonization, as well as changes in the gastrointestinal flora caused by the use of antibiotics and nosocomially transmitted bacteria. A greater predominance of aerobic bacteria including *K. pneumoniae*, *Enterobacter* spp., *Streptococcus* spp., and *S. epidermidis* (Bradley, 1985) have been seen in neonatal abscesses, although anaerobes, including *C. difficile* were also isolated (Brook, 1989b).

Abscesses arising from the stomach, liver, and biliary tract have a predominance of coliform bacteria, although anaerobes are also present, whereas abscesses arising from the ileum and colon have a predominance of anaerobes. Although there are 400 to 500 species found in the colon, only a few of these species are pathogenic. Most abscesses are polymicrobial and contain both anaerobic and aerobic bacteria. The anaerobic bacteria usually found in these abscesses are *B. fragilis, P. melaninogenicus, Peptococcus, Peptostreptococcus, Fusobacterium,* and *Clostridium* spp. The aerobic and facultative organisms most commonly cultured are *E. coli,* alpha- and gamma-hemolytic streptococci, enterococci, *K. pneumoniae,* and *P. aeruginosa* (Brook, 1980b; Brook, 1987). Most of the *B. fragilis* species and many *E. coli* isolates produce β-lactamases.

Infected cerebrospinal fluid at the peritoneal tip of a ventriculo-peritoneal (VP) shunt may result in an abscess. Bacteria within the abscess, usually *S. epidermidis,* will reflect that which is infecting the VP shunt itself.

Clinical Manifestations. Abscesses may form within several days after a perforation of a viscus or may occur several weeks after diffuse peritonitis (Wilson, 1982a). Fever, usually low grade initially, becomes persistent, rising and often spiking in nature. There is usually anorexia, nausea, and vomiting. The presence of chills implies either bacteremia seeding from the abscess or impending perforation or extension of the abscess to adjacent organs.

The clinical presentation of the intraabdominal abscess depends to a great extent on the location of the abscess (Wilson, 1982a). Abscesses located in the subphrenic and intermesenteric spaces often have few localizing signs, whereas abscesses in the pelvis often present with nonspecific lower abdominal pain, diarrhea caused by irritation of the rectum, rectal pain, and urinary urgency caused by pressure on the bladder.

Diagnosis. An intraabdominal abscess should be suspected in a patient who has recently undergone abdominal surgery or has a history of bowel disease and now presents with abdominal pain, diaphragmatic symptoms, and fever. The nonimmunosuppressed patient will have a leukocytosis.

The location of intraabdominal abscess is often determined by history, symptoms, and localizing peritoneal signs. The abdominal peritoneum is segmentally innervated by the same nerves that also innervate muscles and skin (lower six thoracic and first lumbar nerves) overlying the abdomen. Irritation of the parietal abdominal peritoneum produces pain and abdominal rigidity reflecting the underlying pathology. It is important to remember that children who are receiving steroids or antibiotics may have minimal symptoms attributable to an intraabdominal abscess.

However, subphrenic, intermesenteric, and pelvic abscess may be difficult to diagnose because of their location, although certain signs may be helpful in determining their presence (Wilson, 1982a).

Subphrenic abscesses produce dyspnea; chest pain; and short, shallow breathing caused by pain on motion of the diaphragm. Decreased breath sounds and dullness to percussion at the lung base because of pleural effusion, atelectasis, pneumonitis, or empyema will often be present. Prominence of signs attributable to the chest often confuses the diagnosis. If the abscess is located between the liver and the diaphragm, referred shoulder pain may be present. An anteriorly located subphrenic abscess will produce upper abdominal tenderness and peritoneal signs. However, if the subphrenic abscess is in the lesser sac, it is posterior to the liver and, therefore, separated from the anterior abdominal wall. These patients will have upper and midabdominal pain that radiates to the back and no peritoneal signs until the abscess is very large. Patients with intermesenteric abscesses may have fever but often do not have localizing signs, although most of the patients will have a paralytic ileus with decreased bowel sounds and abdominal distention. Pelvic abscesses do not produce lower abdominal rigidity, because the pelvic parietal peritoneum is supplied by the obturator nerve (L2, 3, and 4), which does not innervate the overlying pelvic abdominal musculature. Therefore, on examination of the lower abdomen, there are few signs, although tenderness to deep palpation may be found. The most important part of the physical examination in a child with suspected pelvic infection is the rectal (or vaginal) exam. A bimanual exam permits palpation of a mass in the pelvis through the anterior abdominal wall and the rectum. A tender, bulging mass may be felt through the anterior rectal wall. Repeated daily rectal or vaginal exams may have to be done if it is unclear whether the patient has a pelvic abscess or an inflammatory mass without fluctuance.

Abscesses should be distinguished from other pathologic conditions that cause fever and vague abdominal pain. These include appendicitis, tumor or hematoma, salpingitis, and tuboovarian abscess.

Aerobic and anaerobic blood cultures should be obtained from any child with a suspected intraabdominal abscess and fever. Cultures obtained at the time of abscess drainage should be placed in a syringe that is tightly capped after removal of air and transported to the microbiology laboratory for anaerobic and aerobic culturing within 2 hours. Culture for fungus should also be done, because *Candida* species can be overgrown in the gut of a patient who has recently been on broad-spectrum antibiotics.

CT is a highly accurate radiologic procedure in determining the presence of an abscess (Knochel et al., 1980; Kuhn and Berger, 1980). Opacification of the bowel with oral contrast agent is important in distinguishing air-fluid levels in the GI tract from that in an abscess cavity. Water-soluble contrast agent should be used in cases of suspected leakage of intraluminal contents. Intravenous contrast helps distinguish abscess from hematoma by enhancing the abscess capsule, which should be used to distinguish these two entities. CT scanning has an added advantage in percutaneous drainage of an accessible abscess because of its excellent visualization of the abscess and the surrounding anatomy. MRI also gives exquisite anatomic detail without the requirement of contrast (Baker et al., 1985; Cammoun et al., 1985), but it may not be available at all healthcare facilities and is more costly. Young children often require sedation for either procedure.

The chest radiographs, anterior-posterior and lateral views, may be helpful in determining the presence of a subphrenic abscess. A basal pneumonic process, pleural effusion and fixed elevation of the diaphragm, and in advanced cases an air-fluid level below the diaphragm not attributable to the stomach air bubble may be present. Unfortunately, plain chest radiographs may lead to the misdiagnosis of a primary pneumonic process. The abdominal films may show bowel displacement only if an intermesenteric abscess is large.

Ultrasonography at the bedside is useful in those patients too ill to be transported to a CT scanner or those who require emergent diagnosis. Problems with ultrasonography include the requirement of the transducing probe to make contact with the skin, which may not be possible in patients who have recently undergone abdominal surgery, decreased resolution of the images because of the presence of bowel gas, and accuracy that to a great degree depends on the skill of the radiologist. For visualization of a pelvic abscess, the bladder must be filled to displace bowel loops from the pelvis.

Radionuclide scanning (Froelich and Krasicky, 1985) with gallium citrate or indium-111–labeled leukocytes is useful in determining the presence and location of an intraabdominal abscess. These tests, however, are not useful within the first 2 weeks after either a peritoneal infection or surgery, because the isotopes will localize to inflamed peritoneal and incisional areas. Problems with gallium citrate imaging are uptake of the isotope by certain tumors and excretion by the colon, potentially masking the presence of abscesses. Patient must be able to wait 48 to 72 hours for completion and interpretation of the images. Indium-111 has the advantages of not being excreted into the colon and reduced time for interpretation. However, labeled leukocytes must be able to retain their ability to accumulate at sites of inflammation.

Treatment. In addition to supportive therapy, treatment consists of administration of empiric antibiotics, followed by abscess drainage as soon as possible because most abscesses will not resolve with antibiotic treatment alone (Levison and Bush, 1995). The drainage procedure depends on the location and number of abscesses. Surgical exploration may be required if several abscesses are suspected or if they are inaccessible to percutaneous catheter drainage. Percutaneous drainage of intraabdominal abscesses may be possible in certain patients (Stanley et al., 1984; Pruitt and Simmons, 1988; Levison and Bush, 1995). The criteria for percutaneous drainage is precise definition of the abscess location and accessibility. Patients with ongoing signs of intraabdominal sepsis may require exploration of the abdomen to determine whether several abscesses or a continued source of bacterial contamination is present. Pelvic abscesses can be drained percutaneously through the anterior rectal wall or posterior vaginal vault. All septa within the abscess cavity must be disrupted and a drain placed in the abscess cavity so that complete drainage is achieved.

Empiric antibiotic regimen, such as metronidazole or clindamycin plus aminoglycoside or third-generation cephalosporin or monobactam will adequately cover aerobic and anaerobic bowel flora in the abscess (Solomkin et al., 1984; Levison and Bush, 1995). Imipenem/cilastin or ampicillin/sulbactam alone provides adequate coverage, providing the child is 12 years old or greater (Study Group of Intraabdominal Infections, 1986; Solomkin et al., 1990). The choice of antibiotics after abscess drainage should be determined by the organisms isolated at the time of drainage and their antibiotic susceptibilities. Recent hospitalization and antibiotic treatment increase the risk of infection with multiply resistant bacteria, as well as fungal agents, most often *Candida* spp.

Complications and Prognosis. Early diagnosis and treatment have improved the outcome of intraperitoneal abscesses (Saini et al., 1983). However, life-threatening complications of untreated intraperitoneal abscesses still occur. Extension of the abscess into an adjacent structure or perforation

of a hollow viscus can complicate abscesses. Subphrenic abscesses can rupture through the diaphragm into the pleural space or bronchus. Abscesses located in the pelvis can spread along various fascial planes, resulting in retroperitoneal and ischiorectal abscesses, as well as necrotizing infections in the buttocks, hips, and thighs. An abscess can serve as a source of ongoing intraabdominal sepsis, leading to septic shock, multiple system failure, and death. Infertility from adhesion formation may result from pelvic abscesses involving uterine tubes or ovaries.

Prolonged hospitalizations, occasionally greater than a month, are often required for the treatment of intraperitoneal abscesses (Altemeier et al., 1973). Rapid diagnosis, adequate drainage, and appropriate antibiotic therapy usually result in a favorable prognosis. Abscesses located in the subphrenic space, lesser sac, or pelvis carry a higher mortality because of delayed recognition and treatment.

Peritonitis

Anatomy and Physiology. The peritoneum encases the largest cavity in the body, with a surface area of about 1.7 m^2 in an adult, which is equivalent to that of the skin (Wilson et al., 1982). The peritoneum acts as a passive, semipermeable barrier to bidirectional diffusion of water and solutes and is well equipped to eliminate contaminated fluids from the peritoneal cavity. Normally the peritoneal membrane secretes several milliliters of sterile fluid, which lubricates the surface, allowing the intraperitoneal structures to slide past each other. Normal peritoneal fluid is serous in appearance with a solute concentration similar to that of plasma, a specific gravity of <1.016, protein content of <3 gm/dl, and few leukocytes.

Fluid and small contaminating particles within the peritoneal cavity are removed through stomata located in the peritoneal surface of the diaphragm (Wilson et al., 1982). These openings lead to lymphatics within the diaphragm that drain into substernal lymph nodes and ultimately into the thoracic duct. The flow of intraperitoneal fluid to the diaphragmatic lymphatics depends on flow of fluid upward toward the subphrenic spaces, movement of the diaphragm, and intraabdominal pressure. Diaphragmatic contraction and relaxation increase flow to the lymphatics, while general anesthesia and paralytic ileus decrease clearance of fluids.

The large surface area of the peritoneum and its ability to allow bidirectional diffusion of water and solutes has great physiologic implications in diffuse peritonitis. Injury to such a large, permeable surface area is comparable to that of an extensive burn to the skin and can lead to severe fluid losses with potentially fatal hemodynamic consequences.

Epidemiology. In the neonate, most cases of peritonitis are caused by perforation of the gut from a variety of conditions that cause bowel ischemia and/or perforation (Lister, 1991). These conditions include necrotizing enterocolitis, bowel obstruction caused by atresia or stenosis, meconium ileus or Hirschsprung's disease, and gastric or duodenal perforation. In the older child, peritonitis becomes more frequent because of the increased incidence of appendicitis. The adolescent female with gonococcal pelvic inflammatory disease may develop gonococcal peritonitis if direct extension to the peritoneum occurs.

An increased frequency of peritonitis occurs in patients undergoing peritoneal dialysis and in patients such as those with nephrotic syndrome or cirrhosis, who have decreased opsonic activity in preexisting ascitic fluid (Levison and Bush, 1995). Splenectomized children are at risk for the development of peritonitis with encapsulated bacteria. Primary (spontaneous) peritonitis in children may occur in both immunocompetent and immunocompromised children, although immunocompromised children are at greater risk.

Pathogenesis and Pathophysiology. Processes that introduce bacteria, foreign material, and fluid into the peritoneal cavity (bowel perforation) and prevent its clearing (diaphragmatic paralysis caused by general anesthesia) predispose to the development of peritonitis (Maddaus et al., 1988). Early responses of the peritoneum to infection include nonspecific inflammation that results in vasodilation, increased capillary permeability, edema, fluid transudation into the peritoneal cavity, and influx of neutrophils. Bacteria and their toxins are often absorbed via the lymphatics and capillaries, causing bacteria and toxemia. Accumulation of products such as complement, immunoglobulins, clotting factors, and fibrin occurs. The fibrin results in the eventual formation of adhesions, an attempt to localize infection.

As infection continues, massive fluid loss into the peritoneal cavity occurs because of extensive transudation of fluid from the plasma into the layer of peritoneal connective tissue, peritoneal cavity, and lumen of the paralytic bowel (third-space ef-

fect). An adult with untreated peritonitis can lose several liters of fluid in 24 hours, resulting in hemodynamic and electrolyte abnormalities that, if not corrected, can result in death.

Etiology. Infection of the peritoneal cavity secondary to rupture of an abdominal viscus most often involves aerobic and anaerobic bacteria found in the gastrointestinal tract.

Peritonitis in the neonate caused by rupture of an abdominal viscus involves those bacteria that colonize the gut of the neonate, which includes *E. coli, K. pneumoniae, Enterobacter* spp., *S. aureus* and *Candida* spp., as well as anaerobic bacteria such as *Clostridium* spp. and *B. fragilis* (Bell, 1985). In addition, *S. epidermidis* has been found in the peritoneal fluid in some infants with peritonitis associated with necrotizing enterocolitis (Mollitt et al., 1988). Peritonitis due to extension of omphalitis through the clotted umbilical vessels is predominantly caused by *S. aureus,* group A streptococci, *E. coli, K. pneumoniae,* and *P. mirabilis* (Brook, 1980a), although these infections can also be mixed aerobic and anaerobic infections and, less commonly, anaerobic alone. In neonates, the peritoneum can also be seeded during bacteremia with organisms such as group B streptococci (Chadwick et al., 1983).

Primary (spontaneous) peritonitis results from hematogenous spread of bacteria to the peritoneal cavity (Fowler, 1971; McDougal et al., 1975). In the young female child, it is monomicrobial, associated most often with *S. pneumoniae* and group A streptococci. Children with nephrotic syndrome develop peritonitis because of such organisms as staphylococci, streptococci, and gram-negative bacteria (Speck et al., 1974). Patients with cirrhosis may develop peritoneal infections with bowel flora such as *E. coli* and *Bacteroides* and *Clostridium* spp. Splenectomized children may develop peritonitis with encapsulated bacteria such as *H. influenzae* and pneumococcus. Immunosuppressed patients with lymphomas and leukemias and children who receive high-dose steroid treatment may develop peritonitis caused by gram-negative enteric bacteria, which include *Klebsiella, Enterobacter, Serratia,* and *Pseudomonas* spp., as well as streptococci, enterococci, *Candida* spp., and fungi. Gonococcal peritonitis can occur in the adolescent female if direct extension of gonococcal pelvic inflammatory disease to the peritoneum occurs.

Peritonitis occurring in the setting of peritoneal dialysis is often caused by skin flora, enteric bacteria, or environmental organisms (Rubin et al.,

1980; Powell et al., 1985). Most often *S. aureus,* coagulase-negative staphylococci, and streptococci are isolated from the dialysate fluid. Gram-negative bacteria such as *E. coli, Candida* spp., and, less commonly, atypical mycobacteria may also be found.

Clinical Manifestations. Peritonitis in the newborn usually occurs within the first few days of life, because most of the predisposing conditions, such as bowel obstruction, are present at birth. The diagnosis of peritonitis may be difficult because of the paucity of localizing signs. The neonate is ill appearing, often with hypothermia, vomiting, and abdominal distention. If gross contamination of the peritoneal cavity has occurred, inflammation of the abdominal wall may be present. Shock develops as the infection progresses. Signs and symptoms of the underlying condition will also be present.

In the older child, abdominal pain, nausea and vomiting, distention, high fever, and toxemia will be evident. Early in the disease process, diffuse abdominal guarding, rigidity and rebound tenderness, tympanitic abdomen, and decreased bowel sounds will be detected on physical examination. Rectal or vaginal examination will reveal signs of pelvic tenderness. Initially, the child with normal immune function will have leukocytosis, often greater than 20,000 cells/mm^3, with a predominance of neutrophils. However, as septic shock develops, low white blood cell count, anemia, and signs of disseminated intravascular coagulation are seen. Fluid and electrolyte abnormalities and decreased urine output because of "third spacing" will develop with disease progression. If untreated, metabolic acidosis caused by depression of cardiac function and vasoconstriction occurs. Eventually, capillary leak syndrome occurs, leading to pulmonary edema, decreased ventilatory ability and, eventually, ARDS.

In the adolescent female with gonococcal peritonitis, right upper quadrant tenderness caused by gonococcal perihepatitis (Fitz-Hugh–Curtis syndrome) will be present. Peritonitis caused by contamination of the dialysis catheter will be accompanied by cloudy peritoneal dialysate fluid and tachycardia, hyperventilation, and fever. Patients who are receiving high-dose steroid treatment or have severe neutropenia may not be febrile and may have little or no abdominal tenderness and rebound. These patients, however, will have decreased bowel activity and may have evidence of sepsis.

Diagnosis. Diagnosis of peritonitis is made by assessing clinical manifestations and physical findings. Plain radiographs, which should include upright, supine, and left lateral decubitus positions of the abdomen, may be helpful in demonstrating free air in the peritoneal cavity. Free air will be evident under the diaphragm in the upright film and between the right lobe of the liver and the right diaphragm in the left lateral decubitus film. A paralytic ileus, as well as fluid between bowel loops, may also be seen. CT and ultrasonography are helpful in determining the presence of increased peritoneal fluid.

Peritoneal fluid, obtained during paracentesis, laparotomy, or from the dialysis catheter in the patient undergoing continuous ambulatory peritoneal dialysis will be cloudy fluid and contain an abundance of neutrophils, if normal immune function is present, as well as bacteria (Schumer et al., 1964). Aerobic and anaerobic cultures of blood and peritoneal fluid should be obtained. Gram stain, stains for fungus, and acid fast bacilli of peritoneal fluid are often very helpful in determining empiric antibiotics. Mycobacteria cultures should be done if the patient is receiving peritoneal dialysis or has had exposure to an individual with tuberculosis. If tuberculous peritonitis is suspected, a peritoneal biopsy to search for granulomas and tuberculous organisms may be necessary if the peritoneal fluid does not yield the organism by special stain or culture. All organisms isolated should be tested for antimicrobial sensitivities.

Differential Diagnosis. In the neonate, abdominal processes, such as necrotizing enterocolitis, without spillage of bowel contents into the abdominal cavity, may be indistinguishable from peritonitis. Noninfectious processes that cause peritoneal irritation and abdominal pain can mimic peritonitis. These include meconium peritonitis in the neonate, familial Mediterranean fever, porphyria, lead toxicity, and chylous ascites.

Treatment. Treatment consists of prompt and aggressive correction of hemodynamic and respiratory abnormalities, determination of the source of peritoneal contamination, removal of contaminating intraperitoneal material and foreign bodies, débridement of necrotic tissue (which is essential), and institution of empiric antibiotics. Intraoperative peritoneal irrigation may be helpful in decreasing the intraperitoneal bacterial burden (Wilson, 1982b).

Empiric antimicrobials should be determined by the suspected source of contamination (i.e., secondary bacterial peritonitis, primary peritonitis, peritonitis secondary to contamination of an intraperitoneal foreign body [Gorbach, 1984]). Peritonitis caused by bowel contamination should be treated with antibiotics active against bowel flora. Previously hospitalized children who have developed peritonitis because of a ruptured abdominal viscus, however, may be colonized with highly drug-resistant nosocomial pathogens, such as *Pseudomonas* spp. or *Enterococcus* spp. The antibiotic resistance patterns for these pathogens at the medical institution should be obtained from the hospital epidemiology service, and children should be treated appropriately with agents active against these bacteria. In these cases, a combination of ceftazidime (coverage of resistant *Pseudomonas* spp. and other gram-negative bacilli), vancomycin and gentamicin (coverage *Enterococcus* spp. resistant to ampicillin), and clindamycin or metronidazole (anaerobic coverage) may be needed. Vancomycin, in addition to gentamicin and clindamycin, should be considered for empiric therapy for the neonate with necrotizing enterocolitis and peritonitis because of the incidence of *S. epidermidis* in neonatal peritonitis.

The child with primary peritonitis should be treated with antimicrobials that are active against the most likely organisms. For the immunocompetent child, the antimicrobial coverage should be active against staphylococci, streptococci, and gram-negative enteric organisms. An acceptable regimen is oxacillin and gentamicin or a third-generation cephalosporin. The immunocompromised child with primary peritonitis should have additional coverage of anaerobic bacteria and enterococci. In this case, ampicillin, gentamicin, or a third-generation cephalosporin and clindamycin is an acceptable choice. Vancomycin should be added to the antimicrobial regimen for the child with peritonitis secondary to peritoneal dialysis for additional coverage of methicillin-resistant staphylococci. Identification of fungi and yeast from peritoneal fluid by stain and culture should prompt treatment with amphotericin B. Acid fast bacilli identified in dialysate fluid may be treated initially with amikacin and cefoxitin. Treatment for tuberculous peritonitis should be instituted under the guidance of the infectious diseases service. Adjustments in the antimicrobial regimen should be made in all cases as soon as the identification and antibiotic sensitivities of the isolated organisms are known.

Complications and Prognosis. Peritonitis is a life-threatening condition that rapidly leads to septic shock, multiorgan system failure, intraabdominal abscesses requiring reoperation and repeat drainage procedures, postsurgical abdominal wound infection, and adhesions and prolonged hospital stay (Machiedo et al., 1985). The rapid institution of antibiotics, supportive therapy, and surgery for secondary bacterial peritonitis after bowel perforation has lead to a decrease in mortality from 70% to about 30%.

Primary peritonitis is associated with a mortality of less than 10% in children and 50% in neonates with the use of antibiotics. Immunocompromised patients have a high mortality because of the paucity of physical findings and difficulty in making the diagnosis of peritonitis, leading to delay in institution of appropriate treatment.

Acute Appendicitis

Epidemiology. Acute appendicitis is the most common acute surgical disease of the abdomen (Janik and Firor, 1979). Although it is found in children of all ages, it is rare during the first year of life. Approximately 4% of cases of appendicitis in children occur before the age of 3. The highest frequency of appendicitis is between ages 12 and 20.

Pathogenesis and Etiology. Obstruction of the appendiceal lumen is a major contributor to the development of appendicitis. Obstruction may be caused by fecaliths, concretions of fecal material, hypertrophy of the lymphoid tissue within the appendix because of a concurrent viral infection such as measles and adenovirus, ingested foreign material such as seeds of vegetables and fruits, and intestinal parasites such as *Ascaris,* pinworm *(Enterobius vermicularis)* and whipworm *(Trichuris trichiura).* Luminal obstruction results in the accumulation of mucosal secretions, which causes a rapid rise in intraluminal pressure, venous congestion, and compression of blood vessels that supply the distal appendix. Conditions result that favor multiplication of bacteria in the lumen and subsequent bacterial invasion and, potentially, rupture of the ischemic wall of the appendix. Appendiceal rupture and release of its intraluminal contents into the intraperitoneal cavity may occur in 10% of patients with acute appendicitis within the first 24 hours and in 50% within the first 48 hours after the onset of symptoms. Once rupture occurs, infection can spread to the pelvic recess and the right subhepatic space via the normal flow of peritoneal fluid.

The infection may be localized through the formation of adhesions between the cecum and the ileum, and migration of part of the greater omentum to the inflamed appendix, which wraps itself around the organ, localization of the infection, if appendicitis develops over a longer period of time, resulting in an inflammatory appendiceal phlegmon, and later, as the phlegmon matures, an abscess. Because the greater omentum is poorly developed in children less than 2 years of age, localization of infection may not occur.

Polymicrobial flora reflecting normal bowel flora are usually found within in the inflamed appendix and after appendiceal rupture. The organisms include *B. fragilis, Peptococcus* spp., *Peptostreptococcus* spp., *Fusobacterium* spp., *P. melaninogenicus, Clostridium spp., E. coli,* alpha- and gamma-hemolytic streptococci, enterococci, and *P. aeruginosa* (Brook, 1980a). *Streptococcus pneumoniae* has also been isolated from several cases of appendicitis (Heltber et al., 1984).

Clinical Manifestations. The presentation of appendicitis is influenced by the age of the child and the position of the appendix. The presentation in infants and toddlers is nonspecific, and the diagnosis is often not entertained because of infrequency in these age groups (Snyder and Chaffin, 1952). Infants usually present with an acute abdominal process with abdominal distention, fever, bilious vomiting, and diarrhea. A tender abdomen with guarding and, less commonly, erythema, edema, or cellulitis over the right lower quadrant with a palpable mass in that region will be found.

In the older child, colicky or diffuse abdominal pain is the most constant presentation of acute appendicitis. Appendicular distention results in pain that usually begins in the periumbilical or epigastric region, shifts to McBurney's point in the right lower quadrant within several hours, and becomes constant and severe. In some patients pain may begin in the right lower quadrant. Loss of appetite, nausea, and vomiting are common. Diarrhea or constipation and diarrhea are less common. Fever usually appears within 24 hours after the onset of pain. Shallow, rapid breathing may be present because of pain on diaphragmatic movement during respirations. Tenderness and guarding localized to the right iliac fossa are often present if the appendix is retrocecal, its most common position. The iliopsoas muscle also becomes irritated, causing the child to experience pain on extension of the right thigh when the patient is lying on the left side (psoas test). A tender, palpable mass in the right lower quadrant may be present if a localized abscess is forming around the appendix. Rebound tenderness is a reliable test to use if the diagnosis of appendicitis is unclear. A sudden decrease in abdominal pain that lasts about an hour is very ominous and indicates rupture of the appendix. If diffuse peritonitis results from rupture, generalized tenderness with guarding will be found.

Atypical presentations of appendicitis may occur if the inflamed appendix is directed downward to the pelvis. Early symptoms of appendiceal distention are present but the pain does not localize typically, often leading to delayed diagnosis. Pyuria and psoas irritation may be present when the appendix lies in the right iliac fossa. Pain does not localize in the right lower quadrant when the inflamed appendix is directed toward the pelvis, because it does not come in contact with the parietal peritoneum. However, epigastric pain is often present and will remain until appendiceal distention is relieved by perforation. The inflammed pelvic appendix may cause rectal irritation and bladder irritation, occasionally resulting in diarrhea and pyuria. In these cases it may be difficult to distinguish acute appendicitis from gastroenteritis or urinary tract infection. Rectal or vaginal examination is very helpful, revealing right pelvic tenderness and often a mass against the pelvic wall on the right. A positive obdurator test (rotation of the flexed thigh, especially internal rotation with pain referred to the hypogastrium) can be elicited because the obdurator internus muscle becomes irritated by the overlying inflamed appendix. Occasionally a retroileal appendicitis may not be revealed by localizing signs, and a laparotomy may need to be performed to confirm the diagnosis and avoid perforation of the appendix.

Diagnosis. Because the diagnosis of appendicitis is complicated by the nonspecific presentations of young children; atypical presentations in the older child; the wide variety of nonsurgical conditions that mimic appendicitis; and the lack of a definitive, diagnostic laboratory test, all children with abdominal pain greater than 6 hours should be carefully observed by the pediatrician for continued or worsening abdominal pain. Preliminary laboratory studies, such as white blood cell count and urinalysis, can be done in the physician's office and frequent contact with the patient should be made. Leukocytosis may not be helpful because it is present in only two thirds of cases of appendicitis, although pyuria with bacteriuria suggests a urinary tract infection. Pathologic conditions that need to be considered in the differential diagnosis of acute appendicitis (Knight and Vassay, 1981) include acute mesenteric adenitis, respiratory infections, renal disease, psoas abscess, hepatitis A and B, diseases of the terminal ileum, a variety of other abdominal surgical conditions, and diseases of the female genital tract. In the granulocytopenic child, necrotizing enterocolitis of the cecum (typhilitis or neutropenic enterocolitis) may also present with a picture similar to that of acute appendicitis.

Once the diagnosis of appendicitis is entertained, a surgical evaluation should be made in a timely manner. In cases of atypical presentation or in young children, CT imaging with oral soluble contrast will be very helpful in making the diagnosis of appendicitis (Shapiro et al., 1989). Appendiceal thickening and dilation and surrounding inflammation will be seen. In addition, CT imaging will allow differentiation of an appendiceal abscess from a phlegmon and will also provides accurate information on the location and extent of disease. The use of CT imaging for the detection of appendicitis, however, requires that the child be able to ingest contrast material so that the GI tract is adequately opacified. Other radiologic studies are less helpful. Plain abdominal radiographs may show a calcified appendicolith or a mass displacing the intestine, but they are usually nondiagnostic. Although a barium enema may show nonfilling of the appendix and extrinsic mass effect on the cecum, terminal ileum, and ascending colon, these findings may be caused by other pathologic processes involving the right side of the abdomen. High resolution ultrasonography with graded compression is highly sensitive and specific, but its accuracy is operator dependent and only a limited field can be visualized. Once appendiceal rupture has occurred and intraabdominal abscesses are suspected, both CT and ultrasonography provide a high accuracy and sensitivity in detection of abscesses. However, bowel gas and mesenteric fat decreases the ability of ultrasound to detect midabdominal abscesses (Mendelson and Lindsell, 1987).

Treatment. Treatment with an antibiotic regimen such as clindamycin, gentamicin, and ampicillin should begin immediately if perforation is suspected and should be continued for 5 to 10 days (Elmore et al., 1987) postoperatively. Appendectomy should be performed without delay for unruptured appendicitis or ruptured appendicitis with peritonitis. Aerobic and anaerobic culture results from specimens taken from the inflammed appendix, periappendiceal area, and peritoneal fluid obtained during surgery should guide the final choice of antibiotics. Perioperative prophylactic antibiotics to prevent wound infection (Busuttil et al., 1981; Winslow et al., 1983) such as clindamycin plus an aminoglycoside or third-generation cephalosporin or cefoxitin alone (Bauer et al., 1989) should be administered approximately 30 minutes before surgery (Bates et al., 1989) and discontinued in 24 hours in cases of unruptured appendicitis.

Management of appendiceal mass in children is controversial. Surgical removal of an appendiceal abscess results in a complication rate of 30% because of wound infection, fecal fistula, small bowel obstruction, prolonged ileus, and recurrent abscess (Bradley and Isaacs, 1978). Therefore, if infection is localized and there are no signs of peritonitis, conservative management, consisting of intravenous fluids, antibiotic therapy, and careful observation for signs of spread of infection, is often practiced (Skoubo-Kristensen and Hvid, 1982; Bagi et al., 1987). Appendectomy is performed 4 to 6 weeks later. Recently, percutaneous catheter drainage of appendiceal abscesses under ultrasound or CT guidance (Bagi et al., 1987; Shapiro et al., 1989) has been shown to be a safe and effective alternative to surgery or conservative management. Patients with an appendiceal phlegmon may also be managed conservatively (Skoubo-Kristensen and Hvid, 1982). These children are observed carefully, treated with intravenous antibiotic therapy until resolution of infection, and undergo appendectomy 2 to 3 months later.

Complications and Prognosis. Very few complications occur from unruptured appendicitis when surgical removal is performed without delay following the onset of symptoms. The mortality for acute appendicitis with prompt diagnosis and removal of the unruptured appendix is about 0.1% (Luckmann, 1989). However, unrecognized appendicitis leads to appendiceal perforation in 15% to 37% of children, resulting in diffuse peritonitis and intraperitoneal abscess formation (Janik and Firor, 1979) and adhesion formation. Generalized peritonitis with resulting multisystem failure carries a high mortality of up to 50%.

Bacteremia and fistula formation between the appendix and the bladder may occur if the appendix perforates. Portal vein thrombophlebitis with subsequent development of pyogenic liver abscesses and cholangitis may occur if appendicitis remains untreated. This complication, which carries a high mortality, is now very rare. Postoperative wound infections complicate surgical treatment of appendicitis with rates of 5% in cases of uncomplicated appendicitis, rising to 30% if rupture has occurred.

PYOGENIC LIVER ABSCESS
Epidemiology

Pyogenic liver abscess is a potentially life-threatening infection (Dehner and Kissane, 1969) that is, fortunately, uncommon. A recent study has shown an incidence in children of 25 per 100,000 hospital admissions (Pineiro-Carrero and Andres, 1989). Although children with immunosuppressive states (Pineiro-Carrero and Andres, 1989) such as chronic granulomatous disease, leukemia, liver transplantation (Kusne et al., 1988), and those who have had procedures such as hepaticojejunostomy or choledochojejunostomy (Ecoffey et al., 1987) for correction of biliary atresia or choledochal cysts are at higher risk of hepatic infection, many cases are cryptogenic (Ecoffey et al., 1987).

Pathogenesis

Bacteria may reach the liver by several different routes. Hematogenous spread of bacteria to the liver through the hepatic artery occurs during episodes of bacteremia (Dehner and Kissane, 1969). Bacteria can travel to the liver via the portal veins. This may occur in neonates who develop infection of the umbilical vein after omphalitis or umbilical vein catheterization (Brook, 1989b) or in older children with infectious or inflammatory diseases of the bowel such as appendicitis or Crohn's disease (regional enteritis). In the latter two cases, bacteria can reach the liver through the portal venous system. Liver abscesses may occur from contiguous spread of infection or via lymphatics from pathologic processes such as appendicitis. Infection of the liver may also occur after penetrating or blunt trauma to the liver.

Etiology

S. aureus is the most commonly isolated pathogen in childhood liver abscesses (Pineiro-Carrero and Andres, 1989; Arditi and Yogev, 1990). Gram-negative bacilli, including *E. coli, Klebsiella* spp., *Enterobacter* spp., *Pseudomonas* spp., *Proteus* spp., and anaerobes account for the majority of the remaining isolated pathogens (Brook, 1989b). Immunosuppressed patients may have multiple *candidal* microabscesses (Sobel, 1988). Amebic liver abscess should be considered in a patient with liver abscess, because, worldwide, liver abscess is more frequently caused by infection with *Entamoeba histolytica* than bacteria. Although uncommon, hydatid cysts in liver caused by infection with *Echinococcus* may also be responsible for nonpyogenic hepatic abscesses in the appropriate clinical setting.

Clinical Manifestations

Patients often present with nonspecific signs and symptoms, making the diagnosis of liver abscess difficult. Children with solitary liver abscesses may have a subacute course, whereas those with multiple hepatic abscesses often have spiking fevers, chills, nausea, vomiting, anorexia, malaise, and weakness. Hepatomegaly and liver tenderness may be present. Abscesses located in the right lobe may cause pleuritic pain.

Diagnosis

Blood cultures may be positive in patients with liver abscesses. Alkaline phosphatase is usually elevated and, less commonly, liver transaminases. Nonspecific laboratory abnormalities include leukocytosis, anemia, and an elevated erythrocyte sedimentation rate. Sensitive radiologic imaging techniques that can be employed are CT or MRI scanning, ultrasonography, and radioisotopic scanning (Pineiro-Carrero and Andres, 1989). Crohn's disease should be considered in any nonimmunosuppressed child who presents with liver abscess (Teague et al., 1988).

Treatment

Antimicrobial therapy and drainage of pyogenic liver abscesses are both required for a good outcome (Gerzof et al., 1985; McCorkell and Niles, 1985). Drainage may be achieved by ultrasound or CT-guided percutaneous catheter placement (Do et al., 1991), although a poor clinical response after percutaneous drainage will require an open drainage procedure (Barnes et al., 1987).

Empiric antibiotics should be directed at the expected organisms. Coverage for *S. aureus*, gram-negative bacilli, and anaerobes should be provided and tailored after microbiologic examination of the abscess aspirate. Antibiotics, such as mezlocillin and cefoperazone, that have increased bile penetration should be used in combination with oxacillin and metronidazole or clindamycin. Extended antibiotic treatment of 4 to 6 weeks is often necessary (Barnes et al., 1987). Response should be monitored by ultrasonography, CT, or MRI scanning. Antifungal therapy should be considered in immunosuppressed patients.

Complications and Prognosis

Improved diagnostic techniques and percutaneous drainage procedures have markedly decreased the mortality of pyogenic liver abscesses. Morbidity and mortality, however, remain high in neonates (Brook, 1989b), in children who have serious underlying disease, and in those whose diagnosis has been delayed.

SPLENIC ABSCESS
Epidemiology

Splenic abscesses are uncommon in a healthy individual. Conditions in the spleen that predispose to abscess formation are necrosis caused by embolic phenomenon or hematoma caused by trauma. Disease states such as sickle cell anemia can cause bland infarcts within the spleen, and endocarditis or sepsis originating in a distant site can send infected emboli to the spleen (Chun et al., 1980). Patients with an immunodeficiency that prevents the spleen from performing its normal role of clearing organisms are also predisposed to splenic infection. An enlarging spleen that develops subcapsular infarcts can be seeded by pathogenic organisms.

Pathogenesis and Etiology

Infection can reach the spleen by several different routes. The most common route is hematogenous seeding of organisms from a remote site via the splenic artery. Bacteria from remote sites seed and proliferate with the areas of infarct or hematoma. In about 75% of patients with infection of the spleen, multiple abscesses are found in other organs (Simson, 1980), including the liver, brain, and kidneys.

Streptococci and staphylococci are the most common bacteria isolated from splenic abscesses. *Salmonella* spp. can cause splenic abscesses in patients with diseases that predispose to splenic infarction (such as sickle cell anemia) and decreased phagocytic and opsonizing ability. *M. tuberculosis* reaches the spleen during the initial lymphohematogenous spread. In children with hematologic malignancies, fungi, most commonly *Candida* and *Aspergillus* spp., may enter the spleen during periods of fungemia, resulting in microabscesses. Bacteria in splenic abscesses that result from extension of a subphrenic abscess will reflect the aerobic and anaerobic organisms found in that abscess. Rarely, splenic abscesses can be caused by *Brucella* spp.

Clinical Manifestations

Splenic microabscesses that are deep within the spleen often have few manifestations directly attributable to infection of the spleen. Localizing signs such as left-sided pleuritic pain in the lower chest, upper abdomen, or costovertebral angle and pain that radiates to the left shoulder occur only after splenic abscesses enlarge, producing splenomegaly and splenic capsule irritation.

Most patients will be febrile and may have left upper quadrant tenderness. In advanced disease, cachexia, tachycardia, and constant pain may be present. In many cases, extracting symptoms caused by splenic abscess from those of the underlying disease state may be difficult.

Diagnosis

The diagnosis of splenic abscess should be considered in any patient with a history of fever and left chest, upper abdominal, flank, or shoulder pain, especially in the setting of splenic trauma (Sands et al., 1986), abnormal heart valves, sickle cell anemia, or any other conditions that predispose to splenic infection.

Leukocytosis is often present, unless neutropenia from an underlying disease is present. Blood cultures for aerobic and anaerobic bacteria or fungi may yield organisms if the splenic abscess is serving as a source of continued bacteremia or fungemia. A rise in *Brucella* serum antibody titers suggests brucellosis. Aerobic, including *Brucella* spp., anaerobic, acid-fast bacilli, and fungal cultures of splenic abscesses may reveal the etiology and suggest the primary source of infection.

Ultrasonography, CT, and MRI are the most sensitive radiologic procedures for the detection of splenic abscesses. On CT scan, splenic abscesses can be seen as focal lesions with lower density than the surrounding tissue. Splenic lesions caused by fungi, tuberculosis, and brucellosis each have a characteristic appearance on CT (Berlow et al., 1984). In addition, CT can be used to determine the presence of other intraabdominal foci of infection.

Treatment

Until the infecting organism(s), the source, and extrasplenic foci of infection have been determined, empiric intravenous antibiotics should be started promptly after blood cultures are obtained. The patient's clinical history and presentation will be helpful in determining which antibiotics to use. Splenic abscess after development of an intraabdominal abscess should be treated with antibiotics that are active against bowel flora, whereas those occurring after trauma should be treated with an agent that provides coverage of *S. aureus* and streptococci. Once the microbial etiology has been determined, antimicrobial treatment should be directed against these organisms. For patients with a hematologic malignancy, fungal disease and antifungal therapy with amphotericin B should be considered.

CT-guided catheter drainage of splenic abscesses may be an effective method of diagnosis and treatment, although splenectomy has been the treatment of choice for an isolated splenic abscess (Berkman et al., 1983; Lerner and Spataro, 1984).

Complications and Prognosis

Although most splenic abscesses remain localized in the spleen, intermittent bacteremia caused by release of the organisms from the infected splenic focus can occur, leading to seeding of other distant sites. Rupture of abscesses into the pleural space through the diaphragm, causing a thoracic empyema, or into the abdomen, causing a subphrenic abscess or generalized peritonitis, can occur. Hemorrhage into an abscess cavity may also complicate these abscesses. Untreated splenic abscesses carry a grave mortality because of the many serious complications and underlying disease (Linos et al., 1983). Solitary splenic abscess carries a more favorable prognosis, because two thirds of these patients have lesions confined to the spleen.

RETROPERITONEAL ABSCESS
Epidemiology

Retroperitoneal abscesses are uncommon in both the adult and pediatric population but carry a high mortality because of the difficulty in diagnosis and delay in treatment (Neuhof and Arheim, 1944; Altemeier and Alexander, 1961).

Anatomy and Pathogenesis

The retroperitoneum is a complex anatomic region consisting of potential spaces located between the posterior parietal peritoneum and the posterior part transversalis fascia (Simons et al., 1983). This space extends superiorly to the undersurface of the diaphragm and inferiorly to the pelvic rim. The lateral borders of the retroperitoneum extend to the margins of the lateral borders of the quadratus lumborum muscles.

The retroperitoneum is anatomically divided into three potential spaces, the space anterior to the kidneys (the anterior retroperitoneal or pararenal space), the perirenal space, and the space posterior to the kidneys (the posterior retroperitoneal or pararenal space). The anterior retroperitoneal space, located between the posterior peritoneum and the fascia that surrounds the kidney anteriorly, contains the retroperitoneal portions of the duodenum, ascending and descending colon, pancreas, and retrocecally located appendix. Thus, infection involving any of these organs and viscera may cause retroperitoneal abscesses (Altemeier and Alexander, 1961; Evans et al., 1971; Sheinfeld et al., 1987). In addition, anatomic communications between the perirenal space and the psoas space, between the posterior retroperitoneal space and the lateral abdominal wall, and between adjacent retroperitoneal compartments allow the spread of infection to and from the retroperitoneal space.

Etiology

Retroperitoneal abscesses resulting from perinephric infection may be caused by *S. aureus* or gram-negative organisms such as *E. coli* and *Proteus* spp. (Altemeier and Alexander, 1961). Abscesses following appendiceal perforation will contain anaerobic and aerobic bowel flora.

Clinical Manifestations

Patients with retroperitoneal infections have few localizing symptoms and are often ill out of proportion to the complaints and physical findings. Fever; chills; nonlocalized abdominal pain; flank pain; abdominal distention; weakness and pain in the ipsilateral hip, thigh, or knee; and psoas spasm may be present (Altemeier and Alexander, 1961). Symptoms may be present for weeks before a diagnosis is made. The chronicity of illness often results in anorexia, weight loss, and malaise.

Diagnosis

On physical examination, a tender mass, representing the abscess if sufficiently large, as well as flank tenderness, may be present. If the psoas space is involved, the child will have pain on extension of the ipsilateral thigh (psoas sign). Leukocytosis with a left shift is usually present and, if the disease is long standing, anemia of chronic disease. If a perinephric abscess is present, proteinuria, pyuria, and bacteriuria may be seen (Altemeier and Alexander, 1961). Anaerobic and aerobic blood cultures may be positive if the abscess is seeding the blood.

CT (Gerzof and Gale, 1982; Simons et al., 1983) and MRI imaging provide precise anatomic localization of retroperitoneal abscesses. If not available, other less helpful imaging studies may be used. Plain x-rays may show an abnormal psoas shadow, scoliosis, and, if present, gas within the abscess. An abnormal intravenous pyelogram will determine if the kidneys are involved. Radioisotopic imaging allows localization of an infectious process but entails a delay in the diagnosis (Simons et al., 1983). Ultrasonography is useful in establishing the presence of an abscess, especially in a child who is too ill to be taken to a CT or MRI scanner (Gerzof and Gale, 1982).

Treatment

The ill-appearing patient should be treated with antibiotics such as oxacillin, clindamycin, and gentamicin that have activity against *S. aureus,* gramnegative organisms, and anaerobic bowel flora.

Surgical (Altemeier and Alexander, 1961) or CT-guided drainage (Gerzof and Gale, 1982) should be performed, and abscess material should be cultured for aerobic and anaerobic organisms. Parenteral antibiotics should be directed against the isolated organisms and should be continued for 2 to 3 weeks after drainage. The underlying conditions leading to abscess should be determined and corrected.

Complications and Prognosis

Abscesses can rupture into the intraperitoneal space and can extend long distances along the fascial plane superiorly to the subdiaphragmatic space, mediastinum, and thoracic cavity; laterally to the anterior abdominal wall and subcutaneous tissue of the flank; and inferiorly to the thigh, hip, and psoas muscle (Altemeier and Alexander, 1961). These complications are now rarely seen because of improved diagnostic techniques and earlier intervention. The prognosis is favorable in those retroperitoneal infections that are treated early. Diagnostic delays often result in complications that confer higher morbidity and mortality.

PSOAS ABSCESS
Epidemiology

Psoas abscesses, either primary or secondary to extension from an adjacent focus, are uncommon infections in children. Primary infection of the psoas muscle occurs more often in male children younger than age 15 (Stephenson et al., 1991).

Anatomy and Pathogenesis

The psoas muscle is the major muscle of the anterior wall of the back (Gordin et al., 1983). It is invested in fascia and contains fibers that originate from the transverse processes of the twelfth tho-

racic vertebra and the five lumbar vertebrae and courses inferiorly through the crura of the diaphragm on either side of the vertebral column to merge with the iliacus muscle (Simons et al., 1983; Bresee and Edwards, 1990). The iliopsoas muscle then crosses the sacroiliac joint and passes beneath the inguinal ligament and inserts into the lesser trochanter of the femur. Over its long course from the mediastinum to the femur, it makes contact with or is in close proximity to several key anatomic structures that include the iliacus muscle, sacroiliac joint, inguinal ligament, inguinal lymph nodes, hip joint, and trochanteric bursa. The psoas muscle is also in direct communication with the posterior retroperitoneal (pararenal) space. Thus the psoas muscle can provide a pathway for and be involved in inflammatory processes of mediastinum, the thigh, and the posterior retroperitoneal space.

In children, primary infection of psoas abscesses occurs far more frequently than those caused by a secondary source (Bresee and Edwards, 1990). Often no source of a psoas abscess can be found in children, suggesting that psoas abscess may result from hematogenous seeding of the muscle from a skin or upper respiratory infection (Firor, 1972; Stephenson et al., 1991). Secondary infection of the psoas muscle may occur following retrocecal appendiceal rupture, Crohn's disease, or a perirenal abscess. In addition, infectious process such as vertebral osteomyelitis and discitis involving the twelfth thoracic vertebra and the five lumbar vertebrae areas, septic arthritis of the sacroiliac joint, and osteomyelitis of the ileum can perforate the psoas fascia and cause a psoas abscess (von Dyke et al., 1987). Suppurating bacterial infection of the inguinal nodes has also been reported to extend to the underlying psoas muscle (Maull and Sachatello, 1974).

Etiology

Before the decreasing incidence of tuberculous infection of the spine, Pott's disease, psoas abscesses were often caused by *M. tuberculosis* (Schwaitzberg et al., 1985). Currently, *S. aureus* is the most commonly isolated pathogen from primary psoas abscesses (Firor, 1972; Stephenson et al., 1991) and abscesses originating from vertebral, sacroileal, and many perirenal infections. However, if the primary source of the psoas abscess is from a perirenal infection caused by obstructive pyelonephritis, gram-negative bacteria such as *E. coli* and *Proteus* spp. may be isolated. Aerobic and anaerobic bowel flora may be found in psoas abscesses that occur following perforations of retroperitoneal abdominal structures (Bresee and Edwards, 1990).

Clinical Manifestations

The symptoms of psoas abscess are often vague because of the posterior location of the psoas muscle. The child often has fever and anorexia and weight loss if the infection is chronic. A history of a limp or decreased use of the leg is often reported and the child may complain of pain in the abdomen, flank, back, iliac fossa, over the groin, and in the thigh, in addition to psoas muscle pain. On examination, the child is often found to keep the ipsilateral hip in flexion and externally rotated because this position releases tension of the psoas muscle. Scoliosis, caused by the child leaning toward the side of the infected psoas muscle in an attempt to relieve the pain, is also often seen. Pain on straight leg raising can be elicited, and a tender mass may often be felt in the iliac fossa (Bresee and Edwards, 1990).

Diagnosis

The neutrophil count and erythrocyte sedimentation rate are often elevated. An abnormal urinalysis may be found if the child has renal disease. Sterile pyuria may be seen on occasion, however, without renal disease because the ureter, which lies over the psoas muscle, may become ureteral inflamed. Blood cultures are often positive in children with primary psoas abscesses. If a history of TB exposure is elicited, skin testing with PPD and an anergy control panel should be performed and a chest x-ray should be obtained.

Plain radiographs of the abdomen may show nonspecific signs of infection that include a bulging or obliterated psoas shadow and scoliosis. If the infection has originated from the vertebral column, bony changes may be seen. An IVP may show medial deviation of the lower third of the ureter on the affected side. Radioisotopic scanning with gallium or indium-labeled white blood cells are helpful in localizing the lesion, but there is a delay in obtaining results, especially with gallium scanning. Ultrasonography may show changes in the psoas muscle consistent with abscess CT with intravenous contrast (Lee and Glaser, 1986) and MRI (Gordin et al., 1983; Lee and Glaser, 1986; Stephenson et al., 1991) scans are the most powerful radiographic tools available for detection of psoas abscesses. They provide the clearest anatomic details of the psoas muscle and surrounding tissues and allow detection of infection from an adjacent organ.

The differential diagnosis of psoas abscess is broad and includes septic hip, osteomyelitis of the femoral head or ileum, sacroiliitis, vertebral osteomyelitis (pyogenic or tuberculous), discitis, paraspinal abscess and retroperitoneal abscess, noninfectious diseases such as Perthes' disease, hip dislocation, and tumor.

Treatment

Febrile and ill-appearing children with psoas abscess should be treated with antibiotics that are active against the most common organisms associated with these abscesses. The antibiotics should provide coverage for *S. aureus,* gram-negative bacilli, and anaerobic bowel flora until further microbiologic data and information on the possible source of infection are available. An appropriate initial antibiotic regimen is oxacillin, gentamicin, and clindamycin. Drainage of the psoas muscle abscess, either surgically or by CT-guided percutaneous aspiration (Gordin et al., 1983; Mueller et al., 1984), may be necessary for microbiologic diagnosis or if the patient does not respond to empiric antibiotic treatment. Parenteral antibiotics directed against the organisms isolated from the blood and abscess should be continued for 2 to 3 weeks after defervescence or drainage (Gordin et al., 1983). An underlying source of secondary psoas abscesses should be sought and corrected.

Complications and Prognosis

Infection from psoas abscess may rarely extend anteriorly into the retrofascial space or spread within the fascial plane of the psoas muscle, resulting in vertebral or hip osteomyelitis. With early diagnosis and treatment, a favorable outcome of uncomplicated psoas abscesses is expected. However, delayed detection and treatment or psoas disease that has been caused by extension of infection at another site has a less favorable prognosis.

ANORECTAL ABSCESSES
Epidemiology

Anorectal abscesses occur more frequently in males and children under 2 years of age, with the greatest incidence in neonates and infants (Arminski and Mclean, 1965). Although the incidence of anorectal abscesses in children is not known, one large study showed that 2.5% of children with proctologic disease had an anorectal abscess (Mentzer, 1956). Immunosuppression and neutropenia increase the risk of developing anorectal abscesses (Arditi and Yogev, 1990). Children with ulcerative colitis and Crohn's disease, diabetes mellitus, chronic granulomatous disease, recent rectal surgery, and high-dose steroids are also at risk for this disease (Arditi and Yogev, 1990).

Pathogenesis

Anorectal abscesses may occur by extension of bacteria through the normally intact mucosal barrier (Arditi and Yogev, 1990). Small tears, abrasions, or fissures in the anal mucosa that may occur during bouts of diarrhea or constipation result in the invasion of bowel organisms through the anal mucosa. Infection within the anal canals can lead to abscess formation anywhere along the path of the anal ducts from the anal mucosa to the intersphincteric space. Disease can extend laterally through the external sphincter muscle into the fat contained within the ischiorectal fossa (Howard, 1987) or inferiorly to form a perianal abscess, which may exit via a fistula-in-ano at the anal skin (Arditi and Yogev, 1990). Infection can also spread superiorly to the space between the internal sphincter and the levator ani, a space that lies just inferiorly to the pelvic peritoneum.

Etiology

The majority of anorectal abscesses contain multiple organisms with a predominance of anaerobic bacteria. The most frequently isolated bacteria include *Bacteroides* spp., *P. melaninogenicus, Peptostreptococcus* spp., *E. coli, K. pneumoniae,* and *S. aureus* (Brook and Martin, 1980; Arditi and Yogev, 1990).

Clinical Manifestations

Abscess location influences the clinical presentation of anorectal abscesses. The older child with a superficial abscess (perianal abscess) usually complains of pain when sitting and walking, may refuse to walk or may have an abnormal gait, and will have redness and swelling in the perianal area. An enlarging perianal abscess may produce pain with defecation, coughing, and sneezing. However, abscesses located in the deeper anorectal tissue, such as those in the ischiorectal fossa or in the pelvirectal region, often have poorly localized, deep, throbbing pain and are often associated with rigors, fever, malaise, decreased appetite, and lower abdominal pain.

On physical examination, perianal abscesses present as erythematous, tender, indurated regions near the anus with fluctuance. Digital exam will reveal no pain in the anal canal beyond the superficial lesion. It is important to distinguish early perianal abscess formation from cellulitis of the perianal skin caused by group A beta-hemolytic streptococci and hidradenitis suppurativa, because these diseases do not require surgical treatment. Perianal abscesses should also be distinguished from an anorectal fistula that extends from the anorectal abscess. These fistulous tracts, located in the perianal region, discharge pus or mucus into the anorectal canal and are important clues to the presence of a deeper abscess. Often deep abscesses are difficult to detect. Aside from a fistulous tract, often the only evidence of these abscesses is brawny edema of the perianal area on the affected side and a tender mass deep to the rectal wall on rectal examination. Because of diagnostic and treatment delay, these patients are often febrile and ill appearing by the time the diagnosis is made.

Diagnosis

Elevation of the white blood cell count is usually present unless the child is neutropenic. Bacteremia may be present in children with signs of systemic toxicity. Imaging studies are usually not indicated in children with abscesses detectable by rectal exam. However, in systemically ill children who are thought to have deep abscesses, CT imaging will be helpful in the diagnosis.

Treatment

Patients should be treated empirically with antibiotics that are active against aerobic and anaerobic bowel flora and *S. aureus.* A combination of clindamycin plus an aminoglycoside will provide coverage for these organisms (Arditi and Yogev, 1990).

Prompt surgical drainage or aspiration of the abscess is the required treatment of these lesions, even if local fluctuance is not palpable, in the immunocompetent child (Arditi and Yogev, 1990). Material obtained from drainage or aspiration of the abscesses should be sent for Gram stain and aerobic and anaerobic culture. Culture results should guide further antibiotic therapy.

Treatment of anorectal abscesses in the immunocompromised host remains controversial. A parenteral antibiotic regimen described earlier can be given initially to those immunocompromised patients who do not have fluctuance, extensive infection, or sepsis. Incision and drainage, however, may be necessary if there is disease progression (Shaked et al., 1986; Arditi and Yogev, 1990).

Complications and Prognosis

A 40% complication rate results from anorectal abscesses but is much higher in immunocompromised children because of their underlying disease and inability to localize infection (Glenn et al., 1988). Complications include development of anorectal fistulae, recurrence of the abscess, and bacteremia (Arditi and Yogev, 1990). Fistulae may develop even with appropriate surgical and antibiotic treatment. Less commonly, life-threatening septicemia and necrotizing fasciitis can occur (Howard, 1987), especially in the immunocompromised host (Glenn et al., 1988).

BIBLIOGRAPHY

Adams J, et al. Fournier's gangrene in children. Urology 1990;35:439.

Altemeier W, Alexander JW. Retroperitoneal abscess. Arch Surg 1961;83:512-524.

Altemeier W, Culbertson WR, Fuller W, Shook C. Intra-abdominal abscesses. Am J Surg 1973;125:70-79.

Arditi M, Yogev R. Perirectal abscess in infants and children: report of 52 cases and review of literature. Pediatr Infect Dis J 1990;9:411-415.

Arminski T, Mclean DW. Proctologic problems in children. JAMA 1965;194:137-139.

Bagi P, Dueholm S, Karstrup S. Percutaneous drainage of appendiceal abscess. Dis Colon Rectum 1987;30:352.

Baker H, Berquist TN, Kispert DB, et al. Magnetic resonance imaging in a routine clinical setting. Mayo Clin Proc 1985;60:75-90.

Barker F, et al. Streptococcal necrotizing fasciitis: comparison between histological and clinical features. J Clin Pathol 1987;40:335-341.

Barnes P, DeLock KM, Reynolds TN, et al. A comparison of amebic and pyogenic abscess of the liver. Medicine 1987;66:472-483.

Bates T, et al. Timing of prophylactic antibiotics in abdominal surgery. Br J Surg 1989;76:52-56.

Bauer T, et al. Antibiotic prophylaxis in acute nonperforated appendicitis. Ann Surg 1989;209:307-311.

Baxter C. Surgical management of soft tissue infections. Surg Clin North Am 1972;52:1483-1499.

Bell MJ. Peritonitis in the newborn—current concepts. Pediatr Clin North Am 1985;32:1181-1201.

Berkman W, Harris SA, Bernadina MER. Nonsurgical drainage of splenic abscesses. AJR 1983;141:395-396.

Berlow M, Spirt BA, Weil J. CT follow-up of hepatic and splenic fungal microabscesses. J Comput Assist Tomogr 1984;8:42-45.

Bessman A, Wagner W. Nonclostridial gas gangrene. JAMA 1975;233:958.

Bornstein D, Weinberg AN, Swartz MN, et al. Anaerobic infections: a review of current experience. Medicine 1964;43:207.

Bradley J. Neonatal infections. Pediatr Infect Dis 1985;4:315-320.

Bradley E, Isaacs J. Appendiceal abscess revisited. Arch Surg 1978;113:130.

Bresee J, Edwards MS. Psoas abscess in children. Pediatr Infect Dis J 1990;9:201-206.

Britt R, Enzmann DR. Clinical stages of human brain abscesses on serial CT scans after contrast infusion. Computerized tomographic, neuropathological, and clinical correlations. J Neurosurg 1983;59:972-989.

Britt R, Enzmann DR, Yeager AS. Neuropathological and computerized tomographic findings in experimental brain abscess. J Neurosurg 1981;55:590-603.

Brook I. Aerobic and anaerobic bacteriology of intracranial abscesses. Pediatr Neurol 1992;8:210-214.

Brook I. Anaerobic bacteremia in children. Am J Dis Child 1980a;143:1052.

Brook I. Anaerobic infections in children with neurological impairments. Am J Ment Retard 1995;99:579-594.

Brook I. Bacterial studies of peritoneal cavity and postoperative wound drainage following perforated appendix in children. Ann Surg 1980b;192:208-212.

Brook I. Microbiology of infected epidermal cysts. Arch Dermatol 1989a;125:1658.

Brook I. Microbiology of intraabdominal abscesses in children. Am J Dis Child 1987;141:1148.

Brook I. Pediatric anaerobic infection, ed. 2. St. Louis: Mosby, 1989b.

Brook I, Frazier EH. Aerobic and anaerobic bacteriology of wounds and cutaneous abscesses. Arch Surg 1990;125:1445-1451.

Brook I, Martin WJ. Aerobic and anaerobic bacteriology of perirectal abscess in children. Pediatrics 1980;66:282-284.

Brook I, et al. Recovery of anaerobic bacteria from pediatric patients: a one-year experience. Am J Dis Child 1979;133:1020.

Bryan L, Van Den Elzen HM. Streptomycin accumulation in susceptible and resistant strains of *Escherichia coli* and *Pseudomonas aeruginosa*. Antimicrob Agents Chemother 1976;9:928.

Busuttil R, et al. Effect of prophylactic antibiotics in acute nonperforated appendicitis: a prospective, randomized, double-blind clinical study. Ann Surg 1981;194:502.

Cammoun D, Hendee WR, Davis KA. Clinical application of magnetic resonance imaging—current status. West J Med 1985;143:793-803.

Chadwick E, Shulman S, Yogev R. Peritonitis as a late manifestation of group B streptococcal disease in newborns. J Pediatr Infect Dis 1983;2:142.

Chun C, Johnson JD, Hofstetter M, Raff M. Brain abscess, a study of 45 consecutive cases. Medicine 1986;65:415-431.

Chun C, Raff LJ, Contreras L, et al. Splenic abscess. Medicine 1980;59:50.

Citron D, Goldstein EJC, Kenner MA, et al. Activity of ampicillin/sulbactam, ticarcillin/clavulanate, clarithromycin, and eleven other antimicrobial agents against anaerobic bacteria isolated from infections in children. Clin Infect Dis 1995;20(suppl 2):S356-S360.

Cruse P, Foord R. A five year prospective study of 23,649 surgical wounds. Arch Surg 1976;107:206.

Darke S, King AM, Slack WK. Gas gangrene and related infection: classification, clinical features and aetiology, management and mortality. A report of 88 cases. Br J Surg 1977;64:104-112.

Dehner L, Kissane JM. Pyogenic hepatic abscesses in infancy and childhood. J Pediatr 1969;74:763-773.

Dineen P. A critical study of 100 consecutive wound infections. Surg Gynecol Obstet 1961;113:91-96.

Do H, Lambiase RE, Deyoe L, et al. Percutaneous drainage of hepatic abscesses: comparison of results in abscesses with and without intrahepatic biliary communication. Am J Roentgenol 1991;157:1209-1212.

Donald F. Treatment of brain abscess. J Antimicrob Chemother 1990;25:310.

Dunkle L, Brotherton MS, Feigin RD. Anaerobic infections in children: a prospective study. Pediatrics 1976;57:311.

Ecoffey C, Rothman E, Bernard O, et al. Bacterial cholangitis after surgery for biliary atresia. J Pediatr 1987;111:824-829.

Elmore J, Dibbins AW, Curci MR. The treatment of complicated appendicitis in children: what is the gold standard? Arch Surg 1987;122:424.

Evans J, Meyers MA, Bosniak MA. Acute renal and perirenal infections. Semin Roentgenol 1971;6:274-291.

Fairbanks P, Milmoe GJ. The diagnosis and management of sinusitis in children. Complications and sequelae: an otolaryngologist's perspective. Pediatr Infect Dis 1985;4(suppl 6): 375-379.

Falcone P, Pricolo VE, Edstrom LE. Necrotizing fasciitis as a complication of chicken pox. Clin Pediatr 1988;27:339.

Farmer T, Wise GR. Subdural empyema in infants, children, and adults. Neurology 1973;23:254.

Finegold S, et al. Management of anaerobic infections. Ann Intern Med 1985;83:375-389.

Finland M, McGowan JE Jr. Nosocomial infections in surgical patients. Arch Surg 1976:143.

Firor H. Acute psoas abscess in children. Clin Pediatr 1972;11:228-231.

Fischbein C, Rosenthal A, Fischer EG, et al. Risk factors for brain abscess in patients with congenital heart disease. Am J Cardiol 1981;34:97-102.

Forster M, et al. A randomized comparative study of sulbactam plus ampicillin vs metronidazole plus cefotaxime in the management of acute appendicitis in children. Rev Infect Dis 1986;8(suppl 5):S634-S638.

Fowler R. Primary peritonitis: changing aspects 1956-1970. Aust Paediatr J 1971;7:73-83.

Foy P, Skarr M. Cerebral abscesses in children after pencil-tip injuries. Lancet 1980;2:662-663.

Froelich J, Krasicky GA. Radionuclide imaging of abdominal infections. Curr Concepts Diagn Nucl Med 1985;2:12-16.

Fromm D, Silen W. Postoperative clostridial sepsis of the abdominal wall. Am J Surgery 1969;118:517-520.

Garfield J. Management of supratentorial intracranial abscess: a review of 200 cases. Br Med J 1969;2:7-11.

Gerzof S, Johnson WC, Robbins AH, et al. Intrahepatic pyogenic abscesses: treatment by percutaneous drainage. Am J Surg 1985;149:487-494.

Gerzof S, Gale ME. Computed tomography and ultrasonography for diagnosis and treatment of renal and retroperitoneal abscesses. Urol Clin North Am 1982;9:185-193.

Glenn J, Cotton D, Wesley R, Pizzo P. Anorectal infections in patients with malignant diseases. Rev Infect Dis 1988;10: 42-52.

Goldstein E. Bite wounds and infection. Clin Infect Dis 1992;14:633-640.

Gorbach SL. Antimicrobial prophylaxis for appendectomy and colorectal surgery. Rev Infect Dis 1991;13(suppl 10):S815-S820.

Gorbach SL. Treatment of intraabdominal infection. Am J Med 1984;7(suppl):107.

Gordin F, Stamler C, Mills J. Pyogenic psoas abscesses: noninvasive diagnostic techniques and review of the literature. Rev Infect Dis 1983;5:1003-1011.

Gower D, McGuirt WF. Intracranial complication of acute and chronic infectious ear disease: a problem still with us. Laryngoscope 1983;93:1028-1033.

Greenlee J. Epidural abscess. In Mandell G, Bennett JE, Dolin R (eds). Principal and practice of infectious diseases. New York: Churchill Livingstone, 1995a.

Greenlee J. Subdural empyema. In Mandell G, Bennett JE, Dolin R (eds). Principal and practice of infectious diseases. New York: Churchill Livingstone, 1995b.

Griego R, et al. Dog, cat, and human bites: a review. J Am Acad Dermatol. 1995;33:1019-1029.

Guiliano A, Lewis F, Hadley K, Blaisdell FW. Bacteriology of necrotizing fasciitis. Am J Surg 1977;134:5256.

Haimes A, et al. MR imaging of brain abscesses. AJNR 1989;10:279.

Hart G, Lamb RC, Strauss MB. Gas gangrene: I. A collective review. J Trauma 1983;23:991-1000.

Heltber O, Korner B, Schouenborg P. Six cases of acute appendicitis with secondary peritonitis caused by *Streptococcus pneumoniae*. Eur J Clin Microbiol 1984;3:141-143.

Hlavin M, et al. Intracranial suppuration: a modern decade of postoperative subdural empyema and epidural abscess. Neurosurgery 1994;34:974-981.

Hollin S, Hayashi H, Gross SW. Intracranial abscesses of odontogenic origin. Oral Surg 1967;23:277-293.

Howard R. Anal and perianal infections. In Howard R, Simmons R (eds). Surgical infectious diseases. Norwalk, Conn: Appleton and Lange, 1987.

Jadavji T, Humphreys RP, Prober CG. Brain abscess in infants and children. Pediatr Infect Dis 1985;4:394-398.

Janik J, Firor HV. A 20-year study of 1,640 children at Cook County (Illinois) Hospital. Arch Surg 1979;114:717.

Kaufman D, Litman N, Miller MH. Sinusitis: induced subdural empyema. Neurology 1983;33:123-132.

Keren GT. Nonsurgical treatment of brain abscesses: report of two cases. Pediatr Infect Dis 1984;3:331-334.

Klempner M. Interactions of polymorphonuclear leukocytes with anaerobic bacteria. Rev Infect Dis 1984;6:S40-S44.

Knight P, Vassy LE. Specific diseases mimicking appendicitis in childhood. J Pediatr Surg 1981;116:744.

Knochel JQ, Koehler PR, Lee TG, et al. Radiology. Diagnosis of abdominal abscesses with computed tomography, ultrasound, and 111-indium-leukocyte scans. Radiology 1980; 137:425.

Kramer P, Griffith RS, Campbell RL. Antibiotic penetration of the brain: a comparative study. J Neurosurg 1969;31:295.

Kuhn JP, Berger PE. Computed tomographic diagnosis of abdominal abscesses in children. Ann Radiol (Paris) 1980; 23:153-158.

Kusne S, Dummer JS, Singh N, et al. Infections after liver transplantation. An analysis of 101 consecutive cases. Medicine 1988;67:132-143.

LeBeau J, Creissard P, Harispe L, et al. Surgical treatment of brain abscess and subdural empyema. J Neurosurg 1973;38:198-203.

Lee J, Glaser HS. Psoas muscle disorder: magnetic resonance imaging. Radiology 1986;160:683-687.

Leigh D, Simmons K, Norman E. Bacterial flora of the appendix fossa in appendicitis and postoperative wound infection. J Clin Pathol 1974;27:997-1000.

Lerner R, Spataro RF. Splenic abscess: percutaneous drainage. Radiology 1984;153:643-645.

Levison M, Bush LM. Peritonitis and other intra-abdominal infections. In Mandell G, Bennett JE, Dolin R (eds). Principal and practice of infectious diseases. New York: Churchill Livingstone, 1995.

Lew DS, Mongomery WW, et al. Sphenoid sinusitis: a review of 30 cases. N Engl J Med 1983;309:1149-1154.

Linos D, Nogarney DM, Mcilrath DC. Splenic abscess—the importance of early diagnosis. Mayo Clin Proc 1983;58:261-264.

Lister J. Meconium and bacterial peritonitis. In Lister J (ed). Neonatal surgery, ed. 3. London: Butterworths, 1991.

Loesche W. Oxygen sensitivity of various anaerobic bacteria. Appl Microbiol 1969;18:723-727.

Lorber B. *Bacteroides, Prevotella,* and *Fusobacterium* species (and other medically important anaerobic gram-negative bacilli). In Mandell G, Bennett JE, Dolin R (eds). Principal and practice of infectious diseases, ed. 4. New York: Churchill Livingstone, 1995.

Luckmann R. Incidence and case fatality rates for acute appendicitis in California: a population-based study of the effects of age. Am J Epidemiol 1989;129:905-918.

Lunsford L, Nelson PB. Stereotactic exploration of the brain in the era of computed tomography. Surg Neurol 1984;22:222-230.

Machiedo GW, Tikellis J, Suval W, et al. Reoperation for sepsis. Am Surg 1985;51:149.

Mackenzie MF, Young DG. Subphrenic abscess in children. Br J Surg 1975;62:305-308.

MacLennan J. The histotoxic clostridial infections of man. Bact Rev 1962;26:177.

Maddaus MA, Ahrenholz D, Simmons RL. The biology of peritonitis and implications for treatment Surg Clin North Am 1988;68:431-443.

Mason W, et al. Omphalitis in the newborn infant. Pediatr Infect Dis J 1989;8:521.

Maull K, Sachatello CR. Retroperitoneal iliac fossa abscess. A complication of suppurative lymphadenitis. Am J Surg 1974;127:270-274.

McCorkell S, Niles NC. Pyogenic liver abscess: another look at medical management. Lancet 1985;1:803-806.

McDougal WS, Izant RJ Jr, Zollinger RM Jr. Primary peritonitis in infancy and childhood. Ann Surg 1975;181:310.

Meleny F. A differential diagnosis between certain types of infectious gangrene of the skin with particular reference to hemolytic streptococcus gangrene and bacterial synergistic gangrene. Surg Gynecol Obstet 1933;56:847.

Mendelson R, Lindsell DR. Ultrasound examination of the paediatric acute abdomen. Br J Radiology 1987;60:414-416.

Mentzer C. Anorectal disease. Pediatr Clin North Am 1956;3:113-125.

Meyers M. Dynamic radiology of the abdomen: normal and pathologic anatomy, ed. 2. New York: Springer-Verlag, 1987.

Mollitt DL, Tepas JJ, Talbert JL. The role of coagulase-negative staphylococcus in neonatal necrotizing enterocolitis. J Pediatr Surg 1988;23:60-63.

Mueller P, Ferrucci JT, Wittenberg J, et al. Iliopsoas abscess: treatment by CT-guided percutaneous catheter drainage. AJR 1984;142:359-362.

Neuhof H, Arheim EE. Acute retroperitoneal abscess and phlegmon: a study of sixty-five cases. Ann Surg 1944;119:741-758.

Nichols R. Infections following gastrointestinal surgery: intraabdominal abscess. Surg Clin North Am 1980;60:197-212.

Nichols R, et al. Risk of infection after penetrating abdominal trauma. N Engl J Med 1984;311:1065.

Nielse HG, Harmsen A. Aetiology and pathogenesis, symptoms, diagnosis and treatment. Acta Neurol Scand 1982;65:609-622.

O'Keefe J, Tally FP, Barza M, et al. Inactivation of penicillin G during experimental infection with *Bacteroides fragilis*. J Infect Dis 1978;137:437.

Olafsson S, Khan MA. Musculoskeletal features of acne, hidradenitis suppurativa, and dissecting cellulitis of the scalp. Rheum Dis Clin North Am 1992;18:215.

Onderdonk A, Markham RB, Zaleznik DF, et al. Evidence for T cell-dependent immunity to *Bacteroides fragilis* in an intraabdominal abscess model. J Clin Invest 1982;69:9-16.

Pineiro-Carrero V, Andres JM. Morbidity and mortality in children with pyogenic liver abscess. AJDC 1989;143:1424-1427.

Powell D, san Luis E, Calvin S, et al. Peritonitis in children undergoing continuous ambulatory peritoneal dialysis. Am J Dis Child 1985;139:29-32.

Pruitt T, Simmons RL. Status of percutaneous catheter drainage of abscesses. Surg Clin North Am 1988;68:89-105.

Rotstein O. Interactions between leukocytes and anaerobic bacteria in polymicrobial surgical infections. Clin Infect Dis 1993;16:S190-S194.

Rubin J, Rogers WA, Taylor HM, Everett ED, et al. Peritonitis during continuous ambulatory peritoneal dialysis. Ann Intern Med 1980;92:7-13.

Saini S, Kellum JM, O'Leary MP, et al. Improved localization and survival in patients with intra-abdominal abscesses. Am J Surg 1983;145:136.

Sands M, Page D, Brown RB. Splenic abscess following nonoperative management of splenic rupture. J Pediatr Surg 1986;21:900-901.

Schumer W, Lee DK, Jones B. Peritoneal lavage in postoperative therapy of late peritoneal sepsis. Preliminary report. Surgery 1964;55:841.

Schwaitzberg S, Porkorny WJ, Thurston RS, et al. Psoas abscess in children. J Pediatr Surg 1985;20:339.

Shaked A, Shinar E, Fruend H. Managing the granulocytopenic patient with acute perianal inflammatory disease. Am J Surg 1986;152:510-512.

Shapiro M, Gale ME, Gerzof SG. CT of appendicitis. Radiol Clin North Am 1989;27:753-762.

Sheinfeld J, Erturk E, Spatoro RF, Cockett ATK. Perinephric abscess: current concepts. J Urol 1987;137:191-194.

Simons G, Sty JR, Starshak RJ. Retroperitoneal and retrofascial abscess: a review. J Bone Joint Surg (Am) 1983;65:1041-1057.

Simson J. Solitary abscess of the spleen. Br J Surg 1980;67.

Sjoln J, Lilja A, Ericsson N, et al. Treatment of brain abscess with cefotaxime and metronidazole: prospective study on 15 consecutive patients. Clin Infect Dis 1993;17:857-863.

Skoubo-Kristensen E, Hvid I. The appendiceal mass. Results of conservative management. Ann Surg 1982;196:584-587.

Smith H, Hendrick EB. Subdural empyema and epidural abscess in children. J Neurosurg 1983;58:392.

Snyder W, Chaffin L. Appendicitis during the first two years of life: report on twenty-one cases and review of four hundred forty-seven cases from the literature. Arch Surg 1952;64:549.

Sobel J. *Candida* infections in the intensive care unit. Crit Care Clin North Am 1988;4:325-344.

Solomkin J, Dellinger EP, Christou NV, et al. Results of a multicenter trial comparing imipenem cilastatin to tobramycin-clindamycin for intra-abdominal infections. Ann Surg 1990;212:581-591.

Solomkin J, et al. Antibiotic trials in intraabdominal infections: a critical evaluation of study design and outcome reporting. Ann Surg 1984;200:29.

Sondenaa K, et al. Bacteriology and complications of chronic pilonidal sinus treated with excision and primary suture. Int J Colorect Dis 1995;10:161-166.

Speck WT, Dresdale SS, McMillan RW. Primary peritonitis and the nephrotic syndrome. Am J Surg 1974;127:267.

Spires J, Smith RJH, Catlin FI. Brain abscesses in the young. Otolaryngol Head Neck Surg 1985;93:468-474.

Stamenkovic M, Lew PD. Early recognition of potentially fatal necrotizing fasciitis. The use of frozen-section biopsy. N Engl J Med 1984;310:1689-1693.

Stanley P, Atkinson JB, Reid BS, Gilsanz V. Percutaneous drainage of abdominal fluid collections in children. AJR 1984;142:813-816.

Stepanov S. Surgical treatment of brain abscess. Neurosurg 1988;22:724-730.

Stephenson C, Seibert JJ, Golladay ES, et al. Abscess of the iliopsoas muscle diagnosed by magnetic resonance imaging and ultrasonography. South Med J 1991;84:509-511.

Study Group of Intraabdominal Infections. A randomized controlled trial of ampicillin plus sulbactam vs gentamicin plus clindamycin in the treatment of intraabdominal infections. Rev Infect Dis 1986;8(suppl):S533-S588.

Styrt B, Gorbach SL. Recent developments in the understanding of the pathogenesis and treatment of anaerobic infections. N Engl J Med 1989;321:240-246.

Tay J, Garland JS. Serious head injuries from lawn darts. Pediatrics 1987;79.

Teague M, Baddour LM, Wruble LD. Liver abscess: a harbinger of Crohn's disease. Am J Gastroenterol 1988;83:1412.

Theophilo F, Markikis E, Theophilo L, et al. Brain abscess in childhood. Child Nerv Syst 1985;1:324-328.

Thirmuoothi M, Keen BM, Dajani AS. Anaerobic infections in children: a prospective study. J Clin Microbiol 1976;3:318.

van Dyke J, Holley HC, Anderson DS. Review of iliopsoas anatomy and pathology. Radiographics 1987;7:53-84.

Wang S, Wilson SE. Subphrenic abscess. The new epidemiology. Arch Surg 1977;112:934.

Wilson S. Intraabdominal abscess: subphrenic, lesser sac, intermesenteric, and pelvic. In Wilson SE, Finegold SM, Williams RA (eds). Intra-abdominal infection. New York: McGraw-Hill, 1982a.

Wilson SE. Secondary bacterial peritonitis. In Wilson SE, Finegold SM, Williams RA (eds). Intra-abdominal infections. New York: McGraw-Hill, 1982b.

Wilson SE, Serota AI, Williams RA. Anatomy and physiology of the peritoneum. In Wilson SE, Finegold SM, Williams RA (eds). Intra-abdominal infection. New York: McGraw-Hill, 1982.

Winslow R, Dean RE, Harley JW. Acute nonperforation appendicitis. Efficacy of brief antibiotic prophylaxis. Arch Surg 1983;118:651-655.

Wispelwey B, Scheld WM. Brain abscess. In Mandell G, Bennett JE, Dolin R (eds). Principal and practice of infectious diseases. New York: Churchill Livingstone, 1995.

Zaleznik D, Finberg RW, Shapiro ME, et al. A soluble suppressor T cell factor protects against experimental intraabdominal abscesses. J Clin Invest 1985;75:1023-1027.

Zaleznik D, Kasper DL. The role of anaerobic bacteria in abscess formation. Ann Rev Med 1982;33:217-229.

Zook E, et al. Successful treatment protocol for canine fang injuries. J Trauma 1980;20:243-246.

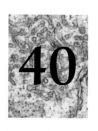

40 DIAGNOSIS OF ACUTE EXANTHEMATOUS DISEASES

SAUL KRUGMAN

EFFECTS OF DIAGNOSIS

Under certain circumstances a physician who examines a patient with a rash is charged with a grave responsibility. An error in diagnosis may have a profound effect on the patient, the contacts, and the community. The following examples (effect on the patient, effect on contacts, and effect on the community) will serve as illustrations.

Effect on the Patient

The disease of a patient with meningococcemia was mistakenly diagnosed as measles. Specific therapy was not started early; however, a potential fatality was averted when the disease was finally recognized and treated. Another patient with scarlet fever was said to have rubella. Complicating otitis media could have been prevented if the correct diagnosis had been made and appropriate treatment had been instituted.

Effect on Contacts

A classic clinical picture of exanthem subitum in an infant was erroneously labeled as rubella. Under normal circumstances this mistake would have been of little consequence. In this instance, however, the patient's mother was 2 months pregnant and had never had rubella. The error in diagnosis created an unnecessary period of anxiety for the parents, who had visions of the future birth of a congenitally malformed infant.

A child with mild measles was said to have rubella. A young sibling contact developed severe measles complicated by pneumonia. This situation could have been prevented by a correct diagnosis, which would have dictated the use of immune globulin to attenuate the sibling's disease.

Effect on the Community

On March 5, 1947, a 47-year-old businessman was admitted to Bellevue Hospital in New York City because of fever and rash. The initial diagnosis was toxic eruption, and the patient was admitted to a dermatology ward. On March 8 he was transferred to a communicable disease hospital, where he subsequently died. The proven cause of his death was smallpox. A small outbreak of the disease was initiated in the general hospital, spreading out from this focus. In the end there were twelve cases of smallpox and two deaths. There were several additional deaths among the 5 million persons who were vaccinated in New York City. The cost in time, effort, and money was incalculable, and the affairs of the entire city and its inhabitants were seriously disrupted. It is unlikely that a similar situation will occur again, since smallpox has been eradicated worldwide. However, occasionally an adult with severe hemorrhagic varicella may be erroneously diagnosed as having smallpox.

DIFFERENTIAL DIAGNOSIS

The rashes of various exanthematous diseases are so similar in appearance that they may be clinically indistinguishable. On the other hand, each disease has a characteristic total clinical picture that is distinctive. The differential diagnosis of the acute exanthems is based on a number of factors, including (1) the past history of infectious disease and immunization, (2) type of prodromal period, (3) features of the rash, (4) presence of pathognomonic or other diagnostic signs, and (5) laboratory diagnostic tests.

An attack of many of the exanthematous diseases is followed by permanent immunity. Consequently, a past history of measles, for example, might preclude that diagnosis. However, the history is only as reliable as the memory of the patient or the parent or the accuracy of the original diagnosis.

The character and duration of the prodromal period are also important. Some diseases have a prolonged (4 or more days) prodromal period before the rash appears; in others it may be short or absent.

In certain diseases the prodrome is characterized by respiratory tract symptoms; in others, influenza-like symptoms predominate.

The character, distribution, and duration of the rash require evaluation. An eruption may be discrete or confluent and central or peripheral in distribution, and it may persist for 1 to 2 weeks or disappear within 1 day.

Pathognomonic and other signs are always helpful diagnostic clues. Koplik's spots, for example, simplify the recognition of measles.

The final diagnosis in many instances cannot be made on clinical grounds alone. Laboratory diagnostic tests must be used for identification of the causative agent or for demonstration of the development of specific antibodies.

CLASSIFICATION OF ACUTE EXANTHEMATOUS DISEASES

The acute exanthematous diseases may be conveniently separated into two categories: those characterized by an erythematous maculopapular or punctiform eruption and those characterized by a papulovesicular eruption. These two types of rash are associated with many conditions other than the acute exanthematous diseases. These diseases and other conditions are given in the accompanying lists.

The following diseases and conditions are characterized by a *maculopapular eruption*:

Measles
Atypical measles
Rubella
Scarlet fever
Staphylococcal scalded skin syndrome
Staphylococcal toxic shock syndrome
Meningococcemia
Typhus and tick fevers
Toxoplasmosis
Cytomegalovirus infection
Erythema infectiosum
Roseola infantum
Enteroviral infections
Infectious mononucleosis
Toxic erythemas
Drug eruptions
Sunburn
Miliaria
Mucocutaneous lymph node syndrome (Kawasaki disease)

The following diseases and conditions are characterized by a *papulovesicular eruption*:

Varicella-zoster infections
Smallpox
Eczema herpeticum
Eczema vaccinatum
Coxsackievirus infections
Atypical measles
Rickettsialpox
Impetigo
Insect bites
Papular urticaria
Drug eruptions
Molluscum contagiosum
Dermatitis herpetiformis

The preceding lists do not include all the conditions associated with a rash.

DIFFERENTIAL DIAGNOSIS OF MACULOPAPULAR ERUPTIONS

The acute exanthems and other conditions listed previously are frequently or occasionally characterized by a maculopapular eruption. These diseases may be differentiated by a complete evaluation of four of the categories described in this discussion of differential diagnosis: (1) prodromal period, (2) rash, (3) presence of pathognomonic or other diagnostic signs, and (4) laboratory diagnostic tests.

Prodromal Period

Measles. As indicated in Fig. 40-1, the rash of measles is preceded by a 3- or 4-day prodromal period of fever, conjunctivitis, coryza, and cough.

Atypical Measles. The prodromal period of atypical measles is usually characterized by fever, cough, headache, myalgia, and occasionally pleuritic chest pain preceding the onset of rash by 2 to 4 days.

Rubella. In rubella in children there is usually no prodromal period (see Fig. 40-1). The appearance of the rash may be the first obvious sign of illness. Lymphadenopathy that precedes the rash is usually asymptomatic in children. Adolescents and adults may have a variable 1- to 4-day period of malaise and low-grade fever before the rash appears. The temperature may be normal.

Scarlet Fever. The rash of scarlet fever occurs within 12 hours of the onset of fever, sore throat, and vomiting. Occasionally the prodromal period may be prolonged to 2 days (see Fig. 40-1).

Staphylococcal Scalded Skin Syndrome. Fever and irritability occur at the time of onset of rash in patients with staphylococcal scalded skin syndrome; there is no prodromal period.

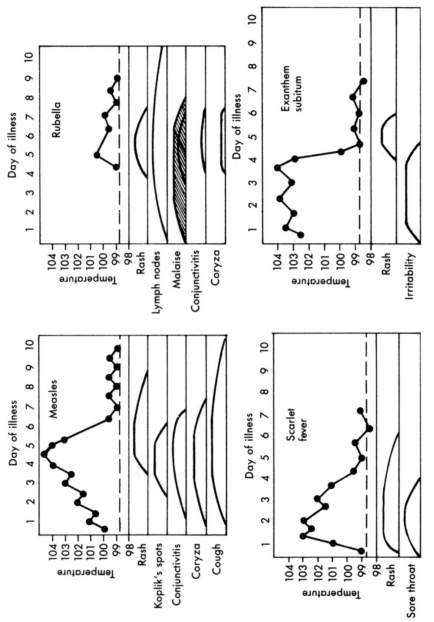

FIG. 40-1 Schematic diagrams illustrating differences between four acute exanthems characterized by maculopapular eruptions.

Staphylococcal Toxic Shock Syndrome. High fever, headache, confusion, sore throat, vomiting, diarrhea, and shock may precede or may be associated with the rash of staphylococcal toxic shock syndrome.

Meningococcemia with or without Meningitis. The prodrome of meningococcemia with or without meningitis is variable. Usually the rash appears within 24 hours. The initial symptoms are fever, vomiting, malaise, irritability, and possibly a stiff neck.

Epidemic and Murine Typhus. A 4- to 6-day prodromal period precedes the appearance of the rash of epidemic and murine typhus. It is characterized by high fever, chills, headache, and generalized aches and pains.

Rocky Mountain Spotted Fever. In patients with Rocky Mountain spotted fever the onset of rash is preceded by a 3- to 4-day period of fever, chills, headache, malaise, and anorexia.

Erythema Infectiosum. In patients with erythema infectiosum no prodromal period is typically present. Usually the first sign of the illness is the appearance of the rash.

Roseola Infantum. A 3- or 4-day prodromal period of high fever and irritability precedes the rash of exanthem subitum, which appears as the temperature falls to normal by crisis (see Fig. 40-1).

Enteroviral Infections. Echovirus type 16 infection (Boston exanthem) may have a prodromal period resembling that of exanthem subitum, but the fever tends to be lower. Fever and constitutional symptoms in Echovirus types 4, 6, and 9 and in coxsackievirus infections may precede but usually coincide with the appearance of the rash.

Mucocutaneous Lymph Node Syndrome (Kawasaki Disease). A nonspecific febrile illness with sore throat precedes the rash of mucocutaneous lymph node syndrome by 2 to 5 days.

Toxic Erythemas, Drug Eruptions, Sunburn, and Miliaria. Toxic erythemas, drug eruptions, sunburn, miliaria, and other noninfectious conditions with a maculopapular eruption do not have prodromal periods.

Rash

Measles. The rash of measles is reddish brown, appears on the face and neck first, and progresses downward to involve the trunk and extremities in sequence. As indicated in Fig. 40-2, the eruption is generalized by the third day. The lesions on the face, neck, and upper trunk tend to be confluent; those on the lower trunk and extremities are usually discrete. The eruption fades by the fifth or sixth day, with brownish staining first, followed by branny desquamation. The hands and feet do *not* desquamate.

Atypical Measles. The rash of atypical measles associated with previous immunization with killed measles vaccine resembles Rocky Mountain spotted fever more than typical measles. The eruption is characterized by erythematous, urticarial, papular, petechial, and purpuric lesions with a predilection for the extremities, especially the hands, wrists, feet, and ankles; occasionally the lesions may be vesicular.

Rubella. The rash of rubella is pink, begins on the face and neck, and progresses downward to the trunk and extremities more rapidly than in measles; it becomes generalized within 24 to 48 hours. The lesions are usually discrete rather than confluent, and those that develop first are the earliest to fade. Consequently, on the third day the face is usually clear, and only the extremities may be involved. The eruption usually disappears by the end of the third day, and as a rule it does not desquamate. The striking contrast between the distribution of measles and rubella rashes on the third day of eruption is illustrated in Fig. 40-2.

Scarlet Fever. The rash of scarlet fever is an erythematous punctiform eruption that blanches on pressure. It appears first on the flexor surfaces and rapidly becomes generalized, usually within 24 hours. The forehead and cheeks are smooth, red, and flushed, but the area around the mouth is pale (circumoral pallor). The lesions are most intense and prominent in the neck, axillary, inguinal, and popliteal skin folds (see Fig. 40-2). Desquamation is characteristic, and, in contrast to measles, it involves the hands and feet.

Staphylococcal Scalded Skin Syndrome. In staphylococcal scalded skin syndrome the rash is a generalized, erythematous, scarlatiniform eruption; it has a sandpaper-like texture. The erythema

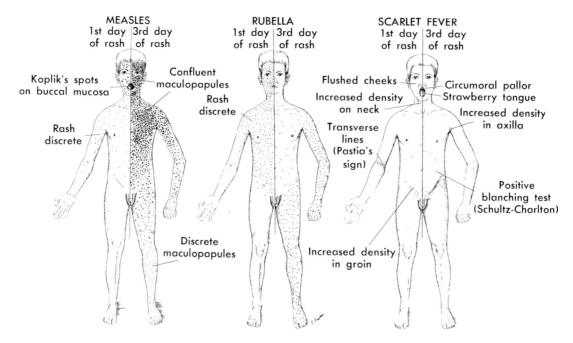

Fig. 40-2 Schematic drawings illustrating differences in appearance, distribution, and progression of rashes of measles, rubella, and scarlet fever.

is accentuated in the skin folds, simulating Pastia's lines. The skin is tender. The course of the rash is different from that of scarlet fever. Within 1 to 2 days bullae may appear, and the epidermis may separate into large sheets, revealing a moist, red, shiny surface beneath. In contrast, the pattern of desquamation is different in scarlet fever; it occurs 1 to 2 weeks later and is characterized by fine, branny flakes or thin sheets of skin.

Staphylococcal Toxic Shock Syndrome. The rash of staphylococcal toxic shock syndrome is scarlatiniform in appearance; it occurs most prominently on the trunk and extremities and is associated with edema of the face and limbs and desquamation.

Meningococcemia. In patients with meningococcemia an early, transient maculopapular eruption may precede the petechial, purpuric rash, which often is present when the patient seeks medical attention. In contrast to measles, this early exanthem has no regular, predictable distribution.

Epidemic and Murine Typhus. The characteristic rash of epidemic and murine typhus is a maculopapular and petechial eruption that has a *central* distribution. The face, palms, and soles are not involved as a rule.

Rocky Mountain Spotted Fever. The eruption of Rocky Mountain spotted fever is maculopapular and petechial, with a *peripheral* distribution. The palms and soles usually are involved, and occasionally the face also may be affected.

Erythema Infectiosum. The afebrile patient with asymptomatic erythema infectiosum develops a characteristic rash that erupts in three stages, in the following sequence: (1) red, flushed cheeks with circumoral pallor (slapped-cheek appearance); (2) maculopapular eruption over upper and lower extremities (the rash assumes a lacelike appearance as it fades); and (3) an evanescent stage characterized by subsidence of the eruption, followed by a recurrence precipitated by a variety of skin irritants.

Roseola Infantum. The lesions of exanthem subitum are typically discrete rose-red maculopapules that frequently appear on the chest and trunk first and then spread to involve the face and extremities. The eruption usually disappears within 2 days. Occasionally it fades within several hours.

Enteroviral Infections. The rashes of echovirus and coxsackievirus infections are often rubella-like in appearance. The lesions are usually maculopapular, discrete, nonpruritic, and generalized. Unlike in measles, desquamation and staining do not occur. Petechial lesions suggesting meningococcemia may rarely be noted in echovirus type 9 and coxsackievirus A type 9 infections.

Mucocutaneous Lymph Node Syndrome (Kawasaki Disease). In patients with mucocutaneous lymph node syndrome there is a generalized erythematous rash with elements of macules and papules. The palms and soles are swollen and reddened, eventually peeling after several days or weeks. Dryness with erythema of the lips, mouth, and tongue accompanies bilateral conjunctival injection (see Chapter 15).

Drug Eruptions and Toxic Erythemas. Drug eruptions and toxic erythemas may be characterized by maculopapular eruptions that may simulate any of the diseases listed previously.

Sunburn. Sunburn may be confused with the rash of scarlet fever, particularly if there is a coincident sore throat. The eruption is confined to the area not protected by a bathing suit.

Miliaria. The fine punctiform lesions of miliaria are chiefly confined to the flexor areas. The rash is usually not generalized, and it does not desquamate as a rule.

Presence of Pathognomonic or Other Diagnostic Signs

Measles. Koplik's spots are pathognomonic for measles.

Atypical Measles. Atypical measles is frequently associated with radiographic evidence of pneumonia and occasionally with pleural effusion.

Rubella. In patients with rubella, lymphadenopathy (particularly postauricular and occipital) is a common manifestation, but it also occurs in other diseases.

Scarlet Fever. A strawberry tongue and exudative or membranous tonsillitis are typical of scarlet fever.

Staphylococcal Scalded Skin Syndrome. An associated staphylococcal infection such as impetigo or purulent conjunctivitis may be present with staphylococcal scalded skin syndrome. Nikolsky's sign is present.

Staphylococcal Toxic Shock Syndrome. The scarlatiniform eruption of staphylococcal toxic shock syndrome is associated with high fever, toxicity, and a shocklike state.

Meningococcemia. A petechial purpuric eruption associated with meningeal signs would point to meningococcemia.

Epidemic and Murine Typhus. A maculopapular petechial eruption centrally distributed in a person living in an area where epidemic typhus is endemic is suggestive of the disease.

Rocky Mountain Spotted Fever. A history of a recent tick bite in a person with a maculopapular, petechial, peripherally distributed eruption is characteristic of Rocky Mountain spotted fever.

Toxoplasmosis. The acquired infection of toxoplasmosis may be characterized by one or more of the following syndromes: (1) fever, pneumonitis, and rash; (2) lymphadenopathy; (3) encephalitis; and (4) chorioretinitis.

Erythema Infectiosum. Erythema infectiosum is suggested by the slapped-face appearance in a well child.

Enteroviral Infections. The rash of enteroviral infections may be associated with aseptic meningitis. The infections occur most commonly during the summer and fall months.

Infectious Mononucleosis. A triad of membranous tonsillitis, lymphadenopathy, and splenomegaly suggests infectious mononucleosis as a possibility.

Laboratory Diagnostic Tests

Measles. The measles hemagglutination-inhibition (HI) test is the most practical diagnostic test. The pattern of appearance of antibody is shown in Fig. 16-4. A fourfold or greater rise in measles HI antibody is detected during convalescence; the peak titer usually ranges between 1:256 and 1:1024. The blood picture typically shows leukopenia.

Atypical Measles. Extraordinary rises in measles HI antibody have been detected within 2 weeks after onset of atypical measles. The titers may exceed 1:100,000.

Rubella. As indicated in Fig. 26-4 a positive throat culture for rubella virus and evidence of a rise in antibody level are helpful diagnostic aids. The blood picture shows either a normal or low white blood cell count.

Scarlet Fever. Group A hemolytic streptococci may be cultured from the nasopharynx. There is usually a rise in antistreptolysin O titer.

Staphylococcal Scalded Skin Syndrome. A culture of skin or other sites of infection is positive for phage group II staphylococci in staphylococcal scalded skin syndrome.

Staphylococcal Toxic Shock Syndrome. Cultures of various mucosal surfaces or purulent lesions should be positive for *Staphylococcus aureus*.

Meningococcemia. The microorganism causing meningococcemia may be observed on Gram stain and recovered from the blood, spinal fluid, or petechiae.

Epidemic and Murine Typhus. The Weil-Felix agglutination reaction with *Proteus* OX-19 is positive. Specific antibody tests are available for epidemic and murine typhus.

Rocky Mountain Spotted Fever. The Weil-Felix agglutination reaction with *Proteus* OX-19 and OX-2 is positive. Thrombocytopenia, hyponatremia, and hypoalbuminemia are common. Specific Rocky Mountain spotted fever antibody tests are available.

Toxoplasmosis. A rise in *Toxoplasma* antibody titer during convalescence indicates acute toxoplasmosis.

Erythema Infectiosum. Diagnostic testing for erythema infectiosum is discussed in Chapter 22, pages 331-332. In the future, standardized serologic tests to confirm parvovirus B-19 infection will become more available.

Roseola Infantum. There is no diagnostic test for roseola infantum at present. As yet, specific virologic and serologic tests to detect human herpesvirus type 6 are not commercially available (see Chapter 13, p. 208). The blood picture shows leukopenia when the rash appears.

Enteroviral Infections. Echoviruses and coxsackieviruses may be recovered from stools, throat, blood, or cerebrospinal fluid (CSF). The diagnosis is confirmed by demonstrating a rise in neutralizing antibody titer to the specific virus.

Infectious Mononucleosis. In patients with infectious mononucleosis the blood smear is positive for abnormal lymphocytes. The monospot test and heterophil agglutination test are positive. Results of liver function tests such as for aminotransferases are abnormal. Epstein-Barr virus antibody appears during convalescence (Chapter 8).

DIFFERENTIAL DIAGNOSIS OF PAPULOVESICULAR ERUPTIONS

The acute exanthems and other conditions listed on p. 591 are usually characterized by a papulovesicular eruption. The following differential criteria are similar to those used for the maculopapular eruptions.

Prodromal Period

Varicella. As indicated in Fig. 40-3, a prodromal period is usually absent in patients with chickenpox. The rash and constitutional symptoms, particularly in children, occur simultaneously. In adolescents and adults, however, there may be a 1- or 2-day prodromal period of fever, headache, malaise, and anorexia.

Smallpox. The smallpox rash is preceded by a 3-day period of chills, headache, backache, and severe malaise (see Fig. 40-3). A transient rash with bathing-trunk distribution may occur during the prodrome.

Herpes Simplex, Herpes Zoster, and Vaccinia. Herpes simplex, herpes zoster, and vaccinia occur without any prodromal period (eczema vaccinatum and herpeticum, see Fig. 40-3).

Rickettsialpox. In patients with rickettsialpox a generalized papulovesicular eruption is preceded by the development of (1) an initial lesion (an eschar), and (2) an influenza-like syndrome (see Fig. 40-3).

Rash

Varicella. The rash of chickenpox is characterized by (1) *rapid* evolution of macules to papules to vesicles to crusts; (2) central distribution of lesions, which appear in crops (Fig. 40-4); (3) presence of lesions in all stages in any one anatomic

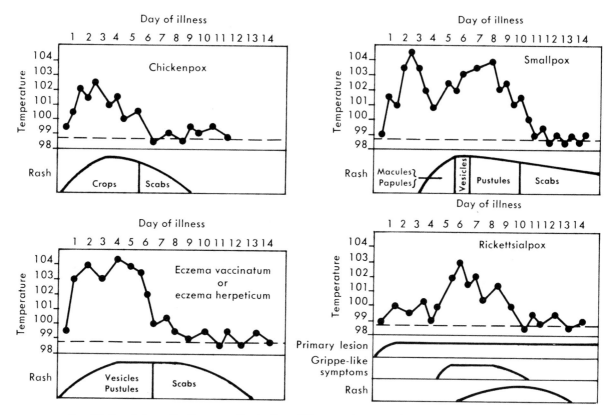

FIG. 40-3 Schematic diagrams illustrating differences between four acute exanthems characterized by papulovesicular eruptions.

area; (4) presence of scalp and mucous membrane lesions; and (5) eventual crusting of nearly all the skin lesions.

Smallpox. The rash of smallpox is characterized by (1) *slow* evolution of macules to papules to vesicles to pustules to crusts; (2) peripheral distribution of lesions, which are most prominent on the exposed skin surfaces (see Fig. 40-4); (3) presence of lesions in the same stage in any one anatomic area; and (4) skin lesions that are more deep seated than those of varicella.

Eczema Herpeticum and Vaccinatum. In patients with eczema herpeticum and vaccinatum the vesicular and pustular lesions are most profuse on the sites of eczema. Mouth and scalp lesions are generally absent. (See Plate 6.)

Herpes Zoster. The lesions of herpes zoster are unilateral and distributed along the line of the affected nerves; vesicles are grouped together and tend to become confluent.

Atypical Measles. The papulovesicular lesions of atypical measles may appear on the face and the trunk. During the crusting phase they resemble varicella. This eruption may or may not be associated with the characteristic maculopapular eruption that resembles Rocky Mountain spotted fever in its peripheral distribution.

Rickettsialpox. The primary lesion of rickettsialpox is an eschar that measures 1.5 cm or more in diameter. The generalized papulovesicular eruption is composed of tiny vesicles superimposed on a firm papule. The vesicles are much smaller than those of chickenpox. Many lesions do not crust.

Impetigo. The lesions of impetigo, at first vesicular, become confluent and rapidly progress to the pustular and crusting stage. They do not appear in crops, they commonly involve the nasolabial area and other sites available for scratching, and they do not involve the oral mucous membranes.

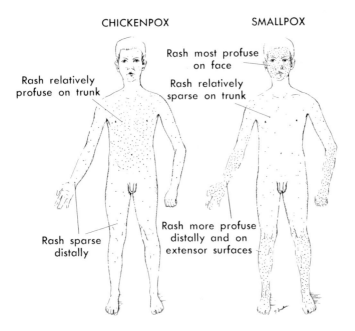

FIG. 40-4 Schematic drawings illustrating differences in distribution of rashes of chickenpox and smallpox.

Insect Bites and Papular Urticaria. Insect bites and papular urticaria do not have a typical vesicular appearance and do not involve the scalp or mucous membranes.

Molluscum Contagiosum. The lesions of molluscum contagiosum are scattered, discrete, firm, small nodular elevations without any surrounding red areolae.

Dermatitis Herpetiformis. Dermatitis herpetiformis is characterized by erythematous papulovesicular lesions that are symmetrical in distribution, by a chronic course, and by healing with residual pigmentation.

Laboratory Diagnostic Tests

Varicella. The virus of varicella is isolated from vesicular fluid or may be identified on smears by indirect immunofluorescence. Detection of specific varicella-zoster antibody during convalescence is accomplished by means of one of the following tests: fluorescent antibody to membrane antigen (FAMA), enzyme-linked immunosorbent assay (ELISA), and latex agglutination (LA) (see Chapter 37).

Smallpox. The virus of smallpox may be identified by electron microscopy or gel diffusion.

Eczema Herpeticum. Herpes simplex virus may be isolated in tissue culture, and the viral antigen may be identified in smears by indirect immunofluorescence. In eczema herpeticum, a rise in the level of antibodies during convalescence may be demonstrated.

Eczema Vaccinatum. The laboratory tests for eczema vaccinatum are the same as those for smallpox.

Herpes Zoster. The laboratory tests for herpes zoster are the same as those for chickenpox.

Rickettsialpox. The isolation of *Rickettsia akari* from the blood can be achieved by inoculation of the yolk sac of embryonated eggs. The rise in the level of rickettsialpox and Rocky Mountain spotted fever antibodies occurs during convalescence.

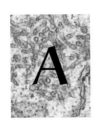

A ANTIMICROBIAL DRUGS

(Tables A-1 to A-3 reprinted with permission from *The Medical Letter Handbook of Antimicrobial Therapy*, 1996, The Medical Letter, Inc., New Rochelle, New York.)

Table A-1 Systemic drugs for fungal infections

Infection/drug of choice	Dosage[1]	Alternatives
Aspergillosis		
Amphotericin B[2]	1-1.5 mg/kg IV[3]	Intraconazole 200 mg PO bid
Blastomycosis[4]		
Itraconazole	200 mg PO once or bid	Ketoconazole 400 mg PO once or bid
or Amphotericin B[2]	0.5-0.6 mg/kg IV	
Candidiasis		
oropharyngeal, esophageal[5]		
Fluconazole[6]	100-200 mg/day PO	Ketoconazole 200-400 mg/day PO
		Itraconazole 200 mg/day PO
deep		
Amphotericin B[2]	0.5-1 mg/kg IV[7]	Fluconazole 400-800 mg IV or PO qd
±Flucytosine	100 mg/kg/day PO[8]	
Coccidioidomycosis[4]		
Fluconazole[9]	400-800 mg/day PO	Itraconazole 200 mg PO bid
or Amphotericin B[2]	0.5 mg/kg IV	Ketoconazole 400 mg PO once or bid
Cryptococcosis		
Amphotericin B[2]	0.3-0.7 mg/kg IV[10]	Fluconazole 400 mg PO qd
±Flucytosine	100 mg/kg/day PO[8]	Itraconazole 200 mg PO bid
chronic suppression[11]		
Fluconazole	200 mg/day PO	Amphotericin B 0.5-1 mg/kg IV weekly
Histoplasmosis[4]		
Itraconazole	200 mg PO bid	Ketoconazole 400 mg PO once or bid
or Amphotericin B[2]	0.5-0.6 mg/kg IV	
chronic suppression[11]		
Itraconazole	200 mg PO once or bid	Amphotericin B 0.5-0.8 mg/kg IV weekly
Mucormycosis		
Amphotericin B[2]	1-1.5 mg/kg/day IV	No dependable alternative
Paracoccidioidomycosis[4]		
Itraconazole	100-200 mg/day PO	Ketoconazole 200-400 mg/day PO
or Amphotericin B[2]	0.4-0.5 mg/kg IV	

1. The optimal duration of treatment with the oral azole drugs is unclear. Depending on the disease, these drugs are continued for weeks or months or, particularly in AIDS patients, indefinitely. With ketoconazole and itraconazole, AIDS patients may have lower serum concentrations.

2. Amphotericin B is given IV over about a 2- to 4-hour interval once a day or in double doses (up to a maximum of 1.5 mg/kg) every other day. The duration of therapy with the drug usually ranges from 4 to 12 weeks. To decrease the severity of the initial reaction to the drug, if the patient is not dangerously ill, some clinicians begin with a 1-mg test dose, followed in 2 to 4 hours, if no severe reaction occurs, by a full therapeutic dose. Pretreatment with acetaminophen (Tylenol and others), aspirin, or 25 mg hydrocortisone IV can decrease the severity of the reaction. Treatment with meperidine (Demerol and others), 25 mg IV, can shorten the duration of fever and chills.

3. Lower doses can be used for indolent infections.

4. Patients with severe illness should receive amphotericin B.

5. For patients with oropharyngeal disease, clotrimazole troches 5 times daily or nystatin solution (100,000 U/ml), 5 ml qid, may be effective and are relatively inexpensive. For patients with fluconazole-resistant esophageal disease, amphotericin B, 0.3 mg/kg IV, can be used.

6. *Candida krusei* infections are usually resistant to fluconazole. *Candida glabrata* infections are often resistant.

7. Bladder irrigation with 50 μg/ml of amphotericin B in sterile water has been used to treat *Candida* cystitis.

8. Given in 4 doses q6h. Dosage must be decreased in patients with diminished renal function. When given with amphotericin B, some experts recommend beginning flucytosine in dosage of 75 mg/kg/day, given in 4 doses q6h, until the degree of amphotericin nephrotoxicity becomes clear or blood levels can be determined.

9. Drug of choice for coccidioidal meningitis; patients who do not respond may require intrathecal amphotericin B.

10. Lower doses are used when given with flucytosine and higher doses when given alone.

11. For patients with AIDS.

Table A-1 Systemic drugs for fungal infections—cont'd

Infection/drug of choice	Dosage[1]	Alternatives
Pseudallescheriasis		
Ketoconazole	400-800 mg/day PO	Miconazole[12] 600 mg q8h
or Itraconazole	200 mg PO bid	
Sporotrichosis		
cutaneous		
Itraconazole	100-200 mg/day PO	Potassium iodide 1-5 ml tid
systemic		
Amphotericin B[2]	0.5 mg/kg/day IV	Itraconazole 200 mg PO bid

12. Monistat IV.

Table A-2 Drugs for treatment of parasitic infections

Infection		Drug	Adult dosage	Pediatric dosage
Amebiasis *(Entamoeba histolytica)*[1]				
Asymptomatic				
Drug of choice:		Iodoquinol[2]	650 mg tid × 20 days	30-40 mg/kg/day in 3 doses × 20 days
	OR	Paromomycin	25-35 mg/kg/day in 3 doses × 7 days	25-35 mg/kg/day in 3 doses × 7 days
Alternative:		Diloxanide furoate[3]	500 mg tid × 10 days	20 mg/kg/day in 3 doses × 10 days
Mild to moderate intestinal disease				
Drug of choice:[4]		Metronidazole	750 mg tid × 10 days	35-50 mg/kg/day in 3 doses × 10 days
	OR	Tinidazole[5]	2 grams/day × 3 days	50 mg/kg (max. 2 grams) qd × 3 days
Severe intestinal disease, hepatic abscess				
Drug of choice:[4]		Metronidazole	750 mg tid × 10 days	35-50 mg/kg/day in 3 doses × 10 days
	OR	Tinidazole[5]	600 mg bid or 800 mg tid × 5 days	50 mg/kg or 60 mg/kg (max. 2 grams) qd × 3 days
Amebic *(Acanthamoeba)* **keratitis**				
Drug of choice:		See footnote 6		

1. *Entamoeba histolytica* and *E. dispar,* until recently termed *pathogenic* and *nonpathogenic E. histolytica,* respectively, are morphologically indistinguishable.

2. Dosage and duration of administration should not be exceeded because of possibility of causing optic neuritis; maximum dosage is 2 grams/day.

3. In the United States, this drug is available from the CDC Drug Service, Centers for Disease Control and Prevention, Atlanta, Georgia 30333; telephone: 404-639-3670 (evenings, weekends, and holidays: 404-639-2888).

4. Treatment should be followed by a course of iodoquinol or one of the other intraluminal drugs used to treat asymptomatic amebiasis.

5. A nitro-imidazole similar to metronidazole, but not marketed in the United States, tinidazole appears to be at least as effective as metronidazole and better tolerated. Ornidazole, a similar drug, is also used outside the United States. Higher dosage is for hepatic abscess.

6. Trophozoites and cysts of *Acanthamoeba* from infected corneas, contact lenses, and their cases are susceptible in vitro to chlorhexidine, polyhexamethylene biguanide, propamidine, pentamidine, diminazine, and neomycin and, especially, to combinations of these drugs (J Hay et al., Eye 1994; 8:555). For treatment of keratitis caused by *Acanthamoeba,* concurrent topical use of 0.1% propamidine isethionate (Brolene–Rhône-Poulenc Rorer, Canda) plus neomycin, or oral itraconazole plus topical miconazole, have been successful (Moore et al., Br J Ophthalmol 1989; 73:271; Ishabashi et al., Am J Ophthalmol 1990; 109:121). Recently, 0.02% topical polyhexamethylene biguanide (PHMB) has been used successfully in a large number of patients (Elder et al., Lancet 1995; 345:791). PHMB is available as *Baquacil* (ICI America), a swimming pool disinfectant (Yee and Winarko, Am J Hosp Pharm 1993; 50:2523).

Continued

Table A-2   Drugs for treatment of parasitic infections—cont'd

Infection	Drug	Adult dosage	Pediatric dosage
Amebic meningoencephalitis, primary			
Naegleria			
Drug of choice:	Amphotericin B[7,8]	1 mg/kg/day IV, uncertain duration	1 mg/kg/day IV, uncertain duration
Acanthamoeba			
Drug of choice:	See footnote 9		
Ancylostoma caninum (Eosinophilic enterocolitis)			
Drug of choice:	Mebendazole	100 mg bid × 3 days	100 mg bid × 3 days
OR	Pyrantel pamoate[8]	11 mg/kg (max. 1 gram) × 3 days	11 mg/kg (max. 1 gram) × 3 days
OR	Albendazole	400 mg once	400 mg once
Ancylostoma duodenals, see HOOKWORM			
Angiostrongyliasis			
Angiostrongylus cantonensis			
Drug of choice:[10]	Mebendazole[8]	100 mg bid × 5 days	100 mg bid × 5 days
Angiostrongylus costaricensis			
Drug of choice:	Thiabendazole[8]	75 mg/kg/day in 3 doses × 3 days (max. 3 grams/day)[11]	75 mg/kg/day in 3 doses × 3 days (max. 3 grams/day)[11]
Alternative:	Mebendazole	200-400 mg tid × 10 days	200-400 mg tid × 10 days
Anisakiasis (*Anisakis*)			
Treatment of choice:	Surgical or endoscopic removal		
Ascariasis (*Ascaris lumbricoides,* roundworm)			
Drug of choice:	Mebendazole	100 mg bid × 3 days	100 mg bid × 3 days
OR	Pyrantel pamoate	11 mg/kg once (max. 1 gram)	11 mg/kg once (max. 1 gram)
OR	Albendazole	400 mg once	400 mg once
Babesiosis (*Babesia* spp.)			
Drugs of choice:[12]	Clindamycin[8]	1.2 grams bid IV or 600 mg tid PO × 7 days	20-40 mg/kg/day in 3 doses × 7 days
	plus quinine	650 mg tid PO × 7 days	25 mg/kg/day in 3 doses × 7 days

7. Naegleria infections have been treated successfully with amphotericin B, rifampin, and chloramphenicol (Wang et al., Clin Neurol Neurosurg 1993; 95:249), amphotericin B, oral rifampin, and oral ketoconazole (Poungvarin et al., J Med Assoc Thailand 1991; 74:112), and amphotericin B alone (Brown, Arch Intern Med 1992; 152:1330).

8. An approved drug, but considered investigational for this condition by the U.S. Food and Drug Administration

9. Strains of *Acanthamoeba* isolated from fatal granulomatous amebic encephalitis are usually susceptible in vitro to pentamidine, ketoconazole *(Nizoral),* flucytosine, and (less so) to amphotericin B. One patient with disseminated infection was treated successfully with intravenous pentamidine isethionate, topical chlorhexidine and 2% ketoconazole cream, followed by oral itraconazole (Slater et al., N Engl J Med 1994; 331:85).

10. Most patients recover spontaneously without antiparasitic drug therapy. Analgesics, corticosteroids, and careful removal of CSF at frequent intervals can relieve symptoms (Koo et al., Rev Infect Dis 1988; 10:1155). Albendazole, levamisole (Ergamisol), or ivermectin has also been used successfully in animals.

11. This dose is likely to be toxic and may have to be decreased.

12. Atovaquone suspension, 750 mg bid, plus azithromycin, 500 to 1000 mg daily, may be effective when quinine and clindamycin fail. Exchange transfusion has been used in severely ill patients with high (>10%) parasitemia (Iacopino and Earnhart, Arch Intern Med 1990; 150:1527). One report indicates that azithromycin, 500-1000 mg daily, plus quinine may also be effective (Weiss et al., J Infect Dis 1993; 168:1289). Concurrent use of pentamidine and trimethoprim-sulfamethoxazole has been reported to cure an infection with *B. divergens* (Raoult et al., Ann Intern Med 1987; 107:944).

Table A–2   Drugs for treatment of parasitic infections—cont'd

Infection	Drug	Adult dosage	Pediatric dosage
Balantidiasis (*Balantidium coli*)			
Drug of choice:	Tetracycline[8]	500 mg qid × 10 days	40 mg/kg/day in 4 doses × 10 days (max. 2 grams/day)[13]
Alternatives:	Iodoquinol[2,8]	650 mg tid × 20 days	40 mg/kg/day in 3 doses × 20 days
	Metronidazole[8]	750 mg tid × 5 days	35-50 mg/kg/day in 3 doses × 5 days
Baylisascariasis (*Baylisascaris procyonis*)			
Drug of choice:	See footnote 14		
Blastocystis *hominis* infection			
Drug of choice:	See footnote 15		
Capillariasis (*Capillaria philippinensis*)			
Drug of choice:	Mebendazole[8]	200 mg bid × 20 days	200 mg bid × 20 days
Alternatives:	Albendazole	200 mg bid × 10 days	200 mg bid × 10 days
	Thiabendazole[8]	25 mg/kg/day in 2 doses × 30 days	25 mg/kg/day in 2 doses × 30 days
Chagas' disease, see TRYPANOSOMIASIS			
Clonorchis sinensis, see FLUKE infection			
Cryptosporidiosis (*Cryptosporidium*)			
Drug of choice:[16]	Paromomycin	500-750 mg qid	
Cutaneous larva migrans (creeping eruption, dog and cat hookworm)			
Drug of Choice:[17]	Thiabendazole	Topically ± 50 mg/kg/day PO in 2 doses (max. 3 grams/day) × 2-5 days[11]	Topically ± 50 mg/kg/day PO in 2 doses (max. 3 grams/day) × 2-5 days[11]
OR	Ivermectin	150-200 µg/kg once	150-200 µg/kg once
OR	Albendazole	200 mg bid × 3 days	200 mg bid × 3 days
Cyclospora infection			
Drug of choice:	Trimethoprim-sulfamethoxazole[18]	TMP 160 mg, SMX 800 mg bid × 7 days	TMP 5 mg/kg, SMX 25 mg/kg bid × 7 days

13. Not recommended for use in children less than 8 years old.

14. Drugs that could be tried include albendazole, mebendazole, thiabendazole, levamisole (Ergamisol), and ivermectin. Steroid therapy may be helpful, especially in eye and CNS infections. Ocular baylisascariasis has been treated successfully using laser photocoagulation therapy to destroy the intraretinal larvae.

15. Clinical significance of these organisms is controversial, but metronidazole 750 mg tid × 10 days or iodoquinol 650 mg tid × 20 days anecdotally has been reported to be effective (Boreham and Stenzel, Adv Parasitol 1993; 32:2; Keystone and Markell, Clin Infect Dis 1995; 21:102-104).

16. Infection is self-limited in immunocompetent patients. In HIV-infected patients, paromomycin has limited effectiveness (White et al., J Infect Dis 1994; 170:419; Bissuel, Clin Infect Dis 1994; 18:447). In unpublished clinical trials, azithromycin 1250 mg daily for 2 weeks followed by 500 mg daily has apparently been effective in some patients.

17. Caumes et al., Am J Trop Med Hyg 1993; 49:641, Wolf et al., Hautarzt 1993; 44:462; Davies et al., Arch Dermatol 1993; 129:588.

18. HIV-infected patients may need higher dosage and long-term maintenance (Pape et al., Ann Intern Med 1994; 121:654).

Continued

Table A-2 Drugs for treatment of parasitic infections—cont'd

Infection		Drug	Adult dosage	Pediatric dosage
Cysticercosis, see TAPEWORM infection				
***Dientamoeba fragilis* infection**				
Drug of choice:		Iodoquinol[2]	650 mg tid × 20 days	40 mg/kg/day in 3 doses × 20 days
	OR	Paromomycin	25-30 mg/kg/day in 3 doses × 7 days	25-30 mg/kg/day in 3 doses × 7 days
	OR	Tetracycline[8]	500 mg qid × 10 days	40 mg/kg/day (max. 2 grams/day) in 4 doses × 10 days[13]
***Diphyllobothrium latum,* see TAPEWORM infection**				
***Dracunculus medinensis* (guinea worm) infection**				
Drug of choice:		Metronidazole[8,19]	250 mg tid × 10 days	25 mg/kg/day (max. 750 mg/day) in 3 doses × 10 days
Alternative:		Thiabendazole[8,19]	50-75 mg/kg/day in 2 doses × 3 days[11]	50-75 mg/kg/day in 2 doses × 3 days[11]
Echinococcus, see TAPEWORM infection				
***Entamoeba histolytica,* see AMEBIASIS**				
***Entamoeba polecki* infection**				
Drug of choice:		Metronidzole[8]	750 mg tid × 10 days	35-50 mg/kg/day in 3 doses × 10 days
***Enterobius vermicularis* (pinworm) infection**				
Drug of choice:		Pyrantel pamoate	11 mg/kg once (max. 1 gram); repeat after 2 weeks	11 mg/kg once (max. 1 gram); repeat after 2 weeks
	OR	Mebendazole	A single dose of 100 mg; repeat after 2 weeks	A single dose of 100 mg; repeat after 2 weeks
	OR	Albendazole	400 mg once; repeat in 2 weeks	400 mg once; repeat in 2 weeks
***Fasciola hepatica,* see FLUKE infection**				
Filariasis				
Wuchereria bancrofti, Brugia malayi				
Drug of choice:[20]		Diethylcarbama-zine[21]	Day 1: 50 mg, p.c. Day 2: 50 mg tid Day 3: 100 mg tid Days 4 through 21: 6 mg/kg/day in 3 doses[22]	Day 1: 1 mg/kg p.c. Day 2: 1 mg/kg tid Day 3: 1-2 mg/kg tid Days 4 through 21: 6 mg/kg/day in 3 doses[22]

19. Not curative, but decreases inflammation and facilitates removing the worm. Mebendazole 400-800 mg/day for 6 days has been reported to kill the worm directly.

20. A single dose of ivermectin, 20-200 μg/kg, has been reported to be effective for treatment of microfilaremia (Kar et al, Southeast Asian J Trop Med Public Health 1993; 24:80).

21. Antihistamines or corticosteroids may be required to decrease allergic reactions caused by disintegration of microfilariae in treatment of filarial infections, especially those caused by *Loa loa.*

22. For patients with no microfilariae in the blood, full doses can be given from day one.

Table A-2 Drugs for treatment of parasitic infections—cont'd

Infection	Drug	Adult dosage	Pediatric dosage
Filariasis—cont'd			
Loa loa			
Drug of choice:[23]	Diethylcarbama-zine[21]	Day 1: 50 mg, oral, p.c. Day 2: 50 mg tid Day 3: 100 mg tid Days 4 through 21: 9 mg/kg/day in 3 doses[22]	Day 1: 1 mg/kg, oral, p.c. Day 2: 1 mg/kg tid Day 3: 1-2 mg/kg tid Days 4 through 21: 9 mg/kg/day in 3 doses[22]
Mansonella ozzardi			
Drug of choice:	See footnote 24		
Mansonella perstans			
Drug of choice:	Mebendazole[8]	100 mg bid × 30 days	
Tropical pulmonary eosinophilia (TPE)			
Drug of choice:	Diethylcarbama-zine	6 mg/kg/day in 3 doses × 21 days	6 mg/kg/day in 3 doses × 21 days
Onchocerca volvulus			
Drug of choice:	Ivermectin[3]	150 μg/kg once, re-peated every 3 to 12 months	150 μg/kg once, re-peated every 3 to 12 months
Fluke, hermaphroditic, infection			
Clonorchis sinensis **(Chinese liver fluke)**			
Drug of choice:	Praziquantel	75 mg/kg/day in 3 doses × 1 day	75 mg/kg/day in 3 doses × 1 day
OR	Albendazole	10 mg/kg × 7 days	
Fasciola hepatica **(sheep liver fluke)**			
Drug of choice:[25]	Bithionol[3]	30-50 mg/kg on alter-nate days × 10-15 doses	30-50 mg/kg on alter-nate days × 10-15 doses
Fasciolopsis buski **(intestinal fluke)**			
Drug of choice:	Praziquantel[8]	75 mg/kg/day in 3 doses × 1 day	75 mg/kg/day in 3 doses × 1 day
Heterophyes heterophyes **(intestinal fluke)**			
Drug of choice:	Praziquantel[8]	75 mg/kg/day in 3 doses × 1 day	75 mg/kg/day in 3 doses × 1 day
Metagonimus yokagawai **(intestinal fluke)**			
Drug of choice:	Praziquantel[8]	75 mg/kg/day in 3 doses × 1 day	75 mg/kg/day in 3 doses × 1 day

23. Diethylcarbamazine should be administered with special caution in heavy infections with *Loa loa* because rapid killing of micro-filariae can provoke an encephalopathy. Ivermectin or albendazole has been used to reduce microfilaremia (Martin-Prevel et al, Am J Trop Med Hyg 1993; 48:186; Klion et al., J Infect Dis 1993; 168:202). Apheresis has been reported to be effective in lowering micro-filarial counts in patients heavily infected with *Loa loa* (Ottesen, Infect Dis Clin North Am 1993: 7:619). Diethylcarbamazine, 300 mg once weekly, has been recommended for prevention of loiasis (Nutman et al., N Engl J Med 1988; 319:752).

24. Diethylcarbamazine has no effect. Ivermectin, 150 μg/kg, may be effective (Nutman et al., J Infect Dis 1987; 156:622).

25. Unlike infections with other flukes, *Fasciola hepatica* infections may not respond to praziquantel. Recent data indicate that tri-clabendazole (Fasinex), a veterinary fasciolide, is safe and effective in a single oral dose of 10 mg/kg (Apt et al, Am J Trop Med Hyg, 1995; 52:532).

Continued

Table A-2   Drugs for treatment of parasitic infections—cont'd

Infection	Drug	Adult dosage	Pediatric dosage
Fluke, hermaphroditic, infection—cont'd			
Nanophyetus salmincola			
Drug of choice:	Praziquantel[8]	60 mg/kg/day in 3 doses × 1 day	60 mg/kg/day in 3 doses × 1 day
***Opisthorchis viverrini* (liver fluke)**			
Drug of choice:	Praziquantel[8]	75 mg/kg/day in 3 doses × 1 day	75 mg/kg/day in 3 doses × 1 day
***Paragonimus westermani* (lung fluke)**			
Drug of choice:	Praziquantel[8]	75 mg/kg/day in 3 doses × 2 days	75 mg/kg/day in 3 doses × 2 days
Alternative:[26]	Bithionol[3]	30-50 mg/kg on alternate days × 10-15 doses	30-50 mg/kg on alternate days × 10-15 doses
Giardiasis (*Giardia lamblia*)			
Drug of choice:	Metronidazole[8]	250 mg tid × 5 days	15 mg/kg/day in 3 doses × 5 days
Alternatives:[27]	Tinidazole[5]	2 grams once	50 mg/kg once (max. 2 grams)
	Furazolidone	100 mg qid × 7-10 days	6 mg/kg/day in 4 doses × 7-10 days
	Paromomycin[28]	25-35 mg/kg/day in 3 doses × 7 days	
Gnathostomiasis (*Gnathostoma spinigerum*)			
Treatment of choice:[29]	Surgical removal		
plus	Albendazole[30]	400-800 mg qd × 21 days	
Hookworm infection (*Ancylostoma duodenale, Necator americanus*)			
Drug of choice:	Mebendazole	100 mg bid × 3 days	100 mg bid × 3 days
OR	Pyrantel pamoate[8]	11 mg/kg (max. 1 gram) × 3 days	11 mg/kg (max. 1 gram) × 3 days
OR	Albendazole	400 mg once	400 mg once
Hydatid cyst, see TAPEWORM infection			
Hymenolepis nana, see TAPEWORM infection			
Isosporiasis (*Isospora belli*)			
Drug of choice:	Trimethoprim-sulfamethoxazole[8,31]	160 mg TMP, 800 mg SMX qid × 10 days, then bid × 3 wk	

26. Unpublished data indicate triclabendazole (Fasinex), a veterinary fasciolide, may be effective in a dosage of 5 mg/kg once daily for 3 days or 10 mg/kg twice in one day.

27. Furazolidone has been reported to be mutagenic and carcinogenic. Albendazole 400 mg daily × 5 days may be effective (Hall and Nahar, Trans R Soc Trop Med Hyg 1993; 87:84). Bacitracin zinc or bacitracin 120,000 U bid for 10 days may also be effective (Andrews et al., Am J Trop Med Hyg 1995; 52:318).

28. Not absorbed and not highly effective, but may be useful for treatment of giardiasis in pregnancy.

29. Ivermectin has been reported to be effective in animals (Anantaphruti et al., Trop Med Parasitol 1992; 43:65).

30. Kraivichian et al., Trans R Soc Trop Med Hyg 1992; 86:418).

31. In sulfonamide-sensitive patients, such as some HIV-infected patients, pyrimethamine 50-75 mg daily has been effective (Weiss et al, Ann Intern Med 1988; 109:474). In immunocompromised patients, it may be necessary to continue therapy indefinitely.

Table A-2   Drugs for treatment of parasitic infections—cont'd

Infection		Drug	Adult dosage	Pediatric dosage
Leishmaniasis *(L. mexicana, L. tropica, L. major, L. braziliensis, L. donovani [Kala-azar])*				
Drug of choice:		Sodium stibogluconate[3]	20 mg Sb/kg/day IV or IM × 20-28 days[32]	20 mg Sb/kg/day IV or IM × 20-28 days[32]
	OR	Meglumine antimonate	20 mg Sb/kg/day × 20-28 days[32]	20 mg Sb/kg/day × 20-28 days[32]
Alternatives:[33]		Amphotericin B[8]	0.25 to 1 mg/kg by slow infusion daily or every 2 days for up to 8 wk	0.25 to 1 mg/kg by slow infusion daily or every 2 days for up to 8 wk
		Pentamidine isethionate[8]	2-4 mg/kg daily or every 2 days IM for up to 15 doses[32]	2-4 mg/kg daily or every 2 days IM for up to 15 doses[32]
Lice infestation *(Pediculus humanus, capitis, Phthirus pubis)*[34]				
Drug of choice:		1% Permethrin[35]	Topically	Topically
	OR	0.5% Malathion	Topically	Topically
Alternative:		Pyrethrins with piperonyl butoxide	Topically[36]	Topically[36]
Loa loa, see FILARIASIS				
Malaria, treatment of *(Plasmodium falciparum, P. ovale, P. vivax,* and *P. malariae)*				
Chloroquine-resistant *P. falciparum*[37]				
ORAL				
Drugs of choice:		Quinine sulfate **plus**	650 mg q8h × 3-7 days[38]	25 mg/kg/day in 3 doses × 3-7 days[38]
		pyrimethamine-sulfadoxine[39]	3 tablets at once on last day of quinine	<1 yr: ¼ tablet 1-3 yrs: ½ tablet 4-8 yrs: 1 tablet 9-14 yrs: 2 tablets
	OR	**plus** tetracycline[8]	250 mg qid × 7 days	20 mg/kg day in 4 doses × 7 days[13]
	OR[40]	**plus** clindamycin[8]	900 mg tid × 3-5 days	20-40 mg/kg/day in 3 doses × 3-5 days

32. May be repeated or continued. A longer duration may be needed for some forms of visceral leishmaniasis.

33. Limited data indicate that ketoconazole (Nizoral), 400 to 600 mg daily for 4 to 8 weeks, may be effective for treatment of cutaneous leishmaniasis (Saenz et al., Am J Med 1990; 89:147). Some studies indicate that *L. donovani* resistant to sodium stibogluconate or meglumine antimonate may respond to recombinant human gamma interferon in addition to antimony (Badaro and Johnson, J Infect Dis 1993; 167(suppl 1): S13), or pentamidine followed by a course of antimony (Thakur et al., Am J Trop Med Hyg 1991; 45:435). Liposomal encapsulated amphotericin B (AmBisome, Vestar, San Dimas, CA) has been used successfully to treat multiple drug–resistant visceral leishmaniasis (Davidson et al., Q J Med 1994; 87:75; Dietze et al., Clin Infect Dis 1993; 17:891). Recently the combination of aminosidine (chemically identical to paromomycin) and sodium stibogluconate has been used to decrease the time to clinical cure of kala-azar (Thakur et al., Trans R. Soc Trop Med Hyg, 1995; 89:219) and to cure diffuse cutaneous leishmaniasis caused by *L. aethiopica* (Teklemariam et al., Trans R. Soc Trop Med Hyg 1994; 88:334). In addition, preliminary studies suggest the aminosidine ointment appears to be effective in the treatment of cutaneous Old World leishmaniasis (Bryceson et al., Trans R Soc Trop Med Hyg 1994; 88:226).

34. For infestation of eyelashes with crab lice, use petrolatum.

35. FDA-approved only for head lice.

36. Some consultants recommend a second application 1 week later to kill hatching progeny.

37. Chloroquine-resistant *P. falciparum* infections occur in all malarious areas except Central America west of the Panama Canal Zone, Mexico, Haiti, the Dominican Republic, and most of the Middle East (chloroquine resistance has been reported in Yemen, Oman, and Iran).

38. In Southeast Asia and possibly in other areas, such as South America, relative resistance to quinine has increased and the treatment should be continued for 7 days.

39. Fansidar tablets contain 25 mg of pyrimethamine and 500 mg of sulfadoxine. Resistance to pyrimethamine-sulfadoxine has been reported from Southeast Asia, the Amazon basin, East Africa, Bangladesh, and Oceania.

40. In pregnancy.

Continued

Table A-2 Drugs for treatment of parasitic infections—cont'd

Infection	Drug	Adult dosage	Pediatric dosage
Malaria, treatment of—cont'd			
Alternatives:[41]	Mefloquine[42,43]	1250 mg[44]	25 mg/kg once[45] (<45 kg)
	Halofantrine[46]	500 mg q6h × 3 doses; repeat in 1 week	8 mg/kg q6h × 3 doses (<40 kg); repeat in 1 week
PARENTERAL			
Drug of choice:[47,48]	Quinidine gluconate[49,50]	10 mg/kg loading dose (max. 600 mg) in normal saline slowly over 1 to 2 hr, followed by continuous infusion of 0.02 mg/kg/min until oral therapy can be started	Same as adult dose
OR	Quinine dihydrochloride[50,51]	20 mg/kg loading dose in 10 mg/kg 5% dextrose over 4 hr, followed by 10 mg/kg over 2-4 hr q8h (max. 1800 mg/day) until oral therapy can be started	Same as adult dose

41. For treatment of multiple drug–resistant *P. falciparum* in Southeast Asia, especially Thailand, where resistance to mefloquine and halofantrine frequently occur, a 7-day course of quinine and tetracycline is recommended (Watt et al., Am J Trop Med Hyg 1992; 47:108). Combinations of artesunate plus mefloquine (Luxemburger et al., Trans R Soc Trop Med Hyg, 1994; 88:213), artemether plus mefloquine (Karbwang et al., Trans R. Soc Trop Med Hyg 1995; 89:296), or mefloquine plus tetracycline are also used to treat multiple drug–resistant *P. falciparum*.

42. At this dosage, adverse effects including nausea, vomiting, diarrhea, dizziness, disturbed sense of balance, toxic psychosis, and seizures can occur. Mefloquine is teratogenic in animals and it has not been approved for use in pregnancy, but mefloquine prophylaxis has been reported to be safe and effective when used during the second half of pregnancy (Nosten et al., J Infect Dis 1994; 169:595). Limited studies also have demonstrated its efficacy in treating *P. falciparum* malaria during pregnancy (Na Bangchang et al., Trans R Soc Trop Med Hyg, 1994; 88:321). It should not be given together with quinine or quinidine, and caution is required in using quinine or quinidine to treat patients with malaria who have taken mefloquine for prophylaxis. The pediatric dosage has not been approved by the FDA. Resistance to mefloquine has been reported in some areas, such as the Thailand–Myanmar border and the Amazon region, where 25 mg/kg should be used.

43. In the United States a 250-mg tablet of mefloquine contains 228 mg of mefloquine base. Outside the United States each 275-mg tablet contains 250 mg base.

44. 750 mg followed 6-8 hours later by 500 mg.

45. White, Eur J Clin Pharmacol 1988; 34:1.

46. May be effective in multiple drug–resistant *P. falciparum* malaria, but treatment failures and resistance have been reported, and the drug causes consistent dose-related lengthening of the PR and QTC intervals (Castot et al., Lancet 1993; 341:1541). Several patients have developed first-degree block (Nosten et al., Lancet 1993; 341:1054). The micronized form of halofantrine has improved its bioavailability, but variability in absorption remains an important problem (Karbwang et al., Clin Pharmacokinet 1994; 27:104). It should not be taken 1 hour before to 3 hours after meals and should not be used for patients with cardiac conduction defects. Cardiac monitoring is recommended.

47. One study found artemether, a Chinese drug, effective for parenteral treatment of severe malaria in children (White et al, Lancet 1992; 339:317).

48. Exchange transfusion has been helpful for some patients with high-density (>10%) parasitemia, altered mental status, pulmonary edema, or renal complications (Zucker and Campbell, Infect Dis Clin North Am 1993; 7:547).

49. Continuous EKG, blood pressure, and glucose monitoring are recommended.

50. Quinidine may have greater antimalarial activity than quinine. The loading dose should be decreased or omitted in those patients who have received quinine or mefloquine. If more than 48 hours of parenteral treatment is required, the quinine or quinidine dose should be reduced by 1/3 to 1/2.

51. Not available in the United States. With IV administration of quinine dihydrochloride, monitoring of EKG and blood pressure is recommended. Use of parenteral quinine or quinidine may also lead to severe hypoglycemia; blood glucose should be monitored.

Table A-2 Drugs for treatment of parasitic infections—cont'd

Infection	Drug	Adult dosage	Pediatric dosage
Malaria, treatment of—cont'd			
All *Plasmodium* except Chloroquine-resistant *P. falciparum*[37]			
ORAL			
Drug of choice:	Chloroquine phosphate[52,53]	1 gram (600 mg base); then 500 mg (300 mg base) 6 hr later, then 500 mg (300 mg base) at 24 and 48 hr	10 mg base/kg (max. 600 mg base), then 5 mg base/kg 6 hr later, then 5 mg base/kg at 24 and 48 hr
PARENTERAL			
Drug of choice:[48]	Quinidine gluconate[49,50]	same as above	same as above
OR	Quinine dihydrochloride[50,51]	same as above	same as above
Prevention of relapses: *P. vivax* and *P. ovale* only			
Drug of choice:	Primaquine phosphate[54,55]	26.3 mg (15 mg base)/day × 14 days or 79 mg (45 mg base)/wk × 8 wk	0.3 mg base/kg/day × 14 days
Malaria, prevention of[56,57]			
Chloroquine-sensitive areas			
Drug of choice:	Chloroquine phosphate[58]	500 mg (300 mg base), once/week[59]	5 mg/kg base once/week, up to adult dose of 300 mg base

52. If chloroquine phosphate is not available, hydroxychloroquine sulfate is as effective; 400 mg of hydroxychloroquine sulfate is equivalent to 500 mg of chloroquine phosphate.

53. In *P. falciparum* malaria, if the patient has not shown a response to conventional doses of chloroquine in 48-72 hours, parasitic resistance to this drug should be considered. *P. vivax* with decreased susceptibility to chloroquine has been reported from Papua-New Guinea, Brazil, Myanmar, India, Colombia, and Indonesia; a single dose of mefloquine, 15 mg/kg, has been recommended to treat these infections.

54. Some relapses have been reported with this regimen; relapses should be treated with chloroquine plus primaquine, 22.5 to 30 mg base/day × 14 days.

55. Primaquine phosphate can cause hemolytic anemia, especially in patients whose red cells are deficient in glucose-6-phosphate dehydrogenase. This deficiency is most common in African, Asian, and Mediterranean peoples. Patients should be screened for G-6-PD deficiency before treatment. Primaquine should not be used during pregnancy.

56. No drug regimen guarantees protection against malaria. If fever develops within a year (particularly within the first 2 months) after travel to malarious areas, travelers should be advised to seek medical attention. Insect repellents, insecticide-impregnated bed nets, and proper clothing are important adjuncts for malaria prophylaxis.

57. In pregnancy, chloroquine prophylaxis has been used extensively and safely, but the safety of other prophylactic antimalarial agents in pregnancy is unclear. Therefore, travel during pregnancy to chloroquine-resistant areas should be discouraged. (See footnote 42.)

58. For prevention of attack after departure from areas where *P. vivax* and *P. ovale* are endemic, which includes almost all areas where malaria is found (except Haiti), some experts prescribe in addition primaquine phosphate 15 mg base (26.3 mg)/day or, for children, 0.3 mg base/kg/day during the last 2 weeks of prophylaxis. Others prefer to avoid the toxicity of primaquine and rely on surveillance to detect cases when they occur, particularly when exposure was limited or doubtful. See also footnote 54 and 55.

59. Beginning 1 week before travel and continuing weekly for the duration of stay and for 4 weeks after leaving.

Continued

Table A-2   Drugs for treatment of parasitic infections—cont'd

Infection	Drug	Adult dosage	Pediatric dosage
Malaria, prevention of—cont'd			
Chloroquine-resistant areas[37]			
Drug of choice:[60]	Mefloquine[43,58,61]	250 mg once/week[59]	15-19 kg: ¼ tablet 20-30 kg: ½ tablet 31-45 kg: ¾ tablet >45 kg: 1 tablet
OR	Doxycycline[58,62]	100 mg daily[62]	>8 years of age: 2 mg/kg/day, up to 100 mg/day
Alternatives:	Chloroquine phosphate[58]	same as above	same as above
	plus pyrimethamine- sulfadoxine[39] for presumptive treatment or	Carry a single dose (3 tablets) for self- treatment of febrile illness when medical care is not immedi- ately available	<1 yr: ¼ tablet 1-3 yr: ½ tablet 4-8 yr: 1 tablet 9-14 yr: 2 tablets
plus	proguanil[63] (in Africa south of the Sahara)	200 mg daily	<2 yr: 50 mg daily 2-6 yr: 100 mg 7-10 yr: 150 mg >10 yr: 200 mg
Microsporidiosis			
Ocular (*Encephalitozoon hellem, Vittaforma corneae [Nosema corneum]*)			
Drug of choice:	See footnote 64		
Intestinal (*Enterocytozoon bieneusi, Septata [Encephalitozoon] intestinalis*)			
Drug of choice:	See footnote 65		
Disseminated (*Encephalitozoon hellem, Encephalitozoon cuniculi, Pleistophora sp.*)			
Drug of choice:	See footnote 66		

60. Several recent studies have shown that daily primaquine provides effective prophylaxis against chloroquine-resistant *P. falciparum* (Weiss et al., J Infect Dis 1995; 171:1569).

61. The pediatric dosage has not been approved by the FDA, and the drug has not been approved for use during pregnancy. Women should take contraceptive precautions while taking mefloquine and for 2 months after the last dose. Mefloquine is not recommended for patients with cardiac conduction abnormalities. Patients with a history of seizures or psychiatric disorders and those whose occupation requires fine coordination or spatial discrimination should probably avoid mefloquine (Medical Letter 1990; 32:13). Resistance to mefloquine has been reported in some areas, such as Thailand; in these areas, doxycycline should be used for prophylaxis.

62. Beginning 1 day before travel and continuing for the duration of stay and for 4 weeks after leaving. Use of tetracyclines is contraindicated in pregnancy and in children less than 8 years old. Doxycycline can cause gastrointestinal disturbances, vaginal moniliasis, and photosensitivity reactions.

63. Proguanil (Paludrine-Ayerst, Canada; ICI, England), which is not available in the United States but is widely available overseas, is recommended mainly for use in Africa south of the Sahara. Prophylaxis is recommended during exposure and for 4 weeks afterwards. Failures in prophylaxis with chloroquine and proguanil have been reported in travelers to Kenya (Barnes, Lancet 1991; 338:1338).

64. Ocular lesions caused by *E. hellem* in HIV-infected patients have responded to fumagillin eyedrops prepared from *Fumidil-B*, a commercial product used to control a microsporidial disease of honey bees, available from Mid-Continent Agrimarketing, Inc., Lenexa, Kansas 66215 (Diesenhouse, Am J Ophthalmol 1993; 115:293). Fumagillin from other sources has also been used successfully (Rosberger et al., Cornea 1993;12:261). In one report a keratopathy caused by *E. hellem* in an HIV-infected patient was treated successfully with surgical debridement, topical antibiotics, and itraconazole (Yee et al., Ophthalmology 1991; 98:196). For lesions caused by *V. corneae,* topical therapy is generally not effective and keratoplasty may be required (Davis et al., Ophthalmology 1990; 97:953).

65. Albendazole, 400 mg bid may be effective for *S. intestinalis* infections (Blanshard et al., AIDS 1992; 6:311) and may be helpful for *E. bieneusi* infections (Dieterich et al., J Infect Dis 1994; 169:178). Octreotide (Sandostatin) has provided symptomatic relief in some patients with large volume diarrhea.

66. Albendazole 400 mg bid may be effective for *E. hellem* and *E. cuniculi.* There is no established treatment for *Pleistophora.*

Table A-2   Drugs for treatment of parasitic infections—cont'd

Infection	Drug	Adult dosage	Pediatric dosage
Mites, see SCABIES			
Moniliformis moniliformis infection			
Drug of choice:	Pyrantel pamoate[8]	11 mg/kg once, repeat twice, 2 wk apart	11 mg/kg once, repeat twice, 2 wk apart
Naegleria **species,** see AMEBIC MENINGOENCEPHALITIS, PRIMARY			
Necator americanus, see HOOKWORM infection			
Oesophagostomum bifurcum			
Drug of choice:	See footnote 67		
Onchocera volvulus, see FILARIASIS			
Opisthorchis viverrini, see FLUKE infection			
Paragonimus westermani, see FLUKE infection			
Pediculus capitis, humanus, Phthirus pubis, see LICE			
Pinworm, see ENTEROBIUS			
Pneumocystis carinii pneumonia[68]			
Drug of choice:	Trimethoprim-sulfamethoxazole	TMP 15 mg/kg/day SMX 75 mg/kg/day oral or IV in 3 or 4 doses × 14-21 days[69]	Same as adult dose
Alternatives:[70]	Pentamidine	3-4 mg/kg IV qd × 14-21 days[69]	Same as adult dose
	Trimetrexate	45 mg/m² IV qd × 21 days	
	plus folinic acid	20 mg/m² PO or IV q6h × 21 days	
	Trimethoprim[8]	5 mg/kg PO tid × 21 days	
	plus dapsone[8]	100 mg PO qd × 21 days	
	Atovaquone suspension	750 mg bid PO × 21 days	
	Primaquine[8,55]	15 mg base PO qd × 21 days	
	plus clindamycin[8]	600 mg IV q6h × 21 days, or 300-450 mg PO q6h × 21 days	
Primary and secondary prophylaxis			
Drug of Choice:	Trimethoprim-sulfamethoxazole	1 DS tab (160 mg TMP, 800 mg SMX) PO qd or 3×/week	TMP 150 mg, SMX 750 mg in 2 doses PO 3×/week
Alternatives:	Dapsone[8]	50-100 mg PO qd, or 100 mg PO 2×/week	2 mg/kg PO qd
	±Pyrimethamine[71]	50 mg PO 2×/week	
	Pentamidine aerosol	300 mg inhaled monthly via *Respirgard II* nebulizer	>5 yr: same as adult dose

67. Albendazole or pyrantel pamoate may be effective (Krepel et al., Trans R Soc Trop Med Hyg 1993; 87:87).
68. In severe disease with room air PO_2 ≤70 mmHg or Aa gradient ≥ 35 mmHg, prednisone should also be used.
69. HIV-infected patients should be treated for 21 days.
70. For patients who have failed or are intolerant to trimethoprim-sulfamethoxazole.
71. Plus folinic acid, 10 mg, with each dose of pyrimethamine.

Continued

Table A–2   Drugs for treatment of parasitic infections—cont'd

Infection	Drug	Adult dosage	Pediatric dosage
Roundworm, see ASCARIASIS			
Scabies *(Sarcoptes scabiei)*			
Drug of choice:	5% Permethrin	Topically	Topically
Alternatives:	Ivermectin	200 μg/kg PO once	200 μg/kg PO once
	10% Crotamiton	Topically	Topically
Schistosomiasis *(Bilharziasis)*			
S. haematobium			
Drug of choice:	Praziquantel	40 mg/kg/day in 2 doses × 1 day	40 mg/kg/day in 2 doses × 1 day
S. japonicum			
Drug of choice:	Praziquantel	60 mg/kg/day in 3 doses × 1 day	60 mg/kg/day in 3 doses × 1 day
S. mansoni			
Drug of choice:	Praziquantel	40 mg/kg/day in 2 doses × 1 day	40 mg/kg/day in 2 doses × 1 day
Alternative:	Oxamniquine[72]	15 mg/kg once[73]	20 mg/kg/day in 2 doses × 1 day[73]
S. mekongi			
Drug of chioce:	Praziquantel	60 mg/kg/day in 3 doses × 1 day	60 mg/kg/day in 3 doses × 1 day
Sleeping sickness, see TRYPANOSOMIASIS			
Strongyloidiasis *(Strongyloides stercoralis)*			
Drug of choice:[74]	Thiabendazole	50 mg/kg/day in 2 doses (max. 3 grams/day) × 2 days[11,75]	50 mg/kg/day in 2 doses (max. 3 grams/day) × 2 days[11,75]
OR	Ivermectin[76]	200 μg/kg/day × 1-2 days	200 μg/kg/day × 1-2 days
Tapeworm infection—**Adult (intestinal stage)**			
***Diphyllobothrium latum* (fish), *Taenia saginata* (beef), *Taenia solium* (pork), *Dipylidium caninum* (dog)**			
Drug of choice:	Praziquantel[8]	5-10 mg/kg once	5-10 mg/kg once
***Hymenolepsis nana* (dwarf tapeworm)**			
Drug of choice:	Praziquantel[8]	25 mg/kg once	25 mg/kg once
—Larval (tissue stage)			
***Echinococcus granulosus* (hydatid cyst)**			
Drug of choice:	Albendazole[77,78]	400 mg bid × 28 days, repeated as necessary	15 mg/kg/day × 28 days, repeated as necessary
Echinococcus multilocularis			
Treatment of choice:	See footnote 79		

72. Neuropsychiatric disturbances and seizures have been reported in some patients (Stokvis et al., Am J Trop Med Hyg 1986; 35:330).

73. In East Africa the dose should be increased to 30 mg/kg, and in Egypt and South Africa, 30 mg/kg/day × 2 days). Some experts recommend 40-60 mg/kg over 2-3 days in all of Africa (Shekhar, Drugs 1991; 42:379).

74. In immunocompromised patients it may be necessary to prolong therapy or use other agents.

75. In disseminated strongyloidiasis, thiabendazole therapy should be continued for at least 5 days.

76. Naquira et al., Am J Trop Med Hyg 1989; 40:304; Lyagoubi et al., Trans R Soc Trop Med Hyg 1992; 86:541; Gann et al., J Infect Dis 1994; 169:1076.

77. With a fatty meal to enhance absorption. Some patients may benefit from or require surgical resection of cysts (Tompkins, Mayo Clin Proc 1991; 66:1281). Praziquantel may also be useful preoperatively or in case of spill during surgery.

78. Percutaneous drainage with ultrasound guidance plus albendazole therapy has been effective for management of hepatic hydatid cyst disease (Khuroo et al., Gastroenterology 1993; 104:1452).

79. Surgical excision is the only reliable means of treatment, although some reports have suggested use of albendazole or mebedazole (Hao et al., Trans R Soc Trop Med Hyg, 1994; 88:340).

Table A-2   Drugs for treatment of parasitic infections—cont'd

Infection	Drug	Adult dosage	Pediatric dosage
Tapeworm infection—**Adult (intestinal stage)**—cont'd			
Cysticercus cellulosae **(cysticercosis)**			
Drug of choice:[80]	Albendazole[81]	15 mg/kg/day in 2-3 doses × 8-28 days, repeated as necessary	15 mg/kg/day in 2-3 doses × 8-28 days, repeated as necessary
OR	Praziquantel[8]	50 mg/kg/day in 3 doses × 15 days	50 mg/kg/day in 3 doses × 15 days
Alternative:	Surgery		
Toxocariasis, see VISCERAL LARVA MIGRANS			
Toxoplasmosis *(Toxoplasma gondii)*[82]			
Drugs of choice:[83]	Pyrimethamine[71]	25-100 mg/day × 3-4 wk	2 mg/kg/day × 3 days, then 1 mg/kg/day (max. 25 mg/day) × 4 wks[84]
	plus sulfdiazine	1-1.5 grams qid × 3-4 wk	100-200 mg/kg/day × 3-4 wk
Alternative:	Spiramycin[85]	3-4 grams/day	50-100 mg/kg/day × 3-4 wk
Trichinosis *(Trichinella spiralis)*			
Drugs of choice:	Steroids for severe symptoms		
	plus mebendazole[8,86]	200-400 mg tid × 3 days, then 400-500 mg tid × 10 days	
Trichomoniasis *(Trichomonas vaginalis)*			
Drug of choice:[87]	Metronidazole	2 grams once or 250 mg tid or 375 mg bid PO × 7 days	15 mg/kg/day orally in 3 doses × 7 days
OR	Tinidazole[5]	2 grams once	50 mg/kg once (max. 2 grams)
Trichostrongylus infection			
Drug of choice:	Pyrantel pamoate[8]	11 mg/kg once (max. 1 gram)	11 mg/kg once (max. 1 gram)
Alternative:	Mebendazole[8]	100 mg bid × 3 days	100 mg bid × 3 days
OR	Albendazole	400 mg once	400 mg once

80. Corticosteroids should be given for 2 to 3 days before and during drug therapy for neurocysticercosis. Any cysticercocidal drug may cause irreparable damage when used to treat ocular or spinal cysts, even when corticosteroids are used.

81. Albendazole should be taken with a fatty meal to enhance absorption.

82. In ocular toxoplasmosis, corticosteroids should also be used for an antiinflammatory effect on the eyes.

83. To treat CNS toxoplasmosis in HIV-infected patients, some clinicians have used pyrimethamine 50 to 100 mg daily after a loading dose of 200 mg with a sulfonamide and, when sulfonamide sensitivity developed, have given clindamycin 1.8 to 2.4 g/day in divided doses instead of the sulfonamide (Remington et al., Lancet 1991; 338:1142; Luft et al., N Engl J Med 1993; 329:995). Atovaquone plus pyrimethamine appears to be an effective alternative in sulfa-intolerant patients (Kovacs et al., Lancet 1992; 340:637). Dapsone-pyrimethamine can prevent first episodes of toxoplasmosis (Girard et al., N Engl J Med 1993; 328:1514).

84. Congenitally infected newborns should be treated with pyrimethamine every 2 or 3 days and a sulfonamide daily for about 1 year (Remington and Desmonts in JS Remington and JO Klein (eds), *Infectious Disease of the Fetus and Newborn Infant* (ed 4), Philadelphia: WB Saunders, 1995, p 140).

85. For use during pregnancy, continue the drug until delivery. If it has been determined that transmission has occurred in utero, then therapy with pyrimethamine and sulfadiazine should be started.

86. Albendazole or flubendazole (not available in the United States) may also be effective.

87. Sexual partners should be treated simultaneously. Outside the United States, ornidazole has also been used for this condition. Metronidazole-resistant strains have been reported; higher doses of metronidazole for longer periods are sometimes effective against these strains (Lossick, Rev Infect Dis 1990; 12:S665). Experimental studies suggest that bacitracin and bacitracin zinc have microbicidal activity against multiple isolates of *T. vaginalis* (Andrews et al., Trans R Soc Trop Med Hyg 1994; 88:704).

Continued

Table A-2 Drugs for treatment of parasitic infections—cont'd

Infection		Drug	Adult dosage	Pediatric dosage
Trichuriasis *(Trichuris trichiura,* whipworm)				
Drug of choice:		Mebendazole	100 mg bid × 3 days	100 mg bid × 3 days
	OR	Albendazole	400 mg once[88]	400 mg once[88]
Trypanosomiasis				
T. cruzi (American trypanosomiasis, Chagas' disease)				
Drug of choice:		Nifurtimox[3,89]	8-10 mg/kg/day in 4 doses × 120 days	1-10 yr: 15-20 mg/kg/day in 4 doses × 90 days; 11-16 yr: 12.5-15 mg/kg/day in 4 doses × 90 days
Alternative:		Benznidazole[90]	5-7 mg/kg/days × 30-120 days	
T. brucei gambiense; T. b. rhodesiense (African trypanosomiasis, sleeping sickness) hemolymphatic stage				
Drug of choice:		Suramin[3]	100-200 mg (test dose) IV, then 1 gram IV on days 1,3,7,14 and 21	20 mg/kg on days 1,3,7,14, and 21
	OR	Eflornithine	See footnote 91	
Alternative:		Pentamidine isethionate[8]	4 mg/kg/day IM × 10 days	4 mg/kg/day IM × 10 days
late disease with CNS involvement				
Drug of choice:		Melarsoprol[3,92]	2-3.6 mg/kg/day IV × 3 days; after 1 wk 3.6 mg/kg per day IV × 3 days; repeat again after 10-21 days	18-25 mg/kg total over 1 month; initial dose of 0.36 mg/kg IV, increasing gradually to max. 3.6 mg/kg at intervals of 1-5 days for total of 9-10 doses
	OR	Eflornithine	See footnote 91	
Alternatives: (*T.b. gambiense* only)		Tryparsamide	One injection of 30 mg/kg (max. 2 g) IV every 5 days to total of 12 injections; may be repeated after 1 month	
		plus suramin[3]	One injection of 10 mg/kg IV every 5 days to total of 12 injections; may be repeated after 1 month	

88. In heavy infection it may be necessary to extend therapy for 3 days.

89. The addition of gamma interferon to nifurtimox for 20 days in a limited number of patients and in experimental animals appears to have shortened the acute phase of Chagas' disease (McCabe et al., J Infect Dis 1991; 163:912).

90. Limited data.

91. In *T. b. gambiense* infections, eflornithine is highly effective in both the hemolymphatic and CNS stages. Its effectiveness in *T. b. rhodesiense* infections has been variable. Some clinicians have given 400 mg/kg/day IV in 4 divided doses for 14 days, followed by oral treatment with 300 mg/kg/day for 3-4 wk (Milord et al., Lancet 1992; 340:652).

92. In frail patients, begin with as little as 18 mg and increase the dose progressively. Pretreatment with suramin has been advocated for debilitated patients. Corticosteroids have been used to prevent arsenical encephalopathy (Pepin et al., Trans R Soc Trop Med Hyg, 1995; 89:92).

Table A-2   Drugs for treatment of parasitic infections—cont'd

Infection	Drug	Adult dosage	Pediatric dosage
Visceral larva migrans[93] (*Toxocariasis*)			
Drug of choice:	Diethyl-carbamazine[8]	6 mg/kg/day in 3 doses × 7-10 days	6 mg/kg/day in 3 doses × 7-10 days
Alternatives:	Albendazole	400 mg bid × 3-5 days	400 mg bid × 3-5 days
	Mebendazole[8]	100-200 mg bid × 5 days	100-200 mg bid × 5 days

Whipworm, see TRICHURIASIS

Wuchereria bancrofti, see FILARIASIS

93. For severe symptoms or eye involvement, corticosteroids can be used in addition.

Manufacturers of antiparasitic drugs

* albendazole—Zental (SmithKline Beecham)
** aminosidine (paromomycin)
atovaquone—Mepron (Glaxo-Wellcome)
bacitracin—many manufacturers
** bacitracin-zinc (Apothekernes Laboratorium A.S., Oslo, Norway)
** benznidazole—Rochagan (Roche, Brazil)
† bithionol—Bitin (Tanabe, Japan)
chloroquine—Aralen (Sanofi Winthop), others
crotamiton—Eurax (Westwood-Squibb)
dapsone (Jacobus)
* diethylcarbamazine—Hetrazan (Wyeth-Ayerst)
† diloxanide furoate—Furamide (Boots, England)
* eflornithine (difluoromethylornithine, DFMO)—Ornidyl (Merrell Dow)
** flubendazole—(Janssen)
furazolidone—Furoxone (Roberts)
** halofantrine—Halfan (SmithKline Beecham)
hydroxychloroquine—Plaquenil (Sanofi Winthrop)
iodoquinol (diiodohydroxyquin)—Yodoxin (Glenwood), others
† ivermectin—Mectizan (Merck)
** malathion—Prioderm
mebendazole—Vermox (Janssen)
mefloquine—Lariam (Roche)
** meglumine antimonate—Glucantime (Rhône-Poulenc Rorer, France)
† melarsoprol—Arsobal (Rhône-Poulenc Rorer, France)
metronidazole—Flagyl (Searle), others

† nifurtimox—Lampit (Bayer, Germany)
** ornidazole—Tiberal (Hoffman-LaRoche, Switzerland)
oxamniquine—Vansil (Pfizer)
paromomycin—Humatin (Parke-Davis)
pentamidine isethionate—Pentam 300 (Fujisawa), NebuPent (Fujisawa)
permethrin—Nix (Glaxo-Wellcome), Elimite (Herbert), Lyclear (Canada)
praziquantel—Biltricide (Miles)
primaquine phosphate—(Sanofi Winthrop)
** proguanil—Paludrine (Ayerst, Canada, ICI, England)
pyrantel pamoate—Antiminth (Pfizer)
pyrethrins and piperonyl butoxide—RID (Pfizer), others
pyrimethamine—Daraprim (Glaxo-Wellcome)
pyrimethamine-sulfadoxine—Fansidar (Roche)
quinidine gluconate—(Lilly)
** quinine dihydrochloride
quinine sulfate—many manufacturers
† sodium stibogluconate (antimony sodium gluconate)—Pentostam (Glaxo-Wellcome, England)
* spiramycin—Rovamycine (Rhône-Poulenc Rorer)
sulfadiazine—(Eon Labs, and others)
† suramin—(Bayer, Germany)
thiabendazole—Mintezol (Merck)
** tinidazole—Fasigyn (Pfizer)
** trichlabendazole—(Ciba-Geigy)
trimetrexate—Neutrexin (U.S. Bioscience)
** tryparsamide

*Available in the United States only from the manufacturer.
**Not available in the United States.
†Available from the CDC Drug Service, Centers for Disease Control and Prevention, Atlanta, Georgia 30333; 404-639-3670 (evenings, weekends, or holidays: 404-639-2888).

Table A-3 Antimicrobial Drug Dosage†

	Adults		Children	
	Oral	**Parenteral**	**Oral**	**Parenteral**
Acyclovir	200-800 mg q4h×5 or 400-800 mg q8h[1]	5-10 mg/kg q8h	20 mg/kg q6h	5-10 mg/kg q8h
Amantadine	100 mg q12-24h		4.4 mg/kg q12-24h	
Amikacin[2]		5 mg/kg q8h or 7.5 mg/kg q12h		5 mg/kg q8h or 7.5 mg/kg q12h
Amoxicillin	250-500 mg q8h		6.6-13.3 mg/kg q8h	
Amoxicillin clavulanic acid	250-500 mg[3] q8h or 500-875 mg[3] q12h		6.6-13.3 mg/kg[3] q8h	
Amphotericin B		0.3-1.5 mg/kg[4] q24h		0.3-1.5 mg/kg[4] q24h
Ampicillin	500 mg-1 g q6h	1-2 g q4-6h	12.5-25 mg/kg q6h	25-50 mg/kg q6h[7]
Ampicillin/ sulbactam		1-2 g[8] q6h		
Azithromycin	250-1000 mg[9] q24h		5-12 mg/kg[9] q24h	
Aztreonam		1-2 g q6-8h		
Bacampicillin	400-800 mg q12h		12.5-25 mg/kg q12h	
Carbenicillin indanyl sodium	1-2 tablets[10] q6h		7.5-12.5 mg/kg q6h	
Cefaclor	250-500 mg q8h		6.6-13.3 mg/kg q8h	
Cefadroxil	1g q12-24h		15 mg/kg q12h	
Cefamandole		500 mg-2g q4-8h		50-150 mg/kg/day, divided q4-8h
Cefazolin		500 mg-1.5 g q6-8h		25-100 mg/kg/day, divided q6-8h

† Antiparasitic and antituberculosis drug dosages are found in the articles on these subjects. The articles on antiviral and antifungal drugs, prophylaxis, sexually transmitted diseases, and AIDS also include dosage recommendations.

1. For treatment of genital herpes. For suppression of genital herpes, 400 mg q12h is used. For treatment of varicella, 800 mg q6h is recommended.

2. Some clinicians give selected patients the total daily dose in one large dose (Shamrock GT et al, Pharmacotherapy 1995; 15:201; Bloser J and König C, Eur J Microbiol Infect Dis 1995; 14:1029; Hatala R et al., Ann Intern Med, 1996; 124:717).

3. Dosage based on amoxicillin content. For doses of 500 or 875 mg, 500-mg or 875-mg tablets should be used, because multiple smaller tablets wound contain too much clavulanic acid. The 875-mg, 500-mg, and 250-mg tablets each contain 125 mg clavulanic acid. 125-mg chewable tablets and 125 mg/5 ml oral suspension both contain 31.25 mg clavulanic acid; 250-mg chewable tablets and 250-mg/5-ml oral suspension both contain 62.5 mg clavulanic acid.

4. Give intravenously once a day, over a period of 2 to 4 hours.

5. OR up to 1.5 mg/kg given every other day.

Usual Maximum Dose/Day	Dose	Adult Dosage in Renal Failure For Creatinine Clearance (ml/min)			Extra Dose After Hemodialysis
		80–50	50–10	<10	
4 g oral 30 mg/kg IV	5 mg/kg	q8h	q12-24h	2.5 mg/kg q24h	yes
200 mg	100 mg	q24h	100–200 mg/d alternate days to every 7 days		no
1.5 g	5-7.5 mg/kg	q12h	q24-36h	q36-48h	yes
3 g	250-500 mg	q8h	q12h	q12-24h	yes
1.5 g	250-500 mg	q8h	q12h	q12-24h	yes
1 mg/kg[5]		Change not required[6]			no
12 g	1-2 g	q8h	q8h	q12h	yes
12 g	1.5-3 g	q6-8h	q8-12h	q24h	yes
500 mg		Change not required			Unknown
8 g	0.5-2 g	See package insert			See package insert
1600 mg	400-800 mg	q12h	q12h	q24h	yes
3 g		See package insert			
4 g	250-500 mg	Change not required			yes
2 g	0.5-1 g	q12-24h	q12-24h	q36h	yes
12 g	0.5-2 g	1-2 g q6h	1-2 g q8h	0.5-1g q8-12h	yes
6 g	0.5-1.5q	q8h	0.5-1 g q8-12h	0.5-1 g q24h	yes

6. Amphotericin B is potentially nephrotoxic; temporary interruption of therapy may be required when the serum creatinine exceeds 3 mg/dl.

7. For meningitis in children caused by ampicillin-sensitive *H. influenzae* type b, Medical Letter consultants recommend up 400 mg/kg/day. Meningitis should be treated q4h.

8. Dosage based on ampicillin content.

9. For adults: 500 mg on day 1 and 250 mg/day on days 2-5. I gram once for *C. trachomatis* urethritis. For children: 10 mg/kg on day 1 and 5 mg/kg on days 2 to 5 for acute otitis media and 12 mg/kg for 5 days for pharyngitis/tonsilitis.

10. Tablets contain 382 mg of indanyl sodium carbenicillin.

Continued

Table A-3   Antimicrobial Drug Dosage—cont'd

	Adults		Children	
	Oral	Parenteral	Oral	Parenteral
Cefixime	200 mg q12h or 400 mg q24h		4 mg/kg q12h or 8 mg/kg q24h	
Cefmetazole		2 g q6-12h		
Cefonicid		500 mg-2 g q24h		
Cefoperazone		500 mg-4g q6-12h		25-100 mg/kg q12h
Cefotaxime		1-2 g q4-12h		50-180 mg/kg/day divided q4-6h
Cefotetan		500 mg-3 g q12h		
Cefoxitin		1-3 g q4-6h		80-160 mg/kg/day, divided q4-6h-
Cefpodoxime	100-400 mg q12h		10 mg/kg q24h or 5 mg/kg q12h	
Cefprozil	250-500 mg q12h		15 mg/kg q12h	
Ceftazidime		250 mg-2 g q8-12h		30-50 mg/kg q8h
Ceftibuten	400 mg q24h		9 mg/kg q24h	
Ceftizoxime		500 mg-4 g q8-12h		50 mg/kg q6-8h
Ceftriaxone		1-2 g q12-24h		50-100 mg/kg/day, divided q12-24h
Cefuroxime		750 mg-1.5 g q8h		50-150 mg/kg/day divided q6-8h
Cefuroxime axetil	125-500 mg q12h		10-15 mg/kg q12h	
Cephalexin	250 mg-1 g q6h		6.25-25 mg/kg q6h	
Cephalothin		500 mg-2 g q4-6h		80-160 mg/kg/day, divided q4-6h
Cephapirin		500 mg-2 g q4-6h		40-80 mg/kg/day, divided q4-6h
Cephradine	250 mg-1 g q6h or 500 mg-1 g q12h	500 mg-2 g q6h	6.25-25 mg/kg q6h or 12.5-50 mg/kg q12h	12.5-25 mg/kg q6h

Usual Maximum Dose/Day	Dose	Adult Dosage in Renal Failure For Creatinine Clearance (ml/min)			Extra Dose After Hemodialysis
		80–50	50–10	<10	
400 mg	200-400 mg	q24h	q24h	200 mg q24h	no
8 g	1-2 g	q8h	q16h	q48h	no*
2 g	0.5-2g	0.5-1.5 g q24h	0.25-1 g q24-48h	0.25-1 g q3-5 days	no
12 g		Change not required			no*
12 g	1-2 g	q4-8h	q6-12h	q12h	yes
6 g	1-3 g	q12h	q12-24h	q48h	yes
12 g	0.5-2 g	1-2 g q8h	1-2 g q12h	0.5-1g q12-24h	yes
800 mg	200-400 mg	q12h	q24h	q24h	yes
1000 mg	250-500 mg	No change	q24h	q24h	yes
6 g	0.5-2 g	q8-12h	1 g q12-24h	0.5 g q24-48h	yes
400 mg	400 mg	q24h	100-200 mg q24h	100 mg q24h	no*
12 g	0.25-1.5 g	0.5-1.5 g q8h	0.25-1 g q12h	0.25-1 g q24-48h	yes
4 g		Change not required			no
9 g	0.75-1.5 g	q8h	q8-12h	q24h	yes
1000 mg	250-500 mg	Change not required			yes
4 g	0.25-1 g	q6h	q8-12h	q12-48h	yes
12 g	0.5-2g	q6h	q6-8h	500 mg q6-8h	yes
12 g	0.5-2 g	q6h	q8h	q12h	yes
8 g	1-2 g	q6h	q8h	q12-72h	yes

*But give usual dose after dialysis.

Continued

Table A-3   Antimicrobial Drug Dosage—cont'd

	Adults		Children	
	Oral	**Parenteral**	**Oral**	**Parenteral**
Chloram- phenicol	12.5-25 mg/kg q6h	12.5-25 mg/kg[11] q6h	12.5-25 mg/kg q6h	12.5-25 mg/kg[11] q6h
Cinoxacin	250 mg q6h or 500 mg q12h			
Ciprofloxacin	250-750 mg q12h	200-400 mg q12h		
Clarithromycin	250-500 mg q12h		7.5 mg/kg q12h	
Clindamycin	150-450 mg q6h	150-900 mg q6-8h	2-8 mg/kg q6-8h	2.5-10 mg/kg q6h
Cloxacillin	500 mg-1 g q6h		12.5-25 mg/kg q6h	
Dicloxacillin	125-500 mg q6h		3.125-6.25 mg/kg q6h	
Didanosine[12] (ddl)	≥60 kg:200 mg q12h <60 kg:125 mg q 12h		1.1-1.4m^2:100 mg q12h 0.8-1m^2:75 mg q12h 0.5-0.7m^2:50 mg q12h ≤0.4 m^2:25 mg q12h	
Dirithromycin	500 mg q24h			
Enoxacin	200-400 mg q12h			
Erythromycin	250-500 mg q6h	250 mg-1 g IV[13] q6h	7.5-12.5 mg/kg q6h	3.75-12.5 mg/kg IV[13] q6h
Famciclovir	500 mg q8h[14]			
Fluconazole	50-400 mg q24h	100-400 mg q24h		
Flucytosine	12.5-37.5 mg/kg q6h		12.5-37.5 mg/kg q6h	
Foscarnet		60 mg/kg q8h or 90 mg/kg q12h[16]		
Ganciclovir	1000 mg q8h or 500 mg 6x	5 mg/kg q12h[17]		5 mg/kg q12h[17]

11. Intravenous administration; dosage should be adjusted according to serum concentration.

12. Refers to chewable, dispersible tablets. For adults and children more than 1 year old, each dose should include two tablets to supply adequate buffer.

13. By slow intermittent infusion to minimize thrombophlebitis.

14. For herpes zoster. For first episode genital herpes, the dosage is 250 mg q8h. For genital herpes recurrence, it is 125 mg q12h.

15. If treatment is essential, begin with 15-25 mg/kg q24h and adjust daily dose to maintain the plasma concentration between 50 and 75 μg/ml.

16. For CMV, given over at least 1 hour for induction; for maintenance, 90-120 mg/kg daily over two hours. For HSV or VZV, 40 mg/kg q8h.

17. For CMV induction, give IV at constant rate over 1 hour; for maintenance, 5 mg/kg 7 days/week or 6 mg/kg 5 days/week.

Usual Maximum Dose/Day	Dose	Adult Dosage in Renal Failure For Creatinine Clearance (ml/min)			Extra Dose After Hemodialysis
		80–50	50–10	<10	
4 g		Change not required			no*
1 g	250-500 mg	250 mg q8h	250 mg q12-24h	250 mg q24h	no
2 g	250-750 mg	q12h	250-500 mg q12-18h	250-500 mg q24h	no*
1 g	250-500 mg	q12h	q24h	Unknown	Unknown
4.8 g		Change not required			no
4 g		Change not required			no
4 g		Change not required			no
400 mg	125-200 mg	Reduction advised	Reduction advised	100 mg q24h	yes
500 mg		Change not required			no
800 mg	200-400 mg	q12h	q12h	q24h	no
4 g		Change not required			no
1.5 g	500 mg	q12h	q24h	Not recommended	yes
400 mg	100-400 mg	q24h	q48h	≥q72h	yes
150 mg/kg	12.5-37.5 mg/kg	q6h	q12-24h	Not recommended[15]	yes
		See package insert			Unknown
10 mg/kg	5 mg/kg IV	2.5 mg/kg q12h	1.25-2.5 mg/kg q24h	1.25 mg/kg q24h	no*
	500 mg or 1000 mg PO	500-1000 mg q8h	500 mg once or q12h	500 mg 3x/week	no*

*But give usual dose after dialysis.

Continued

Table A-3 Antimicrobial Drug Dosage–cont'd

	Adults		Children	
	Oral	Parenteral	Oral	Parenteral
Gentamicin[2]		1-1.7 mg/kg q8h		1-2.5 mg/kg q8h
Griseofulvin Microsize	500-1000 mg q24h		11 mg/kg q24h	
Ultra-microsize	330-660 mg q24h		7.25 mg/kg q24h	
Imipenem		250 mg-1 g[18] q6-8h		15-25 mg/kg[18] q6h
Indinavir	800 mg q8h			
Itraconazole	100-200 mg q12-24h			
Kanamycin[2]		5 mg/kg q8h or 7.5 mg/kg q12 h		5 mg/kg/q8h or 7.5 mg/kg/q12h
Ketoconazole	200-400 mg q12-24h		3.3-6.6 mg/kg q24h	
Lamivudine[20]	≥50 kg;150 mg q12h <50 kg:2 mg/kg q12h		4 mg/kg q12h	
Lomefloxacin	400 mg q24h			
Loracarbef	200-400 mg q12h		7.5-15 mg/kg q12h	
Methenamine hippurate[22]	1 g q12h		12.5-25 mg/kg q12h	
Methanamine mandelate[22]	1 g q6h		12.5-18.75 mg/kg q6h	
Methicillin		1-2 g q4-6h		25-33.3 mg/kg q4-6h
Metronidazole[23]	7.5 mg/kg q6h	7.5 mg/kg q6h	7.5 mg/kg q6h	7.5 mg/kg q6h
Mezlocillin		1.5-4 g q4-6h		50 mg/kg q4-6h
Miconazole[24]		600 mg-1.2 g q8h		6.6-13.3 mg/kg q8h
Nafcillin	500 mg-1 g q6h	500 mg-1.5 g q4-6h	12.5-25 mg/kg q6h	25-50 mg/kg q6h
Nalidixic acid	1g q6h		Not recom-mended	

*But give usual dose after dialysis.

18. Doses are for imipenem, which is combined with equal weight of cilastatin as *Primaxin.*

19. Maximum dosage should be 4 grams or 50 mg/kg, whichever is less.

20. Concurrently with zidovudine.

21. After initial loading dose of 400 mg, 200 mg q24h.

22. Usually given with an acidifying agent

23. Dosage for anaerobic bacterial infections. First dose should be 15 mg/kg loading dose. Dosage should be decreased in patients with severe hepatic disease.

24. The manufacturer recommends an initial test dose of 200 mg.

Usual Maximum Dose/Day	Dose	Adult Dosage in Renal Failure For Creatinine Clearance (ml/min)			Extra Dose After Hemodialysis
		80–50	50–10	<10	
5 mg/kg	1.5 mg/kg	q8-12h	q12-24h	q24-48h	yes
		Change not required			
		Change not required			
4 g[19]	250-500 mg	q6-8h	q8-12h	q12h	yes
		Unknown			
400 mg		Change not required			
1.5 g	5-7.5 mg/kg	q24h	q24-72h	q72-96h	yes
1 g		Change not required			no
300 mg	150 mg	q12h	See package insert		
400 mg	400 mg	q24h	See footnote 21		no
800 mg	200-400 mg	q12h	q24h	q3-5 days	yes
4 g	1 g	q12h	Not recommended		
4 g	1 g	q6h	Not recommended		
12 g	1-2 g	q6h	q8h	q12h	no
4 g	7.5 mg/kg	Change not required			no*
24 g	1.5-4g	q4-6h	q6-8h	q8-12h	yes
3.6 g		Change not required			no
12g		Change not required			no
4 g	1 g	q6h	q6h	Not recommended	

Table A-3 Antimicrobial Drug Dosage—cont'd

	Adults		Children	
	Oral	Parenteral	Oral	Parenteral
Netilmicin[2]		1.5-3.25 mg/kg q12h or 1.3-2.2 mg/kg q8h		2.7-4 mg/kg q12h or 1.8-2.7 mg/kg q8h
Nitrofurantoin	50-100 mg q6h	Not recommended	1.25-1.75 mg/kg q6h	Not recommended
Norfloxacin	400 mg q12h			
Ofloxacin	200-400 mg q12h	200-400 mg q12h		
Oxacillin	500 mg-1 g q6h	500 mg-2 g q4-6h	12.5-25 mg/kg q6h	25-50 mg/kg q6h
Penicillin G[25]	250-500 mg q6h	1.2-24 million U/day, divided q2-12h[26]	6.25-12.5 mg/kg q6h	100,000-250,000 U/kg/day, divided q2-12h[26]
Penicillin V[25]	250-500 mg q6h		6.25-12.5 mg/kg q6h	
Piperacillin		3-4 g q4-6h		200-300 mg/kg/day, divided q4-6h
Piperacillin/ tazobactam[28]		3-4 g q6h		
Rifabutin	150 mg q 12h or 300 mg once			
Rifampin[29]	600 mg/day	600 mg/day	10-20 mg/kg/day	10-20 mg/kg/day
Rimantadine	100 mg once or q12h		5 mg/kg once	
Ritonavir	600 mg bid			
Saquinavir[30]	600 mg q8h			
Spectinomycin		2 g once		40 mg/kg once
Stavudine	≥60 kg: 40 mg q12h <60 kg: 30 mg q12h			
Streptomycin		500 mg-1 g q12h		10-15 mg/kg q12h

25. One mg is equal to 1600 units.

26. The interval between parenteral doses can be as short as 2 hours for initial intravenous treatment of meningococcemia, or as long as 12 hours between intramuscular doses of penicillin G procaine.

27. Patients with severe renal insufficiency should be given no more than one third to one half the maximum daily dosage, that is, instead of giving 24 million units per day, 10 million units could be given. Patients on lower doses usually tolerate full dosage even with severe renal insufficiency.

28. Dosage based on piperacillin content. Piperacillin/tazobactam is supplied a 2 gm piperacillin/250 mg tazobactam, 3 gm piperacillin/375 mg tazobactam, and 4 gm piperacillin/500 mg tazobactam.

Usual Maximum Dose/Day	Dose	Adult Dosage in Renal Failure For Creatinine Clearance (ml/min)			Extra Dose After Hemodialysis
		80–50	50–10	<10	
6.5 mg/kg	1.3-2.2 mg/kg	q8-12h	q12-24h	q24-48h	yes
400 mg	50-100 mg	q6h	Not recommended		
800 mg	200-400 mg	q12h	q12-24h	q24h	no
800 mg	200-400 mg	q12h	q24h	half dose q24h	no
12 g		Change not required			no
24 million units		Change not required; see note 27			yes
4 g	250-500 mg	Change not required			yes
24 g	3-4 g	q4-6h	q6-12h	q12h	yes
16 g	2 g/250 mg-3 g/375 mg	No change	2 g/250 mg q6h	2 g/250 mg q8h	yes
300 mg	300 mg	q24h	q24h	Unknown	no
600 mg		Change not required			no
200 mg		Change not required			no
		Change not required			no
1800 mg	600 mg	Unknown			
		No change	Not recommended		
80 mg	40 mg	q12h	20 mg q12-24h	Not recommended	
	30 mg	q12h	15 mg q12-24h		
2 g	0.5-1 g	q24h	q24-72h	q72-96h	yes

29. For meningococcal carriers, dosage is 600 mg bid × two days for adults, 10 mg/kg q12h × two days for children more than one month old, and 5 mg/kg q12h × two days for infants less than one month old.

30. Concurrently with zidovudine or zalcitabine

Continued

Table A-3   Antimicrobial Drug Dosage—cont'd

	Adults		Children	
	Oral	**Parenteral**	**Oral**	**Parenteral**
Sulfisoxazole	500 mg-1 g q6h	25 mg/kg q6h	150 mg/kg/day divided q4-6h	100 mg/kg/day divided q6-8h
Tetracyclines[31]	250-500 mg q6h		6.25-12.5 mg/kg q6h	
Ticarcillin		200-300 mg/kg/day, divided q4-6h		200-300 mg/kg/day, divided q4-6h
Ticarcillin/ clavulanic acid		3 g[33] q4-8h		200-300 mg/kg/day, divided q4-8h[34]
Tobramycin[2]		1-1.7 mg/kg q8h		6-7.5 mg/kg/day, divided q6-8h
Trimethoprim	100 mg q12h or 200 mg once		2 mg/kg q12h[34]	
Trimethoprim-sulfamethox-azole (TMP-SMX)	1 tablet[35] q6h or 2 tablets q12h[35]	4-5 mg/kg (TMP) q6-12h	4-5 mg/kg (TMP) q6-12h	4-5 mg/kg (TMP) q6-12h
Valacyclovir	1 g q8h[37]			
Vancomycin[38]	125-500 mg q6h[39]	500 mg IV q6h or 1 g IV q12h	12.5 mg/kg q6h[39]	10 mg/kg IV q6h[40,41]
Zalcitabine (ddC)	0.375-0.75 mg q8h			
Zidovudine (AZT)	100 mg q4h 3-5x/day or 200 mg q8h		180 mg/m² q6h (max. 200 mg)	

31. Tetracycline or oxytetracycline. The oral dose of demeclocycline for adults is 600 mg daily in two to four divided doses. The oral dose of doxycycline for adults is 100 mg once or twice a day. The oral dose of minocycline for adults is 100 mg twice a day. The parenteral dose of doxycycline or minocycline is 100-200 mg/day, in one or two doses.

32. Doxycycline can be given in the usual dosage in patients with renal insufficiency, but is not recommended for urinary tract infections in such patients.

33. A 3.1-gram vial contains 3 grams of ticarcillin and 0.1 gram clavulanic acid; a 3.2-gram vial contains 3 grams of ticarcillin and 0.2 grams clavulanic acid.

34. Not recommended by manufacturer for children less than 12 years old.

35. Each tablet contains 80 mg trimethoprim and 400 mg sulfamethoxazole. Double-strength tablets are also available; the usual dosage of these is 1 tablet q12h. Suspension contains 40 mg trimethoprim and 200 mg sulfamethoxazole per 5 ml.

36. The usual maximum daily dose is 4 tablets orally or 1200 mg trimethoprim with 6000 mg sulfamethoxazole intravenously.

37. For herpes zoster. For a first episode of genital herpes, the dosage is 1 g q12h. For recurrence of genital herpes, it is 500 mg q12h.

38. Vancomycin should be infused over a period of at least 60 minutes.

39. Only for treatment of pseudomembranous colitis

40. Sixty mg/kg/day may be needed for staphylococcal central nervous system infections.

41. Peak serum concentrations should be monitored.

42. Alternatively, see nomogram in package insert.

Usual Maximum Dose/Day	Dose	Adult Dosage in Renal Failure For Creatinine Clearance (ml/min)			Extra Dose After Hemodialysis
		80–50	50–10	<10	
8 g	0.5-1 g	q6-8h	q8-12h	q12-24h	yes
2 g		Not recommended[32]			
24-30 g	2-3 g	q4-6h	q6-8h	2 g q12h	yes
18 g	2-3.1 g	3.1 g q4h	2 g q4-8h	2 g q12h	yes
5 mg/kg	1-1.66 mg/kg	q8-12h	q12-24h	q24-48h	yes
200 mg	100 mg	q12h	q18-24h	Not recommended	
See note 36	4-5 mg/kg (TMP)	q12h	q18h	Not recommended	yes
3 g	1 g	q8h	See package insert		
2 g	1 g	q24-72h[42]	q3-7 days[42]	q5-10 days[42]	no
2.25 mg	0.75 mg	No change	q12h	q24h	Unknown
1.2 g	100 mg	No change	No change	Unknown	yes

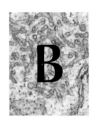

B EMERGING INFECTIONS

Box B-1 Emerging agents identified in the past 25 years infecting humans and causing illness

Box B-2 Agents with problems of antimicrobial resistance

For more than two decades, attention has been focused on new microbial agents responsible for infectious diseases of humans, as well as new behaviors of "old" agents providing new threats to the health and welfare of the populace. Much attention has been paid to these agents in the medical, scientific and popular press under the rubric of "emerging infections." The Institute of Medicine of the National Academy of Sciences organized a committee on "Emerging Microbial Threats to Health" and published a 294-page report in 1992. A new quarterly journal—*Emerging Infectious Diseases*—was initiated in 1995 by the National Center for Infectious Diseases of the Centers for Disease Control and Prevention. Conferences and symposia have been held worldwide to discuss the problems of new and resurgent infections.

Because infectious diseases remain the leading cause of both morbidity and mortality throughout the world, the appearance of new agents has special importance. When the resultant illness is of remarkable severity, such as that caused by the Ebola virus, it tends to generate extensive coverage in the media even though the numbers of patients are few compared to many other infectious diseases. Advances in diagnostic technology have permitted more rapid identification of such agents and epidemiologic surveillance of their origin, extent, and spectrum of illness. Although the recognition of HIV and AIDS in 1985 has had the most major global impact on public awareness, a list of new agents and illnesses in the past 25 years demonstrates the continuing appearance of previously unrecognized human pathogens (Box B-1). Multiple

influences have changed the patterns of disease spread, including international travel, urbanization, altered human behavior, economic development and land utilization, and diminishing support for the public health infrastructure. An ominous warning has been cited by those who prophesy global warming with climate changes such that arthropod vectors may penetrate regions of the world from which they are currently absent, bringing with them the viruses and parasites so common in warmer climates.

In contrast to the newly emerged agents, another facet of the emerging infection focus has been the altered behavior of "old" agents. The emergence of drug-resistant strains of virus, bacterium, fungus, and parasite presents a serious challenge to the infectious disease community. The ability of microbes to select, adapt, and mutate both naturally and under the pressure of antibiotics in their environment is exemplified by organisms listed in Box B-2. Antibiotic resistance is not something new but has been observed for at least 50 years, beginning with the detection of staphylococci producing β-lactamase. Although many antibiotic-resistant organisms were first observed in hospital, where the interactions of multiple antibiotic use and immunocompromised patients provided a fertile substrate, community-acquired infections have more recently been due to antibiotic-resistant organisms with increasing frequency. In addition to hospitals, a number of other settings have proven conducive to the spread of new agents and of drug' resistant organisms: day-care centers for children, nursing homes, prisons, and homeless shelters. These pathogens are most prevalent in the respiratory tract and in sexually transmitted infections. As each new antibiotic has been introduced and its use extended more widely, the suppression of susceptible strains and the selection of naturally resistant ones has progressed. In addition to the problem of primary

744

BOX B-1

EMERGING AGENTS IDENTIFIED IN THE PAST 25 YEARS INFECTING HUMANS AND CAUSING ILLNESS

Rotaviruses
Parvovirus B-19
Cryptosporidium parvum
Ebola virus
Legionella pneumophila
Hantaan virus
Campylobacter jejuni
HTLV-1
HTLV-II
E. coli 0157:H7
Borrelia burgdorferi
HIV-1
HIV-2

Helicobacter pylori
HHV-6, -7, and -8
Ehrlichia chaffeensis
Hepatitis C, E, and G
Vibrio cholerae 0139
Bartonella henselae
Streptococcus iniae
Cyclospora cayetanensis
Haemophilus influenzae aegyptius
Barmah Forest virus
Equine morbillivirus
Guanarito virus
Sabia virus

BOX B-2

SOME AGENTS WITH PROBLEMS OF ANTIMICROBIAL RESISTANCE

Streptococcus pneumoniae (esp. types 6, 14, 19, 23)
Staphylococcus aureus
Staphylococcus coagulase-negative
Pseudomonas aeruginosa
Enterococci
Mycobacterium tuberculosis
Neisseria gonorrheae
Klebsiella pneumoniae

Escherichia coli
Salmonella species
Shigella species
Enterobacter cloacae
Serratia marcescens
Herpes simplex 1, 2
HIV-1
Candida species
Plasmodium falciparum

---

antimicrobial resistance, the added liability of those organisms that depend for transmission on vectors has been the resistance to insecticides developed by many of these species.

With the ease, speed, and extent of international jet travel, the world is increasingly becoming a "global community" where microorganisms arising in any sector of the globe can readily be transported to any other part of the world by an infected host within an incubation period, whether that host is symptomatic or not. Because so much of the food supply brought to temperate areas during the non–growing season is cultivated in more tropical or semitropical environments, infectious agents contaminating the produce can readily accompany them. Recent outbreaks of cyclosporiasis in at least five states (California, Florida, Nevada, New York, Texas) have been attributed to contaminated rasp-

berries imported from Guatemala. The source of infection is uncertain but may be caused by a closely related agent that causes diarrhea in birds whose seasonal migrations may bring them to the berry fields during each spring. Outbreaks in Canada in 1995 and 1996 of serious illness including bacteremia, cellulitis, endocarditis, meningitis, and arthritis were traced to tilapia cultivated in U.S. fish farms and carrying an unusual organism, *Streptococcus iniae,* a fish pathogen previously unassociated with human illness. The complexities of these agricultural and food consumption patterns exemplify the multiple factors that may be involved in introduction of an "emerging infection" into the human cycle. In January 1997 President Clinton declared an initiative to monitor the safety of the U.S. food supply by coordinating local, state, and federal agencies. Contaminated municipal water supplies (e.g., cryptosporidia affecting 400,000 residents of Milwaukee in 1993) have initiated citywide outbreaks in addition to their responsibility for chronic diarrhea in immunocompromised patients.

Many of the agents in Boxes B-1 and B-2 are discussed in the relevant chapters and sections of the main text of this book. A few more "exotic" microbes may not be covered.

BIBLIOGRAPHY

Centers for Disease Control and Prevention. Addressing emerging infectious disease threats. Atlanta: U.S. Dept. HEW, 1994.

Garrett L. The coming plague: newly emerging diseases in a world out of balance. New York: Farrar, Strausss & Giroux, 1994.

Gold HS, Moellering RC Jr. Antimicrobial-drug resistance. N Engl J Med 1997; 335:1445-53.

Lederberg J, Shope RE, Oaks SC Jr (eds). Emerging infections: microbial threats to health in the United States. Washington, DC: National Academy Press, 1992.

Osterholm MT. Cyclosporiasis and raspberries: lessons for the future. N Engl J Med 1997; 336:1597-1599.

Peters CJ, Olshaker M. Virus hunter: thirty years of battling hot viruses around the world. New York: Anchor Books/Doubleday, 1997.

Tenover FC, Hughes JM. The challenges of emerging infectious diseases. JAMA 1996;275-300-304.

Vidaver AK. Emerging and reemerging infectious diseases. Perspectives on plants, animals, and humans. ASM News 1996, 62:583-585.

Walker DH, Barbour AG, Oliver JH, et al. Emerging bacterial zoonotic and vector-borne diseases. JAMA 1996; 275: 463-469.

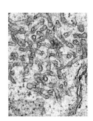

INDEX